AF527267

DIAGNOSTIC RADIOLOGY
Genitourinary Imaging

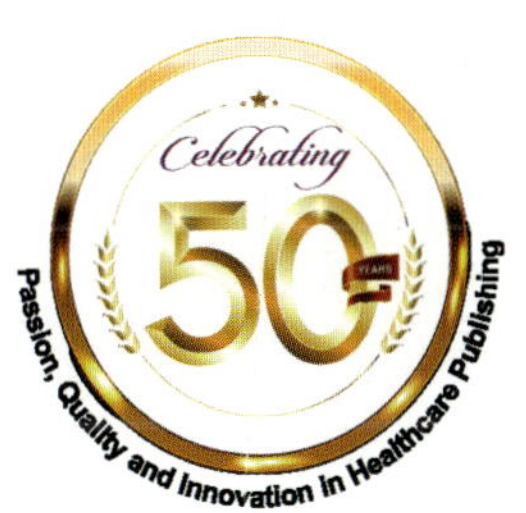

PIONEERS OF AIIMS-MAMC-PGI IMAGING SERIES

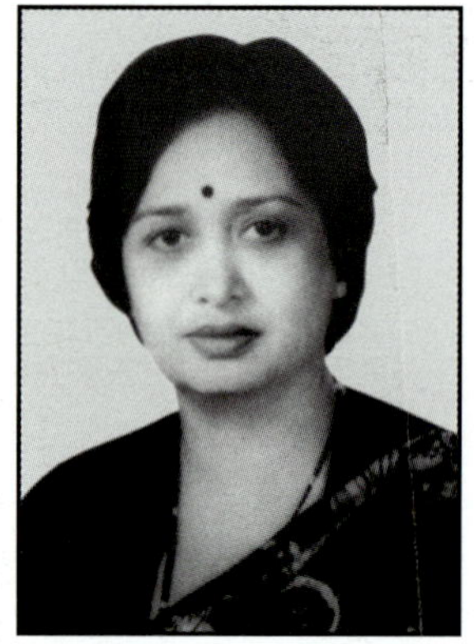

Manorama Berry

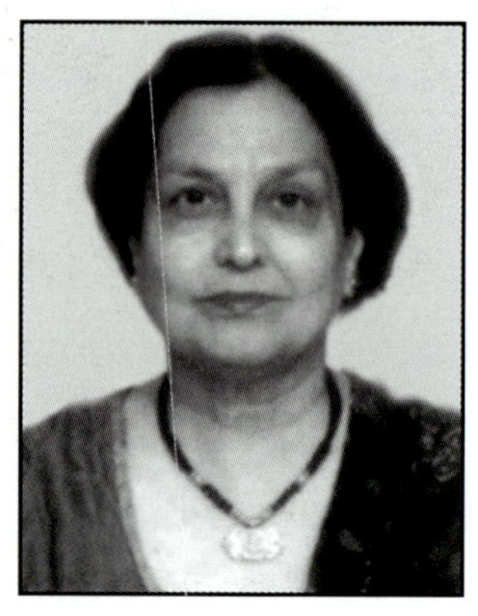

Sudha Suri

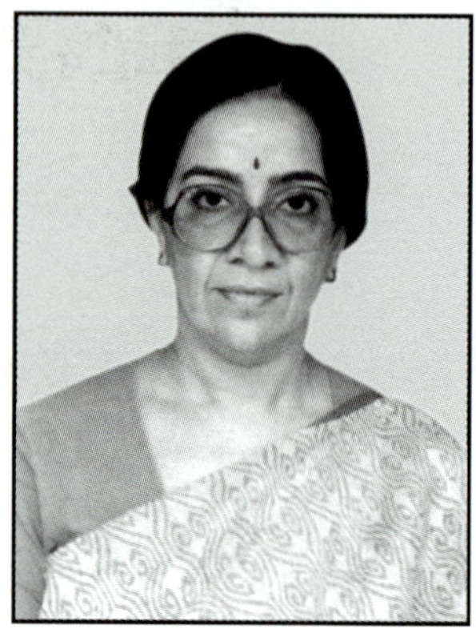

Veena Chowdhury

PAST EDITORS

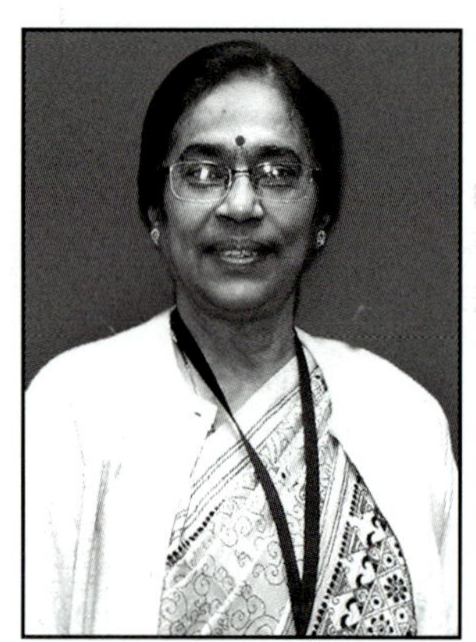

Sima Mukhopadhyay

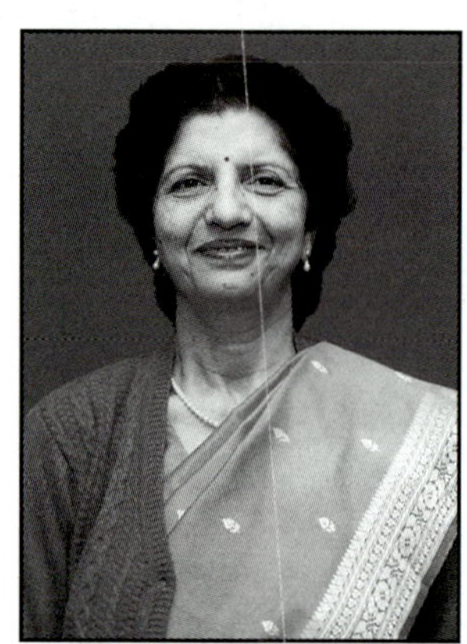

Sushma Vashisht

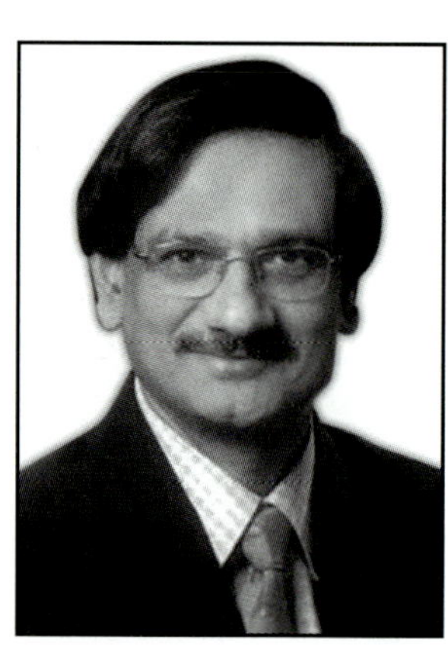

Niranjan Khandelwal

AIIMS-MAMC-PGI IMAGING SERIES

DIAGNOSTIC RADIOLOGY

Genitourinary Imaging

Fourth Edition

Editors

Anju Garg MD
Director Professor and Head
Department of Radiodiagnosis
Maulana Azad Medical College
New Delhi, India

Manavjit Singh Sandhu MD FICR
Professor and Head
Department of Radiodiagnosis
Postgraduate Institute of
Medical Education and Research
Chandigarh, India

Arun Kumar Gupta MD FAMS
Professor and Head
Department of Radiodiagnosis
All India Institute of Medical Sciences
New Delhi, India

Associate Editors

Gaurav Shanker Pradhan MBBS DMRD DNB
Director Professor
Department of Radiodiagnosis
Maulana Azad Medical College
New Delhi, India

Alpana Manchanda MD
Director Professor
Department of Radiodiagnosis
Maulana Azad Medical College
New Delhi, India

Sapna Singh MD DNB MNAMS
Professor
Department of Radiodiagnosis
Maulana Azad Medical College
New Delhi, India

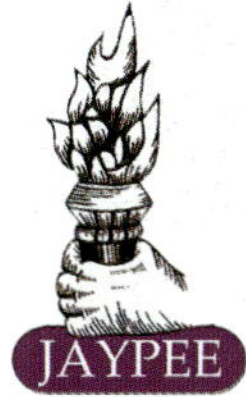

JAYPEE BROTHERS MEDICAL PUBLISHERS

The Health Sciences Publisher

New Delhi | London

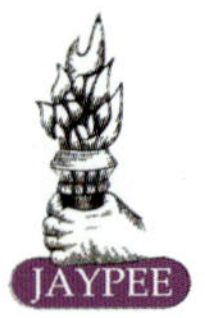

Jaypee Brothers Medical Publishers (P) Ltd.

Headquarters
Jaypee Brothers Medical Publishers (P) Ltd
4838/24, Ansari Road, Daryaganj
New Delhi 110 002, India
Phone: +91-11-43574357
Fax: +91-11-43574314
Email: jaypee@jaypeebrothers.com

Overseas Office
J.P. Medical Ltd
83 Victoria Street, London
SW1H 0HW (UK)
Phone: +44 20 3170 8910
Fax: +44 (0)20 3008 6180
Email: info@jpmedpub.com

Website: www.jaypeebrothers.com
Website: www.jaypeedigital.com

Diagnostic Radiology: Genitourinary Imaging

First Edition: 1996
Second Edition: 2003
Third Edition: 2009
Fourth Edition: **2020**

ISBN: 978-93-89587-36-4

Printed at: Samrat Offset Pvt. Ltd.

Contributors

Ajay Gulati MD MAMS
Additional Professor
Department of Radiodiagnosis
Postgraduate Institute of Medical Education and Research
Chandigarh, India

Ajay Kumar MD
Professor
Department of Radiodiagnosis
Postgraduate Institute of Medical Education and Research
Chandigarh, India

Alpana Manchanda MD
Director Professor
Department of Radiodiagnosis
Maulana Azad Medical College
New Delhi, India

Anindita Sinha MD MAMS
Additional Professor
Department of Radiodiagnosis
Postgraduate Institute of Medical Education and Research
Chandigarh, India

Anjali Prakash DMRD DNB MNAMS
Director Professor
Department of Radiodiagnosis
Maulana Azad Medical College
New Delhi, India

Anju Garg MD
Director Professor and Head
Department of Radiodiagnosis
Maulana Azad Medical College
New Delhi, India

Ankur Goyal MD DNB MNAMS
Associate Professor
Department of Radiodiagnosis
All India Institute of Medical Sciences
New Delhi, India

Anmol Bhatia MD
Assistant Professor
Department of Radiodiagnosis
Postgraduate Institute of Medical Education and Research
Chandigarh, India

Anupam Lal MD
Professor
Department of Radiodiagnosis
Postgraduate Institute of Medical Education and Research
Chandigarh, India

Arun Kumar Gupta MD FAMS
Professor and Head
Department of Radiodiagnosis
All India Institute of Medical Sciences
New Delhi, India

Ashu Seith Bhalla MD MAMS FICR
Professor
Department of Radiodiagnosis
All India Institute of Medical Sciences
New Delhi, India

Atin Kumar MD DNB MNAMS FICR
Professor
Department of Radiodiagnosis
(Trauma Centre Division)
All India Institute of Medical Sciences
New Delhi, India

Chandan J Das
MD DNB MAMS FICR FRCP (Edin)
Additional Professor
Department of Radiodiagnosis
All India Institute of Medical Sciences
New Delhi, India

Deep Narayan Srivastava
MD MBA FAMS FICR
Professor
Department of Radiodiagnosis
All India Institute of Medical Sciences
New Delhi, India

Devasenathipathy Kandasamy
MD DNB FRCR
Additional Professor
Department of Radiodiagnosis
All India Institute of Medical Sciences
New Delhi, India

Ekta Dhamija MD
Associate Professor
Department of Radiodiagnosis
(BRA IRCH division)
All India Institute of Medical Sciences
New Delhi, India

Gaurav Shanker Pradhan
MBBS DMRD DNB
Director Professor
Department of Radiodiagnosis
Maulana Azad Medical College
New Delhi, India

Harish Bhujade MD
Assistant Professor
Department of Radiodiagnosis
Postgraduate Institute of Medical Education and Research
Chandigarh, India

Jyoti Kumar MD DNB MNAMS FICR
Professor
Department of Radiodiagnosis
Maulana Azad Medical College
New Delhi, India

Madhavi Tripathi
MD DNB (Nuclear Medicine)
Additional Professor
Department of Nuclear Medicine and Positron Emission Tomography (PET)
All India Institute of Medical Sciences
New Delhi, India

Mahesh Prakash MD FICR
Professor
Department of Radiodiagnosis
Postgraduate Institute of Medical Education and Research
Chandigarh, India

Manavjit Singh Sandhu MD FICR
Professor and Head
Department of Radiodiagnosis
Postgraduate Institute of Medical Education and Research
Chandigarh, India

Mandeep Kang MD FICR MAMS
Professor
Department of Radiodiagnosis
Postgraduate Institute of Medical Education and Research
Chandigarh, India

Manisha Jana MD DNB FRCR
Additional Professor
Department of Radiodiagnosis
All India Institute of Medical Sciences
New Delhi, India

Manphool Singhal MD DNB MAMS
Additional Professor
Department of Radiodiagnosis
Postgraduate Institute of Medical Education and Research
Chandigarh, India

Naveen Kalra MD FICR MAMS
Professor
Department of Radiodiagnosis
Postgraduate Institute of Medical Education and Research
Chandigarh, India

Paramjeet Singh MD
Professor
Department of Radiodiagnosis
Postgraduate Institute of Medical Education and Research
Chandigarh, India

Priyanka Naranje MD DNB MNAMS
Associate Professor
Department of Radiodiagnosis
All India Institute of Medical Sciences
New Delhi, India

Radhika Batra MD DNB
Assistant Professor
Department of Radiodiagnosis
Maulana Azad Medical College
New Delhi, India

Raju Sharma MD MAMS FICR
Professor
Department of Radiodiagnosis
All India Institute of Medical Sciences
New Delhi, India

Rakesh Kumar DRM DNB PhD
Professor
Diagnostic Nuclear Medicine Division
Department of Nuclear Medicine and Positron Emission Tomography (PET)
All India Institute of Medical Sciences
New Delhi, India

Rashmi Dixit MD
Director Professor
Department of Radiodiagnosis
Maulana Azad Medical College
New Delhi, India

Sameer Vyas
MD DM (Neuroradiology) MAMS
Additional Professor
Department of Radiodiagnosis
Postgraduate Institute of Medical Education and Research
Chandigarh, India

Sanjay Sharma
MD DNB MNAMS FRCR FICR
Professor
Department of Radiodiagnosis
(Division at Rajendra Prasad Center for Ophthalmic Sciences)
All India Institute of Medical Sciences
New Delhi, India

Sanjeev Kumar MD
Associate Professor
Department of Cardiovascular Radiology and Endovascular Intervention
All India Institute of Medical Sciences
New Delhi, India

Sanjiv Sharma MD
Professor and Head
Department of Cardiovascular Radiology and Endovascular Intervention
All India Institute of Medical Sciences
New Delhi, India

Sapna Singh MD DNB MNAMS
Professor
Department of Radiodiagnosis
Maulana Azad Medical College
New Delhi, India

Satyam DNB MNAMS
Specialist
Department of Radiodiagnosis
Lok Nayak Hospital and Associated Maulana Azad Medical College
New Delhi, India

Shivanand Gamanagatti
MD MAMS FICR
Professor
Department of Radiodiagnosis
(Trauma Centre Division)
All India Institute of Medical Sciences
New Delhi, India

Smita Manchanda MD DNB
Associate Professor
Department of Radiodiagnosis
All India Institute of Medical Sciences
New Delhi, India

Smriti Hari MD MAMS
Professor
Department of Radiodiagnosis
All India Institute of Medical Sciences
New Delhi, India

Sreedhara BC MD
Assistant Professor
Department of Radiodiagnosis
Postgraduate Institute of Medical Education and Research
Chandigarh, India

Surabhi Vyas MD DNB MNAMS
Additional Professor
Department of Radiodiagnosis
All India Institute of Medical Sciences
New Delhi, India

Swati Gupta MD DNB FRCR
Assistant Professor
Department of Radiodiagnosis
Maulana Azad Medical College
New Delhi, India

Tulika Singh MD
Additional Professor
Department of Radiodiagnosis
Postgraduate Institute of Medical Education and Research
Chandigarh, India

Ujjwal Gorsi MD
Associate Professor
Department of Radiodiagnosis
Postgraduate Institute of Medical Education and Research
Chandigarh, India

Uma Debi MD
Associate Professor
Department Radiodiagnosis
Postgraduate Institute of Medical Education and Research
Chandigarh, India

Vineeta Ojha MD DNB
DM Senior Resident
Department of Cardiovascular Radiology and Endovascular Intervention
All India Institute of Medical Sciences
New Delhi, India

Preface to the Fourth Edition

The first edition of *Diagnostic Radiology on Genitourinary Imaging* was published in 1996, the second in 2003, followed by the third edition in 2009, which was almost ten years back. In this decade long gap there have been many technological advances in all the various imaging modalities. Advancements in detector technology for CT, dual energy CT, additional field strength and pulse sequences in MR systems, along with a ubiquitous use of functional MR imaging sequences, besides the conventional sequences and 3D, 4D and contrast enhanced ultrasound. All these have led to an improved image resolution with rapid acquisition of three dimensional images in virtually any plane giving us structural and functional information for most disease conditions.

There have been many changes in the imaging evaluation of diverse pathologies including the workup of neoplastic conditions, especially in the staging of urogenital malignancies. The increased use of neoadjuvant chemoradiotherapy in the various genitourinary malignancies has shifted the focus of imaging from diagnosis to staging, prognostication, surveillance and follow up evaluation.

This book incorporates the basics—individual chapters on radiological anatomy and radiological techniques for genital and urinary systems—to advanced imaging including the latest revisions in management recommendations and guidelines. Systematic algorithmic imaging approaches have been incorporated to simplify reporting in an objective and universal manner.

Image-guided interventions in this field have been updated and are outlined in the section on intervention.

The 4th edition has been designed keeping in mind the postgraduate students, residents and the consultants. It aims to be a comprehensive and thoroughly updated book covering recent advances and imaging appearances of various genitourinary pathologies, to be used as a one-stop shop for the same.

We also wish to take this opportunity to thank all our faculty from All India Institute of Medical Sciences (AIIMS), New Delhi; Postgraduate Institute of Medical Education and Research (PGIMER), Chandigarh; and Maulana Azad Medical College (MAMC), New Delhi, for their contribution and support without which this endeavor would not have been possible.

We would also like to thank Shri Jitendar P Vij (Group Chairman), Mr Ankit Vij (Managing Director), Mr MS Mani (Group President), Ms Chetna Malhotra Vohra (Associate Director—Content Strategy), Ms Pooja Bhandari (Production Head) and Ms Kritika Dua (Senior Development Editor) of M/s Jaypee Brothers Medical Publishers (P) Ltd, New Delhi, India, for their professional help and cooperation in publishing this book in the present form.

Anju Garg
Manavjit Singh Sandhu
Arun Kumar Gupta
Gaurav Shanker Pradhan
Alpana Manchanda
Sapna Singh

Preface to the First Edition

Urogenital radiology is practiced today quite differently in many ways than a decade ago. This is mainly due to the technological advances in ultrasound (US), computed tomography (CT) and magnetic resonance imaging (MRI). With the ever-increasing number of diagnostic techniques, the radiologists and the referring clinicians are faced with the dilemma of determining the most appropriate test or tests for a given clinical problem.

Keeping this in view, the present book aims to present the most current information on the role of various techniques, viz conventional radiology, ultrasound, computed tomography and magnetic resonance imaging in the urogenital practice, their merits and limitations and to determine the approach to complex problems in this decade. The comprehensive discussions on the indications of various imaging techniques in urogenital practice are presented throughout the text. Recommendations are offered regarding the role of each technique in various clinical situations based on the collective experience of the Faculties of Radiology, All India Institute of Medical Sciences (AIIMS), Maulana Azad Medical College (MAMC), New Delhi Postgraduate Institute of Medical Education and Research (PGIMER), Chandigarh, India and other renowned Indian radiologists.

We hope this book will help the postgraduate students, practicing radiologists and internists develop an in-depth understanding and appreciation of the contemporary radiologic evaluations of the urogenital tract.

We wish to take this opportunity to thank the authors for their cooperation and prompt submission of their contributions to this volume.

Manorama Berry
Sushma Vashisht
Veena Chowdhury

Contents

SECTION 1
UPPER URINARY TRACT

SECTION 2
LOWER URINARY TRACT

SECTION 3

FEMALE GENITAL TRACT

SECTION 4

MALE GENITAL TRACT

SECTION 5

MISCELLANEOUS

SECTION 6

INTERVENTIONS

SECTION 1

Upper Urinary Tract

Chapter 1

Imaging Techniques and Radiological Anatomy of the Upper Urinary Tract

Sapna Singh, Jyoti Kumar, Anjali Prakash

ANATOMY OF THE UPPER URINARY TRACT

The upper urinary tract consists of paired kidneys and the ureters. The kidneys develop from three structures—the pronephros, the mesonephric, and metanephric ducts in that order. The pronephros regresses by 4th to 8th week of gestation leaving no adult correlate while the mesonephric duct forms the male genital structures. The ureteric bud and the metanephric blastema arise from the metanephric duct in the 5th week of gestation. The metanephric blastema develops into Bowman's capsule, the convoluted tubules, and loop of Henle while the ureteric bud develops into ureter, the renal pelvis, calyces, and the collecting ducts. The calyces arise due to repeated divisions of the upper end of the ureteric bud and this forms the basis of the lobar structure of the kidney, each lobe consisting of a calyx and the associated collecting ducts and renal cortex. The lobar outline becomes smooth by around 5 years of age owing to multiplication of the renal cortical cells. However, in about 5% of the individuals, there is persistence of the lobar outline into adulthood.

It is during the 4th to 8th week of gestation that the kidneys migrate cranially from the pelvic region where they develop. The cranial migration is due to the lengthening of the lumbar and sacral spine during development so that the normal final position of the kidneys is upper lumbar region. They also rotate medially by around 90° so that the renal pelvis lies on the anteromedial aspect of the kidneys.[1] The lateral sacral branches of the aorta supply the pelvic kidneys but during ascent they acquire higher lateral branches of the aorta. The definitive renal arteries are seen at the first lumbar disc (L1-L2) level. If the inferior arteries do not regress, accessory renal arteries can be seen. Accessory unilateral renal arteries are seen in 30% population and bilateral are seen in 10% with a higher frequency seen with anomalies of ascent.[2]

The kidneys come to lie in the retroperitoneal space with the right kidney lower in position than the left owing to the presence of the liver on the right. The normal kidneys should be 12–14 cm in length and the difference between the two should not be more than 1 cm. In quiet respiration, the kidneys move up and down 2–3 cm and much more in deep inspiration. The renal hilum is a vertical opening on the medial aspect which contains the renal pelvis and renal vessels. The renal veins lie anterior to the renal arteries which in-turn lie anterior to the renal pelves. In addition, the hilum also contains fat, nerve fibers, and lymphatic channels which drain into the lateral aortic lymph nodal group.

Each kidney is divided into an outer renal cortex and an inner renal medulla.[3] The medulla consists of 8–16 renal pyramids **(Fig. 1)**. Each renal pyramid in-turn contains the

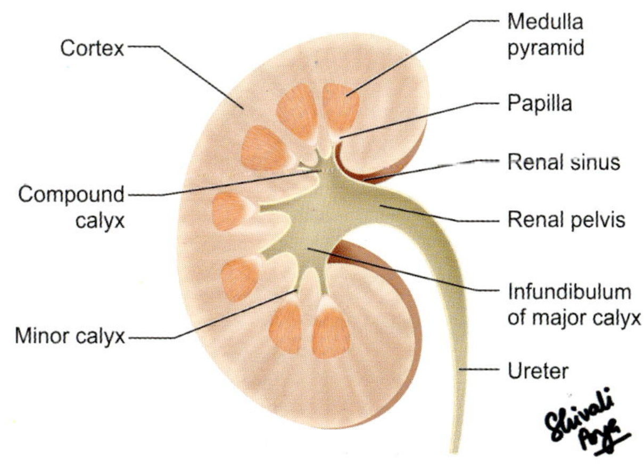

Fig. 1: Schematic diagram of the structure of the kidney.

ascending and descending limbs of the loop of Henle and the collecting ducts. The cortex contains the glomerulus and the proximal and distal convoluted tubules. The apex of the renal pyramid projects into a calyx at the renal papilla. The renal collecting system consists of 10–14 concave-shaped minor calyces. The lateral extensions of the calyces is called the forniceal angle. Two to four minor calyces join together to form the superior, middle, and inferior major calyces respectively from superior to inferior. The minor calyces drain into the major calyx by a narrow neck/infundibulum. The major calyces in-turn drain into the renal pelvis which continues as the ureter at the pelviureteric junction (PUJ).

Variants of the Calyceal Anatomy

- *Compound calyx*: Here, the multiple single calyces fail to divide and form a single large calyx known as the compound calyx. Here, several renal papillae which represent the apices of the renal pyramids drain into a single calyx. Compound calyces are usually seen at the polar region, i.e. at the upper or lower poles and are prone to reflux nephropathy.
- *Complex renal calyces and megacalycosis*: In megacalycosis, there is a greater number of calyces than normal (>15). There is dilatation of some or all renal calyces with normal renal pelvis and ureter. Renal calyces may have a blunted morphology, but this condition should not be confused with papillary necrosis in which the number of calyces is not increased and necrosis tends to be dissimilar from calyx to calyx.
- *Calyceal diverticulum*: It represents a focal extrinsic dilatation of a renal calyx. A calyceal diverticulum connects to the calyceal fornix and projects into the cortex rather than the medulla.

Retroperitoneal Spaces

The kidneys have a tough fibrous capsule closely applied to the renal cortex all around except at the hilum.

The kidneys are retroperitoneal organs and lie in a space called the *perinephric space* or the *perineal space*. The perinephric space is a space bound by layers of fascia and is an important determinant of the direction of disease spread. The fascia anterior to the kidneys is called the Gerota's fascia while the posterior fascia is called the fascia of Zuckerkandl. The space enclosed between the anterior and posterior fascia is called the *perinephric space* **(Fig. 2)**. In addition to the kidneys, the space contains the adrenal gland, the upper ureter and the perinephric fat. As the kidneys ascend from the pelvis to the abdomen, the perinephric fascia forms a cone with its apex pointing superiorly, the apex being closed.[3,4]

The transversalis fascia lines the inferior aspect of the diaphragm, the inside of the abdominopelvic cavity, anterolateral abdominal wall, the anterior aspect of the spinal column, the psoas and paraspinal muscles, and the superior aspect of the pelvic diaphragm. There is a potential space between the posterior perinephric fascia and the adjacent transversalis fascia. This space is called the *posterior pararenal space* and contains only fat **(Fig. 2)**. The posterior pararenal space is of interest to the radiologist as a guidewire may kink in this area or a drain intended for the pelvicalyceal system may be accidently positioned here. The *anterior pararenal space*, on the other hand, is the space between the anterior perinephric fascia and posterior layer of the peritoneum. In the center of the anterior pararenal space lie the pancreas and duodenum, the ascending colon lies to the right and descending colon to the left. These organs are hence in direct contact with the anterior perinephric fascia.[4]

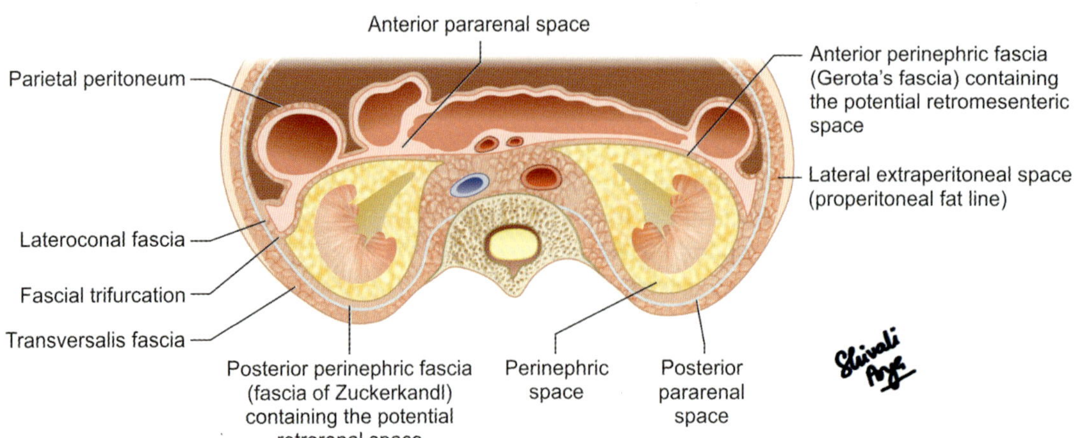

Fig. 2: Diagram showing the retroperitoneal fascial spaces.

Laterally, the anterior and posterior perirenal fascia fuse with the lateroconal fascia at the fascial trifurcation. While the posterior pararenal space is continuous laterally with the lateral extraperitoneal space (the properitoneal line) lying between the parietal peritoneum and transversalis fascia, this space is closed medially. Medially, the posterior perinephric fascia fuses with the transversalis fascia over the paraspinal muscles, that is the psoas muscle and the quadratus lumborum. The posterior perinephric space hence lies directly over the psoas muscle being separated only by the transversalis fascia. Thus, any inflammation process of the kidneys can spread rapidly into the psoas muscles and from there into the iliacus muscle, iliopsoas, and the pelvis.

Thus, superiorly the renal fascia fuses with the diaphragmatic fascia. Laterally, the renal fascia fuses with the lateroconal fascia and inferiorly with the iliac fascia blending loosely with the periureteric connective tissue. Owing to the loose blending of the fascia, the inferomedial angle adjacent to the ureter is the weakest point of the perinephric compartment through which urine or perinephric effusion escapes most easily. The posterior renal fascia fuses with the psoas and quadratus lumborum fascia medially.

The perineal spaces also communicate with each other across the midline and with the retroperitoneal vascular space. The pararenal spaces communicate caudally and with the extraperitoneal spaces including the prevesical space. Infections from one space can hence spread to the other subsequently. The *anterior interfascial or the retromesenteric space* and the *posterior interfascial or retrorenal space* are potential spaces within the laminated anterior perinephric and posterior perinephric fasciae, respectively **(*see* Fig. 2)**.[5] The perirenal space contains thin septations called the Kumin's septa. These septae may arise from the renal capsule and extend to the anterior and posterior renal fascia. Some may arise from the renal capsule and run parallel to the renal surface. The renorenal bridging septum is the most consistent which arises from the posterior renal capsule and runs parallel to the posterior surface of the kidney. These septae thicken consequent to a disease process, what is referred to as perinephric stranding. These fibrous septae act as potential conduits between the perinephric and interfascial spaces. Fluid and collections may track from any of these potential spaces to the other and also via the fascial trifurcation into the lateroconal fascia.

Relations of the Kidneys

The right kidney is related anteriorly with the inferior surface of the liver and the second part of the duodenum while the anterior relations of the left kidney are the pancreatic tail, the spleen, the stomach, the small bowel, the splenic flexure, and the left colon **(Fig. 3)**.[4] Posteriorly, the diaphragm, psoas muscle, aponeurosis of the transverses abdominis muscle, and the lumbar muscles are related to the kidneys. Both the kidneys are related superiorly with the adrenal glands while inferiorly the hepatorenal pouch/Morrison's pouch separates the right kidney from the inferior surface of the liver.

Vascular Anatomy

The renal arteries arise from the aorta, slightly below the origin of the superior mesenteric artery (SMA). The right renal artery (RRA) arises from the anterolateral aspect of the aorta and then passes posterior to the inferior vena cava (IVC) as it courses toward the right renal hilum. The left renal artery (LRA) arises from the lateral or posterolateral aspect of the aorta and follows a posterolateral course to the left renal hilum. Accessory renal arteries may arise from the aorta in as many as 20% individuals, either superior or inferior to the main renal

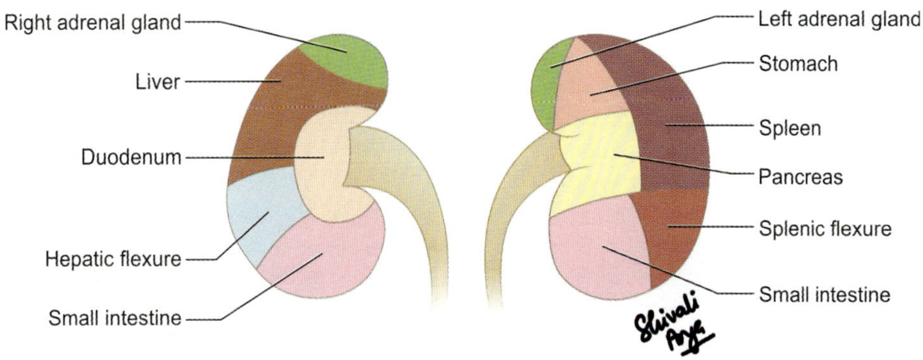

Fig. 3: Schematic diagram of the anterior relations of the right and left kidney.

artery. The renal arteries typically divide into anterior and posterior divisions that lie anterior and posterior to the renal pelvis, respectively. These divisions give rise to the segmental arteries which branch further within the renal sinus, forming interlobar arteries that penetrate the renal parenchyma. These terminate in arcuate arteries that curve around the corticomedullary junction giving rise to cortical branches.[3,4]

Each renal vein is formed from tributaries that coalesce in the renal hilum. The left renal vein passes anterior to the aorta and posterior to SMA, to enter the left side of IVC. The right renal vein, which is shorter, extends directly to the IVC from the right renal hilum.

The lymphatic drainage is to the lateral aortic lymph nodes around the origin of the renal arteries.

Ureters

The ureter runs down the anterior aspect of the psoas muscle, the transversalis fascia separating the two. The ureters run within 1 cm of the lateral margin of the vertebral transverse processes. At the level of the sacroiliac joint, it crosses over the anterior aspect of the bifurcation of the common iliac artery as it enters the pelvis. It then runs along the lateral pelvic wall just medial to the obturator internus muscle. At the level of the ischial spine, it runs anteromedially until it enters the superolateral angle of the bladder base. In males, the vas deferens crosses over the ureter just before it enters the bladder wall. The ureters run obliquely for around 2 cm through the bladder wall.[4]

The ureters have three normal constrictions which act as points of temporary peristaltic arrest which are as follows:

1. At the ureteropelvic junction
2. Crossing the iliac vessels
3. At the pelvic inlet.

IMAGING TECHNIQUES OF THE UPPER URINARY TRACT

CONVENTIONAL RADIOGRAPHY

The conventional plain radiography of the abdomen is an imaging technique for the kidneys ureter and bladder also known as the kidney, ureter, and bladder (KUB) film.[6] The kidneys are visible on the plain radiograph due to natural contrast provided by the perirenal fat. An idea about the renal shape, margins, dimensions, and localization can be made on the plain radiograph. It can also be used to identify renal calculi, calcifications or transparencies due to fat or gas.[7] The psoas shadow can also be seen on the plain radiograph. Radiopacities seen on the plain radiographs correspond to the renal stones or calcifications due to tuberculosis, vascular structures or traumatic lesions like hematoma **(Figs. 4A and B)**. Calcifications seen in solid or cystic neoplasms may also be seen on plain radiograph **(Table 1)**. The radiolucencies

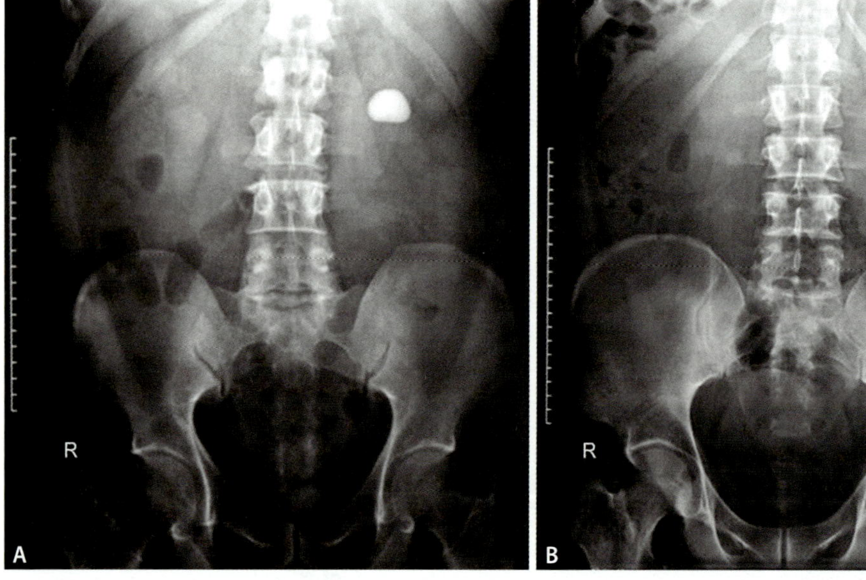

Figs. 4A and B: (A) Plain X-ray of kidney, ureter, and bladder (KUB) showing a large radiodensity in the left renal area suggestive of a left renal calculus; (B) Another plain film showing multiple radiopacities in the left renal area suggestive of multiple renal calculi.

Table 1: Calcification on the KUB.[4]
Urinary tract
Renal: Calculi, tuberculosis, renal cell carcinoma, and arterial atheroma or aneurysm *Ureter*: Calculi, tuberculosis, and schistosomiasis *Bladder*: Calculi, transitional cell carcinoma, and schistosomiasis
Outside the urinary tract
Hepatobiliary: Gallstones and hepatic granuloma *Spleen*: Granuloma *Pancreas*: Chronic pancreatitis *Adrenal*: Tuberculosis and Addison's disease *Aorta*: Atheroma and aneurysm *Venous*: Phlebolith *Musculoskeletal*: Costal cartilage calcification *Uterine*: Fibroid *Lymphatic*: Calcified lymph nodes (presumed postinfective)
(KUB: kidney, ureter and bladder)

correspond to gas, e.g. emphysematous pyelonephritis or fat, i.e. large angiomyolipoma (AML) or liposarcoma.

INTRAVENOUS UROGRAPHY

Intravenous urography (IVU), also known as the excretory urogram is a time-tested technique of uroradiology providing a global view of the renal parenchyma and collecting system.[8]

Indications:

- Urolithiasis
- Ureteric fistulae/strictures
- Renal infections, e.g. tuberculosis. IVU still remains the gold standard in the imaging of renal tuberculosis. It is the only modality that can detect early changes in the renal calyces in tuberculosis, e.g. early fuzziness, irregularity of calyces, papillary necrosis, etc.
- Persistent or frank hematuria.

Normal Physiology Giving Rise to the Appearances on IVU

Intravenous urography consists of a series of plain films following intravenous injection of water soluble iodinated contrast medium.[9] The contrast reaches the renal arteries 12–20 seconds following contrast injection. The concentration of the contrast material is maximum in the vascular compartment at this stage, but it begins to fall rapidly as it enters the extracellular compartment. It also undergoes glomerular filtration and enters the renal tubules. Hence, in the first minute following contrast injection, there is a diffuse enhancement referred to as the nephrogram phase provided the kidneys are healthy with the patient having a normal cardiovascular system. The renal size and outline are best evaluated in the *nephrogram phase*, the normal renal length being at least three lumbar vertebrae and not exceeding four. Contrast then begins to appear in the calyces around 1 minute which subsequently drains into the pelvis and ureter referred to as the *pyelogram phase*. The normal ureters demonstrate continued peristalsis and it may not be possible to visualize the entire length of both (or even one) ureters in a single film. In most cases, partial visualization of the ureters is acceptable.

Technique

Traditionally, patients were deprived of fluid before an IVU examination with the belief that it would lead to a better opacification of the collecting system. However, it has long been established that dehydration is associated with an increased risk of nephrotoxicity and should be completely avoided. In fact, if the patient is dehydrated before the IVU, it needs to be corrected first. Food should be avoided 4–6 hours prior to the examination and bowel preparation (using laxatives) is preferable to avoid gases overlying the renal shadows. The patient is called fasting (4–6 hours) and with adequate bowel preparation but should be well hydrated. A plain radiograph (KUB) is must as it gives an idea of the bowel preparation and is needed to follow up a previously proven calculus. A preliminary KUB also gives an idea of exposure factors, correct positioning/centering, and any obvious pathology, most common of which is urinary tract calcification.

Blood urea and serum creatinine levels should be checked before contrast administration as the risk of contrast-induced nephropathy is increased if serum creatinine is greater than 1.5 mg/dL. Also, in patients with impaired renal function (serum creatinine greater than 3.5 mg/dL), the excretion of the contrast material and subsequent renal and ureteric visualization are limited.

If the patient is fit to undergo the examination, contrast is injected at the dose of 1 mg/kg body weight. The standard dose is usually 50 mL of 350–370 mg l/mL water soluble iodinated contrast medium. Although usually safe there is a small risk of reactions.[10] The most severe reaction that can occur following contrast administration is anaphylactoid type hypersensitivity reaction. Hence, before injection of contrast medium, a history of allergy to any previous contrast exposure should be elicited.[11] The injection should be administered through an indwelling cannula that can be kept in place for the entire duration of the investigation. This would allow any emergency treatment to be given in case of an eventuality. Also, in cases of poor contrast opacification, a further dose of contrast medium can be administered. Most contrast reactions take place within the first few minutes following contrast injection. Emergency drugs, oxygen, and resuscitation should be available in the IVU room. The radiologist should be available in the X-ray room for the entire duration of the procedure.

Sequence of films taken

Film	Purpose
5-minute film	- Opacification of the pelvicalyceal system
15-minute compression film	- Calyceal distention
15-minute release film in supine position (full length films)	- Visualization of the pelvicalyceal system and ureters
15-minute prone film (full length films)	
Post-micturition film	- Residual urine volume

Abdominal compression is applied after the 5-minute film to improve the distention of the pelvicalyceal system by inhibiting ureteric drainage. However, compression should not be applied in children, in patients of hypertension/aortic aneurysm, those with recent abdominal surgery or abdominal pain or tenderness. After 15-minute film with compression, the compression is removed and full length films are taken in the supine and prone positions, the prone position allowing a better visualization of the pelvic ureters **(Figs. 5A to C)**.

At times, a delayed film needs to be taken in cases of significant acute obstruction where there is a delay in the opacification of the pelvicalyceal system. This follow-up IVU needs to be done till a time when the contralateral kidney has completely excreted the contrast.

With the advent of cross-sectional imaging, the utility of IVU is a topic of considerable debate.[12] Computed tomography (CT) scores over IVU for urolithiasis with a sensitivity of 100% versus 52–69% for IVU.[13] In one review, patient acceptability, superior diagnostic performance of CT versus IVU, equivalent radiation doses using low-dose techniques in CT were the factors for recommending CT over IVU.[14] CT is also superior to IVU for urinary tract tumor detection with sensitivities of only 21%, 52%, and 85% for masses less than 2, 2–3, and greater than 3 cm, respectively on IVU.[15] However, a blanket substitution of IVU by cross-sectional imaging is not feasible due to cost and availability factors.

DIGITAL TOMOSYNTHESIS

Digital tomosynthesis (DT) is a technique that enables visualization of stones from multiple angles rather than simply anterior to posterior. The technique involves acquisition of images at regular intervals at different angles during a single linear or arc sweep of the X-ray tube. The images can then be reconstructed providing better

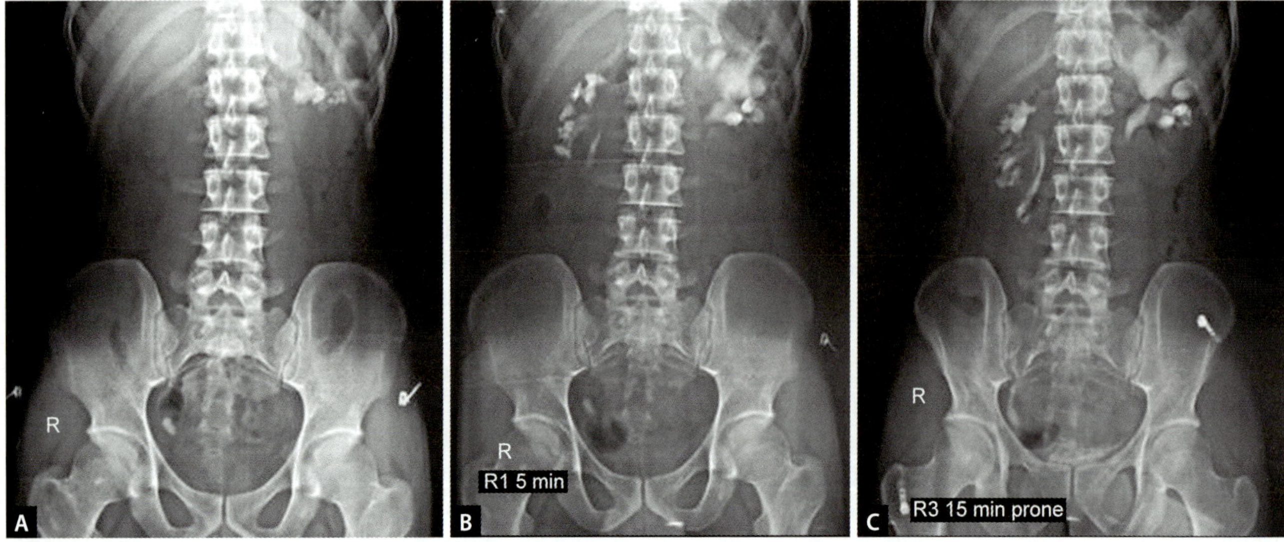

Figs. 5A to C: (A) Plain X-ray of kidney, ureter, and bladder (KUB) showing multiple left renal calculi and radiodensity in the line of the right ureter suggestive of left ureteric calculus; (B and C) Intravenous urography images showing renal calculi as filling defects within the opacified left pelvicalyceal system and the right ureteric calculus. Note is made of the upper ureter being dilated and tortuous with a characteristic medial angulation suggestive of retrocaval ureter.

resolution than conventional radiography. Compared with CT, DT offers a reduced radiation exposure, higher in plane resolution, easier availability, and lower cost. In a study done to evaluate the accuracy of IVU using DT, a significant improvement was seen from 46.5% for conventional IVU to 95.5% for IVU with DT.[16] There was a dose reduction of 56% and a decrease in the length of the procedure.[16] This technique may be useful in situations such as evaluation of residual stone after percutaneous lithotripsy, that is, in situations where a detailed imaging of the renal parenchyma is not required. DT is currently an experimental technique and may play a role in KUB radiography remaining an important technique in kidney stone imaging in the future.

RETROGRADE PYELOGRAPHY

Retrograde pyelography (RGP) involves opacification of the pelvicalyceal system retrogradely by instillation of contrast medium into a ureteric catheter placed by cystoscopy. With the advent of multidetector computed tomography (MDCT) with isotropic data acquisition and multiplanar reconstruction, the role of RGP is limited.[17]

The indications include:

- As a problem-solving tool in cases of persistent diagnostic uncertainty, especially if there is hematuria and/or suspicious cytology.[18]
- To confirm or negate the presence of one or more filling defects within the collecting system.
- To demonstrate the lower end of an obstructed ureter.

Technique

Catheters are positioned within one or both ureters cystoscopically by the urologist. Under fluoroscopic screening, 5–20 mL of water-soluble iodinated contrast medium is injected via the catheter. Care should be taken so as to not inject air bubbles as these can be mistaken for filling defects. The ureters and pelvicalyceal system are hence opacified retrogradely. These should be opacified adequately but not overdistended as a forceful and excessive contrast injection can lead to reflux of contrast into the collecting ducts (pyelotubular reflux), contrast extravasation into the renal sinus (pyelosinus reflux), forniceal rupture, and even into the regional lymphatics or veins (pyelolymphatic and pyelovenous reflux).

ANTEGRADE PYELOGRAPHY

It is a simple invasive procedure used to evaluate the cause and level of ureteric obstruction where other imaging modalities have failed to do so. The technique involves positioning the patient 45° semiprone and puncturing the pelvicalyceal system with a fine (22 gauge) needle under fluoroscopy or ultrasound guidance. The puncture should be directed through the renal parenchyma into a suitable calyx and then into the pelvis.[4] Aspiration of urine can confirm the cannulation. Water-soluble contrast medium is then injected to opacify the pelvicalyceal system. A series of spot films of the ureter down to the level of obstruction can be taken.

NEPHROSTOGRAM

A nephrostomy tube is usually positioned for therapeutic purposes but contrast can be instilled through it and a nephrostogram can be performed. It is indicated to assess the continued presence of calculus or any obstructing lesion or determine the cause of obstruction if it has not been demonstrated. Nephrostogram is also done in post-operative patients of PUJ obstruction to check the patency.[4] It is used to monitor the status of fistulas. Spot films of the ureter are taken down to the level of obstruction.

GRAYSCALE ULTRASOUND

Ultrasound is a reliable technique for the evaluation of upper urinary tract. It is noninvasive, easily available, accurate, safe, and does not require exposure to ionizing radiation. It can be performed bedside for sick patients and interventions can be performed under ultrasound guidance.

Indications for sonography in upper urinary tract:[19]

- Diagnosing dilatation of the collecting system and to search for renal obstruction.
- Excellent modality for evaluation of cystic renal lesions. Their architecture including internal septations, wall thickening, calcifications, presence or absence of solid components (in order to assign a Bosniak grade) can all be evaluated on ultrasound.
- Assessment of congenital anomalies and renal infections as ultrasound is a safe method for evaluating the urinary tract particularly in pediatric patients as high resolution sonography is easily feasible and radiation can be avoided.[20,21]
- Postnatal ultrasound for the evaluation of urinary tract in documented prenatal fetal hydronephrosis.
- Characterization of renal masses.
- Detection of nephrolithiasis and resultant back pressure changes, if any.
- Painless hematuria in low- and medium-risk patients.[22]

- Guidance for therapeutic and interventional procedures.

Technique

Positioning and Access

A 3–5 MHz curvilinear/linear transducer is used to scan the kidneys and ureter. A supine or lateral decubitus position can be adopted for kidneys. The right kidney is usually examined first where the liver is used as an acoustic window **(Figs. 6A and B)**. The transducer is placed in subcostal or intercostal position. Owing to gases from the small bowel and splenic flexure visualization of the left kidney becomes difficult at times via anterior or anterolateral approach. In such situations, a posterolateral approach can be adopted for the left kidney with the left side of the patient raised by approximately 45°.[23] The spleen provides an acoustic window on the left side. If even after raising left side of the body by 45°, visualization is not successful, a full right lateral decubitus with the pillow under the right flank and the left arm extended over the head may allow visualization of the left kidney. Prone position is usually adopted for young children for adequate visualization of the kidneys. A prone position is useful in adults in ultrasound-guided procedures.[24]

Renal Size

The longest craniocaudal length should be measured by rotating the probe around its vertical axis. The longest length should be measured as false low measurements are obtained at times due to ellipsoidal shape of the kidney. Renal length which gives an estimate of the overall renal size is quick and easy to measure. The determination of renal size with ultrasound is more accurate than with IVU because the kidney is imaged without magnification and contrast-induced osmotic diuresis. As a result renal size is approximately 15% smaller. Renal size is related to sex, age, and built of the patient. The length of the normal adult kidney is usually 10–12 cm but can range from 7 cm to 14 cm in patients with normal renal function **(Table 2)**. Length can also vary in the same individual depending on the state of hydration.

Where an absolute accurate estimate of the size of the kidneys is necessary, the renal volume can be measured. This can be achieved by measuring the area of the kidney in serial slices and calculating the volume but this method is very time consuming. A modified three-dimensional (3D) ellipsoidal formula is utilized where the length, anteroposterior diameter, and transverse diameters are multiplied by a constant which is approximately 0.5.[19] Volume measurements are done in postnephrectomy, patients to look for compensatory hypertrophy and in the assessment of renal transplants.

Emamian et al. measured the renal size in 665 healthy adult volunteers and showed that the parenchymal volume of the right kidney is smaller than the left.[26] Possible explanation for this could be: (1) The spleen is

Table 2: Normal kidney length in adults.[25]

Adult female (cm)	*Adult male (cm)*
Left kidney 11 (9.9–12.1)	11.5 (10.4–12.6)
Right kidney 10.7 (9.5–12)	11.2 (10.1–12.4)

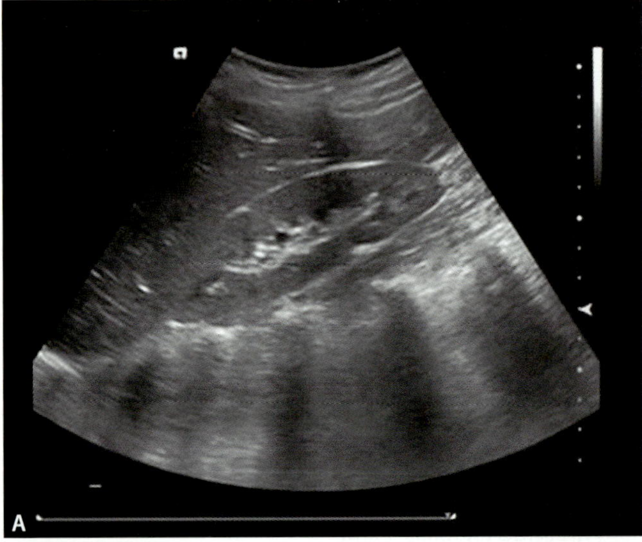

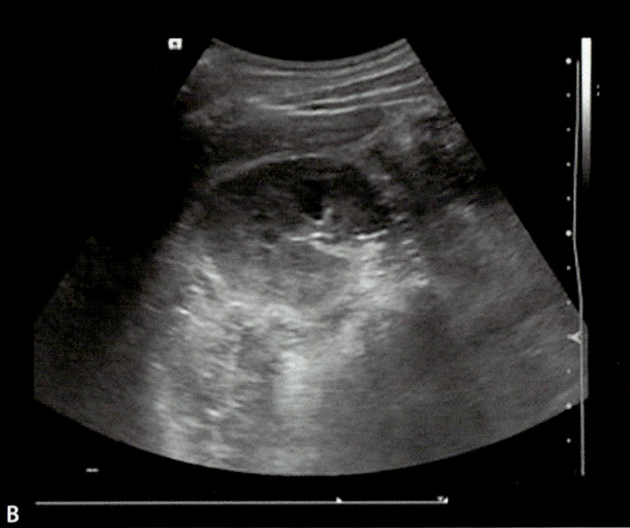

Figs. 6A and B: (A) Longitudinal and (B) transverse views of the kidney on ultrasound showing bright central sinus echoes, the cortex, and the hypoechoic medulla.

smaller than the liver and so there is more space for left kidney growth and (2) The LRA is shorter than the right and, therefore, increased blood flow on the left results in an increase in renal volume.

Cortical and Parenchymal Thickness

The cortical thickness is the distance between the renal capsule and outer margin of the renal pyramids while parenchymal thickness is the distance between renal capsule and margin of the sinus echoes **(Fig. 7)**.

Perirenal Structures

An assessment of the perirenal fat, pararenal areas, and adrenal areas should be done. At times, in case of any renal abnormality, liver, pancreas, lining of ureters, pelvis, and bladder may need to be examined.

An important point while examining the kidneys on sonography is to take care that the whole length of the kidney is included otherwise peripheral abnormalities may be missed. When longitudinal examination is complete, turning the transducer through 90° ensures that kidney is examined in transverse plane from top to bottom. In addition to the size and shape of kidney, its cortical reflectivity as compared to the liver and spleen, the degree of corticomedullary differentiation and the appearance of medullary pyramids should be taken into account.

Normal Appearances on Ultrasound

Identification of kidneys on sonography is easy owing to the difference in reflectivity between parenchyma and surrounding fat. The outer cortical margin is well-defined due to the renal capsule, but the renal parenchyma adjacent to the renal sinus echo is less well-defined. The reflectivity of the kidneys can be compared with that of the liver and spleen on the right and left side, respectively. The renal cortex has a lower reflectivity than the adjacent liver and spleen. This difference in reflectivity may vary as it is dependent on the equipment to some extent and may be less obvious with some makes or scanners or pre- and postprocessing settings. However, if the renal cortex has a higher reflectivity, that is, it is brighter than the adjacent visceral organs, it is highly suggestive of renal parenchymal disease.[27] The medullary pyramids are seen as echo-poor oval structures evenly distributed around the inner margins of the cortical parenchyma **(Fig. 8)**. The pyramids are less reflective as compared to the cortex. The well-defined margin between the pyramids and the adjacent cortex is responsible for the corticomedullary differentiation which gets lost in the presence of generalized parenchymal inflammation and edema.

The renal sinus contains the calyces, infundibulum, a portion of the renal pelvis, fibrous tissue, fat, vessels, and lymphatics. On ultrasound, the renal sinus appears as a central hyperechoic area, largely because of its fat content.[28] When collapsed, the collecting system merges with the echoes of the renal sinus. However, in well-hydrated patients, it may be slightly distended with echo-free urine.

The *neonatal kidney* is sonographically more echogenic than that of the older infant and adults **(Figs. 9A and B)**.[29] Echogenicity is equal to or greater than the adjacent liver.

Fig. 7: Ultrasound image showing the normal cortical thickness (++) measured from the renal capsule to the outer margin of the medullary pyramids and the parenchymal thickness (xx) from the capsule to the margin of the sinus. The parenchymal thickness is more than the cortical thickness.

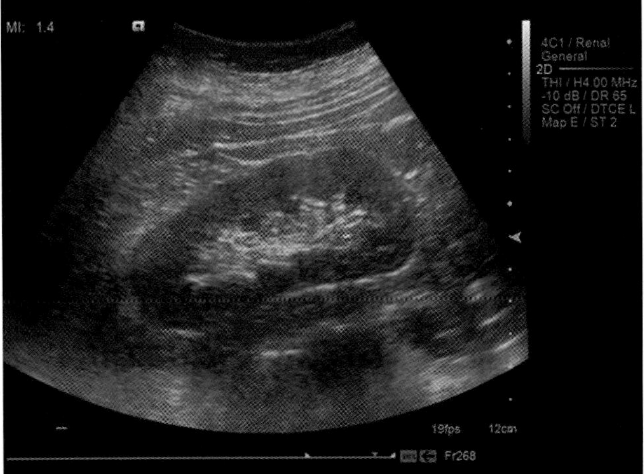

Fig. 8: Ultrasound scan of the kidney showing the corticomedullary differentiation well with the medulla seen as echopoor oval areas evenly distributed around the inner margin of the cortex. Arcuate vessels seen as echogenic foci mark the corticomedullary junction.

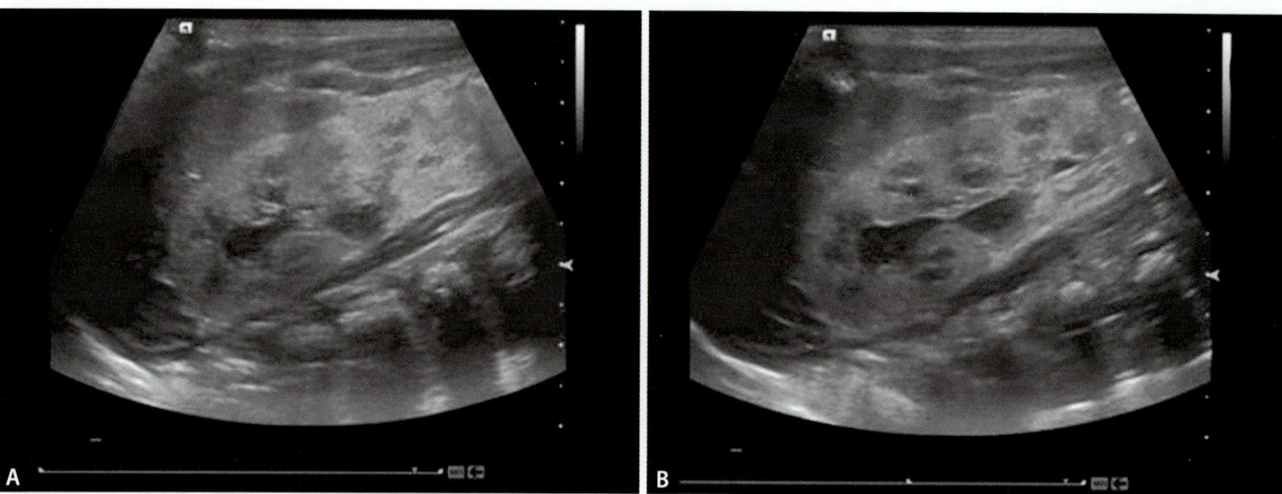

Figs. 9A and B: Ultrasound images showing the normal neonatal kidney. The cortex is thin and highly reflective while the medulla is large out of proportion and very poorly reflective. The renal sinus is also echopoor.

It assumes the adult appearance by 2-3 months of age. Other differences are tabulated in **Table 3**.

Table 3: Differences between neonatal and adult kidney.[30,31]

	Neonatal	*Adult*
Contour	Lobed	Smooth
Cortex reflectivity	++	+
Medullary reflectivity	—	—
Sinus	Echopoor	Echogenic
Collecting system	Apparent	Inapparent

Normal Variations

The kidneys may vary in *position* due to ptosis or an ectopic location. The most common site for the ectopic kidney is the pelvis, where it may be difficult to detect, as it can be obscured by bowel gas. *Renal duplication* is common and spans a range from complete to minimal. However, sonography may only show an elongated kidney perhaps with separation of the renal sinus into two parts. A double pelvis may be visualized when the collecting system is distended. Residual *fetal lobulations* may be seen. A *dromedary hump* can be seen sometimes which is a bulge along the lateral border of the left kidney due to molding by the adjacent spleen.

A *hypertrophied column of Bertin* is a normal variant and represents unresorbed polar parenchyma from one or both of the two subkidneys that fuse to form the normal kidney. Sonographic criteria to diagnose a hypertrophied column of Bertin include isoechogenicity and continuity with rest of the renal cortex, lack of mass effect, indentation of renal sinus laterally, generally less than 3 cm in size with a normal vascular pattern on Doppler.[32] Occasionally, it may be difficult to differentiate a small avascular tumor from a hypertrophied column of Bertin when further investigations may be required. A wedge-shaped echogenic defect or an echogenic line, the *intervesicular fissure or parenchymal junctional defect*, may sometimes be seen running obliquely from the sinus to the capsule in upper anterior or lower posterior part of the kidney.[33] It was thought to represent connective tissue at the junction of the development of anterior and posterior components of the kidney. However, subsequent reassessment suggests that this line represents an extension into the parenchyma of hilar/sinus fat in patients with a deep renal sinus, rather than a true plane of fusion between embryological components. It may mimic a scar or rarely a small echogenic tumor.[34]

The *renal sinus thickness* is normally equal to the parenchymal thickness. However, it may vary depending on the fat content of the sinus. An increase in fat content of the renal sinus can occur in obese individuals, in renal sinus lipomatosis, and in cases of parenchymal atrophy. It is decreased in neonates and in cachectic patients.

A mild distension of the collecting system can occur due to physiological filling. This can be seen in a fluid-loaded subject, a patient on diuretics, diabetics, recovery phase of acute tubular necrosis (ATN), single kidney, neonatal kidney, and patients with an overdistended bladder.

DOPPLER EVALUATION

Indications

- Renovascular hypertension
- Characterization of mass lesions

- Differentiation between obstructive and non-obstructive hydronephrosis
- Evaluation of transplant kidney
- Renal vein thrombosis
- Miscellaneous, e.g. trauma, arteriovenous malformation (AVM), etc.

Technique

With the patient supine, the RRA can be identified arising approximately 1 cm below the origin of the SMA. Occasionally, LRA can be identified at its origin from the posterolateral or lateral surface of aorta. Both renal veins and their junction with the IVC can usually be demonstrated in this plane. In slim patients, it is occasionally possible to follow the renal artery and vein into the hilum of the kidney.[35] The right and left posterior oblique positions can also be used to identify the vessels in the midline. Throughout the course of examination of renal vessels, color Doppler is frequently switched on to confirm the nature and direction of flow **(Fig. 10)**. The optimum pulse repetition frequency is selected to detect moderate flow velocities, although it may need to be modified to detect high velocities if a stenosis with aliasing of color signals is present.[36] With the system set to detect low or moderate flow velocities, flow can be identified in almost all patients in the vessels at the renal hilum. Angling of the probe medially from the right or left flank will allow assessment of the intrarenal vessels. Though the hilar and interlobar vessels are demonstrated in all patients, the arcuate and striate arteries may be seen only in slimmer patients. Power Doppler can show smaller vessels with slow flow, though with loss of directional information **(Fig. 11)**. Contrast-enhanced ultrasound (CEUS) can further enhance visualization of parenchymal vessels.

Normal Doppler Pattern

There is a rapid systolic upstroke, which is occasionally followed by a secondary slower rise to peak systole. Subsequently, there is a gradual diastolic decay but with persistent forward flow in diastole. Spectral indices are measured in the renal artery at proximal, middle, and at the hilum. Normal range of values is shown in **Table 4**.[36] Further, indices should also be measured in the intrarenal vessels at the superior, middle, and inferior pole of the kidney. The resistive index (RI) and pulsatility index (PI) values measured in healthy subjects show a significant dependence on age and the area sampled. The values in the main artery are higher than in the more distal smaller arteries and they are lowest in the interlobular arteries.

The renal vein spectra are often different for right and left veins. The RRV is short and often mirrors the pulsatility of the IVC, while the left, particularly if it is sampled to the left of the SMA, may show only slight variability of flow velocities.

Ureters on Ultrasound

The ureter is a long (25 cm) mucosal lined tube varying in diameter from 2 mm to 8 mm. The normal ureters are usually difficult to visualize as they are thin and collapsed structures. However, dilated ureters can be imaged in their proximal and distal parts. The proximal ureters are best visualized in a coronal oblique view, using the kidney as a window. An attempt can be made to follow the ureter up

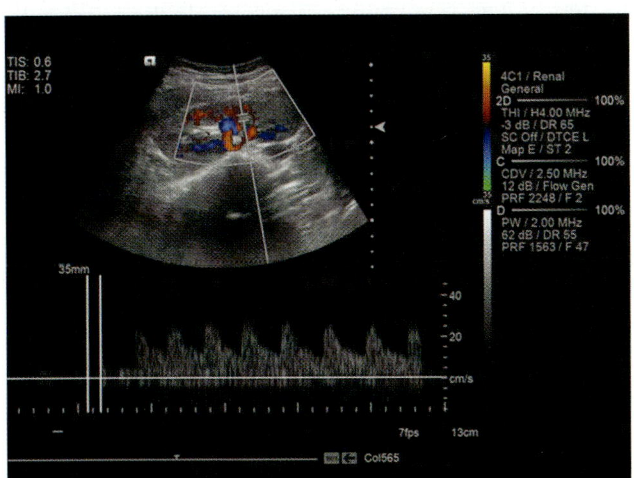

Fig. 10: Normal renal spectral pattern on color Doppler showing steep systolic peak and a good diastolic end flow.

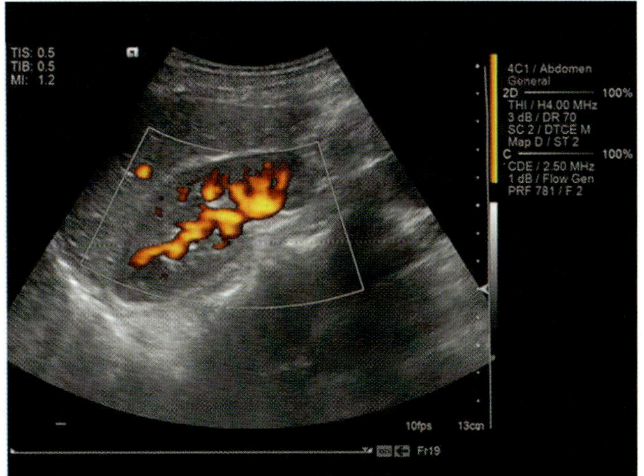

Fig. 11: Power Doppler image of the normal vasculature of the kidney.

Table 4: Normal renal indices.[36]

Index	*Range*
Pulsatility index	0.7–1.4
Resistance index	0.56–0.7
Peak systolic velocity (PSV)	60–140 cm/sec (<180)
Renal artery/aorta ratio (RAR)	< 3.5
Acceleration time	0.04–0.05 sec
Acceleration index	2.5–3.8 m/sec^2

to the bladder using the same approach. The distal ureters can be seen suprapubically through the full bladder.

CONTRAST-ENHANCED ULTRASOUND

Contrast-enhanced ultrasound is an emerging technology for evaluation of the genitourinary system with no known nephrotoxicity. It has a role in the characterization of indeterminate renal lesions, especially among those with chronic kidney disease (CKD). Iodinated contrast medium should be completely withheld in patients with later stages of CKD [glomerular filtration rate (GFR) <30 mL/min]. Similarly, gadolinium-based contrast agents should not be administered in severe renal insufficiency owing to the risk of nephrogenic systemic fibrosis (NSF). CEUS is safe in that it causes no nephrotoxicity. Microbubbles used in CEUS consist of a high molecular weight gas core surrounded by a lipid or albumin shell. The microbubbles are not excreted or secreted in the urinary tract but are exhaled out via the lungs and hence have no adverse effect on the kidneys. According to the 2011 European Federation for the Society of Ultrasound in Medicine and Biology Guidelines, the use of CEUS for renal indications include:[37]

- Characterization of indeterminate lesions when conventional ultrasound is equivocal
- Renal infarcts and cortical necrosis
- Abscesses
- Determination of surgical strategy for complex cystic masses
- Follow-up imaging of nonsurgical complex masses
- Tumor ablation under ultrasound guidance.

SonoVue, Optison, and Sonazoid are some of the ultrasound contrast agents available in the US for intravenous use while SonoVue is available in India. CEUS has shown promising results and its sensitivity has been reported comparable to that of contrast-enhanced CT in the characterization of renal lesions.[38] The sensitivity in detection of renal malignancy has been found to be about 90% in several studies with a moderate specificity of 79–90%.[39] An exciting new frontier in CEUS research is the use of targeted microbubbles where antibodies can be tagged to the outer shell. The antibodies get adhered to their molecular target and on imaging this is seen as persistence of enhancement. This is helpful in the detection of diseases and holds the prospect of delivering therapy specifically at these locations reducing the systemic toxic effects of the chemotherapeutic drugs.

ULTRASOUND ELASTOGRAPHY

Elastography can be used to diagnose kidney diseases and provides a more accurate estimate of the functional impairment than blood tests or kidney dimensions. Intrarenal fibrosis is a final common pathway for all chronic kidney diseases and it has been seen that the degree of fibrosis correlates with the severity of the disease. Renal biopsy can determine the degree of fibrosis and hence the severity of the renal parenchymal disease but it is invasive, is subject to sampling errors and samples a small fraction of the renal parenchyma leading to an inaccurate assessment.

Shear wave elastography (SWE) is an emerging technique which permits a noninvasive measurement of tissue stiffness. SWE uses focused acoustic energy pulses to produce shear waves which travel perpendicular to the tissue. As they progress through the tissue, they can be tracked sonographically. Stiffer the tissue, more is the shear wave velocity. Higher values of shear wave velocity thus correlate with higher degrees of renal fibrosis. Studies have shown that SWE is a low cost way to provide diagnostic information in patients with CKD and a correlation has been found between SWE, estimated renal stiffness, and renal fibrosis severity.[40] Hence, SWE-derived estimates of tissue stiffness may serve as a noninvasive biomarker of healthy and diseased renal parenchyma in the near future.

COMPUTED TOMOGRAPHY OF THE UPPER URINARY TRACT

The cross-sectional imaging modalities such as CT and magnetic resonance imaging (MRI) allow a noninvasive visualization and a better understanding of the genitourinary tract. The anatomical characteristics of the renal and perirenal regions can be visualized objectively and accurately. Perfusion characteristics of the kidney can also be studied. CT plays a vital role in evaluating patients with renal cystic diseases, renal tumors, infections, and flank pain. Lesions containing fat or calcium are best assessed on CT.

MDCT allows volumetric data acquisition and submillimeter excellent quality images can be reconstructed in any plane. MDCT with its 3D postprocessing capabilities is highly accurate in the evaluation of renal masses and a noninvasive evaluation of vascular pedicle by CT angiography. MDCT reduces the diagnosis of indeterminate masses by enabling an improved characterization of renal masses, thus allowing a better therapeutic management. The faster scanning times, improved spatial and temporal resolution, and greater volume coverage with the MDCT scanners allow detection and characterization of small renal masses, display of vasculature similar to conventional angiography, and improved visualization of the collecting system and ureters with better demonstration of both intraluminal and extraluminal pathology.[41,42] MDCT allows images to be obtained in different phases of enhancement of the renal parenchyma including the excretory phase (EP) and images simulating excretory urography can be obtained.[43] Excellent quality multiplanar reformation (MPR) images and 3D rendering of any plane is possible owing to increased temporal resolution and acquisition of thin slices with isotropic voxels.[44]

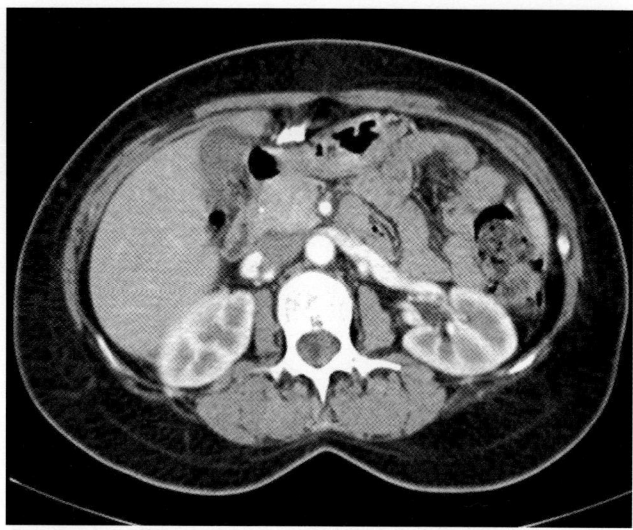

Fig. 12: Contrast-enhanced axial scans showing the kidneys as smooth and oval structures with an anteromedial break in the region of hilum where the vascular pedicle enters. The longer left renal vein is seen crossing anterior to the aorta and posterior to the superior mesenteric artery to enter the inferior vena cava at the level of the uncinate process of the pancreas.

Normal Appearance of the Upper Urinary Tract on CT

On the axial sections, the kidneys appear smooth and oval. The vascular pedicle enters the renal hilum which is seen as an anteromedial break **(Fig. 12)**. The vascular pedicle lies anterior to the renal pelvis. Differentiation between renal artery and vein may not be possible on conventional scans. The renal veins are larger than the renal artery. Of the veins, the left renal vein is larger than the right owing to the aorta and SMA pinching the left renal vein.

The ureters are best visualized after intravenous administration of iodinated contrast material. The ureters are anterior to the common iliac artery, lateral to the external iliac artery, and anteromedial to the psoas major at the level of the sacral promontory. The ureters then reach the midportion of the internal obturator muscle coursing medially and posteriorly to the external iliac arteries. They then course anteromedially to reach the trigone of the urinary bladder **(Figs. 13A to D)**.

Examination Technique and Imaging Protocols of MDCT of Kidney

A multiphasic CT is the preferred imaging technique in the evaluation of the upper urinary tract. It includes an unenhanced scan followed by scanning the kidneys in the corticomedullary, nephrographic, and EPs after rapid bolus injection of contrast (100–120 mL of 300 mgI/mL of contrast) at the rate of 3–4 mL/sec.[45] Use of dense oral contrast medium is not recommended for renal CT as the contrast in the bowel may obscure small ureteral stones making their detection difficult. The dense oral contrast medium poses a major problem in 3D-CT angiography and to avoid major overlay in the postprocessed images,[46] it is recommended that negative oral contrast medium/ water should be administered. And 500–750 mL of water can be given over a 15–20-minute period before the start of a renal CT examination.[47]

Noncontrast

This phase is useful for baseline density measurements of renal masses and diagnosis of areas of hemorrhage/renal hematoma.[48] Areas of renal parenchymal calcification, fat attenuation, and calcification in a renal mass can all be detected on the noncontrast scan. These are also helpful to differentiate a renal solid mass from hyperdense cyst. Noncontrast CT is regarded as the primary imaging modality to detect urinary tract calculi.[49] The American Association and Endourological Society Guidelines for the Surgical Management of stones specifically recommend that clinicians should obtain a noncontrast CT before performing percutaneous nephrolithotomy (PCNL) in adults and children.[50] Low-dose computed tomography (LDCT) and ultralow-dose computed tomography (ULDCT) have been proposed to reduce radiation risks for the detection of urolithiasis.[51,52]

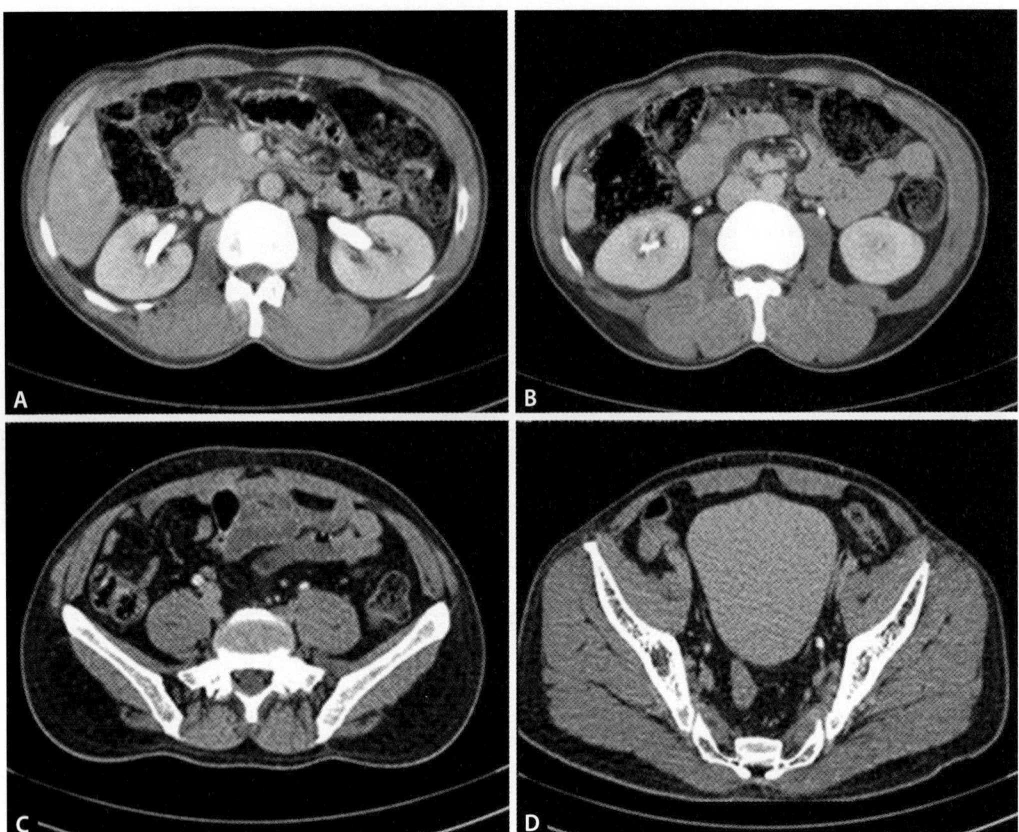

Figs. 13A to D: Axial CT sections showing the normal anatomy of the urinary structures from superior to inferior: (A) The renal pelvis; (B) Upper ureters; (C) Mid ureters; (D) Distal ureters.

Normal CT Nephrogram

The first phase is the corticomedullary phase (CMP) and it is seen 25–80 seconds following contrast administration. In this phase, the lumen of the proximal tubules fills up with contrast which then enters the cortical capillaries and peritubular capillary spaces. In this phase, the renal cortex is distinctly differentiated from the unenhanced medulla **(Fig. 14)**.[53] The nephrographic phase (NP) is the second phase and begins 90–120 seconds after contrast injection. The contrast passes through the renal tubules during this phase. In the nephrogram phase, there is a homogeneous enhancement of the renal parenchyma with loss of the corticomedullary differentiation **(Fig. 15)**. The excretory phase (EP) begins with the excretion of the contrast material into the collecting system and is seen best 3–5 minutes after contrast administration **(Fig. 16)**.

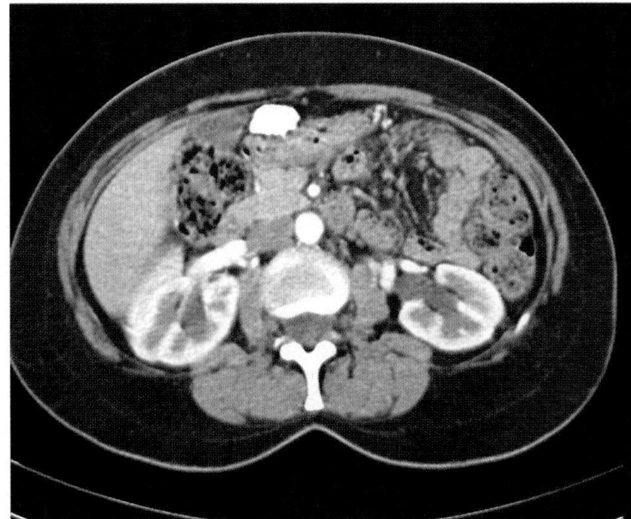

Fig. 14: Contrast-enhanced CT scan of the kidney in the corticomedullary phase showing dense cortical enhancement, the renal cortex is distinctly differentiated from the unenhanced medulla in this phase.

Corticomedullary Phase

This phase is important for the evaluation of tumor hypervascularity and differentiation of normal variants and pseudotumors from renal masses. This phase is also the best phase for the diagnosis of tumor extension in the renal vein as maximum opacification of the renal vein and arteries occur during this time **(Figs. 17A and B)**. However, scanning the kidney only in the CMP may lead to errors as

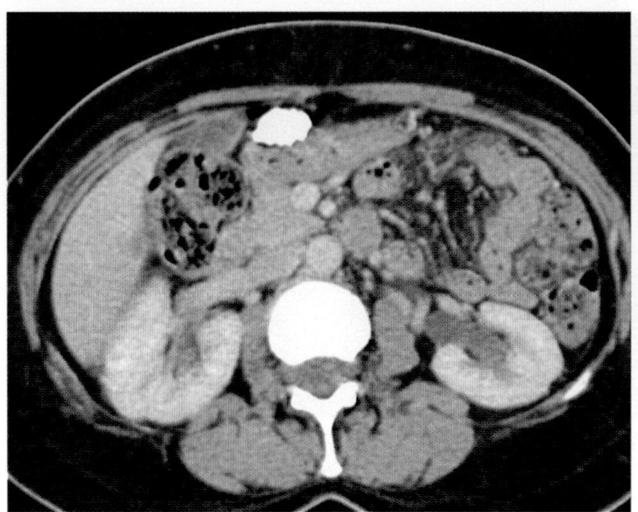

Fig. 15: Contrast-enhanced CT of the kidney in the nephrogram phase showing dense homogeneous parenchymal enhancement. The corticomedullary differentiation disappears during this phase.

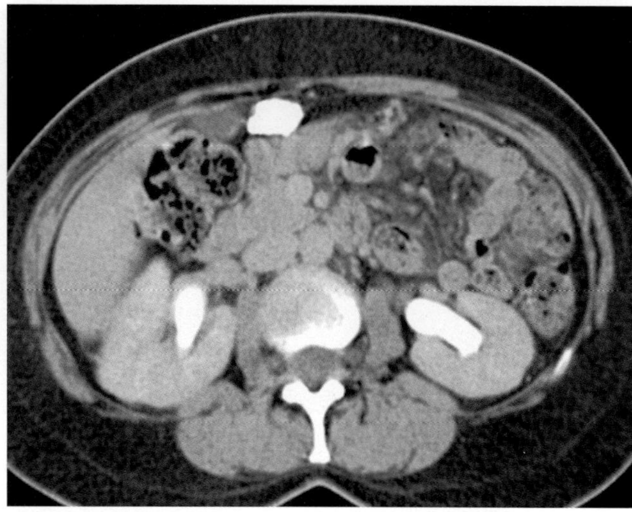

Fig. 16: Excretory phase images showing opacification of the pelvicalyceal system.

hypervascular cortical renal cell carcinomas (RCCs) may enhance to the same degree as the normal cortex and thus may be obscured. Also, small hypovascular tumors of the renal medulla may not enhance sufficiently and may be missed.[54] It is therefore essential to scan the kidney in the NP following the CMP.

Nephrographic Phase

Nephrographic phase is considered as the optimum phase for not only detection but also characterization of renal masses. In this phase, there is a homogeneous enhancement of both the cortex and medulla. This phase is useful particularly for the lesions <3 cm.[55] Any enhancement >20 HU is considered suggestive of malignancy and this lesion enhancement is usually best visualized on the NP.[56] Renal infarction, traumatic parenchymal lesions, and acute pyelonephritis is also best visualized on the NP as the lesions stand out as hypodense areas against the enhanced renal parenchyma **(Figs. 18A and B)**.

Excretory Phase

This provides a good delineation and visualization of the pelvicalyceal system. The excretory phase (EP) images

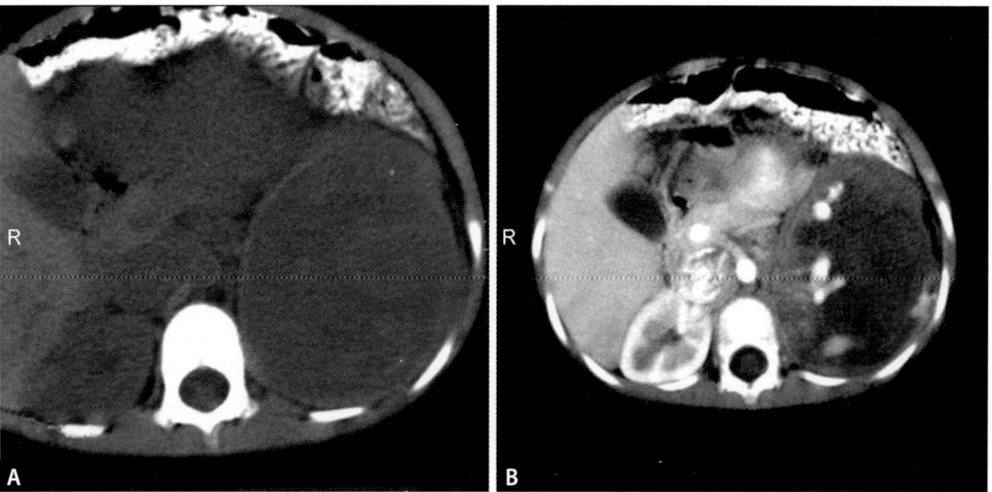

Figs. 17A and B: (A) Noncontrast axial CT showing a large hypodense mass replacing the left kidney. (B) The corticomedullary phase shows multiple tortuous feeder vessels depicting tumor hypervascularity. Thrombus is also seen in inferior vena cava in the case of Wilms' tumor, the corticomedullary phase being excellent for the depiction.

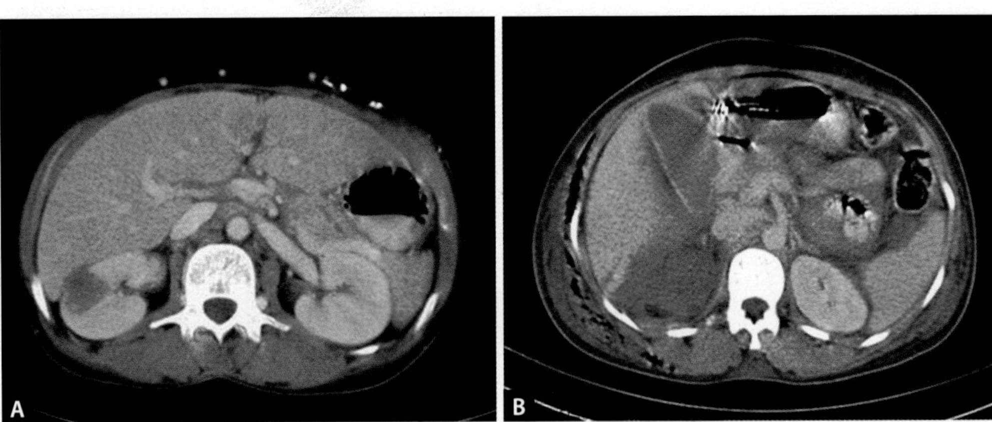

Figs. 18A and B: (A) Nephrogram phase showing a wedge-shaped area of hypoattenuation against the enhanced right renal parenchyma suggestive of renal infarct; (B) Image in another case showing complete lack of nephrogram suggesting devascularization of the right renal parenchyma in a case of trauma. The normal nephrogram with homogeneous enhancement of the renal parenchyma is seen on the left side.

are useful for evaluation of urothelial lesions including urothelial neoplasms, calyceal deformities, papillary necrosis, and strictures and inflammatory changes of the collecting system and ureters.[57]

Pathological CT Nephrogram

Renal infarctions, blunt renal trauma, and acute pyelonephritis account for a pathological nephrogram. These conditions result in impaired renal perfusion with a focal reduction of the nephrogram. A segmental/ total lack of the nephrogram is seen in cases of blunt renal trauma owing to devascularization. In acute pyelonephritis, inflammatory obstruction results in reduced tubule transit rate. The delayed perfusion of the renal tubule system is seen as a "striated nephrogram" pattern.[58] Conditions like acute ureteric obstruction, acute obstruction of the renal vein, and significant stenosis of the main renal artery result in reduced density and slowed temporal progression of the three phases of the nephrogram. Conditions like shock/ severe systemic hypotension result in a bilaterally reduced density and persistence of nephrogram due to a reduced GFR and tubular stasis.

MDCT in Renal Masses

A multiphasic MDCT is necessary for optimal evaluation of renal masses.[59] Noncontrast CT is used to detect calcifications and the precontrast attenuation value allows quantification of enhancement on the postcontrast scans. The CMP best shows the extension of the tumoral tissue into the renal vein and IVC which is important for staging. A hypodense, filling defect within the renal vein which is usually dilated is suggestive of a thrombus. Heterogeneous enhancement of the thrombus with evidence of neovascularity favors a tumor thrombus over a bland thrombus. The neovascularity, arterial feeders, and the entire arterial anatomy is best seen on the CMP. Accurate demonstration of the arterial anatomy is essential to plan a nephron sparing surgery. The NP is the most useful for characterization of indeterminate masses. An enhancement value >20 HU is considered highly suggestive of a RCC as these are hypervascular and enhance on the postcontrast scans.[60] The EP is useful for demonstrating the relationship of a centrally located mass with the pelvicalyceal system. Involvement of the renal pelvis and calyces can also be best seen on the EP. Transitional cell carcinomas (TCCs) are also best detected during this phase as subtle hypodense filling defects within the renal pelvis, calyces or the ureters. A washout >15 HU seen in a mass on the EP is also highly suggestive of a RCC as these show a significant washout as well **(Figs. 19A to C)**.[61] A hyperdense renal cyst, on the contrary, will show no change in density between the corticomedullary and the excretory/delayed images.[61]

Three-dimensional CT (3DCT) along with CT angiography is useful to define the tumor and its relationship to the renal surface, the pelvicalyceal system and the adjacent organs. Viewing in multiple planes and orientations can be done to obtain all the information needed to plan a surgical resection. A display of the arterial and venous anatomy is possible prior to surgery.

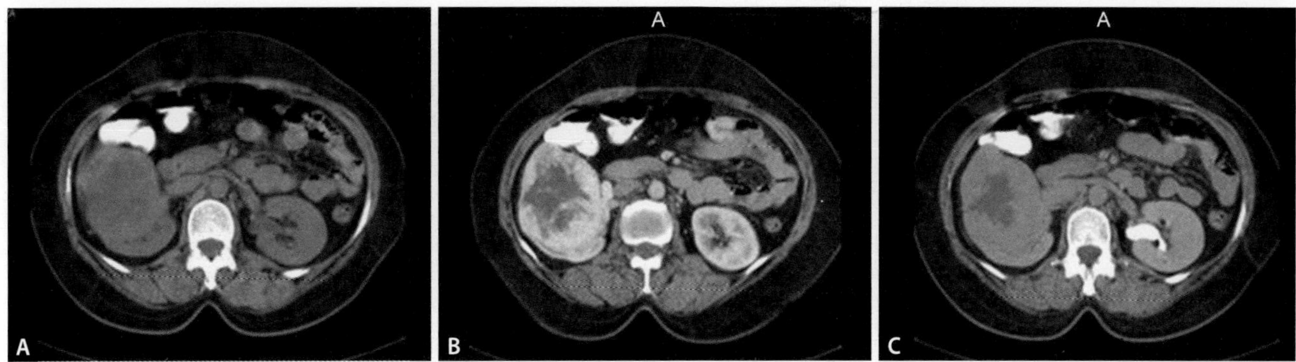

Figs. 19A to C: (A) Noncontrast; and (B and C) contrast-enhanced axial scans showing a large heterogeneous mass in the right kidney with enhancement >20 HU and washout >15 HU suggestive of a malignant renal mass. Areas of necrosis are also noted.

MDCT in Urolithiasis and Acute Flank Pain

A noncontrast CT of the abdomen is the most sensitive and specific test for the detection of urinary tract calculi. A 98% sensitivity and 100% specificity for their detection has been reported by Fielding et al.[62] Noncontrast thin collimation scans (3–5 mm) are obtained from the upper pole of the kidneys to the pubic symphysis for the detection of urolithiasis which may be a cause of hematuria as well. Irrespective of the calcium content, almost all calculi are seen as radiopaque densities on noncontrast CT. Identification of a stone within the ureter is the most specific diagnostic finding of urolithiasis. A "rim sign" may also be seen in cases of calculi owing to the ureteral wall edema that develops at the site of impaction.[63] This is seen as an area of soft tissue thickening (1–2 mm thickness) around the calculus. A decreased density of the renal parenchyma, hydronephrosis, hydroureter, and perinephric stranding are the other features seen in cases of calculi. A decreased attenuation of the renal parenchyma on the obstructed side by 5–14 HU is considered an objective finding of obstruction **(Figs. 20A to C)**.[64] CT can also differentiate calculi from phleboliths. Calculi have a dense center while phleboliths have a central lucency. A "comet tail sign" which is a linear or curvilinear soft tissue density extending from an abdominal/pelvic calcification is highly suggestive of a phlebolith.[65] MDCT is also useful for detecting the cause of pain other than stone such as appendicitis, biliary colic, diverticulitis, etc.[66]

MDCT in Blunt Renal Trauma

In patients with trauma, a noncontrast scan followed by multiphasic scanning needs to be done. The CMP is the best phase to show injuries of the renal arteries including internal injuries which are nonocclusive in nature. Renal vein thrombosis can also be seen. Contrast extravasations which occur during the CMP are due to hemorrhage as compared to contrast extravasations that occur during the EP which are due to rupture of the pelvicalyceal system **(Figs. 21A to C)**. Contained hemorrhage or pseudoaneurysm is seen as a well-defined lesion within the area of laceration. Active hemorrhage is seen as ill-defined or flame-shaped area with bright enhancement close to an artery.[67] NP is the best to demonstrate areas of renal infarction/nonperfused parenchymal injuries. EP images are the best to show contrast extravasation in urinomas indicating an injury to the collecting system.[68]

MDCT in Renal Infections

Multidetector computed tomography is a more useful modality than IVU or ultrasound in the assessment of renal infection. The nature and extent of the disease process as well as complications such as gas forming infections, abscess formation, and urinary obstruction can all be well seen on CT.[69] The most characteristic finding of acute pyelonephritis is poorly defined low attenuating areas of decreased attenuation which are wedge-shaped radiating from the medulla to the cortical surface. These wedge-shaped areas are best seen in the NP. A nephrogram pattern consisting of alternating linear bands of hyper- and hypoattenuation, the so called "striated nephrogram" is another characteristic finding of acute pyelonephritis. Other findings include focal or diffuse enlargement of the kidney, diminished concentration of contrast in the tubules due to the inflammatory process, stranding of the perinephric fat, thickening of Gerota's fascia, and obliteration of renal sinus.[70] A focal thinning of the cortex may result from scarring in chronic cases.

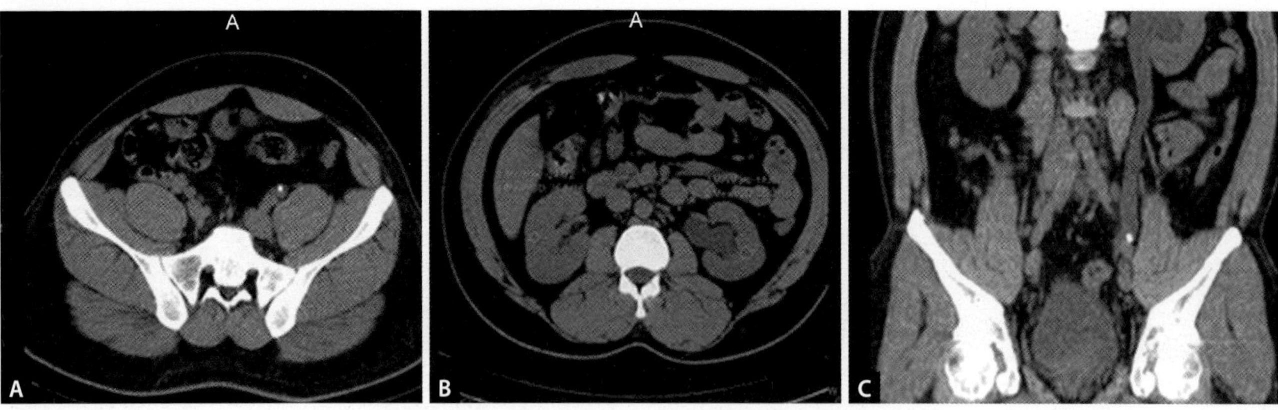

Figs. 20A to C: Noncontrast axial scans (A and B) of the abdomen showing a left ureteric calculus with soft tissue edema around, i.e. the rim sign (A) and the left hydronephrosis (B). The hydronephrotic left kidney has a lower attenuation than the normal right kidney. Curved multiplanar reformation displaying the left ureteric calculus, the consequent hydronephrosis, and the entire dilated left ureter proximal to it regardless of opacification (C).

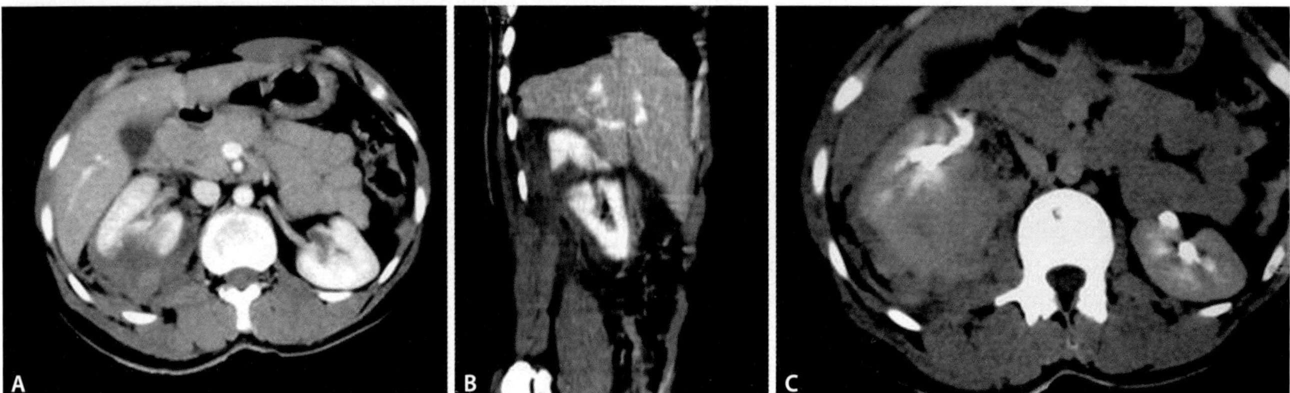

Figs. 21A to C: (A) Nephrogram phase image showing laceration of the right renal parenchyma with perinephric hematoma; (B) Sagittal multiplanar reformation image showing fracture of the kidney; (C) Excretory phase showing extravasation of contrast in the perinephric hematoma suggesting rupture of the pelvicalyceal system.

Image Processing and Postprocessing Techniques on Computed Tomography

The various 3D visualization techniques in the evaluation of the urinary tract are MPR, maximum intensity projection (MIP), shaded surface display (SSD), and volume-rendered techniques (VRTs).

Multiplanar Reformation

Multiplanar reformation (MPR) represents a simple reordering of the image voxel. For MPR, the structures must be in the same plane, hence it cannot be generated for structures not in the same plane. Pseudostenoses are created as structures course in and out of the MPR. Curved multiplanar reformations (CPRs) are useful to overcome this problem.[71] CPR images can be obtained by drawing a line over the structure of interest, it can also be produced by a dedicated software automatically or semiautomatically. CPR is useful in the demonstration of vessels of small diameter or structures with tortuous anatomy like the ureters **(Figs. 22A to C)**.[72] The limitation, however, is the dependence on accuracy of the curve generated.

Maximum Intensity Projection

Maximum intensity projection (MIP) displays the maximum voxel intensity along a line in a given volume. Structures with high density such as the contrast opacified collecting system and vessels are well demonstrated on MIP images. Angiograms and urograms are examples where this technique is used **(Figs. 23A to C)**. However, the major limitation is obscuration of the area of interest by high density material like bone, calcium, and oral contrast medium. MIP also lacks depth orientation.[73]

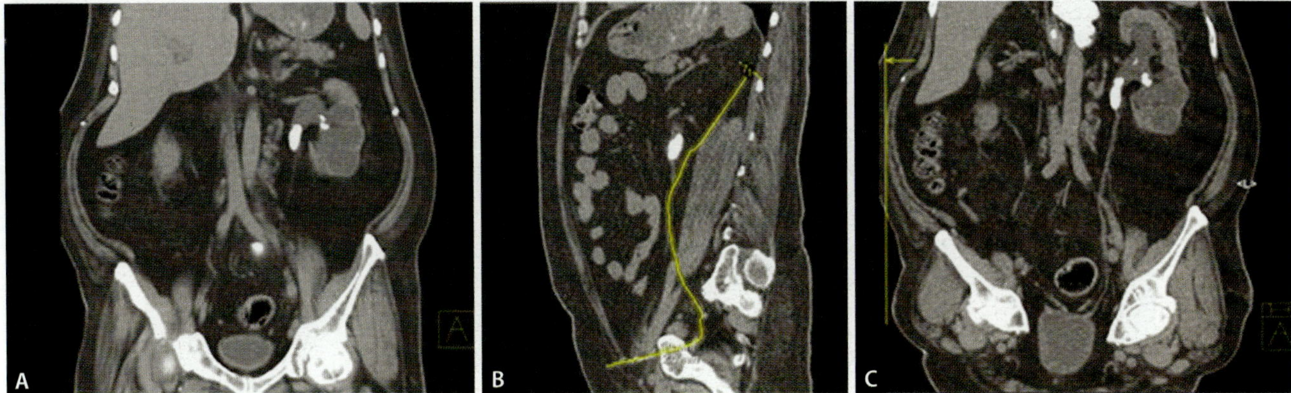

Figs. 22A to C: (A) Coronal multiplanar reformation (MPR) image showing a left ureteric calculus and the dilated pelvicalyceal proximal to it; (B and C) Curved multiplanar images show the left ureter in its entirety.

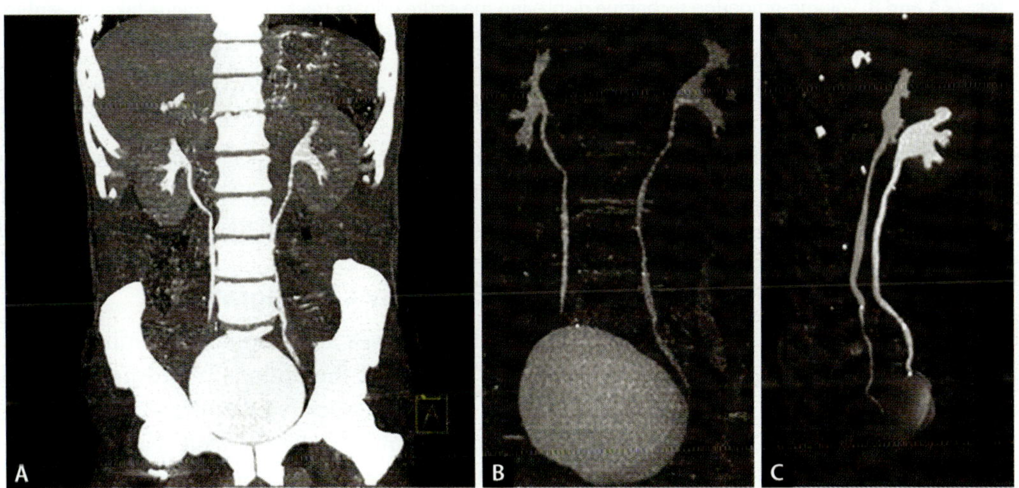

Figs. 23A to C: Maximum intensity projection (MIP) in the excretory phase demonstrating the normally opacified calyces, the ureters, and the bladder. This technique displays the maximum voxel value along a line of viewer and projection through a given volume and a rotational viewing of multiple projections can be done (A to C).

Shaded Surface Display

Shaded surface display (SSD) enables an accurate 3D representation of anatomy. It relies on the gray scale to yield surface reflections of structures. Though it provides a depth orientation, its major limitation lies in the dependence on user selected threshold setting.

Volume Rendered Technique

Volume rendered technique takes the entire volume of data and displays anatomic structures with different levels of opacity/attenuation. All attenuation values within a voxel are used to obtain the final image with each voxel contributing color, brightness, and opacity to the final image. The renal parenchyma, renal vasculature, and the pelvicalyceal system have different levels of opacity and can be seen simultaneously using this technique. VRT is an excellent 3D technique that provides a roadmap to the surgeon and produces images with[72] which the clinicians are familiar with. By editing out bone and other areas that overlie the area of interest excellent 3D images can be generated in the desired orientation **(Figs. 24A and B)**.

MULTIDETECTOR CT UROGRAPHY

It is an examination of the urinary tract in the EP following intravenous contrast on MDCT. CT urography can examine the entire genitourinary tract in a single study. It is a comprehensive examination that allows evaluation of both the renal parenchyma and the urothelium. Multidetector computed tomography urography (MDCTU) can be used as a "one-stop imaging test" for the entire urinary tract.[74]

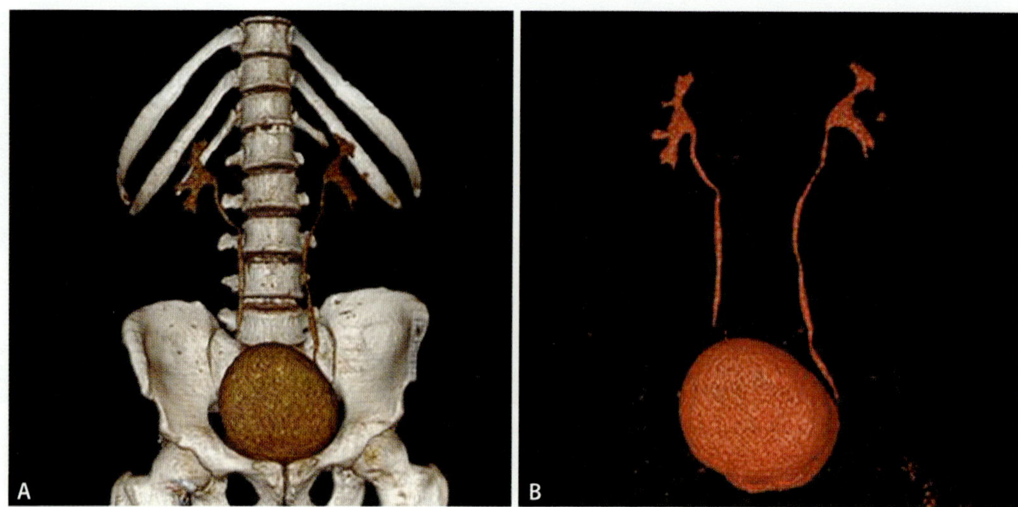

Figs. 24A and B: Volume-rendering technique displaying the entire urinary tract. This technique takes the entire volume of data and displays anatomic structures with different levels of opacity/attenuation.

The two approaches to perform a CT urography include:

1. CT hybrid urography
2. CT—only CT urography.

CT HYBRID UROGRAPHY

This technique combines CT and IVU into a single comprehensive examination. No CT postprocessing is necessary as images are obtained in a coronal reformatted form familiar to the clinicians. CT hybrid urography may entail imaging the patient in two different locations. Conventional urography images can be acquired in an IVU room followed by transferring the patient to the CT room and imaging the patient without an additional dose of contrast medium.[75] However, the disadvantages involved in moving the patient from one place to another involve longer time, additional resources, and inadequate opacification of the pelvicalyceal system during acquisition because of the time elapsed in moving the patient.[76] In some centers, this problem has been solved by installing a ceiling mounted X-ray tube above the CT table and a special tabletop that allows insertion of a screen film system beneath the patient.[77] With this technique, an abdominal radiograph, a noncontrast CT followed by a multiphasic CT followed by overhead excretory urography and postvoid films can be acquired. However, by the use of CT scanned projection radiography (CTSPR) which is also known as topogram or scannogram, the technique can be performed on any MDCT scanner.[78] CTSPR images do not require a ceiling mounted X-ray tube. In this, a combination of axial CT scans and enhanced CTSPR images are obtained. The spatial resolution of CTSPR, however, is inferior to that of conventional radiographs.

CT—Only CT Urography

This involves acquisition of unenhanced and enhanced CT scans of the abdomen and pelvis including the EP. Caoili and associated performed a four phase CT urogram comprising an unenhanced scan, NP and two EPs, one at 5 minutes and the other at 7.5 minutes.[79] However, a four phase protocol consisting of two EPs (at 5 minutes and 7.5 minutes) is usually not recommended because of radiation issues. A three phase protocol is usually followed in most institutions consisting of the unenhanced phase, a NP and an EP.[80] The NP is acquired at 90–100 sec following contrast administration (100–150 mL of 300 mg/mL iodine concentration at the rate of 2–4 mL/sec). The excretory/pyelographic phase is usually taken 12–15 minutes following contrast administration to evaluate the urothelium from the pelvicalyceal system to the bladder.

Techniques to Improve Urinary Tract Distension

- *Diuretic administration*: A diuretic like 10 mg of furosemide given 1 minute before contrast administration has been reported to increase ureteric distension. It also allows for a less dense homogeneous opacification of the collecting system.[81]
- *Oral contrast*: About 1,000 mL of water can be given orally within 15–20 minutes to cause sufficient distension of the collecting system in most cases.

- *Saline infusion*: Saline infusion technique, that is, 250 mL saline chase after administration of IV contrast helps in a better opacification of the distal ureters which are the most difficult segments to visualize.[82,83]
- *Compression*: External compression is not a part of MDCTU protocol because it causes patient discomfort and has not been shown to improve the percentage of visualized segments.[83]
- *Patient positioning*: A MDCTU performed in the prone position achieves a higher opacification of mid and distal ureters than supine position. However, being cumbersome, it is not advocated for routine use. Scanning is done in the supine position for computed tomography urography (CTU).[84]
- *Image interpretation*: MPR, MIP, and VRT images are most commonly used.[85] The reformats show the urinary tract in entirety and are useful for characterization of renal masses, presence of calculi, evaluation of ureter, and localization of the exact level of abnormality.

Split Bolus MDCT Urography with Synchronous NP and EP Enhancement

A split bolus technique has been proposed by Chow and colleagues to minimize radiation dose as well as minimize the number of images generated.[86] This is a two-phase technique in which an unenhanced series of images is followed by the "nephropyelographic phase", that is, there is a simultaneous acquisition of the nephrographic and pyelographic phases. In this technique, following the noncontrast scan, 30 cc of nonionic contrast is infused intravenously which is the first bolus. The patient is then removed from the CT table and allowed to walk around for 10 minutes. 10–15 minutes later a contrast-enhanced CT is performed following a second bolus of contrast injection. 100 cc of nonionic contrast is injected intravenously and scanning is done after a delay of 100 seconds. By allowing the contrast bolus to be split, 30 cc (1st bolus) followed by 100 cc (2nd bolus), the nephrographic and pyelographic phases can be acquired simultaneously. In this single nephropyelographic phase, both the renal parenchyma (NP) and the collecting system (pyelographic phase) can be assessed.

Triple Bolus CT Urography

In this, the bolus is split into three and then a combined corticomedullary, nephrographic, and EP is acquired.[87] The first bolus is 30 mL given at 2 mL/sec used for the opacification of the excretory system followed 7 minutes later by the second bolus of 50 mL at 1.5 mL/sec for the renal parenchyma and finally a third bolus 20 seconds later of 65 mL at 3 mL/sec for arterial information. The three phases are then acquired in a single scan, obtained some 510 seconds after start of first bolus. A triple bolus technique further reduces radiation dose as compared to the split bolus.[87,88]

Indications for CT urography are as follows:

- Hematuria
- Urothelial lesions
- Calculi
- Renal tumors
- Ureteral lesions
- Pelviureteric junction obstruction
- Congenital anomalies.

Hematuria

Computed tomography urography (CTU) has an overall sensitivity of 92.4–100% and specificity of 89–97.4% in detection of the causes of hematuria.[89,90] CTU can be justified as a first line test in hematuria patients with a high probability for TCCs.[91] For the lower risk patients, CTU is a problem-solving modality if the work-up remains negative and hematuria persists.[92]

The algorithm for the evaluation of painless microscopic/macroscopic hematuria is given in **Table 5**.[91]

Table 5: Evaluation of painless microscopic and macroscopic hematuria.[91]

ProbabilityTCC Hematuria Patient age First line tests	Lowest Micro <40 years CYS US ↓	Low Macro <40 years CYS US ↓	Medium Micro >40 years CYS US ↓	High Macro >40 years CYS CTU ↓
Follow-up	Watch and wait If negative	IVU if US and CYS negative and symptoms persist	IVU or CTU if US and CYS negative and symptoms persist	Specialist referral

(TCC: transitional cell carcinoma; US: ultrasound; IVU: intravenous urogram; CTU: computed tomography urography; CYS: cystatin)

Urothelial Lesions

Computed tomography urogram is excellent in the depiction of urothelial lesions with a high sensitivity and specificity. CTU is superior not only to IVU but also to retrograde ureterography, an imaging technique considered superior to IVU in the evaluation of the pelvicalyceal system and ureters.[93] MDCTU is an accurate technique for detection and staging of TCCs of the upper urinary tract. The TCC occurs most commonly in elderly men and risk factors include chemical carcinogens, smoking, cyclophosphamide or phenacetin use. The entire urinary tract is susceptible to malignant transformation owing to the field effect of these carcinogens. As a result, TCCs are often multifocal at presentation and the entire urinary tract should be screened even if a single lesion is detected **(Figs. 25A to D)**. MDCTU is the imaging modality that provides a screening of the entire urinary tract for synchronous and metachronous lesions in TCC.[94] Synchronous lesions are discrete TCC foci identified on a single study while metachronous lesions are those detected on follow-up imaging. MDCTU is the first line imaging modality when noninvasive imaging is needed for the detection and surveillance of urothelial lesions of the upper urinary tract.[95]

Calculi

Computed tomography urogram has an advantage over intravenous urogram (IVU) in detecting extraurinary pathologies that may mimic calculi **(Figs. 26A and B)**.[96] It is more accurate than intravenous urogram in detecting presence, size, and location of the calculi, can detect calculi in unusual positions such as in a calyceal diverticulum. Like intravenous urogram, CT urogram provides physiological information about the function of kidneys. A delayed excretion of contrast which is an index of obstruction, hydronephrosis, and hydroureter can all be well seen on the CT urogram images.

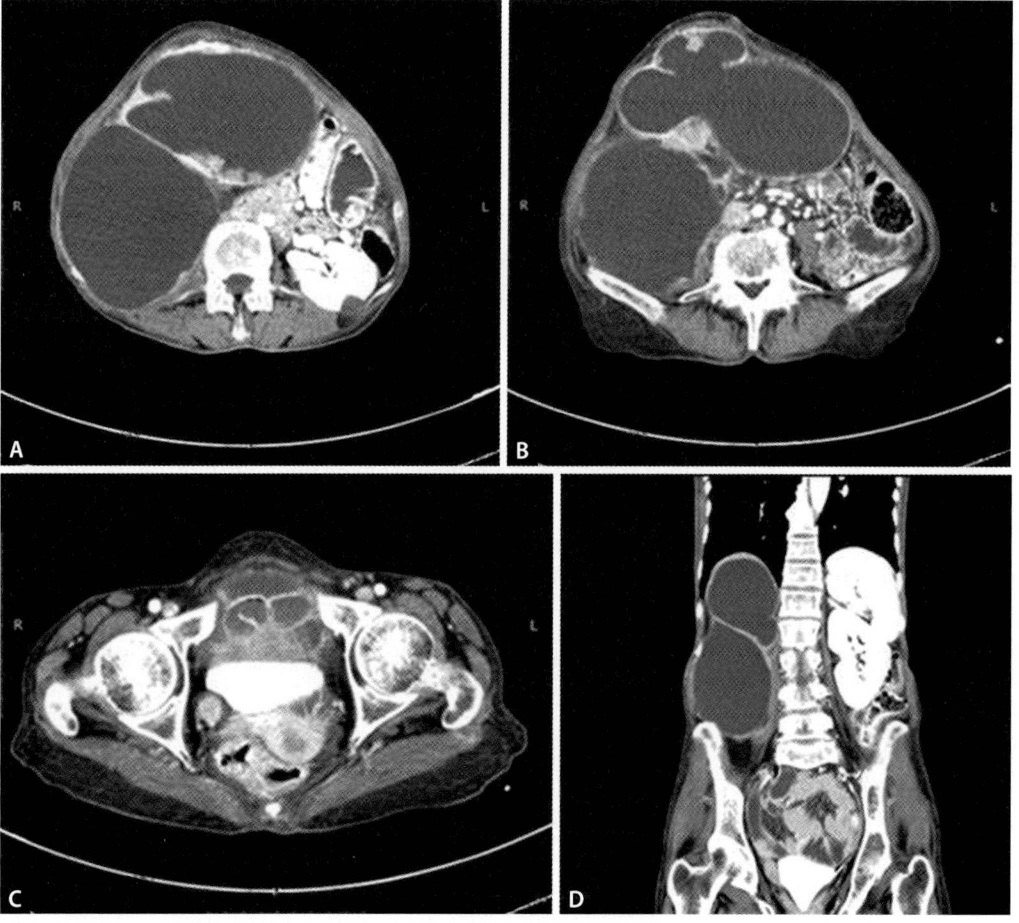

Figs. 25A to D: (A to C) Contrast-enhanced axial and (D) coronal images on CT scan showing a grossly hydronephrotic right kidney with small polypoidal masses within. Note is made of diffuse circumferential thickening of the right ureter at the ureterovesical junction—multifocal transitional cell carcinoma.

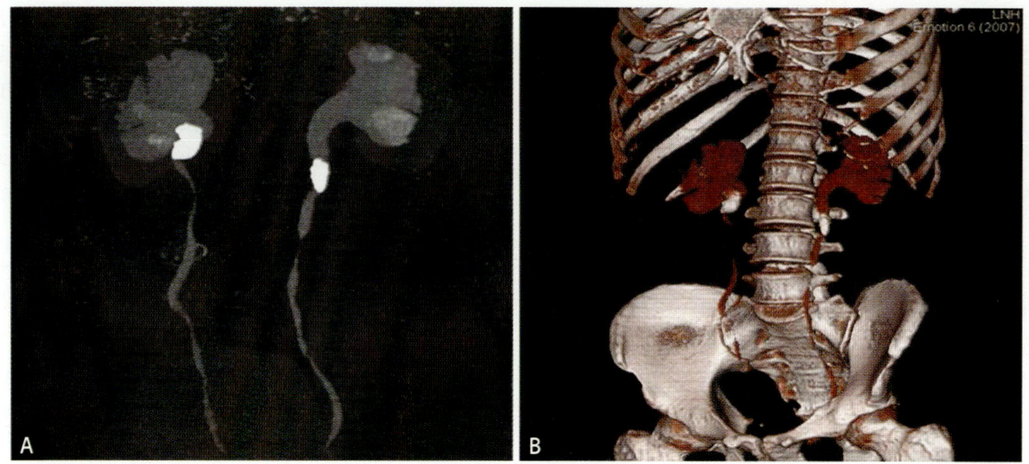

Figs. 26A and B: (A) CT urogram using maximum intensity projection technique depicting a calculus at the pelviureteric junction on the right side and a calculus in the proximal left ureter. There are back pressure changes on both sides; (B) Volume-rendering technique image displaying the same.

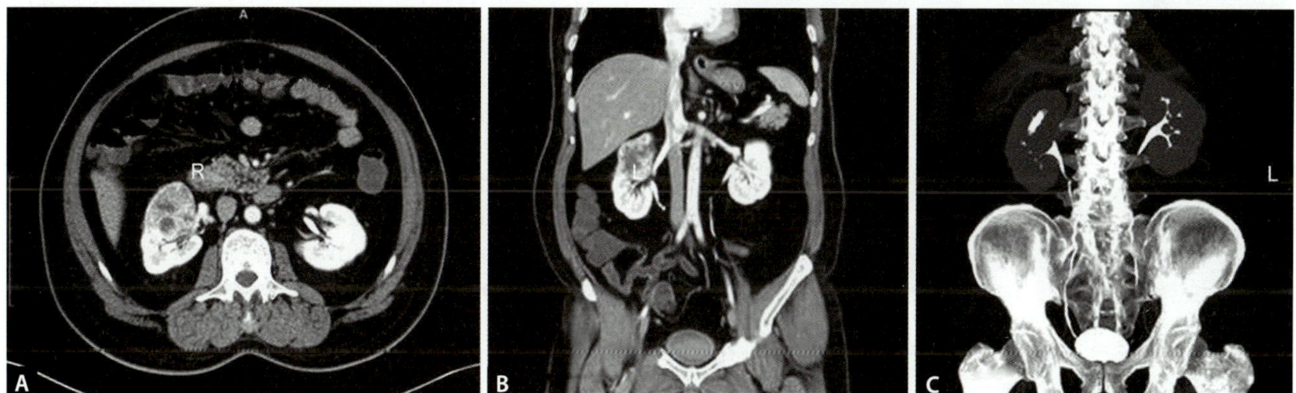

Figs. 27A to C: (A) Contrast-enhanced axial; and (B) coronal images showing a heterogeneous mass in the upper pole of right kidney; (C) CT urogram using maximum intensity projection technique (MIP) showing distortion and amputation of the infundibula of the calyces suggestive of a malignant mass—right renal cell carcinoma.

Renal Tumors

A precise depiction of the tumor and its relation to the collecting system is required in cases of nephron-sparing surgery. CT urogram delineates not only the collecting system, shows distortion splaying, and amputation of the calyces in RCCs but also the renal, perirenal, and the vascular tissues **(Figs. 27A to C)**.[97]

Ureteric Lesions

Computed tomography urography has a role in the depiction of traumatic and iatrogenic ureteral injury. MDCTU scores over intravenous urogram in differentiating extrinsic from intrinsic causes of ureteric obstruction.[98] CTU can show benign ureteric strictures, short segment malignant strictures, mural thickening, retroperitoneal masses, lymphadenopathy, retroperitoneal fibrosis, and iatrogenic causes of ureteric strictures. An infiltration of the ureter due to malignant pelvic masses is also well seen on MDCTU **(Fig. 28)**.[99]

Pelviureteric Junction Obstruction

Visualization of crossing vessels along with narrowing of ureter in the same sets of images helps in establishing the etiology and diagnosis of PUJ obstruction.[100]

Congenital Anomalies

In a duplicated system, CT urogram shows both the functioning and nonfunctioning components in contrast to intravenous urogram which shows only the functioning moiety. It shows the entire course of both upper and lower moiety along with the ectopic opening of the upper moiety which is often hydronephrotic.[101] Crossed fused renal ectopia, horseshoe kidney, and renal ectopia are all well seen on CTU **(Figs. 29A to C)**. In cases of retrocaval ureter, CT urogram shows not only the ureteric compression but also the cause of the compression which is the IVC.

Radiation Dose of CT Urography

There are differing amounts of radiation exposure according to the different techniques used. While a radiation dose of 23.4 mSv is attributed to three phasic CTU, a triple bolus CTU involves lower dose of radiation about 13.2 mSv.[87] Overall a split bolus or a triple bolus technique reduces the radiation dose by 15–45% compared to a three phasic study.[102] Where dual energy computed tomography (DECT) is available, further reduction of radiation dose can be achieved by acquiring virtual nonenhanced scan from DECT and omitting unenhanced scan.[103] In several studies with CTU protocol using iterative reconstruction further reductions in radiation dosage to the tune of 6.1 mSv have been achieved.[104,105]

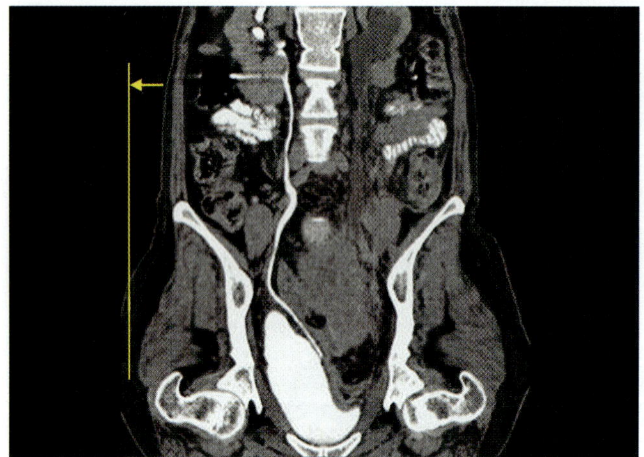

Fig. 28: Curved multiplanar reformation image depicting infiltration of left ureter via cervical mass and consequent proximal hydroureteronephrosis. Delayed opacification of the pelvicalyceal system is seen on the left as compared to the normal well-opacified pelvicalyceal system and ureter on the right side.

DUAL ENERGY CT IN THE UPPER URINARY TRACT

Acquisition of high and low energy datasets can be achieved by either a dual source dual energy scanner or a single source dual energy scanner with rapid alteration of high and low kilovoltage settings, that is, a dual energy scanner with fast kilovoltage switching, with acquisition usually at 80 kVp and 140 kVp. Two types of images are obtained on DECT which are as follows:

1. Material density images which provide material specific information.
2. Monochromatic images which provide energy selective information.

The commonly selected DECT basis material pairs are: (1) Iodine and water; (2) Iodine and calcium. Iodine has a high atomic number while water has a low atomic number. When iodine is paired with water, two sets of images are produced. One set is that of iodine density images and the other of water density. Voxels that show an attenuation similar to that of iodine attenuation are removed from the water density images and represented on the iodine density images. Virtual unenhanced images are produced which provide the same information as a noncontrast scan. The iodine density images give information about the degree of enhancement which can even be quantified

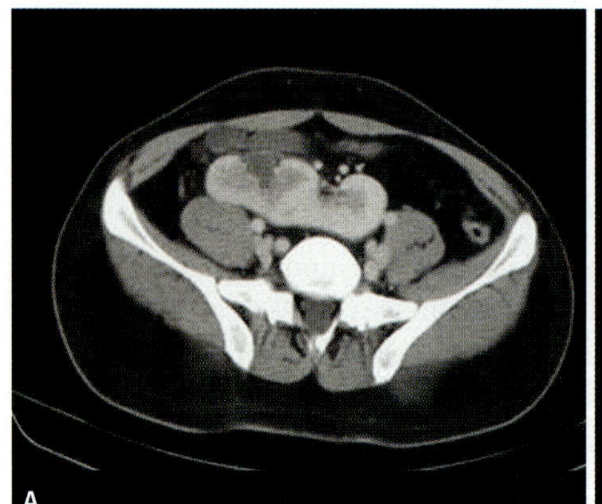

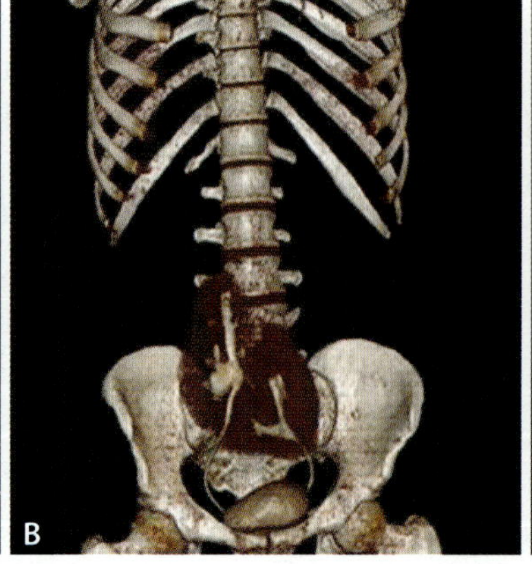

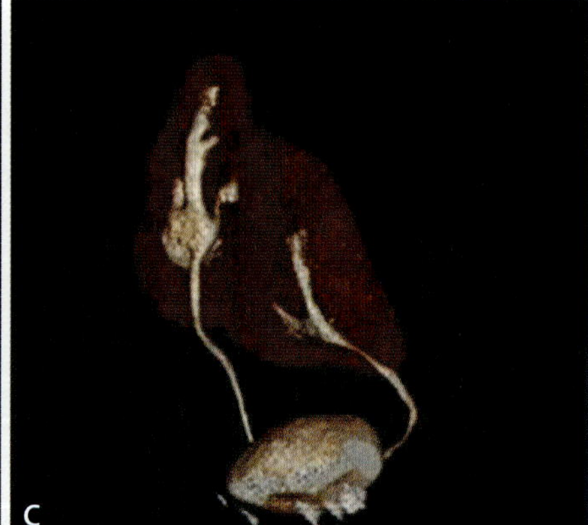

Figs. 29A to C: (A) Contrast-enhanced axial scans revealing a low lying ectopic kidney with fusion of renal parenchyma of both the kidneys; (B) volume-rendered image in the excretory phase depicting the fused low lying ectopic kidney; (C) Volume-rendered image with the bone edited out revealing the same—ectopic pancake kidney.

by placing a region of interest (ROI) over the lesion. Color-coded overlay images can also be generated.[106] A color can be assigned to the voxels containing the selected material and the voxels can be superimposed on the monochromatic images.

Characterization of Renal Masses on Dual Energy CT

Enhancement is an important criterion for differentiating hyperattenuating renal cysts from solid masses. The attenuation measurements of the two may be quite similar on the contrast-enhanced CT images. On iodine density images, voxels containing iodine appear bright and renal masses appear brighter than proteinaceous cysts on these images. The iodine density can be measured in absolute quantitative terms (milligrams/milliliter) and the degree of enhancement in renal masses can be quantified. The water density images can be used as virtual unenhanced images and can be used to detect calcifications/hemorrhage within a renal mass.[107] Also, in cases where surgery cannot be undertaken and thermal ablation is done for renal masses a follow-up can be done by DECT since it involves a single phase of scanning and limits the radiation dose received by the patient.

Characterization of Renal Stones by Dual Energy CT

The different types of calculi cannot be differentiated when scanned at a single energy level owing to a similar attenuation. DECT helps in differentiating uric acid from nonuric acid calculi.[108] Calcium and uric acid density images can be generated depicting the respective calculi. A plot of effective atomic numbers versus monochromatic image-based attenuation values can distinguish the various types of calculi (calcium, struvite, uric acid, and cystine).[109] This differentiation is important because of the different lines of management, for example, uric acid calculi are amenable to oral medications, struvite can be managed by extracorporeal shock wave lithotripsy (ESWL) while the cysteine ones are resistant to fragmentation with lithotripsy.

Dual Energy CT in CT Urography

All CT urography protocols include an unenhanced scan to detect calculi followed by contrast-enhanced scans.[110] The generation of virtual unenhanced images on DECT urography can obviate the need for an unenhanced scan and hence reduce radiation dosages.

CT ANGIOGRAM OF RENAL ARTERIES

Indications of CT angiogram of the renal arteries include:[111]

- Evaluation of renal artery stenosis (RAS).
- Preoperative assessment of the number and course of renal arteries in renal donors.
- Assessment of renal vessels crossing the PUJ prior to repair of obstruction. It is important to know about a crossing vessel because the postsurgical outcome of endopyelotomy is worse in patients with a crossing vessel than those without it.
- Evaluation of renal artery involvement in abdominal aortic aneurysms.
- Detection of renal artery aneurysms.

Technique

The renal arteries have a small diameter and have a parallel or near parallel course to the imaging plane. Hence, nominal section thickness of 1.25 mm and overlapping reconstructions are necessary. A bolus injection of 150 mL of contrast material (300 mg Iodine/mL) with a flow rate of 4 mL/sec produces good opacification of the renal arteries. The ROI for the scan volume is determined by the initial topogram/axial scans. Conventionally, the region between the SMA and lower border of L3 is chosen. This allows the sites of origin of accessory renal arteries to be included. Delay time is determined through prior time density curves of dynamic scanning and patient is instructed to hold breath at time of acquisition. A real-time bolus tracking/care bolus technique can be adopted where acquisition is triggered with the arrival of contrast in the aorta.

Maximum intensity projection (MIP) and volume rendering (VRT) display modes are most commonly used **(Fig. 30)**.[112] Depth, surface, and relative X-ray attenuation

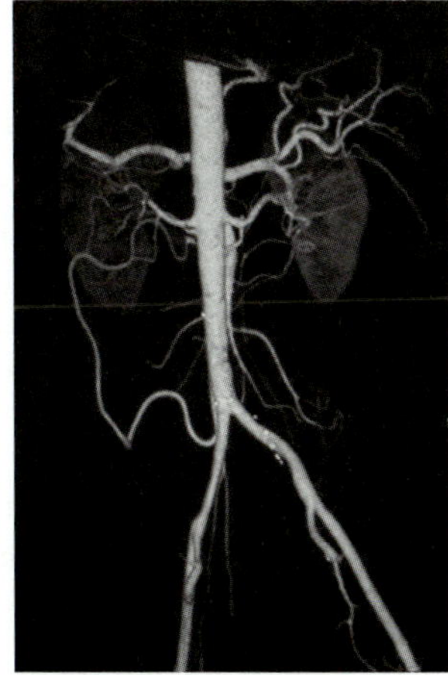

Fig. 30: CT angiogram using volume-rendering technique depicting the normal renal arteries on both sides.

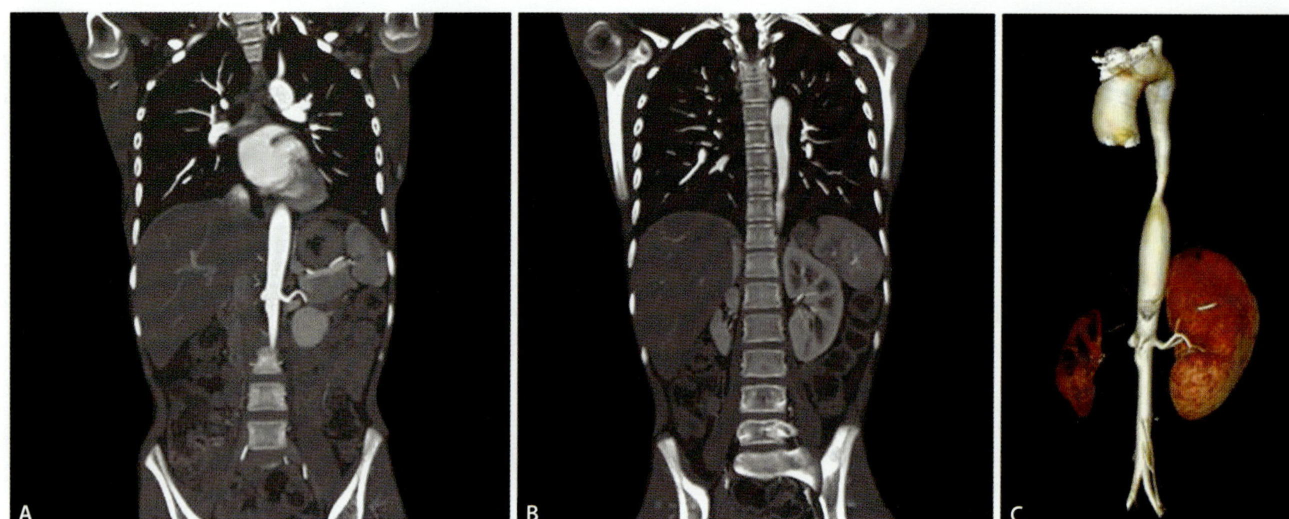

Figs. 31A to C: CT angiogram maximum intensity projection images (A and B) showing stenosis of the right renal artery with the left renal artery being normal in caliber. Volume-rendered image (C) showing narrowing of the abdominal aorta with stenosis of the right renal artery—involvement of the right renal artery in a case of aortoarteritis.

are all conveyed with VRT. The structures adjacent to the vessels can be displayed and the 3D dataset can be modified in any orientation to optimize depiction of the renal vascular anatomy **(Figs. 31A to C)**. MIP images provide useful information about atherosclerotic burden, vascular stenosis, and vascular stents, and are used in conjunction with VRT. Perspective rendering can also be used to produce angioscopic views which are helpful in identifying a vascular orifice and stenosis.

The sensitivity of computed tomography angiogram (CTA) for determination and location of main renal artery approaches 100%.[113] Arterial branches can be identified accurately till the segmental level.[114] Limitation for detection occurs with vessels smaller than 2 mm in size. It is not only the arterial anatomy but renal venous anatomy is also well documented on CTA. The renal venous anatomy is important to document for patients undergoing laparoscopic donor nephrectomy. Tributaries into the left renal vein, especially the posterior lumbar branches, are well displayed on the CTA. If enlarged, this is of potential surgical importance.

MAGNETIC RESONANCE IMAGING OF THE UPPER URINARY TRACT

A growing need for radiation dose reduction combined with advances in MRI has led to the increasing use of MRI for assessment of the urinary tract in recent times. While contrast resolution is a major advantage of MRI over other imaging modalities, the limited temporal and spatial resolution coupled with poor sensitivity for detecting calcifications has impeded this modality to emerge as the single most important modality for evaluation of the urogenital tract.[115] However, the advent of 3 Tesla MRI has changed the scenario. And 3 Tesla MRI provides a significant improvement in signal-to-noise ratio (SNR) which can in turn be used to obtain higher spatial resolution or faster imaging, i.e. imaging times can be reduced while maintaining acceptable SNR. A two-fold increase in SNR can be achieved by 3 Tesla MRI but a major drawback is the increase in magnetic susceptibility artefacts. MRI is the preferred modality:[116,117]

- For determining the cephalic extent of an intracaval tumor in a case of RCC when the superior extent cannot be determined by CT.
- Characterization of small renal masses that are indeterminate on CT or US.
- Differentiation between hemorrhagic renal cysts and renal masses by use of subtraction imaging. In this, a nonenhanced T_1 weighted image is subtracted from a contrast-enhanced T_1 weighted sequence which cancels the native T_1 sequence and leaves behind only the enhancing portion. Thus, subtraction images are useful in identifying true enhancement in complex renal cysts.
- Evaluation of renal donors.
- Evaluation of transplanted kidneys.

- In screening patients with inherited conditions such as Von Hippel–Lindau disease which is characterized by renal cysts, angiomas, and RCC.

Technique

Patient Positioning

The patient lies supine with arms raised above the head. Phased array body coils are used. A phased array coil increases SNR, allows faster acquisitions minimizing breathing motion artefacts.[118]

Breath Holding

The motion of the kidneys during respiration leads to degradation of image quality. Hence, fast imaging techniques with rapid sequences are needed which can be acquired in a single breath hold. The preferred motion phase for breath holding is expiration as the kidney position is more constant and more reproducible in this phase. Before scanning the kidneys, it is important to ask the patient to hold his breath. The use of faster sequences such as single shot imaging, half Fourier technique helps to reduce motion artefacts. In addition, a saturation band can be placed over the subcutaneous fat of the anterior abdominal wall to reduce respiratory artefacts. Parallel imaging techniques such as sensitivity encoding and array spatial sensitivity encoding technique can also be used to reduce the acquisition time.[119] Parallel imaging not only reduces the image blurring inherent to very long echo train spin echo sequences but also lowers the specific absorption rate (SAR). A respiratory gating to limit the data acquisition to end expiration or to a particular fixed point of the respiratory cycle can be done to reduce motion artefacts. A navigator which records diaphragmatic motion can also be used to obtain motion correction.

Sequences

Usually both T_1- and T_2-weighted images are acquired in the axial, coronal, and sagittal planes. Due to shorter acquisition times, T_2 fast spin echo (FSE) imaging has almost replaced the conventional spin echo (CSE) T_2-imaging. High resolution good quality T_2-weighted images can be obtained in a short time using FSE sequences. Also, in and opposed phase breath hold T_1-weighted gradient echo sequences provide a good anatomic detail and is useful for detection of intralesional fat, e.g. in AML. Imaging of the kidneys can be done in the corticomedullary, nephrographic, and EPs following contrast administration, similar to that on MDCT. Gradient echo fast low angle shot (FLASH) sequence can be used to obtain postcontrast images. Differentiation between solid masses and complicated cystic lesions can be achieved on comparison between pre- and postcontrast images obtained in corticomedullary and NPs.[120] Delayed postcontrast images depict tumor extension in the perinephric fat and venous structures.

Gadolinium-based contrast agents (GBCAs), however, should be used with caution in patients with renal insufficiency because of risk of development of NSF .[121] Nephronic systemic fibrosis is an acquired idiopathic systemic disorder characterized by indurated plaques and papules most commonly of the extremities and trunks. Besides skin changes, NSF also results in fibrosis of other organs such as myocardium, skeletal muscles, lungs, kidneys, and testes. The condition is potentially fatal and hence gadolinium should not be administered in severe renal insufficiency (GFR < 30 mL/min).[122]

Normal Appearance of the Upper Urinary Tract on MRI

Magnetic resonance (MR) allows visualization of the corticomedullary differentiation on both T_1- and T_2-weighted images. This differentiation is best visualized on T_1 weighted MR images where the cortex has a higher signal intensity than the adjacent medulla **(Figs. 32A and B)**. The cortex has less water than the medulla and has a longer T_1-time and hence is brighter than medulla on a T_1-weighted image.[123] On T_2-weighted images, the cortex appears hypointense to the medulla **(Figs. 33A and B)**. The renal sinus fat shows a high signal on both T_1 and T_2 weighted images. The renal capsule is seen as a hypointense line while the perirenal and pararenal fat shows a bright signal on all pulse sequences.[124] The pelvicalyceal system is not seen in a nondistended state. When distended with urine, the collecting system shows a low signal on T_1- and bright on T_2-weighted images. The renal arteries, veins, aorta, and IVC are seen as flow voids. Like a contrast-enhanced CT, the corticomedullary differentiation is most accentuated *(CMP)* at 20–80 seconds following contrast. At around 90–120 seconds, there is loss of this differentiation with both cortex and medulla-enhancing intensely *(NP)*. This is followed by contrast appearing in the calyces in approximately 180 seconds *(EP)* **(Figs. 34A to C)**.[125]

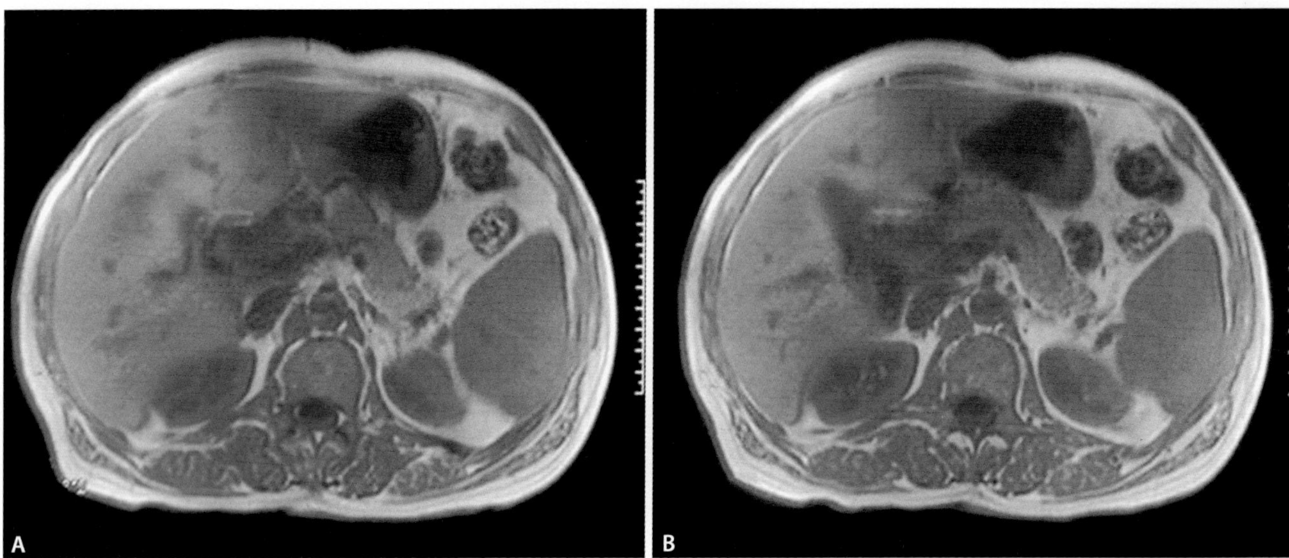

Figs. 32A and B: Axial T1W MR images showing the normal corticomedullary differentiation of the kidneys. The cortex appears brighter than the medulla on T1W image. The pararenal fat also has a bright signal.

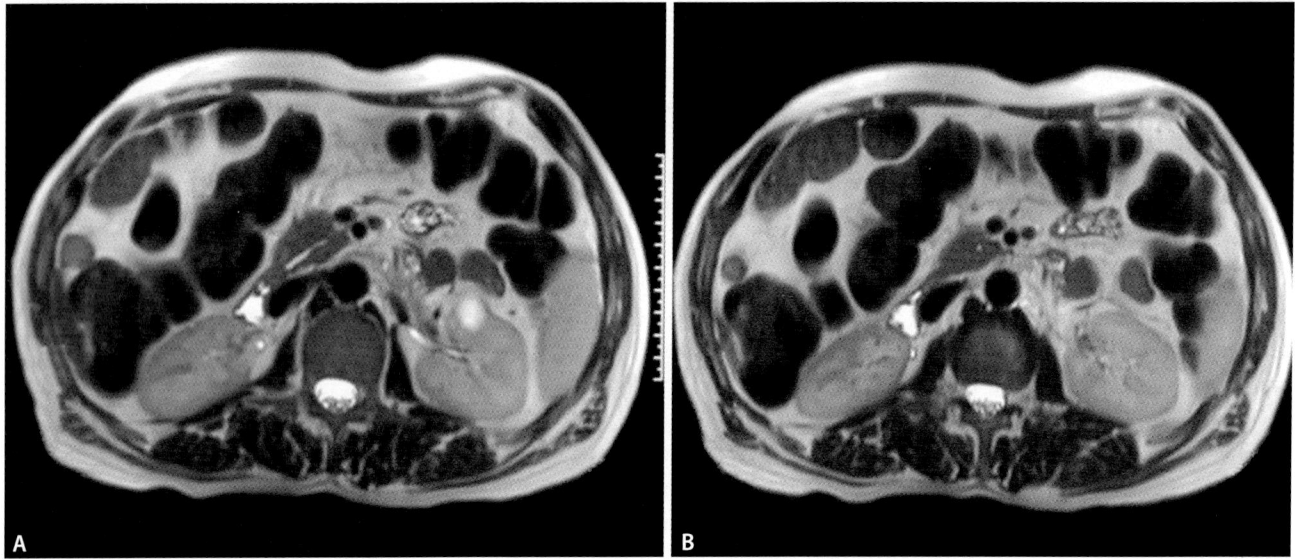

Figs. 33A and B: Axial T2W MR images showing the medulla to be brighter than the renal cortex. The renal sinus is also bright due to fat while the pararenal fat also shows a bright signal.

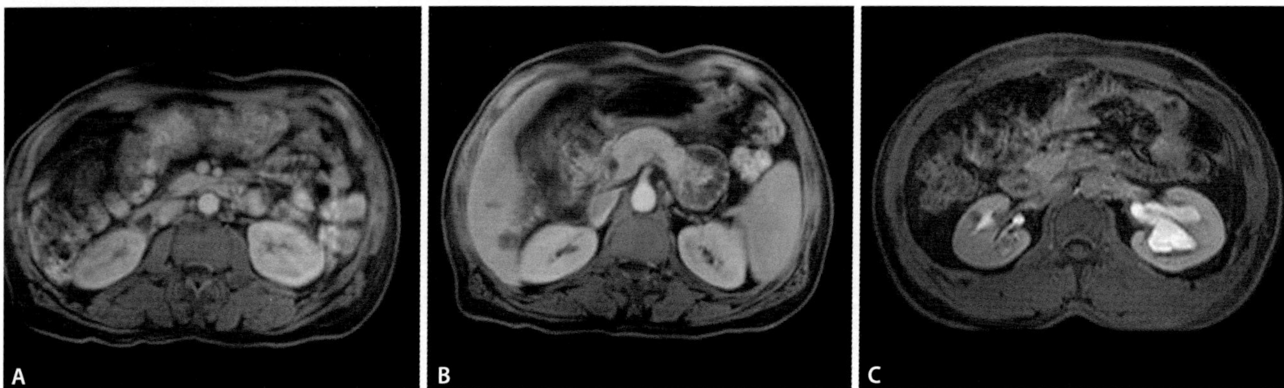

Figs. 34A to C: Postcontrast dynamic axial scans showing (A) the normal corticomedullary phase where the cortex can be distinctly differentiated from the medulla; (B) the nephrogram where there is a homogeneous opacification of the renal parenchyma; and (C) the excretory phase where there is appearance of the contrast into the pelvicalyceal system.

MAGNETIC RESONANCE UROGRAPHY

Magnetic resonance urography (MRU) allows a complete evaluation of the urinary tract. It can be performed with a static fluid or an excretory technique.[126]

Static Fluid MR Urography

In this, no contrast is administered. This technique exploits the long T_2-relaxation time of urine. Heavily T_2-weighted sequences are used to generate high signal intensity images from static fluid in the collecting system.[127] The low signal intensity images of the background tissue are suppressed. Heavily T_2-weighted sequences such as rapid acquisition with relaxation enhancement (RARE) and half Fourier acquisition single shot turbo spin echo (HASTE) are very fast and can be acquired in a single breath-hold. The fat in the background is suppressed. 3D respiratory triggered sequences can also be used to obtain volume rendering (VR) and MIP images. For the evaluation of urinary tract peristalsis and narrowing, stenosis or stricture, multiple images obtained can be played as a cine loop. Static fluid MRU can evaluate the urinary tract course and diameter, even when the kidneys are poorly excreting or it is an obstructed system.

Excretory MR Urogram

Excretory MR urogram is performed using a T_1-weighted gadolinium-enhanced 3D gradient echo fat suppression sequence like 3D FLASH. A standard dose of gadolinium (0.1 mmol/kg) is administered intravenously. Diuretic administration (0.1 mg/kg of furosemide) enhances the urine flow and gives a better dilution and uniform distribution of the contrast agent **(Figs. 35A to C)**.[128] Oral hydration and furosemide administration improve the distension of the ureters and the collecting system. Distension of the upper urinary tracts can be improved by a full urinary bladder, provided the patient can tolerate such an approach. In order to reduce the bowel-related susceptibility effects which are a problem in the region of distal ureters and bladder dome, it is preferable to have patients fast before the examination.

Images are typically acquired in the coronal plane with a field of view that includes the kidneys, ureters, and bladder. As with intravenous urogram, oblique images or multiplanar reconstructions of the collecting system can be undertaken for a better delineation of the anatomy. Excretory MR urography is better at demonstrating a communication between the renal collecting system and a fluid collection than the static MR technique. Since this technique requires excretion of contrast into the collecting system, it is better at delineating nonobstructed ureters and does not have much role in obstructed or poorly excreting kidneys.[129] Excretory MRU is not recommended in patients with severe renal insufficiency due to the risk of NSF and also because the kidneys will not be able to excrete the contrast material.[130]

Clinical Applications of MR Urography

- Magnetic resonance urogram is useful in delineating the level of urinary tract obstruction. About 90% of ureteral stones can be detected by gadolinium-enhanced 3D gradient echo excretory MR urography combined with T_2-weighted sequences. Persistent dilatation of the ureters above a filling defect and high signal intensity perinephric edema on T_2-weighted images constitute the signs of acute calculus

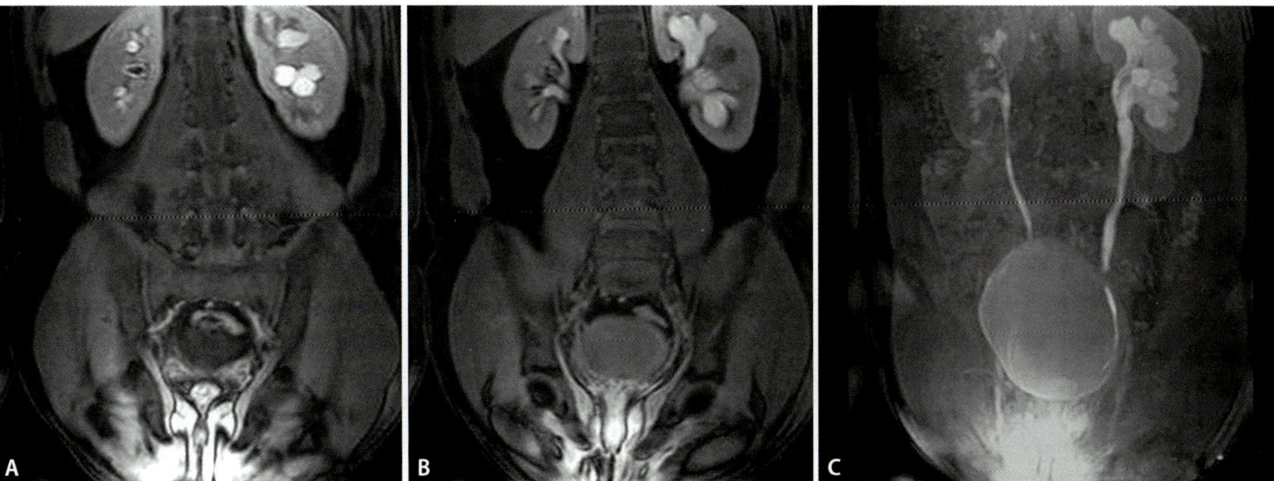

Figs. 35A to C: MR urogram image obtained using contrast administration showing a stricture in the left ureter with proximal hydronephrosis. A filling defect suggestive of calculus is seen in the right pelvicalyceal system—right renal calculus with left ureteric stricture.

obstruction. Persistence of the CMP of enhancement and delayed excretion of contrast can be present when the obstruction is severe.

- Magnetic resonance urography has a role in the detection of urothelial carcinomas. Intravenous GBCAs help in delineating the extent of tumor.[131]
- Extrinsic compressions of the ureters such as in prostate or uterine carcinomas or in retroperitoneal fibrosis can be depicted on MRU.
- Magnetic resonance urography can assess the various congenital urinary tract anomalies accurately such as duplex systems, PUJ obstruction, and insertion of an ectopic ureter.[132]
- Functional data can also be obtained from excretory MRU including renal transit time, differential renal function, and estimated GFR.[133]
- Magnetic resonance urography is useful in the evaluation of potential renal transplant donors and in the assessment of urologic complications following renal transplantation as it avoids the use of potentially nephrotoxic-iodinated contrast material of CT urogram.

Limitations of MR Urograms

- Lower spatial resolution as compared to CT
- Long imaging time
- Motion sensitivity
- Lower sensitivity in detection of calcification as compared to CT.

Magnetic resonance urography is indicated in patients who cannot receive iodinated contrast material or where exposure to ionizing radiation is undesirable. Owing to these limitations of MRU, CT urography still continues to be the test of choice for evaluation of patients with hematuria though MR urography is commonly indicated in children and pregnant patients with a dilated collecting system.[134] In pregnant patients, physiological dilatations of the ureter can be distinguished from obstructive uropathy. Static fluid MRI is quick and easy to perform, does not use contrast medium and hence is well tolerated even in advanced stages of pregnancy.

MAGNETIC RESONANCE ANGIOGRAM

Magnetic resonance angiogram (MRA) can be performed without the use of contrast by techniques such as gradient time of flight (TOF), TRUFISP or the phase contrast (PC).[135] These techniques render the flowing blood bright. However, there are several limitations such as overestimation of stenosis due to turbulent jets leading to signal loss, fresh thrombus giving a bright signal, motion artefacts, nonvisualization of small vessels, and slow flow resulting in poor quality images. Hence, contrast-enhanced MRA (CEMRA) is the preferred technique as it is free of flow-related phenomenon, has high spatial resolution, and assesses the true lumen of vessels.[136] Both the arterial and venous vasculature can be well visualized on the CEMRA images. An ultrafast 3D T_1 gradient echo sequence like FLASH is used to obtain thin slices which are reconstructed as MIP to yield angiographic images **(Fig. 36)**.

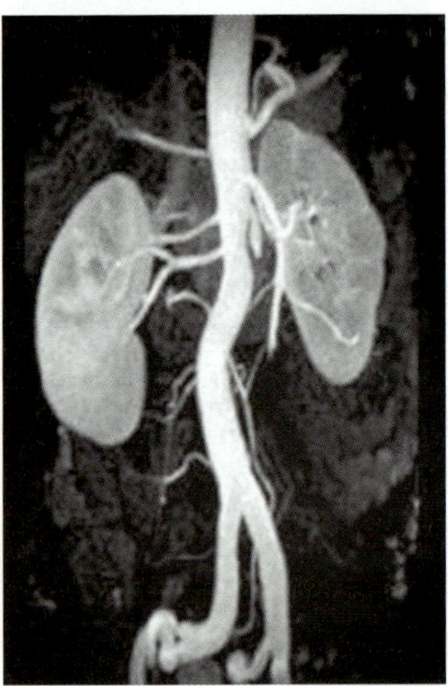

Fig. 36: MR angiogram image showing the normal renal arteries on both sides. An accessory renal artery is seen on the right side.

FUNCTIONAL MRI OF THE KIDNEYS

The primary role of the kidney is to maintain homeostatic balance by filtering out metabolites and minerals from the blood and excreting them along with water in the urine. The most commonly used measure of renal function is serum creatinine. This is, however, a late marker of renal dysfunction, it is often deranged late in the course of the disease and at times when irreversible damage to the kidneys has taken place. Functional impairment occurs much before the anatomic manifestations such as atrophy in cases of renal failure and hence an early detection of functional loss allows for an early institution of therapy to halt the progression.[137] The various techniques for functional imaging include the following as described here.

Contrast-enhanced MR Renography[138]

Dynamic contrast-enhanced MR of the kidneys is called MR renography. This technique measures the transit of contrast material, usually a gadolinium chelate, through the renal cortex, the renal medulla, and the collecting system. The technique involves acquiring images before, during, and after administration of the contrast material, converting the signal intensity of the renal tissues to gadolinium concentration and plotting of the time signal intensity curves.[139] As these gadolinium-contrast agents pass through capillaries and renal tubules, they cause the signal intensity of the renal tissues to increase. By analyzing the enhancement of the renal tissues as a function of time parameters such as renal blood flow, medullary blood volume GFR can be determined. Perfusion maps can then be generated.

Clinical applications of the MR renography:[140]

- *Renovascular hypertension*: Angiotensin-converting enzyme (ACE) inhibitor injection is helpful in differentiating hemodynamically significant stenosis from insignificant stenosis. Those with a significant stenosis have a decrease in GFR following administration of ACE inhibitor while no change in GFR values is noted in those with insignificant stenosis.
- *Allograft dysfunction*: The major complication in renal transplanted kidneys is ATN which is an ischemic injury to renal tubules. While acute rejection shows a reduced cortical and medullary perfusion, ATN shows a maintained perfusion. Thus, MR perfusion maps generated can help differentiate between these conditions obviating the need for an invasive renal biopsy.
- *Functional urinary obstruction*: The renal transit time which is defined as the time between tracer appearance in the kidney and in the ureter can be used to differentiate between normal and obstructed kidneys.[141]

Diffusion Weighted MRI

Diffusion weighted imaging (DWI) which measures the Brownian motion of water molecules in tissues has been historically used for stroke imaging. However, with improvements in hardware and software including parallel imaging, it is being used for abdominal applications. DWI is used for the detection and characterization of focal renal lesions as benign or malignant, in the assessment of nuclear grade and renal cancer subtype as well as in the assessment of malignant lymph nodes from urogenital tumors. It is also being used to assess treatment response in patients with renal cell cancer undergoing targeted chemotherapy. DWI is also being used in the evaluation of renal function. Single shot echoplanar imaging is the sequence most commonly used for DWI. Quantification of diffusion can be done by apparent diffusion coefficient (ADC) values. DWI has a role in:[142]

- *Renal insufficiency*: It has been seen in various studies that patient with acute and chronic renal failure showed lower ADC values in both the cortex and medulla of their kidneys as compared to normal healthy kidneys. DWI also provides split function information unlike the blood parameters which do not provide information about the function of each kidney separately though conditions like RAS and ureteric obstruction are usually unilateral. Studies have also shown that hydronephrotic kidney with impaired renal function has lower ADC values as compared to obstructed kidneys with normal function. DWI thus has a potential role in the evaluation of renal dysfunction.
- *Renal allograft*: DWI has a role in the evaluation of renal allografts. A decrease in cortical ADC value is attributed to allograft dysfunction.
- *Renal artery stenosis*: Patients with significant RAS had lower values of ADC, thus opening the possibility of it being diagnosed without the use of contrast-enhanced MR angiography.

Diffusion Tensor Imaging

The renal medulla is composed of radially oriented compactly arranged renal tubules. Fractional anisotropy (FA) can provide structural and flow information. The role of diffusion tensor imaging in renal imaging is under investigation.[143]

Blood Oxygen Level Dependent MRI

Blood oxygen level dependent (BOLD) imaging is a technique to noninvasively measure renal oxygenation. It utilizes the paramagnetic effects of deoxyhemoglobin to obtain images sensitive to local oxygen concentration. A multiple gradient recalled echo (GRE) sequence is the most widely used sequence for BOLD MRI. Deoxyhemoglobin induces a magnetic susceptibility effect that disturbs the local magnetic field and increases the spin-spin relaxation time (R_2*) of surrounding water. A high R_2* value corresponds to low tissue oxygenation.[144]

Applications of BOLD

- *Renal artery stenosis*: BOLD imaging can detect changes of renal hypoxia. It has been seen that kidneys with maintained functional reserve showed a low R_2* value (higher oxygenation) following administration of furosemide as compared to those with atrophic kidneys with total arterial occlusion.

- *Diabetic nephropathy*: A significant increase in oxygenation of renal medulla has been found in normal healthy kidney in response to water diuresis, while this response is absent in diabetic patients.
- *Renal transplant*: BOLD imaging can help differentiate cases of acute rejection from ATN.

Arterial Spin Labeling: Noncontrast Perfusion Imaging

It is a method of performing perfusion studies without the use of exogenous contrast. Arterial spin labeling (ASL) uses magnetically labeled protons in arteries and is noninvasive. The main applications are assessment of response to antiangiogenic drugs in renal tumor, differentiation between renal tumors and measurement of renal function, and perfusion in CKD.

^{23}Na MRI

This is a promising noninvasive method for physiologic imaging of the human kidneys. The technique allows quantification of ^{23}Na concentration of the cortex and medulla and evaluates the changes which occur under different physiologic conditions.[145]

MR Elastography

In recent years, there is a great interest in the study of tissue stiffness of the kidneys for many disease processes affecting the kidneys. It has been seen in some studies that the stiffness of the renal parenchyma is lower in a diseased kidney as compared to the normal kidneys.[146] Magnetic resonance elastography (MRE) of the kidneys is challenging and holds promise in the evaluation of chronic renal disease and renal allografts.

CONCLUSION

A clear understanding of the anatomy and physiology of the urogenital system is essential for a better understanding of the disease processes. The advanced visualization techniques do not create data over and above the cross-sections, but using the tools to display data in new ways that simulate 3D anatomy creates additional visual information about the patient. An attempt should be made by every radiologist to reach an accurate diagnosis thereby improving patient care and justifying the additional effort and expense.

REFERENCES

1. Nino-Murcia M, de Vries PA, Friedland GW. Congenital anomalies of the kidney. In: Pollack HM, McClennan BL (Eds). Clinical Urography. Philadelphia: Saunders; 2000. pp. 690-763.
2. Satyapal KS, Haffejee AA, Singh B, et al. Additional renal arteries incidence and morphometry. Surg Radiol Anat. 2001;23(1):33-8.
3. Bhatt S, Dogra VS. Kidney. In: Haaga JR, Boll DT (Eds). CT and MRI of the whole body, 6th edition. Philadelphia, PA: Elsevier; 2016. pp. 1781-861.
4. Kabala JE. The urogenital tract: Anatomy and investigations. In: Sutton D (Ed). Textbook of radiology and imaging, 7th edition. London: Churchill Livingstone; 2003. pp. 885-928.
5. Gore RM, Balfe DM, Aizenstein RI, et al. The great escape: interfascial decompression planes of the retroperitoneum. AJR Am J Roentgenol. 2000;175(2):363-70.
6. Kabala J. Attempting to increase the sensitivity of the plain film for ureteric calculi. Use of the full bladder. Br J Radiol. 1991;64(768):1151-3.
7. Levine JA, Neitlich J, Verga M, et al. Ureteral calculi in patients with flank pain: correlation of plain radiography with unenhanced helical CT. Radiology. 1997;204(1):27-31.
8. Dyer RB, Chen MY, Zagoria RJ. Intravenous urography: technique and interpretation. Radiographics. 2001;21(4):799-824.
9. Katzberg RW. Urography into the 21st century: new contrast media, renal handling, imaging characteristics and nephrotoxicity. Radiology. 1997;204(2):297-312.
10. Stacul F. Current iodinated contrast media. Eur Radiol. 2001;11(4):690-7.
11. Katayama H, Yamaguchi K, Kozuka T, et al. Adverse reactions to ionic and nonionic contrast media: a report from the Japanese Committee on the Safety of Contrast Media. Radiology. 1990;175(3):621-8.
12. Dalla Palma L. What is left of i.v. urography? Eur Radiol. 2001;11(6):931-9.
13. Kohli A. Has the time come to write the EPITAPH for the intravenous urogram? Ind J Radiol Imaging. 2005;15(2):161-4.
14. Shine S. Urinary calculus: IVU vs CT renal stone? A critically appraised topic. Abdom Imaging. 2008;33(1):41-3.
15. Warshauer DM, McCarthy SM, Street L, et al. Detection of renal masses: sensitivities and specificities of excretory urography/linear tomography, US, and CT. Radiology. 1988;169(2):363-5.
16. Wells ITP, Raju VM, Rowberry BK, et al. Digital tomosynthesis: a new lease of life for the intravenous urogram. Br J Radiol. 2011;84(1001):464-8.
17. Caoili EM, Cohan RH, Inampudi P, et al. MDCT urography of upper tract urothelial neoplasms. Am J Roentgenol. 2005; 184(6):1873-81.
18. Taylor RJ, Bennett AH, Schwentker FN, et al. Use and abuse of retrograde pyelography. Urology. 1979;14(5):536-9.
19. Paul A. The normal kidney. In: Meire HB, Cosgrove D, Dewbury KC, Tarrant P (Eds). Abdominal and General Ultrasound. Edinburgh: Churchill Livingstone; 2001. pp. 515-27.
20. Greenfield SP, Williot P, Kaplan D. Gross hematuria in children: a ten-year review. Urology. 2007;69(1):166-9.
21. Hulton SA. Evaluation of urinary tract calculi in children. Arch Dis Child. 2001;84(4):320-3.
22. Grossfeld GD, Litwin MS, Wolf JS, et al. Evaluation of asymptomatic microscopic hematuria in adults: the American Urological Association Best Practice Policy. Part I: definition, detection, prevalence and etiology. Urology. 2001:57(4):599-603.
23. Bazzocchi M, Rizzatto G. The value of the posterior oblique longitudinal scan in renal ultrasonography. Urol Radiol. 1980;1:221.

24. Thurston W, Wilson R. The Urinary Tract. In: Rumack CM, Wilson SR, Charboneau JW (Eds). Diagnostic Ultrasound, 5th edition, Maryland Heights: Elseiver Mosby; 2017. pp. 321-93.
25. Purohit K, Purohit A, Satpathy G. Measurement of normal kidney length by sonography and its relation to age, sex and body habitus. IJAR. 2017;5(4.3):4668-73.
26. Emamian SA, Nielsen MB, Pedersen JF, et al. Kidney dimensions at sonography: correlation with age, sex and habitus in 665 adult volunteers. Am J Roentgenol. 1993;160(1):83-6.
27. Marchal G, Verbeken E, Oyen R, et al. Ultrasound of the normal kidney: a sonographic, anatomic and histologic correlation. Ultrasound in Med and Biol. 1986;12:999-1009.
28. Rosenfield AT, Taylor KJ, Dembner AG, et al. Ultrasound of renal sinus: new observations. Am J Roentgenol. 1979;133(3):441-8.
29. Hricak H, Slovis TL, Callen CW, et al. Neonatal kidneys: sonographic anatomic correlation. Radiology. 1983;147(3):699-702.
30. Swischuk LE. Genitourinary Tract and Adrenal Glands. In: Imaging of the Newborn, Infant and Young Child, 5th edition. Philadelphia: Lippincott Williams & Wilkins; 2004. pp. 590-724.
31. Han BK, Babcock DS. Sonographic measurements and appearance of normal kidneys in children. Am J Roentgenol. 1985;145:611-6.
32. Lafortune M, Constantin A, Breton G, et al. Sonography of the hypertrophied column of Bertin. Am J Roentgenol. 1986;146:53-6.
33. Carter AR, Horgan JG, Jennings TA, et al. The junctional parenchymal defect: a sonographic variant of renal anatomy. Radiology. 1985;154:499-502.
34. Hoffer FA, Hanabergh AM, Teele RL. The interrenicular junction: a mimic of renal scarring on normal pediatric sonograms. Am J Roentgenol. 1985;145(5):1075-8.
35. Fine H, Keen EN. The arteries of the human kidney. J Anat. 1966;100:881-94.
36. Dubbins PA. The kidney. In: Allan PL, Dubbins PA, Pozniak M, Mc Dicken WN (Eds). Clinical Doppler Ultrasound. London. Churchill Livingstone; 2000. pp. 169-90.
37. Chang EH. An introduction to contrast-enhanced ultrasound for nephrologists. Nephron. 2018;138(3):176-85.
38. Seguel AP, Perez MM, Gonzalez TR, et al. Evaluation of upper tract urothelial carcinomas by contrast-enhanced ultrasound. Radiologia. 2018;60(6):496-503.
39. Chang EH, Chong WK, Kasoji SK, et al. Diagnostic accuracy of contrast-enhanced ultrasound for characterization of kidney lesions in patients with and without chronic disease. BMC Nephrol. 2017;18(1):266.
40. Leong SS, Wong JHD, Md Shah MN, et al. Shear wave elastography in the evaluation of renal parenchymal stiffness in patients with chronic kidney disease. Br J Radiol. 2018;91(1089):20180235.
41. Schreyer H, Uggowitzer M, Ruppert Kohlmayr A. Helical CT of the urinary organs. Eur Radiol. 2002;12:575-91.
42. Foley WD. Special focus session. Multidetector CT: Abdominal visceral imaging. Radiographics. 2002;22(3):701-19.
43. Wolin EA, Hartman DS, Olson JR. Nephrographic and pyelographic analysis of CT urography: principles, patterns and pathophysiology. Am J Roentgenol. 2013;200(6):1210-14.
44. Kocakoc E, Bhatt S, Dogra VS. Renal multidetector row CT. Radiol Clin N Am. 2005;43:1021-47.
45. Yuh BI, Cohan RH. Different phases of renal enhancement: role in detecting and characterizing renal masses during helical CT. Am J Roentgenol. 1999;173(3):747-55.
46. Wintersperger BJ, Nikolaou K, Becker CR. Multidetector row CT angiography of the aorta and visceral arteries. Semin Ultrasound CT MR. 2004;25:25-40.
47. Sheth S, Fishman EK. Multidetector row CT of the kidneys and urinary tract: techniques and applications in the diagnosis of benign diseases. Radiographics. 2004;24(2):e20.
48. Tunaci A, Yekeler E. Multidetector row CT of the kidneys. Eur J Radiol. 2004;52:56-66.
49. Villa L, Giusti G, Knoll T, et al. Imaging for urinary stones: update in 2015. Eur Urol Focus. 2016;2(2):122-9.
50. Assimos D, Krambeck A, Miller NL, et al. Surgical management of stones: American Urological Association/Endourological Society Guideline. Part I. J Urol. 2016;196(4):1153-60.
51. Lukasiewicz A, Bhargavan Chatfield M, Coombs L, et al. Radiation dose index of renal colic protocol CT studies in the United States: a report from the American College of Radiology: National Radiology Data Registry. Radiology. 2014;27(12):445-51.
52. Kluner C, Hein PA, Gralla O, et al. Does ultra-low dose CT with a radiation dose equivalent to that of KUB suffice to detect renal and ureteral calculi? J Comput Assist Tomogr. 2006;30(1):44-50.
53. Saunders HS, Dyer RB, Shifrin RY, et al. The CT nephrogram: implications for evaluation of urinary tract disease. Radiographics. 1995;15(5):1069-85.
54. Szolar DH, Kammerhuber F, Altziebler S, et al. Multiphasic helical CT of the kidney: increased conspicuity for detection and characterization of small (<3 cm) renal masses. Radiology. 1997;202(1):211-7.
55. Urban BA. The small renal mass: What is the role of multiphasic helical scanning? Radiology. 1997;202(1):22-3.
56. Hilton S, Jones LP. Recent advances in imaging cancer of the kidney and urinary tract. Surg Oncol Clin N Am. 2014;23:863-910.
57. Cowan NC, Turney BW, Taylor NJ, et al. Multidetector computed tomography urography for diagnosing upper urinary tract urothelial tumour. BJU Int. 2007;99(6):1363-70.
58. Kawashima A, LeRoy AJ. Radiologic evaluation of patients with renal infections. Inf Dis Clin North Am. 2003;17:433-56.
59. Sheth S, Scatarige JC, Horton KM, et al. Current concepts in the diagnosis and management of renal cell carcinoma: Role of multidetector CT and three-dimensional CT. Radiographics. 2001;21:S237-54.
60. Zagoria RJ. Imaging of small renal masses: A medical success story. AJR Am J Roentgenol. 2000;175(4):945-55.
61. Macari M, Bosniak MA. Delayed CT to evaluate renal masses incidentally discovered at contrast-enhanced CT: demonstration of vascularity with de-enhancement. Radiology. 1999;213:674-80.
62. Fielding JR, Steele G, Fox LA, et al. Spiral computerized tomography in the evaluation of acute flank pain: a replacement for excretory urography. J Urol. 1997;157:2071-3.
63. Heneghan JP, Dalrymple NC, Verga M, et al. Soft tissue "rim" sign in the diagnosis of ureteral calculi with use of unenhanced helical CT. Radiology. 1997;202:709-11.
64. Georgiades CS, Moore CJ, Smith DP. Differences of renal parenchymal attenuation for acutely obstructed and unobstructed kidneys on unenhanced helical CT: a useful secondary sign. Am J Roentgenol. 2001;176:965-8.
65. Bell TV, Fenlon HM, Davison BD, et al. Unenhanced helical CT criteria to differentiate distal ureteral calculi from pelvic phleboliths. Radiology. 1998;207(2):363-7.

66. Smith RC, Verga M, McCarthy S, et al. Diagnosis of acute flank pain: value of unenhanced helical CT. Am J Roentgenol. 1996;166:97-101.
67. Willmann JK, Roos JE, Platz A, et al. Multidetector CT: Detection of active hemorrhage in patients with blunt abdominal trauma. Am J Roentgenol. 2002;179:437-44.
68. McNicholas MM, Raptopoulos VD, Schwartz RK, et al. Excretory phase CT urography for opacification of the urinary collecting system. Am J Roentgenol. 1998;170:1261-7.
69. Kundra V, Silverman PM. Impact of multislice CT on imaging of acute abdominal disease. Radiol Clin North Am. 2003;41(6):1083-93.
70. Kawashima A, Sandler CM, Goldman SM, et al. CT of renal inflammatory disease. Radiographics. 1997;17:851-66.
71. RubinGD.3-DimagingwithMDCT.EurJRadiol.2003;45(Suppl1): S37-41.
72. Lockhart ME, Smith JK. Technical considerations in renal CT. Radiol Clin North Am. 2003;41:863-75.
73. Rydberg J, Buckwalter KA, Caldemeyer KS, et al. Multisection CT: Scanning techniques and clinical applications. Radiographics. 2000;20:1787-806.
74. Dillman JR, Caoili EM, Cohan RH. Multidetector CT urography: a one stop renal and urinary tract imaging modality. Abdom Imaging. 2007;32(4):519-29.
75. Herts BR. The current status of CT Urography. Crit Rev Comput Tomogr. 2002;43(3):219-41.
76. Vrtiska TJ, King BF, LeRoy AJ, et al. CT urography: analysis of techniques and comparison with IVU (abstr). Radiology. 2000;217(P):225.
77. McCollough CH, Daly TR, King Jr BF, et al. An auxiliary CT table top for radiography at the time of CT. J Comput Assist Tomogr. 2001;25(6):876-80.
78. Kawashima A, Vrtiska TJ, LeRoy AJ. CT scanned projection radiographs (SPR) utilizing enhanced algorithms: applications in CT urography (abstr). Radiology. 2002;225(P):690.
79. Caoili EM, Cohan RH, Korobkin M, et al. Urinary tract abnormalities: Initial experience with multidetector row CT urography. Radiology. 2002;222(2):353-60.
80. Kawashima A, Vrtiska TJ, LeRoy AJ, et al. CT urography. Radiographics. 2004;24:S35-54.
81. Sanyal R, Deshmukh A, Sheorain VS, et al. CT urography: a comparison of strategies for upper urinary tract opacification. Eur Radiol. 2007;17(5):1262-6.
82. Silverman SG, Akbar SA, Mortele KJ, et al. Multidetector-row CT urography: comparison of furosemide and saline as adjuncts to contrast medium for depicting the normal urinary collecting system. Radiology. 2006;240:749-55.
83. Caoili EM, Inampudi P, Cohan RH, et al. Optimization of multidetector row CT urography: effect of compression, saline administration and prolongation of acquisition delay. Radiology. 2005;235:116-23.
84. McTavish JD, Jinzaki M, Zou KH, et al. Multidetector row CT urography: Comparison of strategies for depicting the normal urinary collecting system. Radiology. 2002;225:783-90.
85. Jinzaki M, McTavish JD, Zou KH, et al. Evaluation of small (≤3 cm) renal masses with MDCT: benefits of thin overlapping reconstructions. Am J Roentgenol. 2004;183(1):223-8.
86. Chow LC, Kwan SW, Olcott EW, et al. Split bolus MDCT urography with synchronous nephrographic and excretory phase enhancement. Am J Roentgenol. 2007;189:314-22.
87. Kekelidze M, Dwarkasing RS, Dijkshoorn ML, et al. Kidney and urinary tract imaging: triple bolus multidetector CT urography as a one stop shop: protocol design, opacification, and image quality analysis. Radiology. 2010;255(2):508-16.
88. Abedi G, Okhunov Z, Lall C, et al. Comparison of radiation dose from conventional and triple bolus computed tomography urography protocols in the diagnosis and management of patients with renal cortical neoplasms. Urology. 2014;84(4):875-80.
89. Lang EK, Thomas R, Davis R, et al. Multiphasic helical computerized tomography for the assessment of microscopic hematuria: a prospective study. J Urol. 2004;171(1):237-43.
90. Albani JM, Ciaschini MW, Streem SB, et al. The role of computerized tomographic urography in the initial evaluation of hematuria. J Urol. 2007;177(2):644-8.
91. Van Der Molen AJ, Cowan NC, Mueller-Lisse UG, et al. CT Urography Working Group of the European Society of Urogenital Radiology (ESUR). CT urography: definition, indications and techniques. A guideline for clinical practice. Eur Radiol. 2008;18(1):4-17.
92. Khadra MH, Pickard RS, Charlton M, et al. A prospective analysis of 1930 patients with hematuria to evaluate current diagnostic practice. J Urol. 2000;163(2):524-7.
93. Raman SP, Fishman EK. Upper and lower tract urothelial imaging using computed tomography urography. Urol Clin N Am. 2018;45:389-405.
94. Vikram R, Sandler CM, Ng CS. Imaging and staging of transitional cell carcinoma: part 2. Upper urinary tract. Am J Roentgenol. 2009;192(6):1488-93.
95. Chlapoutakis K, Theocharopoulos N, Yarmenitis S, et al. Performance of computed tomographic urography in diagnosis of upper urinary tract urothelial carcinoma, in patients presenting with hematuria: systematic review and meta-analysis. Eur J Radiol. 2010;73(2):334-8.
96. Chai RY, Jhaveri K, Saini S, et al. Comprehensive evaluation of patients with haematuria on multi-slice computed tomography scanner: protocol design and preliminary observations. Australas Radiol. 2001;45:536-8.
97. Joffe SA, Servaes S, Okon S, et al. Multidetector row CT urography in the evaluation of hematuria. Radiographics. 2003;23(6):1441-55.
98. Potenta SE, D'Agostino R, Sternberg KM, et al. CT Urography for Evaluation of the Ureter. Radiographics. 2015;35:709-26.
99. Patel RC, Newman RC. Ureteroscopic management of ureteral and ureteroenteral strictures. Urol Clin North Am. 2004;31(1):107-13.
100. Lawler LP, Jarret TW, Corl FM, et al. Adult ureteropelvic junction obstruction: insights with three dimensional multidetector row CT. Radiographics. 2005;25(1):121-34.
101. Berrocal T, López-Pereira P, Arjonilla A, et al. Anomalies of the distal ureter, bladder and urethra in children: embryologic, radiologic and pathologic features. Radiographics. 2002;22(5):1139-64.
102. Lupescu IG, Marica OL. CT urography. How when why? Rev Rom Urol. 2012;11(4):17-20.
103. Kaza RK, Platt JF, Cohan RH, et al. Dual-energy CT with single and dual source scanners: current applications in evaluating the genitourinary tract. Radiographics. 2012;32(2):353-69.
104. Juri H, Matsuki M, Itou Y, et al. Initial experience with adaptive iterative dose reduction 3D to reduce radiation dose in computed tomographic urography. J Comput Assist Tomogr. 2013;37(1):52-7.
105. Van der Molen AJ, Miclea RL, Geleijns J, et al. A survey of radiation doses in CT urography before and after

implementation of iterative reconstruction. Am J Roentgenol. 2015;205(3):572-7.
106. Jepperson MA, Cernigliaro JG, Sella D, et al. Dual-energy CT for the evaluation of urinary calculi: image interpretation, pitfalls and stone mimics. Clin Radiol. 2013;68:e707-14.
107. Kaza RK, Caoili EM, Cohan RH, et al. Distinguishing enhancing from nonenhancing renal lesions with fast kilovoltage switching dual energy CT. Am J Roentgenol. 2011;197(6):1375-81.
108. Primak AN, Fletcher JG, Vrtiska TJ, et al. Noninvasive differentiation of uric acid versus non-uric acid kidney stones using dual-energy CT. Acad Radiol. 2007;14(12):1441-7.
109. Eliahou R, Hidas G, Duvdevani M, et al. Determination of renal stone composition with dual-energy computed tomography: an emerging application. Semin Ultrasound CT MR. 2010;31(4):315-20.
110. Takahashi N, Vrtiska TJ, Kawashima A, et al. Detectability of urinary stones on virtual nonenhanced images generated at pyelographic phase dual energy CT. Radiology. 2010;256(1):184-90.
111. Kim TS, Chung JW, Park JH, et al. Renal artery evaluation: comparison of spiral CT angiography to intra-arterial DSA. J Vasc Inter Radiol. 1998;9:553-9.
112. Napoli A, Fleischmann D, Chan FP, et al. Computed tomography angiography: state of the art imaging using multidetector row technology. J Comput Assist Tomogra. 2004;28:S32-45.
113. Türkvatan A, Özdemir M, Cumhur T, et al. Multidetector CT angiography of renal vasculature: normal anatomy and variants. Eur Radiol. 2009;19:236-44.
114. Yeh BM, Coakley FV, Meng MV, et al. Precaval right renal arteries: prevalence and morphologic associations at spiral CT. Radiology. 2004;230:429-33.
115. Merkle EM, Dale BM, Paulson EK. Abdominal MR imaging at 3T. Magn Reson Imaging Clin N Am. 2006;14:17-26.
116. Nikken JJ, Krestin GP. MRI of the kidney: State of the art. Eur Radiol. 2007;17:2780-93.
117. Pedrosa I, Sun MR, Spencer M, et al. MR imaging of renal masses: correlation with findings at surgery and pathologic analysis. Radiographics. 2008;28:985-1003.
118. Zhang J, Pedrosa I, Rofsky NM. MR techniques for renal imaging. Radiol Clin North Am. 2003;41:877-907.
119. Glockner JF, Hu HH, Stanley DW, et al. Parallel MR imaging: a user's guide. Radiographics. 2005;25(5):1279-97.
120. Israel GM, Bosniak MA. Pitfalls in renal mass evaluation and how to avoid them. Radiographics. 2008;28(5):1325-38.
121. Schieda N, Krishna S, Davenport MS. Update on Gadolinium Based Contrast Agent-Enhanced Imaging in the Genitourinary System. Am J Roentgenol. 2019;212(6):1223-33.
122. Perez-Rodriguez J, Lai S, Ehst BD, et al. Nephrogenic systemic fibrosis: incidence, associations and effect of risk factor assessment—report of 33 cases. Radiology. 2009;250(2):371-7.
123. Bassignani MJ. Understanding and interpreting MRI of the genitourinary tract. Urol Clin N Am. 2006;33(3):301-17.
124. Probert JL, Glew D, Gillatt DA. Magnetic resonance imaging in urology. BJU Int. 1999;83(3):201-14.
125. Prasad SR, Dalrymple NC, Surabhi VR. Cross-sectional imaging evaluation of renal masses. Radiol Clin North Am. 2008;46(1):95-111.
126. O'Connor OJ, McLaughlin P, Maher MM. MR urography. Am J Roentgenol. 2010;195(3):W201-6.
127. Leyendecker JR, Gianini JW. Magnetic resonance urography. Abdom Imaging. 2009;34(4):527-40.
128. Ergen FB, Hussain HK, Carlos RC, et al. 3D excretory MR urography: improved image quality with intravenous saline and diuretic administration. J Mag Reson Imaging. 2007;25(4):783-9.
129. Silverman SG, Leyendecker JR, Amis Jr ES. What is the current role of CT urography and MR urography in the evaluation of the urinary tract? Radiology. 2009;250(2):309-23.
130. Nolte-Ernsting CC, Staatz G, Tacke J, et al. MR urography today. Abdom Imaging. 2003;28(2):191-209.
131. Takahashi N, Kawashima A, Glockner JF, et al. Small (<2 cm) upper tract urothelial carcinoma: evaluation with gadolinium enhanced three dimensional spoiled gradient recalled echo MR urography. Radiology. 2008;247(2):451-7.
132. Dickerson EC, Dillman JR, Smith EA, et al. Pediatric MR urography: Indications, techniques and approach to review. Radiographics. 2015;35(4):1208-30.
133. Jones RA, Perez-Brayfield MR, Kirsch AJ, et al. Renal transit time with MR urography in children. Radiology. 2004;233(1):41-50.
134. Grattan-Smith JD, Little SB, Jones RA. MR urography evaluation of obstructive uropathy. Pediatr Radiol. 2008;38(Suppl 1):S49-69.
135. Michaely HJ, Schoenberg SO, Rieger JR, et al. MR angiography in patients with renal disease. Magn Reson Imaging Clin N Am. 2005;13(1):131-51.
136. Leiner T, Michaely H. Advances in contrast-enhanced MR angiography of the renal arteries. Magn Reson Imaging Clin N Am. 2008;16(4):561-72.
137. Zhang JL. Functional magnetic resonance imaging of the kidneys—with and without gadolinium based contrast. Adv Chronic Kidney Dis. 2017;24(3):162-8.
138. Zhang JL, Rusinek H, Chandarana H, et al. Functional MRI of the kidneys. J Magn Reson Imaging. 2013;37(2):282-93.
139. Michaely HJ, Kramer H, Oesingmann N, et al. Intraindividual comparison of MR-renal perfusion imaging at 1.5 T and 3.0 T. Invest Radiol. 2007;42(6):406-11.
140. Chu WC, Lam WW, Chan KW, et al. Dynamic gadolinium enhanced magnetic resonance urography for assessing drainage in dilated pelvicalyceal systems with moderate renal function: preliminary results and comparison with diuresis renography. BJU Int. 2004;93(6):830-4.
141. Shokeir AA, El-Diasty T, Eassa W, et al. Diagnosis of ureteral obstruction in patients with compromised renal function: the role of noninvasive imaging modalities. J Urol. 2004;171:2303-6.
142. Mürtz P, Krautmacher C, Träber F, et al. Diffusion-weighted whole body MR imaging with background body signal suppression: a feasibility study at 3.0 Tesla. Eur Radiol. 2007;17:3031-7.
143. Notohamiprodjo M, Dietrich O, Horger W, et al. Diffusion tensor imaging (DTI) of the kidney at 3 Tesla–feasibility, protocol evaluation and comparison to 1.5 Tesla. Invest Radiol. 2010;45(5):245-54.
144. Gloviczki ML, Glockner J, Gomez SI, et al. Comparison of 1.5 and 3T BOLD MR to study oxygenation of kidney cortex and medulla in human renovascular disease. Invest Radiol. 2009;44(9):566-71.
145. Maril N, Rosen Y, Reynolds GH, et al. Sodium MRI of the human kidney at 3 Tesla. Magn Reson Med. 2006;56(6):1229-34.
146. Bensamoun SF, Robert L, Leclerc GE, et al. Stiffness imaging of the kidney and adjacent abdominal tissues measured simultaneously using magnetic resonance elastography. Clin Imaging. 2011;35(4):284-7.

Chapter 2

Current Status of Nuclear Medicine in Urinary Tract Imaging

Rakesh Kumar, Madhavi Tripathi

INTRODUCTION

Nuclear medicine techniques play a complimentary role in the functional evaluation of genitourinary tract. In fact, they have been effectively included in the management algorithm of conditions like congenital hydronephrosis and urinary tract infections (UTI). Radiopharmaceuticals evaluate various aspects of renal function like glomerular filtration rate (GFR) and clearance and provide a wealth of information to the nephrologist and urologist. Besides being highly sensitive, these procedures are noninvasive, simple, nontoxic, and most importantly, do not interfere with normal physiology and function. Using these techniques, it has now become possible to assess split renal function, evaluate perfusion, especially of transplant kidneys, evaluate upper urinary tract dilatation, and diagnose urinary tract obstruction, detect the presence of kidneys, which are poorly functioning and ectopic and monitor renal function in renal failure.

The nuclear medicine investigations for evaluation of nephro-urological disorders can be broadly classified into: (1) Dynamic renography, (2) renal cortical scintigraphy, (3) radionuclide cystography and voiding cystography, and (4) Clearance studies, i.e. glomerular filtration rate (GFR) estimation, effective renal plasma flow (ERPF) estimation, etc. Various interventions like Lasix diuresis and angiotensin-converting enzyme inhibitors (captopril/losartan) have further enhanced the diagnosis of obstruction and renovascular hypertension using radionuclide studies.

RENAL POSITRON EMISSION TOMOGRAPHY

Positron emission tomography (PET) radiotracers for functional renal imaging have recently been developed, in particular focusing on Fluorine-18 (^{18}F)- and Gallium-68 (^{68}Ga)-labeled agents. Several of these PET imaging probes such as ^{68}Ga ethylenediaminetetraacetic acid (^{68}Ga EDTA), ^{68}Ga-IR-Dye800-tilmanocept, and 2-deoxy-2-[^{18}F] fluorodeoxysorbitol (^{18}F-FDS) have been evaluated for assessment of GFR and the diagnostic performance of ^{68}Ga EDTA has been demonstrated in a clinical trial.[1-4] ^{68}Ga-IR-Dye800-tilmanocept shows receptor-mediated binding to glomerular mesangial cells, which in turn may allow the monitoring of progression of diabetic nephropathy. ^{18}F-FDS shows excellent kidney extraction and excretion in rats.[5] Further, due to its simple one-step radiosynthesis via the most frequently used PET radiotracer 2-deoxy-2-[^{18}F]fluoro-D-glucose, [^{18}F]FDS could be available at nearly every PET center. A new PET radiotracer for the effective assessment of plasma flow in the kidneys is Re(CO)3-N-([^{18}F]fluoroethyl) iminodiacetic acid (Re(CO)3[^{18}F]FEDA).[6] This compound demonstrates similar pharmacokinetic properties to its ^{99m}Tc-labeled analog [99mTc](CO)3(FEDA). Thus, if there is a shortage of molybdenum-99, Re(CO)3[^{18}F]FEDA would allow a direct comparison with previous ^{99m}Technetium (^{99m}Tc)-based studies. PET radiotracers for renal imaging have tremendous potential for evaluation of kidney function. Further, simultaneously acquired CT images enable precise anatomical coregistration with rapid three-dimensional imaging capability.

RADIOPHARMACEUTICALS

The various radiopharmaceuticals presently used in nephro-urology practice are classified into glomerular agents (filtered a glomerulus), and tubular agents, which are further subdivided into tubular fixation and tubular clearance agents. The prototype glomerular agent is ^{99m}Tc-diethyl triamine pentaacetic acid (DTPA), which is effectively used to measure the global GFR. Tubular clearance agents include ^{99m}Tc-L,L ethylene dicysteine (LLEC), which is the standard agent used for renography studies in India and ^{99m}Tc-mercaptoacetyltriglycine (MAG-3), which is used in the west and is not cost-effective in the Indian context. ^{99m}Tc-glucoheptonate (GHA) undergoes both glomerular filtration and tubular fixation (approximately 10–15% of the injected dose is retained in the renal parenchyma while 65% of the injected dose is eliminated in the urine within 6 hours after injection) and is an agent which can be used both for renal dynamic studies and for renal cortical scintigraphy. The agent which is recommended for renal cortical scintigraphy is ^{99m}Tc-dimercaptosuccinic acid (DMSA) which enables detailed evaluation of the renal parenchyma.

^{99m}Technetium-L,L Ethylene Dicysteine

Currently, it is the most commonly used radiopharmaceutical for renal dynamic studies. It is a metabolite of the brain perfusion tracer ^{99m}Tc-ethylcysteinate dimer (ECD) and is cleared principally through active tubular transport. LLEC has good imaging properties and a higher renal clearance than MAG-3.[7] Labeling EC with ^{99m}Tc does not require boiling and highest labeling yield is obtained at pH of 10–12 (97%). Like ^{123}I-orthoiodohippurate (OIH) and ^{99m}Tc-MAG-3, the secretion of ^{99m}Tc-LLEC occurs in proximal tubule.[8] DD-EC has highest and faster renal clearance while LLEC has lower renal excretion and higher tissue retention.[8,9] Protein binding of DD-EC is 28% and LLEC has 50%. Production of DD-EC form, however, demands HPLC purification, a drawback for clinical use. The clearance of LLEC is about 75%. The disadvantage of EC is unknown amounts of different stereoisomers and forms produced by the different labeling kit, which have different excretion.

^{99m}Technetium-Mercaptoacetyltriglycine

Currently, ^{99m}Tc-MAG 3 is mostly used in Europe and USA. It is cleared principally through active tubular transport.[10] Plasma clearance is in the order of 300 mL/min, approximately 60% of OIH,[11,12] and after 3 hours, approximately 90% of the injected dose can be recovered in the urine. It is more extensively protein bound than ^{123}I-OIH (88% vs 65%) and therefore, its volume of distribution is lower than that of ^{123}I-OIH. Since it is eliminated by tubular secretion and has a high initial renal uptake, the kidney to background ratio provided by this tracer is high. Moreover, the rapid excretion provides good temporal resolution. ^{99m}Tc-MAG 3 is a superior agent for renal dynamic scintigraphy, but a practical limitation to its extensive use is the relatively high cost.

^{99m}Technetium-Diethyl Triamine Pentaacetic Acid

^{99m}Technetium-DTPA has been the tracer of choice for dynamic renal scintigraphy for almost three decades. However, it is has been replaced by ^{99m}Tc-LLEC and ^{99m}Tc-MAG 3 in daily clinical practice. It is excreted primarily by glomerular filtration, at a slightly lower rate than inulin, approximately 90 mL/min.[13,14] This lower rate of filtration is probably due to protein binding, the amount of which varies with the formulation. A maximum concentration in kidneys is usually achieved 3 minutes after intravenous injection. This is the best agent for in vitro GFR studies and for simultaneous renal dynamic study with estimation of GFR.

^{99m}Technetium-Dimercaptosuccinic Acid

^{99m}Technetium-DMSA is currently the agent of choice for cortical renal scintigraphy—planar and single photon emission tomography (SPECT). The renal uptake of this agent is about 50% of the injected dose at 1 hour and about 70% at 24 hours after injection.[15] One hour or more postinjection, the tracer is found principally in the proximal convoluted tubules with very minimal activity elsewhere in the kidney. In most patients, therefore, excellent images of renal cortex can be obtained approximately 4 hours after injection of ^{99m}Tc-DMSA. Here again, patients with obstructive pathology may have tracer retention within the pelvicalyceal system leading to false interpretation. In such cases, Lasix injection is recommended to allow tracer in the urine to be eliminated.

IMAGING TECHNIQUES

Renal Dynamic Scintigraphy

This refers to serial continuous imaging following intravenous injection of radio-tracer. It encompasses three principal techniques—(1) Dynamic renography, (2) diuretic renography, and (3) captopril renography.

Dynamic Renography

Patient preparation: Patient should be well-hydrated before the study and encouraged to drink fluids ad libitum. Before the examination begins, the patients are asked to empty their bladder. In suspected cases of vesicoureteric junction

Table 1: Different radiopharmaceutical and their doses.

Radiopharmaceutical	*Dose (mCi/kg)*	*Minimum dose (mCi)*	*Maximum dose (mCi)*
^{99m}Tc-LLEC	0.15	1	10.0
^{99m}Tc-MAG3	0.15	1	10.0
^{99m}Tc-DTPA	0.15	1	8.0
^{99m}Tc-DMSA	0.05	0.5	3.0
^{123}I-OIH	0.010	0.1	0.5

obstruction, when patients cannot void completely (neurogenic bladder) or in children with vesicoureteral reflux (VUR), the study is recommended with a bladder catheter (Foley's type) in situ so that bladder drainage is maintained throughout the entire duration of the study. An intravenous line is established to avoid extravasation of tracer, which may yield erroneous interpretation.

Radiopharmaceuticals recommended: ^{99m}Tc-LLEC, or ^{99m}Tc-MAG 3, or ^{99m}Tc-DTPA (rarely): The dose administered for each tracer is given in **Table 1**.

Imaging: Patients are examined supine with the gamma-camera positioned underneath the examination table (posteriorly) viewing the kidney and bladder area. In this position, the distance from the skin to each of the kidneys is approximately the same and for calculation of the left/right renal uptake ratio, depth correction is not critical. In renal transplants, however, the camera is placed anteriorly with the patient in supine position, viewing the allograft and bladder. In children with ectopic (including fused ectopia) or horseshoe kidneys dual-head acquisition is preferred so that geometric mean can be used for calculation of the differential function of each unit. In children, appropriate immobilization should be attained during acquisition. Patient must be asked to void immediately before start of study. Once the patient is appropriately positioned, a rapid intravenous bolus of the tracer is injected and acquisition begins simultaneously. One frame per two seconds is recorded for 60 seconds (perfusion phase) followed by one frame per 15 seconds (parenchymal phase) for a total of 20–30 minutes.

Interpretation: A dynamic renal study is evaluated for the parenchymal phase, the cortical transit time, and the drainage phase. The renogram curve generated is evaluated for function and drainage pattern. A cinematic display verifies whether the patient moved during acquisition or not.

- *Parenchymal phase:* Evaluation of this phase is very critical. During the first few minutes of the dynamic study, after the initial vascular distribution of the tracer and before its appearance in the renal collecting system, the tracer is concentrated in the renal parenchyma. At this point there is progressive decrease in the blood level of the tracer with increasing concentration in the parenchyma till a peak is reached, where maximum concentration has been attained. Usual time to peak T_{max} is 2–5 minutes for normally functioning kidneys. After this, the tracer progressively decreases within the parenchyma, marking the beginning of the drainage phase. The parenchymal phase is usually visualized 60–120 seconds after the IV injection and provides the following information:
    - Relative and absolute size of the functional renal units.
    - Relative or split renal function (right vs left).
    - Overall renal morphology.
    - Position of the renal units and axis.

The relative renal size and their placement can be estimated by simple visual observation. Renal dimensions in longitudinal and transverse planes can be measured with a measuring scale provided in the processing station. A qualitative estimate of the renal function can be obtained by visually evaluating the ratio of the renal and background activity. Normally, very little tracer activity should be present in the background, the blood pool and the liver during the parenchymal phase. If a high level of tracer activity is noted within these regions, then the renal uptake shall be low indicating a poor renal function. Split renal function can be assessed visually and also by calculating the individual renal uptake as a fraction of the total renal uptake from renal regions of interests (ROIs). Placement of ROIs should be strictly over the parenchymal region but under certain special circumstances such as hydronephrosis, this may be difficult. Background ROIs (2 pixels wide and 2 pixels away from the renal ROI) should be placed with caution since this step is usually done manually and different size and position can produce different results, a particular problem when renal function is low and/or severe hydronephrosis is present.

Information about intrarenal distribution of radiotracer can be obtained during the parenchymal phase. Hydronephrosis is usually seen as a "photon deficient" area and depending on the severity of hydronephrosis, the cortical uptake appears as a rim of varying thickness. Reduced or absent tracer activity in a relative portion of the kidney such as a malfunctioning upper pole in a duplex kidney, trauma, tumor, or cyst can be detected.

- *Cortical transit time*: Cortical transit time is defined as the time interval between the intravenous injection of the radiotracer and its first appearance within the renal collecting system. Normally, this is about 3–6 minutes. A normal cortical transit time indicates that renal parenchymal function is not compromised, even in the presence of dilatation of the pelvicalyceal system. Conversely, therefore, the poorer the renal function, the longer is the cortical transit time. As the tracer is eliminated into the renal pelvis, there is gradual decline in the parenchymal activity. Even if the cortical transit time appears to be within the normal range, it is important to determine, if it is associated with a decrease of tracer activity from the renal cortex. Cortical retention of tracer activity indicates renal dysfunction. A number of conditions may prolong the cortical time. These include pelviureteric junction obstruction, acute and chronic pyelonephritis, nephrotoxicity, trauma, renal artery stenosis, renal vein thrombosis, acute tubular necrosis, and allograft rejection.
- *Drainage phase*: Drainage phase comprises the passage of the radiotracer from the pelvicalyceal system through the ureter into the bladder. Usually, at the end of 20 minutes of study, much of the tracer would leave the renal parenchyma. At this time, minimal or no tracer should be visible in the renal collecting system. Time activity curves (renogram) are generated from ROI over an entire kidney and reveal a peak time (T_{max}) at 2–5 minutes with subsequent decrease to 30–50% of the peak activity within 10 minutes. Time activity curves should always be interpreted along with careful evaluation of images in the parenchymal phase and drainage phase, keeping in mind the cortical transit time. It is possible to see a normal cortical transit time with complete cortical clearance of tracer by 20 minutes accompanied by a time activity curve that reveals a delayed peak and a high-residual value. Such a pattern indicates delayed drainage without parenchymal dysfunction and is almost always without any clinical significance. The possibility of a VUR of tracer during the drainage phase should also be kept in mind in order to be able to differentiate it from outflow tract obstruction.

Normal dynamic renal study: There is an intense and rapid concentration of tracer in the renal parenchyma by 2–5 minutes post-injection **(Fig. 1)**. Subsequently, the tracer passes into the renal calyces and pelvis by 3–6 minutes. Ureters may be visualized during the dynamic phase in normal patients and in those with slow ureteral transit time. However, a dilated ureter with or without obstruction is always visible in the postvoid phase. The renal parenchyma is usually completely cleared of radiotracer by 20 minutes but a small residual amount may sometimes be present and is usually of no clinical significance. This residual tracer usually clears spontaneously with change in the patient's position or after the patient voids (gravity-assisted drainage). The bladder is seen 3–6 minutes after injection and there is a progressive increase in tracer concentration with time. The background activity is usually a reflection of blood clearance of tracer or rather the renal extraction of tracer from the blood pool, which rapidly decreases with time in a patient with normal renal function. The dynamic acquisition can be terminated at 15–20 minutes, when there is no retention of tracer within the pelvicalyceal system or ureters. If at the end of the initial 20 minutes, there is evidence of tracer retention, then the patient should be asked to get up and move for a few minutes (a small child should be picked up for a few minutes) to encourage postural-gravity assisted drainage (GAD). An additional postvoid image is recommended to determine the tracer clearance, which if adequate, should be considered normal, and the outflow tract not obstructed. A diuretic renogram is indicated, if an obstruction is present or suspected.

Diuretic Renography

Furosemide causes a rapid diuretic response that drains out tracer from dilated nonobstructed system. In significant outflow tract obstruction, tracer in the renal area may decrease slowly or fail to decrease or even increase in response to a diuretic challenge. The urine flow depends not only on the function and amount of renal parenchyma, but also on the ability of the parenchyma to respond to a diuretic. Drainage is directly proportional to urine flow and inversely proportional to the volume of the renal pelvis and ureters; the poorer the function, the longer is the drainage time. Compliance and volume of the pelvicalyceal system are also important; in that a large flaccid renal pelvis usually causes slow drainage of radiotracer. There are several factors that can limit the usefulness of diuretic renography. Severe hydroureteronephrosis may partly or wholly mask the effect of a diuretic on the emptying of the renal pelvis. Other factors include poor response of the renal parenchyma to the diuretic, poor delivery of the diuretic to the kidneys, bladder over distension, complex pelvic surgeries, prune-belly syndrome, dehydration, and ectopic kidney.

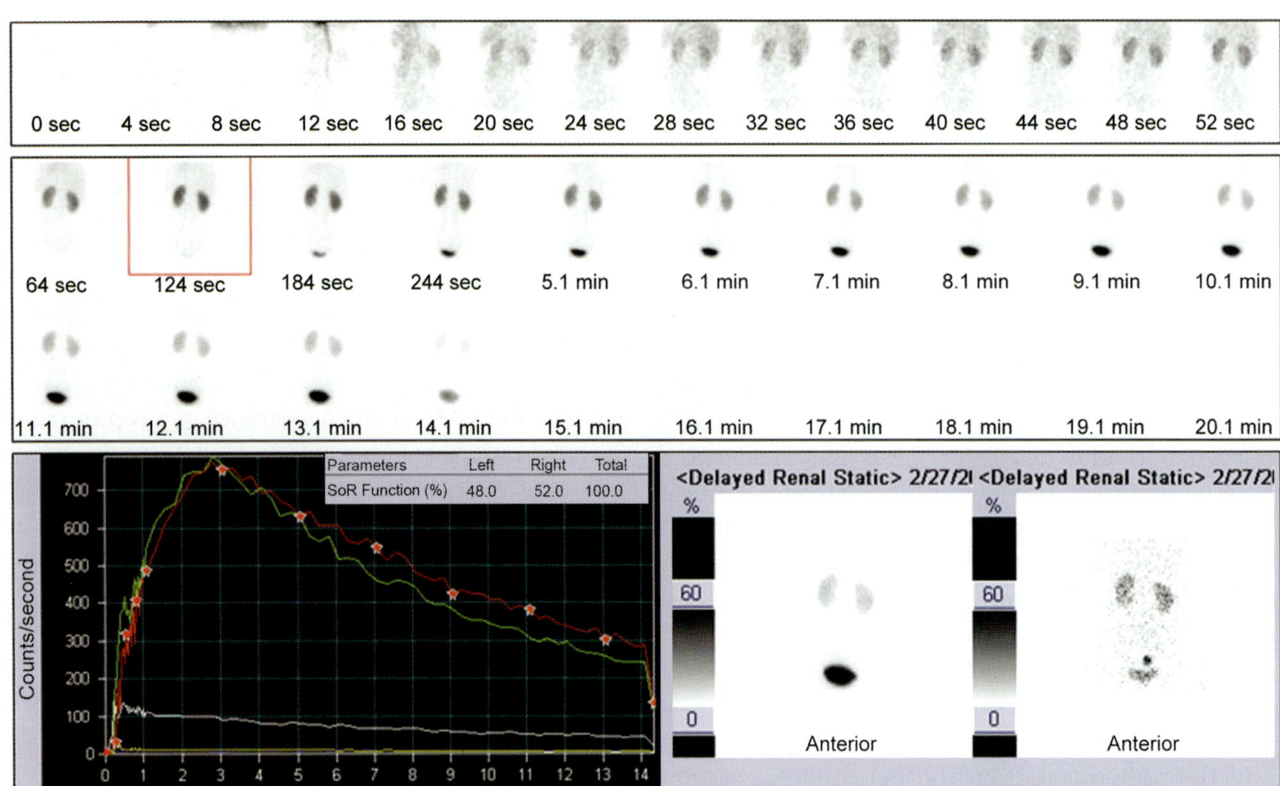

Fig. 1: Normal ^{99m}Tc-LLEC scan: Normal dynamic function images with prompt symmetric radiotracer perfusion (upper row), uptake and rapid clearance (middle row). Normal time activity curves with steep uptake slope, distinct peak, and rapid clearance (left lower row) with normal early and delayed static images (right lower row).

Imaging: Diuretic renography can be performed using the same radiopharmaceuticals mentioned earlier. It is important to ensure that tracer has filled the renal pelvis and postural drainage has not occurred before the diuretic is administered. The diuretic can be administered 15 minutes postinjection (F+15) or simultaneously with the radiotracer (F0).[16] The diuretic effect usually starts within 1-2 minutes after administration of furosemide. Patients with intermittent hydronephrosis who complain of intermittent flank pain may have reproduction of pain on administration of diuretic. It is important to note that in patients with urinary diversions, even in the absence of obstruction, flow dynamics may be slow, making the diagnosis of obstruction difficult. Overlap of kidney and an ileal or colonic diversion may give rise to confusing images. Imaging in various projections, removal or replacement of external urine collecting devices and attempts at postural drainage may sometimes be helpful.

Interpretation: Careful evaluation of the dynamic renal study preceding a diuretic administration is important during interpretation. In the absence of obstruction, rapid and complete washout of radiotracer occurs from the pelvicalyceal system **(Fig. 2)**. On the other side of the spectrum is an obstructed system with slow or no drainage of radiotracer following a diuretic challenge **(Figs. 3 and 4)**. Interpretation of equivocal diuretic renography patterns is difficult. F-15 diuresis (Lasix is administered 15 minutes prior to the tracer injection and at the start of renography) is recommended to unmask obstruction in such curves by performing study with peak diuresis.

The diuretic washout $T_{1/2}$ is estimated using an exponential interpolation between a point on the initial descent of the time activity curve and another point on the downward slope while the curve is decaying monotonically. The diuretic $T_{1/2}$ should be only one of the several factors, which are considered while assessing urinary obstruction. Although there may be many variations in the time of diuretic injection and subsequent time of acquisition following a diuretic response, the overall sensitivity of a diuretic renography for the detection of obstruction in children has been estimated at 93%.[17]

Drainage pattern of renogram: O' Reilly et al. (1978) classified patients on the basis of the renogram curve of ^{99m}Tc-DTPA with diuretic.[18]

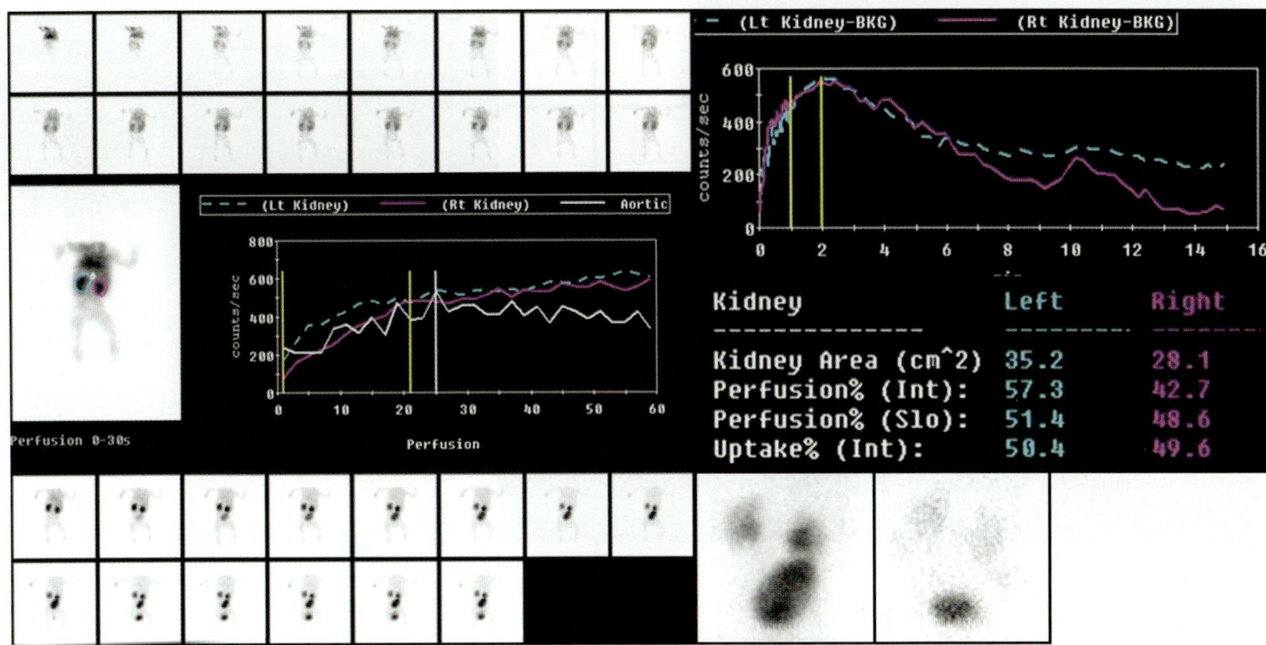

Fig. 2: ^{99m}Tc-LLEC scan in nonobstructive hydronephrosis: Dynamic and static renal images shows right-sided hydronephrosis with good clearance on delayed images; findings are consistent with nonobstructive hydronephrosis (Lt: left; Rt: right).

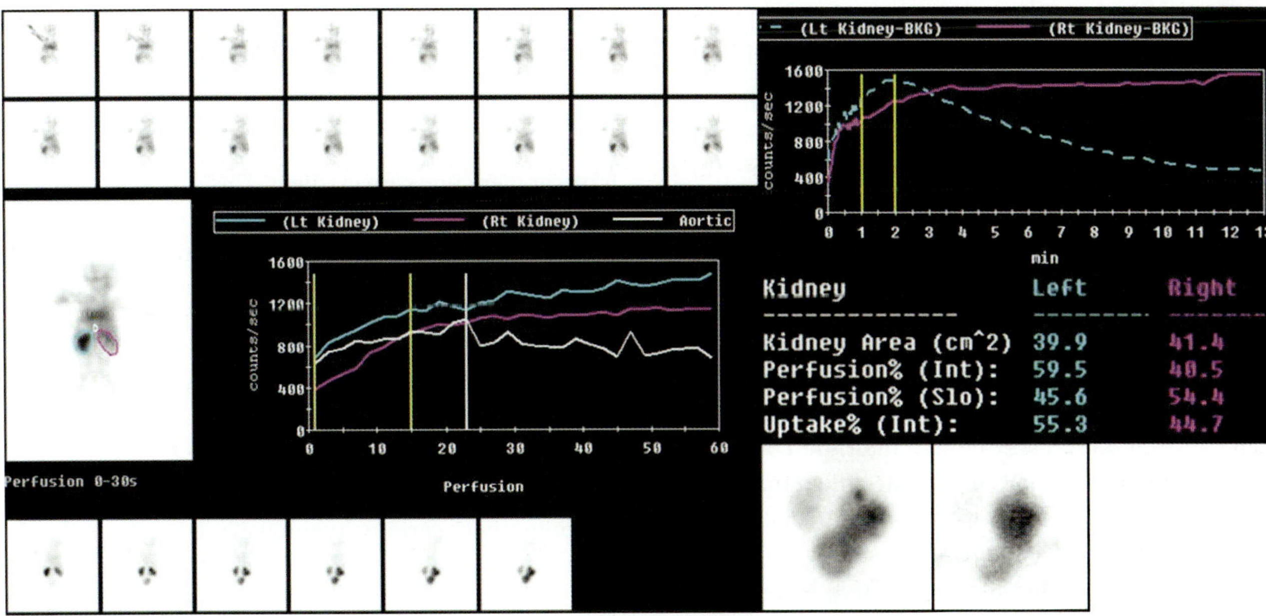

Fig. 3: ^{99m}Tc-LLEC scan in obstructive hydronephrosis: Progressive filling of dilated pelvicalyceal system (PCS) is seen on right side, whereas the left kidney clears normally. Time activity curves show washout on the left side and obstructed pattern on right side. Early and delayed static images show persistent activity in dilated PCS without any clearance on right side (Lt: left; Rt: right).

Response I: Normal initial renography and remained so after diuretics.

Response II: Obstructive initial renography and remained so after diuretics.

Response IIIa: Obstructive initial renography and showed rapid clearance after diuretics.

Response IIIb: Obstructive initial renography and showed mild/partial clearance after diuretics.

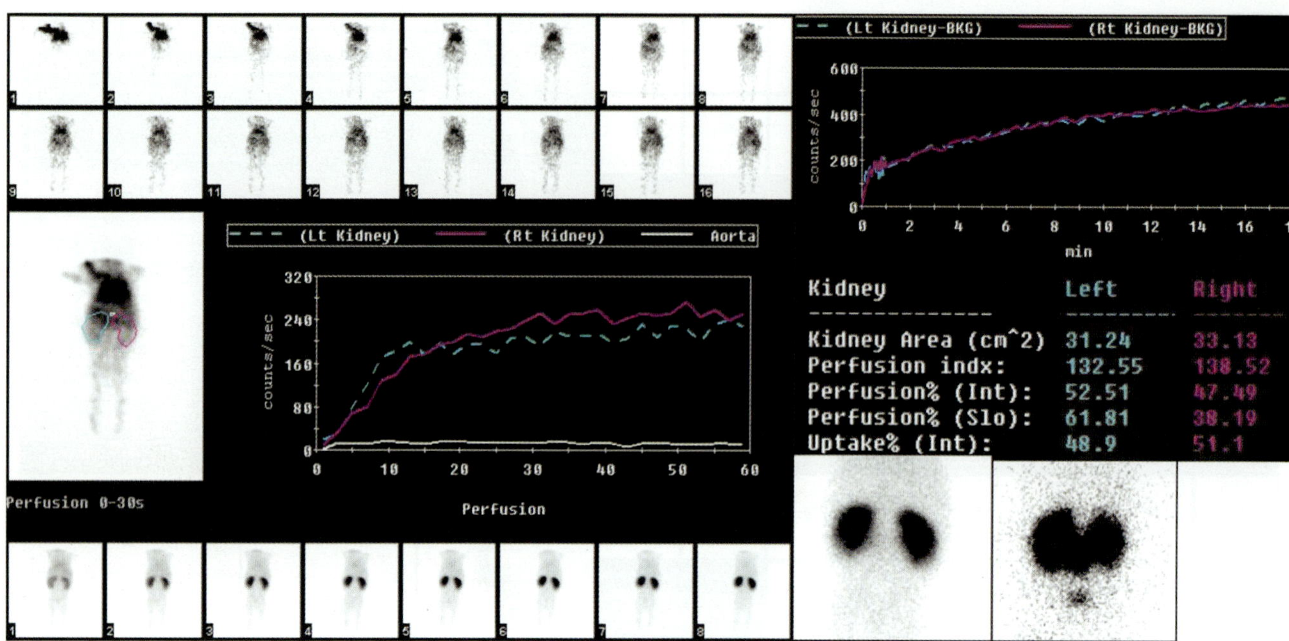

Fig. 4: ^{99m}Tc-LLEC scan in bilateral pelviureteric junction obstruction: Dynamic images shows progressive filling of dilated collecting system seen on both side. Time activity curves show obstructed pattern on both side. Early and delayed static images show persistent activity in dilated pelvicalyceal system (PCS) (Lt: left; Rt: right).

Captopril Renography

Secondary hypertension is more common in children and renal disease is perhaps the most common cause in this group. In a study conducted by Londe S et al. in 1978,[19] 563 pediatric patients with secondary hypertension were evaluated. 78% had renal abnormalities and 12% had renal artery disease. Secondary hypertension may be caused less frequently by endocrinal, cardiovascular, or nervous system disorders. The renal causes of hypertension are infarction, postpyelonephritic scarring, posttraumatic lesions and renal artery stenosis. Conventional renal dynamic scintigraphy usually shows the affected kidney to be smaller with lesser uptake than the contralateral normal kidney. The more severe the affliction, the lower is the renal uptake of tracer. ^{99m}Tc-DMSA scintigraphy in patients with renovascular hypertension typically reveals renal asymmetry. The affected kidney is smaller and shows lesser tracer uptake than the normal one. In the presence of unilateral renal artery stenosis, there may be reduced renal perfusion and function on the affected side. However, sometimes the same kidney may remain adequately perfused and owing to the autoregulation mechanism, the radionuclide study may remain normal in a significant number of cases. Thus conventional radionuclide studies are not reliable screening tests for the diagnosis of renovascular hypertension and that angiotensin-converting enzyme (ACE) inhibitor renal scintigraphy is a markedly improved technique.

Angiotensin-converting enzyme inhibitors such as captopril block the formation of angiotensin II, producing dilatation of efferent arterioles and a fall in transcapillary pressure gradient. This causes a significant decrease in GFR of the kidney with renal artery stenosis that can be easily diagnosed by renography.[19-23] Initially ^{99m}Tc-DTPA was used, but presently tubular agents are used. To ensure better absorption of captopril, patients should not take solid food at least 4 hours before the study. Enalapril has a distinct advantage over captopril as this can be administered intravenously, and therefore does not depend on the variations of absorption in the gastrointestinal tract. Caution should be taken about the potentially serious hypotensive episodes following intravenous enalapril. Significant hypotension is also seen after a single dose of captopril, and therefore the patient should be well-hydrated and an intravenous access maintained throughout the study. Blood pressure should be monitored every 5–15 minutes. Diuretics may exaggerate the hypotensive effect and should not be used in conjunction with captopril renography.

A baseline study is obtained followed by a repeat examination either 1 hour after oral captopril (1 mg/kg, up to 50 mg), or 15 minutes after intravenous enalapril (0.03 mg/kg). Some authors obtain the initial study with an ACE inhibitor and repeat later without the ACE inhibitor only, if the first study is abnormal. Since the primary effect of ACE inhibitor is decreased GFR, studies using glomerular agents show decreased extraction of tracer and delayed visualization of the collecting system, whereas with tubular agents prolonged cortical tracer retention is seen. Moreover, detection of cortical retention of tracer is easier to appreciate than focal decreased extraction, tubular agents are probably more effective than glomerular agents in the detection of segmental renal artery stenosis. The typical findings of a positive captopril study (renin-dependent renovascular hypertension) are—a decrease in differential renal uptake, increase in cortical transit time, prolongation of time to peak, and retention of tracer in the renal parenchyma **(Fig. 5)**. The most important parameter, however is the split renal uptake and change

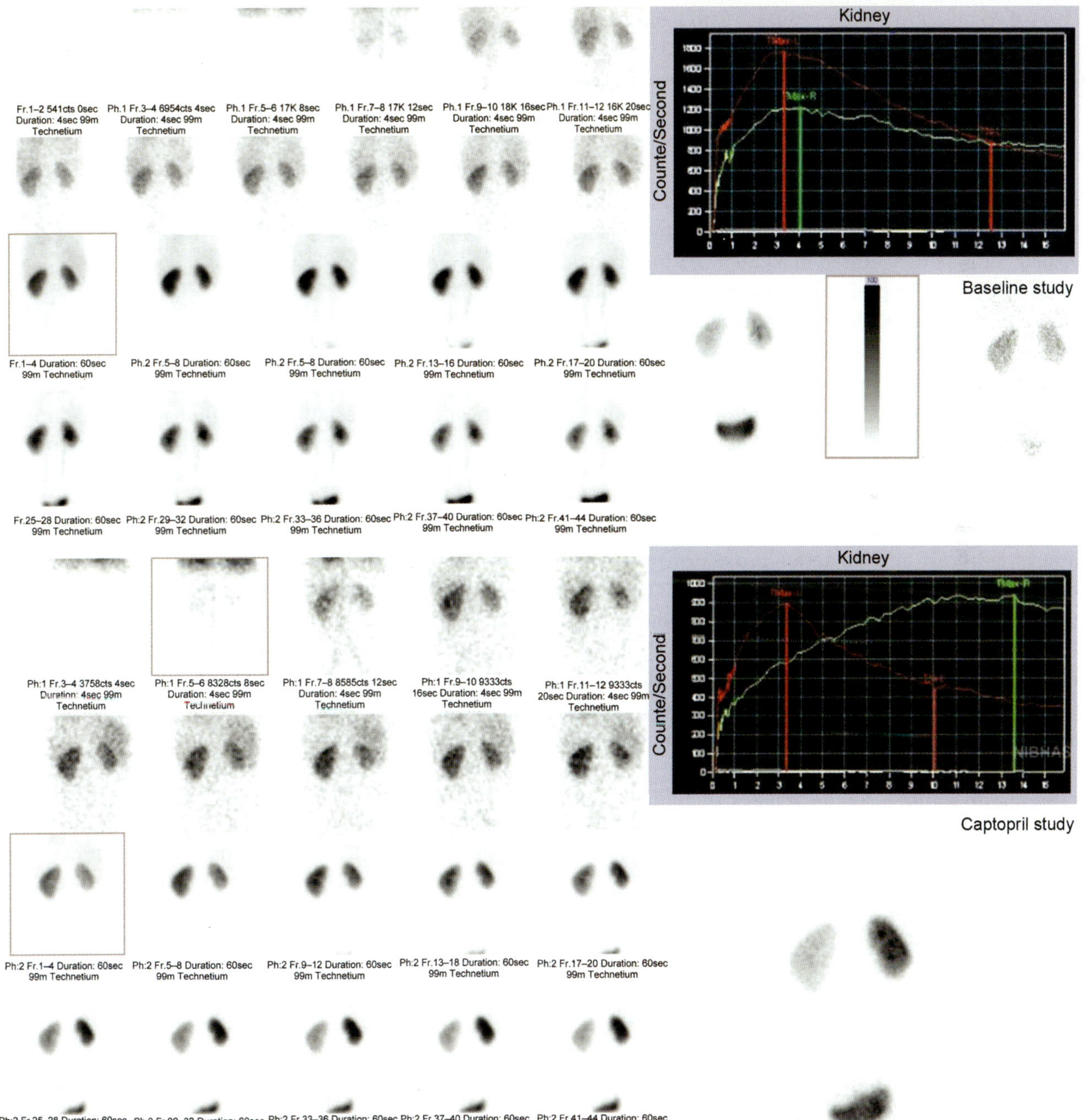

Fig. 5: Positive captopril study with ^{99m}Tc-LLEC: Baseline study (upper) shows normal functioning left kidney and slightly smaller right kidney with preserved function. Captopril study (lower) shows retention of radiotracer on right side and delayed peaking with a change in renogram pattern.

in renogram pattern. In patients with bilateral renal artery stenosis, the narrowing is usually asymmetrical and so is the effect of ACE inhibitor on each kidney. Cases, in which captopril does not induce scintigraphic changes, are usually associated with failure of revascularization or nephrectomy.[24-26]

RENAL CORTICAL SCINTIGRAPHY

^{99m}Technetium-DMSA is administered intravenously, dose of 0.04–0.05 mCi/kg (1.5–1.9 MBq/kg) with a minimum of 0.5 mCi (18.5 MBq) and a maximum of 3 mCi (111 MBq). Imaging is started about 3–4 hours after injection. Planar magnified images and SPECT images are acquired.

Imaging Techniques

Planar renal scintigraphy: Patient is examined supine with the gamma-camera positioned posteriorly and 300,000–500,000 counts are acquired in a 256 × 256 matrix using a high resolution or preferably an ultra high-resolution collimator. Left and right posterior oblique projections are acquired, which sometimes prove useful in the identification of cortical defects. Split renal uptake can be calculated by placing ROIs over posterior and anterior images and calculation of geometric mean. In cases of renal duplication, the upper and lower moieties can be outlined and differential renal function ascertained. In ectopic kidney, crossed renal ectopia and horseshoe kidneys, anterior and posterior projections are taken. Pinhole magnification or zoomed acquisition is mandatory in neonates and infants and may be useful in identification of cortical defects in older children and adults. Cortical defects following pyelonephritis, infarction, duplication and fetal lobulation can be discerned more frequently with pinhole magnification than with parallel hole high-resolution collimators since the former with an internal diameter of 2 mm provide images of higher spatial resolution than the latter.

Single photon positron emission tomography: Mapping of regional functional parenchyma is best done with ^{99m}Tc-DMSA SPECT. The surface and volume rendered SPECT images permit a superior overall view of the functional anatomy of the kidneys. Using the modern multi-headed SPECT cameras, acquiring 120 images over 360° on a 128 × 128 matrix usually requires 15–20 minutes. Proper sedation is mandatory for acquiring SPECT images.[27]

Radionuclide Cystography

This has been accepted as the technique of choice for evaluation and follow-up of children with urinary tract infection and reflux. The estimated gonadal radiation dose is one-hundredth of the voiding cystourethrography. Radionuclide cystography is more sensitive than voiding cystography in detecting vesicoureteric reflux. Other parameters like residual urine volume, bladder volume at the time of reflux and the rate of clearance of refluxed urine can also be calculated. The only disadvantage of radionuclide cystography is poor anatomical resolution of the bladder and urethra.

Clinical Applications

In urology practice, the most important clinical areas, where radionuclide studies may be of particular importance in patient management, can be considered under the following headings:

- Urinary tract obstruction
- Urinary tract infection
- Renovascular hypertension
- Congenital anomalies
- Renal failure
- Renal transplant evaluation.

Urinary tract obstruction: Radionuclide studies may be necessary to establish or confirm the diagnosis of obstruction, to ascertain its site or level, to determine its extent or severity or to measure how well the obstructed kidney is functioning.[16,28] In addition, radionuclide studies may be needed in other situations when any change in the function or condition of the kidney, or of the site and severity of obstruction, is to be determined, if desirable clinically to assess patients prognosis and in differential diagnosis of urinary obstruction. In the differential diagnosis of urinary obstruction, diuretic renography is of immense value, especially in those patients with a nonobstructed dilated collecting system associated with indeterminate flow curve (***see* Fig. 2**). Injection of diuretic is essential, if obstruction at the pelviureteric junction is suspected, as this diagnosis can only be confirmed at high urine flow rate. However, one of the major drawbacks of diuretic renography is a large number of indeterminate results in poorly functioning kidneys. Some progress has been made in this regard by correcting furosemide response for level of renal function. Significant renal function has been reported on radionuclide studies in a large percentage of the patients with nonfunctioning kidneys seen on intravenous urography. Estimation of renal output efficacy (ROE), which is calculated by a technique independent of variations in uptake rate by the kidneys, provides an accurate diagnosis of renal outflow obstruction in patients with significantly impaired renal function.[29]

Urinary tract infection: Renal infection may be clinically obvious, but can be easily overlooked. Clinically, it is frequently difficult or impossible to differentiate infection of the bladder and ureters from the acute renal parenchymal infection. The lack of sensitivity of intravenous urography (IVU) and ultrasonography in the demonstration of early renal infection is well-known. ^{99m}Tc-DMSA is valuable in the identification of renal damage due to early pyelonephritis. Even in the absence of urographic or ultrasonographic abnormalities, regional parenchymal uptake of DMSA may be altered in acute pyelonephritis. ^{99m}Tc-DMSA is also useful to quantify the degree of renal damage, to follow the progress on antibiotic therapy, and to assess recovery and/or residual renal damage.

Imaging with ^{99m}Tc-DMSA facilitates, detection of cortical scarring as a sequelae of pyelonephritis **(Fig. 6)**. Unlike urography, RCS can detect cortical defects that do not deform the renal outline or the collecting system. In the detection of renal scars ^{99m}Tc-DMSA scan is more sensitive (96%) and specific (98%) as compared with IVU.[30] Besides, in patients with chronic pyelonephritis with uncontrolled hypertension, demonstration of a severe segmental scar on a DMSA scan may guide the surgeon in undertaking partial nephrectomy **(Figs. 7 and 8)**.

One of the most common and routinely employed procedures in children with urinary tract infection is the direct radionuclide cystogram (DRCG) in conjunction with RCS **(Figs. 9 to 11)**. In the diagnosis of vesicouretic reflux, this procedure is much superior and the radiation exposure to the patient is much less as compared to micturating cystourethrogram (MCU).[31]

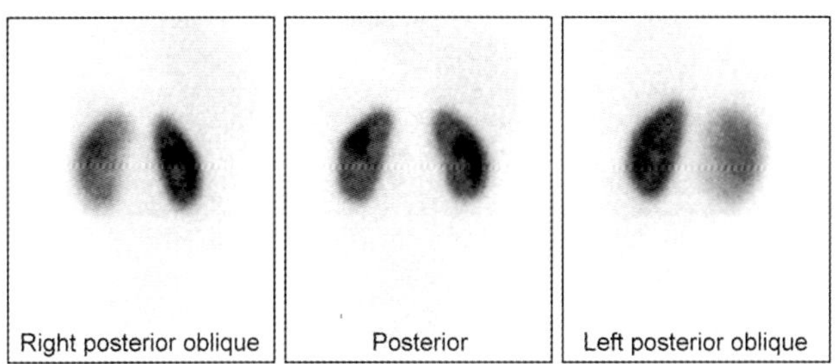

Fig. 6: Normal ^{99m}Technetium-dimer captosuccinic acid scan: Bilateral kidneys are normal in size with smooth cortical outline and normal function.

Renovascular hypertension: Renovascular hypertension is the most common cause of secondary and potentially curable hypertension. Regardless of the problems associated with the routine renogram, availability of gamma-camera computer system has made meaningful pre-intervention renal assessment possible in such patients. This test as a follow-up procedure for evaluating the result of percutaneous angioplasty or surgery on the function in the affected kidney of the patients with renovascular disease is an extremely important but often overlooked application.

A major approach to the nuclear medicine diagnosis of the renovascular hypertension has been the introduction of captopril, an ACE inhibitor. The concept for the use of ACE inhibitors in the differential diagnosis of the renovascular hypertension arose from the observation that patients with bilateral renal artery stenosis (RAS), or patient with solitary kidney having RAS had a tendency to develop acute renal failure when treated with these drugs. The theoretical basis for complication of ACE inhibitor therapy and the rationale for the captopril renography test are essentially the same. The renin-angiotension system is thought to be a compensatory mechanism by which the kidney maintains perfusion, when it is subjected to low perfusion pressure, as may result distal to a renal artery stenosis. ACE inhibitors act to block the step, where angiotensin I is converted to angiotensin II, and as a result prevent the subsequent increase in the efferent arteriolar tone. In the absence of this compensatory mechanism, the glomerular filtration rate (GFR) drops significantly in the affected kidney.[21-23] A normal base line study

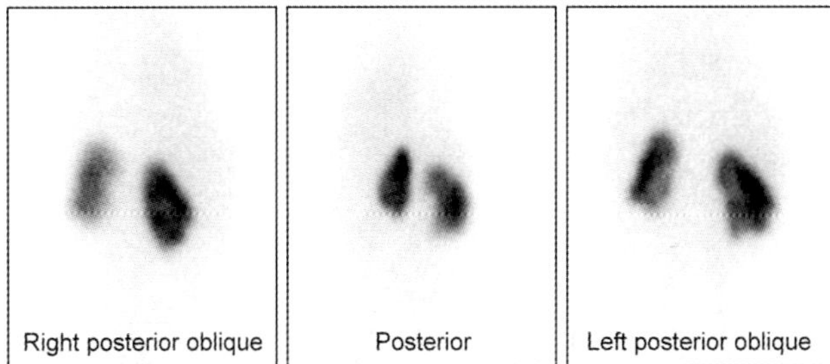

Fig. 7: ^{99m}Technetium-dimer captosuccinic acid (^{99m}Tc-DMSA) study in patient with bilateral vesicouretric reflux. All three views of ^{99m}Tc-DMSA scan show cortical break suggestive of renal scarring (multiple on left side and lower polar on right side).

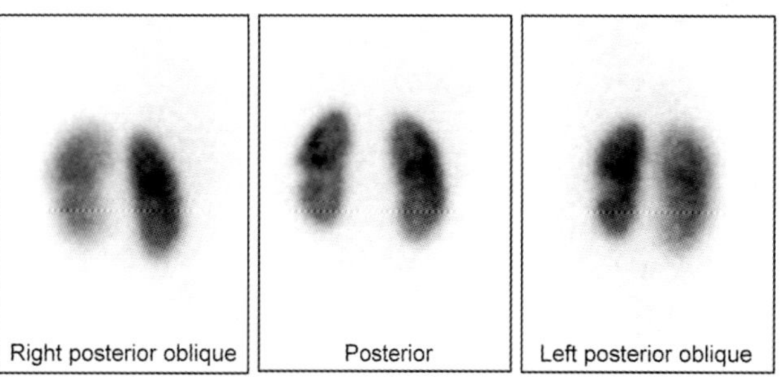

Fig. 8: ^{99m}Technetium-dimer captosuccinic acid (^{99m}Tc-DMSA) study in patient with left vesicouretric reflux. All three views of ^{99m}Tc-DMSA scan show cortical break in left kidney suggestive of left renal scarring.

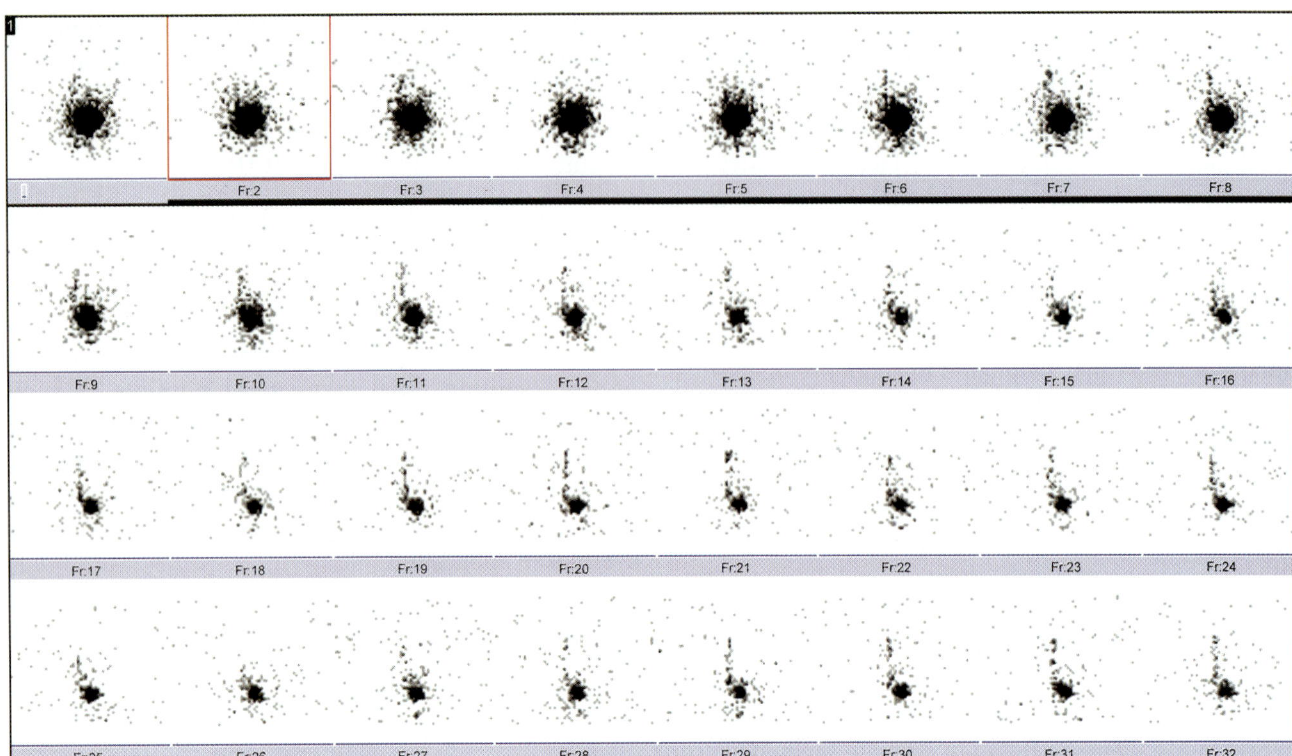

Fig. 9: Direct radionuclide cystogram study: Dynamic images show vesicoureteral reflux from bladder into left ureter (Grade-II).

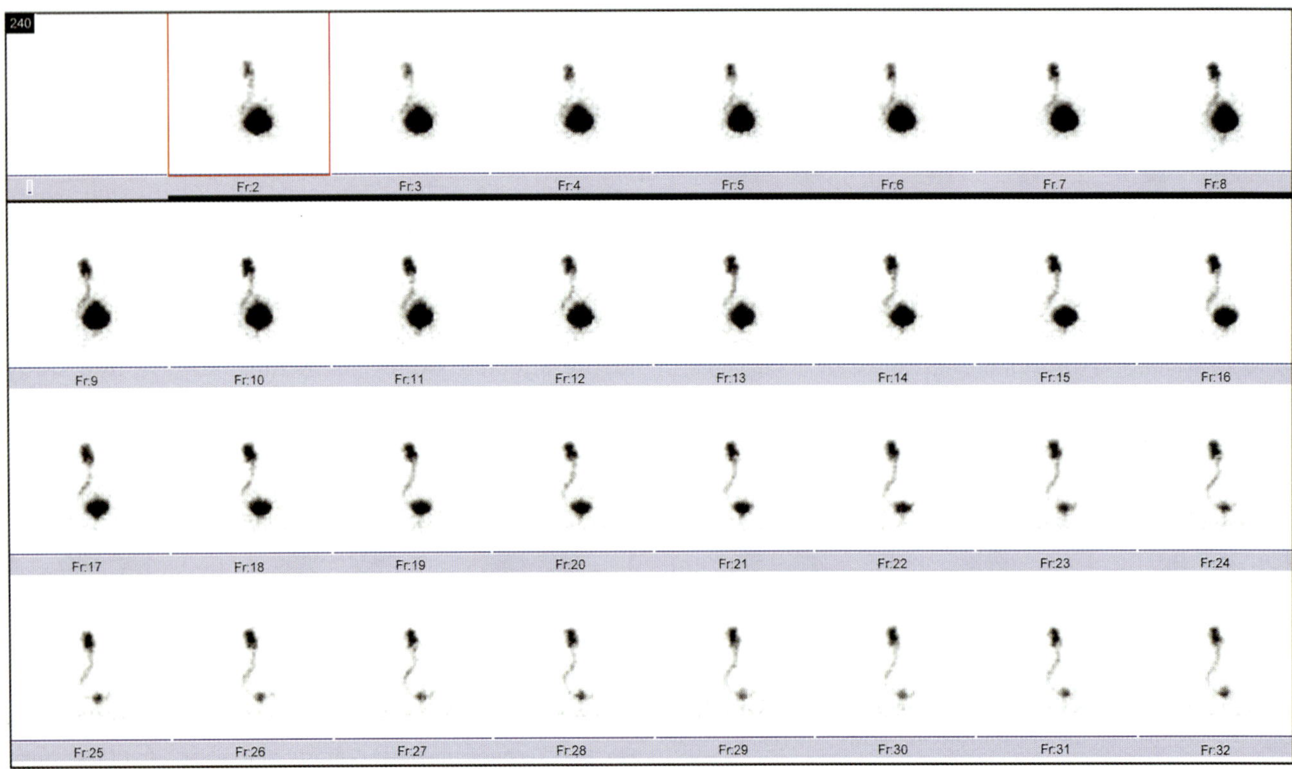

Fig. 10: Direct radionuclide cystogram study in unilateral reflux: Dynamic images show vesicoureteral reflux from bladder into left ureter (Grade-III).

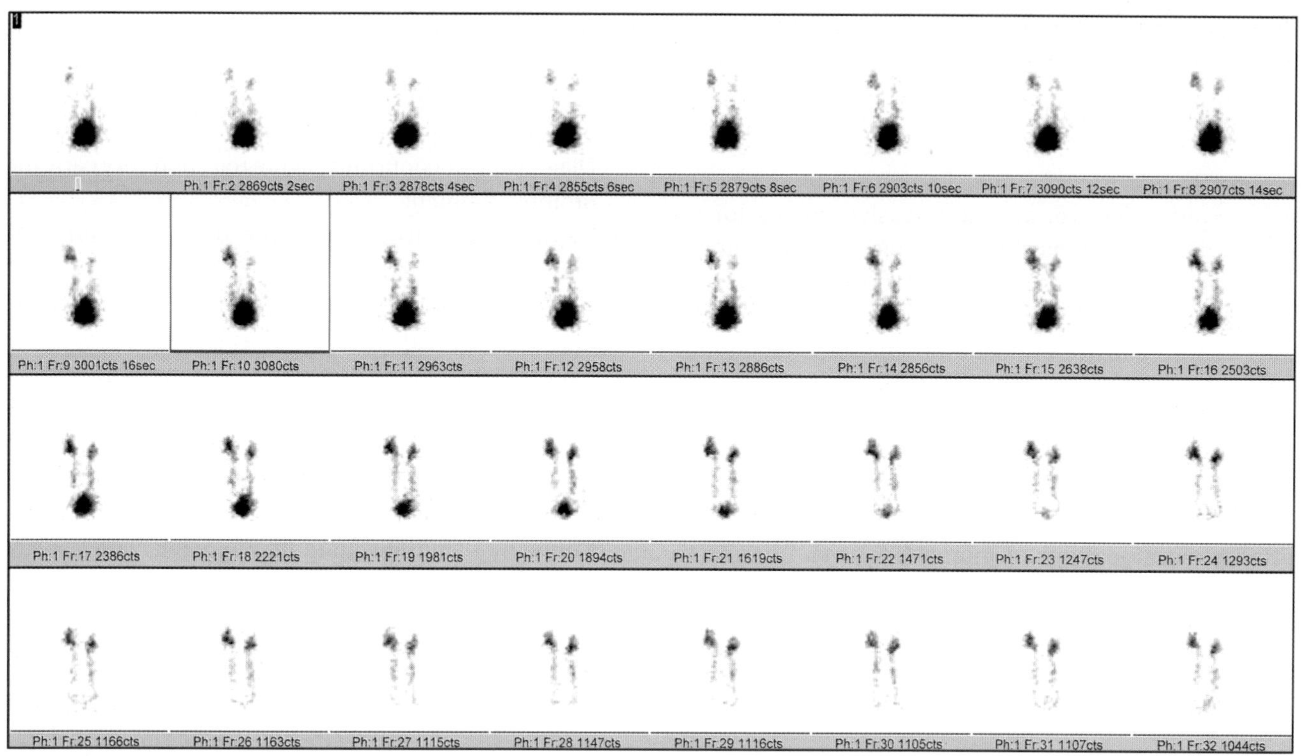

Fig. 11: Direct radionuclide cystogram study shows bilateral vesicoureteral reflux: Dynamic images showing reflux of radiotracer from bladder into both ureters (Grade-III).

followed by unilateral decreased in split renal function are the hallmark of unilateral renovascular hypertension (***see* Fig. 5**). Widespread application of the captopril renography and improved surgical techniques as well as perfection of the catheter techniques for percutaneous transluminal angioplasty, has caused tremendous excitement in the field of renovascular disease, and resulted in sudden repopularization of radioisotope renography. Enalapril is presently used instead of captopril, although the procedure name remains captopril renography.

Congenital anomalies: Renal radionuclide studies are helpful in the diagnosis and functional evaluation of a spectrum of congenital disorders. Serial evaluation of the parenchymal and drainage function may be essential in patients with polycystic kidneys, and in medullary sponge kidneys. Radionuclide investigations have a definite "functional" edge over the urography in the management of ectopic kidneys, horseshoe kidney, crossed ectopias, or malrotated kidneys.[32,33] Radionuclide studies are useful in the evaluation of regional cortical renal function in patients with duplications of the ureters and renal pelvis. Preoperative and serial postoperative functional as well as morphologic evaluation of the kidney, upper urinary tracts, and the urinary bladder can be effectively done in patients with posterior urethral valves by the dynamic renography, RCS, and DRCG studies. Functional evaluation of the kidney and the urinary bladder by radionuclide studies in patients with neurogenic bladder has also been very well-established. Nonfunctioning multicystic dysplastic kidneys are evaluated on DMSA scintigraphy.

Global renal impairment: ^{99m}Tc-DMSA is used for renal imaging in chronic kidney disease (CKD) patients to establish tubulointerstitial disease as the cause for renal impairment.

Radionuclide clearance studies provide valuable information and help in monitoring glomerular or tubular function in nephropathies of various origins, the most important being the diabetic nephropathy. Kidney disease in diabetic patients has a devastating effect on survival, most evident in those with juvenile onset disease. It has been advocated that in such patients, the prospective monitoring of diminishing renal function should include precise measurement of GFR by radionuclide techniques combined with determination of fractional clearance of high molecular weight proteins. This is particular important when the effects of treatment on the early proteinuric phase of the diabetic nephropathy are being evaluated.[34,35] The considerable loss of glomerular filtration capacity at this stage is undetected by inverse creatinine measurement, which remains a valuable tool for monitoring the late stage of nephropathy, when metabolic correction is unlikely to be effective.

Renal transplant evaluation: Radionuclide techniques offer rapid, effective, and noninvasive means for the correct diagnosis of many of the medical and few surgical complications of the renal transplantation. Renal perfusion and function studies using ^{99m}Tc-EC or ^{99m}Tc-MAG3 offer comprehensive evaluation of the renal blood flow, function, and drainage **(Fig. 12)**. Many techniques have been described for establishing the cause of early graft dysfunction, especially for the diagnosis of acute rejection (AR) and acute tubular necrosis (ATN) **(Fig. 13)**. Some of the surgical complications like urinary obstruction, urinary extravasations, urinoma **(Fig. 14)**, nonurinary pelvic collections, e.g. hematoma or lymphocele and VUR can be diagnosed on radionuclide studies. Despite the relative merits and demerits of the radionuclide studies vis-a-vis other noninvasive diagnostic modalities, nuclear medicine has made an impact in clinical practice in at least three ways:

1. By reducing the number of invasive biopsies in transplant patients.
2. Diagnosing or confirming acute rejection very early for prompt treatment.
3. By being able to reassure the transplant surgeon regarding the viability of the allograft in uncomplicated ATN with prolonged periods of oliguria or anuria. With improved techniques and increasing availability of the renal transplantation procedures at many more centers around the country, nuclear medicine is bound to play an important role in evaluation and management of renal transplant.[36,37]

Management of a nephro-urological problem can be best done by a multidisciplinary approach. The various diagnostic modalities like X-ray, CT, US, magnetic resonance urography and nuclear medicine often support and complement each other.[38] However, radionuclide techniques have the most important "functional edge"

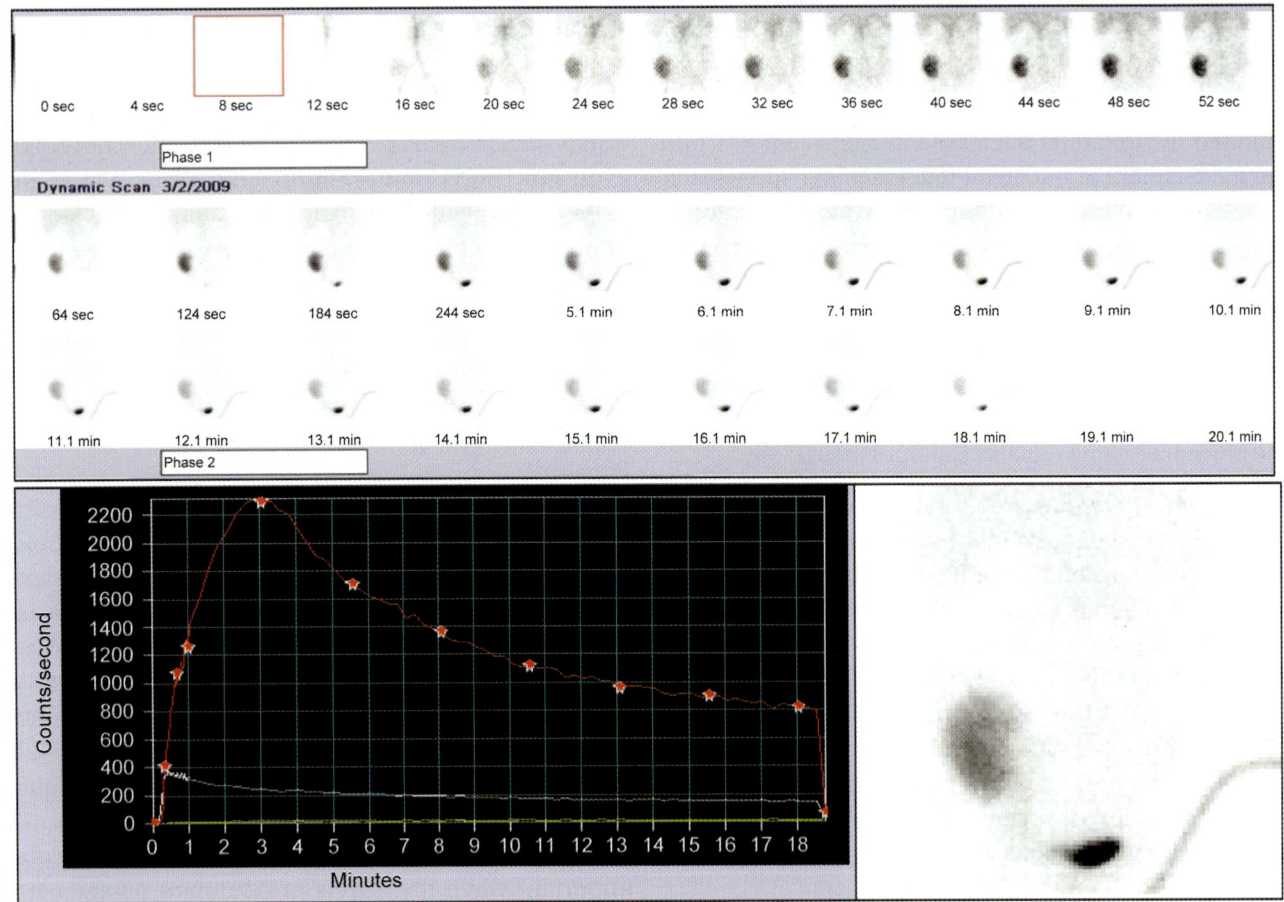

Fig. 12: ^{99m}Tc-LLEC scan in normal functioning transplanted kidney. Dynamic images show normal perfusion and uptake with prompt clearance. Time activity curves show steep uptake, distinct peak, and rapid clearance.

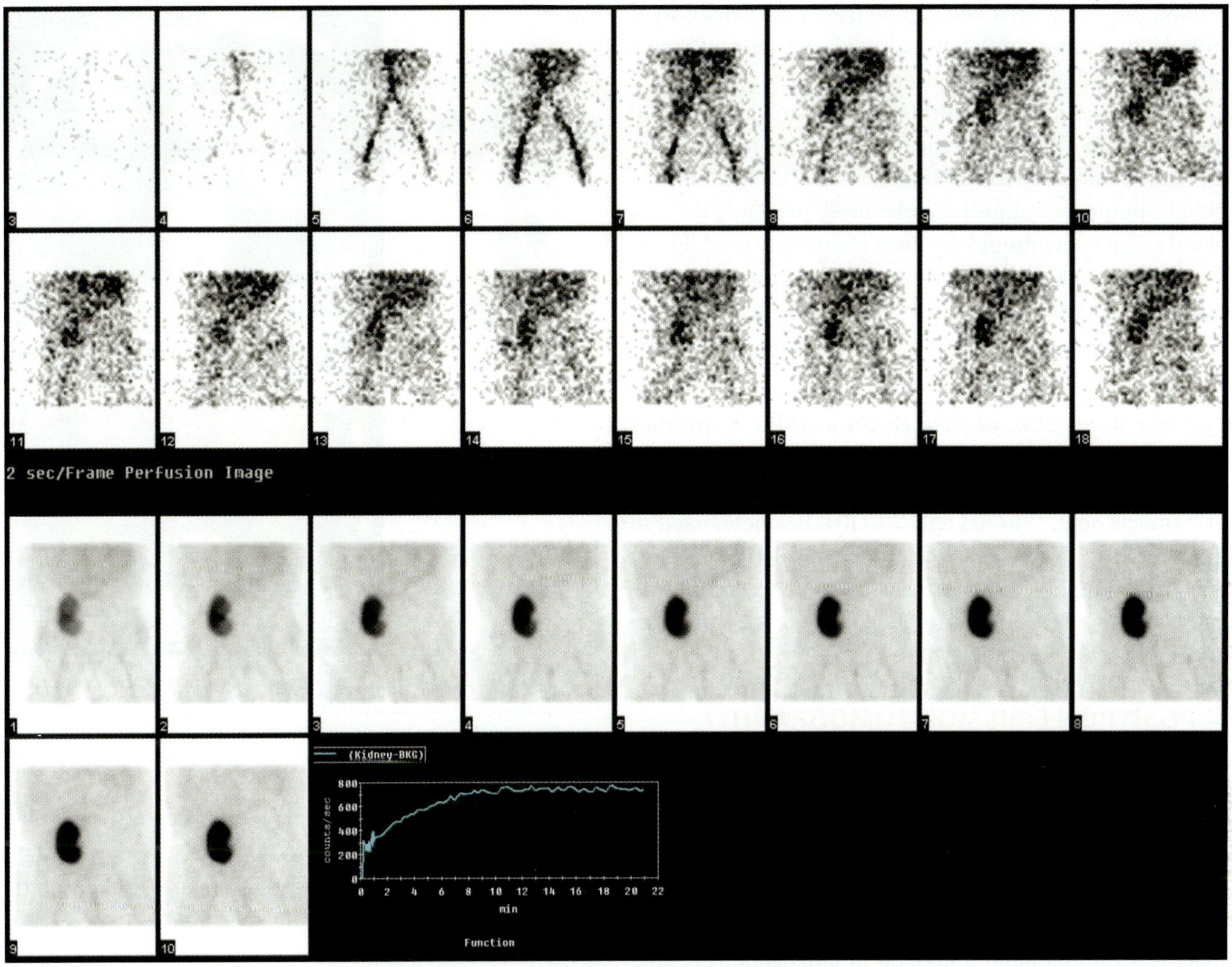

Fig. 13: ^{99m}Tc-LLEC scan in ATN. Baseline images show normal perfusion and uptake but significant retention. Time activity curve show rising trend consistent with ATN.

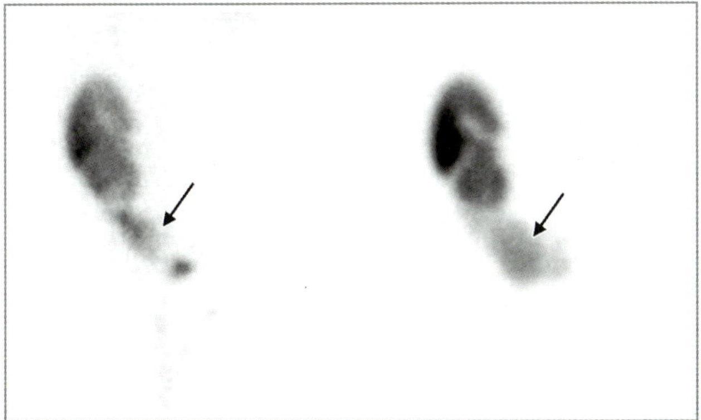

Fig. 14: Renal allograft in right iliac fossa, postvoid (left), and delayed static (right) views show an increasing collection in mid and lower ureteric regions (arrows)—suggestive of urine leak.

over many other diagnostic methods. With further refinements in technology, instrumentation, and radiopharmaceuticals, nuclear medicine is destined to improve more in the future.

Measurement of Renal Function

Glomerular filtration rate: Renal function can be assessed by clinical methods using blood urea nitrogen (BUN) and serum creatinine level but these are relatively crude, as significant decrease in function must occur before changes in BUN and creatinine are seen. Other factors which affect creatinine level are diet, difference in muscle mass, and certain medications.

Glomerular filtration rate is the clearance rate of substance that is excreted from the body by glomerular filtration and not secreted or reabsorbed by tubules, the ideal molecule for this is inulin. Substances which have a complete first pass extraction through kidney are used to calculate renal plasma flow (RPF). Paraamino hippurate is about 90% extracted and can be used for calculation of RPF. As it is not completely excreted, the term effective renal plasma flow (ERPF) is used.

Many radiopharmaceuticals are used to calculate GFR; these include ^{99m}Tc-DTPAand ^{51}CrEDTA. In India, ^{99m}Tc-DTPA is mainly used for GFR calculation. Though multiple blood sample techniques scan be used, presently the two blood sample techniques are most commonly used. Blood samples are taken at 1 hour and 3 hour postinjection. Normal GFR value is approximately 106 ± 27 mL/min/ 1.73 m^2 for adults. In children adult GFR levels are reached by about 2 years of age.

Effective renal plasma flow (ERPF): ERPF is another parameter of renal function and the ideal agent for this is paraaminohippuric acid (PAH). The radiolabeled form of hippuric acid, ^{131}I-OIH and ^{123}I-OIH, has been used to quantify ERPF. The urinary clearance of ^{131}I-OIH is about 85% of the PAH. ^{99m}Tc-EC or MAG-3 can be used for ERPF calculation with a single sample collected at 54 minutes and 44 minutes, respectively.

POSITRON EMISSION TOMOGRAPHY/ COMPUTED TOMOGRAPHY

State-of-art integrated positron emission tomography/ computed tomography (PET/CT) provides functional (metabolic) and structural information in the same setting. At present, 2-deoxy-2-[^{18}F]-fluorodeoxyglucose (FDG) is the workhorse agent for PET/CT imaging. ^{18}F-FDG is a radiolabeled analogue of glucose and is able to detect altered glucose metabolism in various disease conditions. There is a significant upregulation of the GLUT-1 transporters in cancer cells, which results in increased FDG uptake compared with the surrounding normal tissues. The role of FDG-PET in the initial staging, restaging, monitoring response to therapy, and follow-up surveillance of many cancers is well-documented.[39] There are relatively few FDG-PET reports describing its role in assessing primary urologic tumors due to the potential problem of tracer excretion through the kidneys. In recent years, however, special PET/CT techniques have evolved to make PET/CT imaging possible even in patients with primary urinary bladder cancers.[40] Moreover, the introduction of other PET radiotracers, such as ^{11}Carbon (^{11}C)-choline **(Fig. 15)**, ^{11}C-acetate, and Glu-NH-CO-NH-Lys-(Ahx) [Ga-68(HBED-CC)]) (^{68}Ga PSMA) **(Fig. 16)** has enhanced the role of this technique in patients with urologic cancers including prostate cancer.[41] ^{68}Ga PSMA 11 has emerged as a useful tracer not only as a diagnostic agent but also for therapy of metastatic castrate resistant

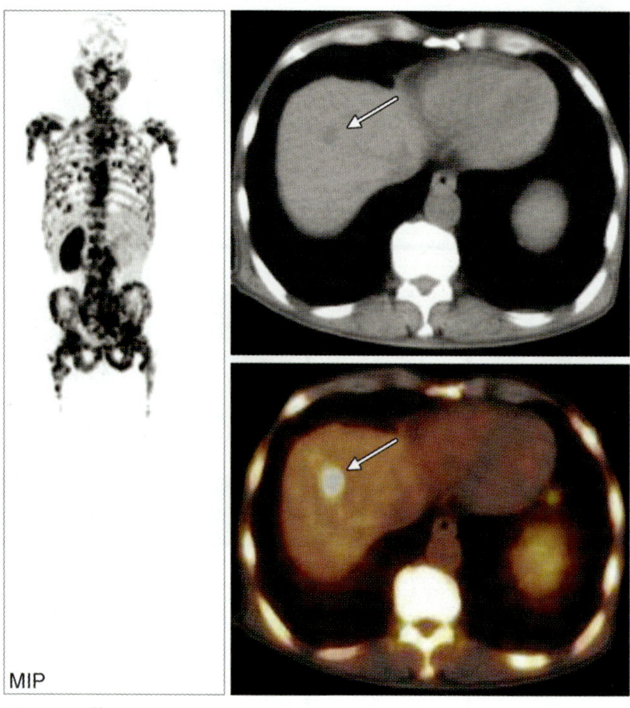

Fig. 15: ^{68}Ga PSMA positron emission tomography/computed tomography (PET/CT) in a patient with extensive skeletal metastases [maximum intensity projection (MIP)], showing in addition PSMA accumulation in a focal liver metastasis with a hypodense lesion on CT (arrow).

prostate cancer with Lutetium-177 PSMA-617 therapy.[42] The main role of PET/CT in urologic malignancies is initial diagnosis and staging, re-staging, evaluation of treatment response, and detection of recurrent/metastatic disease.[39]

Fluorodeoxyglucose-PET also plays a role in the evaluation of posttransplant lymphoproliferative disorders and pyrexia of unknown origin in renal transplant patients. Available studies report promising results with FDG-PET in detection, staging, and therapy evaluation of PTLD patients and PET findings can alter or guide treatment in up to 29% of cases. Concerns remain with regard to occurrence of false negatives due to physiological high background activity and early PTLD lesions as well as false positives due to inflammatory conditions.[43]

Renal Cell Carcinoma

Despite significant uptake and excretion through the kidneys, FDG has been used in the management of renal cell carcinoma (RCC). Bachor et al.[44] studied 29 patients with solid renal masses and found that PET was positive in 20 (77%) of 26 patients of RCC. PET was false positive in an angiomyolipoma, a pericytoma, and a pheochromocytoma. Ramdave et al.[45] evaluated the accuracy of FDG-PET for staging and management of 17

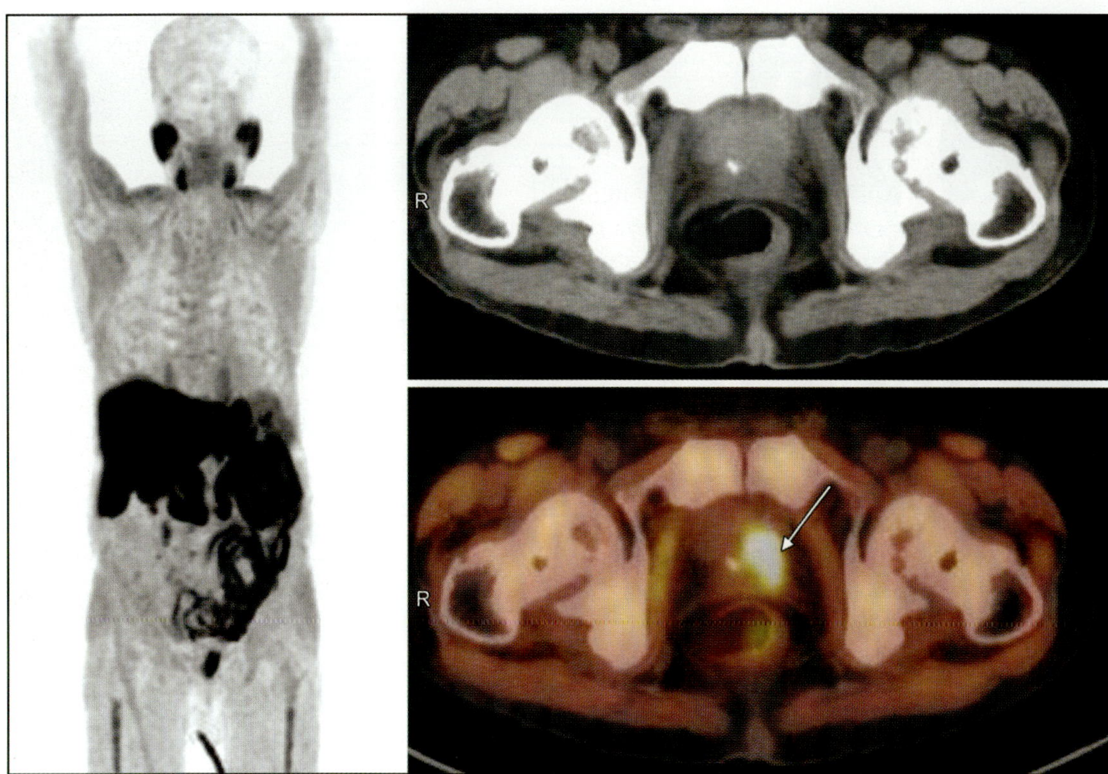

Fig. 16: ^{18}F-Fluorocholine positron emission tomography/computed tomography in a case of prostatic carcinoma with tracer accumulation in the primary in the prostate left side (arrow).

patients with known or suspected RCC. PET and CT had an accuracy of 94%. In addition, PET detected pulmonary metastases in two patients. Miyakita et al.[46]compared biologic characteristics of RCC with FDG and concluded that PET-positive tumors had higher tumor grade and increased GLUT-1 expression. Kumar et al.[47]showed good results with FDG PET in 28 solid renal masses of which 10 were primary (nine malignant, one benign) and 18 were metastatic renal tumors. FDG-PET accurately detected 23 of 27 (85%) malignant renal masses. Of the 10 primary renal tumors **(Fig. 17)**, FDG-PET was true positive in eight of nine (89%), true 28 negative in one and false negative in one. In addition to the characterization of primary tumors, FDG-PET was valuable in 31 primary staging and altered treatment in 30% of patients (3 of 10). Of the 18 metastatic renal 32 masses, FDG-PET was positive in 15 (83%) masses. For detection of recurrent and distant disease, PET was found to have an accuracy of 100% in detecting local recurrence and metastases as compared CT which had accuracy of 88% **(Fig. 18)**. Majhail et al.[48]evaluated FDG-PET in the detection of distant metastases in 24 patients with RCC. FDG-PET results were compared with those abstracted with biopsy in 33 lesions. Overall sensitivity, specificity, and PPV of FDG-PET were 64%, 100% and 100%, respectively.

Urinary Bladder Cancer

Previously, FDG PET was thought to have limited use in diagnosis and management of bladder cancer. However, with modified techniques[40] (after injection of diuretic and delayed imaging) it is possible to image primary as well as recurrent urinary bladder cancer **(Fig. 19)**. Kosuda et al.[49]studied 12 patients with urinary bladder cancers with FDG PET for the evaluation of recurrent or residual disease. PET identified 100% (17 of 17) of distant metastases (lung, bones, and remote lymph nodes) and 67% (2 of 3) of local lymph nodes. Ahlstrom et al.[50] attempted to improve the accuracy of PET by using C11-methionine, which has no urinary excretion. The authors reported a sensitivity of 78% (18 of 23) and there was good correlation of tracer uptake and tumor stage.

In conclusion, PET-CT has shown very encouraging results in a limited number of studies, and has also demonstrated a good sensitivity for initial staging in patients with renal and bladder cancer. FDG-PET seems to be superior to conventional imaging modalities for

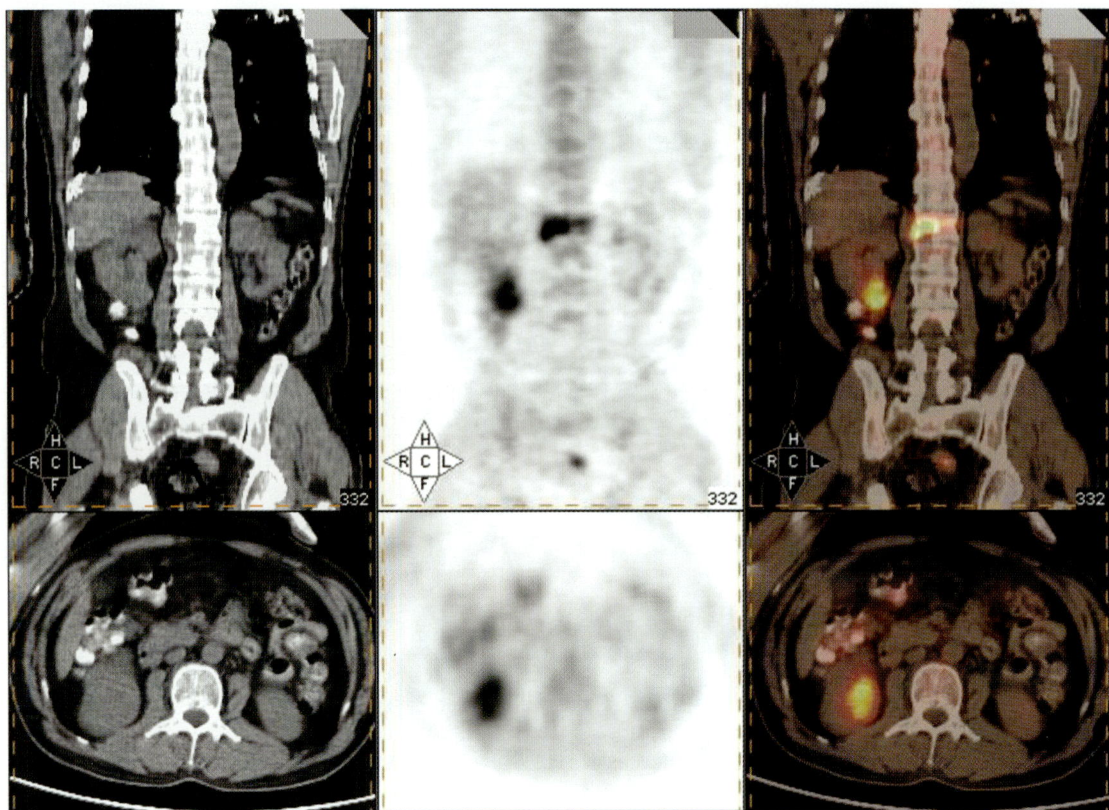

Fig. 17: 2-deoxy-2-[^{18}F]-fluorodeoxyglucose (^{18}F-FDG) positron emission tomography/computed tomography (PET-CT) study: Coronal and axial sections of CT, PET, and PET-CT showing soft tissue mass at lower pole of right kidney. Note FDG Uptake in T12.

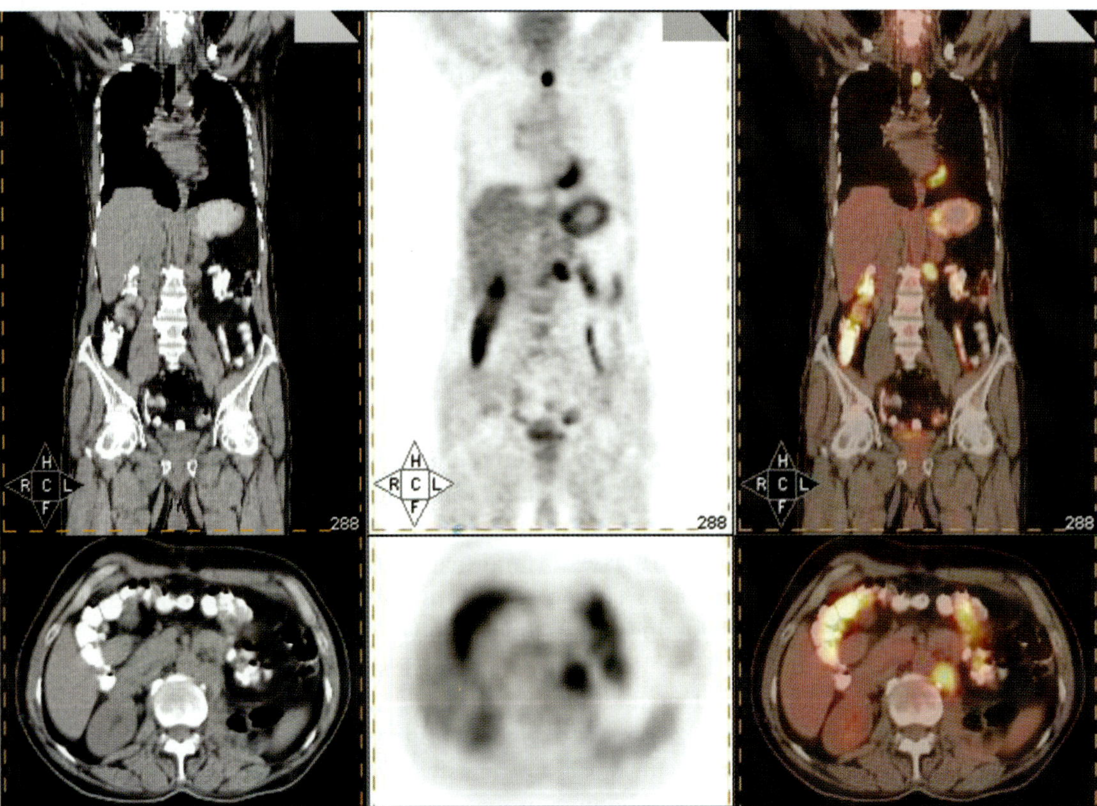

Fig. 18: 2-deoxy-2-[^{18}F]-fluorodeoxyglucose positron emission tomography/computed tomography (PET-CT) study: Coronal and axial sections of CT, PET, and PET-CT showing soft tissue mass in left renal bed suggestive of local recurrence.

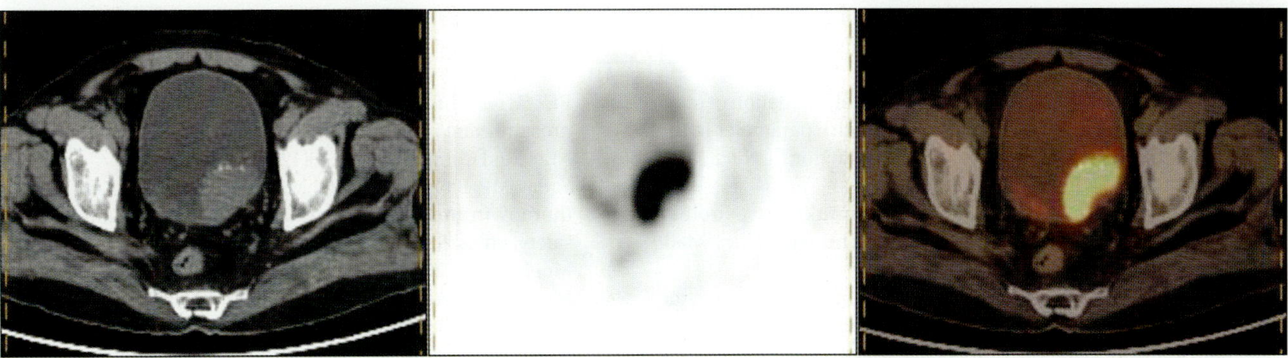

Fig. 19: 2-deoxy-2-[^{18}F]-fluorodeoxyglucose positron emission tomography/computed tomography (^{18}F-FDG PET-CT) study: Axial sections of CT, PET, and PET-CT showing soft-tissue mass in urinary bladder suggestive primary bladder cancer.

detecting local disease and recurrence, and distant metastases.

REFERENCES

1. Werner RA, Chen X, Lapa C, et al. The next era of renal radionuclide imaging: novel PET radiotracers. Eur J Nucl Med Mol Imaging. 2019;46(9):1773-86.
2. Hofman MS, Hicks RJ. Gallium-68 EDTA PET/CT for renal imaging. Semin Nucl Med. 2016;46(5):448-61.
3. Wakabayashi H, Werner RA, Hayakawa N, et al. Initial preclinical evaluation of 18F-fluorodeoxysorbitol PET as a novel functional renal imaging agent. J Nucl Med. 2016;57(10): 1625-8.
4. Werner RA, Wakabayashi H, Chen X, et al. Functional renal imaging with 2-deoxy-2-(18)F-fluorosorbitol PET in rat models of renal disorders. J Nucl Med. 2018;59(5):828-32.
5. Qin Z, Hoh CK, Olson ES, et al. Molecular imaging of the glomerulus via mesangial cell uptake of radiolabeled tilmanocept. J Nucl Med. 2019;16(9):1325-32.
6. Klenc J, Taylor A, Lipowska M. Synthesis and evaluation of 99mTc(CO)3(FEDA): a new dual-purpose 99mTc/18F renal imaging agent. J Nucl Med. 2015;56(Suppl 3):654.
7. Kabasakal L. Tc-99m Ethylene dicysteine: A new renal tubular function agent. Eur J Nucl Med. 2000;27(3):351-7.
8. Gutsche HU, Scheffler M, Muller-Surr R, et al. Micropuncture study on filtration and reabsorption of technium-99m L, L-Ethylenedicysteine in rats. In: Taylor A, Nally JV, Thomsen H (Eds). Radionuclides in nephrourology. Reston, Virbinia: Society of nuclear medicine; 1997. pp. 160-64.
9. Taylor A, Hansen L, Eshima D, et al. Comparison of 99mTc-LL-EC in rats and humans. J Nucl Med. 1997;38(5): 821-26.
10. Berkhin EF, Humphreys MH. Regulation of tubular secretion of organic compounds. Kindney Int. 2001;59(1):17-30.
11. Bubek B, Brandau W, Steinbacher M. Technetium-99m labeled renal function and imaging agent: II. Clinical evaluation of Tc-99m MAG-3(99mTc mercaptoacetylglycylglycylglycine). Nucl Med Biol. 1988;15(1):109-18.
12. Jafri RA, Britton KE, Nimmon CC. Tc-99m MAG-3:A comparison with I-125 and I-131OIH, in patients with renal disorders. J Nucl Med. 1988;29:147-58.
13. Atkins HL, Cardinale KG, Eckelman WC, et al. Evaluation of Tc 99m DTPA prepared by three different methods. Radiology. 1971;98:674-77.
14. Cohen ML, Smith FGJ, Mindell RS, et al. A simple reliable method of measuring glomerular filtration rate using single low dose iothalamate I-131. Pediatrics. 1969;43(3):407-15.
15. Enlander D, Weber PM, dosRemedios LV. Renal cortical imaging in 35 patients: Superior quality with Tc99m-DMSA. J Nucl Med. 1974;15(9):743-49.
16. Tripathi M, Chandrasekhar N, Phom H, et al. Evaluation of dilated upper renal tracts by technetium-99m ethylenedicysteine F+0 diuresisi renography in infants and children. Ann Nucl Med. 2004;18(8):681-7.
17. Meller St, Eckstein HB. Renal scintigraphy: Quantitative assessment of upper urinary tract dilatation in children. J Paeditr Surg. 1981;16(2):123-26.
18. O'Reilly PH, Testa HJ, Lawson RS, et al. Diuresis renography in equivocal urinary tract obstruction. Br J Urol. 1978;50(2):76-80.
19. Londe S. Causes of hypertension in the young. Pediatr Clin North Am. 1978;25(1):55-66.
20. Blaufox MD, Fine EJ, Heller S, et al. Prospective study of simultaneous orthoiodohippurate and diethylenetri-aminepentaacetic acid captopril renography. The Einstein/Cornell Collaborative Hypertension Group. J Nucl Med. 1998;39(3):522-28.
21. Sfaklanakis GN, Sfakiankis E, Bourgoignie J. Lasix captopril renography in the diagnosis of renovascular hypertension. Contrib Nephrol. 1990;79:219-27.
22. Taylor A, Nally J, Aurell M, et al. Consensus Report on Captopril Renogram in Renovascular Hypertension. J Nucl Med. 1996;37:1876-82.
23. Wenting GJ, Tan-Tjiong HI, Derkx FH. Split renal function after captopril in unilateral renal artery stenosis. BMJ. 1984;288(6421):886-90.
24. Dondi M. Captopril renal scintigraphy with 99mTc-mercaptoacetyltriglycine (Tc99m-MAG-3) for detecting renal artery stenosis. Am J Hypertens. 1991;4(12 Pt 2):737S-40S.
25. Kumar R, Padhy AK, Machineni S, et al. Individual kidney GFR in the interpretation of non-diagnostic curves on captopril renography. Nucl Med Commun. 2000;21(7):637-43.
26. Setaro JF, Chenn CC, Hoffer PB, et al. Captopril renography in the diagnosis of renal artery stenosis and the prediction of improvement with revascularisation: The Yale vascular center experience. Am J Hypertens. 1991;4(12 Pt 2):698S-705S.
27. Tripathi M, Agarwal KK, Mukherjee A, et al. Tc-99m DMSA planar imaging versus dual-detector SPECT for the detection of renal cortical scars in patients with CKD-3. Nucl Med Commun. 2016;37(9):911-6.

28. Padhy AK, Gopinath PG, Basu AK. Role of 99mTc-DTPA renal study in children with upper urinary tract dilation. Indian J Med Res. 1985;82:238-47.
29. Chaiwatanrat T, Padhy AK, Bomanji JB, et al. Validation of renal output efficiency as an objective quantitative parameter in the evaluation of upper urinary tract obstruction. J Nucl Med. 1993;34(5):845-48.
30. Sfakianakis GN, Damoulaki-Sfakianaki E. Nuclear medicine in pediatric urology and nephrology. J Nucl Med. 1988;29(9):1287-300.
31. Padhy AK, Gopinath PG, Mitra DK, et al. Direct radionuclide cystogram (DRCG) and urine flowmetry in the evaluation of patients with VUR and/or associated obstructive/neurogenic pathology of lower urinary tract in children. Indian J Paeditr. 1989;56(4):423-92.
32. Sfakianakis GN. Nuclear medicine in congenital urinary tract anomalies. In: LM Freeman (Ed). Nuclear Medicine Annual. New York: Raven Press; 1991. pp. 129-92.
33. Kumar R, Gupta R, Malhotra A. Nephroptosis: the Tc-99m glucoheptonate scan as a diagnostic modality. Clin Nucl Med. 2000;25(6):473.
34. Bell EG, Blaufox MD. Clinical application of renal imaging. In: Gottschalk A, Potchen EJ (Eds). Diagnostic Nuclear Medicine. Baltimore: Williams and Wilkins Co.; 1976. pp. 476-91.
35. Viberti GC, Bilous RW, Mackintosh D, et al. Monitoring Glomerular function in diabetic nephropathy. A prospective study. Am J Med. 1983;74(2):256-64.
36. Padhy AK, Gopinath PG, Mehta SN, et al. Significance of transplant perfusion index in the diagnosis of acute rejection—experience in live-related renal transplant recipients. Indian J Med Res. 1989;90:113-23.
37. Hilson AJW, Maisey MN, Brown CE, et al. Dynamic renal transplant imaging with 99mTc-DTPA (Sn) supplemented by a transplant perfusion index in the management of renal transplants. J Nucl Med. 1978;19(9):994-1000.
38. Padhy AK, Gopinath PG, Mehta SN, et al. Tc-99m renal transplant scintigraphy in the diagnosis of urinoma. Clin Nucl Med. 1989;14:769-71.
39. Kumar R, Zhuang H, Alavi A. PET in the management of urologic malignancies. Radiol Clin North Am. 2004;42(6):1141-53.
40. Nayak B, Dogra PN, Naswa N, et al. Diuretic F-18 FDG PET/CT imaging for the detection and locoregional staging of urinary bladder cancer: prospective evaluation of a novel technique. Eur J Nucl Med Mol Imaging. 2013;40(3):386-93.
41. Tulsyan S, Das CJ, Tripathi M, et al. Comparison of Ga-68 PSMA PET/CT and multiparametric MRI for staging of high-rosk prostate cancer 68Ga-PSMA PET and MRI in prostate cancer. Nucl Med Commun. 2017;38(12):1094-102.
42. Yadav MP, Ballal S, Tripathi M, et al. 177Lu-DKFZ-PSMA-617 therapy in metastatic castration resistant prostate cancer: safety, efficacy and quality of life assessment. Eur J Nucl Med Mol Imaging. 2017;44(1):81-91.
43. Montes de Jesus FM, Kwee TC, Nijland M, et al. Performance of advanced imaging modalities at diagnosis and treatment response evaluation of patients with post-transplant lymphoproliferative disorder: A systematic review and meta-analysis. Crit Rev Oncol Hematol. 2018;132:27-38.
44. Bachor R, Kotzerke J, Gottfried HW, et al. Positron emission tomography in diagnosis of renal cell carcinoma. Urologe A. 1996;35(2):146-50.
45. Ramdave S, Thomas GW, Berlangieri SU, et al. Clinical role of F-18 fluorodeoxyglucose positron emission tomography for detection and management of renal cell carcinoma. J Urol. 2001;166(3):825-30.
46. Miyakita H, Tokunaga M, Onda H, et al. Significance of 18F-fluorodeoxyglucose positron emission tomography (FDG-PET) for detection of renal cell carcinoma and immuno-histochemical glucose transporter 1 (GLUT-1) expression in the cancer. Int J Urol. 2002;9(1):15-8.
47. Kumar R, Chauhan A, Lakhani P, et al. 2-Deoxy-2-[F-18]fluoro-D-glucose-positron emission tomography in characterization of solid renal masses. Mol Imaging Biol. 2005;7(6):431-9.
48. Majhail NS, Urbain JL, Albani JM, et al. F-18 fluorodeoxyglucose positron emission tomography in the evaluation of distant metastases from renal cell carcinoma. J Clin Oncol. 2003;21(21):3995-4000.
49. Kosuda S, Kison PV, Greenough R, et al. Preliminary assessment of fluorine-18 fluorodeoxyglucose positron emission tomography in patients with bladder cancer. Eur J Nucl Med. 1997;24(6):615-20.
50. Ahlstrom H, Malmstrom PU, Letocha H, et al. Positron emission tomography in the diagnosis and staging of urinary bladder cancer. Acta Radiol. 1996;37(2):180-5.

Chapter 3

Renal Calculus Disease and Obstructive Uropathy

Uma Debi, Mahesh Prakash, Mandeep Kang

UROLITHIASIS

INTRODUCTION

Urolithiasis is a common disease entity. The incidence of renal calculus in India varies between different geographical locations.[1] Maharashtra has a high incidence (7.6%). Similarly, Rajasthan reports a high incidence. Southern states, however, report a lower incidence. Recent reports suggest an increasing incidence, with more and more calculi being diagnosed at a younger age. Pregnant patients form a special subset of patients with unique diagnostic and management considerations. Calcium oxalate forms the major constituent by frequency of stones.[2] The other constituents are uric acid, magnesium ammonium phosphate (MAP or struvite), cysteine, xanthine, triamterene, and indinavir. Nephrolithiasis is also a chronic disorder. Even after treatment, the recurrence rates are very high and range from 14% to 52%.[3]

COMPOSITION

Calcium-based stones are the most common (~75%) which can include calcium oxalate (80%) and calcium phosphate (20%). Uric acid and struvite stones are the next in frequency (~10% each), followed by cysteine, indinavir, xanthine, and triamterene stones (<1% each).[4]

ETIOLOGY

Calculi have a multifactorial etiology. The cause also varies for the specific type of calculus. The proposed causative factors for calcium calculi include low urine volume, increased excretion of calcium, oxalate, uric acid, and decreased excretion of citrate. Abnormal urine pH can also lead to precipitation of calculi. For uric acid calculi, decreased urine pH is the most important cause. Surprisingly, hyperuricosuria and low urine volume are less common causes. Struvite calculi are composed of magnesium ammonium phosphate or calcium apatite. Infection with urease positive organisms leads to the development of MAP calculus. Inherited cysteine metabolism defects cause cysteine calculus.

PRESENTATION

Nonobstructive renal calculi are asymptomatic. Pain is the most common presenting symptom for any disorder involving obstruction to the urinary tract. Calculi generally get lodged at sites of narrowing in the urinary tract—the pelviureteric junction (PUJ), ureterovesical junction, and the site of crossing of iliac vessels. The pain can be very severe and incapacitating. Depending on the site of obstruction, pain is referred to the iliac fossae in the case of mid-ureteric obstruction, or may be referred to the groin in cases of obstruction at a lower level. Lower-ureteric obstruction also produces bladder symptoms like frequency, urgency and suprapubic pain.

Nausea, vomiting and rarely fever might be associated. Calculi may also produce hematuria. Calculi in the urinary tract can also predispose to infection.

DIAGNOSTIC EVALUATION

Ultrasonography

Although noncontrast computed tomography (NCCT) scan is considered to be the gold-standard imaging modality to accurately depict the calculus burden, recent studies reflect a greater role for USG in diagnosis and follow-up of stone disease. American Urological Association (AUA), American College of Radiology (ACR) and National Institute for Health and Care Excellence (NICE) guidelines advocate NCCT as the first-line imaging modality in all patients with urolithiasis, except in pediatric and pregnant patients, where USG is recommended.[5,6] However, the recent guidelines by European Association of Urology (EAU) recommend USG as the primary imaging tool in all patients, irrespective of age and gender.[7] Literature reports a wide range of sensitivities and specificities for USG as compared to NCCT. However, most recent studies report a fairly high sensitivity of approximately 60% and specificity of approximately 70–90%.[6,8]

The role of imaging in a patient presenting with symptoms of urolithiasis is to confirm the diagnosis, exclude alternate causes for flank pain/hematuria, measure the stone burden and stone size, assess the exact location of the stone, and finally to guide the subsequent management strategies.[9] In specific circumstances, an USG with kidney ureter and bladder (KUB) radiography might be sufficient to provide all the information required for subsequent management. However, in cases where more information is needed, an NCCT or CT urography is usually required. Currently, apart from calculus visualization, USG is also indicated to look for echogenic contents within the pelvicalyceal system which may suggest pyonephrosis, accurately grade hydronephrosis (HDN), suspect pyelonephritis and to detect complications of urinary tract infection (UTI) like renal/perinephric abscess. In a patient, presenting with obstruction, detection of pyonephrosis is an indication for diversion with percutaneous nephrostomy (PCN).[10]

Sonographic Technique

Ultrasonography has a high sensitivity for detecting calculi in the kidney which are more than 5 mm. Calculi appear as echogenic structures with sharp posterior acoustic shadowing **(Fig. 1A)**. Stone visualization in USG depends on a lot of factors, including patient size, positioning, probe frequency, focal zone, spatial compound imaging, bowel gases, stone size, shape, location, composition, etc. In general, the highest frequency that allows adequate penetration should be selected for imaging. The focal zone should be adjusted to lie at or just posterior to the location of calculus. Spatial compounding (obtaining an average of two or more frames obtained from different angles) should be turned off. Harmonic imaging enhances visualization of the calculus.

Color Doppler evaluation produces twinkling artifact around the calculus which can aid in diagnosis **(Fig. 1B)**. The twinkling artifact is a complex phenomenon which was first described in 1996 by Rahmouni et al.[11] The most accepted theory for the formation of this artifact involves narrow-band noise (called phase or clock jitter) in the Doppler circuitry. Highly reflective, rough surfaces are associated with this artifact. Hence, apart from calculi, these artifacts can also be produced by soft tissue/vascular calcification, ureteral stents, coils, surgical clips, gallstones, and other foreign bodies. Conversely, a very smooth calculus would not produce this artifact.[12] If the focal zone is below the calculus, twinkling artifact is more prominent.

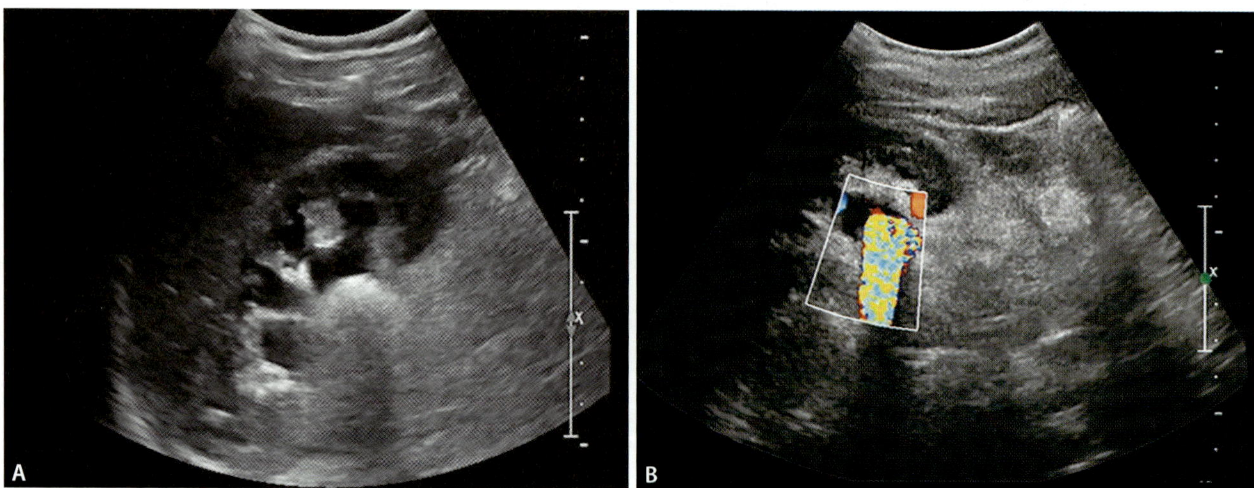

Figs. 1A and B: (A) Ultrasound image shows an echogenic calculus in renal pelvis with distal acoustic shadowing causing hydronephrosis. Noncontrast computed tomography (NCCT) with coronal reconstruction image shows two small hyperdense calculi in lower calyx of right kidney; (B) Color Doppler ultrasound image shows twinkling artifact.

Increasing the grayscale gain, decreases whereas increasing the Doppler gain, increases visualization of the artifact. It has also been suggested that calcium oxalate or calcium phosphate calculi produced this artifact, while calcium oxalate monohydrate and calcium urate calculi did not.[13]

Ureteric stones are more difficult to detect in USG because of bowel gases. The upper ureter can usually be visualized by using the kidney as a sonographic window. Similarly, a well-distended bladder might allow evaluation of the distal ureter using a suprapubic window. A transperineal or transvaginal route may also allow evaluation of the distal ureter and vesicoureteric junction (VUJ). Complete obstruction causes ureteric dilatation which facilitates tracing using the USG probe. Alternatively, ureteric jets can be used as a diagnostic tool. Ureteric jets can be visualized both in B-mode as well as in Doppler. The frequency of ureteric jets varies from person-to-person depending on the state of hydration, but is at least one per minute. The jets are symmetric bilaterally.[14] Ureteric stone with complete obstruction produces an absence of jet on the affected side. Partial obstruction produces low level continuous jet on the affected side (as compared to intermittent bursts of high level jet on the normal side).

Ureteric calculus with complete obstruction also produces hydronephrosis which can be easily detected using USG. The resistivity index [RI = (PSV – EDV)/PSV] of intrarenal arteries has also been described as an indirect indicator of urinary tract obstruction. Acute obstruction increases the back pressure leading to elevated resistive index. An RI of more than 0.70 has been suggested as a cutoff.[15] A difference between the two kidneys of more than 0.10 is also suggestive. However, the RI being more reflective of tissue compliance, rather than tubular pressure within the nephron, is an inaccurate index for routine use.[16]

Various disorders can mimic renal calculi in USG and reduce accuracy. These include intrarenal gas, vascular and parenchymal calcification, calcified renal cell carcinoma/ transitional cell carcinoma (RCC/TCC), calcified papilla, encrusted ureteric stent, and alkaline-encrusted pyelitis.

Kidney Ureter and Bladder Radiography

Kidney ureter and bladder radiography is a low-cost, low-radiation investigation (~0.15 mSv) which is especially useful in nonemergency settings **(Fig. 2)**. It has a sensitivity of approximately 35% for stones less than 5 mm and approximately 85% for stones more than 5 mm. Uric acid, xanthine, indinavir, and triamterene stones are radiolucent and hence are not visualized in KUB radiography. Currently, KUB radiography is mainly used for follow-up of urolithiasis after treatment/medical expulsion therapy.

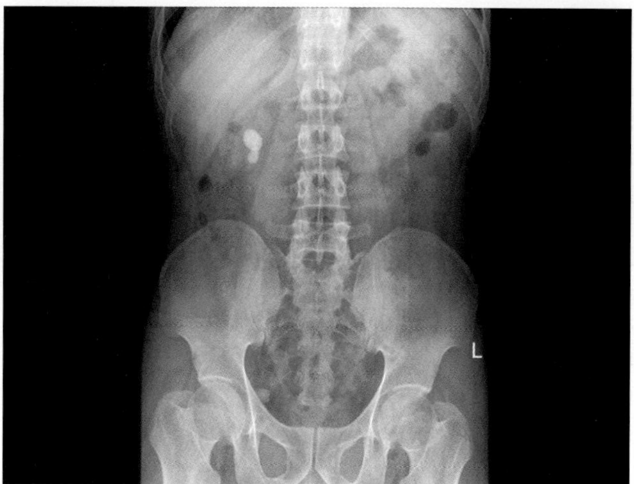

Fig. 2: Plain X-ray of abdomen shows two radiodense calculi in right kidney.

Computed Tomography

Noncontrast CT has the highest sensitivity among all imaging modalities for renal calculus. It can also exclude other causes of flank pain like diverticulitis, cholecystitis, pancreatitis, appendicitis, ovarian torsion, pyelonephritis, bladder outlet obstruction, etc. Hence, it is the modality of choice in urolithiasis.[9,10,17-20] All stones are visualized in CT, except indinavir stones. The Hounsfield unit (HU) value of the calculus gives a rough idea about the composition of the stone, uric acid calculi are usually 200–400 HU, while calcium oxalate calculi are 600–1200 HU **(Fig. 3)**. More importantly, a greater attenuation predicts lesser responsiveness to lithotripsy. Also, a heterogeneous appearance of the stone, with interposed areas of low and high attenuation predicts increased fragility and hence a greater susceptibility for Shockwave lithotripsy (SWL).

The various treatment modalities for urolithiasis include medical expulsion therapy, SWL, ureteroscopy (URS), percutaneous nephrolithotomy (PNL), and surgical open or laparoscopic pyelo/ureterolithotomy. Choosing one treatment modality over the other is a question of multiple considerations including the overall stone burden, size, composition, HU values and site of stone, structural and functional status of the kidneys, obstruction, hydronephrosis, presence or absence of tract infection, obesity, age of the patient, coagulopathy, pregnancy, etc. For instance, an impacted stone of 1 cm in the lower ureter can be easily dealt with using URS, whereas a similar stone in the upper polar calyx with an attenuation of 400 HU and a skin to surface distance less than 10 cm is amenable for SWL. It is hence the duty of the radiologist to give adequate information to ensure proper treatment planning. It is worth mentioning here that for measuring the size of a calculus, bone window should be used, which has a greater accuracy than soft tissue window. Recently, dual-energy CT has been used to characterize the exact composition of calculus, which has a greater potential to alter the management protocols. Uric acid stones can be easily differentiated from nonuric acid stones with 100% accuracy, thus allowing appropriate treatment strategies **(Figs. 4A and B).**[21]

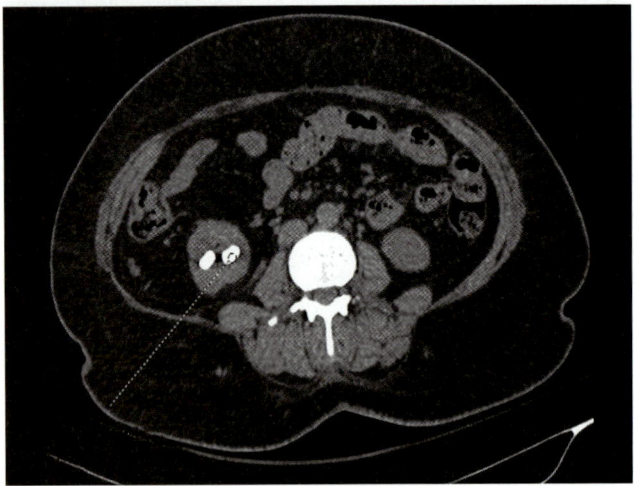

Fig. 3: Low-dose noncontrast CT scan shows two small hyperdense calculi in lower calyx of right kidney.

Technical and Dose Considerations

Current multidetector CT scanners allow complete scanning of the entire KUB region within 10–15 seconds, thus permitting evaluation in a single breath hold. Pitch in helical CT is the length of table fed into the scanner per gantry rotation divided by the beam collimation. If 1 cm of the table is fed per gantry rotation and the total beam collimation is 10 mm, the pitch is 1 mm. A pitch of 2 mm can be used for calculus imaging, which provides images of sufficient diagnostic quality but a reduced radiation exposure (as compared to a pitch of less than 1 mm). A calculus is a high-contrast structure. Therefore, images acquired with low-tube current can sufficiently delineate calculi. For stone imaging, the tube current can be lowered to as low as 30 mA without compromising the image quality. Current generation scanners are also equipped with automated tube modulation with automatically adjusts the tube current based on tissue attenuation. Low-dose CT is a term used for those scans with an effective exposure of less than 3 mSv. AUA recommends low-dose CT for all adult, nonpregnant patients with a BMI of less than 30 kg/m^2. For patients with a higher BMI a standard dose CT is recommended. An ultra-low dose CT with a radiation exposure of <1 mSv can also be used for follow-up scans (it is equivalent to ~5 KUB radiographies).

Imaging Features

The definitive sign of urolithiasis is identification of a calculus in the urinary tract. Using CT, even calculi that are less than 1 mm can be identified. The demonstration

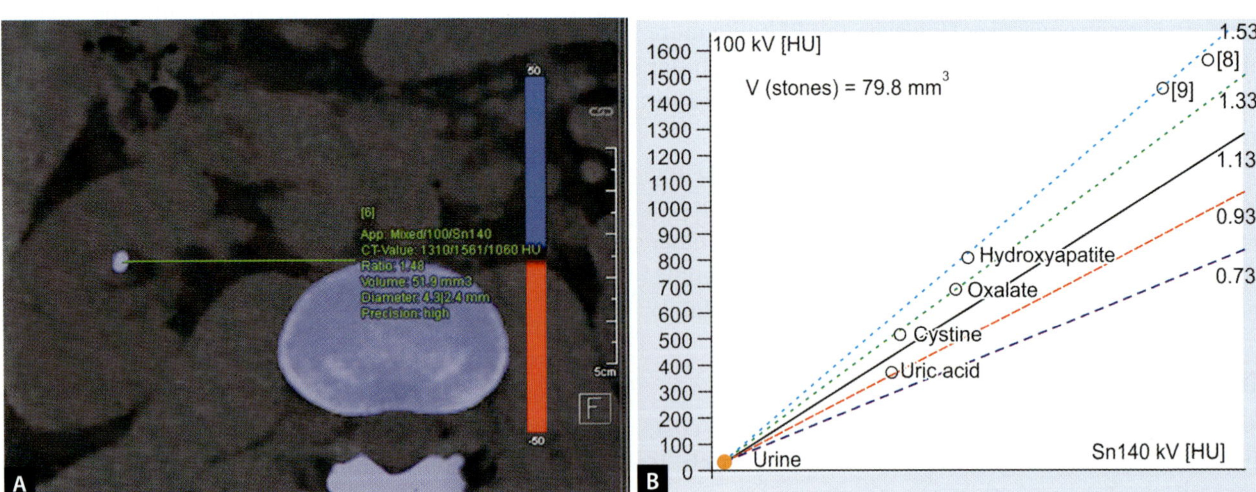

Figs. 4A and B: (A) Color coded axial dual-energy CT image shows a calcified calculus in the middle calyx. All calcified structure including bone of the vertebral body are color coded in blue. Color coding of the calculus is blue based on the dual-energy index. Volume of the calculus is also calculated; (B) Screenshot of the diagram used to adjust the software in the dual-energy setting. Color coding in blue above the slope indicates that it is a calcium containing calculus and in red below the slope which is consist of pure uric acid.

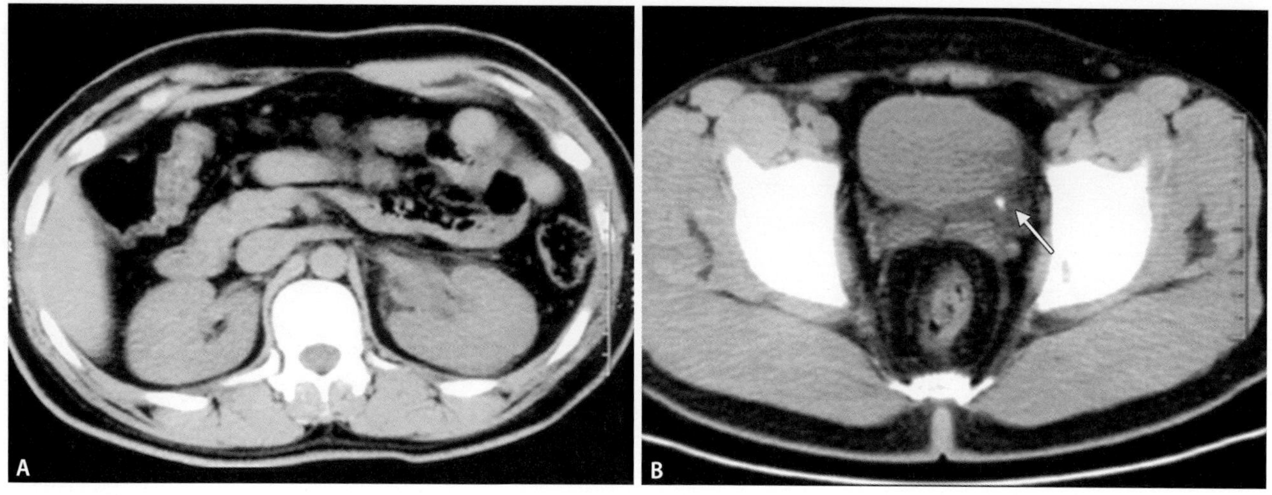

Figs. 5A and B: Low dose noncontrast CT scan of young male presented with acute loin pain. Axial section at the level of kidneys (A) shows minimal calyceal separation and perinephric stranding on left side and lower section at the level of bladder and (B) shows obstructed calculus in lower ureter (arrow).

of calculus within the ureter requires tracing of the tract in contiguous sections. Soft tissue rim sign is produced due to a rim of edematous soft tissue present around an impacted ureteric calculus **(Figs. 5A and B)**. Most ureteric calculi demonstrate this sign. Phleboliths can be a problematic differential, especially in thin patients. Phleboliths are commonly seen in the pelvis. They are produced by calcification of thrombus within veins. Plain radiographs show phleboliths with a radiolucent center while this appearance is uncommon with calculi. Phleboliths demonstrate comet tail sign in CT, which is an eccentric soft tissue present around the phlebolith. The soft tissue is due to the thrombosed vein which leads up to the phleboliths.

Other indirect signs of obstruction include renal enlargement, perinephric stranding, upstream dilatation of the ureter, periureteral stranding, renal sinus fullness causing effacement of fat at the sinus **(Figs. 6A and B)**, thickening of lateroconal fascia and absence of hyperdense medullary pyramids unilaterally. Perinephric stranding is considered to be produced due to lymphatic congestion in the bridging septae. Hyperdense medullary pyramids can be seen in normal individuals as an incidental finding. Its absence on one side may indicate obstruction on that side.

Intravenous Urography

Intravenous urography (IVU) historically has been the initial technique in evaluation of possible urinary obstruction including urolithiasis. The signs indicative of acute obstructive process are: (1) prolonged dense nephrogram, (2) renal enlargement, (3) dilatation of the collecting system, (4) delayed pyelogram, (5) ureteric dilatation, and (6) pyelosinus extravasation **(Figs. 7A to D)**.

If the obstruction is mild, then the nephrogram and calyceal opacification may be normal with minimal dilatation of the ureter. With more severe obstruction, the nephrogram is delayed in onset and becomes more dense and persistent. The nephrogram may demonstrate faint radial striations due to contrast in the collecting ducts and tubules.[22] The kidney is often larger than normal. The opacification of calyces and ureter is delayed and depends upon the degree of obstruction. A completely obstructed kidney that has become anuric may not show any opacification of the collecting system, however, once the opacification of the collecting system begins, additional radiographs are required to demonstrate the site of obstruction. If no contrast appears in the collecting system by 15 minutes after injection, there is little reason to obtain next film until 2 hours later. The collecting system and ureter are mildly dilated in acute obstruction. High obstructions cause more pelvicaliectasis then low ones. Extravasation of contrast medium from the kidney is demonstrated by IVU in up to 24% of obstructed patients.[23] Forniceal rupture occurs and opacified urine dissects through the tissues of the renal sinus. Minimal extravasation of contrast causes a smudged appearance of the calyces; however, when there is extensive leakage, contrast medium tracks around the renal pelvis and along the psoas muscles causing outlining of the ureter. Rarely, pyelolymphatic and pyelosubcapsular extravasation can occur. Unrelieved obstruction with continued extravasation of urine may result to a retroperitoneal collection called urinoma.[23] These collections are best visualized on USG, CT or MRI.

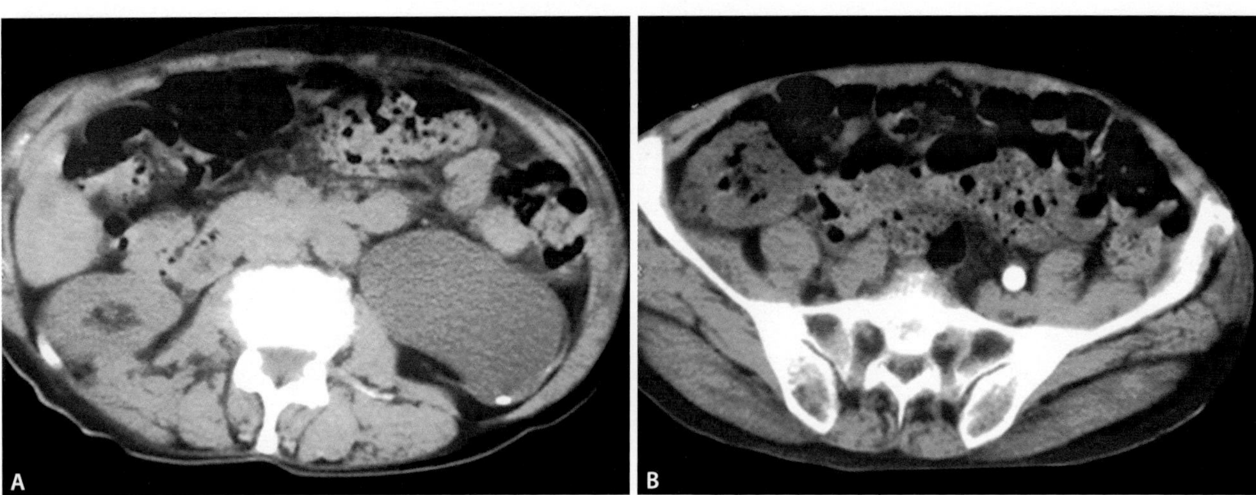

Figs. 6A and B: Noncontrast CT axial images (A) showing gross hydronephrosis with obstructive atrophy and left renal calculus; (B) Lower sections show obstructing calculus in lower ureter.

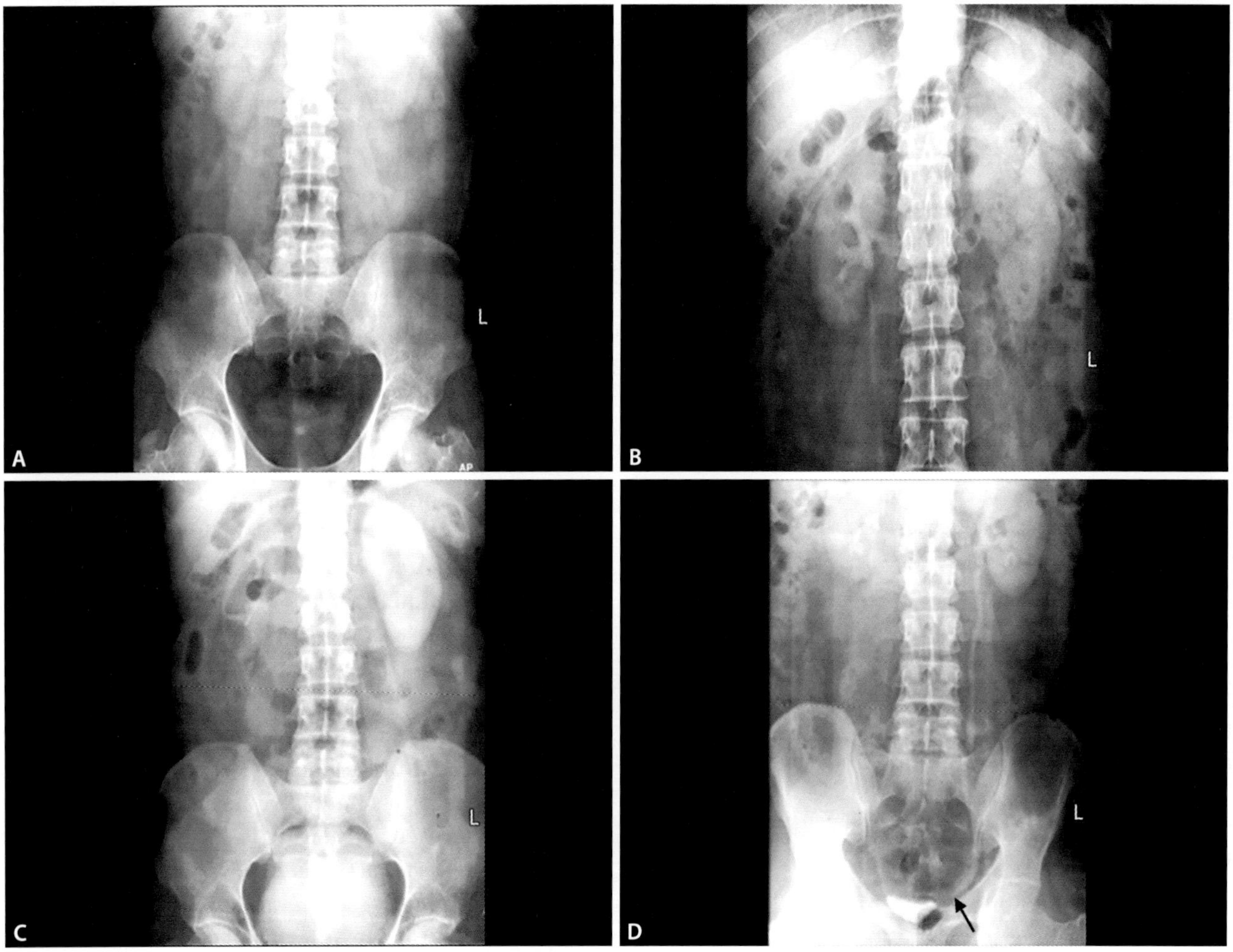

Figs. 7A to D: Serial intravenous urography (IVU) images of acute obstruction showing obstructing nephrogram. (A) Plain film; (B) Five-minute film; (C) 1-hour film shows increasingly dense left nephrogram; (D) Delayed film well depicted the left lower ureter calculus as the cause of obstruction (arrow).

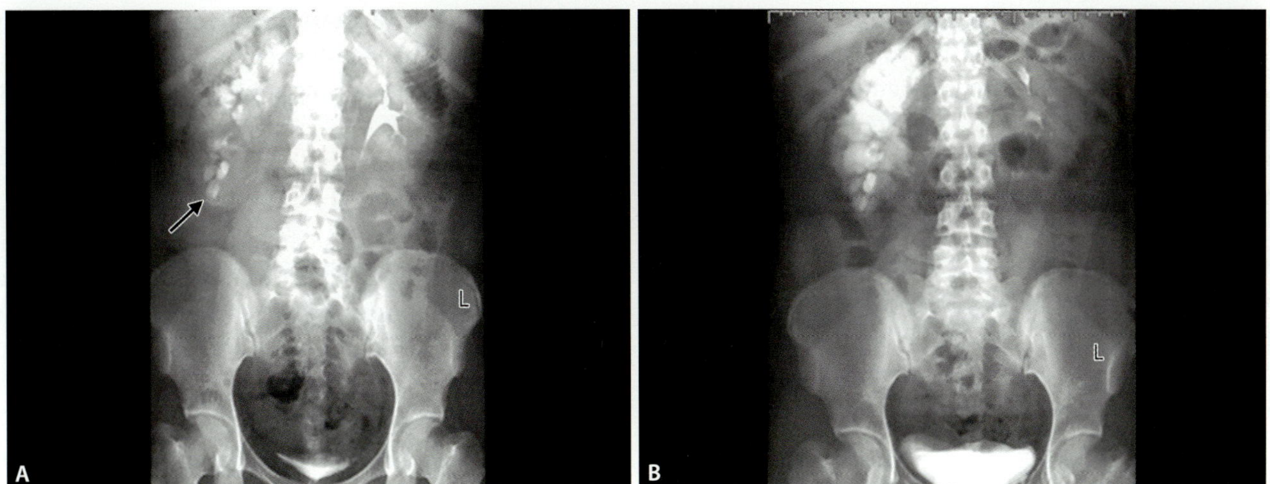

Figs. 8A and B: Intravenous urography study of chronic hydronephrosis due to ureteric stricture. (A) 11-minute film shows crescents (arrow); (B) 1-hour film shows ball pyelogram.

There has been a significant decline in the use of IVU as the dominant imaging technique in acute obstruction. This change has been driven by fear of contrast-induced nephrotoxicity and by growth of renal sonography and particularly low-dose CT. The main drawback of IVU is that it can be time consuming because of the serial delayed films which may be required to be obtained until the level of obstruction is delineated. This may require many hours and repeated films. Acute side effects of iodinated contrast and contrast-induced nephrotoxicity are also partly responsible for the decline in the use of IVU.

The urographic pattern varies in chronic obstruction. The kidney size is small in untreated complete obstruction, however, long-standing partial obstruction can result in enlargement of the collecting system and kidney. The obstructive nephrogram is usually not seen in cases of chronic obstruction as tubular concentrating ability and glomerular filtration rate (GFR) are reduced. The nephrographic density may be normal, faint or none depending upon the residual functioning parenchyma. The renal parenchyma is usually atrophied. When parenchymal thickness is reduced to 1–2 cm, but the renal function is relatively preserved then calyceal crescents are sometimes seen during nephrogram. The crescents are thin, curved collections of contrast denser than the nephrogram, located in the medulla. They represent realigned collecting tubules running perpendicular to their usual orientation.[24] They parallel the cortical margin of the ballooned calyces, located just 1–2 mm peripheral to the calyces. These crescents remain fixed regardless of patient position. The opacification of extremely thin parenchyma over the dilated calyceal sac produces a rim or shell nephrogram.

Chronic obstruction produces varying degree of pyelocalyceal dilatation. As contrast medium enters the dilated system, it glides to the dependent portion of calyces. With the patient supine, rounded puddles of contrast appear separated from the surrounding nephrogram by a boundary of non-radiopaque urine, this picture has been called the ball pyelogram **(Figs. 8A and B)**.

Chronic obstruction may lead to nonvisualized kidney on urogram. The ureter becomes dilated proximal to the obstructing lesion, elongated and tortuous, and in extreme cases it may resemble a segment of small intestine. This is called giant hydroureter or giant megaureter.

Magnetic Resonance Imaging

At present, MRI has limited role to in the evaluation of urinary obstruction. Magnetic resonance urography (MRU) is an ideal technique in pregnancy, where there is contrast allergy, renal failure patients and if radiation dose is an issue.[25] Ureteric abnormalities are poorly defined especially if they are small.

OBSTRUCTIVE UROPATHY

INTRODUCTION

Obstructive uropathy is a general term that describes obstructive changes in any part of the urinary tract. The renal structural and functional alterations caused by obstruction are termed "obstructive nephropathy". Despite remarkable advances in diagnosis and treatment, obstruction remains a leading cause of damage to the urinary tract.[26] Urinary obstruction affects patients of all ages and is responsible for thousands of hospital admissions and surgical procedures. Obstruction predisposes to urinary tract infection and renal failure. Early diagnosis and treatment of urinary obstruction can reverse the renal damage.

PATHOPHYSIOLOGY

When the ureter is acutely obstructed, the pressure of the collecting system proximal to the obstruction rises. Over the next 6–12 hours, the renal blood flow drops due to increase of renal vascular resistance. There are two mechanisms that come into play to temporarily decompress the nephron. First is pyelosinus and pyelovenous backflow and second is enhanced absorption of fluid from the tubules. The preglomerular arteriolar resistance increases in acute obstruction. This RI measure by Doppler has been used with variable success to confirm intrarenal vascular resistance in acute obstruction **(Figs. 9A and B)**.[27] The elevated intrarenal resistance produces diminished diastolic flow eventually causing ischemia. Relief of total but short-lived obstruction leads to full restoration of the GFR. Longer period of total obstruction causes progressive nephron loss called obstructive atrophy. Relief of obstruction that has already caused renal atrophy is followed by improvement in renal function but not to normal levels. The kidney often shrinks in size with blunting of the calyces and impaired ability of urinary concentration and acidification.

These semirecovered kidneys showing the anatomical and functional sequelae are said to exhibit postobstructive atrophy. If the obstruction is partial and chronic, its effect to renal function is less predictable. Structural changes can occur in the medulla with impairment of the ability to concentrate urine. Sometimes partial obstruction can exist for years without causing any functional impairment.

CAUSES OF OBSTRUCTION AND DISEASES OF URETER

In children, obstruction is commonly due to congenital causes whereas in adults most cases are due to acquired causes. Obstruction may also be classified by location as intrarenal, postrenal, supravesical or infravesical.

Congenital Ureteric Obstruction

Primary megaureter and obstruction associated with duplication are common causes of congenital ureteric obstruction.

Ureteropelvic Junction Obstruction

Congenital obstruction of the ureteropelvic junction (UPJ) is a common anomaly of the urinary tract. The proposed etiology includes incomplete recanalization of the ureter during early gestation, aberrant vessel causing extrinsic compression, or other bands/kinks causing PUJ constriction.[28] It results due to deficiency and derangement of the ureteric smooth muscle fibers resulting in failure of normal peristalsis in the affected segment and subsequent functional obstruction. Males and the left side are commonly affected. Dilated renal pelvis and calyces are demonstrated on urography. Delayed radiographs are usually necessary for demonstrating the point of obstruction at UPJ. With long-standing or high-grade obstruction the kidney may become nonfunctional. When there is insufficient contrast excretion or the ureter is not

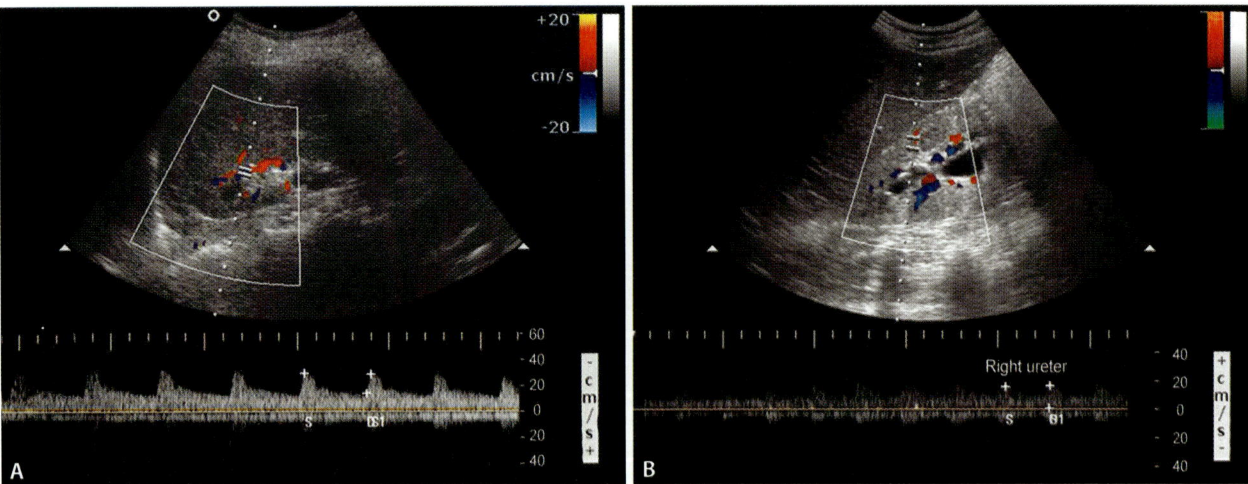

Figs. 9A and B: Doppler tracing of (A) normal kidney and (B) in acute obstruction. The resistive index is increased in acute obstruction.

visualized, the diagnosis can be established by antegrade pyelography. Ultrasound usually shows hydronephrosis and dilated renal pelvis with a nondilated ureter. In patients with equivocal UPJ obstruction, diuresis renography, and Whitaker procedure may be employed to assess functional obstruction.[29]

Primary Megaureter

Primary megaureter or congenital megaureter is an uncommon entity probably caused by functional abnormality of the juxtavesical ureter, which is less distensible and fails to transmit normal peristalsis. Secondary megaureter on the other hand is secondary to causes like neurogenic bladder, vesicoureteric reflux (VUR) or posterior urethral valve (PUV).[30] The differentiation between these causes can be done using micturating cystourethrogram. Primary megaureter may be seen in both children and adults and typically remains asymptomatic in many cases. Males are affected more than females. A characteristic beak-like configuration of the distal ureteral segment is seen on urography with proximal dilatation of ureter **(Fig. 10)**. The dilatation may extend proximally to calyces. Primary megaureter may be associated with UPJ obstruction, contralateral renal agenesis, and VUR. Ultrasound readily detects PCS and ureteral dilatation. This condition is asymptomatic in majority of individuals and can be conservatively managed. Surgical intervention is indicated in cases having recurrent UTIs or falling renal function.

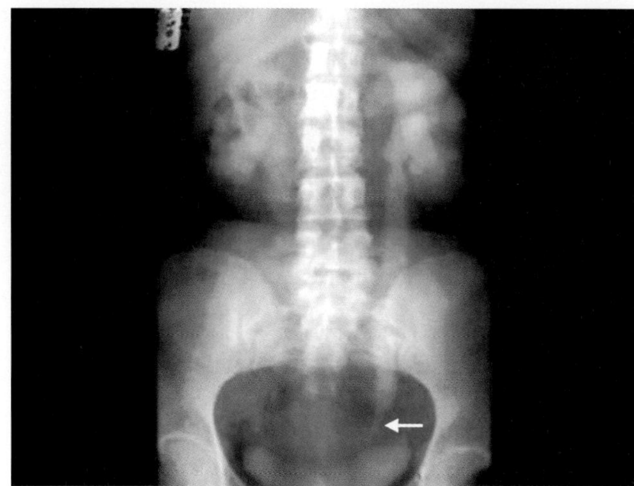

Fig. 10: Delayed intravenous urography image (1-hour film) shows bilateral hydroureteronephrosis with smooth tapering of lower ureter suggestive primary megaureter (arrow).

Ureterocele

The term ureterocele means saccular dilatation of the intramural portion of ureter as it passes through the bladder wall **(Fig. 11)**. It may be of two types—simple (orthotopic) and ectopic. The ureters of a simple ureterocele drain a nonduplex kidney and insert into the bladder at their normal position at the trigone. An ectopic ureterocele frequently occurs in a duplex kidney. In complete duplication, the ureter of the upper moiety generally inserts at a lower/ectopic location. This ureter is generally affected with ureterocele (the lower moiety, on the other hand is predisposed for VUR).[31] Morphologically, ureteroceles can be completely intravesical or extravesical—where the dilated portion extends outside the UB to involve the distal ureter. Ureterocele typically appear on urography and cystography as smooth, rounded or ovoid filling defect in the bladder. The major concern with ureterocele is obstruction, stasis, and UTI. Hence, treatment is directed toward relieving the obstruction using cystoscopy, partial nephrectomy for the nonfunctioning upper moiety and/or ureteric reimplantation for refluxing ureter of lower moiety.

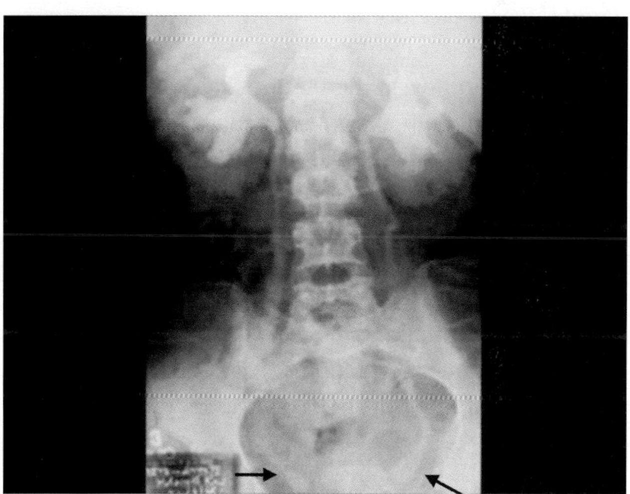

Fig. 11: Intravenous urography (IVU) (30-minute film) shows bilateral hydronephrosis with fusiform dilatation (arrows) of lower most portion of ureters suggestive of ureterocele.

Circumcaval Ureter

Circumcaval ureter results when the supracardinal vein persists and forms the major portion of the inferior vena cava (IVC). Embryonically, the subcardinal vein lies ventral to the ureter. The right ureter is carried medially by the migration of the subcardinal vein toward the developing IVC. The typical pattern on urography is a tortuous, dilated proximal right ureter, and associated hydronephrosis. The proximal ureter has a characteristic reverse-J course before it crosses behind and around the IVC and then descends medial to the ipsilateral lumbar pedicle. The confirmation of the diagnosis can be made with CT, which shows the ureter passing posterior and medial to the IVC.

Acquired Ureteric Obstruction

The causes of acquired ureteric obstruction can be intraluminal or extraluminal.

Intraluminal Causes

Abnormalities may develop within the ureteral lumen without any attachment to the uroepithelial lining. The common causes are calculi, blood clots, tissue slough, fungus ball, and foreign material.

Ureteric calculus: Ureteric calculus has been dealt with in the previous section on urolithiasis.

Blood clots: Blood clots in ureter are secondary to trauma, tumors, nephritis, vasculitis and bleeding disorders. Blood clots exhibit radiographic features that are common to other non-radiopaque lesions. The location of clot varies with time or with change in position of patient. When clot persists as a mass of fibrin, calcification may develop that resembles stones or uroepithelial tumors.[32] Sonography shows a mass-like filing defect with low level echoes. The CT attenuation value of clot varies with time. When the clot is fresh, its attenuation value exceeds that of soft tissue. Within a week its attenuation decreases. Blood clot does not enhance after intravenous contrast administration.

Tissue slough: Necrosed papilla and cholesteatoma can slough and cause obstruction of ureter with proximal dilatation. Urography shows features of nonopaque filling defect. Calcium is sometime deposited along the periphery of a sloughed papilla. Sonography and CT demonstrate hypoechoic and hyperdense mass lesion respectively.

Fungus ball: Most fungus balls or mycetomas are caused by *Candida albicans* and *Aspergillus*. Fungal infection of the urinary tract occurs in the setting of altered host resistance like HIV, steroid intake, severe debilitating disease, and antineoplastic drug intake. The fungus balls fill the renal pelvis or ureter with a nonopaque mass. Sometime contrast material insinuates into the interstices of the mass causing lacelike radiodense pattern during IVU. The fungus ball appears as an echogenic mass on sonography while CT shows soft tissue attenuation filling defects. Neither sonography nor CT can differentiate fungus ball from other intraluminal soft tissue.

Intramural Causes

Ureteral tumors: Primary ureteral tumors are relatively rare, accounting for approximately 1% of all urinary tract tumors. Tumors arising from epithelium are most common, however, they can arise from mesoderm. Males are affected more than females with the usual age of presentation being in the fifth to eighth decades. The most common tumor of ureter is transitional cell carcinoma. Rare tumors include squamous carcinoma, adenocarcinoma, sarcoma, and metastasis.

Transitional cell carcinoma: It occurs more frequently in males and has a peak incidence in the seventh decade. Certain epidemiological factors have been associated with increased risk for development of transitional cell carcinoma. These include exposure to chemicals, dye, petroleum, rubber and cable industries. Tobacco, coffee, artificial sweetener, chronic inflammation, and infection are additional risk factors. There is increased prevalence of TCC in analgesic and Balkan nephropathy. Squamous cell carcinoma occurs in older age and is generally associated with chronic infection and leukoplakia of urinary tract. Adenocarcinoma occurs in patients with severe infection and stone disease.[33]

Radiological findings:

- *Intravenous urography*: The lesion appears as a smooth or lobulated, polypoid filling defect in the ureter which maintains a constant relationship with the ureteric wall **(Fig. 12A)**. There is usually proximal obstruction dilatation of the ureter. The ureter just distal to the tumor is also often slightly dilated. The combination of distal margin of soft tissue mass invaginating into the distended segment of opacified ureter constitutes the Chalice or Bregman's sign.[34] This sign is useful in distinguishing tumor from nonopaque stone as the ureter is not dilated distal to a stone.
- *Sonography*: Tumors of the ureter may be seen as a soft tissue mass situated at the distal end of a slightly dilated ureter.
- *Computed tomography*: CT defines the contour and mural attachment of tumor following ureteral opacification **(Fig. 12B)**. The tumor may enhance after intravenous contrast administration. The tumor may project into the ureteric lumen with circumferential or eccentric mural thickening. The lesion may infiltrate into the periureteric fat. CT is important in the staging of a documented ureteric tumor as it detects periureteral extension as well as lymph node enlargement. MR may be used in patients in whom CT cannot be done.

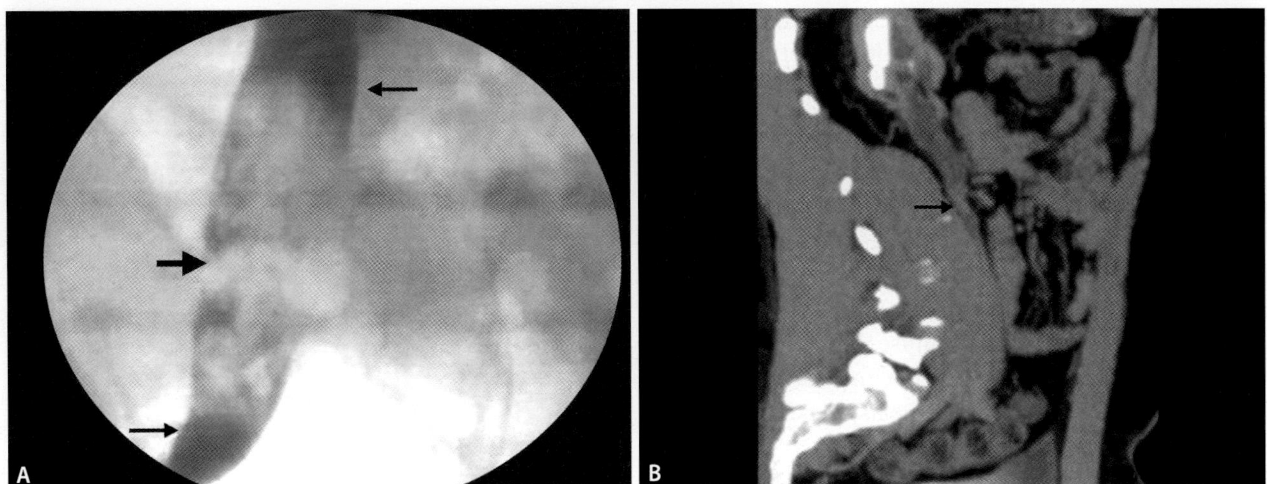

Figs.12A and B: Transitional cell carcinoma (TCC) of ureter. (A) Fluoroscopic spot of nephrostogram shows irregular filling defect (thick arrow) in midureter with dilatation of ureter (thin arrows) proximal as well as distal to the lesion (Bregman's sign). Another patient with TCC: (B) Contrast-enhanced CT with sagittal reconstruction showing circumferential mural thickening (arrow) of ureter with proximal hydroureteronephrosis. These findings may mimic inflammatory lesion of ureter.

Benign tumors: Benign tumors of urothelium constitute approximately 20% of ureteral neoplasms. The most common is a papilloma which presents as a solitary filling defect attached to the ureter by a stalk.

Nonepithelial tumors: Fibroepithelial polyp is the most common nonepithelial tumor. These typically occur in patients in the 20–40 years age group. The usual location is the proximal one-third of the ureter. The lesion is usually solitary but multiple lesions can rarely be seen. The lesion can present as a mobile, smooth, cylindrical, slightly mobile, and filling defect. Sometimes the lesion can be frond like.

Secondary tumors and contiguous infiltration: These are more common than primary ureteric tumors. Direct extension of the tumor from primary sites such as cervix, prostate and bladder can cause ureteric obstruction. Malignant retroperitoneal lymphadenopathy also cause obstruction to the ureter. Rarely, hematogenous malignant deposit can occur to the ureters. The common primaries responsible are melanoma, renal cell carcinoma, breast, lung, and prostate.[35]

Inflammatory Lesions of Ureter

Inflammatory conditions of the ureter include a wide variety of disorders.[36] Primary inflammation of the ureter is rare in the absence of systemic or regional disease in urinary tract, retroperitoneum, pelvis or peritoneum. Inflammation of ureteral wall may originate from inflammatory elements excreted in the urine, hematogenous embolism or contiguous spread from adjacent areas within the urinary tract and abdomen. The general responses of the ureter to inflammation are loss of ureteric peristalsis, dilatation, ulceration, irregularity, pseudopolyposis, edema, and desmoplasia leading to stricture and calcification.

Radiological imaging: Radiology plays an important role in diagnosing and characterizing inflammatory conditions of the ureter. This information supplements that from other clinical diagnostic tools including urinalysis, urine culture, urine cytology, and cystoureteroscopy.

Malakoplakia: It is a benign chronic granulomatous disorder more commonly seen in women than men. It can be seen at any level of the urinary tract but has a predilection for the bladder and lower ureter. It is seen in association with chronic *Escherichia coli* or *Proteus mirabilis* infection and is found more frequently in diabetics and immunosuppressed patients. On urography, the lesions are rounded to flat, coalescent filling defects lending an irregular contour to the ureteral margin. Ureteric obstruction may be present. The imaging features overlap with ureteritis cystica but the lesions are usually rounder and the ureter is not dilated in the latter condition.

Ureteritis cystica: This disease entity is usually asymptomatic but may present with hematuria or symptoms of urinary tract infection. Histologically, this condition consists of multiple, small, subepithelial, fluid-filled cysts in the ureteric wall. Ureteritis cystica does not cause ureteric obstruction. The disease has a slight predilection for the upper ureter. The typical radiographic appearance is that of multiple, small, filling defects with scalloping of the ureteral margin. The differential diagnosis include air bubbles, hemorrhage into ureteric wall, and papillary neoplasm. The condition may or may not regress with treatment of the underlying inflammatory condition.

Leukoplakia: It is a rare inflammatory condition which more commonly involves the urinary bladder than the ureter. It results from squamous metaplasia of the urothelium and is frequently associated with chronic urinary tract infection or long-standing stone disease. The imaging features include diffuse, irregular, and filling defects. There may be ridging of the mucosa with ureteric dilatation. Differentiation from malakoplakia or ureteral malignancy is difficult on imaging.

Schistosomiasis: It is a chronic indolent infestation caused by the trematode *Schistosoma haematobium*. The parasite lays its eggs in the veins of the bladder and lower ureter stimulating chronic inflammatory reaction resulting in cystitis and ureteritis and eventually scarring and calcification. Schistosomiasis commonly affects the bladder and ureteric involvement is seen in one-third of patients. The ureters are bilaterally asymmetrically involved with predominant involvement of the lower ureter. The disease usually affects a younger age group. Imaging findings are characteristic. Calcification of the ureter is seen in 75% of cases which is usually linear or tram-track in appearance. There is a characteristic deformity of the distal ureters consisting of medial and cephalic displacement which may resemble cow's horns. There is varying degree of stenosis and dilatation and the ureter may show a beaded appearance which can resemble tuberculous ureteritis.

Tuberculous ureteritis: Tuberculosis of the urinary tract is usually due to hematogenous dissemination of *Mycobacterium tuberculosis*. Ureteral involvement is usually due to descending renal infection. The symptoms are nonspecific and include constitutional symptoms and lower urinary tract symptoms like frequency, dysuria, and suprapubic pain. The patients may present with hematuria and sterile pyuria. When the infection affects the ureteral wall, the first changes are those of ulceration and wall edema with thickening which progress to strictures and calcification. These changes may lead to proximal dilatation of the ureter and PCS. Plain films of abdomen may show evidence of ureteric calcification with or without calcification of the kidney. Characteristic urographic findings include alternating areas of dilatation and short strictures of the ureter (beaded appearance), long straight stricture (pipestem ureter) or isolated stricture. The ureter is shortened and straightened due to periureteral fibrosis

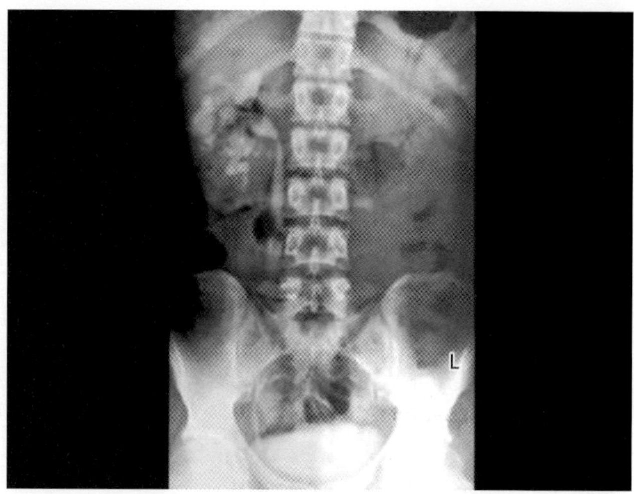

Fig. 13: Intravenous urography (15-minute film) shows hydronephrosis, forniceal stenosis, cavitary changes in right kidney with ureteric narrowing. All these features suggest tubercular involvement of urinary tract.

(Fig. 13). CT scan is useful in demonstrating ureteric wall thickening and presence of lymph nodes if any. The bladder may show poor distensibility owing to irritative spasm or fibrosis within the wall **(Figs. 14A and B)**.

Radiation ureteritis: Radiation can lead to early and late changes in the ureteric wall, ultimately leading to fibrosis and stricture. Fibrosis continues to develop long after radiotherapy has been completed. IVU may demonstrate mucosal irregularity and a short or long distal ureteric stricture. CT may demonstrate these findings as well as thickening and stranding of the wall of the ureter.

Inflammatory bowel disease: Genitoureteric complications may occur in up to one-fourth of patients with inflammatory bowel disease. Obstruction due to direct ureteral involvement is the second most common complication, the first being nephrolithiasis. Ureteric involvement by Crohn's disease is usually at the level of the pelvic brim and the right ureter is more commonly involved. On urography, the ureter shows a smooth area of narrowing with varying degree of obstruction. CT scan shows an inflammatory soft tissue mass with narrowing and mural thickening of the ureter.

Endometriosis: Ureteral involvement generally occurs in cases with widespread pelvic disease, however, cases of isolated ureteral involvement have been reported. Two forms of ureteral endometriosis have been described. Extrinsic involvement is four times more common than the intrinsic variety. The distal ureter is commonly involved. Ureteral involvement may result in narrowing of ureter, hydronephrosis and occasionally an intraluminal mass.

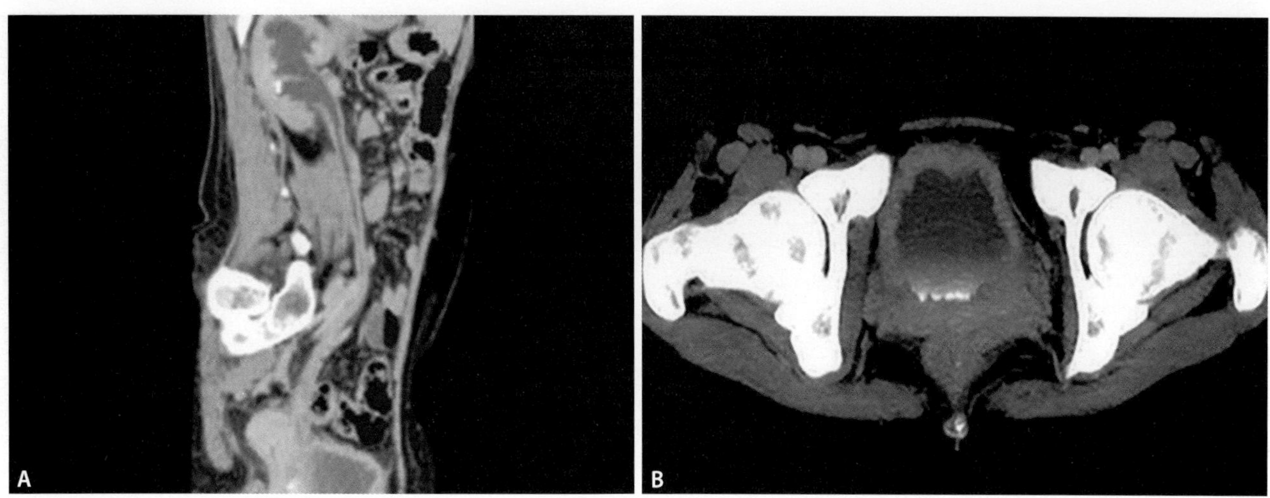

Figs. 14A and B: CT scan of urinary tract tuberculosis. (A) Multiplanar reconstruction (MPR) shows hydronephrosis of kidney with thickened ureteric wall; (B) Irregular thickening of urinary bladder with reduced capacity.

The stricture is usually smooth but abruptly tapered and may show medial sharp angulation. CT may demonstrate a soft tissue mass or endometrioma causing encasement of the ureter **(Figs. 15A to D)**.

Extrinsic Causes of Ureteral Obstruction

Retroperitoneal Fibrosis

Retroperitoneal fibrosis (RPF) is an important cause of obstructive uropathy leading to renal failure.[37] It encompasses a range of diseases characterized by the presence of fibroinflammatory tissue, which usually surrounds the abdominal aorta and iliac arteries and extends into the retroperitoneum to envelop neighboring structures including the ureters. RPF may be idiopathic (Ormond's disease) or secondary to a wide variety of stimuli which includes both benign and neoplastic causes.

The classic triad of delayed renal contrast excretion with unilateral or bilateral (60% of cases) hydronephrosis and proximal hydroureter secondary to ureteral involvement, medial deviation of the middle-third of both ureters and tapering of the ureteral lumen at the L4–L5 vertebral level, though less frequently seen than previously thought, is still useful in the identification of RPF. When there is insufficient contrast excretion on urography, retrograde or antegrade pyelography is required to demonstrate the characteristic ureteral changes. CT scan demonstrates sheet-like soft-tissue mass in retroperitoneum with encasement of ureters. CT may help in the identification of disease activity with the degree of soft-tissue enhancement correlating with the activity of the fibrotic process **(Figs. 16A to C)**. RPF has signal characteristics similar to those of other fibrotic processes, with a tendency toward diffusely low-signal intensity on T1-weighted MRI. T2 signal is a reflection of the degree of associated active inflammation (and thus edema) with high signal indicating early inflammatory phase of benign RPF or malignancy while low signal signifies chronic phase of benign RPF. Chronic, inactive fibrosis will have little edema and thus be visualized as having low signal on both T1- and T2-weighted imaging. This feature may also prove valuable in assessing a patient's response to treatment; decreasing T2-signal indicating a favorable therapeutic response.[38]

Retroperitoneal Neoplasms

Extraureteral malignancies causing obstructive uropathy are much more common than primary ureteral neoplasms. The ureter is very prone to involvement as it is near many structures in the retroperitoneum that frequently harbor malignancies. In many cases, obstruction may result from direct extension of neoplasms from primary sites like the bladder, prostate, endometrium, sigmoid colon, rectum, and cervix. In other cases, there may be metastasis to the periureteral tissues especially the lymph nodes by distant tumors which causes uropathy by direct infiltration of one or both the ureters or by compression and mechanical obstruction. Bulky lymph nodes seen in lymphomas may cause similar manifestations.

Primary retroperitoneal tumors arising in the vicinity of the ureters may also lead to mechanical obstruction. CT scores over sonography in the detection and possible classification of these tumors. Malignancies may incite an intense periureteral desmoplastic reaction resembling retroperitoneal fibrosis leading to ureteral obstruction. This is especially seen in metastases from carcinomas of lung, breast, pancreas, colon, stomach, and sometimes

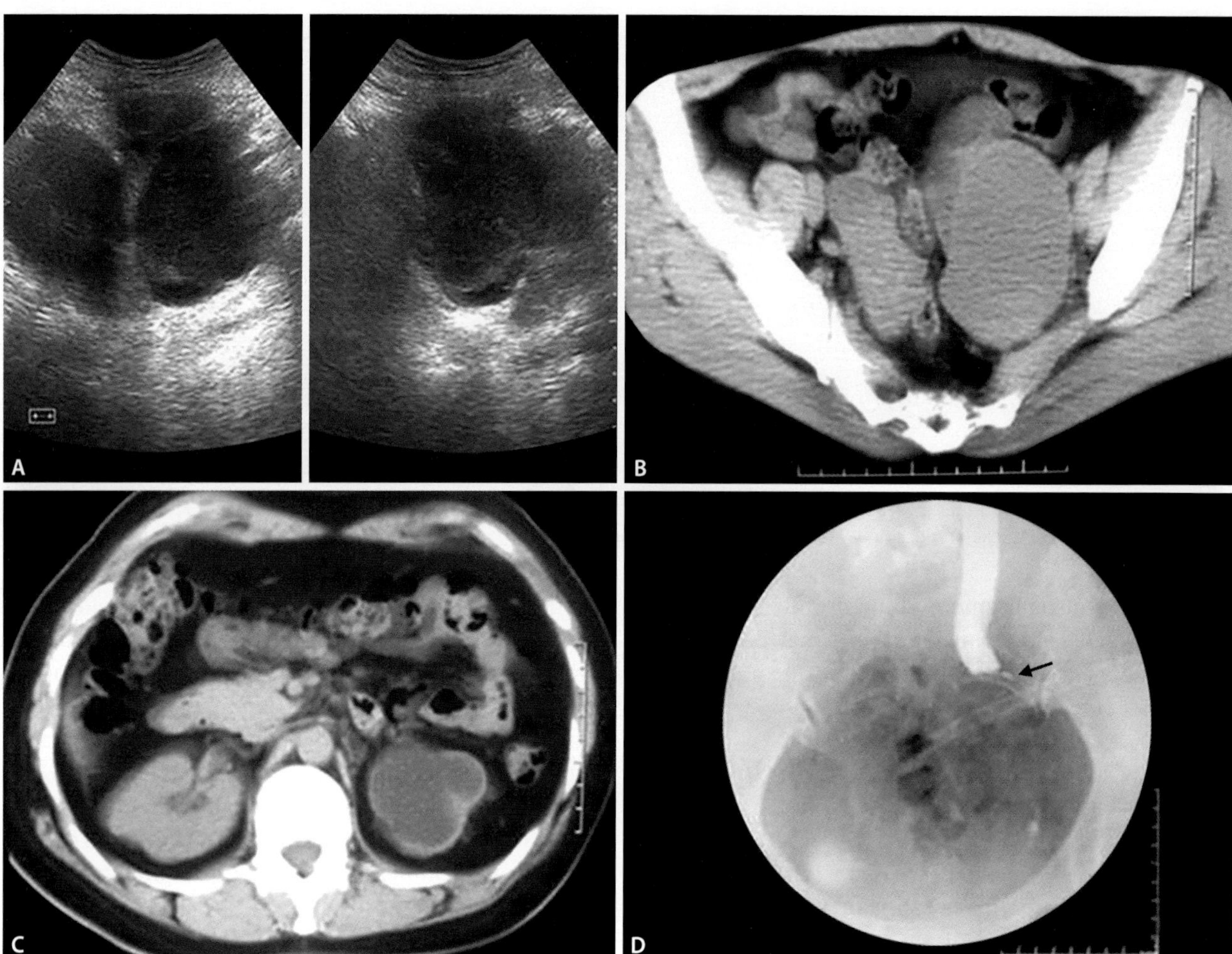

Figs. 15A to D: Obstructive uropathy due to endometriosis. (A) Ultrasound image shows complicated cyst within left adnexa; CT axial scan at the level of pelvis; (B) shows adnexal mass compressing and displacing lower ureter, resulting obstructive atrophy of kidney; (C) The nephrostogram of the same patients shows displacement and stricture of lower ureter (arrow); (D) of the same patients shows displacement and stricture of lower ureter (arrow).

lymphoma. Patients who have received radiation therapy in the vicinity may also experience obstructive symptoms. This was initially thought to be due to radiation-induced ureteric stricture but lately it has been realized that the ureter is relatively resistant to radiation. An obstruction in this case usually means that the tumor had involved the ureteral wall before radiation or there has been a recent relapse.

Pelvic Lipomatosis

It is an unusual disease resulting from proliferation of mature fibroadipose tissue in the pelvis. Usually seen in males, it may require surgery if it is causing obstructive uropathy by ureteral compression. Radiographic findings include relative hyperlucency of the pelvic cavity on plain radiographs. Contrast studies may show displacement and compression of rectosigmoid and urinary bladder leading to "tear drop" or "pear"-shaped bladder. The distal ends of the ureters are displaced medially in the majority of cases with presence of hydroureter or hydroureteronephrosis. Identical appearance of the bladder can also be seen with pelvic lymphadenopathy, diffuse pelvic carcinomatosis, pelvic/perivesical liposarcoma, and pelvic fibrosis (resembling retroperitoneal fibrosis).

Pregnancy-related Dilatation of Ureter

Variable degree of ureteral dilatation is often seen during pregnancy which is most marked in the third trimester with predominant involvement of the right side. In most of the cases, the dilatation progressively disappears in the postpartum period. The ureteral segments below the pelvic brim do not show dilatation indicating that partial mechanical obstruction by the gravid uterus accounts for the major changes of hydroureter seen during pregnancy.

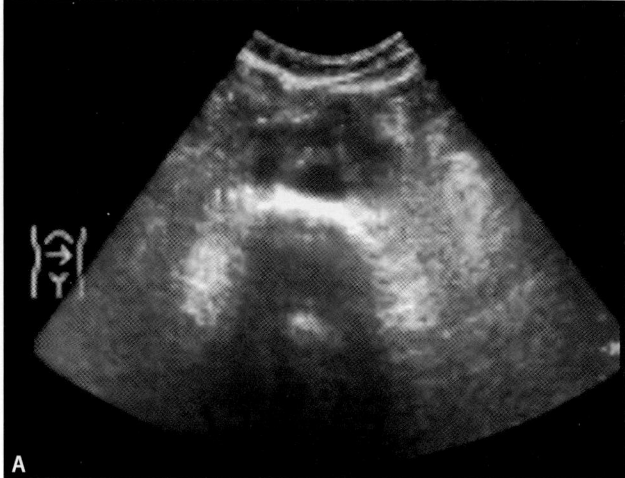
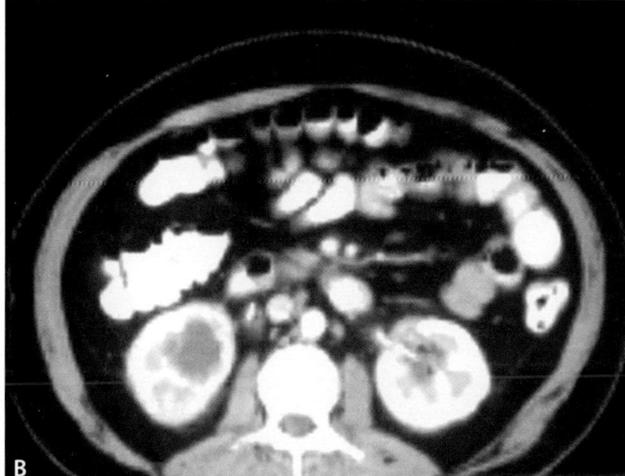
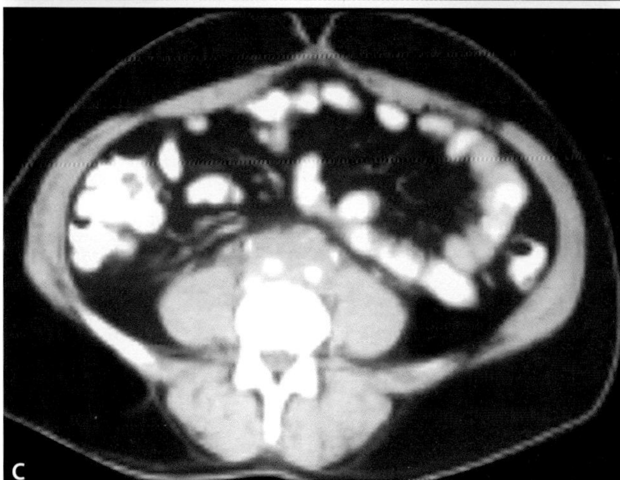

Figs. 16A to C: A young patient of idiopathic retroperitoneal fibrosis presented with obstructive uropathy. (A) Ultrasound image and (B and C) Contrast-enhanced CT scan show retroperitoneal mass encasing major vessels and bilateral ureter. Note made of bilateral double J stents.

Sonography forms the initial and mainstay imaging modality in these conditions. If the sonographic findings are equivocal, MR urography can show tapered narrowing of the lumbar portion of the ureter due to compression by the gravid uterus against the iliac artery at the sacral promontory. An obstructing calculus is usually above or below this level.

Gynecological Causes

Various gynecological disorders may cause extrinsic compression on the ureter leading to proximal dilatation of the urinary system **(Figs. 17A and B)**. Tubo-ovarian abscesses in pelvic inflammatory disease (PID) may cause extrinsic ureteric compression or surround the ureter with inflammation leading to partial obstruction with lateral displacement of the ureter below the pelvic brim. Pneumohydronephrosis may rarely develop due to fistula formation between the abscess and the ureter. Uterine and bladder prolapse are important causes of reversible and preventable renal failure. Obstruction is usually bilateral and is often associated with UTI. Sonography along with IVU helps in the easy identification of the disease. Carcinoma of urinary bladder can extend into the VUJ and distal ureter **(Figs. 18A and B)**.

Miscellaneous Diseases of Ureter

Ureteral Injury

The causes of ureteric injury can be iatrogenic and external trauma. Radical hysterectomy, gynecological surgery, and obstetric trauma are common causes of iatrogenic injury. Penetrating injury and fall from height are common causes for external trauma. Most surgically induced ureteric injuries go unsuspected at the time of injury, because they are often not a direct injury but the result of ischemia. IVU may demonstrate extravasation of urine and hydronephrosis. The complications of ureteric injury include hydronephrosis/pyonephrosis secondary to stricture, calculus formation, ureteric fistula, urinomas, and renal failure **(Figs. 19A and B)**.

Ureteral Herniation

Herniation of ureter is rare. Inguinal, femoral, and sciatic hernias may include the ureter. Herniation of ureter can be recognized on urography, e.g. in sciatic herniation, the pelvic ureter extends laterally through the sacrosciatic notch, producing a hairpin-shaped redundancy.

Ureteral Fistula

The common causes of ureteral fistulae are penetrating trauma, complicated ureteral surgery and inflammatory or malignant disease. Ureteral fistula usually presents

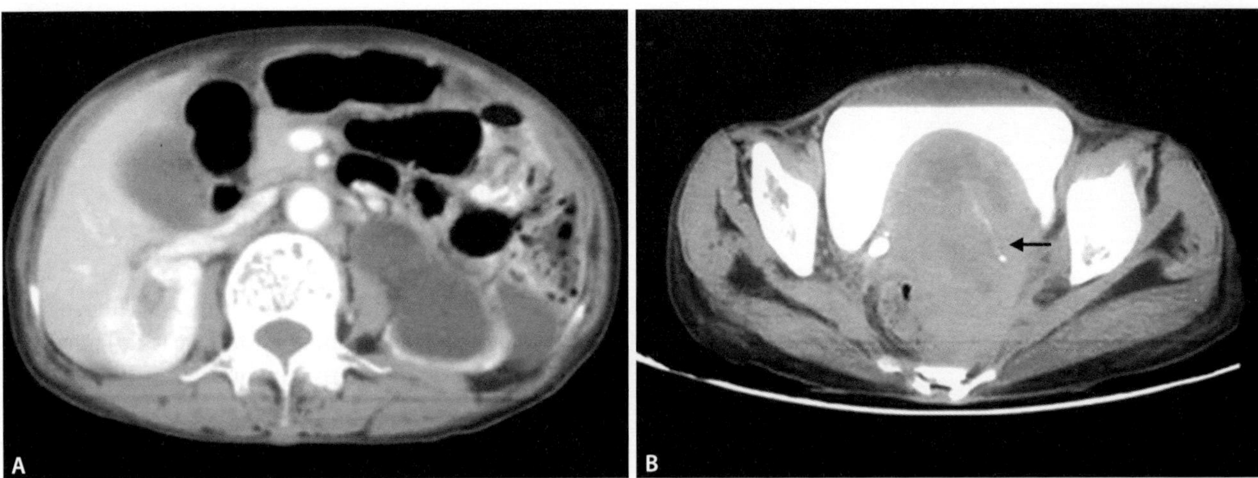

Figs. 17A and B: Carcinoma of cervix causing obstructive uropathy. Contrast-enhanced CT scans: (A) Axial section shows obstructive atrophy of left kidney; (B) Delayed section at the level of pelvis shows large heterogeneous cervical mass causing encasement of lower ureter (arrow).

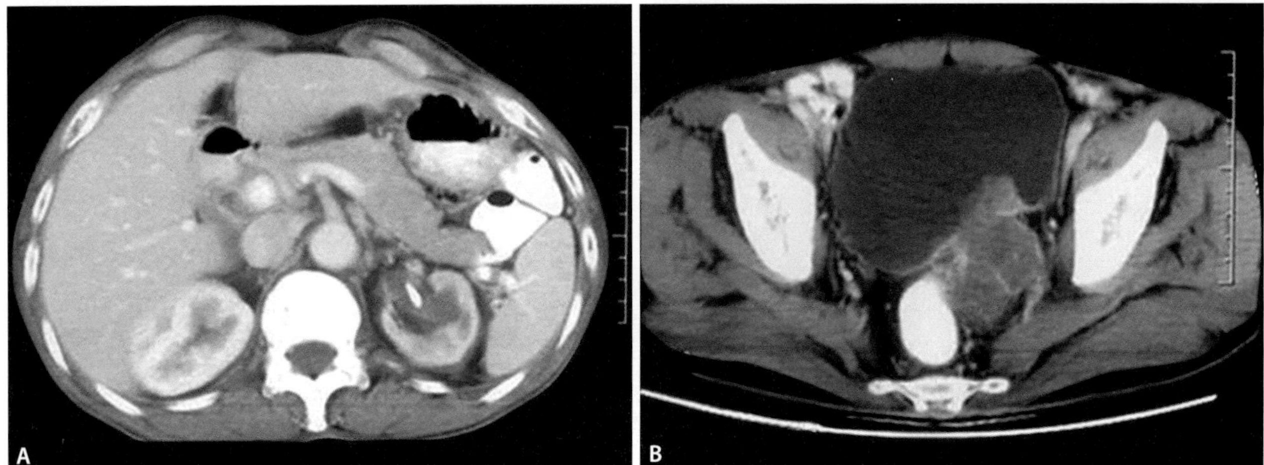

Figs. 18A and B: Ureteric obstruction caused by urinary bladder malignancy. Contrast-enhanced CT scans: (A) Axial section shows left hydroureteronephrosis with large calculus in renal pelvis; (B) Inferior section shows large lobulated mass arising from urinary bladder with exophytic component causing left ureteric involvement.

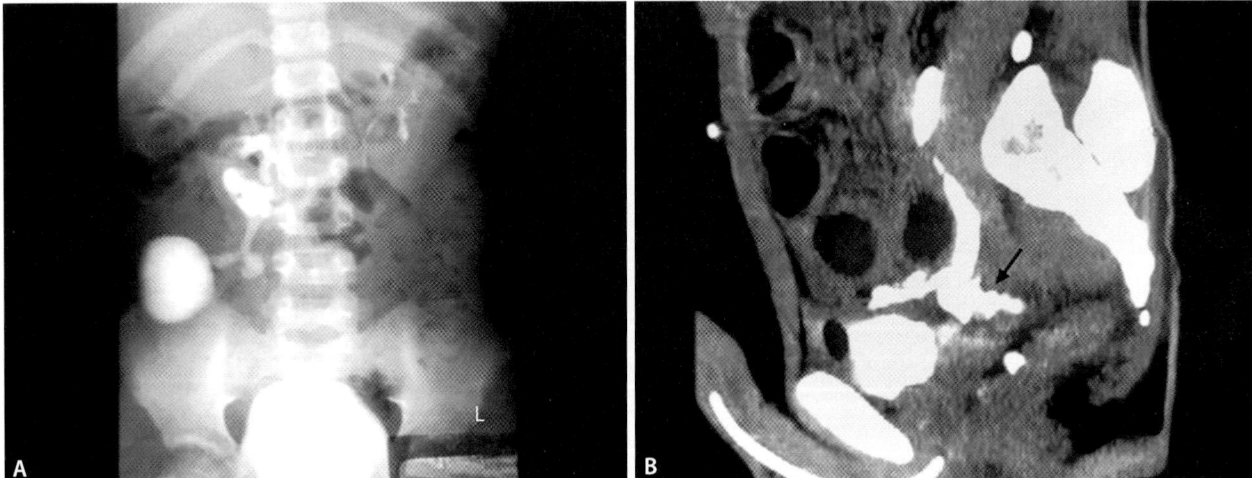

Figs. 19A and B: Ureteric trauma. (A) Delayed IVU film (2-hour film) shows extravasation of contrast from right upper ureter; (B) CT reformation in another patient shows contrast leak from lower ureter suggestive of ureteric trauma (arrow).

with urinary tract infection and clinical evidence of flow through the fistula. The diagnosis of fistula usually made by urography.

REFERENCES

1. Kumari A, Dokwal S, Mittal P, et al. An increase incidence in uric acid nephrolithiasis: changing patterns. J Clin Diagn Res. 2016;10(7):BC01-3.
2. Ansari MS, Gupta NP, Hemal AK, et al. Spectrum of stone composition: structural analysis of 1050 upper urinary tract calculi from northern India. Int J Urol. 2005;12(1):12-6.
3. Uribarri J, Oh MS, Carroll HJ. The first kidney stone. Ann Intern Med. 1989;111(12):1006-9.
4. Shadman A, Bastani B. Kidney calculi: pathophysiology and as a systemic disorder. Iran J Kidney Dis. 2017;11(3):180-91.
5. NICE (2019). Renal and ureteric stones: assessment and management. Guidance: Recommendations. [online] Available from https://www.nice.org.uk/guidance/ng118/chapter/Recommendations#diagnostic-imaging [Last accessed October, 2019].
6. American Urological Association (2012). Clinical Effectiveness Protocols for Imaging in The Management of Ureteral Calculous Disease: AUA Technology Assessment. [online] Available from https://www.auanet.org/guidelines/imaging-for-ureteral-calculous-disease [Last accessed October, 2019].
7. European Association of Urology. Professionals SO. EAU Guidelines: Urolithiasis [online] Available from: https://uroweb.org/guideline/urolithiasis/#3 [Last accessed October, 2019].
8. Smith-Bindman R, Aubin C, Bailitz J, et al. Ultrasonography versus computed tomography for suspected nephrolithiasis. N Engl J Med. 2014;371(12):1100-10.
9. Brisbane W, Bailey MR, Sorensen MD. An overview of kidney stone imaging techniques. Nat Rev Urol. 2016;13(11): 654-62.
10. Ather MH, Jafri AH, Sulaiman MN. Diagnostic accuracy of ultrasonography compared to unenhanced CT for stone and obstruction in patients with renal failure. BMC Med Imaging. 2004;4(1):2.
11. Rahmouni A, Bargoin R, Herment A, et al. Color Doppler twinkling artifact in hyperechoic regions. Radiology. 1996; 199(1):269-71.
12. Gliga ML, Chirila CN, Podeanu DM, et al. Twinkle, twinkle little stone: an artifact improves the ultrasound performance! Med Ultrasound. 2017;19(3):272-5.
13. Alan C, Koçoğlu H, Kosar S, et al. Role of twinkling artifact in characterization of urinary calculi. Actas Urol Esp. 2011;35(7):396-402.
14. Baker SM, Middleton WD. Color Doppler sonography of ureteral jets in normal volunteers: importance of the relative specific gravity of urine in the ureter and bladder. Am J Roentgenol. 1992;159(4):773-5.
15. Bertolotto M, Moro U, Gioulis E, et al. Changes of renal resistive index in response to hydration and diuretic administration in normal subjects and in patients with small ureteral stone. J Ultrasound Med. 1999;18(12):819-25.
16. Tublin ME, Bude RO, Platt JF. The resistive index in renal Doppler sonography: where do we stand? Am J Roentgenol. 2003;180(4):885-92.
17. Motamedinia P, Okhunov Z, Okeke Z, et al. Contemporary assessment of renal stone complexity using cross-sectional imaging. Curr Urol Rep. 2015;16(4):18.
18. Shadman A, Bastani B. Evaluation and management of kidney calculi. Iran J Kidney Dis. 2017;11(6):395-407.
19. Yamashita S, Kohjimoto Y, Iwahashi Y, et al. Noncontrast computed tomography parameters for predicting shock wave lithotripsy outcome in upper urinary tract stone cases. Biomed Res Int. 2018;2018:9253952.
20. McCarthy CJ, Baliyan V, Kordbacheh H, et al. Radiology of renal stone disease. Int J Surg Lond Engl. 2016;36(Pt D):638-46.
21. Karçaaltincaba M, Aktas A. Dual-energy CT revisited with multidetector CT: review of principles and clinical applications. Diagn Interv Radiol. 2011;17(3):181-94.
22. Bigongiari LR, Davis RM, Novak WG, et al. Visualization of the medullary rays on excretory urography in experimental ureteric obstruction. Am J Roentgenol. 1977;129(1):89-93.
23. Bernardino M, Clennan B. High dose urography: incidence and relationship to spontaneous peripelvic extravasation. Am J Roentgenol. 1976;127(3):373-6.
24. Dunbar JS, Nogrady MB. The calyceal crescent—a roentgenographic sign of obstructive hydronephrosis. Am J Roentgenol Radium Ther Nucl Med. 1970;110(3):520-8.
25. Somani BK, Dellis A, Liatsikos E, et al. Review on diagnosis and management of urolithiasis in pregnancy: an ESUT practical guide for urologists. World J Urol. 2017;35(11):1637-49.
26. Nicola R, Menias CO. Urinary obstruction, stone disease, and infection. In: Hodler J, Kubik-Huch RA, von Schulthess GK (Eds). Diseases of the Abdomen and Pelvis 2018-2021: Diagnostic Imaging—IDKD Book. Switzerland: Springer; 2018.
27. Amirthalingam U. Intrarenal Doppler indices in acute ureteric obstruction. J Clin Diagn Res. 2014;8(12):RC11-13.
28. Ramanathan S, Kumar D, Khanna M, et al. Multi-modality imaging review of congenital abnormalities of kidney and upper urinary tract. World J Radiol. 2016;8(2):132-41.
29. Johnston RB, Porter C. The Whitaker test. Urol J. 2014;11(3): 1727-30.
30. Chiodini B, Ghassemi M, Khelif K, et al. Clinical outcome of children with antenatally diagnosed hydronephrosis. Front Pediatr. 2019;7:103.
31. Merlini E, Lelli Chiesa P. Obstructive ureterocele—an ongoing challenge. World J Urol. 2004;22(2):107-14.
32. Thomas J, Steg A, Aboulker P. Calculi on blood clots. J Urol Nephrol (Paris). 1976;82(6):496-505.
33. Soria F, Shariat SF, Lerner SP, et al. Epidemiology, diagnosis, preoperative evaluation and prognostic assessment of upper-tract urothelial carcinoma (UTUC). World J Urol. 2017;35(3): 379-87.
34. Fein AB, McClennan BL. Solitary filling defects of the ureter. Semin Roentgenol. 1986;21(3):201-13.
35. Karaosmanoglu AD, Onur MR, Karcaaltincaba M, et al. Secondary tumors of the urinary system: an imaging conundrum. Korean J Radiol. 2018;19(4):742-51.
36. Moosavi B, Fasih N, Virmani V, et al. Beyond ureterolithiasis: gamut of abnormalities affecting the ureter. Clin Imaging. 2016;40(4):678-90.
37. Kawano M, Saeki T, Nakashima H. IgG4-related kidney disease and retroperitoneal fibrosis: an update. Mod Rheumatol. 2019;29(2):231-9.
38. Cronin CG, Lohan DG, Blake MA, et al. Retroperitoneal fibrosis: a review of clinical features and imaging findings. Am J Roentgenol. 2008;191(2):423-31.

Chapter 4

Renal Parenchymal Disease

Sreedhara BC, Anupam Lal, Anindita Sinha

Disorders of renal function are ubiquitous in contemporary practice of medicine. Kidney disease manifestations may vary from complete asymptomatic cases to life-threatening emergencies. Insight into the causes and consequences of medical renal disease has progressively increased over the last decade, and radiological imaging has played a pivotal role in this improved understanding.

DEFINITION AND CLASSIFICATION OF KIDNEY DISEASE

The term renal failure encompasses the spectrum of diseases from acute and reversible to chronic and irreversible. It is broadly divided into two categories which are described here.

Acute Kidney Injury

Acute kidney injury (AKI), also termed as acute renal failure previously is defined as a rapid deterioration in renal function, characterized by progressive azotemia (best measured by serum creatinine) which may or may not be accompanied by oliguria (urine output <400 mL/day). The cardinal feature of AKI is decline in glomerular filtration rate (GFR). According to Acute Kidney Injury Network (AKIN) criteria,[1] AKI is diagnosed if one of the following is present:

- An abrupt (within 48 hours) reduction in kidney function (defined as an absolute increase in serum creatinine of more than or equal to 0.3 mg/dL (≥26.4 μmol/L), or percentage increase in serum creatinine of more than or equal to 50% (1.5-fold from baseline).
- Reduced urine volume less than 0.5 mL/kg/h for 6 hours. There is sudden and often temporary loss of renal function, which is frequently reversible, with less than 20% cases ultimately requiring renal replacement therapy.[2] Imaging is, therefore, directed at identifying correctable causes of acute renal insult. Most common causes include acute tubular necrosis (ATN), severe dehydration, tubular blockade, infection, and obstruction.

Chronic Kidney Disease

The diagnosis of chronic kidney disease (CKD) implies a persistent abnormality in GFR with a wide range of causes. Slow progressive loss of kidney function over a span of years occurs, resulting in permanent kidney damage. CKD is defined as sustained kidney damage greater than 3 months duration resulting in a GFR of less than 60 mL/min/1.73 m^2.[2]

For purposes of diagnosis and management, renal failure can be divided into three categories which are as follows:

1. *Prerenal*: Diseases caused by any process that decreases perfusion to kidneys in which the integrity of renal parenchymal tissue is preserved.
2. *Intrarenal*: Diseases affecting renal parenchymal tissue (which can be further divided into vascular, glomerular, and tubular diseases).
3. *Postrenal*: Diseases associated with obstruction of the urinary tract or venous blood flow. It is also known as "surgical renal failure" as it is often amenable to correction.

This chapter is designed to give a contemporary insight of the intrarenal causes of acute and chronic kidney disease—"*Medical Renal Diseases*".

Table 1: Causes of acute renal failure.

Prerenal	*Intrarenal*	*Postrenal*
• Hypovolemia • Cardiogenic shock • Anaphylaxis • Sepsis • Renal artery stenosis • Severe dehydration	• *Acute tubular necrosis:* – Hemolysis – Antibiotics – Contrast nephrotoxicity • *Glomerulopathy:* – SLE – HSP – Postinfective glomerulonephritis • Papillary necrosis • *Vascular diseases:* – PAN, scleroderma	• Renal vein thrombosis • *Obstruction due to:* – Calculi – Hemorrhage – Tumor

(SLE: systemic lupus erythematosus; HSP: Henoch-Schönlein purpura)

Table 2: Causes of chronic renal failure.

Prerenal	*Intrarenal*	*Postrenal*
• Renal artery stenosis • Chronic dehydration • Congestive heart failure • Cirrhosis	• *Common causes:* – Diabetic nephropathy – Hypertensive – Glomerulosclerosis • Glomerulonephritis • Congenital ADPKD • Renal tubular acidosis • Drugs • TB • *Systemic diseases:* – FSGS – Gout – AIDS nephropathy – Scleroderma	• Posterior cortical value • Neurogenic bladder • Ureteric/bladder outlet obstruction • Retroperitoneal fibrosis • Tumor encasement

(ADPKD: autosomal dominant polycystic kidney disease; TB: tuberculosis; FSGS: focal segmental glomerulosclerosis)

Various causes of acute and chronic kidney disease are enumerated in **Tables 1 and 2**.[2]

ROLE OF IMAGING IN RENAL FAILURE

Overlapping imaging findings are seen in renal failure. Comprehensive evaluation should be done in a particular case which includes clinical profile, laboratory findings, and histopathology along with imaging to arrive at a conclusive diagnosis.

The role of imaging in renal failure is to segregate the surgical and medical conditions resulting in renal insufficiency.[1] Goals for radiological studies in renal failure are as follows:

- Exclusion of correctable causes of acute renal failure (e.g. obstruction and thrombosis).
- Estimation of renal size to differentiate acute parenchymal disease from chronic parenchymal disease.

Once obstruction is excluded, prerenal and postrenal causes of renal failures can be managed medically.

Radiological Approach to Renal Parenchymal Disease

Most diseases affecting the parenchyma of the kidney may produce lesions detectable only by electron or light microscopy, or by deranged renal function. However, some pathological processes manifest as renal morphological abnormalities and may be diagnosed by radiological imaging.

Morphological criteria are useful to categorize the wide spectrum of renal parenchymal diseases. Evaluation is done based on renal size, contour abnormality, and laterality of involvement **(Flowchart 1)**.

Renal size is an important diagnostic criterion. Large kidneys result from accumulation of fluid, deposition of proteins, inflammatory or neoplastic infiltrates, and hypertrophy secondary to glomerular, microvascular or cellular proliferation. Small kidneys result from loss of renal substance due to atrophy, hypoplasia, necrosis or fibrosis.

Flowchart 1: Morphological criteria to categorize renal parenchymal disease (size, contour, and laterality).

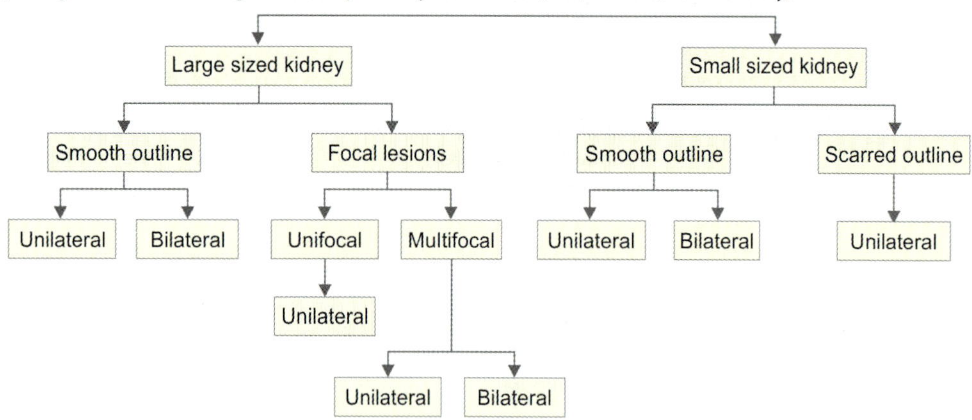

Renal contour is another useful indicator. If a disease causes global reduction in renal mass, parenchymal bulk is uniformly lost and its size decreases with smooth contour. This is ascertained by preserved interpapillary line, which is a useful landmark for evaluating loss of renal parenchyma. Interpapillary line is drawn through the tips of papilla (base of the calyces) **(Fig. 1)**, the distance from this line to lateral surface of kidney is the renal parenchymal thickness which averages to 2.5–3 cm. It is greater at polar calyces ranging up to 3.5 cm. Distances less than 2 cm are suggestive of parenchymal loss while those greater than 3.5 cm indicate mass lesion or infiltration.[4]

Assessment of renal contour may show a deviation when there is focal loss or regional expansion. Laterality indicates nature of the disease. Bilateral renal lesions are usually found in systemic disorders in which total renal mass is affected.[5,6]

Radiological imaging in renal parenchymal disease is usually targeted to reach a set of differential diagnosis, with distinct morphological description. "Bilateral large smooth kidney" constitutes to the group of acute renal parenchymal disease, while "bilateral small smooth kidney" falls into description of chronic renal parenchymal disease.

Imaging Techniques

Recent advancements in all the fields of imaging have led to better evaluation of renal diseases and their improved management. Imaging studies performed for evaluating the kidney diseases can provide anatomic, functional, and metabolic information. To reach a diagnosis for a particular case, it is important to know the benefits and the limitations along with the diagnostic yield of each modality.

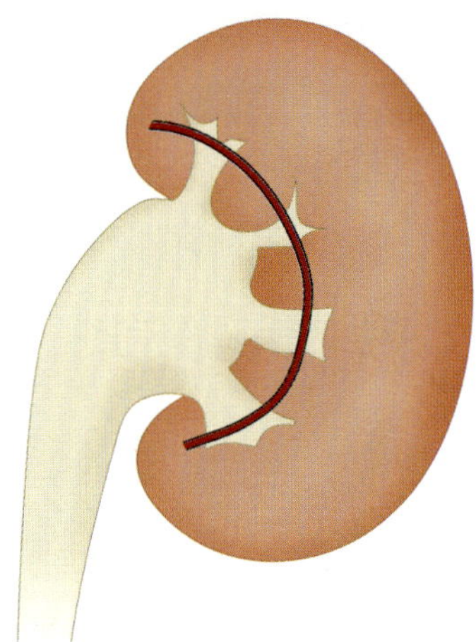

Fig. 1: Schematic diagram of normal interpapillary line. This line is drawn by joining the tips of renal papillae; smooth uninterrupted interpapillary line is seen in normal kidney.

Plain Radiography and Urography

The plain film also known as KUB (kidney, ureter, and bladder), has been used for years as the first step in the evaluation of the kidneys, however it gives little significant information on its own. Role of plain radiography is to detect renal parenchymal calcification and calculi. In an acute emergency setting, plain X-ray can be used to assess perinephric or retroperitoneal air foci, as seen in cases of emphysematous pyelonephritis **(Fig. 2)**. Renal size and contour may be estimated if the renal outlines can be visualized. Renal size is approximately equal to 3–4 lumbar vertebral body height. Normal kidney measures 10–14 cm in men and 9–13 cm in women on conventional radiography and 1–2 cm less on ultrasonography. Generally, right kidney is smaller than the left by about 0.5 cm. In clinical setting, discrepancy in renal size of

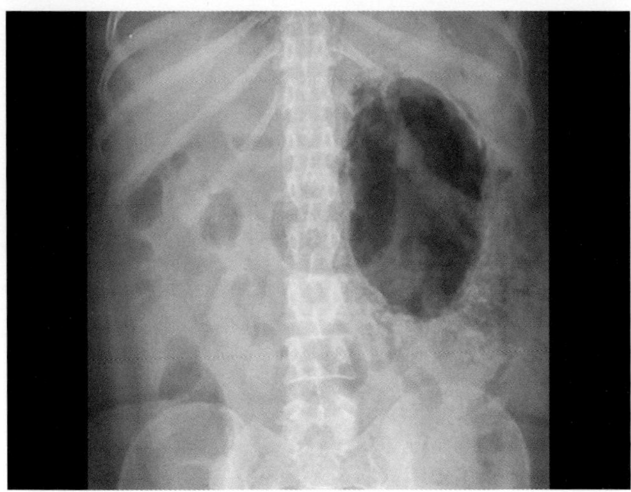

Fig. 2: Extensive gas overlying left renal parenchyma and perinephric space in a case of emphysematous pyelonephritis.

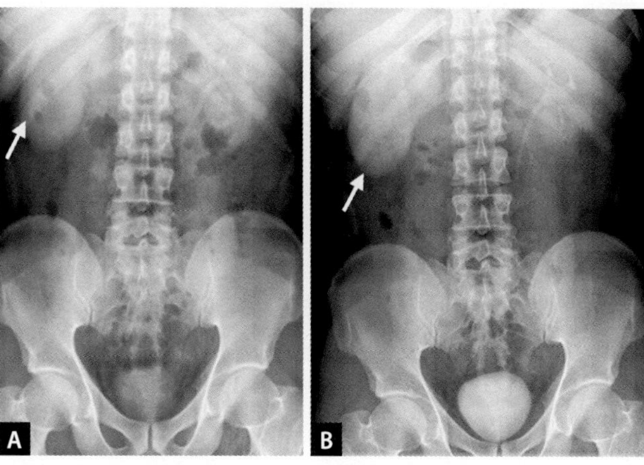

Figs. 3A and B: Increasing dense nephrogram. Intravenous urogram shows increased nephrographic density (arrows) on 2-hour film as compared to 5-minute nephrographic phase. Patient had right-sided urinary obstruction because of a small tumor near the right vesicoureteric junction.

more than 2 cm is considered significant.[3] In this era of cross-sectional imaging, urography is more of historic importance; however, interesting abnormal nephrographic patterns present in certain sets of diseases, were described by Fry and Cattell, which are as follows:[7]

- Immediate faint persistent nephrogram—chronic glomerular disease.
- Increasingly dense nephrogram—acute renal obstruction, hypotension, renal ischemia, acute glomerular disease, intratubular obstruction, and acute renal vein thrombosis **(Figs. 3A and B)**.
- Immediate dense persistent nephrogram—ATN and severe inflammatory renal disease.

Striated nephrogram is a variant of obstructive nephrogram which may also be encountered in other conditions like pyelonephritis, polyarteritis nodosa (PAN), trauma, and medullary cystic kidney disease. Prominent cortical nephrons are seen extending into the medulla as "medullary rays".

Ultrasonography

Ultrasonography is initial imaging modality for azotemia as it is noninvasive and readily differentiates between obstructive (surgical) and nonobstructive (medical) causes of renal failure **(Fig. 4A)**.[6] Renal sizes, cortical thickness, echogenicity of the kidneys, and the presence or absence of hydronephrosis are easily assessed on ultrasonography. Renal size and parenchymal thickness are useful parameters to assess chronicity of renal disease **(Fig. 4B)**. Enlarged kidneys indicate an acute parenchymal lesion while contracted small kidneys suggest a chronic disease. Renal cortical echogenicity is an important indicator for the diagnosis of renal parenchymal disease. Normally the echogenicity of renal cortex is less than liver or spleen; the demonstration of increased echogenicity of the renal cortex under standard scanning techniques may be useful in suggesting the presence of renal parenchymal (medical renal) disease. Renal corticomedullary differentiation (CMD) may be preserved, obliterated or accentuated depending on the severity of renal cortical echoes **(Figs. 4C to F)**.[8,9]

Increased cortical echogenicity with preserved CMD may be seen in glomerulonephritis, nephrosclerosis, amyloidosis, acute leukemia, ATN, and Alport's syndrome while cortical echogenicity is decreased in lymphoma, acute pyelonephritis, and renal vein thrombosis. Increased medullary echotexture is found in gouty nephropathy, medullary nephrocalcinosis, and medullary sponge kidney. Interestingly, some authors recognize the altered state of hydration at the time of scanning as one of determining factors influencing the renal cortical echotexture of the patient.[9,10] An extracapsular hypoechoic rim of edema may surround the kidneys in renal failure. This finding when present is usually bilateral and is called as "kidney sweat sign".[11]

Ultrasound examination is also valuable for assessing the kidneys for follow-up of renal parenchymal disease. Changes in renal size, progression as well as resolution of the disease can easily be monitored on ultrasonography.

Color Doppler

Color Doppler is a handy, easily available, and noninvasive tool for evaluation of renal blood vessels. Normal renal arterial branching pattern is well-appreciated on color

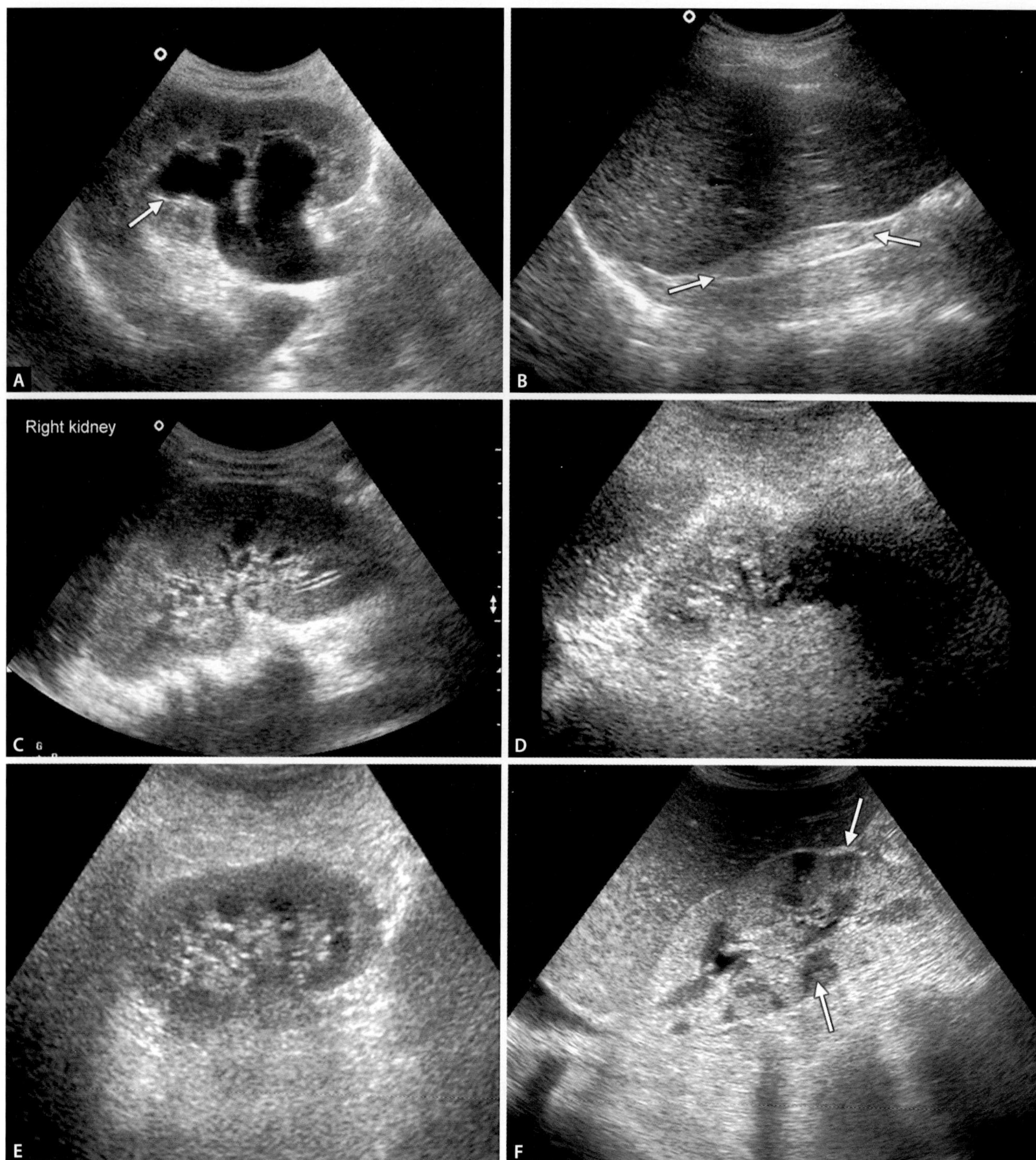

Figs. 4A to F: (A) Obstructive renal failure with distal ureteric calculus: Longitudinal ultrasound (US) image depicts marked dilatation of the pelvicalyceal system (arrow). Note the upper ureter is also dilated. (B) Chronic renal failure: US image shows small smooth kidney with markedly decreased renal parenchymal thickness. (C to F) Acute renal parenchymal disease US images. (C) Slightly raised cortical echogenicity and lack of renal corticomedullary differentiation. (D) Markedly increased parenchymal echoes nearing to that of renal sinus resulting in loss of corticomedullary differentiation. (E) Hyperechoic renal cortex, relatively prominent renal medulla with accentuated corticomedullary differentiation. (F) Complicated pyelonephritis with multiple renal abscesses: Severely raised cortical echoes and few hypoechoic well-defined parenchymal lesions (abscesses) (arrows) with right pleural effusion.

flow imaging. Assessment of spectral wave pattern and flow indices of renal arteries can be done. Vascular resistance (resistive index: RI) and pulsatility (pulsatility index) along with absolute flow velocities of the main, intralobar, and arcuate arteries may be calculated. Out of these indices RI is most commonly used. It is calculated as:

$$\text{Resistive Index} = \frac{\text{Peak systolic velocity} - \text{Lowest diastolic velocity}}{\text{Peak systolic velocity}}$$

Normal RI is less than 0.7. Parenchymal diseases with tubulointerstitial or vascular involvement cause increased RI (>0.7), while glomerular diseases do not cause any significant increase in this parameter.[12] Elevated RI correlates with the severity of disease in systemic lupus erythematosus (SLE), hemolytic uremic syndrome (HUS), diabetes, and hepatorenal syndrome **(Fig. 5)**.[5]

Contrast-enhanced Ultrasound

Contrast-enhanced ultrasound (CEUS) is an alternative imaging modality to contrast-enhanced computed tomography (CECT) in the evaluation of renal parenchymal diseases, urinary tract infections, and associated complications. The elimination properties of microbubbles through lungs make CEUS an attractive nontoxic imaging modality in renal insufficiency patients. It can also be performed at the bedside in sick patients, and a useful modality in assessing claustrophobic patients and children who cannot tolerate CT or magnetic resonance imaging (MRI) without sedation.

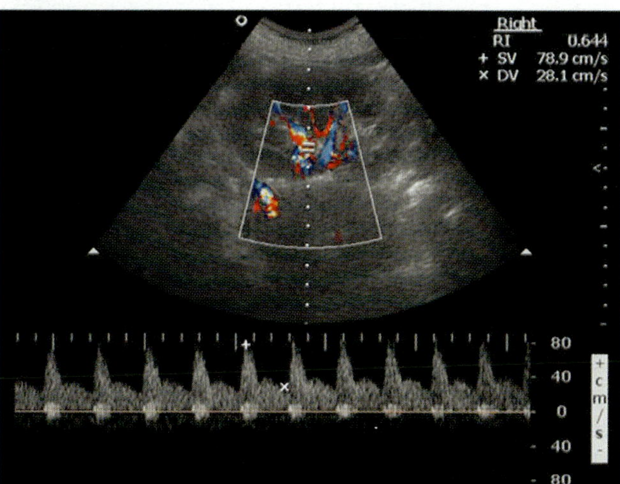

Fig. 5: Normal Doppler ultrasound. Doppler spectra obtained in the area of interlobar arteries show a sharp systolic peak and prominent antegrade flow during diastolic phase. Resistive index in this patient is 0.64, which is normal.

Contrast-enhanced ultrasound showed almost equal sensitivity and specificity to CT in detecting renal parenchymal changes associated with pyelonephritis.[13] CEUS features suggestive of pyelonephritis include peripheral wedge-shaped perfusion defects and heterogeneous enhancement, similar to CECT but without the exposure to radiation. CEUS is also useful in measurement of renal perfusion in AKI, to rule out ischemic perfusion injury, and is more accurate method than Doppler. In postrenal transplant patients with acute rejection, CEUS can detect regional perfusion defects of the allograft.

Computed Tomography

Computed tomography has a specific role in evaluation of renal failure. In acute renal failure noncontrast computed tomography (NCCT) scan of kidneys may show parenchymal calcification. Renal parenchyma, however, appears homogenous in attenuation on NCCT. Various nephrographic patterns are demonstrated after the administration of contrast. Differential diagnosis of the nephrographic patterns used on urography is similarly applied to CT nephrogram. Excretory function can further be assessed on sequential dynamic imaging.[14]

Magnetic Resonance Imaging

Routine MRI evaluation of the kidney includes axial and coronal T1-weighted (T1W) and T2-weighted (T2W) spin echo sequences, with or without fat suppression. CMD is distinctly seen on T1W and T2W images. In normal kidney, the cortex is slightly higher in signal intensity than the medulla on T1W images while renal medulla is hyperintense to cortex on T2W images **(Figs. 6A to D)**. In a normal well-hydrated kidney, sharp CMD is seen on T1W sequence due to high signal of cortex as compared to medulla. Wide variety of renal medical diseases cause decrease in cortical signal and subsequent loss of CMD. Loss of CMD on T1W spin echo sequences is a sensitive indicator of parenchymal diseases and correlates with elevated serum creatinine levels >3.0 mg/dL. Dynamic contrast-enhanced T1W sequences can also be done. CMD is lost on postgadolinium dynamic MRI when serum creatinine is >8.5 mg/dL.[15]

Diffusion-weighted imaging (DWI) is sensitive to changes in the renal interstitium during cellular infiltration or edema, renal fibrosis, and in renal perfusion. The most promising application of DWI so far is in fibrosis estimation in CKD and guidance for biopsy in acute graft dysfunction.[16] Apparent diffusion coefficient (ADC)

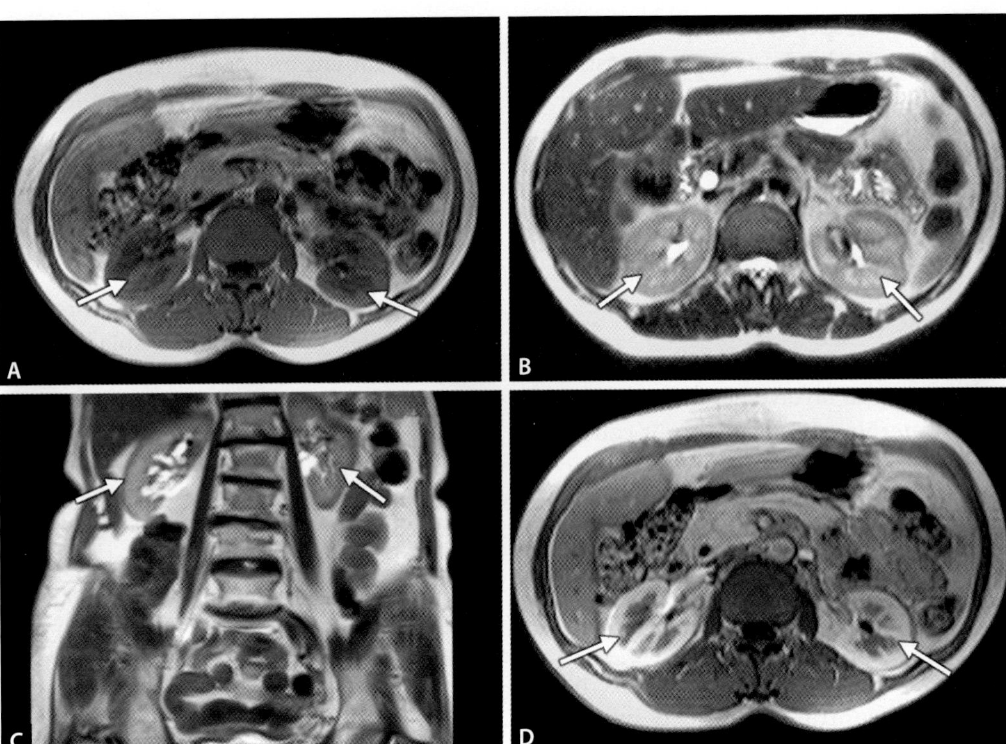

Figs. 6A to D: Normal spin echo magnetic resonance imaging findings: (A) T1-weighted axial image shows corticomedullary differentiation resulting from high signal intensity of normal renal cortex and lower signal intensity of renal medulla (arrows). (B and C) T2-weighted axial and coronal magnetic resonance (MR) images depict the hyperintensity of normal renal medulla as compared to renal cortex (arrows). (D) Postgadolinium dynamic MR in cortical phase reveals the striking distinction between renal cortex and medulla (arrows).

values correlate with renal function, usually estimated by creatinine values. The cortical ADC values show good correlation with cortical fibrosis and chronic lesions (reduction in ADC values with increasing grade of CKD), however, at present no clear cut-off of ADC values can be chosen to differentiate CKD versus healthy kidney due to limitations in image resolution, protocol variability, and interindividual variability. Diffusion tensor imaging (DTI) is another noninvasive tool to assess renal function with medullary fractional anisotropy values significantly lower in patients with CKD than in healthy controls similar to ADC.[17] Arterial spin labeling (ASL) is a powerful tool for noninvasive measurement of regional renal perfusion in humans, with a typical in plane resolution of 2–3 mm. It uses magnetic labeling of water in arterial blood as an endogenous tracer to generate maps of absolute regional perfusion without requiring exogenous contrast. The studies performed so far have shown reproducible measurements of renal perfusion from both renal cortex and medulla, and ASL is highly suited to repeated measurements. The renal perfusion values reduce with increasing stage of CKD and correlates to estimated glomerular filtration rate (eGFR).[18]

Renal Angiography

Renal angiography has limited role in renal parenchymal disease as it is an invasive procedure and usually requires large amount of iodinated contrast medium. Characteristic appearances like aneurysmal dilatation of medium and small-sized vessels on arteriography are seen in conditions like PAN, granulomatosis with polyangiitis, and SLE. Pruned, tortuous vessels with slow flow with thinned renal cortex are demonstrated. Lucent or mottled nephrogram may be seen. Renal artery stenosis is most accurately diagnosed on angiography and can be treated by angioplasty.[19]

Radionuclide Imaging

Scintigraphy provides imaging based diagnostic information on renal structure and function. Radionuclide agents are excreted by kidneys; hence, they should be judiciously employed in patients with renal failure. ^{99m}Tc-DTPA (diethylenetriaminepentaacetic acid) is excreted solely by the glomerular filtration, therefore it should not be used frequently. Tubular secretion of ^{99m}Tc-MAG3 (mercaptoacetyltriglycine) and Hippuran I-131 occurs, hence these may be utilized in severe renal insufficiency.[20]

Contrast-induced Nephropathy

The presence of renal failure may pose some limitations on the choice of an individual imaging modality. Iodinated contrast media may cause exacerbation of renal insufficiency. Contrast-induced nephropathy (CIN) is one of the common causes of hospital-acquired acute renal failure (ARF). The exact mechanism of CIN is still unknown, but it is thought to be multifactorial.[21] CIN is defined as either 0.5 mg/dL (44 μmol/L) increase in absolute serum creatinine value within 48–72 hours or 25% increase in serum creatinine from baseline after administration of intravascular contrast material when no other cause of renal injury is readily apparent.[22] The rise in serum creatinine usually peaks at 3–5 days and return to baseline within 10–14 days. The most important risk factor is pre-existing renal insufficiency (serum creatinine >1.5–2.0 mg/dL), followed by diabetes mellitus, advancing age, congestive heart failure, dehydration, high dose of contrast media, and furosemide. Adequate hydration, dose reduction, and use of nonionic contrast media are recommended as preventive measures.

IMAGING IN RENAL PARENCHYMAL DISEASE

Acute Renal Parenchymal Disease

Radiographic appearance of "bilateral, large, smooth" kidneys is usually seen in the setting of renal failure of recent onset. When obstruction is ruled out a similar picture of enlarged smooth kidneys with normal or effaced collecting system is seen that indicates parenchymal disease of recent origin, which is possibly reversible. **Box 1** and **Table 3** enumerate the causes of renomegaly based on morphological criteria.[4]

However, in some conditions certain characteristic appearances are seen in imaging which shall be discussed in the next section of this chapter. Infections, cystic renal diseases, obstructions, renal vascular diseases, and tumors are not included here as they are covered in other chapters in this book.

Box 1: Causes of bilateral large smooth kidneys.[5]

- Proliferative/necrotizing disorders
- Acute glomerulonephritis
- Polyarteritis nodosa (microscopic form)
- Systemic lupus erythematosus
- Granulomatosis with polyangiitis
- Allergic angiitis
- Diabetic glomerulosclerosis
- Lung hemorrhage and glomerulonephritis (Goodpasture's syndrome)
- Anaphylactoid purpura (Henoch-Schönlein syndrome)
- Thrombotic thrombocytopenic purpura
- Focal glomerulonephritis associated with subacute bacterial endocarditis
- Plasma cell dyscrasias
- Multiple myeloma
- Waldenstrom's macroglobulinemia
- Amyloidosis
- Abnormal glycogen deposition
- von Gierke's disease (Glycogen storage disease type-I)
- Abnormal lipid deposition
- Fabry's disease
- *Abnormal fluid accumulation:*
  - Acute tubular necrosis
  - Acute cortical necrosis
- Leukemia
- Acute interstitial nephritis
- Acute blockage of tubules
- Acute urate nephropathy
- Tamm-Horsfall protein
- Acute myeloma nephropathy
- Acromegaly
- Nephromegaly associated with cirrhosis, hyperalimentation, and diabetes mellitus
- Hemophilia
- Homozygous-S disease
- Tyrosinosis type I
- Infectious mononucleosis
- Autosomal recessive polycystic kidney disease
- Physiological response to contrast material and diuretics

Table 3: Large kidney with focal lesion.[5]

Unifocal unilateral	*Multifocal*	
	Bilateral	*Unilateral*
• Simple cyst • Focal hydronephrosis • *Benign neoplasm:* – Adenoma – Mesenchymal tumor – Inflammatory mass • *Malignant neoplasm:* – RCC – Sarcoma – Metastatic deposit	• Autosomal dominant polycystic kidney disease • Lymphoma • Acquired cystic kidney disease	• Multicystic kidney disease Xanthogranulomatous • Pyelonephritis • Malakoplakia

Acute Tubular Necrosis

Acute tubular necrosis is the most frequent cause of AKI in the renal category. An acute clinical event with ischemic cascade or nephrotoxic agents **(Table 4)** results in ATN.[23] The multicentric observational study concluded with the ischemic ATN as the presumed etiology for ~50% of patients with renal failure, ~12% related to the unresolved prerenal causes, and ~25% were related to the nephrotoxic agents.[24] Generally, ATN follows a pattern of sequential manifestations including the initiation [reduced GFR, with increased creatinine and blood urea nitrogen (BUN)], maintenance (stabilization of low GFR over 1-2 weeks with increased serum creatinine and BUN), and recovery (polyurea with return of serum creatinine and BUN to preinjury level) phases. When the hypoperfusion overwhelms the renal autoregulatory mechanisms, the tubular cell injury (especially at loop of Henle dipping into the medulla) is initiated, but not always, leading to the cellular death. Ischemia leads to the formation of apical blebs and loss of brush border membrane in proximal tubular cells followed by the loss of cell polarity and integrity of tight junctions resulting in ineffective filtration. Cellular casts block the tubular lumen and adds on to the underlying hypoperfusion complex resulting in decreased GFR. Acute tubule or cell damage resulting from the ischemic or nephrotoxic agents follows almost the similar pattern and the altered pathophysiological events.[25]

Imaging Evaluation

Blood tests and urinalysis along with renal ultrasonography findings are useful in identifying the cause for ATN. In ATN, both kidneys are enlarged (especially anteroposterior dimeter) with prominent medulla and smooth in outline. Contrast-enhanced studies are not recommended in ATN. If intravenous (IV) contrast is inadvertently given, persistent dense nephrogram is seen in neurography which may persist for more than 24 hours. As tubules are filled with cellular infiltrates, contrast leaks into the interstitium through the damaged basement membrane, hence, faint or nonopacification of pelvicalyceal system occurs.

Variable appearances of ATN on ultrasonography have been proposed by different authors, which are:[26]

- Normal cortical and medullary echogenicity—ischemic ATN.
- Increase in cortical echogenicity with maintained CMD—drug-related ATN.
- Normal cortical echogenicity with echogenic pyramids—associated with precipitation of Tamm-Horsfall protein. Increased RI (>0.7) on Doppler imaging is present in majority of patients with ATN.[27]

Izumi et al.,[28] proved the superior role of Doppler sonography in evaluation as well as follow-up of the ATN subjects in comparison to the prerenal azotemia with the finding of raised RI (>0.75) and obvious reduction of resistive indices in ATN subjects as compared to the subjects with prerenal azotemia.

Bilateral renomegaly with patchy nephrogram is seen on CT scan. Gadolinium-enhanced MRI demonstrates compartmental renal involvement of cortex, inner and outer medulla, and give complementary information about the pathological condition of the kidney. Perfusion abnormalities were also shown in experimentally induced ATN. Blood-oxygen-level-dependent MRI (BOLD MRI) assesses intrarenal oxygen bioavailability which reflects tissue deoxyhemoglobin levels. Ischemia

Table 4: Etiology of acute tubular necrosis (ATN).

Condition	*Underlying mechanisms*	*Direct causes*
Ischemic ATN	Hypovolemic state	Hemorrhage, fluid loss, burns, and fluid sequestration
	Low cardiac output	Cardiac failure and underlying conditions (arrhythmia, myocardial or pericardial diseases)
	Systemic vasodilatation	Sepsis and anaphylaxis
	Disseminated intravascular coagulation	
Nephrotoxic ATN	Exogenous agents	Aminoglycoside-related toxicity, amphotericin B related toxicity, contrast agents (CIN), cyclosporines, sulfa drugs, etc.
	Endogenous agents	Myoglobinuria (rhabdomyolysis) Hemoglobinuria (transfusion reactions) Acute crystal-induced nephropathy Multiple myeloma

(ATN: acute tubular necrosis; CIN: contrast-induced nephropathy)

and hypoperfusion in ATN results in reduced tissue oxygen bioavailability which is utilized to discriminate between acute rejection and ATN that may follow renal transplantation.[29]

Acute Cortical Necrosis

Acute cortical necrosis (ACN) is a rare form of acute renal failure which is characterized by ischemic necrosis of renal cortex, including renal column of Bertin with sparing of renal medulla, and thin rim of subcapsular cortex. Both kidneys are involved either diffusely or in patchy distribution; in both instances peripheral renal cortex is spared as it is supplied by the preserved capsular vessels.[5]

More than two-thirds of cases are associated with pregnancy and its complications—abruptio placenta, septic abortion, and placenta previa. Other causes include severe trauma with shock, sepsis, transfusion reaction, severe dehydration, burns, peritonitis, and toxins (e.g. snake venom). Although large numbers of conditions are associated with ACN, the pathophysiology unfortunately remains unclear. Ischemia following vasospasm is probably the initiating event which results due to constriction of small intracortical blood vessels. This may follow exposure to toxins, circulating hormones, or neural stimuli.[30]

Diffuse involvement of both the kidneys may result in complete renal failure requiring either dialysis or transplantation for survival, whereas patchy involvement leads to renal insufficiency.

Imaging Features

Imaging findings depend on the stage of illness. In the acute stage, urographic findings are nonspecific. Kidneys are diffusely enlarged with faint opacification of collecting system. For those surviving the early phase, smooth renal shrinkage occurs over several months. Radiographically, distinctive tram-like or egg shell calcification of cortex may be seen which starts appearing as early as 24 days after the onset of disease.

On ultrasonography, enlargement of both kidneys and loss of the normal CMD with a circumferential hypoechoic zone corresponding to the necrotic cortex is seen. Ultrasound is useful for follow-up. Calcification of cortex causes dense cortical echoes with distal acoustic shadowing.

Specific appearance of ACN is described on CECT scan. The three diagnostic features are (a) enhancement of the medulla, (b) nonenhancement of the renal cortex, and (c) lack of excretion of contrast medium into the collecting system. Enhanced subcapsular cortex, the distinctive "Cortical rim sign" on CECT scan suggests the sparing of the most peripheral region of renal cortex **(Figs. 7A and B)**. "Cortical rim sign" is also seen in other conditions which result in hemodynamic derangement like renal infarction, renal vein thrombosis, and ATN.[31-33]

Magnetic resonance imaging also shows these representative findings. Kidneys are enlarged in the early phase. Low signal intensity of the inner renal cortex and the columns of Bertin on every MRI sequence is the major

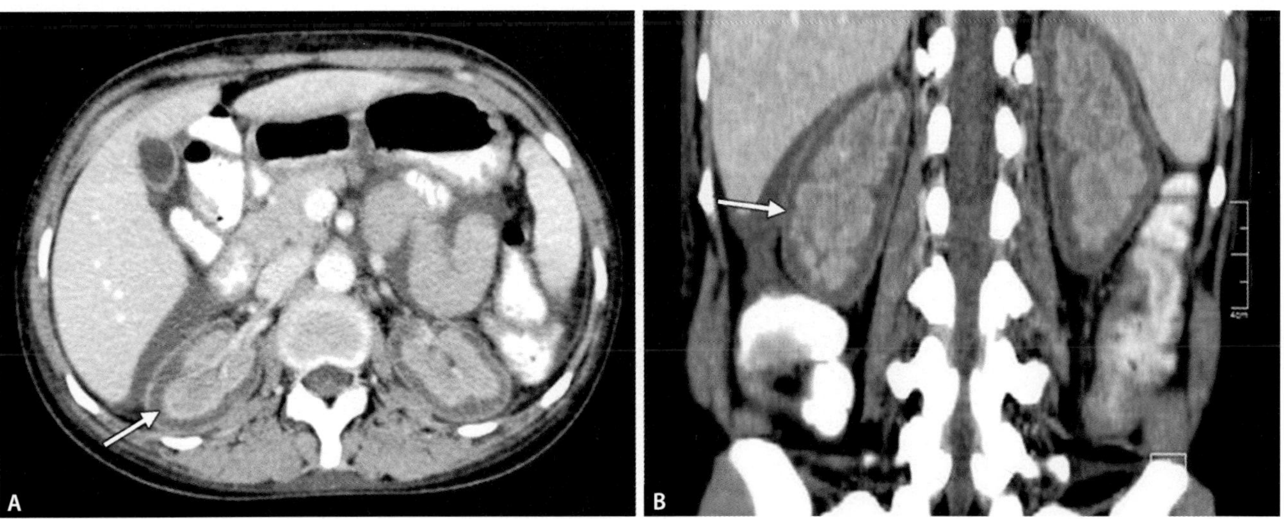

Figs. 7A and B: Acute cortical necrosis in a female patient with septic abortion: Axial and coronal postcontrast computed tomography scans (corticomedullary phase) demonstrate the absence of contrast enhancement in the cortex and relatively hyperdense medulla and subcapsular cortex, the characteristic "cortical rim sign".

characteristic finding of renal cortical necrosis. Swelling of both kidneys with increased signal intensity of the cortex on T2W images instead of T1W images is another feature of renal cortical necrosis at MRI. Later a thin rim of low signal intensity (T1WI and T2WI) may be seen along the border of kidneys due to calcification.[34]

Leukemia

Leukemia (predominantly lymphocytic leukemia) is the most common malignant cause of bilateral renal enlargement in children. Renal enlargement occurs due to infiltration of kidneys by leukemic cells. Usually, markedly large kidneys are seen, however, sometimes asymmetrical renal involvement or focal renal mass may be seen **(Figs. 8A and B)**.

Imaging Features

In leukemic infiltration of kidney, the nephrogram is faint and the collecting system is attenuated. Pelvicalyceal system is often filled with blood clots or uric acid stones which appear as filling defects.[20]

Acute Interstitial Nephritis

Acute interstitial nephritis (AIN) is an acute hypersensitivity reaction, mediated through immunologic mechanisms. It may result following an exposure to drugs, nonrenal infection (e.g. infectious mononucleosis, legionella, and leptospirosis), systemic autoimmune disorders (SLE, Sjögren's syndrome, and sarcoidosis), and tubulointerstitial nephritis and uveitis (TINU syndrome). However, an idiopathic variety is also described. The most common cause of AIN are drugs particularly—antibiotics (methicillin, penicillin, and amphotericin), Nonsteroidal anti-inflammatory drugs (NSAIDs), sulfonamides, phenytoin, and thiazide.[35]

Fever, skin rashes, eosinophilia, oliguria, and proteinuria are the common clinical signs and symptoms of drug-induced AIN which appear between 5 days and 5 weeks of exposure. Patient recovers with the withdrawal of the causative agent.[36]

Imaging Features

Bilateral renomegaly with diminished to normal opacification of collecting system is seen on urography. Ultrasound shows increased cortical echogenicity with renal enlargement. Enhanced uptake of Gallium citrate in the kidneys on renal scintigraphy is also reported.[35] CT shows low attenuation areas in the cortex and corticomedullary junctions **(Fig. 9)**. Kidneys may become shrunken and irregular as the disease progresses to a chronic course. Calcification of renal papillae may occur in analgesic-induced nephritis. Interstitial fibrosis leads to low signal intensity of renal cortex on T1W MRI.

Amyloidosis

Amyloidosis is a diverse group of diseases that have extracellular deposition and accumulation of an insoluble fibrillar proteinaceous substance with a beta sheath configuration, which is characteristically appreciated as apple green birefringence on congo red staining and when viewed under polarized light.

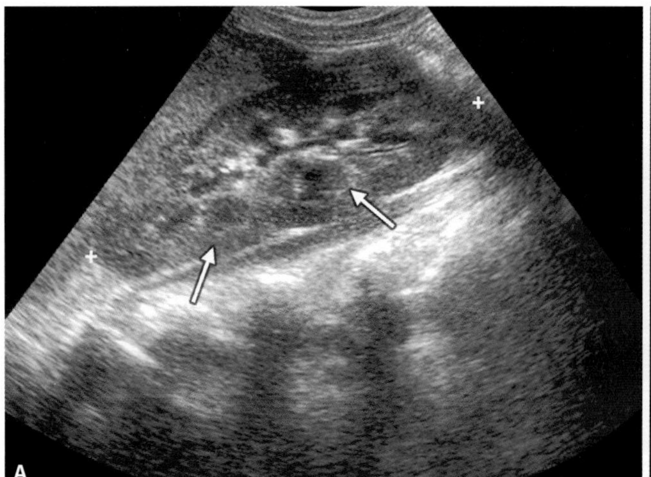

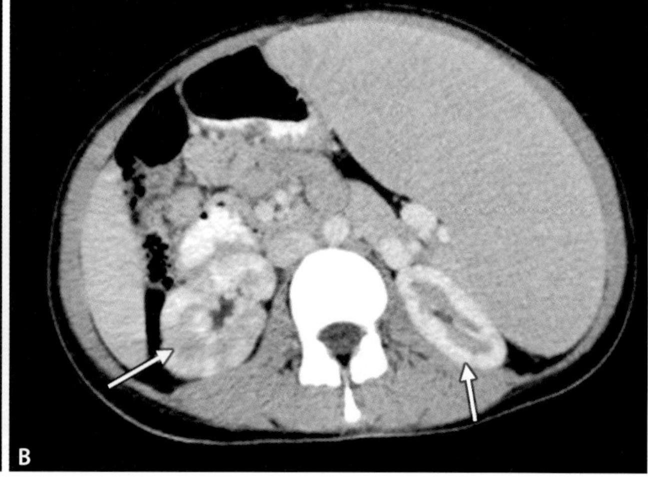

Figs. 8A and B: Renal manifestation of leukemia. (A) Ultrasonography of kidney shows focal, well-defined, and hypoechoic masses; (B) Contrast-enhanced CT axial image in another patient also shows bilateral, multiple, and focal hypodensities suggestive of leukemic deposits. Massive splenomegaly is also seen.

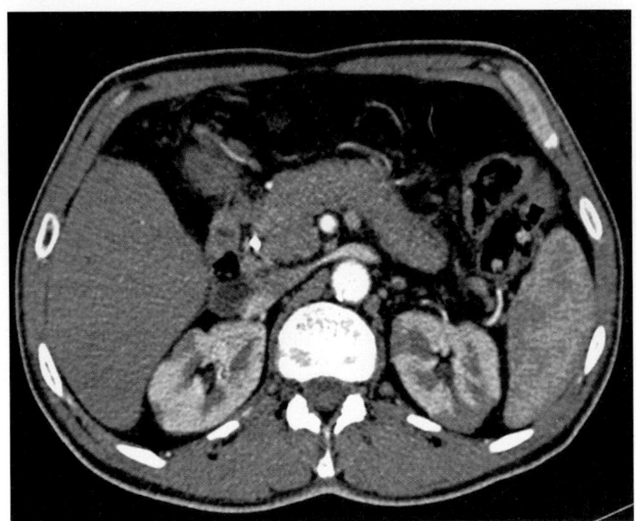

Fig. 9: Acute interstitial nephritis in a case of autoimmune pancreatitis. Multifocal hypodense areas in the cortex of bilateral kidneys.

Amyloidosis can be classified as follows:[37]

- *Primary amyloidosis*: Usually called as primary light chain (AL) amyloidosis resulting from the B-cell or plasma cell dysplasia. Usually involves renal and cardiac organs with poor prognosis. Rarely heavy chain associated amyloidosis is also seen accounting for ~4–6% with no cardiac involvement explaining the good prognosis in affected subjects.
- *Secondary amyloidosis*: Secondary amyloidosis [amyloid-associated disease (AA)] is usually associated with chronic inflammatory conditions such as rheumatoid arthritis, Crohn's disease, tuberculosis, bronchiectasis, and chronic osteomyelitis.

Secondary amyloidosis is more prevalent and more common in underdeveloped countries whereas primary amyloidosis is the most common type of amyloidosis in the Western hemisphere. Other rare familial and senile forms and dialysis-related amyloidosis have also been described.

Older men are more affected than women,[38] usually presenting with nonspecific symptoms like weight loss, fatigue, and weakness. Multiorgan involvement is present in more than 85% of cases. Kidney is affected in 80% patients with secondary amyloidosis and 35–40% patients with primary disease. Isolated involvement of the renal pelvis, ureter bladder, urethra, prostate seminal vesicle, and retroperitoneum can occur.[39]

Imaging Features

Based on the extent of involvement, amyloidosis can also be classified as systemic and localized forms of disease. In acute phase, bilateral renal enlargement is seen. Decrease in size occurs with progression of disease process, smooth outline is, however, maintained. Nephrogram is diminished with variable excretion into normal pelvicalyceal system. Cortical echogenicity is raised as seen in other parenchymal diseases. Rapid deterioration in renal function or sudden onset nephrotic syndrome indicates renal vein thrombosis, a complication of amyloidosis. Thrombosed renal vein is demonstrated on color Doppler, CT scan or MRI. Perinephric soft tissue mass with retroperitoneal and mesenteric extension is seen. CT examination depicts the extent of soft tissue involvement as well as calcification changes resulting from the amyloid proteinaceous material.

Magnetic resonance imaging shows reduced cortical signal intensity on T1W images with subsequent loss of CMD. Bilateral increased delayed uptake of Gallium 67 when other causes of abnormal gallium activity are excluded.[39]

Amyloidosis of renal pelvis-isolated involvement of renal pelvis can occur in amyloidosis. Interesting radiological appearance of calcification or ossification in the amyloid deposits may be seen. These deposits are usually located in the submucosa of the pelvicalyceal system. A lucent band of mucosa separates the IV contrast density from calcification in the pelvis on intravenous urogram (IVU). Other causes for calcification of pelvicalyceal system are tuberculosis, leukoplakia, primary carcinoma of renal pelvis, and renal calculus. Submucosal amyloid deposits appear hypointense on T1W and T2W magnetic resonance images.

Localized forms of amyloidosis are also encountered in the urinary bladder and lower ureter which may mimic chronic granulomatous (tubercular and schistosomiasis) and neoplastic conditions of these organs. It is extremely important to differentiate the systemic form of involvement from the localized variety as therapeutic approaches vary based on the involvement. Biopsy of renal tissue or extra renal tissue, bone marrow biopsy, and urinalysis will aid in establishing and guiding in management of these conditions.

Multiple Myeloma

Multiple myeloma is a plasma cell disorder which originates in the bone marrow and is characterized by involvement of the skeleton at multiple sites. The neoplastic plasma cells produce excess immunoglobulins (Igs) and Bence Jones proteins are characteristically present in the urine. Multiple pathogenic mechanisms contribute to renal injury/failure in multiple myeloma, which include abnormal protein precipitation in renal tubules, secondary to nephrotoxic monoclonal Ig and independent of paraprotein deposition. Myeloma kidney or cast nephropathy is a form of monoclonal Ig-mediated kidney disease. The mechanism of renal injury in myeloma and plasm cell dyscrasias can be broadly classified into monoclonal Ig-dependent and independent **(Table 5)**.[40]

Nausea, vomiting, anorexia, weight loss, and progressive weakness are the presenting features. Nephrocalcinosis resulting from hypercalcemia, uric acid calculi, renal infections, and amyloidosis may further complicate the illness.

Imaging Features

Imaging features are nonspecific and depends on the mechanism of renal injury. The most frequently reported renal manifestation at imaging are perinephric nodules and masses, however, can also present as focal renal masses. Positron emission tomography (PET) CT can demonstrate diffuse medullary and extramedullary (including kidneys) manifestations. Active myeloma lesions show intense FDG (fluorodeoxyglucose) activity unlike renal cell carcinomas (mild FDG activity), which helps to distinguish. Due to Ig-independent mechanism of involvement in certain cases, it may present as medical renal disease on imaging, and ultrasonography shows nephromegaly with reduced cortical echotexture initially, followed by increased cortical echogenicity, progressive loss of CMD, and renal atrophy in later stages.[41] Injection of iodinated contrast media is hazardous in patients of multiple myeloma as it precipitates myeloma proteins in the renal tubules. Dehydration has to be avoided to reduce the risk of complications.

Table 5: Mechanism of renal injury in myeloma and plasma cell dyscrasias.[40]

Mechanism	*Details*
Ig-dependent mechanisms	
Cast nephropathy (known traditionally as myeloma kidney)	Risk factors include light chain myeloma with >10 g/day monoclonal Ig excretion, volume depletion, sepsis, and medications (see below); Ig deposition is primarily in the tubules
Monoclonal Ig deposition disease	Systemic syndrome may be present; Ig deposition can be in the tubules or glomeruli but generally not both
Light chain amyloidosis (AL)	Often associated with nephrotic-range albuminuria and λ-light chains; systemic syndrome may be present, and amyloid deposition is primarily in the glomeruli
GN	Membranoproliferative, diffuse proliferative, crescentic, and cryoglobulinemic all recognized
Tubulointerstitial nephritis	May also result from non-Ig mechanisms
Thrombotic microangiopathy (TMA)	Paraprotein causes endothelial injury with resulting TMA
Hyperviscosity syndrome	More common in cases of IgA, IgG3, or IgM myeloma
Ig-independent mechanisms	
Volume depletion	Can cause prerenal azotemia and acute tubular necrosis and/or contribute to cast nephropathy
Sepsis	
Hypercalcemia	Can cause AKI directly or contribute to cast nephropathy
Tumor lysis syndrome	Uric acid or phosphate nephropathy
Direct parenchymal invasion by plasma cells	Rare cause; associated with advanced or aggressive myeloma
Pyelonephritis	Rare cause; multifactorial from immunodeficiency and deficient Ig and chemotherapy from myeloma

(Ig: immunoglobulin; GN: glomerulonephritis; AKI: acute kidney injury)

Paroxysmal Nocturnal Hemoglobinuria

Paroxysmal Nocturnal Hemoglobinuria (PNH) is a very rare, acquired hematopoietic stem cell disorder caused by an increased sensitivity to complement, resulting in intravascular hemolysis. The complement-mediated erythrocyte damage results in hemolysis with release of hemoglobin in plasma, which passes through glomeruli and reabsorbed in the proximal tubules, and stored as hemosiderin. This can result in chronic renal failure due to repeated episodes of microvascular thrombosis and tubular damage from hemosiderin deposition. Hemolysis is precipitated by infections, drugs immunization, and exercise. Patient presents with hemoglobinuria, iron deficiency anemia, and venous thrombosis.

Imaging Features

Noncontrast computed tomography may show high density of renal cortex due to hemosiderin pigments. Paramagnetic effects of hemosiderin results in markedly reduced signal in the cortex in both T1W and T2W images. Changes are more pronounced on T2W sequences with signal intensity of the renal cortex lower than that of the medulla, causing reversed CMD. Similar imaging features are seen in intravascular hemolysis like in malfunctioning prosthetic valves, sickle cell anemia, hereditary spherocytosis, and thalassemia.[42]

Chronic Renal Parenchymal Disease

In contrast to the capacity of kidney to regain back its function following acute renal insult, renal injury of more prolonged nature often leads to progressive and irreversible loss of nephrons. Such reduction in renal mass subsequently results in bilaterally small smooth kidneys. The uremic kidney shrinks globally reflecting the inherent tissue loss. Renal contour may be smooth or irregular. The echogenicity can be normal or increased. Radiological features, like those in acute renal parenchymal disease are overlapping in most of the causes of chronic renal parenchymal disease. However, some conditions show interesting radiological appearances and are discussed here. The various causes of bilateral small smooth kidneys are listed in **Flowchart 2**, the conditions leading to morphologically small, unilateral kidneys are also cited.[4] **Figures 10 to 13** show imaging in cases of chronic renal failure.

Renal Papillary Necrosis

Renal papillary necrosis is not a specific clinical entity, rather it is a manifestation of multiple renal pathological conditions resulting in prolonged sustained hypoxic injury to the medulla. Necroses of the renal papillae not only have many causes but also many radiological forms. Parenchymal diseases affecting the papillae and calyces are diagnosed on urography. In mild cases, the kidney size and function are normal, and the abnormality is limited to the papillae only. In advanced disease, there is global shrinkage of kidney with impaired renal function. Most common cause of renal papillary necrosis is analgesic abuse nephropathy. Other causes are diabetes, sickle cell nephropathy, obstruction with infection, renal vein thrombosis, dehydration, and prolonged hypotension.[5] (Pneumonic to remember causes of renal papillary necrosis—ADIPOSE: Analgesic nephropathy, diabetes, infant in shock, pyelonephritis, obstruction, sickle cell disease, and ethanol). In early papillary necrosis, ischemia occurs in the renal papillae due to compression of the medullary vessels by inflammatory changes in the interstitium. If the phase of temporary spasm passes, normal circulation is restored and the involved tissues may recover. However, if ischemia continues and perfusion is not restored, irreversible coagulation necrosis, tubular fibrosis, and lobar infarcts result.

Urographic findings during this period of early ischemic change are usually normal. On multidetector computed tomography, the ischemic changes that lead to renal papillary necrosis can be demonstrated best on nephrographic phase as small, poorly marginated areas of diminished enhancement at the tip of the medullary pyramid.

In advanced stage of necrosis, clefts originate from the fornices and extend to the medullary pyramids and papillae, ultimately causing the papillae to slough **(Fig. 14)**.

Flowchart 2: Causes of small kidney.

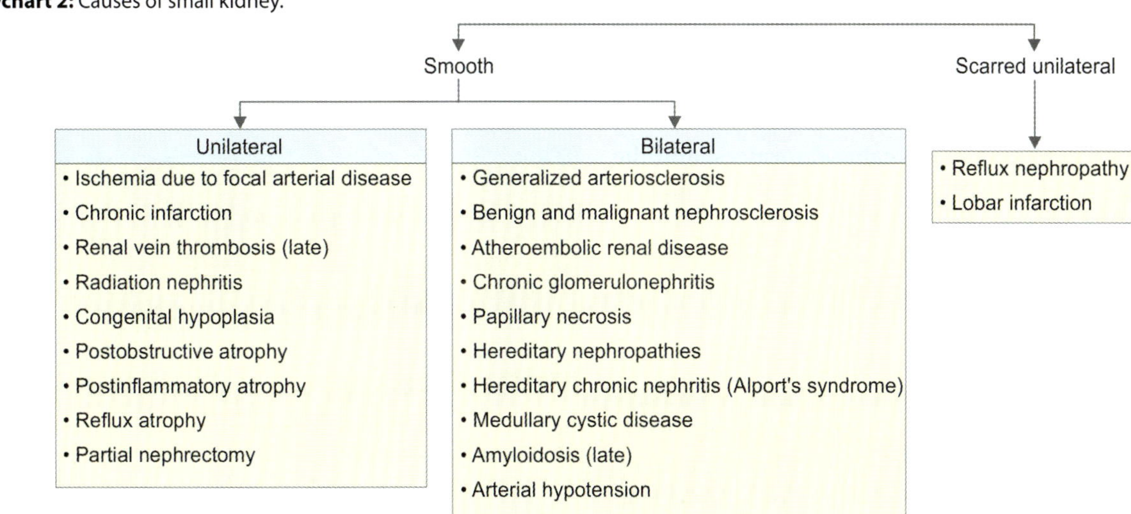

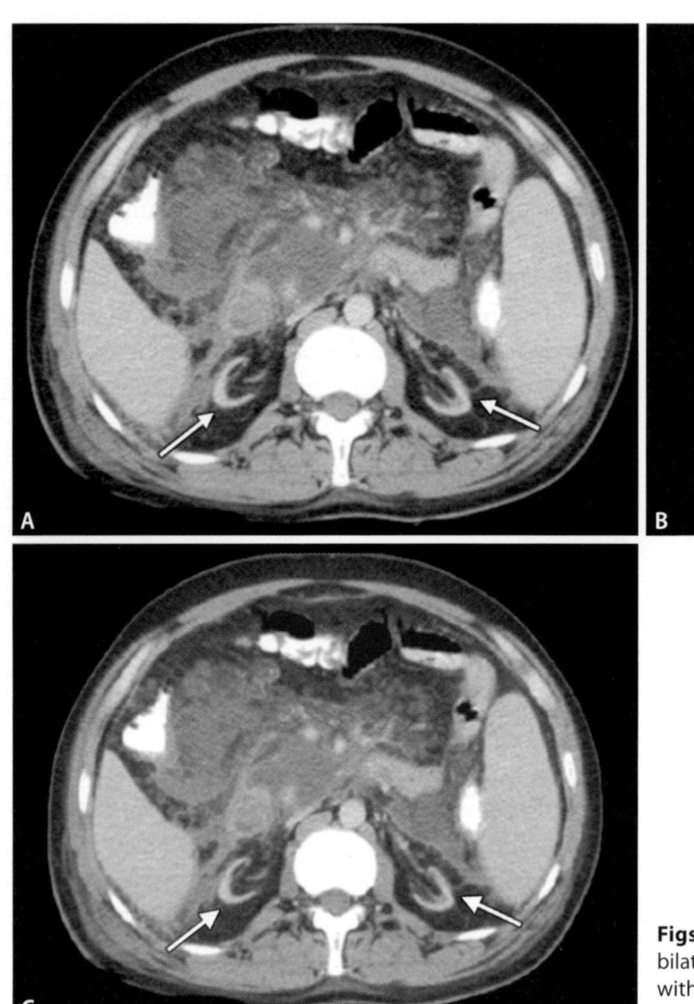

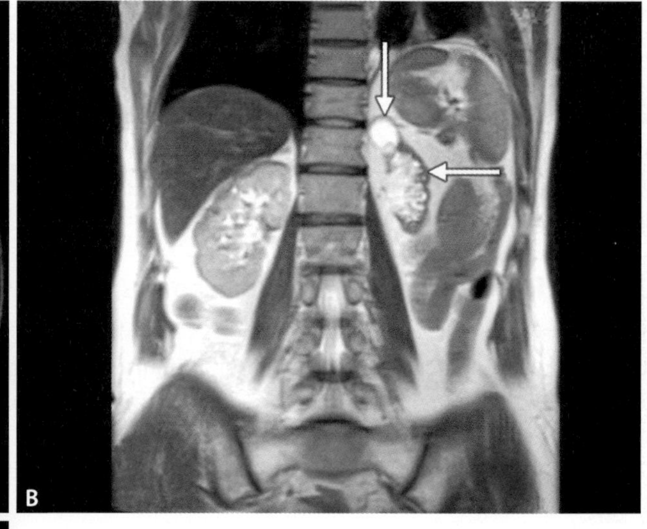

Figs. 10A to C: End-stage renal disease. CECT axial image shows bilateral smooth shrunken kidneys in a patient of chronic renal failure with pancreatitis. Peripancreatic inflammatory fluid collections are also present.

Caliceal deformities in renal papillary necrosis occur in three forms:

1. *Medullary*: Central necrosis takes place at the tip of the pyramid. Detachment of necrotic papillae starts in the central part of the calix, opening into a round or oval cavity.
2. *Papillary*: Detachment of necrotic papillae usually begins in the region of the caliceal fornices, and the resulting defect is triangular in shape also termed as lobster claw appearance.
3. *In situ*: When papillae fail to separate (necrosis *in situ*) calyces appear normal, they later calcify to give appearance of nephrocalcinosis.

In the healing phase, the papilla may epithelialize, and its tip takes a blunted appearance. In addition, shrinkage of the kidney may occur with reduction of parenchymal thickness. This is the common sequel of renal papillary necrosis. Moreover, the loss of renal cortex is associated hypertrophy of the renal columns resulting in a typical

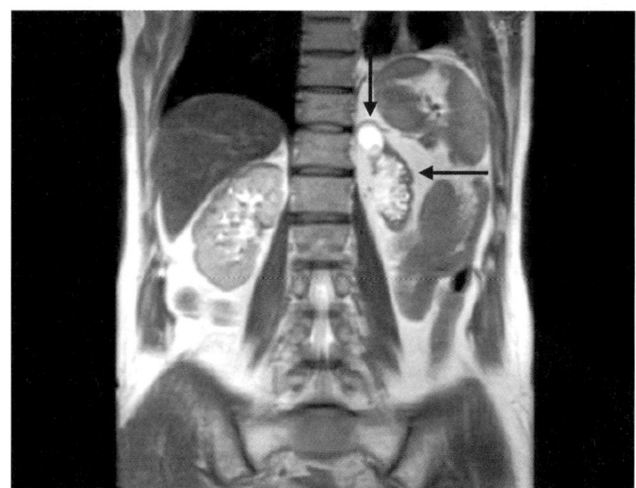

Fig. 11: Unilateral small smooth kidney. T2-weighted coronal MR image reveals small, contracted left kidney with thinned renal parenchyma and indistinct corticomedullary differentiation, subsequent to left renal artery stenosis (arrow). Note made of simple cortical renal cyst in left upper pole (short arrow).

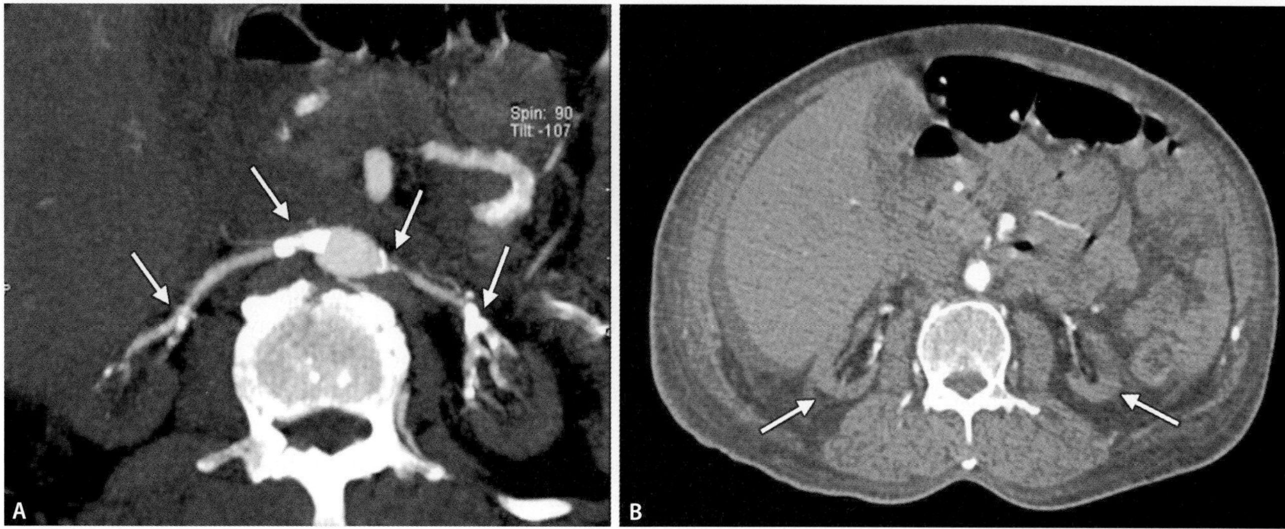

Figs. 12A and B: Bilateral small smooth kidneys. CT angiography (A) shows calcified atherothrombotic plaques involving both main renal arteries and their ostia (B) smooth globally shrunken kidneys, in a patient of severe bilateral renal artery stenosis. Mild perihepatic fluid is seen.

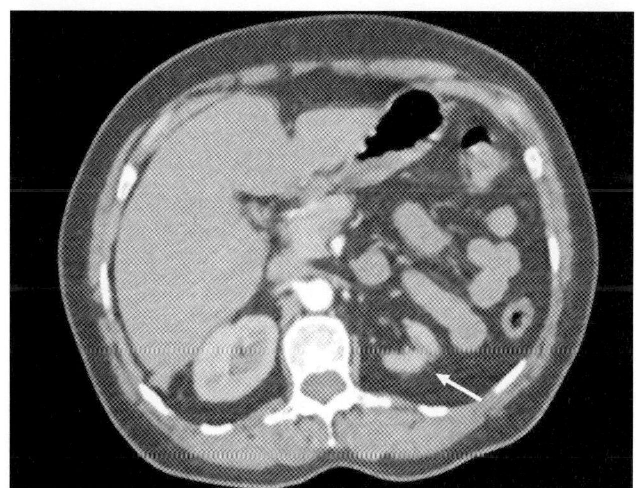

Fig. 13: Unilateral small scarred kidney. CECT axial image in cortical phase of enhancement shows small left kidney with irregular outline with parenchymal defect at interpolar region.

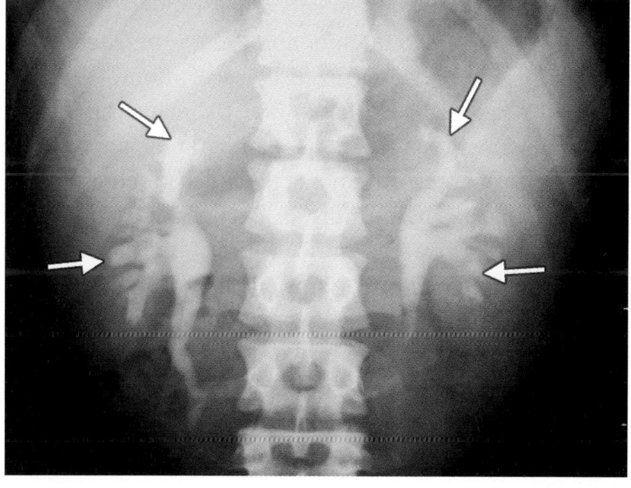

Fig. 14: Renal papillary necrosis. Intravenous urogram film showing irregular and distorted calyces of both kidneys, with contrast excavation and formation of multiple cavities. Few amputated calyces are also seen.

irregular wavy renal outline.[43] In advanced disease, after the sloughing of necrotic papillae, cavities are seen that are continuous with calyces in renal medullary areas. Their differentiation with other cystic lesions in the renal medullae should be done (like hydronephrosis, congenital megacalyces, parapelvic cysts, and caliceal diverticula).[44]

Benign and Malignant Nephrosclerosis

Nephrosclerosis affects the renal arterioles. The disease courses over many years but it rarely leads to kidney failure on its own. Malignant nephrosclerosis, however, progresses very rapidly and damages the arteries. These damaged arteries are unable to provide enough oxygen to the kidney tissues, resulting in kidney failure. The incidence of hypertensive nephrosclerosis increases with advancing age.[45]

Imaging Features

Kidneys are small and smooth in benign nephrosclerosis; occasionally shallow infarcts can be seen. Normal nephrographic opacification, and excretion into pelvicalyceal system is seen on urography.

On ultrasonography, increased central sinus echogenicity due to fat deposition may be seen. Subcapsular and perirenal hemorrhages may be detected as hypoechoic or anechoic fluid collections. High density fluid (blood) can be better detected on noncontrast CT scan. Blood degradation product may also be identified on MRI.[46]

Renal Osteodystrophy

Renal osteodystrophy is complex musculoskeletal abnormalities seen in patients with CKD. The primary radiologic bone changes reflect:

- *Deficiency in active form of vitamin D due to impaired renal function:* Rickets.
- *Impaired clearance of calcium leading to increased parathormone secretion:* Secondary hyperparathyroidism.

The spectrum consists of secondary hyperparathyroidism along with rickets, osteomalacia, osteosclerosis, and osteoporosis.

Inability of the kidney to adequately excrete phosphate, leads to hyperphosphatemia and increased osteoclastic activity. It can be categorized by resorption of bone at subperiosteal, cortical, subchondral, trabecular, endosteal, and subligamentous locations. Radiographic appearance of subperiosteal resorption has been described as a lace-like irregularity of the normal cortical margin, which may progress to areas of scalloping and spiculation. The earliest involvement is often seen along the radial aspects of the middle phalanges of the index and middle fingers, beginning in the proximal metaphyseal region. The terminal tufts may also demonstrate subperiosteal resorption **(Fig. 15)**. Additional sites of subperiosteal bone resorption include the upper medial tibia, humerus, and femur; superior and inferior ribs; and lamina dura.

Loss of trabecular sharpness occurs with trabecular resorption. This is well seen in the skull, described as a granular salt-and-pepper appearance, with loss of distinction between the inner and outer tables. Common sites of subchondral resorption are the distal clavicle and acromioclavicular joint, sacroiliac joint, sternoclavicular joint, symphysis pubis, and posterior patella **(Figs. 16A and B)**.[14] Osseous resorption may also occur at sites of ligamentous and tendinous attachments. Brown tumors are rare.

Osteosclerosis has a strong predilection for the axial skeleton, where cancellous bone predominates over cortical bone. In the vertebral bodies, band-like areas of

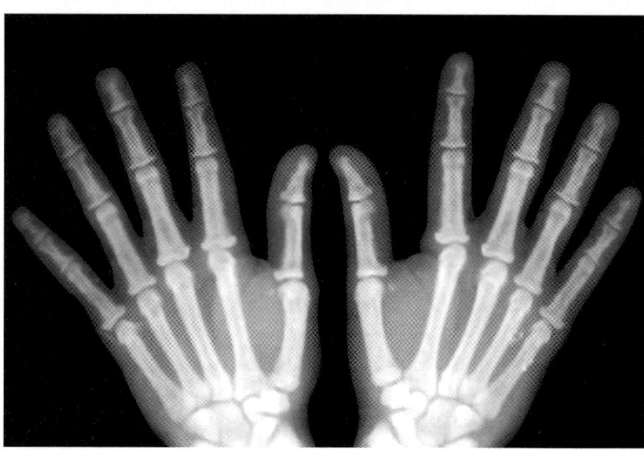

Fig. 15: Radiographs of hands in a patient of hyperparathyroidism in renal osteotrophy. Characteristic subperiosteal resorption phalanges including terminal tufts is seen. Subchondral and intracortical resorptions are also seen.

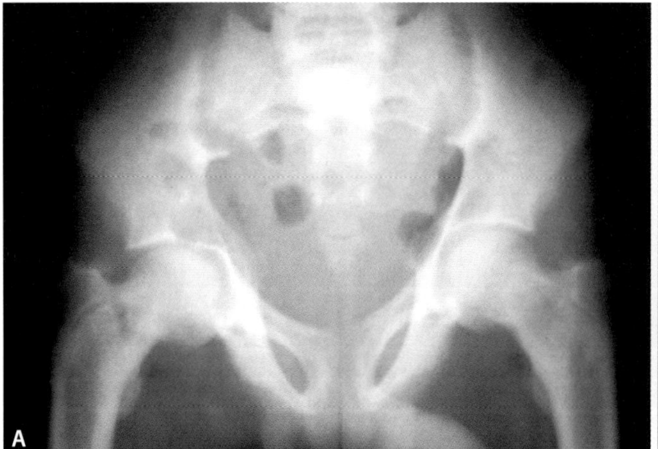

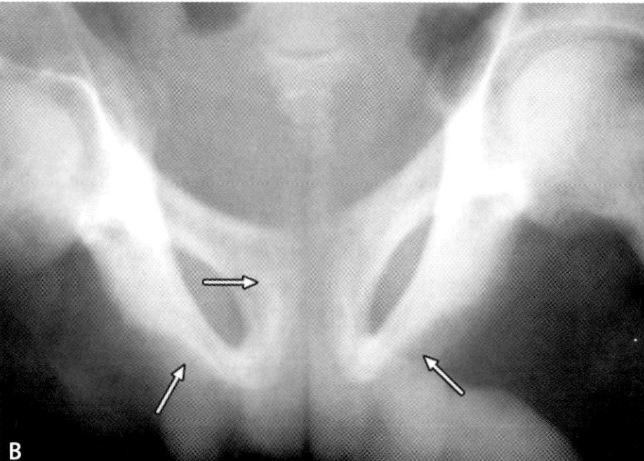

Figs. 16A and B: Renal osteodystrophy in a patient of tuberculosis. Anteroposterior view of pelvis shows osteopenic triradiate pelvis. Subchondral resorption of bone is seen at the pubis symphysis, ischial tuberosities, and sacroiliac joint (arrows).

sclerosis involving the superior and inferior end plates with intervening normal osseous density are classically seen, which resemble the stripes on rugby jerseys called as rugger jersey spine.

Changes of rickets can be seen in children with a general delay in bone age, bowing of long bones, scoliosis, diffuse concave impressions at multiple vertebral end plates, basilar invagination of the skull, "triradiate pelvis" deformity, and rachitic rosary. In children, epiphyseal displacement (slipped epiphysis) in children is also seen. Osteomalacia in adults may manifest as looser zones. Metastatic soft tissue and vascular calcification can be seen in ocular tissues, arteries, subcutaneous and periarticular soft tissues, and viscera.[47]

CONCLUSION

Imaging and management of medical renal diseases and renal failure continues to evolve with the advances in anatomical and functional imaging. Despite these achievements radiological imaging still has limitations in evaluation of renal parenchymal disease and renal failure. Radiological imaging techniques are rapidly expanding and are expected to grow even further, predominantly in advanced MRI. The future possibly holds improved methods to readily identify the causes of reversible acute renal failure and plan treatment strategies to combat chronic renal failure. The combination of better diagnostic methods and management strategies will lead to improved quality of life in patients with renal failure.

REFERENCES

1. Mehta RL, Kellum JA, Shah SV, et al. Acute Kidney Injury Network: report of an initiative to improve outcomes in acute kidney injury. Crit Care. 2007;11:R31.
2. Choyke PL, Zeiessman HA. Imaging of renal failure. In: Pollack HM, McClennan BL (Eds). Clinical Urography, 2nd edition. Philadelphia, PA: WB Saunders; 2000. pp. 3029-31.
3. National Kidney Foundation: K/DOQ1 Clinical practice guidelines for chronic kidney diseases: evaluation, classification, stratification. Am J Kidney Dis. 2002;39(1):S1-266.
4. Friedenberg RM, Dunbar JS. Excretory urography. In: Pollack HM, McClennan BL (Eds). Clinical Urography, 1st edition, Philadelphia, PA: WB Saunders; 1990. pp. 2264-76, 100-245.
5. Davidson AJ, Hartman DS. A systemic approach to Radiological Diagnosis of Renal Parenchymal Disease. In: Davidson AJ, Hartman DS (Eds). Radiology of Kidney and Urinary Tract, 2nd edition. Philadelphia, PA: WB Saunders; 1990. pp. 101-243.
6. Kim SH, Kim B. Renal Parenchymal Disease. In: Pollack HM, McClennan BL (Eds), Clinical Urography, 2nd edition. Philadelphia, PA: WB Saunders; 2000. pp. 2654-84.
7. Fry IK, Cattell WR. The nephrographic pattern during excretion urography. Br Med Bull. 1972;28:227-32.
8. Ritche WW, Vick CW, Glocheski SK, et al. Evaluation of azotemic patients: diagnostic yield of initial US examination. Radiology. 1998;167:245-7.
9. Hungtington DK, Hill SC, Hill MC. Sonographic manifestations of medical renal disease. Semin Ultrasound CT MR. 1991;12:290-307.
10. Manley JA, O'Neill C. How echogenic is echogenic? Quantitative acoustics of the renal cortex. Am J Kidney Dis. 2001;37:706-11.
11. Yasa NA, Peng M, Ralls PW. Perirenal lucency ('Kidney sweat'): A new sign of renal failure. AJR. 1999;173:1075-9.
12. Platt JF, Ellis JH, Rubin JM, et al. Intrarenal arterial Doppler sonography in patients with non-obstructive renal disease: correlation of resistive index with biopsy findings. AJR. 1990;157:1223-7.
13. Mitterberger M, Pinggera GM, Colleselli D, et al. Acute pyelonephritis: comparison of diagnosis with computed tomography and contrast enhanced ultrasonography. BJU Int. 2007;101(3):341-4.
14. Saunder HS, Dyer BB, Shifrin RY, et al. The CT nephrogram: implications of evaluation of urinary tract disease. Radiographics. 1995;15:1069-95.
15. Chung JJ, Semelka RC, Martin DR. Acute renal failure: common occurrences of preservation of corticomedullary differentiation on MR images. Magn Reson Imaging. 2001;19:789-93.
16. Caroli A, Schneider M, Friedli I, et al. Diffusion-weighted magnetic resonance imaging to assess diffuse renal pathology: a systematic review and statement paper. Nephrol Dial Transplant. 2018;33(Suppl 2):ii29-40.
17. Saini S, Kumar V, Koteshwara P, et al. Role of diffusion tensor imaging in renal parenchymal changes. Indian J Radiol Imaging. 2018;28(2):175-81.
18. Odudu A, Nery F, Harteveld AA, et al. Arterial spin labelling MRI to measure renal perfusion: a systematic review and statement paper. Nephrol Dial Transplant. 2018;33(Suppl 2):ii15-21.
19. Abrams HA, Grassi CJ. Renal angiography in hypertension. In: Baums (Ed). Abrams Angiography: Vascular and Interventional Radiology, 4th edition. Boston: Little, Brown and Company; 1997. pp. 1244-89.
20. Maisey M, Briton KE. Nuclear Imaging in Nephrology. In: Davidson AM, Cameron JS, Grunfeld JP, et al. In: Oxford Textbook of Clinical Nephrology, 2nd edition. Oxford: Oxford University Press; 1998. pp. 137-50.
21. Barrett BJ, Cariske EJ. Meta-analysis of relative nephrotoxicity of high- and low-osmolality iodinated contrast media. Radiology. 1993;188:171-8.
22. Fliser D, Laville M, Covic A, et al; Ad-hoc working group of ERBP. A European Renal Best Practice (ERBP) position statement on the Kidney Disease Improving Global Outcomes (KDIGO) clinical practice guidelines on acute kidney injury: part 1: definitions, conservative management and contrast-induced nephropathy. Nephrol Dial Transplant. 2012;27(12):4263-72.
23. Lewington A, Kanagasundaram S. Renal association clinical practice guidelines on acute kidney injury. Nephron Clin Pract. 2011;118(Suppl 1):c349-90.
24. Mehta RL, Pascual MT, Soroko S, et al. Spectrum of acute renal failure in the intensive care unit: the PICARD experience. Kidney Int. 2004;66(4):1613-21.
25. Verghese E, Ricardo SD, Weidenfeld R, et al. Renal primary cilia lengthen after acute tubular necrosis. J Am Soc Nephrol. 2009;20(10):2147-53.

26. Rosenfeld AT, Zeman RK, Cicchetti DV, et al. Experimental acute tubular necrosis: US appearance. Radiology. 1985;157:771-4.
27. Platt JH, Rubin JH, Ellis JH. Acute renal failure: Possible role of duplex Doppler US in distinction between acute pre-renal failure and acute tubular necrosis. Radiology. 1991;179: 419-23.
28. Izumi M, Sugiura T, Nakamura H, et al. Differential diagnosis of prerenal azotemia from acute tubular necrosis and prediction of recovery by Doppler ultrasound. Am J Kidney Dis. 2000;35(4):713-9.
29. Han F, Xiao W, Xu Y, et al. The significance of BOLD MRI in differentiation between renal transplant rejection and acute tubular necrosis. Nephrol Dial Transplant. 2008;23: 2666-72.
30. Gormsen H, Iverson P, Raaschou I. Kidney biopsy in acute anuria: with case of acute, bilateral cortical necrosis. Am J Med. 1955;19:209-11.
31. Jordan J, Low R, Jeffrey RB Jr. CT findings in acute renal cortical necrosis. J Comput Assist Tomogr. 1990;14:155-6.
32. Wang MT, Wu RH, Chen JC. CT findings of acute renal cortical necrosis. Chin J Radiol. 2007;32:103-6.
33. Hnn L, Pfister RC. Renal subcapsular rim sign: new etiologies and pathogenesis. AJR. 1982;138:51-4.
34. Jeong JY, Kim SH, Lee HJ, et al. Atypical low-signal intensity renal parenchyma: causes and patterns. Radiographics. 2002;22:833-46.
35. Ten RM, Torres VE, Milliner DS, et al. Acute interstitial nephritis: immunologic and clinical aspects. Mayo Clin Proc. 1988;63:921-30.
36. Davidson AJ, Hartman DS. Diagnostic set: Large smooth, bilateral. In: Davidson AJ, Hartman DS (Eds), Radiology of Kidney and Urinary Tract, 2nd edition. Philadelphia, PA: WB Saunders; 1990. pp. 157-86.
37. Sipe JD, Cohen AS. Amyloidosis. In: Fauci AS, Braunwald E, Isselbacher KJ, et al. (Eds). Harrison's Principle of Internal Medicine. New York: McGraw-Hill; 1998. pp. 1856-60.
38. Cohen AS: Amyloidosis. In: Pertersdrof RG, Adams RD, Braunwald E, et al. (Eds). Harrison's Principle of Internal Medicine. New York: McGraw-Hill; 1983. pp. 368-71.
39. Amendola RA. Amyloidosis of the urinary tract. In Pollack HM (Ed). Clinical Urography: An Atlas and Textbook of Urologic Imaging, Philadelphia, PA: WB Saunders; 1990. pp. 2493-500.
40. Heher EC, Rennke HG, Laubach JP, et al. Kidney disease and multiple myeloma. Clin J Am Soc Nephrol. 2013;8(11):2007-17.
41. Andrei SP, Antonio CW, Erick MR, et al. Imaging manifestations of hematologic diseases with renal and perinephric involvement. radiographics. 2016;36:1038-54.
42. Kim SH, Han MC, Lee JS, et al. Paroxysmal nocturnal hemoglobinuria: case report of MRI and CT findings. Acta Radiol. 1991;32:315-6.
43. Jung DC, Kim SH, Jung S, et al. Renal papillary necrosis: review and comparison of findings at multi-detector row CT and intravenous urography. Radiographics. 2006;26:1827-36.
44. Davidson A. Chronic renal failure. In: Pollack HM, McClennan BL (Eds). Clinical Urography, 1st edition. Philadelphia, PA: WB Saunders; 1990. pp. 2279-90.
45. Davidson AJ, Hartman DS. Diagnostic set: Small, Smooth, bilateral. In Davidson AJ, Hartman DS (Eds). Radiology of Kidney and Urinary Tract, 2nd edition. Philadelphia, PA: WB Saunders; 1990. pp. 135-86.
46. Ono H, Ono Y. Nephrosclerosis and hypertension. Med Clin North Am. 1997;81(6):1273-88.
47. Murphey MD, Sartoris D, Quale JL, et al. Musculoskeletal manifestations of chronic renal insufficiency. Radiographics. 1993;13:357-79.

Chapter 5

Nontubercular Infections of the Urinary Tract

Ujjwal Gorsi, Naveen Kalra, Ajay Kumar

INTRODUCTION

Nontubercular renal infections can be divided into acute and chronic infections. They can also be divided into uncomplicated and complicated subtypes. The infections which are not associated with permanent damage are usually referred to as uncomplicated pyelonephritis.

Common acute renal infections are acute pyelonephritis and its various complications, renal abscess, and emphysematous pyelonephritis (EPN). Chronic renal infections encountered include chronic pyelonephritis and xanthogranulomatous pyelonephritis (XGPN). In addition, various fungal and parasitic infections can also affect kidneys. Various etiologies of nontubercular renal infections are listed in **Table 1**. Spectrum of renal infections will be discussed in this chapter. Infections affecting the ureters and urinary bladder are dealt with in subsequent chapters.

The diagnosis of urinary tract infection (UTI) is based on typical clinical features and laboratory findings and usually does not warrant radiological imaging in suspected uncomplicated cases.[1-3] Indications of imaging in suspected cases of UTI include unusual severe symptoms, high-risk patients (elderly, diabetics, or immunocompromised), patient not responding to intravenous antibiotics within 72 hours and episodes of multiple repeated infections. The objectives of imaging in renal infections are: (1) to detect the conditions that must be cured immediately to preserve renal function and to avoid septic complications, e.g. pyonephrosis, EPN, and abscesses; (2) to search for primary etiological cause of UTI, i.e. calculus, obstruction, vesicoureteral reflux (VUR), and cyst infection.[1,2]

Table 1: Types of nontubercular renal infections.

Acute infections	*Chronic infections*	*Others infections*
Acute pyelonephritis	Chronic pyelonephritis	Fungal
Acute focal bacterial nephritis	Reflux nephropathy	Parasitic
Renal, perirenal, and pararenal abscess	Xanthogranulomatous pyelonephritis	HIV-associated nephropathy
Emphysematous pyelonephritis	Malacoplakia	
Pyonephrosis		

(HIV: human immunodeficiency virus)

With the availability of ultrasonography (USG), computed tomography (CT), magnetic resonance imaging (MRI), and advances in nuclear medicine and interventional radiology, diagnosis, and management of the renal and perirenal infections have undergone sea changes. USG and CT are most common radiological modalities used in suspected renal infections with ever-decreasing role of once indispensable plain radiograph and intravenous urography (IVU).

IMAGING MODALITIES

Ultrasonography is a sensitive modality in detecting hydronephrosis and can detect underlying stones and obstruction. USG has 98% sensitivity in detection of hydronephrosis.[4] Echogenic debris in hydronephrotic kidney suggest pyonephrosis. Renal abscess and extrarenal fluid collections are easily detected. Sonography is however less sensitive than CT in detecting the subtle changes of inflamed parenchyma, microabscesses, and small calculi. Accuracy of USG can be improved with addition of ultrasound contrast agents (UCAs). US contrast agents are of particular value in patients of renal failure in whom use of iodine-based and gadolinium-based contrast media may be hazardous.[5] USG is radiation free, relatively inexpensive, easily available, and can diagnose many of abnormalities affecting genitourinary system that require specific treatment. It is also commonly used guiding modality for various interventional procedures such as nephrostomy or cyst aspiration.

Plain X-ray may provide diagnostic information such as presence of abnormal gas collection in the renal or perirenal area in patients with EPN and renal abscess or staghorn calculus in a patient suspected to have pyonephrosis. IVU has a limited role and can exclude congenital anomalies, which are important risk factors in patients of recurrent UTIs. Certain conditions such as papillary necrosis and early tuberculosis may still be diagnosed with confidence on IVU.[6]

Contrast-enhanced computed tomography (CECT) is the gold standard for accurate diagnosis of suspected renal infections in which imaging is being contemplated. It can detect anatomic or physiologic factors associated with complicated UTI as well as delineate disease extent accurately. CT without contrast can demonstrate stones, air, hemorrhage, obstruction, and occasionally abscesses.[7] Contrast is needed to demonstrate alterations in renal perfusion, which may be subtle and become evident only after contrast administration.

Magnetic resonance imaging is being increasingly used as an effective modality for both medical and surgical diseases of kidney especially in pregnant women, children, and in diabetics. MRI may demonstrate infected regions of the renal parenchyma to enhance abnormally and to have restricted diffusion and can demonstrate obstruction and abscesses but often fails to reveal small stones. The cost and limited availability precludes its routine use, although it may provide information similar to CT.

Radionuclide studies with cortical scintigraphy agents such as ^{99m}Tc dimercaptosuccinic acid (DMSA) and glucoheptonate have been shown to be the most sensitive techniques for the diagnosis of acute pyelonephritis and detection of the renal scars in reflux nephropathy.[8]

ACUTE PYELONEPHRITIS

Acute pyelonephritis occurs when there is inflammation affecting the collecting system and the renal interstitium. Bacterial organisms such as *Escherichia coli*, *Proteus mirabilis*, and *Klebsiella pneumoniae* are the usual culprits when transmission of infection occurs by the ascending route. Hematogenous infections occur especially in drug addicts and patients with endocarditis. They are usually staphylococcal in origin. Fungal or viral infections may also be encountered. Predisposing factors for acute pyelonephritis are: obstruction, prolonged catheter drainage, reflux, congenital anomalies, pregnancy, and diabetes. 90% of UTIs occur as a single episode where as 10% are recurrent.[3] Pyelonephritis affects sexually active women commonly and a peak is also noticed in men over 60 years as a consequence of prostatic hyperplasia and resultant stasis of urine.[3]

Pathology

The affected kidney is usually increased in size due to edema. Multiple foci of inflammation, which are characteristically patchy and may lead to microabscesses, are noticed. These focal areas of inflammation usually resolve completely without any sequelae with treatment but in the presence of risk factors such as diabetes or immunocompromised status and inadequate treatment, bacterial nephritis may result which may be focal or diffuse and may lead to renal and perirenal abscesses subsequently.

Radiology

Imaging is usually not required for uncomplicated cases of acute pyelonephritis. The role of IVU in acute pyelonephritis has rapidly diminished. Positive IVU findings will be seen only in 25% of acute pyelonephritis.[1,3] IVU may show renal enlargement with decreased, delayed, and persistent nephrogram. Attenuation of the calyces or minimal dilatation of pelvicalyceal system may also be seen on IVU.

Ultrasound may show enlargement of the kidney, which can be focal or diffuse. Changes in echogenicity may mirror underlying pathological changes. Affected kidney may show hypoechoic areas due to edema or hyperechoic areas due to hemorrhage. Loss of corticomedullary differentiation and loss of renal sinus fat may also be seen **(Fig. 1)**. Unfortunately, on routine gray-scale images, interstitial nephritis is not well characterized so it is not unusual to have negative results on USG in clinically suspected pyelonephritis cases. In one prospective study, USG could reveal abnormalities in only 24% of patients whereas other studies reported abnormalities in as low as 20% of patients.[9,10]

Doppler may help in assessing areas of reduced perfusion. Extent of hypoperfusion is defined better by Power Doppler as compared to Color Doppler. Newer

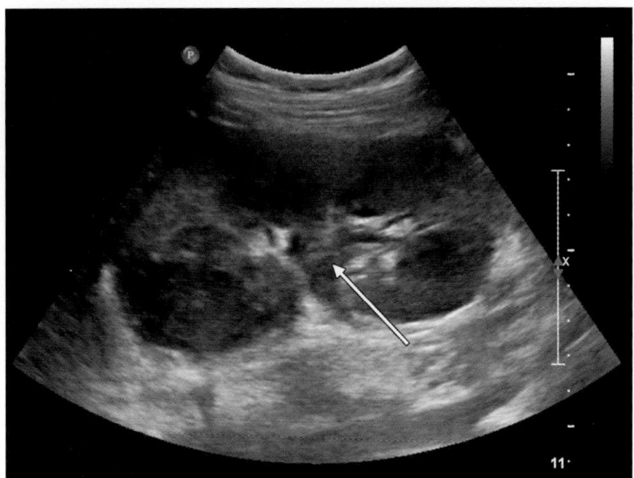

Fig. 1: *Acute pyelonephritis*: Grayscale longitudinal ultrasound scan shows diffusely enlarged kidney with heterogeneous echotexture. Both hypoechoic and hyperechoic areas are appreciated with loss of corticomedullary differentiation. Accompanying urothelial thickening (arrow) is also noticed.

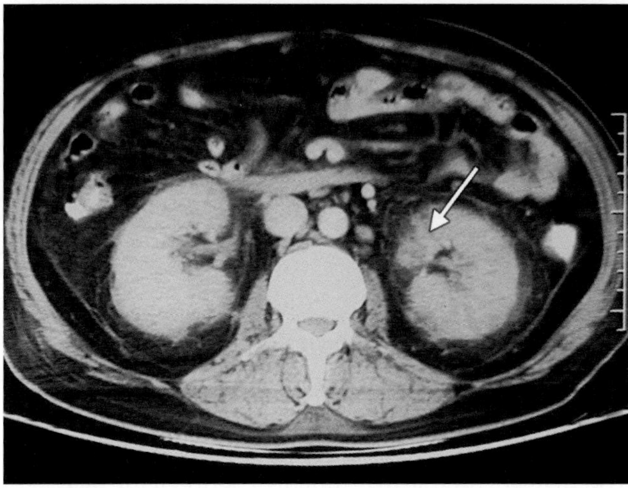

Fig. 2: *Bilateral acute pyelonephritis*: Contrast-enhanced computed tomography scan shows bilaterally enlarged kidneys with striated nephrogram (arrow). There is presence of perinephric stranding and thickening of Gerota's fascia and lateral conal fascia.

tools such as tissue harmonic imaging have improved sensitivities and specificities as high as 97% and 80%, respectively.[11] Areas of poor perfusion related to nephritis may be better demonstrated by US contrast agents.[5]

Multiphasic CECT is superior to both USG and IVU in demonstrating features of inflammation. The recommended phases of CT scan for evaluating renal infections are a noncontrast scan and a nephrographic phase at 50–90 seconds. Excretory phase at 2 minutes is usually acquired only if underlying obstruction is suspected.[3]

On noncontrast computed tomography (NCCT), affected areas may appear hypoattenuating as compared to normal parenchyma due to edema; less frequently, higher attenuation regions may be seen which are likely to represent hemorrhage.[12] However, it is not unusual to have nonenhanced CT images which appear completely normal. Features of acute bacterial nephritis may only be demonstrated after administration of contrast material.

Contrast-enhanced computed tomography may reveal wedge-shaped areas of decreased attenuation radiating from papilla to the cortex due to hypoperfusion in an enlarged kidney **(Fig. 2)**. The transverse areas of alternate bands with increased and decreased density may also be seen and are related to underlying pathophysiology of tubular obstruction caused by inflammatory debris within the lumen, interstitial edema, and vasospasm.[13] Flow of contrast through the tubule is reduced due to these three pathophysiologic disturbances. This tubular obstruction is also the cause of persistent delayed enhancement, which usually is seen 3–6 hours after contrast injection. The wedge-shaped defects, which originally show hypoattenuation during the nephrographic phase show hyperattenuation later due to prolonged accumulation and slow transit of injected contrast through tubules which are compromised.[14]

Diffuse homogeneous involvement of the renal parenchyma in acute pyelonephritis is unusual and is seen if there is ureteric obstruction.[15] Thickening of the walls of the collecting system, which sometimes is seen in renal infections, points toward pyelitis.[15] Antibiotic therapy can alter the CT appearance of pyelonephritis. A rounded or ovoid area of decreased enhancement, which has poorly defined margins, may be seen in patients who are partially treated with antibiotics and undergo CT scan.[15]

Computed tomography is also the best modality for complete evaluation of the secondary signs of renal infections and their complications. Perinephric stranding, thickening of Gerota's fascia, renal, and perirenal abscess formation are very well demonstrated on CT.[16]

Scintigraphic techniques are superior to US and IVU for the diagnosis of acute pyelonephritis.[9] Renal cortical scintigraphy with ^{99m}Tc DMSA will reveal wedge-shaped cortical defects which are characteristic of acute pyelonephritis.

On MRI, the affected regions will have low signal on T1-weighted images (T1WI) and high signal on T2-weighted images (T2WI). Loss of corticomedullary differentiation may also be appreciated. MRI features of pyelonephritis resemble those of CECT.[16] Affected areas show diffusion restriction, and diffusion-weighted (DW) images may be

Box 1: Findings in acute pyelonephritis.

- Diffuse (usually)/focal enlargement
- Striated kidney commonly seen in nephrographic phase
- Areas of increased attenuation in hemorrhagic bacterial nephritis
- Perinephric stranding
- Thickening of Gerota's fascia
- Focal involvement may mimic renal tumor

more sensitive than either T2WI or contrast-enhanced T1WI for detecting regions of pyelonephritis.[15] MRI may also help in differentiating acute infection from chronic scar in problematic cases. The potential pitfalls of MRI are in patients with gas-forming infections and calculi where MRI may not be able to distinguish between the two.[3]

Imaging findings of acute pyelonephritis are summarized in **Box 1**.

ACUTE FOCAL BACTERIAL NEPHRITIS

Acute focal bacterial nephritis (AFBN) is a rare interstitial nephritis, which presents with focal lesions in radiological studies.[17] First described in 1978 by Rosenfield et al,[18] it was earlier known as acute lobar nephronia.

Fever and flank pain are the leading symptoms usually accompanied by leukocytosis. US reveals hypoechoic poorly defined mass, which may be echogenic if there is hemorrhage.

Computed tomography shows focal hypoattenuating area with patchy enhancement. They can be wedge-shaped occasionally and hence difficult to differentiate from acute renal infarction. The cortical rim sign when seen on CECT and contrast-enhanced magnetic resonance imaging (CEMRI) may be useful in distinguishing acute pyelonephritis from a segmental renal infarct **(Fig. 3)**. In AFBN, areas of abnormal hypoenhancement, extends from centrally located medulla to the peripheral renal capsule typically involving a complete wedge of renal parenchyma. In segmental renal infarcts by contrast, wedge-shaped areas of abnormal renal hypoenhancement spare the outermost cortex. This happens due to the fact that outer aspect of the cortex is supplied by perforating branches of the renal capsular artery, which is an early branch of the renal artery.[18,19]

Perinephric fat stranding may also be seen. AFBN can be differentiated from renal abscess by the absence of peripheral contrast enhancement and nonliquefactive center.[18]

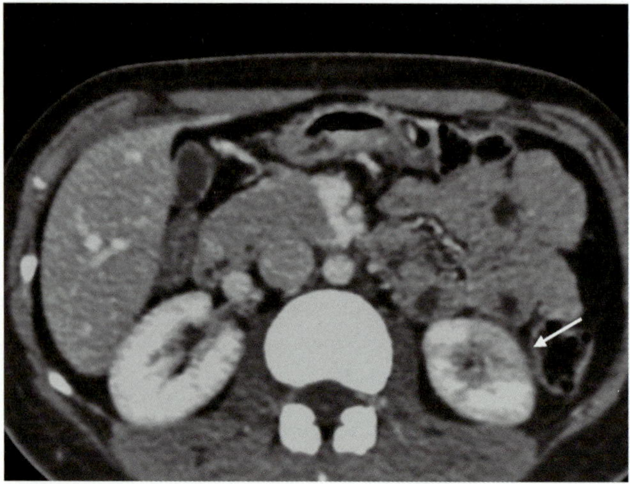

Fig. 3: Acute focal bacterial nephritis: Contrast-enhanced CT scan showing a focal wedge-shaped hypoenhancing area in left kidney reaching till renal capsule with absent cortical rim sign. Subtle perinephric stranding (arrow) is also seen.

RENAL AND PERIRENAL ABSCESSES

Renal and perirenal abscesses usually result as a complication of bacterial pyelonephritis. Other mechanisms that may lead to formation of renal and perirenal abscesses are hematogenous infection and superadded infection in a pre-existing renal cyst. In addition, inflammatory conditions of colon, pancreas, and retroperitoneum may extend into perinephric space.

Plain radiograph and IVU are rarely done in suspected renal and perirenal abscesses in present era of USG and CT. Plain radiograph may show enlarged kidney, rotation and enlargement of affected kidney, presence of mottled gas in renal fossa, and loss of outline of psoas muscle. Poorly or nonfunctioning kidney with calyceal attenuation and compression due to mass affect may be seen on IVU.

Ultrasonography may reveal a well-defined focal lesion with irregular shaggy margins, good sound transmission, and no internal flow **(Fig. 4A)**. Features of accompanying pyelonephritis may also be seen. Echogenic mobile debris within the lesion may help in reaching a correct diagnosis. Cysts with superadded infection or hemorrhage or necrotic tumors may mimic renal abscess on USG.

Computed tomography is the gold standard to assess the renal abscess as well as its extrarenal extent. Changes in the renal size, contour, parenchymal attenuation, enhancement pattern, and accompanying abnormalities such as thickening of the Gerota's fascia, retroperitoneal extension, and involvement of psoas muscle are very well demonstrated on CT. During the earlier course of renal abscess, poorly marginated nonenhancing area of decreased attenuation may be seen suggestive of evolving abscess. Surrounding area may show reduced enhancement due to edema. Later in the course of the disease, as renal abscess matures, it is seen as a well-marginated area of low

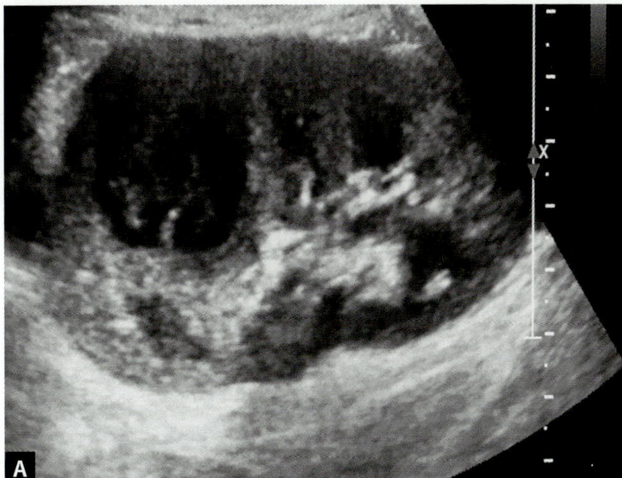

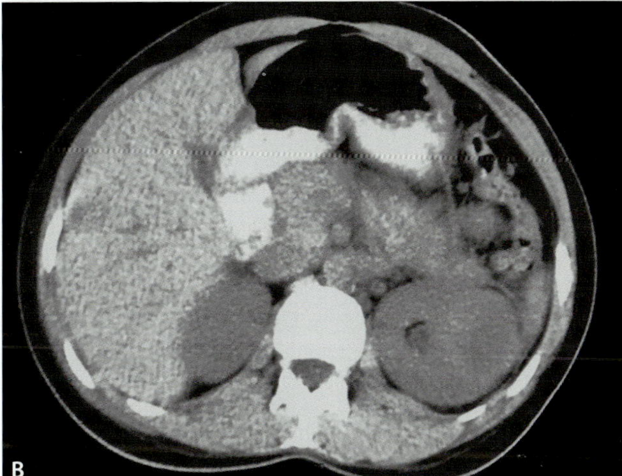

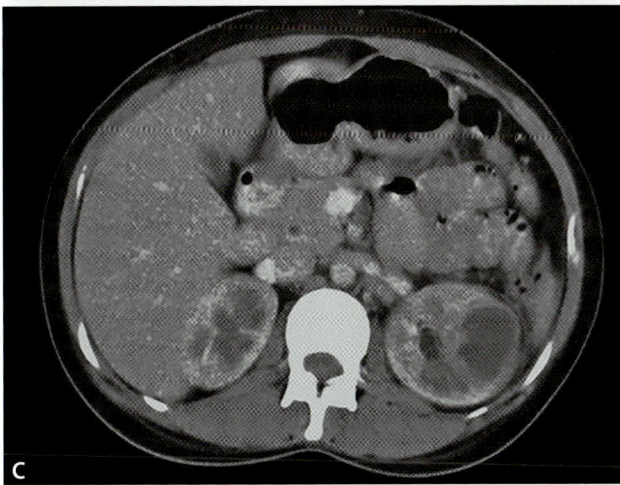

Figs. 4A to C: *Renal abscess*: (A) Longitudinal ultrasound scan of the left kidney shows a cystic lesion with internal debris and thick irregular shaggy margins; Noncontrast (B) and contrast-enhanced (C) CT scan of the same patient shows a well-defined hypodense lesion with peripheral contrast enhancement and perinephric inflammation.

attenuation due to central area of necrosis with a peripheral enhancing rim **(Figs. 4B and C)**. Septations are frequent in perinephric abscess, hence they are more difficult to drain as compared to renal abscess **(Fig. 5)**.

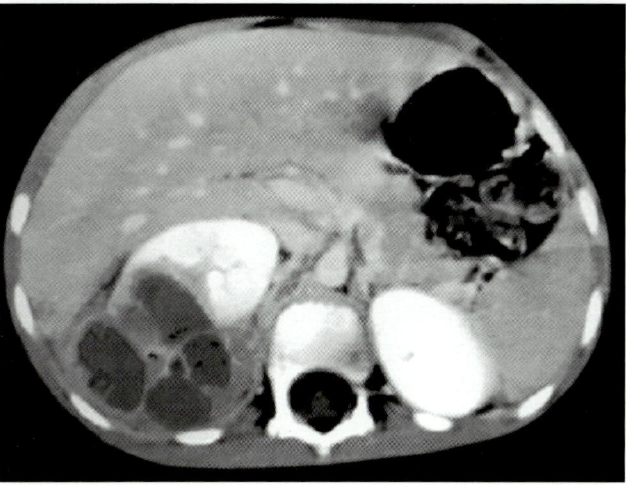

Fig. 5: Contrast-enhanced CT scan showing multiseptated hypodense lesion in the right kidney suggestive of renal abscess with extension into the perinephric space.

On MRI, a renal abscess is seen as a hypointense lesion on T1WI and a hyperintense lesion on T2WI. Diffusion restriction is seen in the central necrotic area and on contrast administration; the lesion shows peripheral rim-like enhancement **(Figs. 6A to F)**. Percutaneous drainage under USG/CT guidance has been successful in reducing mortality with a success rate of 85–95%.[20]

EMPHYSEMATOUS PYELONEPHRITIS

Emphysematous pyelonephritis is a rare but severe form of renal infection caused by gas-forming organisms. The most commonly causative organisms are *E. coli*, *K. pneumoniae* and *P. mirabilis*. Its radiological hallmark is presence of gas in the collecting system and/or renal parenchyma. Approximately 90% of patients have poorly controlled diabetes. Other predisposing factors include immunocompromised status or associated urinary tract obstruction secondary to calculus, sloughed papilla, or tumor. EPN progresses rapidly leading to fulminant sepsis. It is associated with high mortality in absence of prompt therapeutic intervention.[16,21]

Plain X-ray can reveal mottled gas in renal fossa in over 85% of cases **(Fig. 7)**. Crescentic gas collection may also be seen. The crescent-shaped air indicates the extension into perinephric space suggesting the advanced stage. IVU is rarely performed these days, but will show a poorly functioning or nonfunctioning kidney, if performed.

Ultrasound examination reveals coarse echoes with dirty shadowing in intrarenal infection **(Fig. 8A)**. The echogenic foci appear different than those seen in typical stone disease, with the distal shadowing having

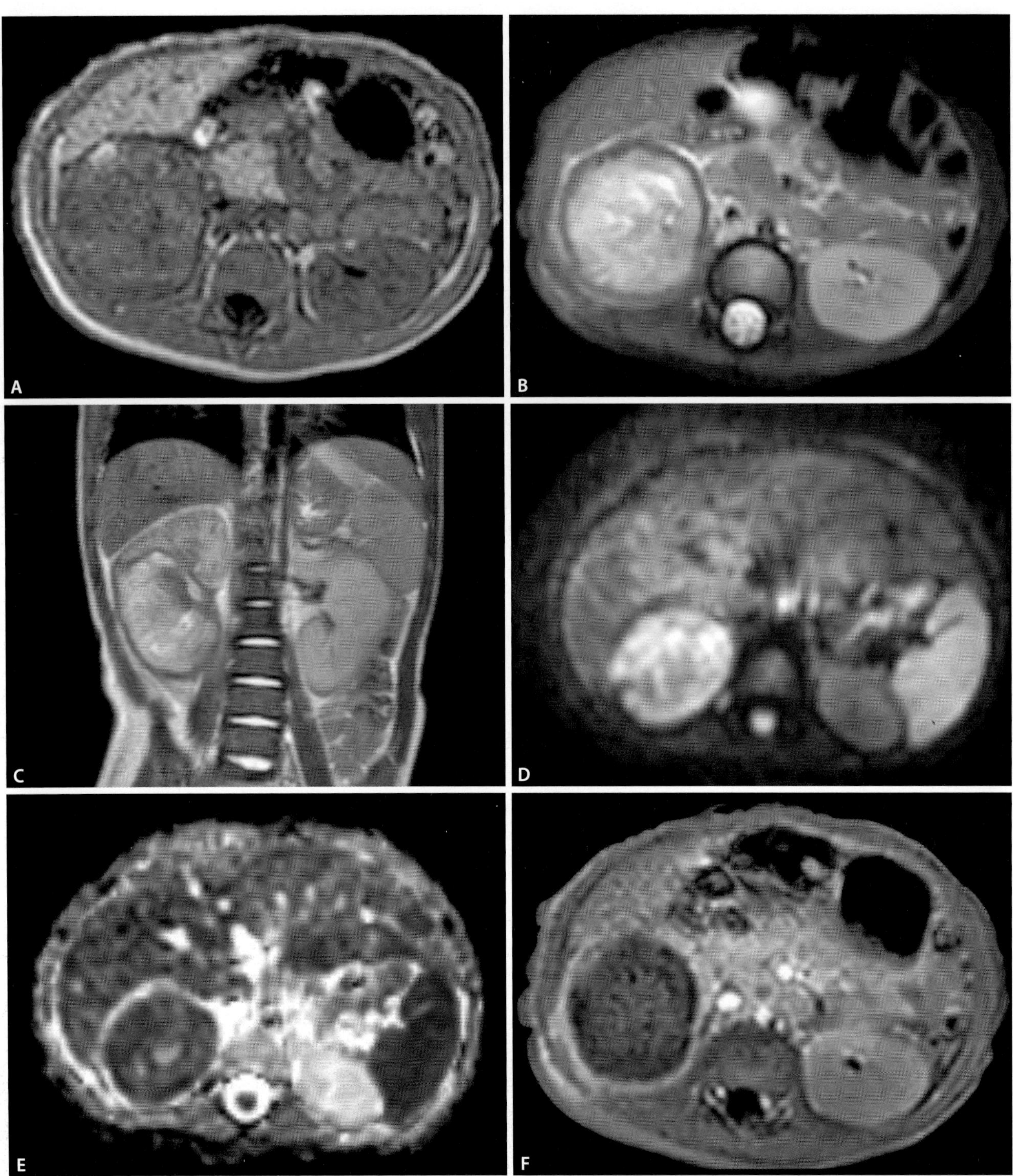

Figs. 6A to F: *Renal abscess in a child*: Axial T1-weighted image (A) shows a large hypointense lesion in right kidney. Axial T2-weighted image (B) and coronal (C) plane shows hyperintense lesion in interpolar and lower polar region. The lesion shows diffusion restriction (D and E). Gadolinium-enhanced axial T1-weighted image (F) shows peripheral irregular rim enhancement.

reverberations/ring down artefacts and low-level echoes that are nicknamed "dirty shadowing". If the gas extends into the perinephric space, kidney may not be seen at all on USG (gassed-out kidney).

Computed tomography is the imaging modality of choice to confirm the diagnosis and to see the renal as well as perirenal extent **(Fig. 8B)**. It detects the presence of air, its precise location within the kidney as well as its extension into the perirenal or pararenal compartments of the retroperitoneal space **(Fig. 9)**. The role of MRI is limited as gas appears as an area of signal loss, which cannot be differentiated from calculi, renal calcification, and flowing blood on T1 and T2WI.

Prognosis appears to correlate with two types of gaseous distribution. In Type 1 EPN, there is greater than one-third renal parenchymal destruction, which is associated with either mottled or streaky areas of gas. Intra- or extrarenal fluid collections are absent. In Type 2 EPN, renal or perirenal fluid collections are present, which are associated with loculated or bubbly gas within the collecting system. Type 1 disease has typically been found to have a more aggressive course, with a shorter duration between initial presentation and death.[22] However, recent literature reports much better results even in Type 1 disease with mortality rates for both types approximately 8%.[23] Aggressive medical treatment along with percutaneous image-guided drainage and partial or complete nephrectomy is advocated to reduce mortality due to either type of EPN.

In addition to this, the Huang-Tseng CT classification system[24] is also followed in EPN and is described in **Box 2**.

Prognosis is worse for higher classes. For localized EPN (classes 1 and 2), percutaneous drainage combined with antibiotic treatment can provide a good outcome with reduced mortality.

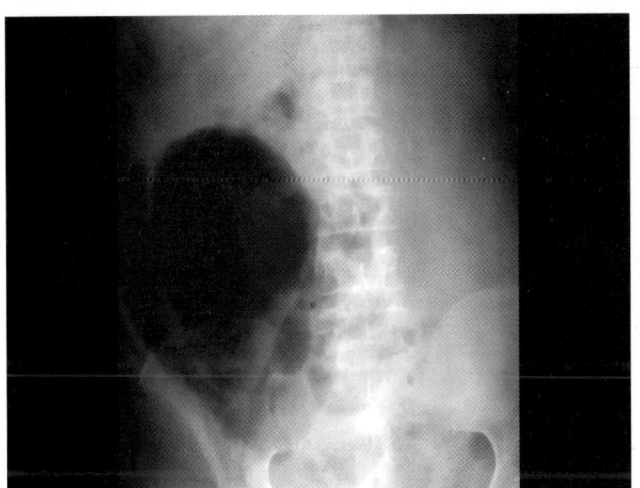

Fig. 7: Plain X-ray of abdomen showing a large loculus of air overlying the right renal fossa in a diabetic patient with extensive emphysematous pyelonephritis.

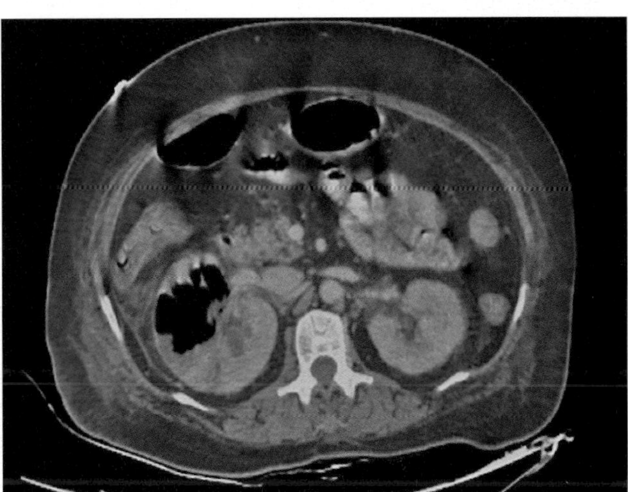

Fig. 9: *Emphysematous pyelonephritis*: Contrast-enhanced computed tomography scan shows large air loculus in right kidney with presence of fluid posteriorly. Thickening of perirenal fascia and associated stranding is also seen.

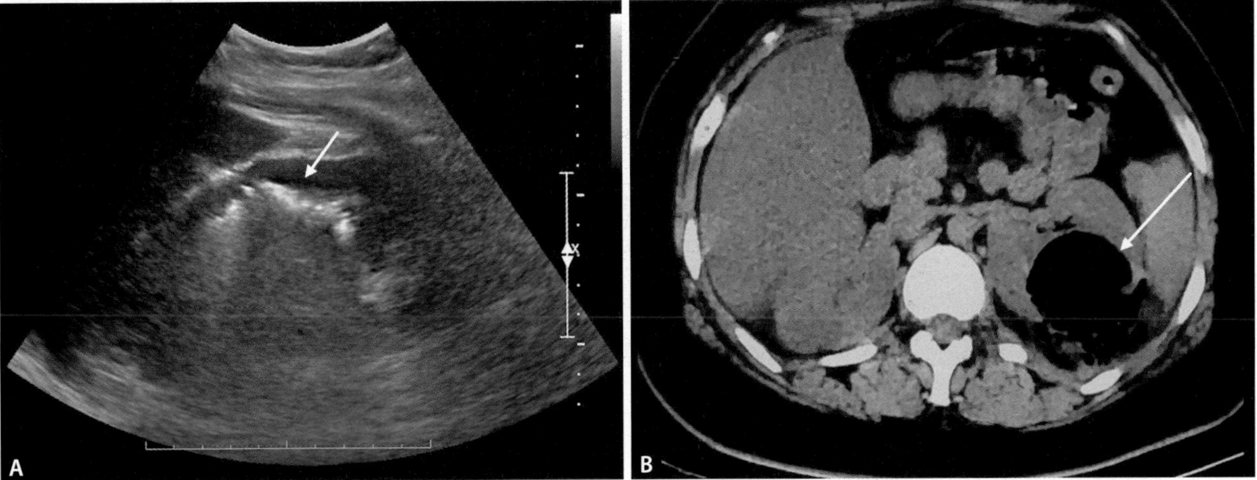

Figs. 8A and B: *Emphysematous pyelonephritis*: (A) Longitudinal ultrasound scan of the left kidney shows coarse echoes (arrow) with posterior dirty shadowing; (B) Noncontrast CT scan of the same patient shows large intraparenchymal air collection with extension into left posterior perinephric space.

PYONEPHROSIS

Pyonephrosis is the term given to infection in an obstructed collecting system, which may lead to suppurative destruction of the renal parenchyma if not treated immediately. Cause of obstruction can be sloughed papilla, stone, stricture, or neoplasm. Early diagnosis is important as untreated pyonephrosis may lead to rapid and irreversible decline in renal function. In addition, patient may develop septic shock if direct, immediate intervention is not undertaken.[16]

Ultrasound is the modality of choice to detect dilated collecting system, which often shows mobile dependent echogenic debris **(Fig. 10)**. Echogenic debris (i.e. the lack of a completely anechoic collecting system) is considered the most reliable sign of pyonephrosis.[16]

On CT, high density of urine in the dilated system can suggest infection in appropriate clinical context. CT, in addition, will often reveal the underlying cause of obstruction, which USG may sometimes fail to reveal. Thickening of the urothelium can be seen both on USG or CT.

Box 2: Classification of emphysematous pyelonephritis.

- *Class 1*: Gas in the collecting system only
- *Class 2*: Gas in renal parenchyma only (without extrarenal extension)
- *Class 3*: Gas in renal parenchyma with extrarenal extension
  - *Class 3a*: Extension of gas or abscess to perinephric space
  - *Class 3b*: Extension of gas or abscess to pararenal space
- *Class 4*: Bilateral emphysematous pyelonephritis or solitary kidney with emphysematous pyelonephritis

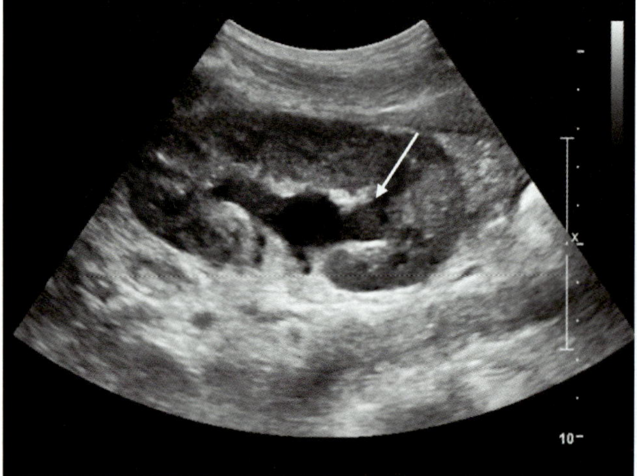

Fig. 10: *Pyonephrosis*: Longitudinal ultrasound scan of the kidney shows echogenic debris (arrow) in pelvicalyceal system. These debris were found to be mobile on continuous scanning. Associated features of pyelonephritis are also apparent in form of heterogeneous echotexture of kidney and poor corticomedullary differentiation.

Magnetic resonance imaging will reveal findings similar to those seen at CT. Dilated pelvicaliceal system, debris within the system are usually noticed. Fluid-fluid levels are also appreciated and underlying cause may also be apparent. DW-MRI may be used as a problem-solving tool in distinguishing hydronephrosis from pyonephrosis as in pyonephrosis-restricted diffusion may be seen.[25]

Ultrasound-guided aspiration may be performed to confirm the diagnosis as well as obtain specimen for culture and sensitivity. Percutaneous nephrostomy may also be performed under USG and fluoroscopic guidance to provide immediate decompression of the collecting system and also as an adjunct prior to definitive surgery. In case of pyonephrosis due to fungal etiology, direct infusion of amphotericin B may be done through the nephrostomy tube in place of systemic amphotericin, which is more toxic.

CHRONIC PYELONEPHRITIS

The term chronic focal atrophic pyelonephritis refers to renal parenchymal scarring, which manifests as focal thinning of both cortex and medulla with blunting of underlying calyces.[15] This renal parenchymal scarring can be due to a number of causes, including severe focal pyelonephritis, VUR, and calyceal calculi. Once the scars have formed, the gross pathologic and radiologic appearance of the affected kidney is identical hence does not allow determination of etiology.[15] Once the radiologic manifestations of chronic pyelonephritis have been established, repeat imaging does not provide any new findings and is usually unnecessary.

The term reflux nephropathy is specifically used, if the etiology is proven to be VUR. Possible mechanism of renal scarring in reflux nephropathy is thought to be the transient increase in hydrostatic pressure in the collecting system due to urine reflux during contractions of urinary bladder. This often-infected urine enters into the collecting tubules of the kidney in retrograde fashion due to pyelotubular reflux. As there are local differences in the papillary openings of the collecting ducts of the renal medullae, this intrarenal reflux occurs in a patchy distribution, which is the probable cause for the focal nature of the resultant scarring.[15] Normal nephrons are replaced by dense fibrous tissue in scarred areas of renal parenchyma.

In middle-aged or elderly patients, calculi are the most common cause of chronic pyelonephritic scarring, whereas in children, reflux is the most common etiology.[15]

Intravenous urography, if done, may reveal spectrum of findings seen in chronic pyelonephritis **(Fig. 11)**. On USG, focal loss of parenchyma is usually apparent, which

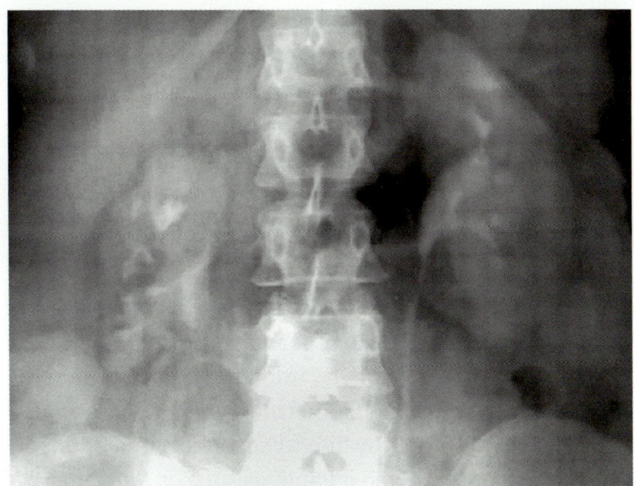

Fig. 11: *Chronic pyelonephritis*: Excretory urogram showing small irregular right kidney with dilated and distorted calyces and thinned out parenchyma especially opposite the polar calyces.

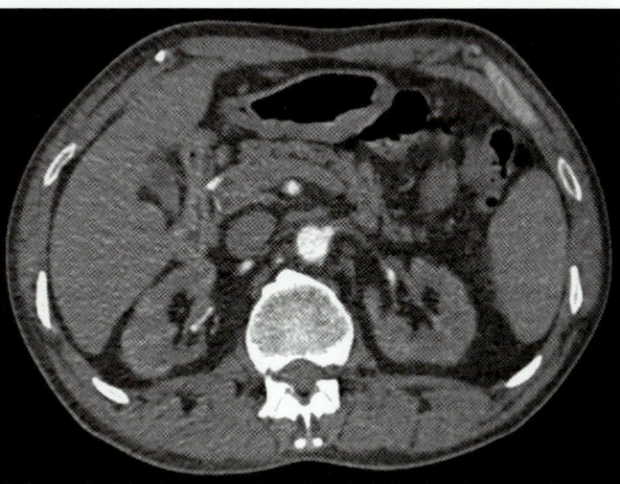

Fig. 12: *Chronic pyelonephritis*: Contrast-enhanced CT showing irregular outline of bilateral kidneys with multifocal areas of parenchymal scarring and distortion of underlying calyces.

can be demonstrated on longitudinal or cross-sectional images. Regions of scars may show increased echogenicity due to underlying fibrosis. The central renal sinus echoes may extend to the periphery of the kidney in the area of abnormality due to underlying volume loss. The process is patchy and focal in contrast to other causes of generalized increased cortical echogenicity.[15]

The radiologic findings of chronic pyelonephritis on cross-sectional imaging whether CT, computed tomographic urography (CTU), and MRI include one or more parenchymal scars overlying a deformed calyx **(Fig. 12)**. Focal areas of compensatory hypertrophy may be apparent adjacent to the areas of cortical scarring if loss of parenchyma has been severe. These focal areas may mimic solid parenchymal tumors but can be distinguished from tumors by observing their enhancement pattern. These pseudotumors enhance to the same degree as adjacent normal parenchyma unlike true tumors.[15] Renal cortical scintigraphy is considered the best technique to detect renal scarring. Other differential diagnoses include fetal lobulation, ischemia, and hypoplastic kidney. In ischemia, the underlying calyx is usually normal. In fetal lobulation, the scars are in between the calyces and in congenital hypoplastic kidney, the number of calyces are less than five.

XANTHOGRANULOMATOUS PYELONEPHRITIS

Xanthogranulomatous pyelonephritis (XGPN) is a rare chronic granulomatous inflammation of the kidney. It is usually seen in patients who have stones and obstruction. In XGPN, there is destruction of renal parenchyma, which is replaced by para-aminosalicylic acid-positive and lipid-laden macrophages (xanthoma cells). In addition to xanthoma cells, other inflammatory cells such as leukocytes, plasma cells, and histiocytes are also present.

Three stages of XGPN have been described depending on the extent of the disease. In Stage I, only kidney is involved; in Stage II, there is extension of inflammatory process into Gerota's fascia; and in Stage III, disease extends into the perinephric spaces.

Women are more affected than men. The presenting features and signs of the disease are nonspecific and similar to any long-standing chronic inflammatory process. Patients may present with fever, malaise, weight loss, pain, or tenderness in flanks. Leukocytosis will be seen in majority of patients. Lower urinary tract symptoms such as dysuria and increased frequency are seen in only one-half of patients.[15] Active UTI is present in almost all the cases with *E. coli*, *P. mirabilis*, *K. pneumoniae*, or *Pseudomonas aeruginosa* alone or in combination being the offending agents. Triad of radiological features consists of: (1) poorly defined renal mass; (2) reduced or absent contrast excretion; and (3) staghorn calculus.[15]

Plain radiograph will reveal the calculus. IVU may show tumefactive-type focal mass or enlarged nonfunctioning kidney. USG reveals global enlargement of the kidney with a central obstructing calculus. The renal parenchyma reveals a diffuse hypoechoic pattern, which represents areas of inflammation or abscess. The calyces may appear as multiple fluid-filled regions with echogenic debris, which may be indistinguishable from pyonephrosis.[15]

Computed tomography findings strongly point towards the correct diagnosis though are not specific. The diffusely enlarged kidney retains its reniform shape. One characteristic feature is poorly defined or normal renal pelvis, unless there is concomitant ureteropelvic junction obstruction. One or more stones are usually present **(Figs. 13A and B)**. Small areas of parenchymal calcification may also be appreciated. Atrophic parenchyma may be seen as hypoattenuating areas at the periphery of the kidneys. Hypoattenuating central areas which represent dilated calyces filled with pus and necrotic material are usually separated by renal column of Bertin. On CECT, hyperemia is seen around the calyces, at the periphery of the kidney and in the renal fascia. Extrarenal extension of inflammatory process is usually evident on CT.[15]

The common form of XGPN causes diffuse involvement of the affected kidney. In the tumefactive form of XGPN, inflammatory process is limited to a portion of the kidney. This appearance may mimic poorly enhancing renal tumor and radiological differentiation may be difficult. Both forms of XGPN usually are associated with extensive perinephric inflammation.[15]

MALACOPLAKIA

Malacoplakia is a rare granulomatous inflammatory condition seen almost exclusively in women and clinically presents as repeated attacks of UTI. Bladder and ureter are most frequently affected. Renal involvement is rare. Radiological features include enlarged poorly functioning kidney with filling defect in the ureter and bladder and may mimic pyeloureteritis cystica or transitional cell carcinoma. Strictures may also develop thus mimicking tuberculosis. Renal involvement leads to focal or multiple masses indistinguishable from renal cell carcinoma or XGPN on US, CT, or IVU. Diagnosis is confirmed on pathology, which reveals Van Hansemann cells and Michaelis-Gutmann bodies in the nodular deposits.[16]

HIV-ASSOCIATED NEPHROPATHY

Human immunodeficiency virus can affect any organ of the body and renal involvement can be seen in variety of disease processes in HIV infection. Kidneys may be involved as a collapsing glomerulopathy (HIV-associated nephropathy, HIVAN) or due to secondary infections by bacteria or opportunistic organisms such as *Pneumocystis carinii* and cytomegalovirus. HIVAN is a serious disorder, which results in rapidly progressive renal failure. It manifests histologically as focal glomerulosclerosis and as membranous, membranoproliferative, and mesangial proliferative glomerulonephritis.[25,26]

Imaging will demonstrate renal enlargement (>13 cm) with increased echogenicity on USG. Atta et al.[27] found that only renal echogenicity and not kidney size has diagnostic utility for HIVAN. On NCCT scan, hyperattenuating medulla may be seen as a result of dilated protein filled tubules. On CECT, enlarged kidneys with striated nephrogram may be evident.[28,29] Imaging findings may suggest the diagnosis of HIVAN but confirmation is on histology. *P. carinii* infection of the kidney will result in punctate areas of calcification within the renal parenchyma similar to those seen with *Mycobacterium avium* intracellulare or cytomegalovirus.[30]

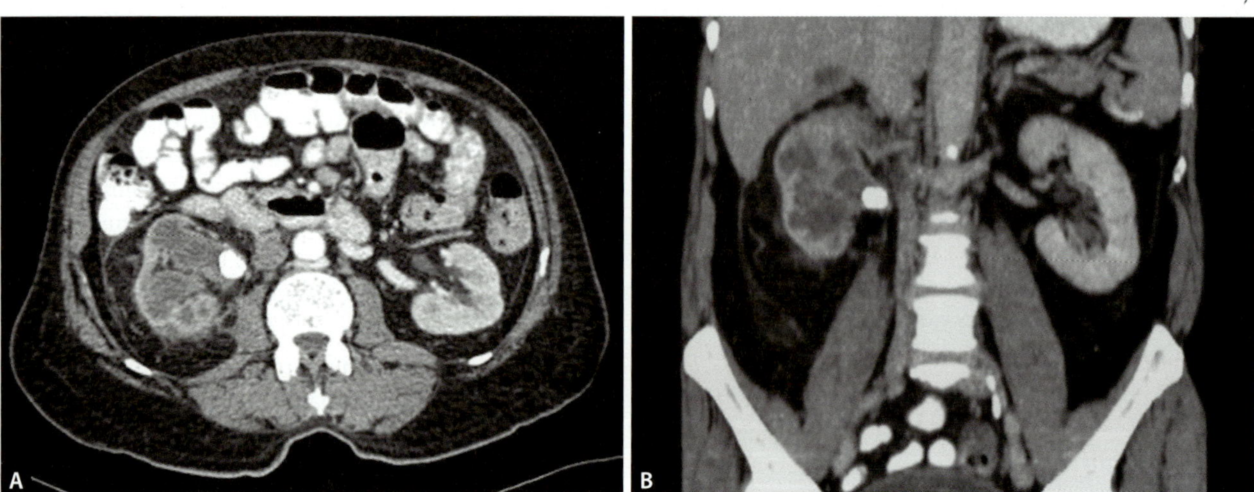

Figs. 13A and B: *Xanthogranulomatous pyelonephritis*: Contrast-enhanced CT scan in arterial phase axial plane (A) and venous phase coronal plane; (B) shows calculus in deformed pelvis of right kidney with dilated collecting system secondary to inflammatory debris. Kidney maintains its reniform shape. Perinephric inflammation is also noted.

FUNGAL INFECTION

Fungal infections of the kidney are rare, usually encountered in patients with deranged immunity such as diabetics, postrenal transplant patients, those with other chronic infections and those on prolonged steroid therapy. Infection by *Aspergillus*, *Candida*, *Cryptococcus*, and mucor has been described. On CT, bilateral poorly functioning or nonfunctioning enlarged kidneys with multiple hyperattenuating areas present both in the cortex and medulla should raise the possibility of the diagnosis of mucormycosis especially in diabetic patients **(Fig. 14)**.[31]

Both *Aspergillus* and mucor are angioinvasive fungi. These fungi cause thrombosis of the large as well as small arteries with resultant infarction and necrosis of the kidneys. The infection usually occurs by hematogenous route resulting in multiple abscesses, which may extend into perinephric space.

PARASITIC INFECTION

Schistosoma usually affects the bladder causing calcification. Renal pelvic striations may be seen. Intrarenal hydatid is rare and occurs in only approximately 2–3% of patients. Within the kidney, the worms form three-layered hydatid cyst that may grow rapidly and destroy the kidney or may progress very slowly, producing minimal clinical symptoms. USG, CT, and MRI show the lesions to be cystic and usually reveal the walls of the daughter cysts. Associated curvilinear mural calcification may be seen **(Figs. 15A to C)**. US may demonstrate internal debris. Cyst walls are of various thicknesses and may enhance slightly on CECT and CEMRI. Extensive renal destruction may result in a nonfunctioning kidney.[15]

Fig. 14: *Bilateral mucormycosis*: Contrast-enhanced CT scan in a diabetic patient shows bilateral globular kidneys with large hypodense nonenhancing areas (arrowheads). There is extensive bilateral perinephric and mesenteric stranding and thickening of fascias. Few enlarged lymph nodes are also seen.

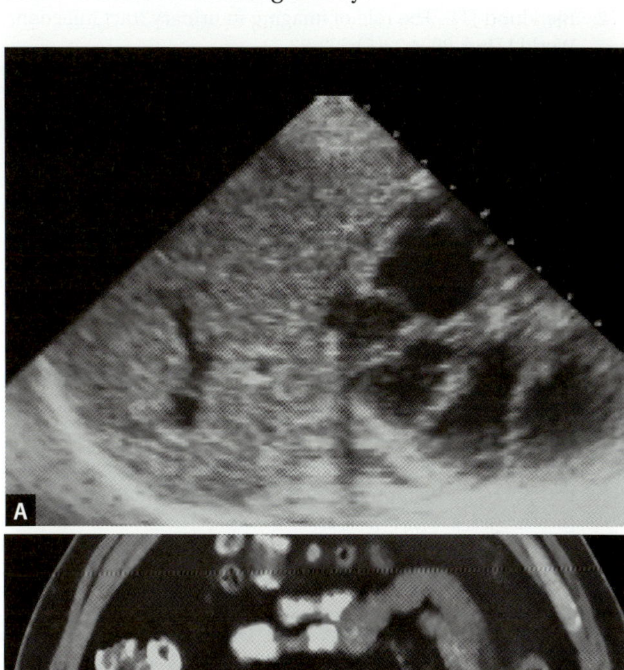

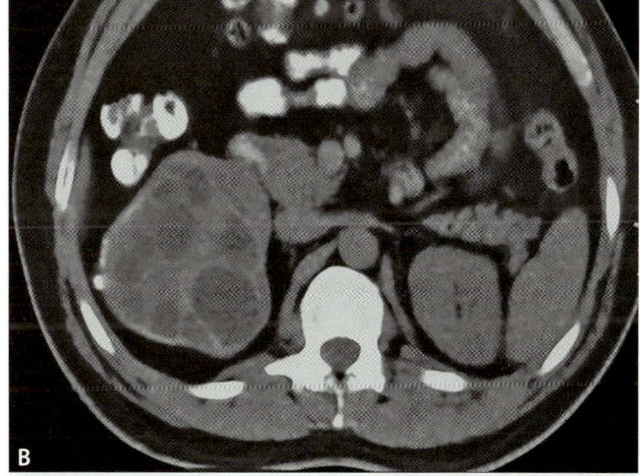

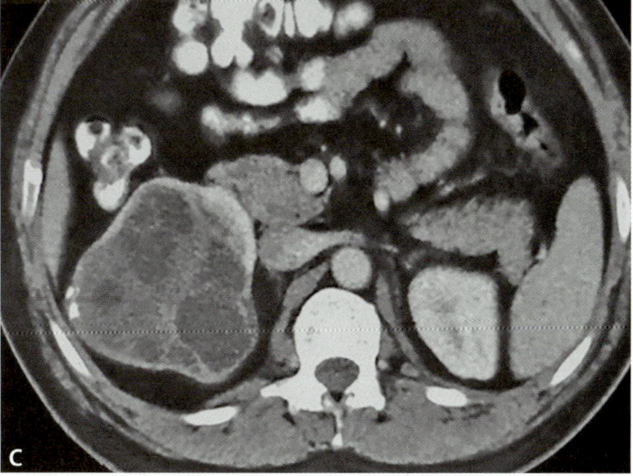

Figs. 15A to C: *Renal hydatid cyst*: Ultrasound (A); Noncontrast CT (B); and contrast-enhanced CT showing characteristic multiloculated appearance of hydatid cyst due to presence of daughter cysts. (C) Peripheral discontinuous calcification is also noted.

REFERENCES

1. Kawashima A, Sandler CM, Goldman SM. Imaging in acute renal infection. BJU Int. 2000;86(Suppl 1):70-9.
2. Bjerklund JTE. The role of imaging in urinary tract infections. World J Urol. 2004;22(5):392-98.
3. Stunell H, Buckley O, Feeney J, et al. Imaging of acute pyelonephritis in the adult. Eur Radiol. 2007;17(7):1820-28.
4. Ellenbogen PH, Schieble FW, Talner LB, et al. Sensitivity of gray scale ultrasound in detecting urinary tract obstruction. AJR. 1978;130(4):731-3.
5. Fontanilla T, Minaya J, Cortes C, et al. Acute complicated pyelonephritis: contrast-enhanced ultrasound. Abdom Imaging. 2012;37(4):639-646.
6. Merenich WM, Popky GL. Radiology of renal infection. Med Clin N Am. 1991;75(2):425-69.
7. Kawashima A, LeRoy AJ. Radiologic evaluation of patients with renal infections. Infect Dis Clin North Am. 2003; 17(2):433-56.
8. Conway JJ. The role of scintigraphy in urinary tract infection. Semin Nucl Med. 1998;18(4):308-19.
9. June CH, Browning MD, Smith LP, et al. Ultrasonography and computed tomography in severe urinary tract infection. Arch Intern Med. 1985;145(5):841-5.
10. Vourganti S, Agarwal PK, Bodner DR, et al. Ultrasonographic evaluation of renal infections. Radiol Clin North Am. 2006; 44(6):763-75.
11. Kim B, Lim HK, Choi MH, et al. Detection of parenchymal abnormalities in acute pyelonephritis by pulse inversion harmonic imaging with or without microbubble ultrasonographic contrast agent: correlation with computed tomography. J Ultrasound Med. 2001;20(1):5-14.
12. Rigsby CM, Rosenfield AT, Glickman MG, et al. Hemorrhagic focal bacterial nephritis: findings on gray-scale sonography and CT. Am J Roentgenol. 1986;146(6):1173-7.
13. Talner LB, Davidson AJ, Lebowitz RL, et al. Acute pyelonephritis: can we agree on terminology? Radiology. 1994;192(2):297-305.
14. Dalla-Palma L, Pozzi-Mucelli R, Pozzi-Mucelli F. Delayed CT in acute renal infection. Semin Ultrasound CT MR. 1997;18(2): 122-8.
15. Dunnick NR, Newhouse JH, Cohan RH, Maturen KE, et al. Renal inflammatory disease. In: Dunnick NR, Newhouse JH, Cohan RH, Maturen KE, et al. (Eds). Genitourinary Radiology. Philadelphia: Wolters Kluwer; 2018. pp. 145-62.
16. Craig WD, Wagner BJ, Travis MD. Pyelonephritis: radiologic-pathologic review. Radiographics. 2008;28(1):255-77; quiz 327-8.
17. Sieger N, Kyriazis I, Schaudinn A, et al. Acute focal bacterial nephritis is associated with invasive diagnostic procedures: a cohort of 138 cases extracted through a systematic review. BMC Infect Dis. 2017;17(1):240.
18. Rosenfield AT, Glickman MG, Taylor KJ, et al. Acute focal bacterial nephritis (acute lobar nephronia). Radiology. 1979; 132(3):553-61.
19. Dyer RB, Chen MY, Zagoria RJ. Classic signs in uroradiology. Radiographics. 2004;24(1):247-80.
20. Van Sonnenberg E, D'Agostino HB, Sanchez RB, et al. Percutaneous abscess drainage. Radiol. 1992;184:27-9.
21. Allen HA, Walsh JW, Brewer WH, et al. Sonography of emphysematous pyelonephritis. J Ultrasound Med. 1984; 3(12):533-7.
22. Wan YL, Lee TY, Bullard MJ, et al. Acute gas-producing bacterial renal infection: correlation between imaging findings and clinical outcome. Radiology. 1996;198(2):433-8.
23. Chen MT, Huang CN, Chou YH, et al. Percutaneous drainage in the treatment of emphysematous pyelonephritis: 10-year experience. J Urol. 1997;157(5):1569-73.
24. Huang JJ, Tseng CC. Emphysematous pyelonephritis: clinicoradiological classification, management, prognosis, and pathogenesis. Arch Intern Med. 2000;160(6):797-805.
25. Cova M, Squillaci E, Stacul F, et al. Diffusion-weighted MRI in the evaluation of renal lesions: preliminary results. Br J Radiol. 2004;77(922):851-7.
26. Symeonidou C, Standish R, Sahdev A, et al. Imaging and histopathologic features of HIV-related renal disease. RadioGraphics. 2008;28(5):1329-54.
27. Atta MG, Longenecker JC, Fine DM, et al. Sonography as a predictor of human immunodeficiency virus-associated nephropathy. J Ultrasound Med. 2004;23(5):603-10.
28. Kuhlman JE, Browne D, Shermak M, et al. Retro-peritoneal and pelvic CT of patients with AIDS: primary and secondary involvement of the genitourinary tract. RadioGraphics. 1991; 11(3):473-83.
29. Miller FH, Parikh S, Gore RM, et al. Renal manifestations of AIDS. RadioGraphics. 1993;13:587-96.
30. Bray HJ, Lail VJ, Cooperberg PL. Tiny echogenic foci in the liver and kidney in patients with AIDS: not always due to disseminated *Pneumocystis carinii*. Am J Roentgenol. 1992;158(1):81-2.
31. Chugh KS, Sakuja V, Gupta KL, et al. Renal mucormycosis: computerized tomographic findings and their diagnostic significance. Am J Kidney Dis. 1993;22(3):393-7.

Chapter 6

Tubercular Infection of the Urinary Tract

Ashu Seith Bhalla, Priyanka Naranje, Arun Kumar Gupta

INTRODUCTION

India continues to remain a high tuberculosis (TB) burden country, with a incidence rate of 204 (140–281) per 100,000 population according to the WHO global TB report of 2018.[1] These cases comprise both pulmonary TB (PTB) and extrapulmonary TB (EPTB). TB of the urinary tract is not uncommon in India. While the lymph nodes are the most common site of EPTB, the genitourinary system is also a common site, accounting for 14–41% of cases.[2,3] Approximately 4 to 8% of patients with PTB will develop clinically significant genitourinary infection.[4] A significant number of patients (10.4%) with PTB may simultaneously, have subclinical forms of urogenital TB.[3] TB occurs in approximately 10% of patients with AIDS and involves at least one extrapulmonary site in nearly 50% of the patients, with kidneys being the most commonly involved genitourinary site.[2,5]

Urinary tract TB is an important clinical problem because of its nonspecific clinical presentation and progression to renal failure if undiagnosed and untreated. It is also a diagnostic problem because of variable imaging features which often resemble many other lesions.

PATHOGENESIS

Renal TB results from hematogenous dissemination of the tubercle bacilli from a primary infection elsewhere.[6] Past or concurrent pulmonary lesion is the most common primary lesion, followed by bone and joint TB. There is a latent period of 5 to 20 years between the pulmonary infection and initial manifestation of clinical kidney involvement. This explains the low incidence of disease in children. The organisms may involve both kidneys in the initial phase, and are lodged in the glomerular and peritubular capillary bed. The subsequent course of the infection is determined by virulence of the organisms and host-resistance factors. Most of the initial lesions heal without sequelae, and only one or a few progress to clinically or radiologically apparent abnormalities. This happens when the bacilli erode out of their initial vascular location and spill into the tubules. This results in granuloma formation along the nephron. Granuloma, caseous necrosis, and cavitation represent stages of progression of the infection. This may communicate with the pelvicalyceal system, and the infection further spreads to the ureter and urinary bladder. The pelvicalyceal and ureteral involvement appears as mucosal ulcerations, focal or generalized dilatation or cicatrization. Fibrosis and calcium depositions represent healing. The pattern of progression and healing is variable and produces asymmetric histologic, microscopic and radiological findings unique to each patient. If the hydronephrotic kidney becomes nonfunctioning, extensive dystrophic (putty like) calcification may form a cast of the kidney, referred to as autonephrectomy. Nonfunctioning kidneys in TB may be due to autonephrectomy or as a sequela of obstruction **(Flowchart 1 and Fig. 1)**. Important complications of renal TB include perinephritis, perinephric abscess, fistulae and psoas abscesses.

CLINICAL PICTURE

The disease is predominant between second and fourth decades of life being distinctly low in children, and less prevalent in fifth and sixth decades. The disease shows a male predominance. Frequency of urination, burning,

Flowchart 1: Pathogenesis of urinary tract tuberculosis.

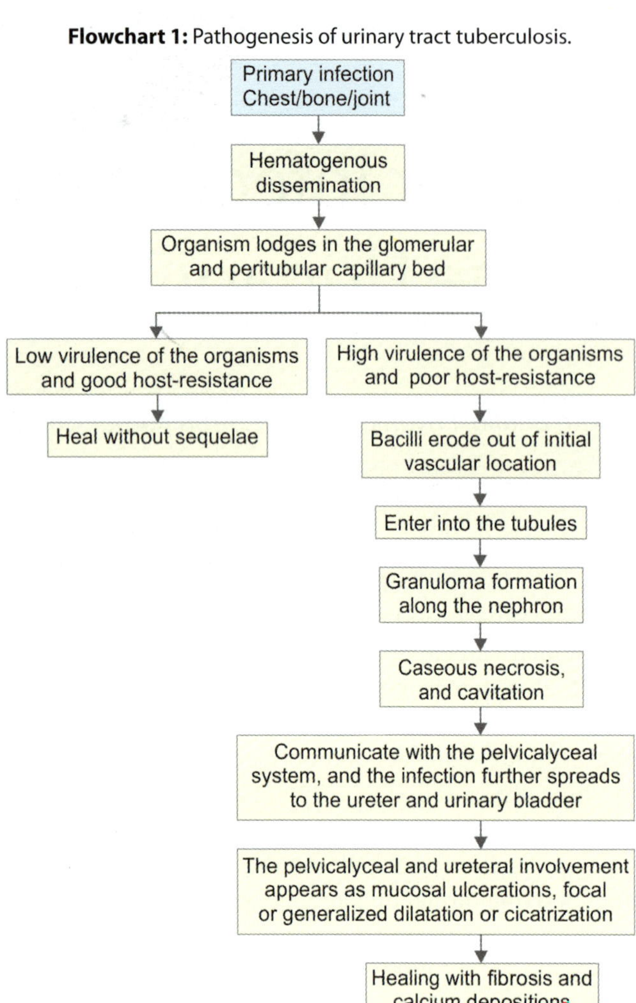

dysuria or urgency are the most common presenting symptoms. Nearly 50% of the patients at sometimes during the course of the disease have hematuria.

Dull or chronic renal pain, even acute colic is not uncommon. Constitutional symptoms like fever, weight loss, and fatigue are present in about 50% of the patients. Obstructive uropathy, and chronic cystitis are not uncommon with TB.[7,8] Patients may develop fistulae particularly in lower urinary tract involvement. The physical examination is often insignificant. Diagnosis of TB should be considered in patients with recurrent urinary tract infection that is not responding to appropriate therapy for typical pathogens.

LABORATORY INVESTIGATIONS

Pyuria which is sterile when cultured on standard media is characteristic. Presence of red blood cells in urine is frequent. The diagnosis is established by demonstration

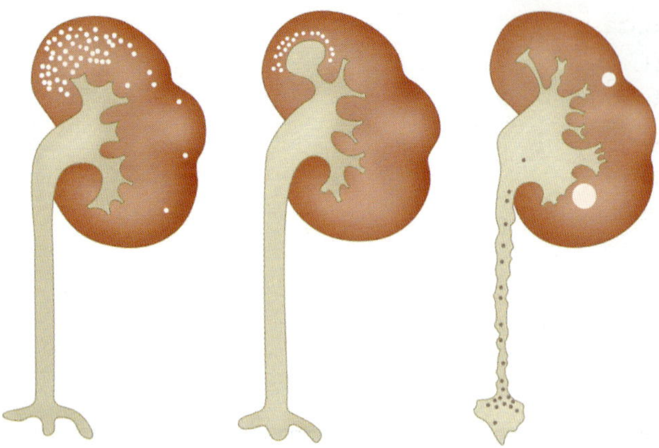

Fig. 1: Schematic diagram showing stages of progression of the disease.

of acid-fast bacilli (AFB) on microscopic examination of urine, urine culture or growth of tubercle bacilli in inoculated guinea-pigs. However, urine culture for acid-fast bacilli is positive in nearly 33%, while soluble antigen fluorescent antibody (SAFA) test is strongly positive in only 13%, and weak or nonreactive in 87% of the patients. Also, routine AFB culture is cumbersome involving a delay of 6–8 weeks with a false negative rate of 10–20%, using LJ media. Newer techniques for recovery of mycobacteria from urine specimens include BACTEC 460 and using the automated Mycobacteria Growth Indicator Tube system (MGIT 960), with mean time of positivity of 20 days.[9] As an alternative, polymerase chain reaction (PCR) technique or US-guided fine needle aspiration cytology (FNAC) can be used. PCR is highly sensitive (up to 94%), provides a quicker diagnosis but has a relatively poor specificity.[10] FNAC is useful in those with a negative culture to define granulomatous nature of the visible lesions.

CYSTOSCOPY

Visualization of tubercle, ulcer or retracted ureteric orifice strongly suggest the diagnosis. Generalized cystitis with reduced capacity is almost diagnostic. Biopsy from ulcer, tubercle or inflammatory lesion, particularly in absence of positive urine culture may provide the only diagnostic evidence of the disease.

IMAGING EVALUATION

A key role is often played by the radiologist in the diagnosis of the disease. The balance between local progress and healing of the disease process manifests many abnormal imaging features. Since, demonstration of the typical calyceal, ureteral and vesical abnormalities is critical to establish the diagnosis of TB, conventional radiological studies remain the procedures of choice, while ultrasonography (US) and computerized tomography (CT) have an adjunct role. Essentially, early findings are best detected on intravenous urography (IVU) while US and CT are useful for late or chronic changes. US and CT are especially valuable in the evaluation of areas of mass effect and of the nonvisualized kidney at IVU.[11] MRI had not found a place in the diagnostic protocol for evaluation till recently. However, MRI can be useful too in evaluation of the nonfunctioning kidney and focal lesions. A study by Navarro et al. found that IVU provided the diagnosis in 87.5% of cases. The average interval between onset of symptoms and diagnosis was 15 months. They in fact state that the current use of imaging studies other than urography and the finding of other microorganisms in urine culture can delay the diagnosis.[12] The most valuable radiologic feature of genitourinary TB is the multiplicity of abnormal findings. Whenever an imaging pattern of chronic renal inflammatory disease is recognized, particularly in the setting of periureteric or peripelvic fibrosis, TB must be considered.[13]

Radiographs

Plain radiograph of abdomen is an important initial examination before IVU and may provide valuable information such as calcification or evidence of skeletal involvement. Small, enlarged or normal renal size; presence of scarring or focal bulge are all nonspecific findings. Deposition of calcium in an attempt to heal and limit the pathological process often provides a diagnostic clue. Calcification is of two types: (1) Amorphous granular associated with granulomatous masses, and (2) Dense punctate calcification representing healed tuberculoma. It varies from a few minute areas to a cast of entire kidney **(Figs. 2A and B)**. The lobar distribution of calcification is quite specific for renal TB. Tubercular calcification of ureter is not as common as renal calcification **(Fig. 2B)**, and calcification of bladder is relatively rare.[14] Plain films may also reveal an evidence of skeletal TB in hip, sacroiliac joint or spine with or without a paraspinal abscess and calcification of abdominal lymph nodes. A co-existing focus of extrarenal TB elsewhere, ranges from 23 to 53% in various series. Chest X-ray is abnormal in about 50% of the patients. However, active PTB is seen in only 5–10% with most patients showing sequelae of past infection.

Intravenous Urography

Even though miliary tubercles involve both kidneys, disease progression and hence radiological abnormalities are confined to a single kidney in over 70% of the patients.

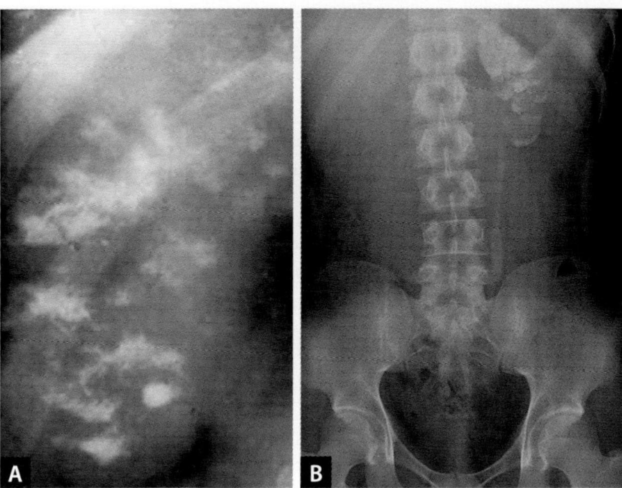

Figs. 2A and B: Patterns of calcification in renal tuberculosis. (A) Plain radiograph abdomen showing amorphous granular calcification involving the right kidney; (B) Extensive calcification involving the entire left kidney with ureteral calcification—auto-nephrectomy.

Intravenous urography is a very useful modality to detect early features of urinary tract TB.[15,16] However, the diagnosis can be made with certainty on urography only if the lesion has ulcerated into the calyx. Hence, IVU may be normal in symptomatic renal TB in the initial stages when the bacilli are lodged in glomerulus and peritubular capillary bed. IVU is essential to assess the extent and severity of involvement, to monitor the response to treatment and to look for complications. The various IVU findings are summarized in **Table 1**.

Kidney

The earliest urographic abnormality is the loss of definition of a minor calyx producing an indistinct feathery outline (smudged papillae), irregularity of the surface of one or more papillae or calyces with normal renal size and contour **(Figs. 3A and B)**.[17]

Progressive involvement of renal parenchyma occurs in three forms, which occur singly or in combination. First is coalescence of granulomas leading to unifocal or multifocal mass lesions. These may enlarge overall renal length or increase thickness of renal substance and cause displacement of adjacent collecting system. Caliectasis occurs with irregularity in contour indicating erosion of the pyramids and cortical necrosis. Depending on the necrosis, a cavity with irregular walls communicates with a deformed calyx **(Figs. 4 and 5)**. Radiographic appearance of this form simulates papillary necrosis of other origins. The second form seen in advanced renal TB

Table 1: Intravenous urography findings of urinary tract tuberculosis.

Region of involvement	*IVU findings*
Kidney	• Irregularities of surface of papillae—"Smudged" papillae • Calyceal erosion (early change)—"Moth-eaten" calyx • Irregular tract formations from calyx into papilla • Large irregular cavities communicating with deformed calyx—"papillary necrosis" • Dilated calices (hydrocalycosis) often with infundibular strictures • Renal calculi • "Hiked up pelvis" due to pelvic scarring • Marked hydronephrosis due to longstanding obstruction • "Putty kidney" extensive parenchymal and PCS calcifications • Autonephrectomy—small shrunken scarred nonfunctioning kidney ± dystrophic calcifications • Infection may extend into peri or pararenal space/psoas
Ureter	• Dilatation—due to atony and prolonged bacilluria • Long segment strictures—most commonly at distal one-third • Beaded/corkscrew ureter • "Pipe stem ureter"—rigid shortened ureter with narrow lumen • Ureteral calcifications (uncommon)
Urinary bladder	• Filling defects—due to tuberculomas in wall • "Thimble bladder"—irregular contracted bladder • Vesicoureteric reflux—fibrosis in trigone region
Urethra	• Stricture at bulbomembranous location (on MCU study)

(MCU: micturating cystourethrogram)

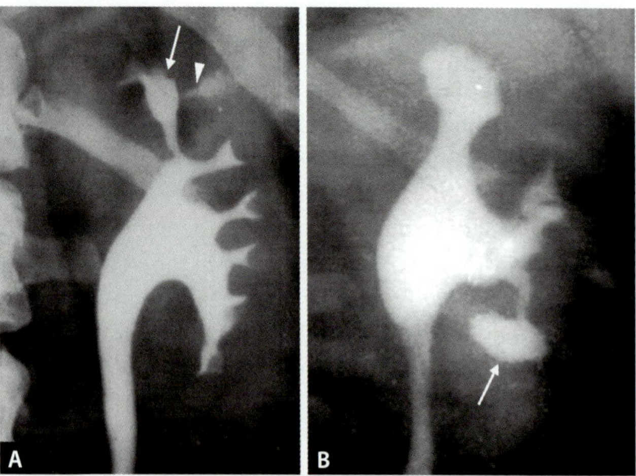

Figs. 3A and B: Intravenous urography findings of calyceal involvement by tuberculosis. (A) Early changes—Fuzzy, moth eaten outline of calyx (arrow) with caliectasis and irregular tracts in papilla (arrowhead); (B) Intravenous urography reveals marked dilatation of the inferior calyx with loss of sharpness and fuzziness of its outline (arrow). Rest of the calyces are also dilated.

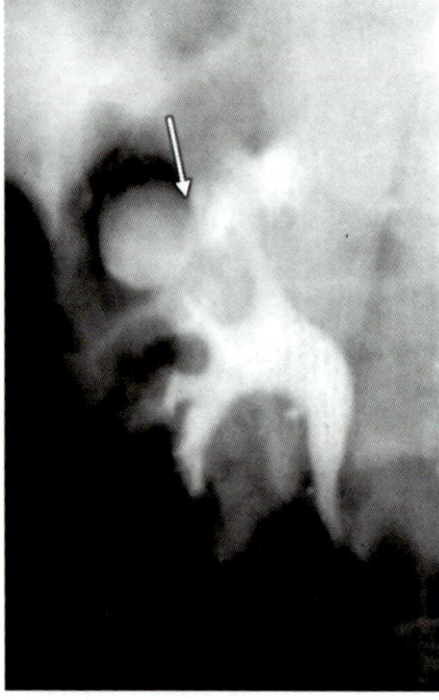

Fig. 4: Intravenous urography findings of calyceal involvement by tuberculosis. IVU shows a large cavity communicating with a dilated, irregular superior calyx (arrow).

is parenchymal surface scarring over retracted papillae and dilated calyces. This may be focal or diffuse involving the entire kidney and occurs due to tissue loss leading to fibrosis. Associated calcification or calculi maybe seen. Radiographic identification of calcification associated with renal TB is becoming less common. Calculus disease is rapidly becoming the most frequent form of calcification associated with renal TB.[18] Due to pelvic scarring the calculi formed also tend to take on this deformed shape. Upward pointing renal pelvic calculi may be seen due to "hiked up" pelvis[18] **(Figs. 6A to C)**. Impaired excretion of contrast is seen in either of these two forms.

A third form is autonephrectomy, which represents end stage disease. It may be of two types: (1) caseo-cavernous type-enlarged sac filled with caseous material, with or without calcification[2] **(Fig. 7)**. This can simulate xanthogranulomatous pyelonephritis; (2) calcified shrunken nonfunctioning kidney.

Following the drainage of a cavity into the collecting system, there is spread of infection to other parts of the urinary tract. Subsequent stimulation of scirrhous reaction causes stenosis and obstruction of parts of the collecting system. The common sites of strictures being the neck of a calyx, pelviureteric junction and lower end of the ureter **(Figs. 8 to 10)**. Depending on the site of

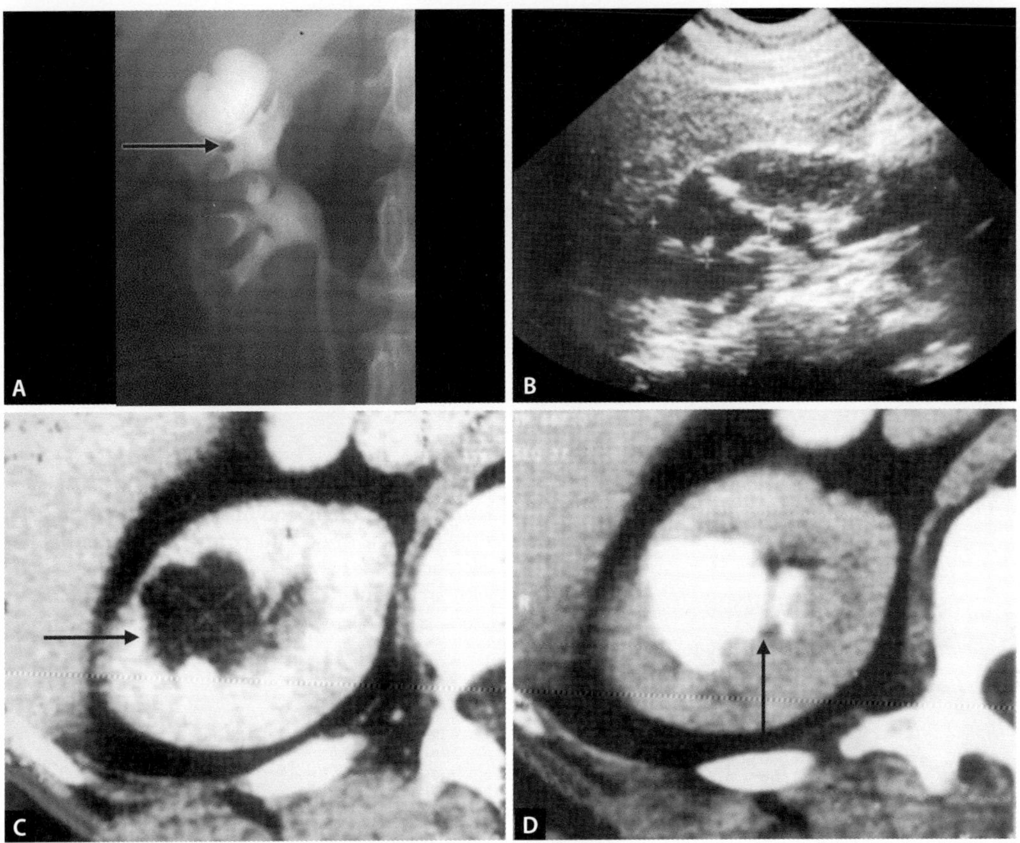

Figs. 5A to D: Papillary necrosis with irregular cavities. (A) IVU reveals a large cavity communicating with the superior calyx of right kidney (arrow); (B) Ultrasonography shows a hypoechoic focal lesion in the upper polar cortex with an echogenic rim; (C) CT confirms the presence of the cavity seen on IVU and US, with pooling of contrast on delayed images, (D) due to communication with the pelvicalyceal system (arrows).

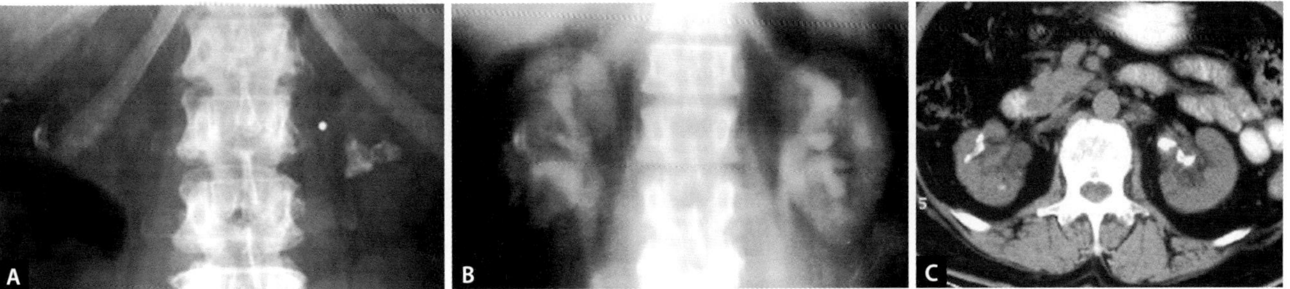

Figs. 6A to C: Renal pelvis involvement in tuberculosis. Plain radiograph (A) reveals deformed calculus in (L) renal pelvis with parenchymal calcification in the right kidney; (B) IVU reveals bilateral small kidneys with calyceal dilatation and parenchymal scarring; (C) CT better demonstrates the calcification and pelvic scarring.

narrowing there is dilatation of a single calyx (hydrocalyx) or regional hydrocalycosis or generalized dilatation of the pelvicalyceal system. A completely stenosed infundibulum or calyx may lead to failure of contrast excretion by the involved parenchyma (phantom calyx). A tiny infundibular stump (amputated calyx) may be seen in such cases. The renal pelvis may be dilated or may show filling defects due to caseous debris and granulation tissue. The involvement progresses to fibrosis with scarring. If the inferior margin of the renal pelvis is involved with resultant cephalic retraction, a characteristic deformity called the "hiked up pelvis" results. In addition, deformity of the pelvicalyceal system may be caused by traction from a strictured infundibulum or parenchymal fibrosis kinking the pelvis

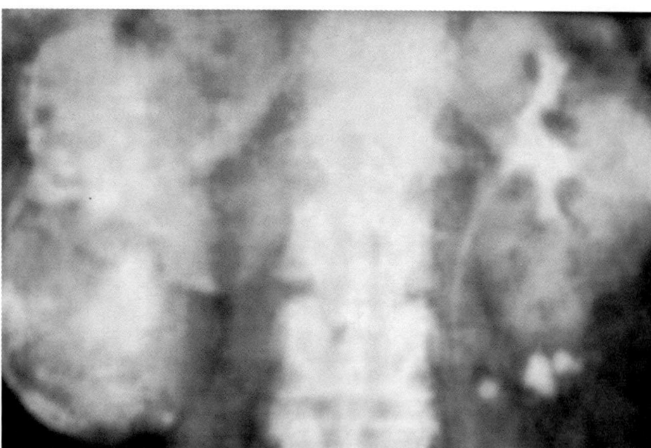
Fig. 7: Advanced disease of caseo-cavernous type. IVU slowing an enlarged, sac like poorly functioning right kidney.

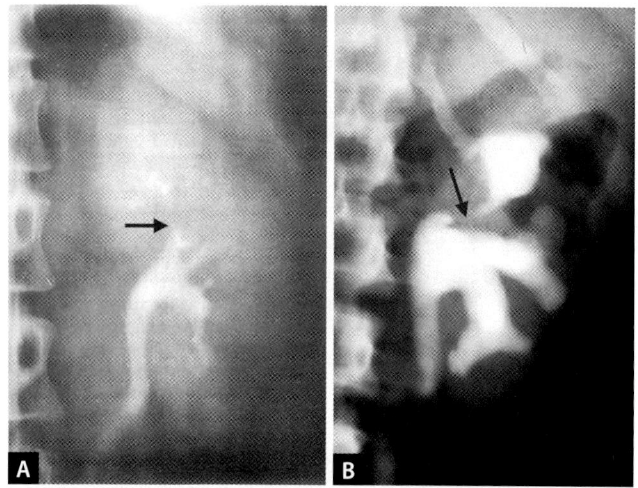
Figs. 8A and B: Infundibular strictures. (A) IVU shows irregularity of the superior calyx with intrarenal reflux and infundibular narrowing (arrow); (B) IVU in a different patient shows infundibular narrowing (arrow) with dilated superior calyx.

(Kerr's kink) and involving areas not directly affected by tuberculous ulcerations. Occasionally, obstruction can be of such a high grade and so prolonged that marked hydronephrosis develops.[19]

Ureter

Ureteral involvement is almost always secondary to renal TB with spread of infection by bacilluria. In the early stages there is dilatation resulting from atony and prolonged bacilluria. With progression of the disease, irregular segments of ureter are seen due to mucosal ulcerations. Further necrosis of ureteral musculature is accompanied by fibrosis resulting in stricture formation. The ureteric

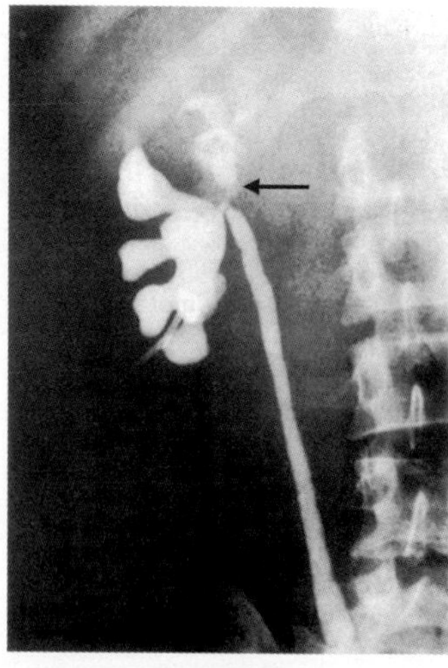
Fig. 9: Renal pelvis and Infundibular strictures. Nephrostogram showing deformed and contracted renal pelvis with proximal dilatation of the pelvicalyceal system. Superior calyx is communicating with an irregular cavity and there is infundibular stenosis (arrow). Ureter is also dilated due to lower end stricture.

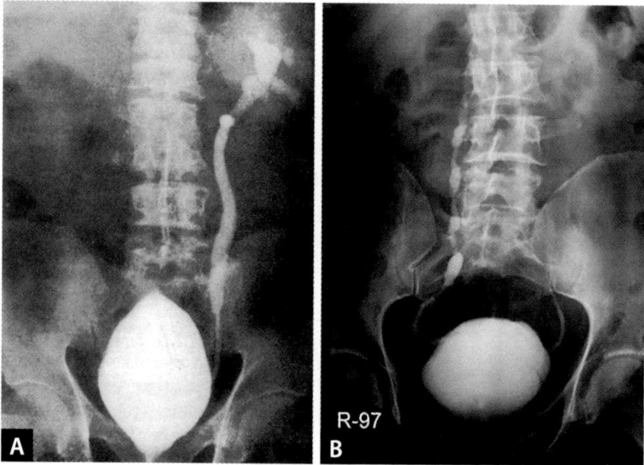

Figs. 10A and B: Ureteric strictures. (A) IVU showing long irregular stricture involving lower end of left ureter with hydroureter, hydronephrosis and infundibular stenosis of inferior calyx of left kidney. Also note changes of tuberculosis involving L2-L3 vertebrae; (B) Beaded appearance of right ureter.

segments which are more superficially involved may heal without stricture formation. This produces a beaded or corkscrew appearance of the ureter.[20] Ureteral strictures have been reported in 10–56% of patients with urinary tract TB.

The terminal segment of the ureter is most commonly involved **(Figs. 10A and B)**. However, any part may be involved with multiple strictures seen in 19% cases. In later stages, severe thickening of the wall produces a rigid shortened ureter with narrow lumen termed as "pipe stem ureter". Renal damage secondary to ureteral strictures may

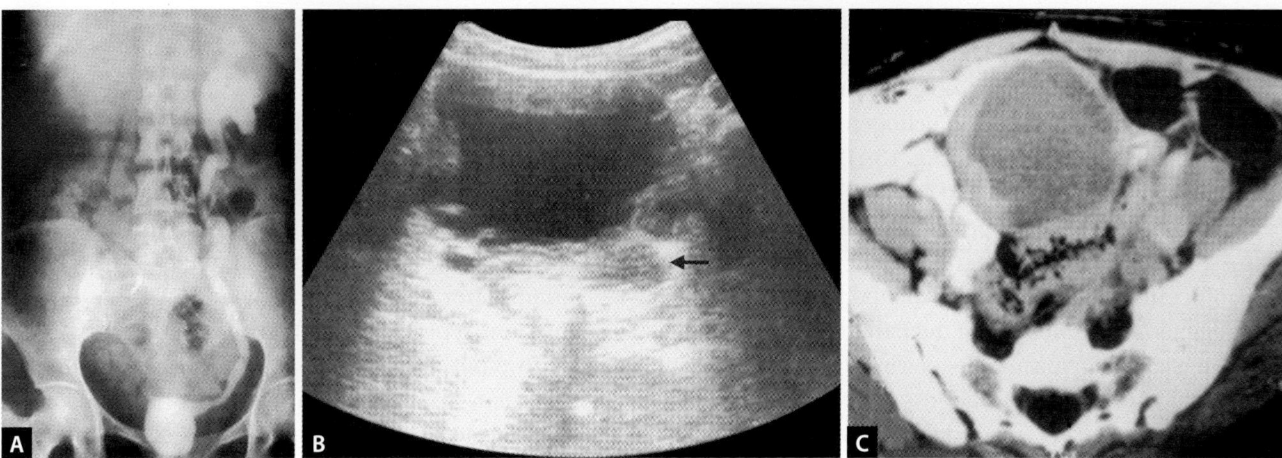

Figs. 11A to C: Urinary bladder TB. (A) IVU reveals a small capacity (thimble) urinary bladder, ureteral stricture with proximal hydroureter and hydronephrosis on left side. Right kidney is nonfunctioning; (B) Ultrasonography shows irregular, asymmetric wall thickening of the urinary bladder with trabeculations. A left adnexal mass is also seen posterior to the bladder (arrow) (C) CT shows a similar appearance of the urinary bladder.

be more severe than the effect of the original parenchymal involvement. Dilatation and stenting of the ureter may restore ureteral patency and salvage a kidney.

Urinary Bladder

Urinary bladder is involved later in the course of the disease in up to one-third of patients of urinary tract TB. Use of bacillus Calmette-Guérin therapy for bladder cancer can cause symptomatic tubercular infections of the lower genitourinary tract.[7] Tubercular cystitis leads to edema of the bladder mucosa. Large tuberculomas in vesical wall can manifest radiologically as filling defects simulating carcinoma.[21] Advanced disease leads to irregular contracture with thick walls and reduction of bladder capacity—the "thimble bladder" **(Figs. 11A to C)**. Fibrosis in the region of the trigone produces gaping of the ureterovesical junction resulting in free vesicoureteric reflux **(Fig. 12)**.

Urethral Tuberculosis

Tuberculosis of the male urethra is uncommon and usually occurs secondary to renal infection. It may also be associated with prostatic abscess, periurethral abscess or fistula formation. It may result in a nonspecific stricture almost always in the bulbomembranous urethra that is indistinguishable on imaging from strictures due to other causes.

Retrograde Pyelography

Retrograde pyelography is particularly indicated in a patient with nonfunctioning kidney to demonstrate ureteric obstruction and cavitation in the kidney.

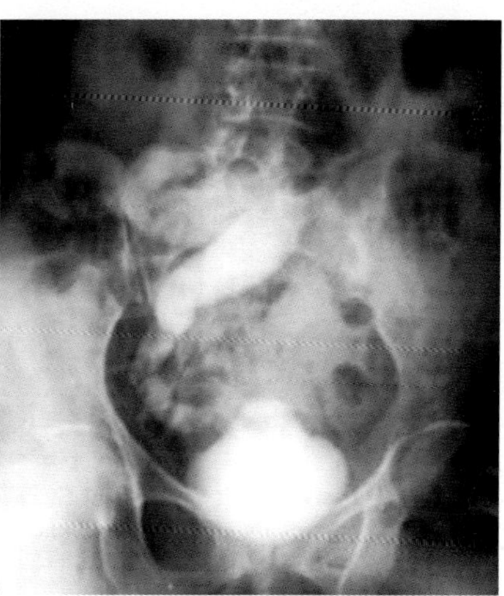

Fig. 12: Urinary bladder tuberculosis with vesicoureteric reflux (VUR). Micturating cystourethrogram (MCU) study reveals a small capacity bladder with reflux into a dilated, tortuous right ureter.

Ultrasonography

Ultrasound is not used as the primary imaging modality for diagnosis of urinary tract TB, as it is unable to show early calyceal changes and does not provide information about renal functional status. However, carefully performed sonogram can show a spectrum of morphological abnormalities.[22,23] The role of sonography is also to provide guidance for the interventional procedures of percutaneous nephrostomy (PCN), antegrade dilatation of ureteral stricture and drainage of the perinephric abscess.

Kidney

A focal renal lesion of varying echogenicity is a frequently encountered sonographic abnormality. In the early

stages US demonstrates papillary lesions as areas of hypoechogenicity or hypoechoic foci with echogenic walls or echogenic nonshadowing lesions **(*see* Fig. 5B)**.[23] A sloughed calyx is seen as an echogenic flap separated from the normal calyceal wall **(Fig. 13A)**. Large liquefying conglomerate cavities or dilated calyces formed as a result of infundibular stricture appear as hypoechoic nodules or masses. The communicating tract from a cavity appears as a sonolucent track entering the dilated calyx **(Fig. 13B)**. Heterogeneous echotexture of the parenchyma or normal appearing parenchyma may be seen in diffuse involvement **(Figs. 14A and B)**. Such patients show poor excretory function on IVU and CT. Following pelvicalyceal system involvement, US may characteristically show uneven caliectasis without renal pelvis dilatation. It may also demonstrate hydronephrosis, parenchymal calcification, and perinephric abscess **(Figs. 15A and B)**.

Xuefang Rui et al.[24] reviewed sonographic features of 258 cases of renal TB. In this series of 258 cases, 152 cases were correctly diagnosed as renal TB by B-mode ultrasonography, and these were classified under 6 types.

Type I: Nephrectasia type (23 cases); type II: Hydrops type, (21 cases); type III: Empyema type (13 cases); type IV: Inflammatory and atrophy type (15 cases); type V: Calcification type (34 cases); type VI: Mixed type (46 cases). In type I (Nephrectasia), the renal capsule was very irregular. In the renal parenchyma and renal sinus, there were one or several anechoic zones, of different sizes with irregular margins and some nebulous light spot echoes within. The type II (Hydrops type) also showed an

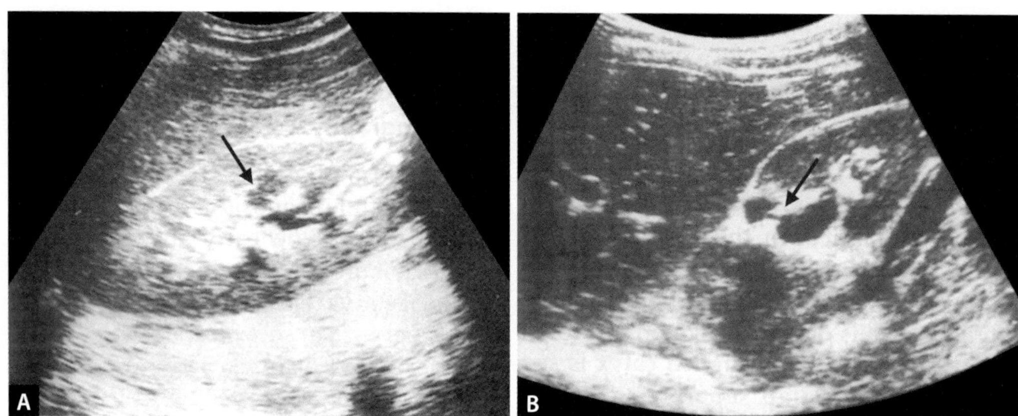

Figs. 13A and B: Ultrasonography findings of renal tuberculosis. (A) US showing echogenic papillary sloughing in the middle calyx of the right kidney (arrow); (B) US of another patient reveals an anechoic cavity in the renal cortex with a sonolucent track (arrow) connecting the cavity and the pelvicalyceal system.

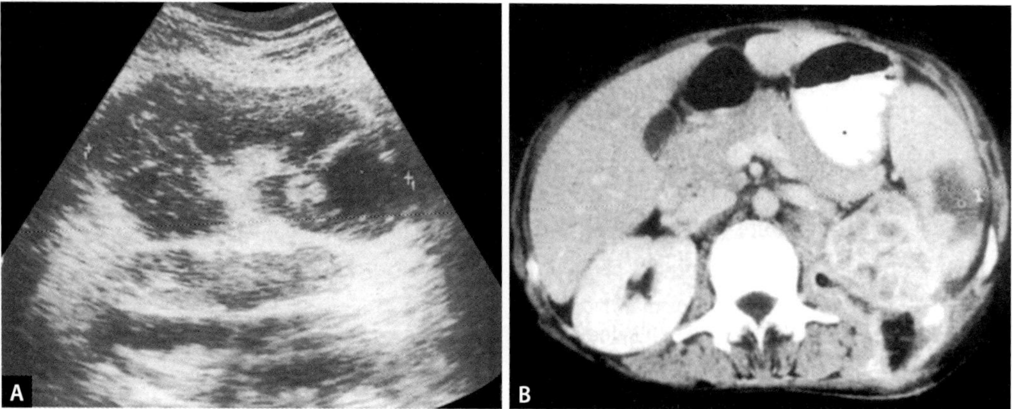

Figs.14A and B: Ultrasonography appearance of diffuse involvement of kidney by tuberculosis. (A) US shows an enlarged heterogeneous left kidney with an anechoic cavity in the lower pole; (B) CECT of the same patient reveals poorly functioning heterogeneous left kidney with hypodense areas within. An irregular hypoattenuating splenic abscess and inflammatory changes in the left posterior renal space, left psoas and posterior parietes are also seen.

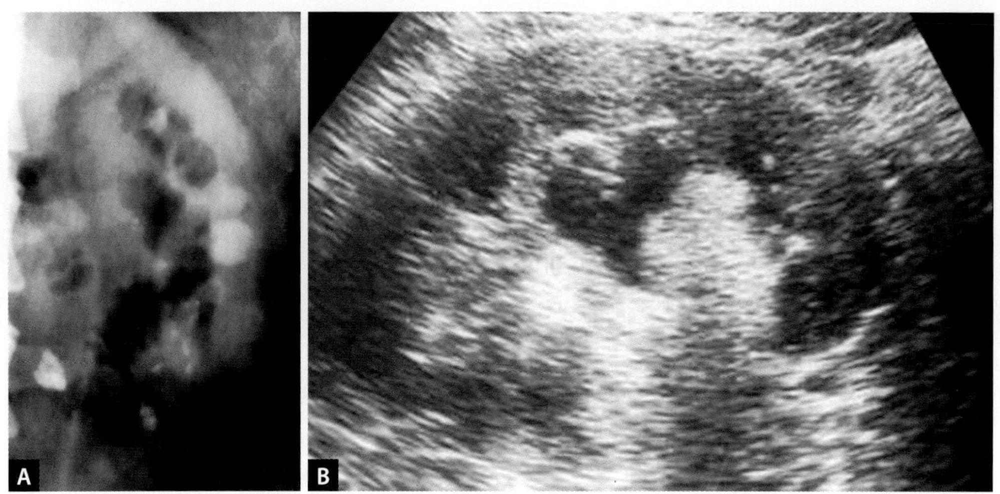

Figs. 15A and B: Uneven caliectasis on ultrasonography. (A) Intravenous urography; and (B) Ultrasound of left kidney of a 28 years old male reveals uneven caliectasis with calcification within.

irregular renal capsule. The renal pelvis and calyces were distended, within which there was an anechoic zone, similar to hydronephrosis. However, the inner wall was rough and uneven. In most cases, the ureter was involved and appeared thickened.

Ureter

Ultrasonography does not play a significant role in the acute phase. It is useful in assessment and follow up of back pressure changes and adjoining retroperitoneal disease.

Urinary Bladder

Ultrasonography may detect focal irregularity or thickening of the bladder wall with reduced capacity. Distension of the bladder may be necessary to gauge the bladder capacity accurately. The deformed bladder shape and focal abnormalities are also better appreciated following distension **(Fig. 11B)**.

Computed Tomography

Over the years, there has been a decrease in the number of IVUs, and a corresponding increase in the number of multidetector CT(MDCTs) being performed even in the setting of urinary tract TB. MDCT with its multiple reconstructions is useful in demonstrating the extent of involvement, length of ureteric stricture, adjoining retroperitoneal disease and associated spinal or solid organ involvement.[25] A combination of corticomedullary, nephrographic and urographic phases allows the delineation of both renal parenchymal as well as urothelial changes. However, the acquisition can be restricted to a single phase in young patients. While IVU is superior to CT in the demonstration of early calyceal changes and papillary necrosis, CT is comparable or better for most abnormalities, it also has the advantage of demonstrating involvement of other abdominal organs. Compared to US, CT is also able to provide better visualization of retroperitoneal structures, more detailed information on presence and pattern of calcification and functional status of the kidney.

Spectrum of Imaging Findings on Computed Tomography

Kidney

Computed tomography may show a spectrum of findings in renal involvement including multiple small poorly enhancing nodules, uneven caliectasis and calcification. In poorly functioning of kidneys the nephrogram effect is much better seen on CT than on IVU.

- *Solid focal lesions*: Representing granulomas, hypodense, variable size. Smaller lesions are often nonenhancing, while larger lesions show rim enhancement. **(Figs. 16A to C)** These have been reported in 12% of cases in a CT based study.[26]
- *Cystic focal lesions*: A cystic lesion adjoining a renal calyx (representing a cavity) is one of the commonest findings (reported in 68% of cases[26]). These often show multiple septations. The overlying cortex is thinned out. Granulomas which caseate and coalesce often appear as complex cystic lesions. On delayed phases, pooling of contrast is seen if the cavity is

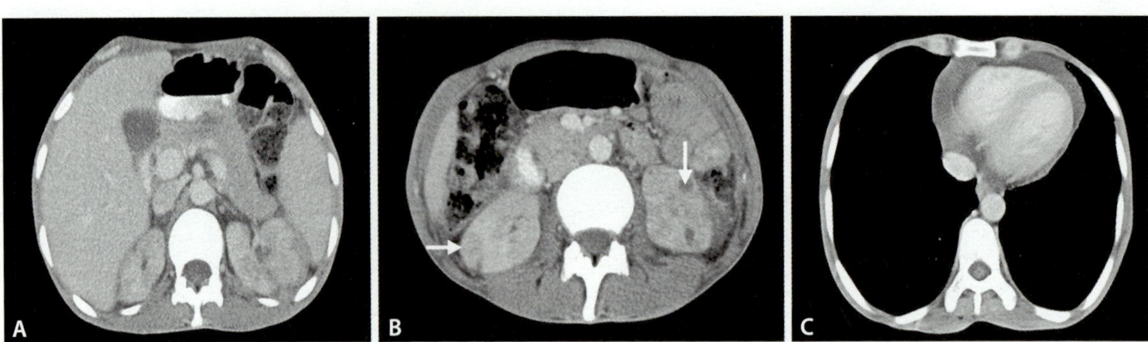

Figs. 16A to C: Solid focal lesions pattern of renal involvement on CT. CECT of a 36 years old male (A and B) showing multiple hypodense lesions in the left kidney with adjoining perinephric collection and fascial thickening. Right kidney reveals a small hypodense lesion (arrows) (C) Patient also had pericardial effusion.

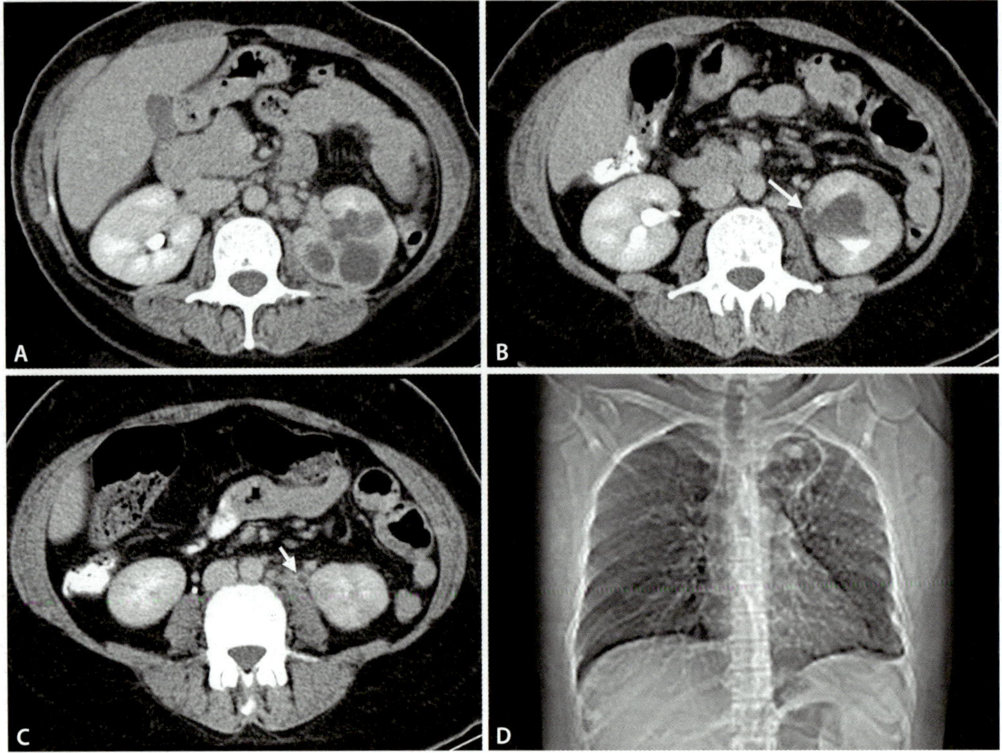

Figs.17A to D: Urothelial involvement. CECT of a young girl reveals a poorly functioning (L) kidney with hydronephrosis. (A) Small retroperitoneal nodes are present; (B) Renal pelvis is contracted with a thickened wall (arrow); (C) The ureteric wall is also thickened (arrow); (D) Topogram reveals a cavity in the left upper lobe of lung.

communicating with the PCS **(Fig. 5C)**. Abscesses often show peripheral enhancement and adjoining inflammation.

- *Focal areas of hypoperfusion*: These are a consequence of vasoconstriction/or small vessel narrowing resulting from active inflammation and edema. This picture resembles acute pyelonephritis.
- *Perinephric inflammation*: Abscess often spread into the perinephric space with thickening of adjoining fasciae **(Figs. 16A and B)**.
- *Urothelial involvement*:
  - Thickening of the wall of pelvis/urothelial thickening leads to narrowing **(Figs. 17 and 18)**.
  - Calyceal irregularity and dilatation may be seen.[27]
  - Uneven caliectasis is characteristic with contracted pelvis **(Figs. 18 and 19)**.
- *Sequelae*:
  - With healing and fibrosis, parenchymal scars develop seen as focal areas of cortical thinning often overlying a dilated or distorted calyx.

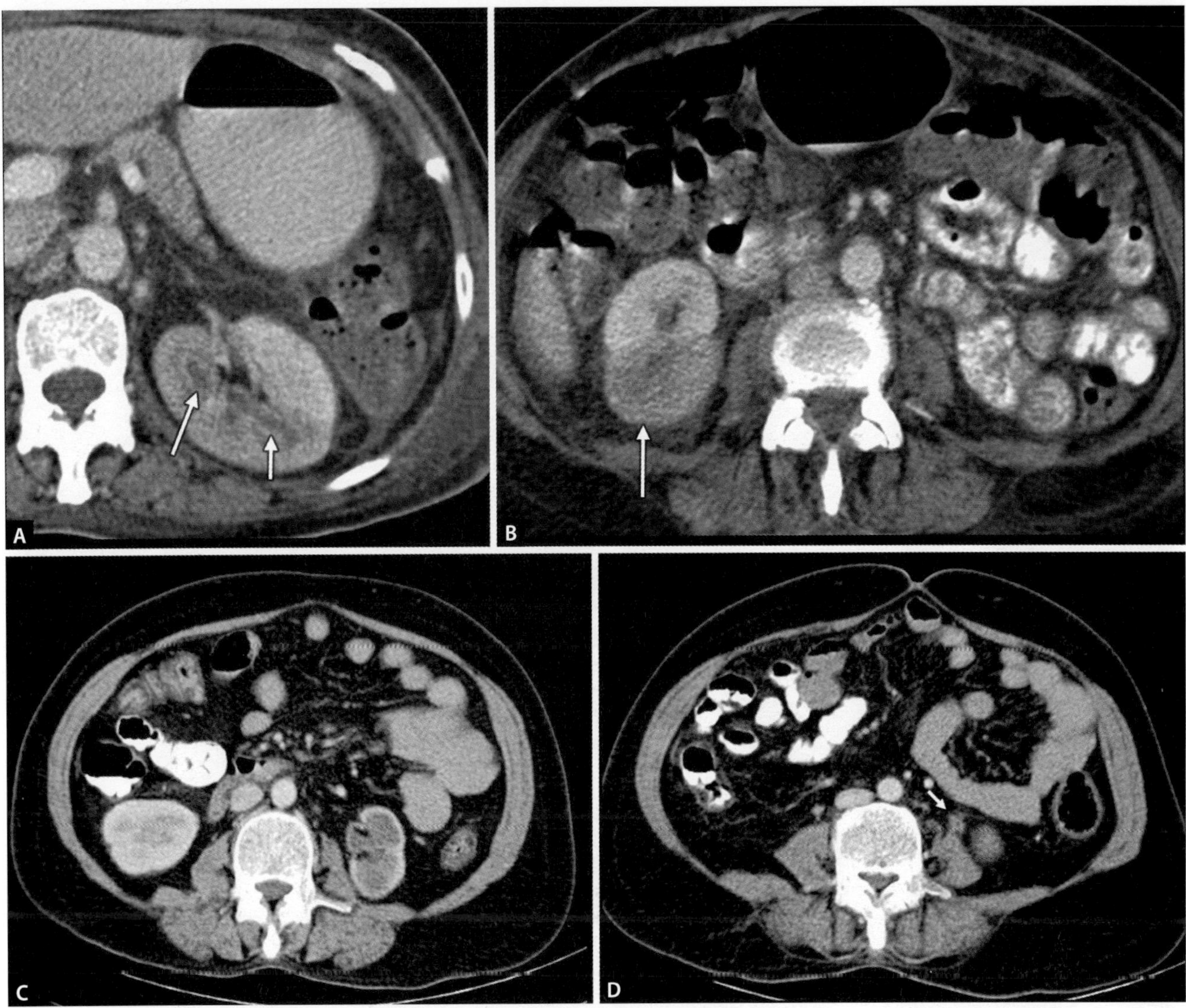

Figs. 18A to D: Pelvicalyceal and ureteric urothelial thickening in two different patients. (A) CECT of 61/F shows thickening of the urothelium of pelvicalyceal system (PCS) of left kidney (arrows); (B) Focal large hypodense area seen in upper pole of right kidney with perinephric stranding (focal pyelonephritis form); (C) CECT of a different patient, a 43 years old female reveals left kidney is shrunken with hydronephrosis, scarred pelvis and parenchymal thinning (C). Wall thickening of ureter (arrow) is present (D).

- *Calcification*: Various patterns including punctate, curvilinear, amorphous or lobar calcification are seen **(Figs. 19A to C)**.

Ureter

Thickening of the ureteric wall is highly suggestive of TB and can be readily identified on CT **(Fig. 18D)**.

Urinary Bladder

Computed tomography delineates the bladder involvement well similar to IVU/USG but offers no additional advantage except for detection of faint calcification and demonstration of adjacent genital tract disease **(Figs. 11C and 19D)**.

Magnetic Resonance Imaging

Although, there are few published studies on the use of MRI in urinary tract TB, it has in recent years evolved as a useful adjunct modality in the evaluation of these patients. MRI provides both morphological and functional information. Noncontrast scans are immensely useful in those with compromised renal functions, especially with addition of MR urography.[28] Contrast-enhanced magnetic resonance (CEMR) not only delineates the extent better, characterizes focal lesions, demonstrates

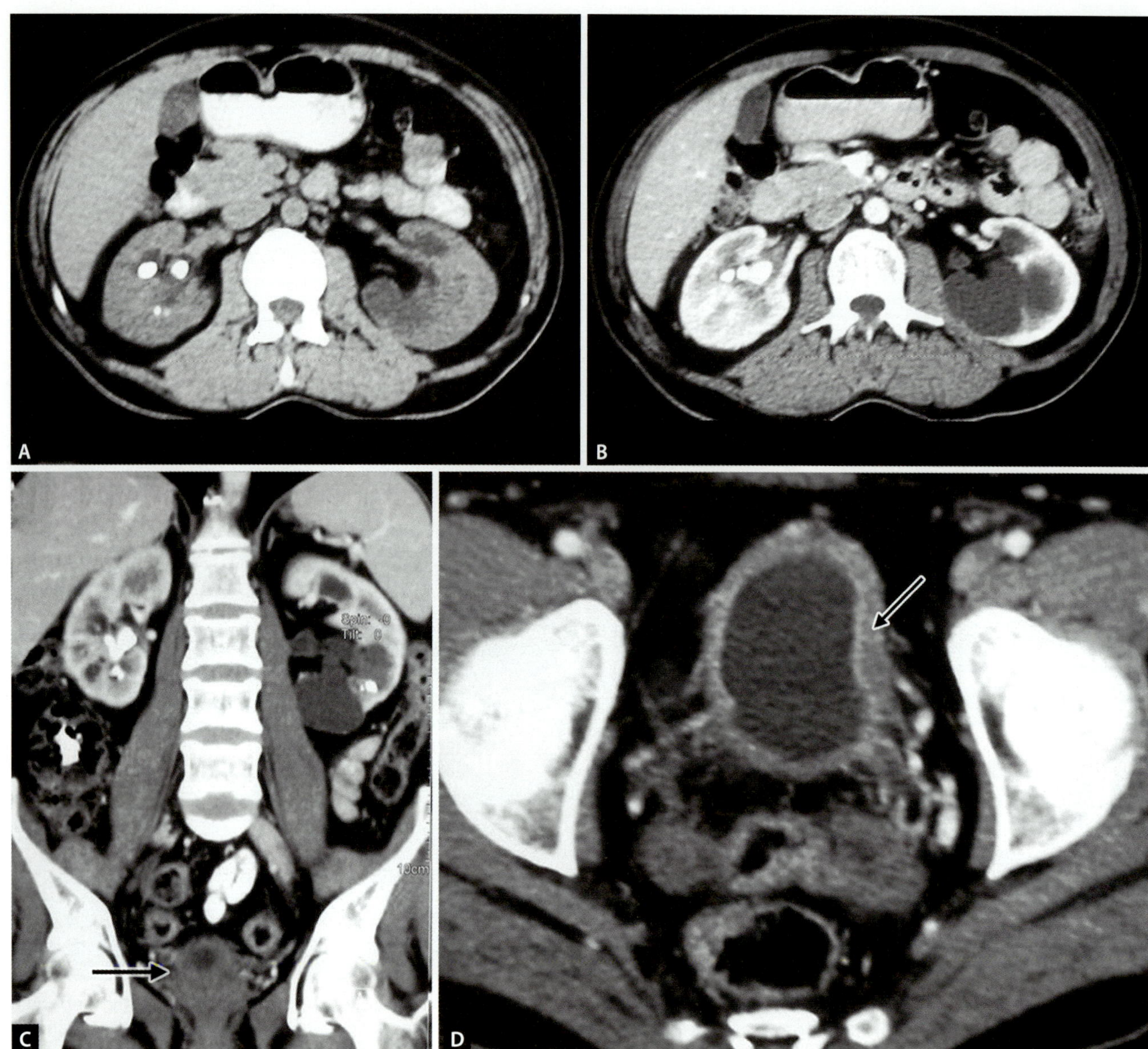

Figs. 19A to D: Uneven caliectasis and bladder involvement on CT. Multidetector computed tomography (MDCT) axial (A and B) and coronal; (C) Show a large cavity with irregular caliectasis and calcification involving the lower pole of left kidney. Right kidney has calculi. Scan through pelvis; (D) reveals urinary bladder wall thickening with small capacity (arrow).

urothelial thickening but can also evaluate renal function **(Figs. 20 and 21)**. Diffusion-weighted imaging (DWI) aids in characterizing the focal renal lesions, differentiates hydronephrosis from pronephrosis; and is an indicator of renal fibrosis. Time-resolved dynamic CEMR urography can be used for the evaluation of ureteral peristalsis.[29]

Key MRI findings of urinary tract TB are summarized in **Table 2**.

COMPLICATIONS

The prominent complications include perinephric inflammation/abscess formation including psoas abscesses **(Figs. 21A to E)**. Fistulae or sinus tracts may develop into adjacent tissues or viscera **(Figs. 22 and 23)**.

DIFFERENTIAL DIAGNOSIS

The differential diagnosis of urinary TB can be varied depending upon the form of involvement. Early renal TB can simulate papillary necrosis. Focal lesions resemble other infections or even neoplasms. Calcification and extensive inflammation can mimic xanthogranulomatous pyelonephritis. Similarly, urinary bladder involvement may be confused with neoplastic involvement.

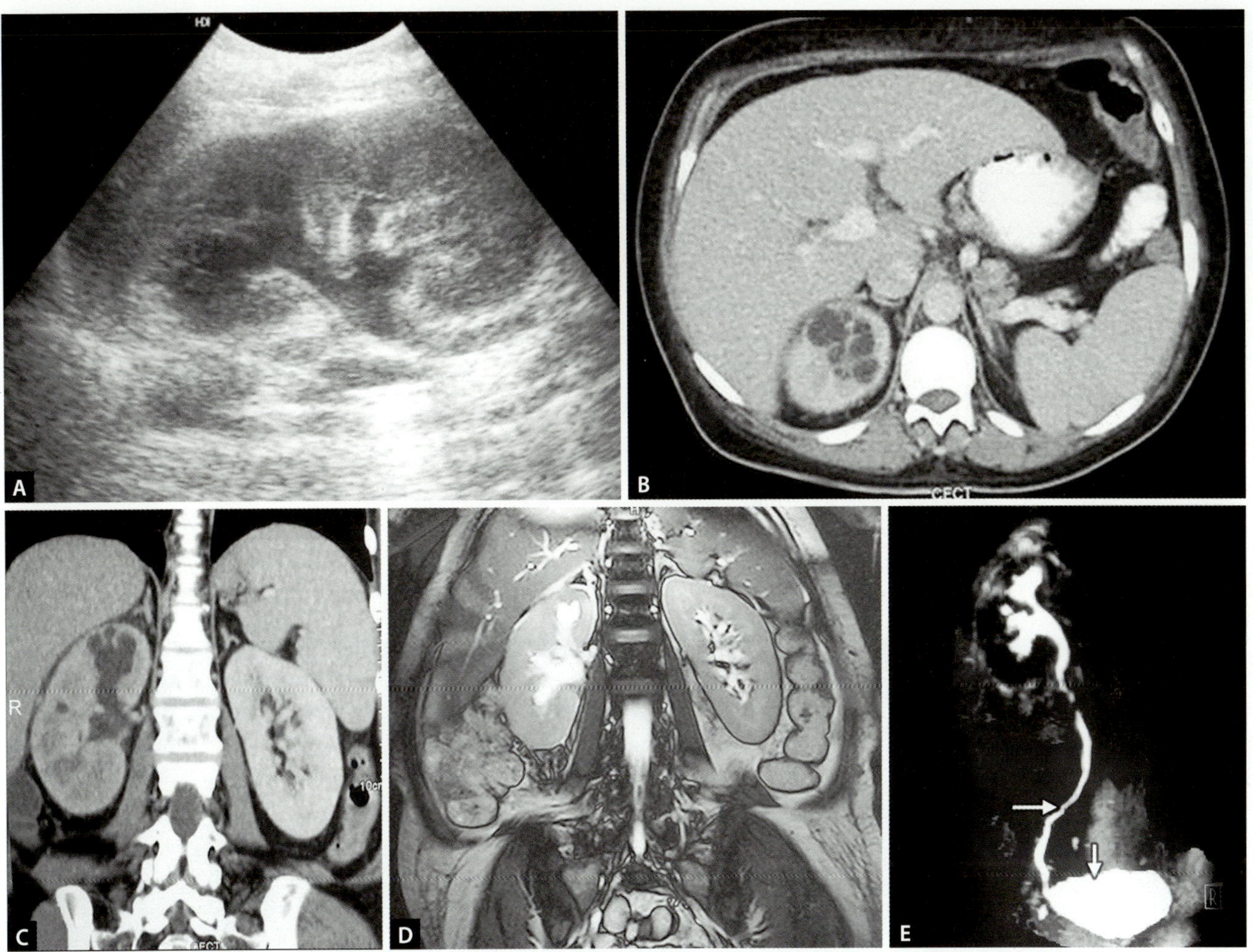

Figs. 20A to E: Utility of MR urography in urinary tract TB. Images of a 49 years female. US (A) reveals caliectasis of the superior calyx. Axial CECT (B) shows multiple cavities involving upper pole of the right kidney. Coronal CECT MPR (C) shows the cavities communicating with the superior calyx with parenchymal atrophy of the upper pole, and poor function of the right kidney. True-FISP coronal MRI (D) reveals increased signal intensity of the right kidney. MR urogram (E), in addition illustrates ureteric and bladder irregularity (arrows).

GENITOURINARY TUBERCULOSIS IN HUMAN IMMUNODEFICIENCY VIRUS

The impact of human immunodeficiency virus (HIV) epidemic on the incidence and clinical presentation of genitourinary TB is largely unknown. Navarro et al.[12] evaluated clinical and epidemiological characteristics of patients diagnosed with genitourinary TB at their center over the last 10 years, found that of the 45 patients analyzed, 33% had a coexisting disease (14 were infected by HIV). In a retrospective study from USA, case records of 16 patients infected with HIV and genitourinary TB were compared with those of 8 patients without HIV infection diagnosed with genitourinary TB. Data abstracted from records included demographics, symptoms, signs, laboratory and radiologic findings, and in-hospital mortality. Of 1,282 patients with TB, 24 patients had positive urine cultures for *Mycobacterium TB*. HIV infection was present in 16 patients (75%). Patients infected with HIV were younger (mean age, 39.1 ± 6.2 versus 53.9 ± 17.2, P = 0.047) but did not differ significantly in clinical presentation from patients who did not have HIV infection.[30]

TUBERCULAR INFECTION OF THE GRAFT KIDNEY

Tuberculosis is a frequent complication in solid organ transplant (SOT) recipients, due to their immunosuppressed status, especially in TB endemic regions. TB involving the transplanted kidney is however rare. TB in graft kidney may either be a consequence of preexisting infection in the donor; or a part of disseminated TB in the recipient.[31] TB in transplant kidney can result

Table 2: Magnetic resonance imaging findings of urinary tract tuberculosis.

Form of involvement	*MRI findings*
Active inflammation	• CEMR: Focal hypoperfusion (D/D acute pyelonephritis) • Loss of interface with adjoining parenchyma • Surrounding fat tissue stranding
Chronic abscess	• Signal characteristic resembling a cyst; with thick walls and internal septae, restricted diffusion • Differential diagnosis cystic neoplasm
Granuloma (depending on size, amount of caseation and calcification)	• *Solid mass (variable size):* – Small lesions—hypointense on both T1WI and T2WI – Central hyperintensity in larger lesions • Caseation—mildly hyperintense on T2WI, fluid debris level • Calcification—hypointense
PCS involvement	• Caliectasis (MRU) • Pelvic scarring • Urothelial thickening (CEMR) • Low ADC in pyonephrosis • Ureteral strictures • Urethral strictures
TB sequelae (Interstitial fibrosis)	• Small size, irregular • Low ADC

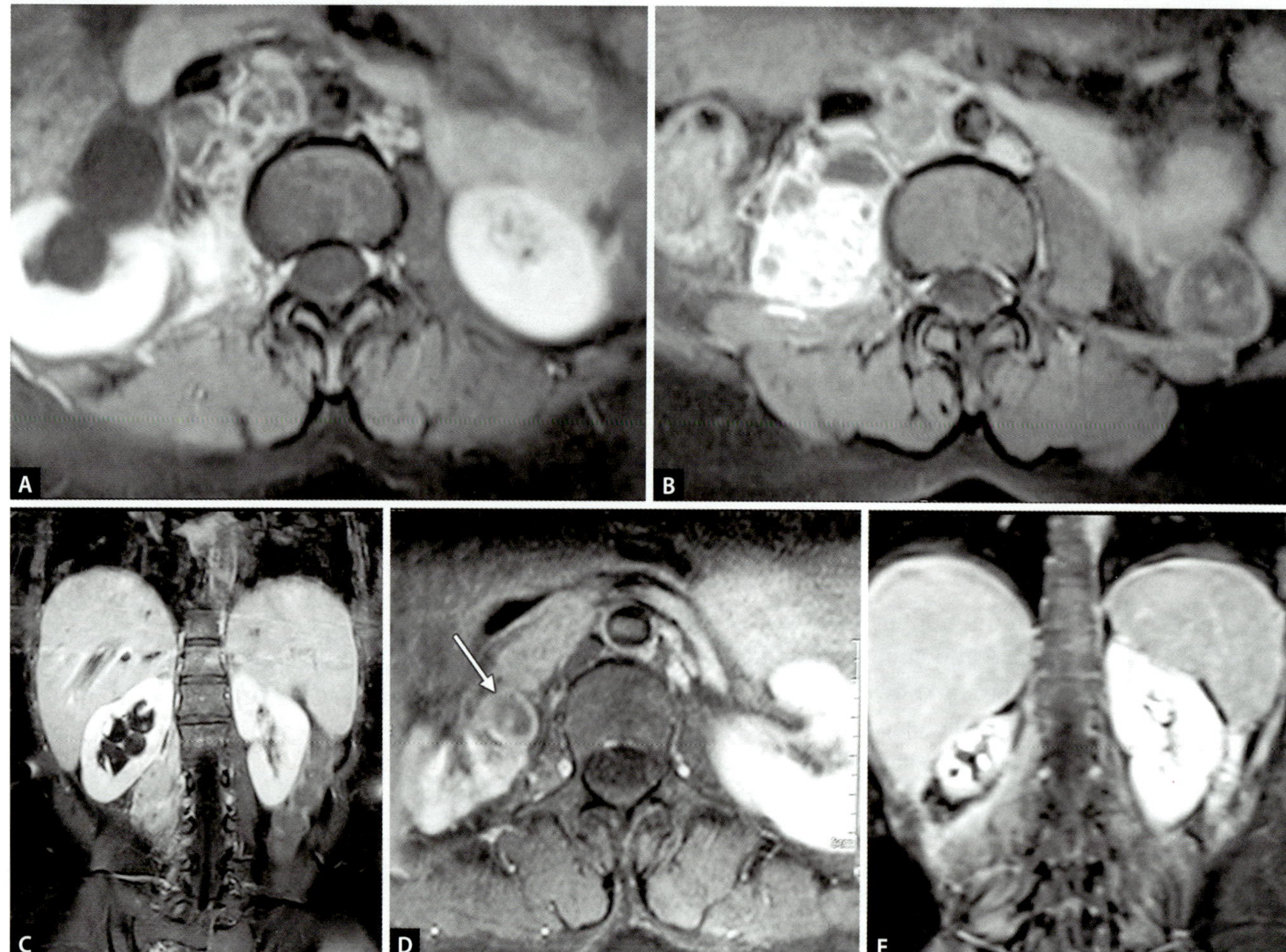

Figs. 21A to E: MRI characterizing focal renal lesion (chronic abscess) and retroperitoneal involvement in TB. Serial gadolinium-enhanced MR images of a 28 years old woman of multidrug resistant tuberculosis. Axial (A and B) and coronal; (C) Post-gadolinium images reveal necrotic retroperitoneal nodes with right psoas abscess encasing the ureter and causing hydronephrosis. MR scan obtained 8 months after second line antitubercular treatment (ATT); (D and E) shows reduction of the lymphadenopathy and psoas abscess. The right kidney is however shrunken and has a rim-enhancing lesion in the renal cortex suggesting an abscess (arrow).

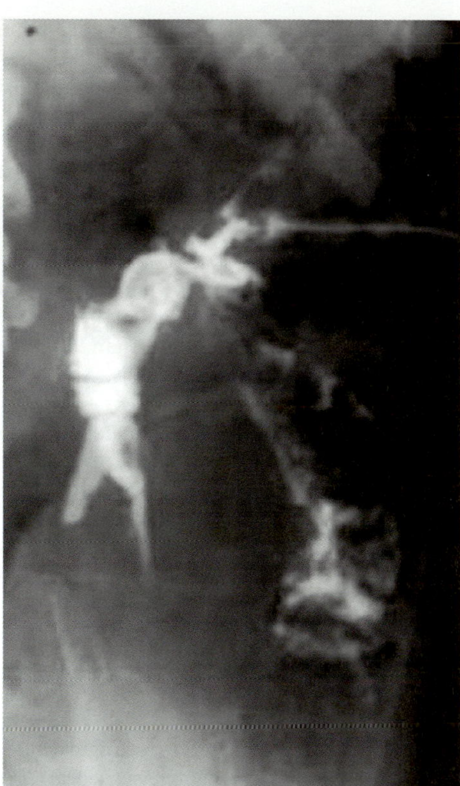

Fig. 22: Sinogram performed in a 28 years old man with a **chronic discharging (L) lumbar sinus** reveals opacification of the pelvicalyceal system.

in graft rejection, and also increases mortality, 17.86% is reported in a series.[32] There are several risk factors that predispose a recipient to develop graft TB. These include: diabetes, use all cyclosporine, mycophenolate mofetil, posttransplant rejection, coexisting chronic liver disease. Renal TB in the graft is often a part of disseminated TB in the recipient, and no characteristic imaging features are described. Also, the findings are often mild and resemble other infections (nonspecific).

The main differences between TB in a graft kidney as compared to TB in an immunocompetent host are enlisted in **Box 1**.

CONCLUSION

In conclusion, diagnosis of urinary tract TB is based on a high index of clinical suspicion supported by a collective evaluation of microbiological, radiological and endoscopic features. While individual radiological features of urinary tract TB can be seen in other diseases such as papillary necrosis due to other causes, infections and neoplasms; the key to diagnosis is pattern recognition. Also, follow-up excretory urography at regular intervals is useful both for assessment of therapeutic response, and for an early detection of the complications.

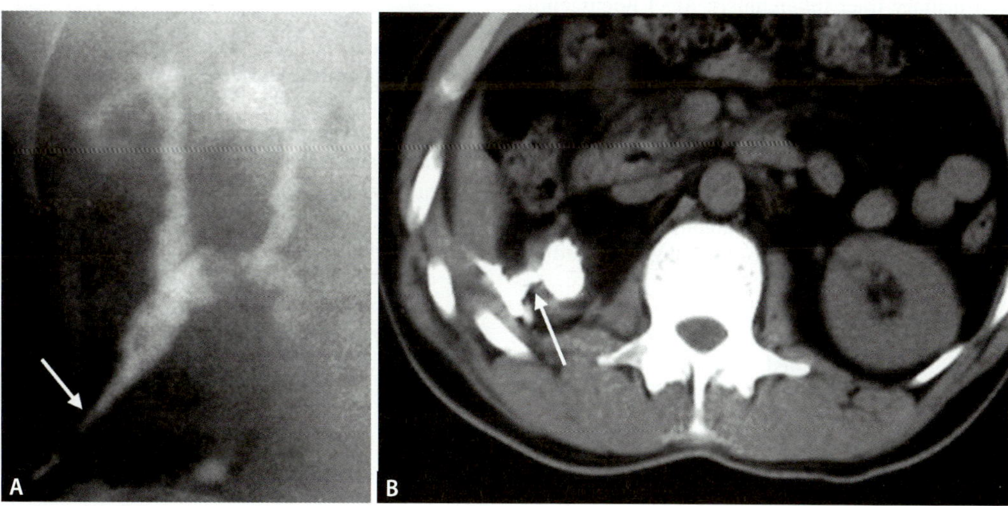

Figs. 23A and B: Sinogram (A) and CT sinogram; (B) of a different patient shows a shrunken right kidney, with **sinus tract** extending from the calyces to the skin (arrows).

Box 1: Graft kidney tuberculosis versus tuberculosis in immunocompetent host.

- No long latency. Typical period of onset is early (often in first 6 months)
- High urine culture positivity
- Urinary tract symptoms are often absent
- Part of disseminated disease
- Imaging findings mild and nonspecific

REFERENCES

1. World Health Organization (2018). Global tuberculosis report 2018. World Health Organization. https://apps.who.int/iris/handle/10665/274453. License: CC BY-NC-SA 3.0 IGO.
2. Merchant S, Bharati A, Merchant N. Tuberculosis of the genitourinary system-urinary tract tuberculosis: renal tuberculosis-part I. Indian J Radiol Imaging. 2013;23(1):46-63.
3. Zachoval R, Nencka P, Vasakova M, et al. The incidence of subclinical forms of urogenital tuberculosis in patients with pulmonary tuberculosis. J Infect Public Health. 2018;11(2):243-5.
4. Leder RA, Low VH. Tuberculosis of the abdomen. Radiol Clin North Am. 1995;33(4):691-705.
5. Naidich DP, Garay SM, Leitman BS, et al. Radiographic manifestations of pulmonary disease in the acquired immunodeficiency syndrome (AIDS). Semin Roentgenol. 1987;22(1):14-30.
6. Chandan D, ankur G. Imaging in urogenital tuberculosis. 1st edition. New Delhi: Jaypee Brothers Medical Publishers; 2019.
7. Wise GJ, Shteynshlyuger A. An update on lower urinary tract tuberculosis. Curr Urol Rep. 2008;9(4):305-13.
8. Wise GJ, Marella VK. Genitourinary manifestations of tuberculosis. Urol Clin North Am. 2003;30(1):111-21.
9. Chan DS, Choy MY, Wang S, et al. An evaluation of the recovery of mycobacteria from urine specimens using the automated Mycobacteria Growth Indicator Tube system (BACTEC MGIT 960). J Med Microbiol. 2008;57(Pt 10):1220-2.
10. Hemal AK, Gupta NP, Rajeev TP, et al. Polymerase chain reaction in clinically suspected genitourinary tuberculosis: comparison with intravenous urography, bladder biopsy, and urine acid fast bacilli culture. Urology. 2000;56(4):570-4.
11. Premkumar A, Lattimer J, Newhouse JH. CT and sonography of advanced urinary tract tuberculosis. Am J Roentgenol. 1987;148(1):65-9.
12. Navarro-Vilasaro M, Font B, Sala M, et al. Genitourinary mycobacteriosis: retrospective study of 45 cases in a general hospital. Enferm Infecc Microbiol Clin. 2008;26(9):540-5.
13. Goldman SM, Fishman EK, Hartman DS, et al. Computed tomography of renal tuberculosis and its pathological correlates. J Comput Assist Tomogr. 1985;9(4):771-6.
14. Pollack HM, McClennan BL. Clinical Urography: Saunders; 2000.
15. Dalla Palma L. What is left of IV urography? Eur Radiol. 2001;11(6):931-9.
16. Kollins SA, Hartman GW, Carr DT, et al. Roentgenographic findings in urinary tract tuberculosis. A 10 year review. Am J Roentgenol Radium Ther Nucl Med. 1974;121(3):487-99.
17. Engin G, Acunas B, Acunas G, et al. Imaging of extrapulmonary tuberculosis. Radiographics. 2000;20(2):471-88.
18. Merchant S, Bharati A, Merchant N. Tuberculosis of the genitourinary system-urinary tract tuberculosis: renal tuberculosis-part II. Indian J Radiol Imaging. 2013;23(1):64-77.
19. Narayana A. Overview of renal tuberculosis. Urology. 1982;19(3):231-7.
20. Wasserman NF. Inflammatory disease of the ureter. Radiol Clin North Am. 1996;34(6):1131-56.
21. Camilien LD, Boyce JG. Diagnostic imaging of gynecological diseases: the clinician's view. Urol Radiol. 1991;13(1):3-8.
22. Das KM, Indudhara R, Vaidyanathan S. Sonographic features of genitourinary tuberculosis. Am J Roentgenol. 1992;158(2):327-9.
23. Schaffer R, Becker JA, Goodman J. Sonography of tuberculous kidney. Urology. 1983;22(2):209-11.
24. Rui X, Li XD, Cai S, et al. Ultrasonographic diagnosis and typing of renal tuberculosis. Int J Urol. 2008;15(2):135-9.
25. Gaudiano C, Tadolini M, Busato F, et al. Multidetector CT urography in urogenital tuberculosis: use of reformatted images for the assessment of the radiological findings. A pictorial essay. Abdom Radiol (NY). 2017;42(9):2314-24.
26. Lu P, Li C, Zhou X. Significance of the CT scan in renal tuberculosis. Zhonghua Jie He He Hu Xi Za Zhi. 2001;24(7):407-9.
27. Lang EK, Macchia RJ, Thomas R, et al. Improved detection of renal pathologic features on multiphasic helical CT compared with IVU in patients presenting with microscopic hematuria. Urology. 2003;61(3):528-32.
28. Leyendecker JR, Barnes CE, Zagoria RJ. MR urography: techniques and clinical applications. Radiographics. 2008;28(1):23-46.
29. Kim S, Jacob JS, Kim DC, et al. Time-resolved dynamic contrast-enhanced MR urography for the evaluation of ureteral peristalsis: initial experience. J Magn Reson Imaging. 2008;28(5):1293-8.
30. Nzerue C, Drayton J, Oster R, et al. Genitourinary tuberculosis in patients with HIV infection: clinical features in an inner-city hospital population. Am J Med Sci. 2000;320(5):299-303.
31. Nayak S, Satish R. Genitourinary tuberculosis after renal transplantation-a report of three cases with a good clinical outcome. Am J Transplant. 2007;7(7):1862-4.
32. Centers for Disease Control and Prevention (CDC). Transplantation-transmitted tuberculosis--Oklahoma and Texas, 2007. MMWR Morb Mortal Wkly Rep. 2008;57(13):333-6.

Chapter 7

Renal Cystic Diseases

Jyoti Kumar, Anjali Prakash, Sapna Singh

INTRODUCTION

Renal cystic lesions are a heterogeneous group of disorders characterized by multiple cysts in the kidneys. The most common cystic disease of the kidney is serous renal cyst, seen with advancing age. These may be simple or get complicated by hemorrhage, infection, or ischemia. These can then be difficult to differentiate from cystic malignancy. Bosniak classification of cysts helps categorize renal cysts to aid in management strategy based on imaging appearances. Although Bosniak classification has been currently described on contrast-enhanced computed tomography (CT) examination, contrast-enhanced ultrasound (US) and magnetic resonance (MR) are also being used to classify renal cysts.

In adults, other causes of renal cystic lesions can be focal or multifocal. Focal lesions include cystic tumors, pyelocalyceal diverticulum, and infection. Multifocal cystic disease of the kidney can also be characterized into heritable and nonheritable diseases. Since cystic lesions of kidney can have overlapping appearances, an understanding of the spectrum of this vast majority of renal cystic lesions can help reach a more specific diagnosis or suggest further relevant imaging recommendations to the clinician.

RENAL CYSTS

Serous Renal Cysts

The most common cystic disease of the kidney is serous renal cysts. These are increasingly seen with advancing age. These cysts can be multiple and variably sized.

On US examination, simple cysts are round and uniformly echo-free internally, with a well-defined posterior wall and strong acoustic shadowing. On Doppler examination, simple cysts show lack of color flow.

Computed tomographic scans show cysts to be masses of water density [0 20 Hounsfield unit (HU)] sharply defined from the adjacent renal parenchyma with no perceptible wall thickness. They are homogeneous and do not show calcification or enhancement after intravenous contrast is administered **(Fig. 1)**.

On MR imaging, simple cysts appear uniformly low-signal intensity on T1- and high-signal intensity on T2-weighted sequences with no contrast enhancement.

Atypical Cysts

Occasionally, simple cysts can get complicated by hemorrhage, infection, or ischemia. In these cysts,

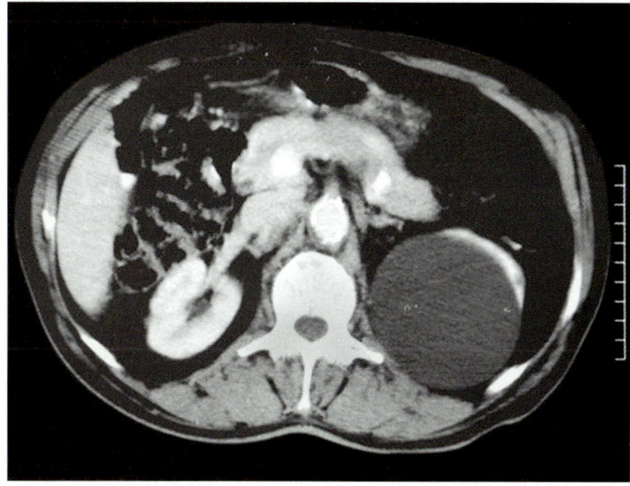

Fig. 1: Contrast-enhanced CT showing a large smoothly marginated lesion of homogeneous fluid density in left kidney with cortical "beak" sign typical of simple cyst. (CT: computed tomography).

Table 1: Bosniak classification.

Category of cyst	*Morphology*	*Management*
Bosniak I	• Simple cysts: No wall thickness, septae, calcification or enhancement	Benign, no follow-up
Bosniak II	• Cysts with pencil-thin wall. May have few fine internal septations (with or without perceived enhancement but no measurable enhancement); minimally thick calcification or short segment of thickened calcification • Homogeneous hyperdense cysts ≤3 cm that are well-defined and nonenhancing	Benign, no follow-up
IIF	• Cysts with mildly thickened wall/ multiple thin septations with no measurable enhancement but may have few thick or nodular calcifications • Homogeneous hyperdense nonenhancing cysts >3 cm that are completely intrarenal	Follow-up
Bosniak III	Cysts with thickened or irregular wall/septae with measurable enhancement	30–100% chances of malignancy. Surgical resection
Bosniak IV	Cyst with enhancing nodule in the wall/septum	Malignant unless proven otherwise. Surgical resection

differentiation from cystic neoplasms, infectious diseases, and other renal cystic disorders may be difficult. In 1986, Bosniak developed a classification system to characterize cystic lesions of the kidney based on CT features. However, it does not take into account the underlying pathophysiology. Changes to this classification were made in 1990s and in 2005 and now five basic categories are recognized.

Bosniak Classification System (Table 1)

Five major categories are recognized:

1. Category I lesions are simple cysts of water density (0–20 HU), sharply defined from the adjacent renal parenchyma with no perceptible wall thickness. They are homogeneous and do not show calcification or contrast enhancement **(Fig. 1)**. Category I lesions are considered benign and do not require follow-up.
2. Category II lesions **(Fig. 2)** are minimally complicated benign cysts. These may have hairline thin septae. There may be fine calcification in the wall/septa. The septae may show perceived but no measurable enhancement. A homogeneous hyperdense cyst >20 HU or ≤3 cm in size, with some extrarenal component, is also classified as category II cysts. The extrarenal component of the cyst helps us to verify the smooth nature of the cyst wall.
Lesions falling into category II are also considered benign and do not require follow-up.

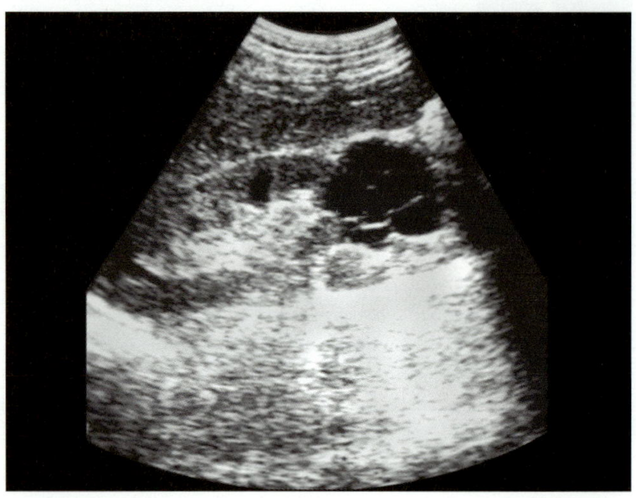

Fig. 2: Gray-scale sonogram of right kidney showing a complicated cyst with few thin internal septations (Bosniak's category II lesion) (CT: computed tomography).

3. *Category IIF cyst (F for follow-up):* These cysts lie in between category II and III lesions. These include cysts with multiple thin internal septations but no measurable enhancement, few nodular calcifications, or a smoothly thickened cyst wall **(Fig. 3)**. Hyperattenuating cysts which are larger than 3 cm or completely intrarenal are also included in category IIF cysts.
The risk of malignancy in these lesions is approximately 5% and these lesions need to be followed up. Recommendations for follow-up vary in the literature from 1 to 4 years depending upon how complex the lesion is.
4. Category III cysts have thick or irregular walls and/or septae that demonstrate measurable enhancement. There may be thick nodular calcification. As the chances of malignancy are high (30–100%), surgical resection is recommended in these lesions. Many of these lesions may prove to be benign, e.g. aggregates of simple cysts, multilocular cystic nephroma, lymphangioma, or hydatid disease.

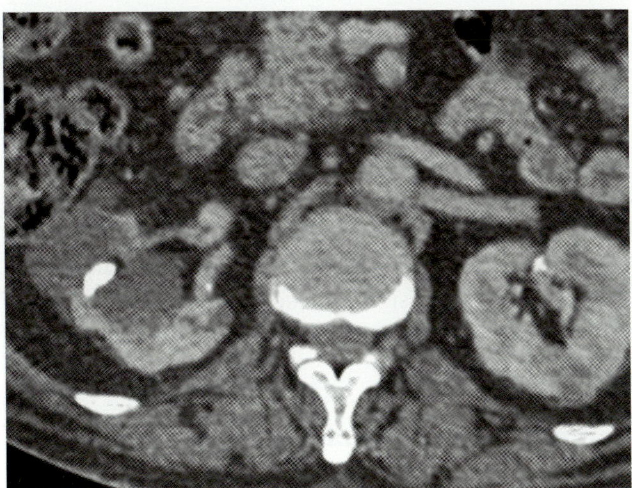

Fig. 3: Contrast-enhanced CT scan showing a cyst in the right kidney with thick nodular calcification (Bosniak's category IIF lesion). (CT: computed tomography).

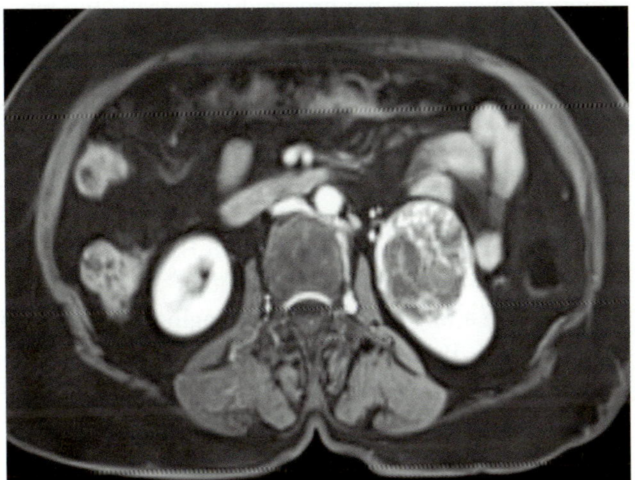

Fig. 4: Contrast-enhanced MR showing a multiloculated cystic mass arising from left kidney with nodular mural thickening and irregularity Bosniak's category IV lesion. (MR: magnetic resonance).

5. Category IV cysts are cysts with a clear enhancing nodule in the wall or in the septa **(Fig. 4)**. The management is surgical resection as they are considered malignant unless proven otherwise. Several associated patient comorbidities are the only factor that warrant against surgery.

Diagnosis and management are clear in category I and IV lesions but difficult in category II and III lesions. The gold standard of surgical resection has come under the scanner owing to the increasing database that mortality rates from renal cell carcinoma (RCC) have risen over the past 20 years despite early detection and resection. Studies also suggest that more and more lesions are being treated surgically which would otherwise have no impact on patient mortality. Hence, there remains the challenge of distinguishing benign Bosniak 2F, 3, and 4 lesions from malignant Bosniak IIF, III, and IV lesions.

Although the size is not a criterion in Bosniak classification, it is believed by various researchers that small-sized lesions (<1.5 cm) in a patient with no risk factor for RCC can be considered benign.

Bosniak Classification Version 2019

In 2019, an updated Bosniak classification of cystic renal masses has been proposed to reduce inter-reader variability, more precisely predict the rate of malignancy within each Bosniak category, and minimize the number of unnecessary surgeries for otherwise benign or indolent malignant cystic masses. This updated Bosniak classification incorporates MRI into the classification and gives more specific definitions for various imaging features that are ambiguous in the previous Bosniak classification. However, this new Bosniak version 2019 needs validation before it is accepted widely.

In the proposed classification, the Bosniak categories are defined as follows:

- *Bosniak version 2019, Class I*: Well-defined lesions with a thin (≤2 mm) smooth wall, which may show enhancement with homogenous internal contents (–9 to 20 HU).
- *Bosniak version 2019, Class II:* Well-defined lesions with thin (≤2 mm) smooth walls. In addition, they may have any of the following features:
    - Thin (≤2 mm) and few (1–3) septa, which may enhance; may have calcification of any type
    - Homogenous hyperattenuating mass (≥70 HU) on noncontrast CT
    - Homogenous nonenhancing mass >20 HU on renal mass protocol CT
    - Homogenous masses –9 to 20 HU at NCCT
    - Homogenous masses 21 to 30 HU at portal venous phase CT
    - Homogenous low attenuation masses too small to characterize
    - Homogenous mass markedly hyperintense on T2-weighted images (similar to cerebrospinal fluid) or markedly hyperintense on T1-weighted images (approximately 2.5 times normal renal parenchyma) on noncontrast MRI.
- *Bosniak version 2019, Class IIF*:
    - Cystic masses with minimally thickened (≥3 mm) enhancing wall or septae
    - Cystic masses with many (>4) smooth thin enhancing septa (≤2 mm).

- *Bosniak version 2019, Class III*: One or more enhancing thick (≥4 mm) septa or enhancing irregular wall/septa (≤3 mm thick protrusion with obtuse margins to the wall septa).
- *Bosniak version 2019, Class IV*: One or more enhancing nodule (≥4 mm convex thickening with obtuse margins to wall/septa or a convex protrusion of any size but with acute margin).

IMAGING MODALITIES

Conventional Radiography

Plain radiography and excretory urography (EU) are indirect imaging modalities and are relatively insensitive in detecting and characterizing renal cysts. EU may show the following imaging findings when renal cysts are present:

- Abnormality of the renal contour or adjacent fascial planes, displacement of bowel loops or splayed ribs
- Curvilinear or rim calcification in the cyst wall
- Filling defects in the opacified cortex during the nephrographic phase of urography
- Splaying and distortion of the opacified collecting system **(Fig. 5)**.

Cross-sectional imaging techniques are more appropriate for investigating a patient of renal cystic disease.

Ultrasonography

Gray-scale, real-time sonography is a noninvasive, multiplanar direct imaging modality, which requires no patient preparation, and unlike EU it shows the mass lesion itself, along with changes in the renal parenchyma and renal sinus. However, obesity and excessive bowel gas can obscure the kidneys. Gray-scale US is useful in characterizing simple cysts but is limited in evaluation of complex cysts **(Fig. 6)**. Color Doppler can aid in assessing blood flow in renal cystic lesions, however with poor sensitivity. As Bosniak classification relies on enhancement, various studies have shown promising results using contrast-enhanced US in the evaluation of renal cystic lesions based on the Bosniak classification system.

Computed Tomography

Computed tomography is the main modality for imaging and characterizing cystic renal lesions. Multiphasic renal CT is obtained including unenhanced CT, corticomedullary phase, nephrographic phase, and excretory phase. The nephrographic phase is the most valuable for detecting mass lesions less than 3 cm which include clinically insignificant renal cysts and RCCs.

A change of less than 10 HU from pre- to postcontrast images is considered typical of a benign cyst. Very rarely, cystic tumors may enhance less than 10 HU. Majority of pathologic lesions enhance more than 15 HU. An enhancement between 10 HU and 15 HU is considered suspicious but not diagnostic of a tumor.

There are a few pitfalls on CT imaging that must be kept in mind. Pseudoenhancement that is defined as an artefactual increase in HU values of >10 on contrast-enhanced CT can result from beam hardening artifact. Also, if the lesion is smaller than twice the slice thickness

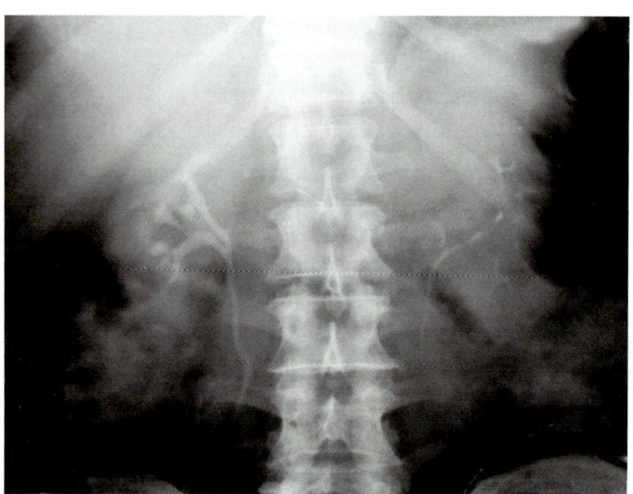

Fig. 5: Excretory urogram showing enlarged kidneys with splaying and stretching of pelvicalyceal system (spidery calyces) in a patient with polycystic kidney disease.

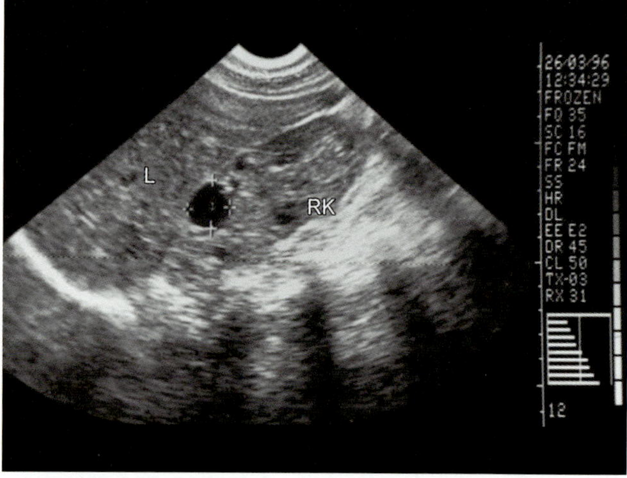

Fig. 6: US of kidney showing a well-marginated anechoic lesion with distal enhancement—simple cortical cyst. (US: ultrasonography).

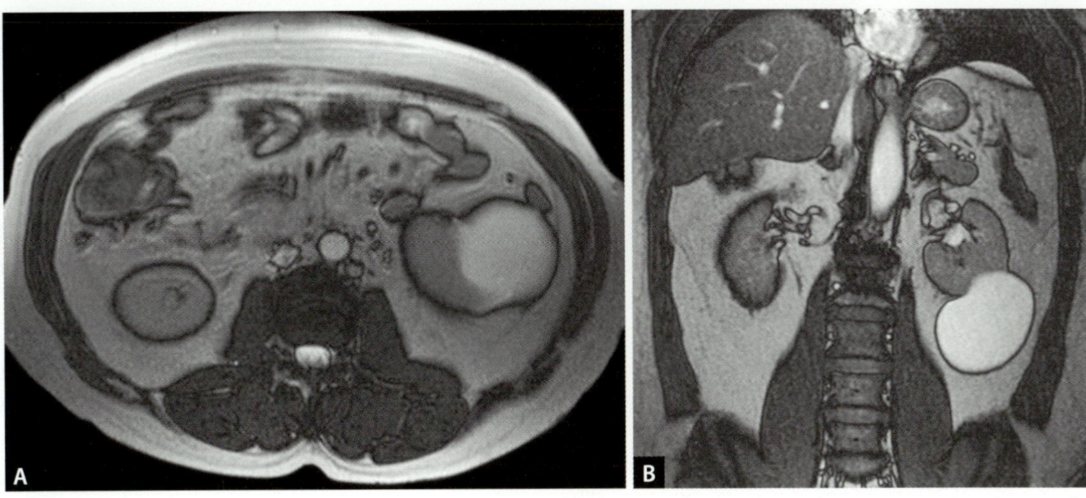

Figs. 7A and B: Steady state free precession sequence axial (A) and coronal (B) MR images reveal a homogenous sharply marginated lesion with imperceptible wall thickness and high signal arising exophytically from the left kidney—an exophytic simple cortical cyst. (MR: magnetic resonance).

used, then partial volume averaging may result in misinterpretation. Virtual monochromatic imaging on dual-energy computed tomography may completely eliminate pseudoenhancement in renal cysts larger than 1.5 cm.

Magnetic Resonance Imaging

Multiplanar imaging capability and angiographic capabilities with excellent soft-tissue contrast resolution have made MRI a useful method for evaluating the kidneys **(Figs. 7A and B)**. High-field strengths, breathhold imaging, fat suppression techniques, and use of MR-contrast agents help in differentiating tumor from cysts. The multiplanar imaging capability of MRI makes it easier to assess polar lesions and coronal images make it simple for the urologist to visualize the relative position of a small lesion if wedge resection or partial nephrectomy is to be planned.

Although the Bosniak classification has been described on CT, various researchers have proven that MR may be equivalent to CT in Bosniak classification of cystic lesions. Calcification is however better picked up on CT than on MR. Owing to increased contrast resolution, there is increased sensitivity of MR for picking up septations and wall thickening on T2-weighted images. This can result in false upgradation of the Bosniak category of the lesion. Other pitfalls include evaluation of enhancement in hemorrhagic and calcified lesions. In these situations, subtraction imaging may be used. The subtraction imaging technique can suffer from misregistration and additional noise.

In few equivocal cases, MR can be problem solving. Postcontrast free breathing 3D fat-suppressed T1 gradient echo (T1 vibe fat sat) sequence allows better evaluation of enhancement which forms the main basis for Bosniak categorization of lesions. Diffusion-weighted imaging can also be of utility in differentiating cystic renal masses from simple cysts.

Angiography

Prior to the advent of newer imaging modalities such as US, CT, and MRI, angiography was commonly used for evaluation of renal mass lesions. However, in the present era it is mainly indicated for interventional procedures of vascular mass lesions of the kidney. Actively bleeding tumors such as angiomyolipomas (AMLs) can be treated with selective angiography by embolization of the intrarenal supply of the tumor.

Biopsy

Biopsy may not give a high yield from cystic lesions owing to paucity of cells within. It is however useful to biopsy or drain cystic lesions which are suspected to be abscesses and may be attempted in patients with suspected malignancy if they are poor surgical candidates.

ADULT RENAL CYSTIC DISEASE: CLASSIFICATION

In adults, apart from simple renal cysts, multifocal renal cystic disease comprises a diverse group of heritable and acquired disorders. Renal infections, tumors, and renal sinus cysts are other miscellaneous conditions that can present as cystic disease. Because of their diverse etiology, histology, and clinical presentation, no single universally accepted

Table 2: Classification of renal cystic disease.	
Multifocal	
Heritable	• Autosomal dominant polycystic kidney disease • Medullary cystic kidney disease • Von Hippel-Lindau disease • Tuberous sclerosis
Acquired	• Acquired renal cystic disease • Medullary sponge kidney disease • Glomerulocystic kidney disease • Lithium-induced nephrotoxicity • Multicystic dysplastic kidney • Localized cystic renal disease • Cyst of renal pelvis
Focal	• Mixed epithelial stromal tumor • Cystic nephroma • Cystic renal cell carcinoma • Pyelocalyceal diverticulum
Infectious causes	• Pyogenic-renal abscess • Tubercular • Parasitic-renal hydatid, echinococcosis • Fungal-renal aspergillosis

classification exists, but a practical working classification composed of major categories and the most clinically significant renal cystic diseases is shown in **Table 2**.

MULTIFOCAL CYSTIC RENAL DISEASE

Heritable Multifocal Cystic Renal Disease

Autosomal Dominant Polycystic Kidney Disease

Autosomal dominant polycystic kidney disease (ADPKD) is the most common of hereditary renal cystic diseases (1 in 400–1,000 live births). Mostly, it shows an autosomal dominant inheritance. Rare cases may result from a spontaneous mutation with no family history. Although multiple bilateral renal cysts are the most important manifestation, ADPKD is really a systemic hereditary disorder that is characterized by cyst formation in ductal organs, the liver being the most common site of extrarenal involvement. Other extrarenal manifestations include cysts in pancreas, spleen, and gonads. The patients may also have intracranial aneurysms, cardiac valve abnormalities, colonic diverticulae, and musculoskeletal abnormalities.

About 85% of cases are due to a dominant gene located on the short arm of chromosome 16 (the *ADPKD-1* gene) whereas 5–10% of cases are due to an abnormal gene located on the long arm of chromosome 4 (the *ADPKD-2* gene), which causes a milder form of the disorder with late onset of disease.

Patients with a positive family history of ADPKD and no imaging evidence of renal cysts can be further evaluated using gene-linkage analysis. It is proposed that the disorder results from failure of union of the branches of ureteral bud with metanephros which, deprived of the organizing influence, form cysts. There is cystic dilatation of nephrons involving all segments from the proximal convoluted tubule to the collecting duct due to epithelial hyperplasia leading to redundancy that predisposes to cyst formation. Hence, cysts may be seen in both renal cortex and medulla.

Most patients are born with normal kidneys. Only 2% patients present before 15 years of age. Most affected individuals present in the fourth or fifth decade with flank pain, palpable masses, hypertension, hematuria, urinary tract infection, proteinuria, or polycythemia. Progressive azotemia ensues as renal parenchyma is destroyed and renal failure occurs in most patients by the age of 60 years. Complications include superimposed infection, cyst hemorrhage, uric acid stones, and hypertension. Renal cell carcinoma is not a complication of ADPKD unless the patient is on prolonged dialysis.

Imaging plays an important role in diagnosis, detection of complications, and follow-up. Conventional radiograph may reveal bilateral enlarged kidneys with lobulated margins causing displacement of the surrounding structures, such as colonic flexures. Calcification may be curvilinear or amorphous and the presence of renal calculi often signifies superimposed infection. The "nephrogram" phase of the EU is characterized by numerous, smoothly marginated radiolucencies throughout the cortex and medulla, which have been likened to the appearance of "Swiss cheese." An appearance of spidery collecting system with stretched and crescentic calyces may be noted.

Ultrasound is the modality of choice for primary evaluation of most patients with suspected ADPKD. On US, cysts of varying sizes are noted in enlarged kidneys, which may result in a lobulated outline **(Figs. 8A and B)**. However, the reniform shape is maintained. Similar cysts may be seen in liver, pancreas, and spleen. Most patients develop renal cysts by their third decade. Antenatal diagnosis is sometimes also possible on demonstration of enlarged cystic kidneys, ascites, and hepatomegaly. The presence of even one cyst in a genetically predisposed child is suspicious of ADPKD.

On CT and MR, variable sized cysts which are usually ≥3 cm in diameter are seen diffusely involving bilateral enlarged kidneys. Imaging also helps to identify infection, hemorrhage, and rupture. On MRI, the renal cysts are hypointense on T1-weighted and hyperintense on T2-weighted images, with infected and proteinaceous

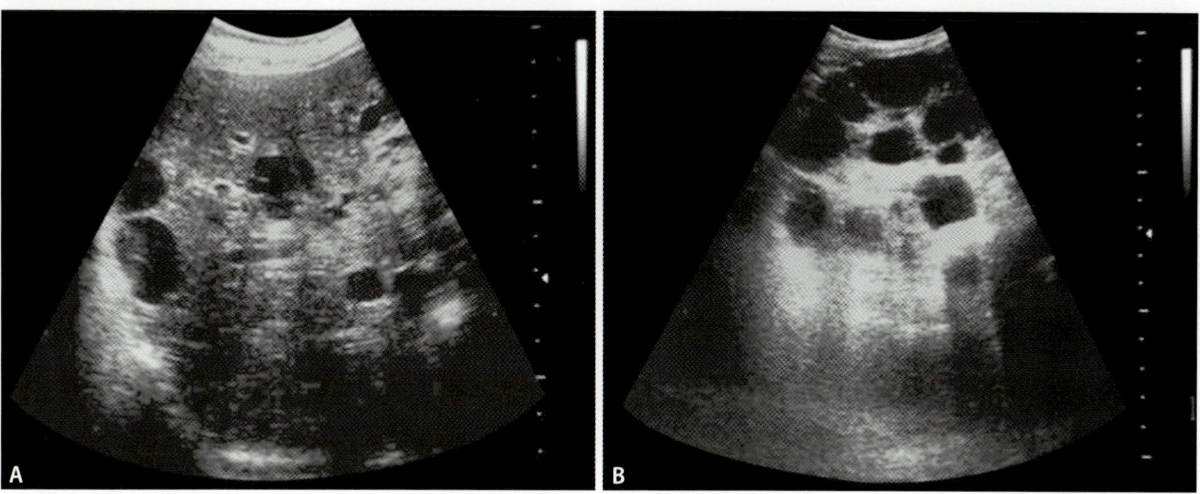

Figs. 8A and B: Sonography showing multiple noncommunicating cysts of varying sizes replacing the renal parenchyma and distorting the central sinus echoes—ADPKD. Cysts are also seen in the liver. (ADPKD: autosomal dominant polycystic kidney disease).

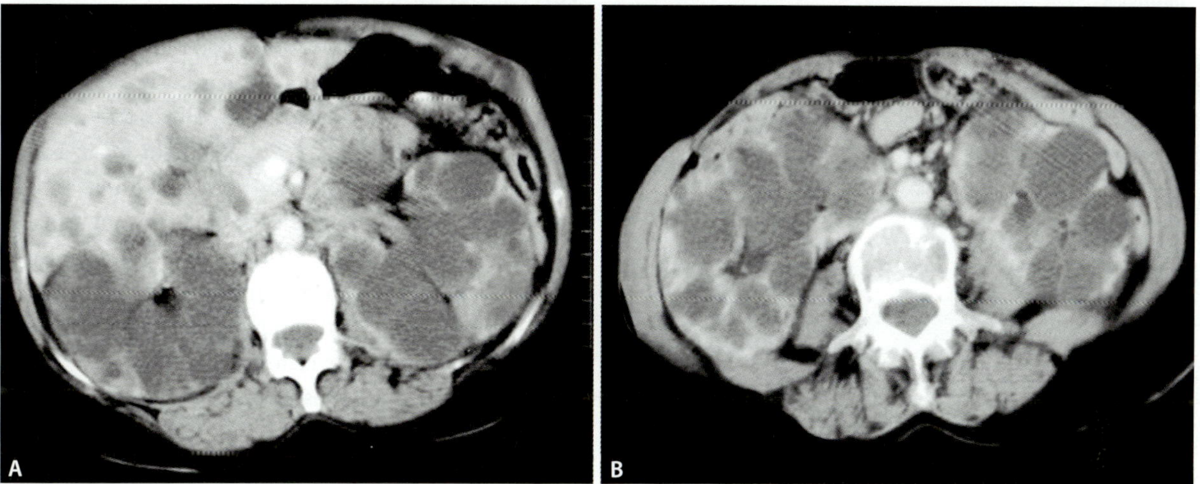

Figs. 9A and B: Contrast-enhanced CT scans revealing multiple noncommunicating cysts in both kidneys. Cysts are also seen in the liver—ADPKD (ADPKD: autosomal dominant polycystic kidney disease; CT: computed tomography).

cysts showing intermediate signal intensities **(Figs. 9 to 11)**. MRI-based renal and cyst volumetry enables assessment of disease progression. With increasing renal volume, the glomerular filtration rate may decline and the patient may present with abdominal pain, hypertension, or hematuria. Renal blood flow may also decrease suggesting progression of the disease.

Imaging is critical in evaluation of patients who have a first-degree relative with ADPKD. It is especially so in evaluation of prospective donors who plan to donate a kidney to their kin with ADPKD. Severe cases can be diagnosed easily on imaging but a milder form of the disease, especially with PKD2 mutation, can be difficult to diagnose. Genetic testing helps in the diagnosis of ADPKD in only 70% cases.

The criteria for diagnosing ADPKD on US in patients with unknown genotype but at high risk of ADPKD (i.e. with a first-degree relative with the disease) are as follows:

- 15–39 years—three renal cysts
- 40–59 years—≥2 cysts in each kidney
- 60 years or more—≥4 cysts in each kidney.

The sensitivity of CT scan is greater than that of ultrasound in detecting renal cysts and thus may establish the diagnosis more definitively at an earlier age.

Nephronophthisis and Medullary Cystic Kidney Disease

Medullary cystic disease complex applies to two tubulointerstitial diseases—nephronophthisis and medullary cystic disease—which are progressive and

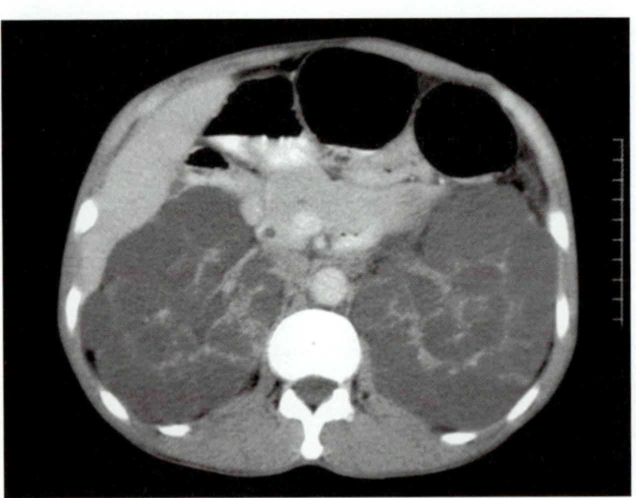

Fig. 10: Contrast-enhanced CT (CECT) scan in another case showing multiple noncommunicating cysts in both kidneys—ADPKD. (ADPKD: autosomal dominant polycystic kidney disease; CT: computed tomography).

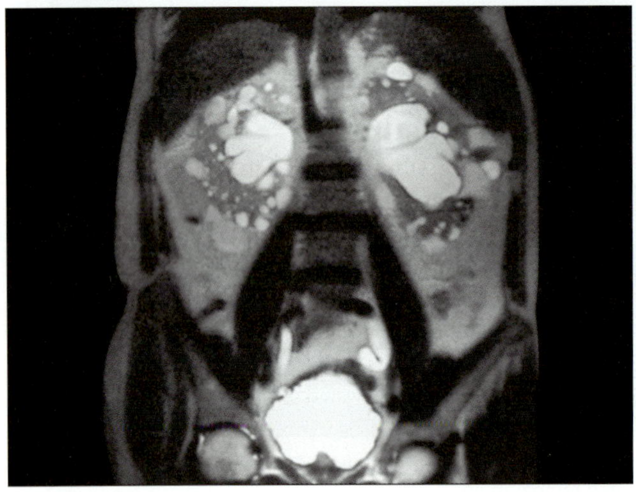

Fig. 11: T2W coronal MR image showing both kidneys to be enlarged with multiple cysts of varying sizes having fluid signal intensity studding the renal parenchyma of both kidneys consistent with polycystic kidney disease. Note is also made of bilateral hydronephrosis and back pressure changes in the bladder due to bladder outflow obstruction. (MR: magnetic resonance).

the most common heritable cause of renal failure in children and young adults. It shows autosomal dominant inheritance. Genetic mutations result in protein derangement which further results in ciliary dysfunction and formation of medullary cysts.

Nephronophthisis has three forms—infantile, juvenile, and adolescent—based on the age of onset. The juvenile form is the most common with presentation at 4–6 years of age. Renal failure can ensue at an average age of 13 years. MCKD presents in young adults. Patients with both the forms of the disease present with polyuria, polydipsia, and salt wasting. They may also develop hyperuricemia and gout.

Imaging features are similar for both the disease entities. At US imaging, kidneys are normal to small sized with increased echogenicity and poor corticomedullary differentiation. Multiple small-sized cysts <3 cm can be seen at the corticomedullary junction and in renal medulla, but these are typically seen after the onset of end-stage renal disease. Renal cysts increase with increasing age. When present, the typical location of the cysts and characteristic clinical findings help to differentiate MCKD from other renal cystic diseases.

Patients progress to renal failure and renal transplantation is the treatment of choice. The disease does not involve the transplanted kidney.

Von Hippel-Lindau Disease

Von Hippel-Lindau (VHL) disease is a relatively rare, autosomal dominant disorder with a prevalence of 1 in 30,000–50,000. It is caused by an abnormal gene on the short arm of chromosome 3. This disorder is associated with hemangioblastomas of the central nervous system (CNS), retinal angiomatosis, pheochromocytomas, cysts and tumors of the kidney, pancreatic cysts and tumors, endolymphatic sac tumors, and papillary cystadenomas of the epididymis. Both males and females are equally affected. The diagnostic criteria include:

- >1 CNS hemangioblastoma
- 1 CNS hemangioblastoma and visceral manifestations of VHL
- Any manifestation of VHL with known family history.

Renal lesions include simple and atypical cysts, cystic RCC, and solid RCC. Clear cell RCCs are the major cause of patient morbidity and mortality, especially in Type 1 and Type 2B VHL disease.

On EU, renal cortical cysts are seen bilaterally, causing distortion of the renal architecture. Extensive disease can mimic ADPKD. USG is highly sensitive for detection of renal cysts; however, small renal tumors may not be seen. CT is more sensitive than USG for detection and characterization of renal masses and small, solid renal masses can be precisely defined **(Fig. 12)**.

MR imaging is indispensable for the diagnosis of neurological neoplasms seen in patients with VHL disease. Furthermore, small RCCs can be detected on contrast-enhanced MR. Large tumors can be evaluated and characterized on nonenhanced scans and tend to be more heterogeneous.

Although RCC in VHL disease is slower growing than in patients without VHL disease, RCC is a significant cause of mortality in VHL disease. In VHL disease, RCC may either arise de novo or within small cysts. Hence, each cyst needs to be carefully assessed in a case of VHL disease and none can be described as free of cancer cells on imaging.

In patients with VHL disease, imaging surveillance is recommended at intervals of 6–12 months. While some cysts enlarge over time, others may involute. Complex cysts and solid tumors can show progressive increase in size. The cutoff size of the solid tumor to be taken for surgery is accepted as 3 cm. When a 3 cm-sized solid nodule is seen, it needs to be resected along with other smaller solid/cystic lesions if possible. Thereafter, surveillance is maintained till a 3 cm nodule is again formed. Treatment is mostly with nephron sparing surgery.

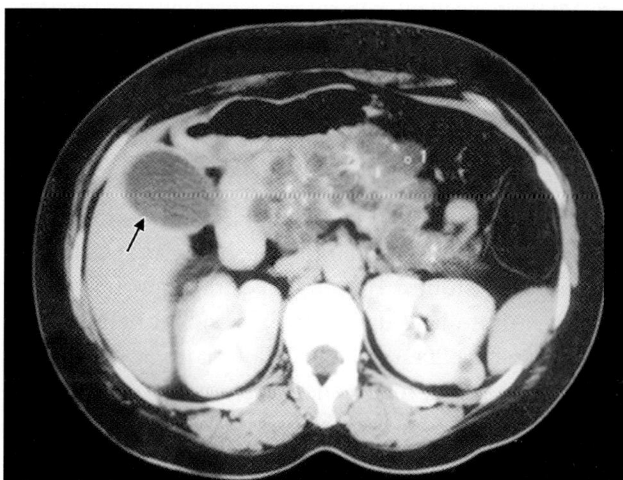

Fig. 12: Contrast-enhanced CT (CECT) sections showing a solid enhancing mass and cyst in the left kidney with multiple cysts and calcifications in the pancreas—von Hippel-Lindau disease. (CT: computed tomography).

Tuberous Sclerosis

Tuberous sclerosis (TSC) is also known as Bourneville disease. It is a genetically transmitted autosomal dominant neurocutaneous syndrome. Genetic markers have been identified at 9q34 (TSC 1) and 16p13 (TSC 2), although they account for only 50% of TSC families. Sporadic occurrence is seen in 50–60% of cases. The true incidence of TSC is difficult to measure though its birth incidence ranges from 1 per 5,800 to 1 per 10,000. It is characterized by mental retardation, seizures, and cutaneous lesions. This disorder is associated with multiple hamartomas in the brain (cortical tubers), retina, skin, heart (rhabdomyomas), kidney (AMLs), and other organs. Renal cysts and AMLs are seen in 50–60% of cases. Occurrence of both AMLs and renal cysts is virtually diagnostic of TSC. Angiomyolipomas are benign masses consisting of varying amounts of abnormal blood vessels, smooth muscle, and fat. These manifest in childhood and increase in size with age.

On abdominal radiography, lucency suggesting fat within an AML can occasionally be detected. On EU, the findings vary with the size and number of renal cysts and the presence of AMLs. Multiple nonopacifying renal masses causing distortion of the collecting system are seen.

On sonographic examination, multiple renal cysts and AMLs, showing hyperechoic reflections, may be seen owing to lesional fat. On CT, fat-containing AMLs with low attenuation values and intralesional hemorrhage may be noted along with renal cysts **(Figs. 13A and B)**. MR

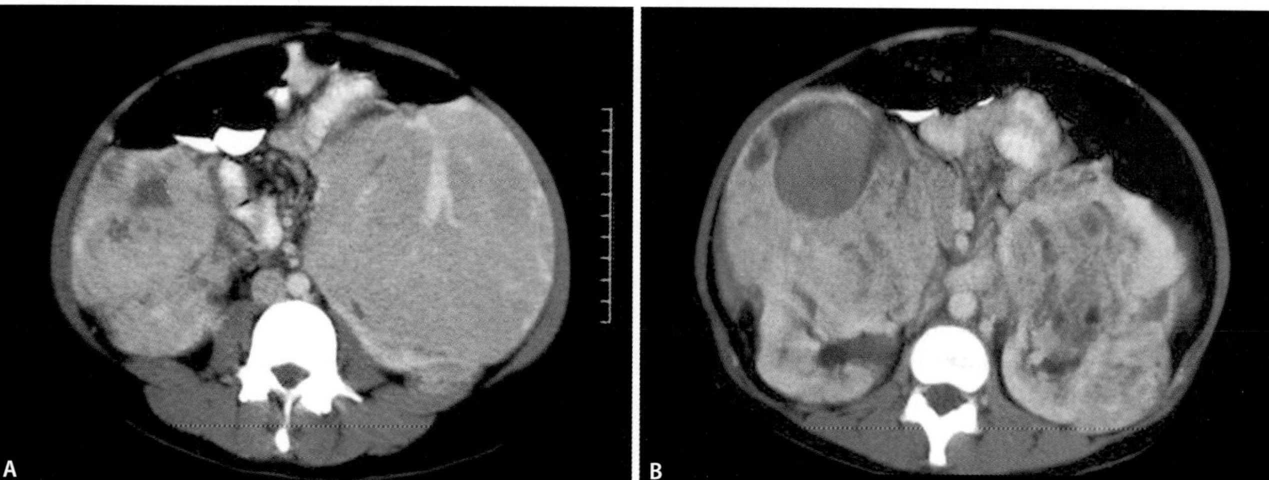

Figs. 13A and B: Contrast-enhanced CT scan showing heterogeneous masses involving both the kidneys. The masses show fat-attenuation values and cystic areas within. The lesions show intralesional vascularity—bilateral angiomyolipomas. (CT: computed tomography).

imaging aids in diagnosing AMLs by showing high-signal intensity on both T1- and T2-weighted images.

Although the risk of RCC in these patients is the same as that in the general population, it occurs at an earlier age. The mean age of RCC in patients with TSC is 28 years compared with 58 years in the general population. Other complications include renal failure and hemorrhage from AML rupture.

Lipid poor AML and RCC can be difficult to differentiate on imaging. Rapid growth and presence of calcification are features that favor RCC over AML. However, biopsy may be needed to confirm the diagnosis.

TSC2-PKD1 is a related condition which has mutations in both *TSC2* and *PKD1* genes. These patients have lesions of both TSC and ADPKD.

Acquired Multifocal Cystic Renal Disease

Acquired Cystic Kidney Disease

Acquired cystic kidney disease (ACKD) is characterized by the formation of multiple renal cysts in patients with end-stage renal disease, who have no history of hereditary cystic disease. Risk factors include male sex and increased duration of time on dialysis. These patients can have acquired cysts even before undergoing dialysis in 8–13% of patients. After 3–5 years of dialysis, the prevalence of ACKD is 40–60% while it rises to 90% after 5–10 years on dialysis. The incidence reaches nearly 100% after 10 years of dialysis. Men are affected three times more often than females. However, there is no relation with the method of dialysis, age, or race of the patient. At least three cysts in each kidney are required to make this diagnosis. US shows atrophic echogenic kidneys with small cysts of varying complexity. CT and MR show small kidneys with variably sized cysts. While US is a good modality for screening, CT and MR are useful in detecting complications. Multiple, bilateral small cysts are seen to involve both the renal cortex and the medulla **(Fig. 14)**.

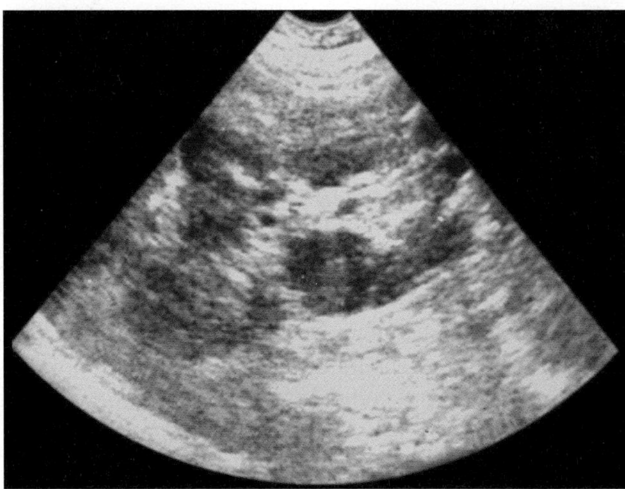

Fig. 14: US in a patient with chronic renal failure on long-term hemodialysis showing shrunken echogenic kidney with loss of corticomedullary differentiation and multiple small renal cysts—ACKD. (ACKD: acquired cystic kidney disease; US: ultrasonography).

ACKD is associated with an increased incidence of renal neoplasms. Risk factors for malignancy in this setting include increasing duration of dialysis, male gender, and kidney weight more than 150 g. Factors causing renal cyst and tumor formation in end-stage renal disease are unknown but the two are interrelated. It is postulated that with progressive destruction of functioning renal tissue, cystogenic substances accumulate and cause hypertrophy and hyperplasia of epithelial cells. The tubular epithelium proliferate and cystic dilatation of tubules occurs. Subsequently, there is a continuum of changes from single-layered epithelial cysts to multilayered cysts to RCCs. Tumors can be multiple and bilateral. Other complications in this setting include cyst infection, hemorrhage, rupture, and ureteral stones. Hemorrhage into cyst may result in cyst rupture leading to retroperitoneal hemorrhage. Asymptomatic patients can be followed up by US whereas complications may require nephrectomy.

In post-transplant cases, true cysts decrease in the native kidney but the risk of malignancy persists, in fact with more aggressiveness owing to ongoing immunosuppression in transplant cases.

Medullary Sponge Kidney

Medullary sponge kidney is also known as Lenarduzzi-Cacchi-Ricci disease. It was first described by Lenarduzzi in 1931. Although it is mostly sporadic, a few cases with autosomal dominant inheritance have also been described.

The most probable cause is disruption in the ureteric bud metanephros interface. It is characterized histologically by ectasia of the renal medullary and papillary collecting ducts with subcentimetric cysts in the medulla. This disease entity may be associated with congenital hemihypertrophy, Beckwith-Wiedemann syndrome, Caroli syndrome, Wilms tumor, or horseshoe kidney.

Patients usually present in the third to fifth decades of life. Although mostly asymptomatic, some patients may present with hematuria, renal colic, or urinary tract infection.

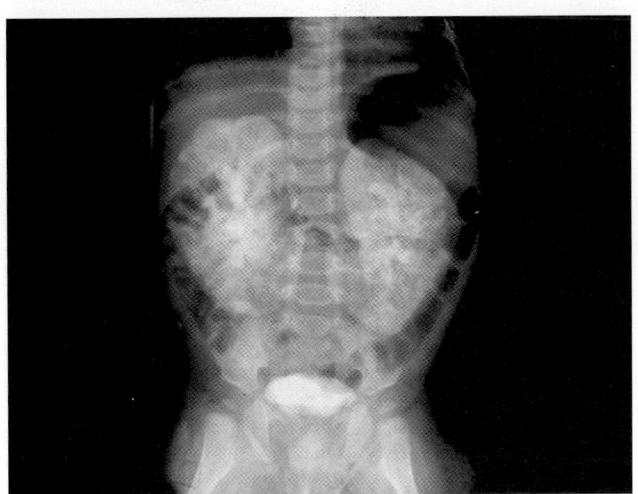

Fig. 15: Excretory urogram in a child with medullary sponge kidneys showing enlarged kidneys with and characteristic "paint brush" appearance owing to dilated medullary collecting ducts.

At EU **(Fig. 15)**, papillary blush is classically noted as contrast pools in the dilated medullary collecting ducts. This gives a classic "paint brush" appearance. Striated appearance of the medullary collecting ducts with calyceal distortion may also be encountered as the disease increases in severity. This entity typically involves both the kidneys. Unilateral or segmental involvement may be seen at times. US examination reveals echogenic medullary pyramids. Tiny calculi can be seen involving the medullary pyramids. On CT examination, the typical papillary blush appearance can be noted in the urographic phase with associated calculi in the dilated collecting ducts suggestive of medullary nephrocalcinosis. CT urography scores over EU in identification of dilated medullary collecting ducts, calculi, obstruction, and infection.

This is a benign disease entity. Severe complications of calculi and infection may result in renal failure in rare circumstances.

Glomerulocystic Kidney Disease

Glomerulocystic kidney disease (GCKD) is a rare cystic disease owing to cystic dilatation of Bowman's capsule. The cysts involve the subcapsular renal cortex and spare nephron tubules. Although many sporadic cases are known, autosomal dominant inheritance has also been reported. This is seen mostly in neonates and young children who may have mild renal failure.

On imaging, kidneys may be normal or small in size. Tiny cysts are seen in the subcapsular location in the cortex. These are difficult to discern on US as well as noncontrast CT. Contrast is usually not administered owing to renal failure. On US, increased cortical echogenicity may be seen owing to the extremely small size of the cysts. T2-weighted MR imaging is the most sensitive sequence in picking up these tiny cysts in the subcapsular location. This location of the cysts helps to differentiate this entity from other multifocal cystic renal diseases like ADPKD, multicystic dysplastic kidney (MCDK).

Lithium-induced Nephrotoxicity

Long-term lithium therapy can result in nephrotoxicity which can manifest in the form of acute toxicity, nephrogenic diabetes insipidus as well as chronic renal disease. While the first two are reversible, chronic interstitial nephritis is progressive and irreversible. Nephrogenic diabetes insipidus is the most common complication.

In the setting of chronic renal disease, microcyst formation results with progressive renal dysfunction in normal sized kidneys. This is seen as numerous 1–2 mm cysts scattered in cortex and medulla of normal sized kidneys. These are best seen on T2W MR images. Based on the imaging findings, the differential diagnosis is ADPKD, GCKD, and *MCKD*. Clinical history, size and distribution of the cysts help to distinguish this entity from others cystic diseases of the kidney. While clinical and laboratory data are sufficient to reach the diagnosis, renal biopsy, if performed, depicts tubular atrophy, interstitial fibrosis and distal tubular ectasia resulting in microcyst formation.

Multicystic Dysplastic Kidney

Multicystic dysplastic kidney is a developmental, nonhereditary anomaly with multiple, smooth noncommunicating cysts. It is one of the most common abdominal masses in the newborn and is typically unilateral and asymptomatic. It has an incidence of 1 in 4,300 live births. The bilateral form of MCDK is usually associated with congenital gastrointestinal and cardiac abnormalities. The bilateral form has a poor outcome due to accompanying oligohydramnios and pulmonary hypoplasia.

The proposed theory of this dysplastic kidney is failure of the ureteric bud to induce development of metanephric blastema. The ureteric bud may be absent or may not integrate with metanephric blastema owing to urinary tract obstruction.

In children, it is seen as a nonreniform mass which is a cluster of noncommunicating cysts replacing the renal parenchyma or sometimes only a part of the renal parenchyma **(Fig. 16)**. The contralateral kidney must be assessed to rule out associations such as vesicoureteric reflux or pelviureteric junction obstruction. It may also be picked up on antenatal USG **(Figs. 17A and B)**.

A few patients present in adulthood. The kidney regresses in size and presents as "renal agenesis" or a small central soft tissue surrounded by peripheral cysts which could be confused with cystic renal neoplasm. The findings that help to reach the correct diagnosis are nonfunctioning kidney with peripheral cysts around central soft tissue along with atrophic pelvicalyceal system, ureter, and renal vessels. With time, the affected kidney involutes and is typically not a source of clinical concern. The contralateral kidney may show compensatory hypertrophy **(Figs. 18A and B)**. There may also be a segmental form involving the upper pole of a duplex kidney and this may be associated with ureterocele of the lower moiety.

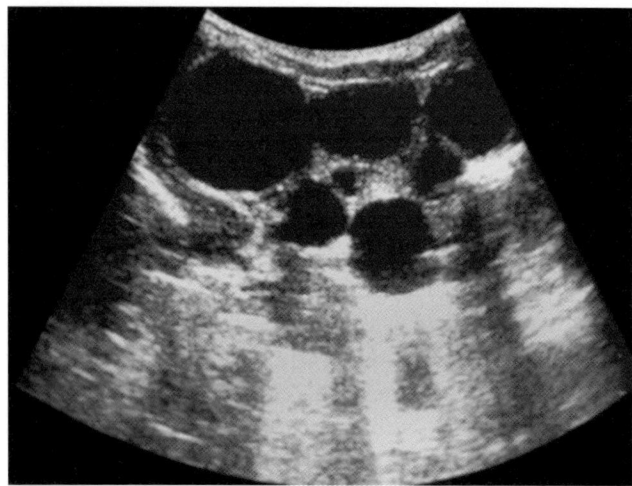

Fig. 16: US of right kidney in a 4-year-old child shows multiple cysts of varying sizes distorting the reniform contour––MCDK. (MCDK: multicystic dysplastic kidney; US: ultrasonography).

Localized Renal Cystic Disease

This is a rare disease where a cluster of tightly packed cysts replaces a portion of the kidney or rarely the entire kidney. It is also known as segmental renal cystic disease and unilateral renal cystic disease. It is a benign, nonprogressive condition. Multiple cysts are seen in one kidney with no cysts in the contralateral kidney or any other organ. Most patients are asymptomatic. Some may present with abdominal pain, hematuria, or hypertension but with intact renal function.

CT and MR show a conglomerate mass of variably sized simple renal cysts with intervening enhancing renal parenchyma involving a portion of one kidney or the entire kidney. There is no surrounding capsule **(Figs. 19A to C)**. The intervening normal parenchyma is usually normal but sometimes atrophic. Remaining renal parenchyma and contralateral kidney are generally normal but can show a few scattered cysts.

Unilateral involvement with no cysts involving other viscera distinguishes this entity from ADPKD. The presence of normal collecting system and renal vessels helps to differentiate it from multicystic dysplastic kidney. Intervening normal parenchyma and absence of capsule differentiate this nonprogressive condition from multilocular cystic RCC and cystic nephroma. As this may be difficult to discern at times, the key remains to identify

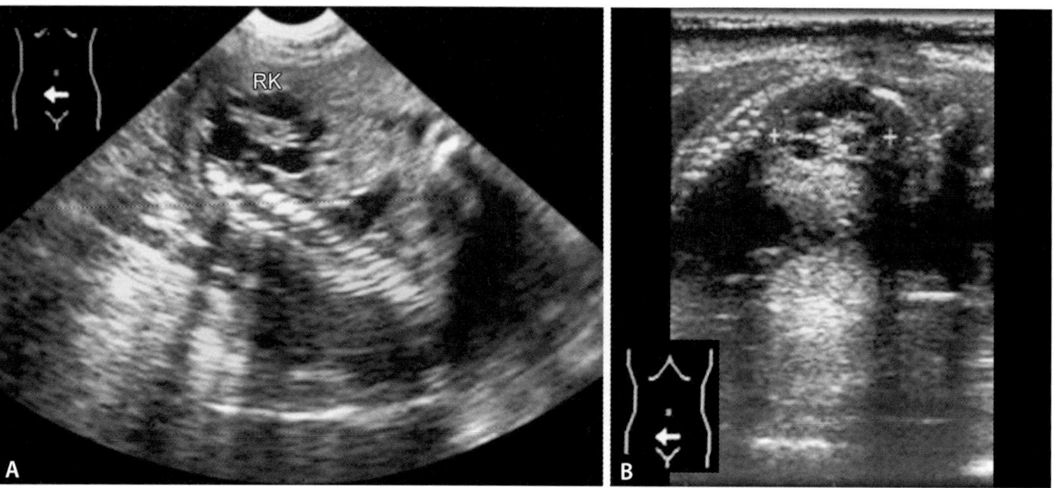

Figs. 17A and B: Antenatal sonogram showing multiple noncommunicating cysts in an enlarged fetal kidney—multicystic dysplasia.

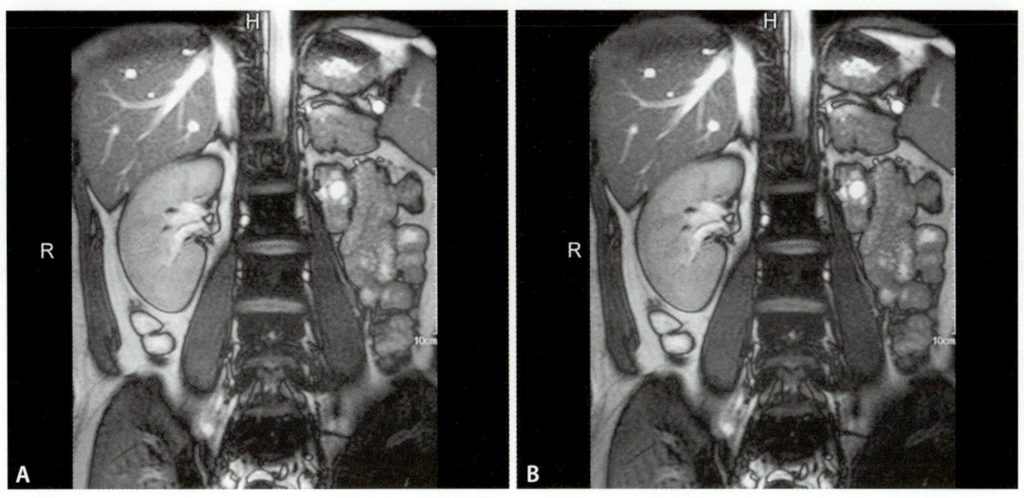

Figs. 18A and B: Coronal steady state MR images reveal a small dysplastic left kidney replaced by multiple noncommunicating cysts showing hyperintensity on T2W image with compensatory hypertrophy of right kidney—adult MCDK. (MCDK: multicystic dysplastic kidney).

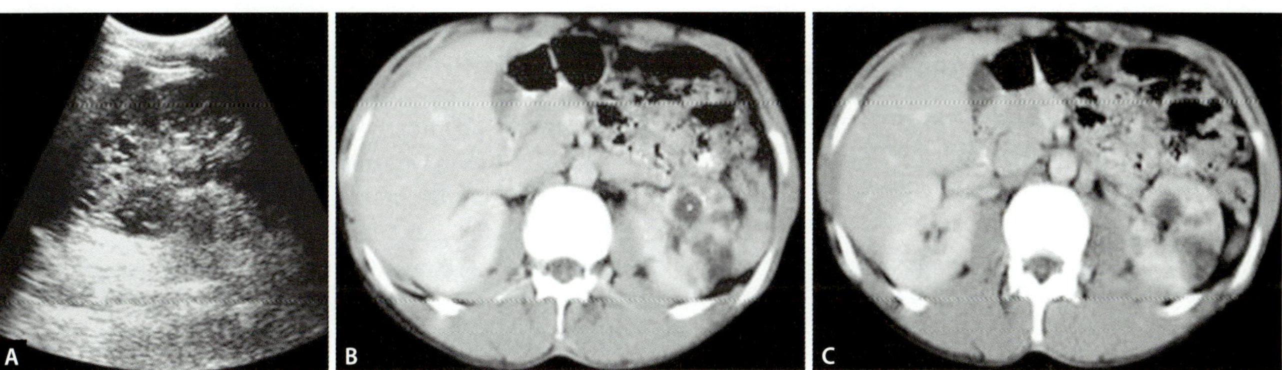

Figs. 19A to C: Sonogram (A) showing multiple small cysts in the upper pole of the left kidney seen as a multiloculated mass. Contrast-enhanced CT scans (B and C) revealing multiple cysts in the upper pole of the left kidney separated by enhancing bands of renal parenchyma—unilateral localized cystic disease. (CT: computed tomography).

at least one cyst which is surrounded by normal renal tissue.

This is a benign condition. Surveillance is however recommended if the patient is symptomatic or imaging findings are equivocal.

Cysts of Renal Pelvis

Cysts of renal pelvis can be of two types:

1. Parapelvic cyst
2. Renal sinus cyst (also called peripelvic cysts).

Parapelvic cysts are cortical cysts that extend into renal sinus **(Fig. 20)**. Mostly, these do not produce any symptoms but sometimes may result in hydronephrosis, hypertension by renal artery compression, pain, and hematuria. These are usually simple cysts on imaging.

Infection and hemorrhage are some of the unusual complications that may occur in these cysts.

Renal sinus cysts are multiple, small, and bilateral cysts in contrast to parapelvic cysts which are usually single and unilateral. These arise from renal sinus lymphatics. The differential diagnosis here is hydronephrosis which can be distinguished on the excretory phase of CT scan where there is no contrast excretion into these cysts.

FOCAL CYSTIC RENAL DISEASE

Mixed epithelial and stromal tumor (MEST) and cystic nephroma are benign cystic lesions that can have imaging appearance ranging from Bosniak category 2F to 4. These can appear similar to cystic RCC and hence end up being surgically treated most often.

Pelvicalyceal diverticulum is another lesion that can present as a focal cystic lesion in the renal cortex but has a distinctive feature of communication with the pelvicalyceal system.

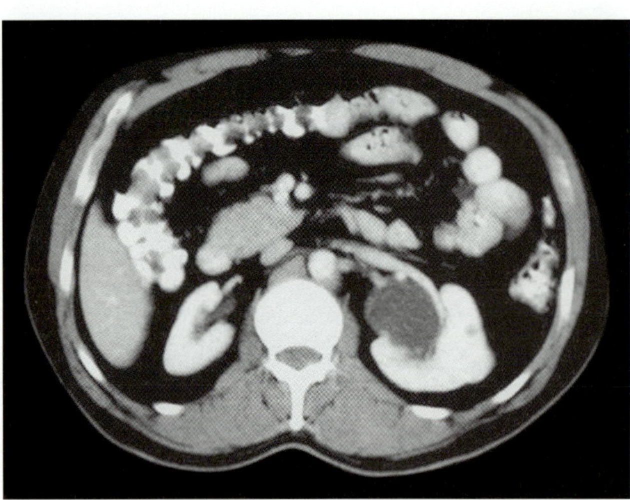

Fig. 20: Contrast-enhanced CT scan showing a solitary fluid-filled lesion in the renal sinus detected as an incidental finding in this patient—a parapelvic cyst. (CT: computed tomography).

Mixed Epithelial and Stromal Tumor

This is relatively a recently described entity that is seen most often in perimenopausal women with an average age of 50 years. Estrogen supplement/contraceptive use has been found to have an association with this tumor. Patients may present with flank mass or hematuria. However, they may also be asymptomatic in nearly one-fourth of the cases. MEST is a cystic and solid neoplasm, with both stromal elements resembling ovarian stroma and epithelial components resulting from cysts with epithelial lining.

This is seen as a multilocular cystic mass that can herniate into the renal pelvis. There may be enhancing solid component or wall calcification. The cysts may have hemorrhage within. Although the lesion is benign, it may be hard to differentiate from cystic RCC and hence is often treated surgically.

Cystic Nephroma

Cystic nephroma is also a rare benign tumor that has a bimodal age and sex distribution, the first peak occurring in boys less than 4 years of age and the second in women aged 40–60 years. In pediatric population, these present as painless abdominal masses while in the adults, they may present with pain and/or hematuria.

On imaging, these are seen as well-defined multilocular cystic masses with enhancing septae and may herniate into the pelvis like MEST. On MRI, the septae and the capsule are hypointense on both T1- and T2-weighted images owing to their fibrous nature. It is actually believed that MEST and cystic nephroma belong to the same spectrum of pathology with more cystic components in cystic nephroma than in MEST. As differentiation from RCC may be difficult on imaging, these lesions are most often treated surgically despite being benign.

Cystic Renal Cell Carcinoma

Multilocular cystic RCC is a low-grade tumor with male predominance that can look like cystic nephroma on imaging. Cystic clear cell RCC also can simulate this appearance (***see* Figs. 8A and B**); however, it is a more malignant lesion. This is discussed in detail elsewhere in the book.

Pyelocalyceal Diverticulum

This is a cyst within the renal cortex that has communication with the renal pelvicalyceal system. Two types have been described. Type1 is more common and seen to communicate with minor calyx while Type 2 communicates with major calyx or pelvis. These are thought to be mostly congenital in origin; however, acquired cases may result from calculi or infections.

These may be picked up on intravenous urogram studies (2.1–4.5 per 1000 IVU examinations). On US and noncontrast CT or nephrographic CT phase, these are seen as renal cysts. However, on contrast administration, these cysts show layering of contrast within them in the excretory phase. They may also be complicated by calculi or milk of calcium. These cysts then show thin layering of hyperattenuation material on noncontrast CT. Typically, these milk of calcium cysts lose connection with the collecting system and hence may not show contrast excretion within them. A large diverticulum may simulate a hydrocalyx due to obstruction. Complications of pyelocalyceal diverticulum include hemorrhage, infection, rupture, and rarely even malignancy.

INFECTIOUS CYSTS

Pyogenic Abscess

This is usually secondary to incompletely treated or untreated acute pyelonephritis. This may also result from hematogenous spread. Risk factors include pregnancy, diabetes, and other forms of immunosuppression.

Excretory urography reveals filling defects or irregular cavities that may communicate with the pelvicalyceal system. On sonography, thick-walled cystic lesions with low-level internal echoes are seen. Apart from imaging features, clinical features also help to distinguish them from renal cysts. Contrast-enhanced CT shows low attenuation masses with rim enhancement and thickening of perirenal fascia. The abscess often shows a thick halo around it. On MR, these are seen as heterogeneous mass with thick walls, hypointense on T1W and hyperintense on T2W images. Diffusion restriction is often seen. Air within the abscess results in susceptibility artifact seen on gradient echo images.

Hydatid Cyst

The kidney can also be involved by hydatid disease; the patient is usually asymptomatic until the cyst has grown large enough to cause pressure symptoms or rupture. Patients may present with flank pain/mass or dysuria. Rupture into the collecting system may result in renal colic and excretion of hydatid cysts in the urine. Hydatid cysts are typically single lesions usually located in the polar regions of either kidney.

Imaging findings are dependent on the stage of the hydatid cyst. Hydatid cysts are categorized into three types depending on the stage of the parasite:

1. *Type 1*: Unilocular cyst seen in the initial stage.
2. *Type 2*: Cyst with multiple daughter cysts seen in the intermediate stage.
3. *Type 3*: Calcified cyst suggestive of parasitic death.

Plain radiography may reveal a localized bulge on the renal contour or evidence of peripheral or curvilinear calcification which is in the pericyst. There may be complete calcification of the cyst in the third type. On EU, presence of hydatid cyst may result in distortion of the pelvicalyceal system. There may also be renal obstruction or impaired renal function.

On cross-sectional imaging, a unilocular cyst is typically seen in the first stage of the disease. In the next stage, when daughter cysts develop, they may be seen as multilocular cysts. The daughter cysts have a lower attenuation than of the mother cyst. These can have a thick enhancing wall and enhancing septae. A thick bilayered wall distinguishes type 2 cyst from multicystic renal disease. Few signs on imaging are considered characteristic of a hydatid cyst. A snowstorm sign can be seen on US when the hydatid sand disperses as the patient is rolled. The floating membrane sign results from separation of the cyst layers from pericyst. In type 3 cyst, when the parasite dies becomes quiescent, the cyst becomes calcified **(Figs. 21A to C)**.

Characteristic imaging findings along with history of stay in the endemic region is diagnostic of hydatid disease of the kidney, although the clinical findings may be nonspecific.

Tuberculosis

The genitourinary system accounts for nearly one-fifth of the extrapulmonary tubercular size. The most common route of spread of *Mycobacterium tuberculosis* to the kidney is hematogenous seeding from the lungs. A tuberculous focus is usually located in the renal cortex and may develop a communication with the tubular system and the pyramids, which can rupture into the calyces. Although the route of spread to kidney is hematogenous, significant disease is usually limited to one kidney. Patients may present with flank pain, dysuria, and hematuria while constitutional symptoms are less common.

On conventional radiographs, the most common finding is that of renal calcification. Extensive calcification

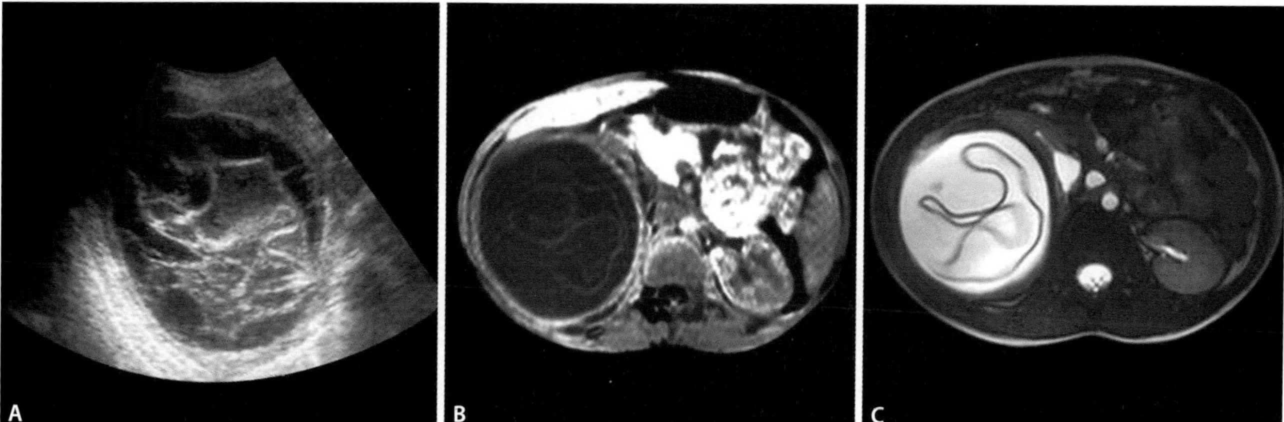

Figs. 21A to C: Sonogram (A) showing a cyst replacing the right kidney with multiple serpentine linear structures/membranes within s/o ruptured hydatid cyst. T1W MR axial image (B) showing the cyst replacing the right kidney. The cyst is hypointense on T1. T2W MR image (C) shows the cyst to have high signal. The membranes are seen as linear areas of low signal within—ruptured hydatid cyst of the right kidney. (MR: magnetic resonance).

in a nonfunctional kidney is a characteristic finding in end-stage tuberculosis and is referred to as putty kidney. EU reveals findings dependent on the severity of infection. 10–15% patients may have normal EU. "Moth eaten" calyx is one of the early findings resulting from papillary necrosis. Papillary cavitation can then result which lead to the formation of medullary cavities that can communicate with the collecting system. These medullary cavities may be large and irregular. End-stage tubercular kidneys usually do not excrete contrast medium at urography. On US, multiple renal cavities can be seen. Focal calyceal changes are seen on CT as calyceal enlargement, pericalyceal areas of early cavitation, infundibular strictures, and loss of perirenal fat planes. Late features of calcification or hydronephrosis secondary to strictures may be seen.

Renal Aspergillosis

Renal aspergillosis is an uncommon renal infection. This is most often seen in the immunocompromised state. Infection may be acquired by the hematogenous route or ascending infection, the former being the more common route. On imaging, renal aspergillosis is difficult to differentiate from a renal abscess. It is seen as a complex cystic renal lesion with thick wall and internal septations. The kidney may show accompanying focal pyelonephritic features. Diagnosis is confirmed on either lesion aspiration or urine analysis.

CONCLUSION

Renal cystic disease in adults comprises a heterogenous group of heritable and nonheritable disorders. The Bosniak classification helps in stratification of renal cysts according to the risk of malignancy. Knowledge of imaging features of various renal cystic diseases can assist the radiologist in providing useful information to the clinician to aid patient management.

SUGGESTED READING

1. Ascenti G, Mazziotti S, Zimbaro G, et al. Complex cystic renal masses: characterization with contrast-enhanced US. Radiology. 2007;243(1):158-65.
2. Avni FE, Garel C, Cassart M, et al. Imaging and classification of congenital cystic renal diseases. Am J Roentgenol. 2012;198(5): 1004-13.
3. Chung EM, Conran RM, Schroeder JW, et al. From the radiologic pathology archives: pediatric polycystic kidney disease and other ciliopathies: radiologic-pathologic correlation. Radiographics. 2014;34(1):155 78.
4. Clevert DA, Minaifar N, Weckbach S, et al. Multislice computed tomography versus contrast-enhanced ultrasound in evaluation of complex cystic renal masses using the Bosniak classification system. Clin Hemorheol Microcirc. 2008; 39(1-4):171-8.
5. Farmer DL. Urinary tract masses. Semin Pediatr Surg. 2000;9(3):109-14.
6. Friedmann W, Vogel M, Dimer JS, et al. Prenatal differential diagnosis of cystic kidney disease and urinary tract obstruction: anatomic, pathologic, ultrasonographic and genetic findings. Eur J Obs Gyn Rep Biol. 2000;89:127-33.
7. Hindman NM. Cystic renal masses. Abdom Radiol. 2016;41:1020-34.
8. Hollenbeck BK, Taub DA, Miller DC, et al. Use of nephrectomy at select medical centers—a case of follow the crowd? J Urol. 2006;175(2):670-4.
9. Hollingsworth JM, Miller DC, Daignault S, et al. Rising incidence of small renal masses: a need to reassess treatment effect. J Natl Cancer Inst. 2006;98(18):1331-4.
10. Howlader N, Noone A, Krapcho M, et al (Eds). SEER Cancer Statistics Review, 1975–2011. Bethesda: National Cancer Institute; 2013.
11. Ignee A, Straub B, Brix D, et al. The value of contrast-enhanced ultrasound (CEUS) in the characterisation of patients with renal masses. Clin Hemorheol Microcirc. 2010;46(4):275-90.
12. Israel GM, Hindman N, Bosniak MA. Evaluation of cystic renal masses: comparison of CT and MR imaging by using the Bosniak classification system. Radiology. 2004;231(2): 365-71.
13. Katabathina VS, Kota G, Dasyam AK, et al. Adult renal cystic disease: a genetic, biological, and developmental primer. Radiographics. 2010;30:1509-23.
14. Lonergan GJ, Rice RR, Suarez ES. Autosomal recessive polycystic kidney disease: radiologic-pathologic correlation. AFIP Archives Radiographics. 2000;20:837-55.
15. Mileto A, Nelson RC, Marin D, et al. Dual-energy multidetector CT for the characterization of incidental adrenal nodules: diagnostic performance of contrast-enhanced material density analysis. Radiology. 2014;274(2):445-54.
16. Narayanasamy S, Krishna S, Shanbhogue AP, et al. Contemporary update on imaging of cystic renal masses with histopathological correlation and emphasis on patient management. Clin Radiol. 2018;74(2):83-94.
17. Park BK, Kim B, Kim SH, et al. Assessment of cystic renal masses based on Bosniak classification: comparison of CT and contrast-enhanced US. Eur J Radiol. 2007;61(2):310-4.
18. Pei Y, Obaji J, Dupuis A, et al. Unified criteria for ultrasonographic diagnosis of ADPKD. J Am Soc Nephrol. 2009;20(1):205-12.
19. Silverman SG, Israel GM, Herts BR, et al. Management of the incidental renal mass. Radiology. 2008;249(1):16-31.
20. Silverman SG, Pedrosa I, Ellis JH, et al. Bosniak classification of cystic renal masses, version 2019: an update proposal and needs assessment. Radiology. 2019;292(2):475-88.
21. Tantravahi JR, Steinman TI. Acquired cystic kidney disease. Semin Dialysis. 2000;13(5):330-4.
22. Wood III CG, Stromberg III LJ, Harmath CB, et al. CT and MR imaging for evaluation of cystic renal lesions and diseases. Radiographics. 2015;35(1):125-41.

Chapter 8

Renal Neoplasms

Anjali Prakash, Gaurav Shanker Pradhan, Rashmi Dixit

INTRODUCTION

Cross-sectional imaging has led not only to an increased detection of incidental renal mass, but also to a more confident diagnosis of its nature. Imaging is required to differentiate clinically significant renal masses from benign or indolent malignant conditions. Noninvasive characterization is possible in a majority of cases, which has a clinical impact by decreasing unnecessary biopsies and/or surgical interventions. A solid renal mass is aggressively pursued for a diagnosis of renal carcinoma, once infective, traumatic or vascular causes have been ruled out, solid masses are more likely than cystic masses to be malignant and management is more aggressive.

Renal tumors constitute a heterogeneous group of tumors with characteristic histology and variable clinicobiological profile.

CLASSIFICATION OF RENAL TUMORS

The World Health Organization has classified renal tumors in 2016 **(Table 1)**. This classification has divided tumors on the basis of cell/tissue of origin (renal cell, mesenchymal, metanephric, neuroendocrine tumors, etc.).[1]

Renal cell carcinoma (RCC) has been further subdivided into various subtypes based on predominant cytoplasmic features (clear cell and chromophobe RCC), architectural features (papillary RCC), anatomic location of tumors (collecting duct, renal medullary carcinoma), based on association with a specific renal disease background (acquired cystic disease-associated RCC). Certain subtypes are based on molecular alterations pathognomonic for RCC subtypes (MiT family translocation, succinate dehydrogenase-deficient renal

Table 1: WHO classification of renal tumors (2016).

- *Renal cell tumors:*
  - Clear cell renal cell carcinoma
  - Multilocular cystic renal neoplasm of low malignant potential
  - Papillary renal cell carcinomas
  - Hereditary leiomyomatosis and renal cell carcinoma-associated renal cell carcinoma
  - Chromophobe renal cell carcinoma
  - Collecting duct carcinoma
  - Renal medullary carcinoma
  - MIT family translocation renal cell carcinomas
  - Succinate dehydrogenase-deficient renal carcinoma
  - Mucinous tubular and spindle cell carcinoma
  - Tubulocystic renal cell carcinoma
  - Acquired cystic disease-associated renal cell carcinoma
  - Renal cell carcinoma, unclassified
  - Papillary adenoma
  - Oncocytoma
- *Metanephric tumors:*
  - Metanephric adenoma
  - Metanephric adenofibroma
  - Metanephric stromal tumor
- *Nephroblastic and cystic tumors occurring mainly in children:*
  - Nephrogenic rests
  - Nephroblastoma
  - Cystic partially differentiated nephroblastoma
  - Pediatric cystic nephroma
- *Mesenchymal tumors:*
  - *Mesenchymal tumors occurring mainly in children:*
    - Clear cell sarcoma
    - Rhabdoid tumor
    - Congenital mesoblastic nephroma
    - Ossifying renal tumor of infancy
  - *Mesenchymal tumors occurring mainly in adults:*
    - Leiomyosarcoma
    - Angiosarcoma
    - Rhabdomyosarcoma
    - Osteosarcoma
    - Synovial sarcoma

Contd...

Contd...

- Ewing's sarcoma
- Angiomyolipoma
- Epithelioid angiomyolipoma
- Leiomyoma
- Hemangioma
- Lymphangioma
- Hemangioblastoma
- Juxtaglomerular cell tumor
- Renomedullary interstitial cell tumor
- Schwannoma
- Solitary fibrous tumor
- *Mixed epithelial and stromal tumor family:*
  - Cystic nephroma
  - Mixed epithelial and stromal tumor
- *Neuroendocrine tumors:*
  - Well-differentiated neuroendocrine tumor
  - Large cell neuroendocrine carcinoma
  - Small cell neuroendocrine carcinoma
  - Pheochromocytoma
- *Miscellaneous tumors:*
  - Renal hematopoietic neoplasms
  - Germ cell tumors
- *Metastatic tumors*

carcinoma), and there are certain familial cancers [hereditary leiomyomatosis and RCC (HLRCC) syndrome-associated RCC].

IMAGING OF RENAL MASS: MODALITIES AND TECHNIQUES

The workup of a renal mass starts with the differentiation of cystic mass from solid renal masses. Up to 90% of solid masses are malignant, with the risk increasing with size of the tumor (50% in size <1 cm to 90% in size >7 cm). The commonly seen malignant solid renal masses are renal cell carcinoma, urothelial carcinoma, lymphoma, and metastasis, whereas the benign lesions seen are angiomyolipoma and oncocytoma.

Ultrasound is used as a first-line imaging test for suspected renal disease. A simple cyst can be confidently diagnosed on ultrasound as a completely anechoic structure with posterior enhancement. Septation, calcification, and solid nodular component are seen in a complicated cyst. The detection of blood flow by Doppler or lesion enhancement after intravenous contrast denotes presence of a solid component.[2]

Any solid lesion or a complicated cyst requires further evaluation by **CT or MRI**. These examinations should be performed with a protocol according meticulous attention to detail to evaluate an indeterminate mass accurately and to stage a possible renal cancer. The recommended protocols for CT and MRI for characterization of renal mass are provided in **Tables 2 and 3**.[3]

Both CT and MRI should have noncontrast imaging with contrast imaging in various phases [corticomedullary (CM), nephrographic, and delayed]. Slice thickness should be 2.5–3 mm with a reconstruction interval of not more than 3 mm.

Renal enhancement occurs in different phases at 20 seconds after administration of contrast, in the *arterial phase*, aorta, and renal arteries enhance. At 60–70 seconds starts the *CM phase*, where the differentiation of cortex and medulla is prominent, pseudotumors like dromedary hump, and hypertrophied column of Bertin can be identified. At 90–120 seconds begins the *nephrographic phase,* when enhancement of cortex fades and medulla enhances homogeneously. This is the most sensitive phase for renal mass detection. At 180 seconds appears the *excretory phase*, where contrast appears in the collecting system. Computed tomography for detection of thrombus requires thin (<5 mm) slices at level of renal vein after pressure injection of contrast. Renal vein enlargement and displacement are not accurate signs for venous invasion, as it may be enlarged due to high flow and displaced due to bulk of tumor. The flow of unenhanced blood from pelvis may be mistaken for inferior vena cava (IVC) thrombus. In these cases, delayed images may be needed for further characterization.

Precontrast imaging in MRI, should include T1 and T2 imaging, chemical shift imaging (in and opposed phase) and diffusion-weighted imaging. A fat suppression technique for detection of macroscopic fat is also required. Dynamic imaging, in at least two phases after administration of intravenous (IV) contrast completes the protocol. Subtraction imaging is required in MRI to demonstrate enhancement, especially in a T1-hyperintense lesion.

DIAGNOSTIC CRITERIA

Balls versus Beans

A useful strategy for the evaluation of renal mass is to divide them on the basis of their growth pattern into ball type or bean type masses. This concept was developed by Hartman and Ros. Most renal masses like cysts, renal cell carcinomas, angiomyolipoma, metastasis, and oncocytoma grow by expansion. These masses are shaped similarly to spheres or balls and they displace and compress the adjacent structure, rather than invade normal structure. As these masses enlarge, they expand from normal parenchymal margins, either peripherally to the kidney or into renal sinus. Other renal lesions like transitional cell carcinoma, squamous cell carcinoma,

Table 2: CT protocol for renal mass characterization.

Phases	*Noncontrast*	**Corticomedullary*	*Nephrographic*	*Excretory*
Phase timing	–	40 seconds	90–120 seconds	5–7 minutes
Coverage	Kidneys	Diaphragm through kidneys	Diaphragm through kidneys	Kidneys
Field of view	Whole body	Whole body	Whole body	Whole body
Reconstructions	Axial: 3 mm	Axial: 3 mm Coronal: 2 mm Sagittal: 2 mm	Axial: 3 mm Coronal: 2 mm Sagittal: 2 mm	Axial: 3 mm Coronal: 2 mm Sagittal: 2 mm

*Contrast 100–150 mL low osmolality (LOCM) at 5 mL/second.

Table 3: Multiparametric magnetic resonance protocol for characterization of renal mass.

Sequences	*Imaging planes*
T1W dual echo gradient (in and opposed phase)	Axial
T2W HASTE	Axial, coronal, sagittal
T2W TSE with fat suppression	Axial
3D fat-saturated T1W SPGR precontrast and postcontrast DCE (corticomedullary, nephrographic, and excretory*)	Axial
Diffusion weighted (b = 50,500,800), ADC map	Axial

*Corticomedullary phase = 40 seconds, nephrographic = 90 seconds, excretory = 3 minutes after IV gadolinium at dose of 0.01 mmol/kg in patients with GFR > 60 mL/min/1.73 m^2 via pressure injector followed by a saline flush.

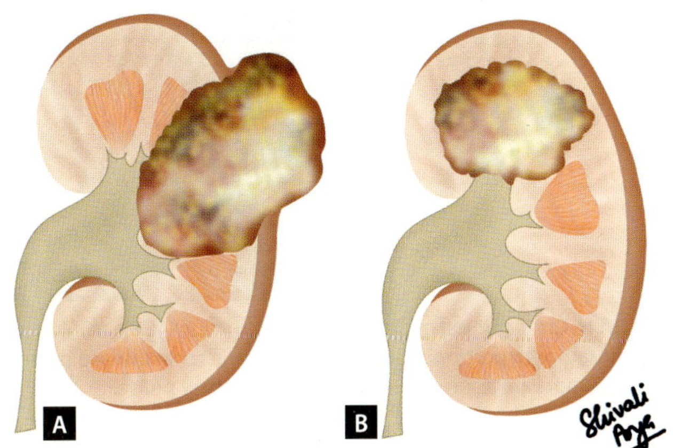

Figs. 1A and B: Ball versus bean concept: (A) Ball type mass grows exophytically, with a contour deformity; (B) Bean type mass uses renal parenchyma as framework for growth with maintained reniform shape. Sinus fat and collecting system elements may be destroyed.

infiltrating carcinoma, lymphoma, and renal medullary carcinoma grow along the latticework of normal renal parenchyma. Infiltrating lesions do not deform the shape, with the kidney retaining the "bean" shape **(Figs. 1A and B)**. These are difficult to detect radiologically since little mass effect is associated.[4-6]

Renal Pseudotumors

It is essential to determine that the detected "mass" is actually a renal neoplasm and not a finding that mimics it. Renal pseudotumors are a diverse group, including congenital and developmental anomalies (fetal lobulations, prominent renal columns of Bertin, dromedary humps), inflammatory lesions (renal abscess, pyelonephritis), and vascular anomalies (renal artery aneurysm, arteriovenous malformation). Renal contusion and hematoma may also mimic a tumor. Many patients with chronic renal disease develop focal nodular compensatory hypertrophy which mimics a tumor. Imaging in CM phase provides the correct answer **(Figs. 2A to C)**. Enhancement, a key feature in the diagnosis of a neoplasm may be seen in infective and vascular lesions. Clinical history (e.g. pain, fever, and pyuria favor infection and not a neoplasm), multiphasic CT/MR examination, and knowledge of the pseudotumors will help to reach a correct diagnosis.[7]

Most solid renal masses measure between 20 and 70 Hounsfield units (HU) on noncontrast CT. Lesions measuring less or more than that are cysts—simple cysts or hyperdense/hemorrhagic cysts, respectively. Indeterminate renal mass is a lesion containing areas that measure 20–70 HU on noncontrast imaging. Homogeneous lesions measuring more than 70 HU can be considered benign, whereas lesions either entirely or partially within the 20–70 HU range should be considered indeterminate and require further evaluation.

Enhancement of a renal mass is considered to be the key in determining the nature of the mass. The main criteria for diagnosing a solid renal mass is to document measurable enhancement on CT/MRI. Any nodular enhancement within a mass confirms some solid

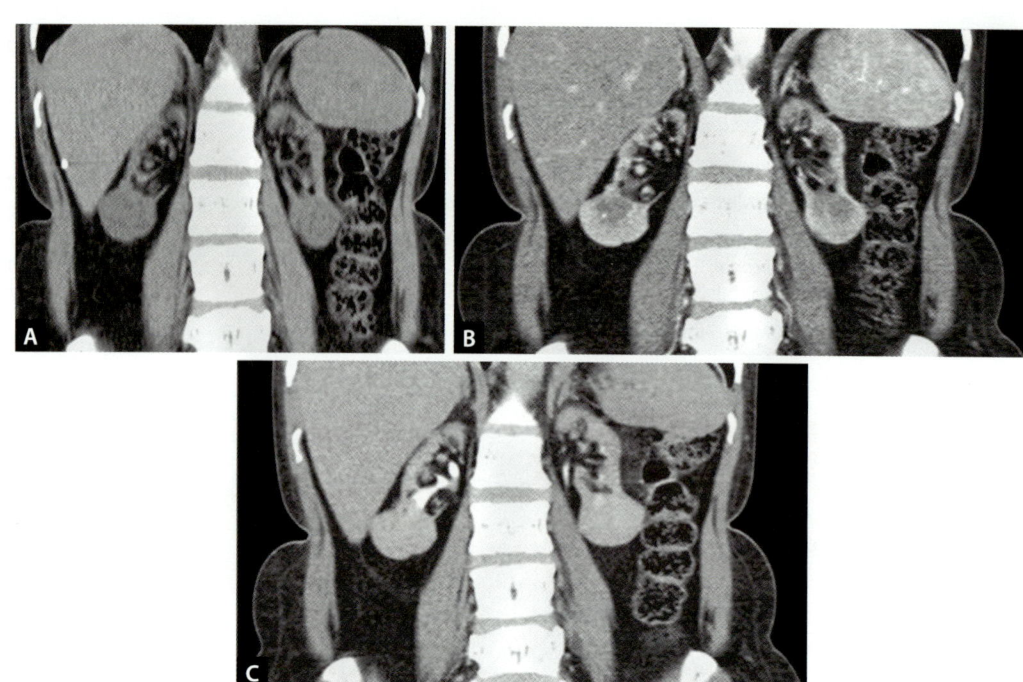

Figs. 2A to C: CT coronal multiphasic reconstruction (MPR): (A) Noncontrast; (B) Corticomedullary phase; (C) Nephrographic phase-focal nodular compensatory hypertrophy in a case of chronic renal disease presenting as "tumor" in lower poles of both kidneys. The true nature of these pseudotumors are appreciated on corticomedullary phase.

component and a high probability of a renal neoplasm. An increase of more than 20 HU on administration of IV contrast is taken as evidence of presence of solid elements while an increase of less than 10 HU is considered as no enhancement. An indeterminate enhancement is an increase of 10–20 HU and requires follow-up or imaging by MRI, which is more sensitive to contrast enhancement than CT.

Enhancement may be incorrectly identified as present on CT due to two reasons. First is *volume averaging*, which occurs when CT image averages part of mass (usually <1.5 cm in size) with the normal enhancing renal parenchyma. To prevent this, the slice thickness should not be more than half the renal mass diameter. The second reason of pseudoenhancement is *beam hardening*. This occurs in small masses or masses completely surrounded by enhancing parenchyma, leading to an increase in attenuation of less than 30 HU. This effect cannot be overcome by decreasing slice thickness.[8,9]

RENAL CELL TUMORS

Renal Cell Carcinoma

Renal cell carcinoma, also called hypernephroma, is the most common primary renal malignancy in adults. It accounts for 85% of all malignant renal tumors and about 3% of all diagnosed neoplasms. RCC is nowadays most commonly discovered incidentally (30%). These are often smaller and of lower grade and staging. RCC may however, present with symptoms like flank pain (37%), hematuria and palpable mass, weight loss, anorexia, fever, gastrointestinal or neurological symptoms, and paraneoplastic syndromes. Superficial tumors can invade and breach the renal capsule and directly involve perirenal fat, adrenal gland, and adjacent organs. Metastases often occurs in regional nodes, invasion of cisterna chyli can lead to hilar and supraclavicular nodes. RCC has a propensity for venous thrombi. Systemic dissemination can take place into liver, bone, adrenal, and opposite kidney or brain in decreasing order of frequency.

Renal cell carcinoma occurs more commonly in males, in the 5th–7th decade. Most cases are sporadic; some may be associated with syndromes such as Von Hippel–Lindau disease (vHL) **(Box 1)**. Risk factors include smoking, hypertension, obesity, acquired renal cystic disease, exposure to petroleum and asbestos, and certain genetic syndromes. Usually RCC is unilateral, 2% are bilateral and 9% are multicentric in the same kidney. Bilateral and multicentric tumors arise in patients of vHL syndromic, familial RCC and in patients on long-term hemodialysis.[10]

Renal cell carcinoma is comprised of different histological subtypes with different disease progression and metastatic potential.

Box 1: Inherited cancer susceptibility syndromes with increased risk of renal cancer.

- BAP1-mutant disease
- Birt-Hogg-Dubé syndrome
- Familial clear cell renal cancer with chromosome 3 translocation
- Hereditary leiomyomatosis and renal cell cancer
- Hereditary papillary renal cancer
- PTEN hamartoma syndrome
- SDH-associated renal cancer
- Tuberous sclerosis complex
- Von Hippel-Lindau disease

Clear cell renal cell carcinoma: *Clear cell RCC* is the most common subtype accounting for 75–85% of cases, which are mostly sporadic in occurrence, 5% are associated with hereditary syndromes, including vHL and tuberous sclerosis. These tumors originate from the proximal convoluted tubules. It typically appears as a variegated, expansile, cortical mass with areas of necrosis, hemorrhage, cystic change, and calcification (15%). Clear cell RCC is a hypervascular tumor and has the greatest metastatic potential with hematogenous metastasis to lung, liver, and bones. There is also a propensity of clear cell RCC for lymphatic, late, and unusual sites of metastasis.[3,11,12]

Papillary renal cell carcinoma: These arise from the epithelium of the proximal convoluted tubule, and are the second most common subtype of RCC. Characterized by papillary or tubopapillary histologic architecture, they account for 10–15% of RCC. These are bilateral in I4% and multifocal in 23% cases.

Papillary RCC usually presents at 40–50 years of age and is a slow-growing tumor. Papillary RCC (pRCC) appears as homogeneous, hypovascular, soft tissue cortical mass with foci of calcification. Papillary RCCs frequently show hemorrhage.[3,11,12]

Chromophobe renal cell carcinoma: It is a subtype of RCC, characterized by large, pale cells with prominent cell membranes. 5–10% of RCCs are of the chromophobe subtype, which arise from intercalated cells of the renal cortex and have the same origin as oncocytoma with overlapping histological and imaging features. They usually occur as a solitary cortical mass. Bilateral and multicentric chromophobe RCCs are found in association with oncocytomas and Birt-Hogg-Dubé syndrome. The tumor is typically large at presentation, homogeneous without necrosis or hemorrhage, and is relatively hypovascular. The chromophobe type is associated with the least malignant potential and best prognosis.[13]

Multicystic renal cell carcinoma: It is a recently described, rare subtype of RCC. The term is used to describe a cystic RCC with a small volume (25% or less) of neoplastic clear cells in the cyst. Multicystic renal cell carcinoma (MCRCC) typically manifests as multiseptated cystic masses with thin septations on imaging. Distinction from other cystic masses is difficult.[14]

Other Subtypes of Renal Cell Carcinoma

Carcinoma of the collecting ducts (CDC) of Bellini: This is a rare subtype of RCC accounting for <1% cases. Slightly more common in males, patients are usually in the mid-50s. This tumor is characterized by its medullary location, infiltrative growth pattern and weak, heterogeneous enhancement.[15]

Renal medullary carcinoma: It is a rapidly growing aggressive subtype, often presenting with metastasis. Seen in young males of African descent with a sickle cell trait, this is usually seen on right side of body, presenting as an infiltrative necrotic mass with caliectasis and lymphadenopathy.[16,17]

Renal carcinoma associated with Xp11.2 translocations/ TFE 3 gene fusions: This carcinoma affects children and young adults. Large size, cystic changes, calcification, lymph node and distant metastasis are indicative of this subtype, especially in a young female patient.[18,19]

Imaging of Renal Cell Carcinoma

Plain radiograph: *It is not used to diagnose a renal mass.* Renal mass may be visible as a soft tissue shadow with displacement of retroperitoneal fat. Calcification can also be detected on plain film **(Fig. 3)**. Pattern of calcification may help in differentiating benign from malignant masses. Renal masses that contain central, irregular calcifications are usually malignant, whereas peripheral rim calcifications are seen in renal cysts.

Intravenous urography: It is an insensitive method of detecting a renal mass, especially central placed ones. It lacks specificity for accurately characterizing a lesion. Expansile masses cause contour abnormalities calyceal splaying, stretching, and draping **(Fig. 4)**. Infiltrating renal mass produce little parenchymal mass effect, and may be seen as a filling defect in the collecting system.

Ultrasound: Ultrasound is usually the initial method of investigation in a renal mass. It can reliably differentiate solid masses from renal cysts.

Renal cell carcinoma has varied appearance on sonography. Mostly solid, RCCs can have a predominant

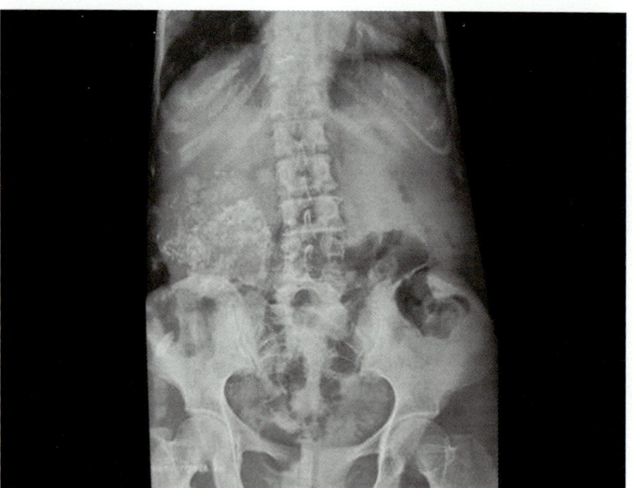

Fig. 3: X-ray abdomen showing soft-tissue mass with calcification in the right renal fossa.

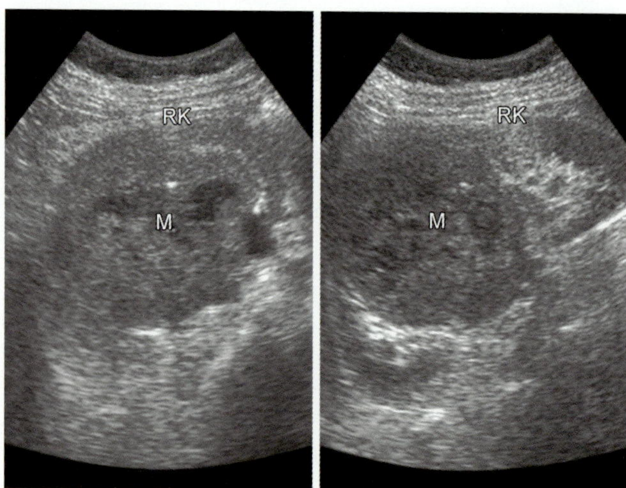

Fig. 5: US—transverse and longitudinal sonogram of the right kidney shows a large well-defined heterogeneous mass arising from the upper pole right kidney—renal cell carcinoma.

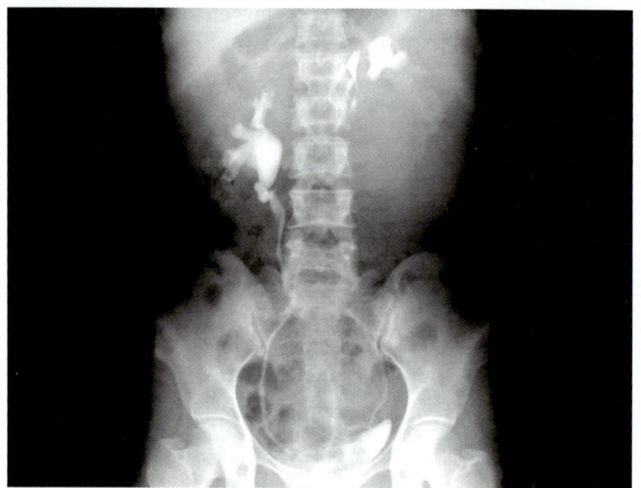

Fig. 4: Intravenous renogram—showing compression and displacement of calyces of the left kidney with focal upper pole hydrocalyx in a case of renal cell carcinoma.

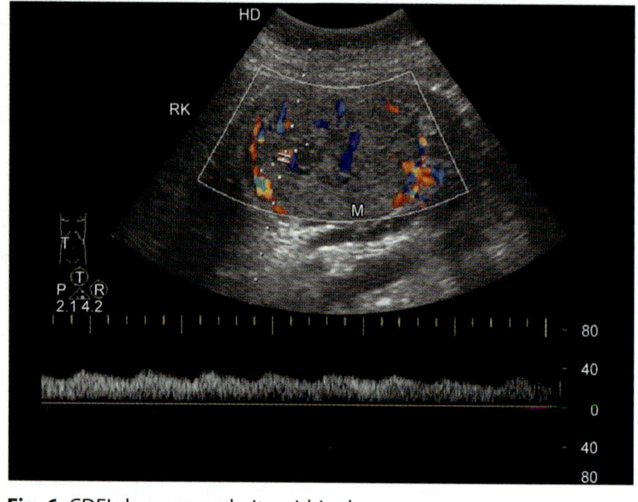

Fig. 6: CDFI shows vascularity within the mass.

cystic component. Usually, hypo- to isoechoic to the renal parenchyma **(Fig. 5)**, they can appear hyperechoic making differentiation from angiomyolipoma difficult. Color Doppler demonstrates neovascularity of tumor. Different patterns of flow have been demonstrated in various subtypes of RCC. High-peak systolic velocity and Doppler shift has been seen in clear cell RCC **(Fig. 6)**. Contrast-enhanced ultrasound (CEUS) is useful to demonstrate presence of vascularity in a renal mass, which is the most important feature of a possible malignant etiology. Clear cell RCC demonstrates strong uptake in arterial phase with a delayed washout. Hypovascularity of a mass compared to the renal cortex is a feature of papillary carcinoma. Presence of a vascularized capsule around a solid renal mass is another suspicious feature. CEUS helps in the workup of indeterminate lesion on CT and has proved useful in dividing these lesions as surgical or nonsurgical.[20]

Computed tomography on unenhanced CT, renal cell carcinomas may be hypodense, isodense, or hyperdense to the unenhanced renal parenchyma. They are often heterogeneous in appearance with low-density necrotic areas. The renal outline is distorted in a majority (94%) of cases, irrespective of tumor size. The presence of calcification is also noted in approximately 25%, CT being the most sensitive modality for the depiction of parenchymal calcification **(Figs. 7A and B)**. Calcification in RCC may be punctate, amorphous, linear or peripheral.

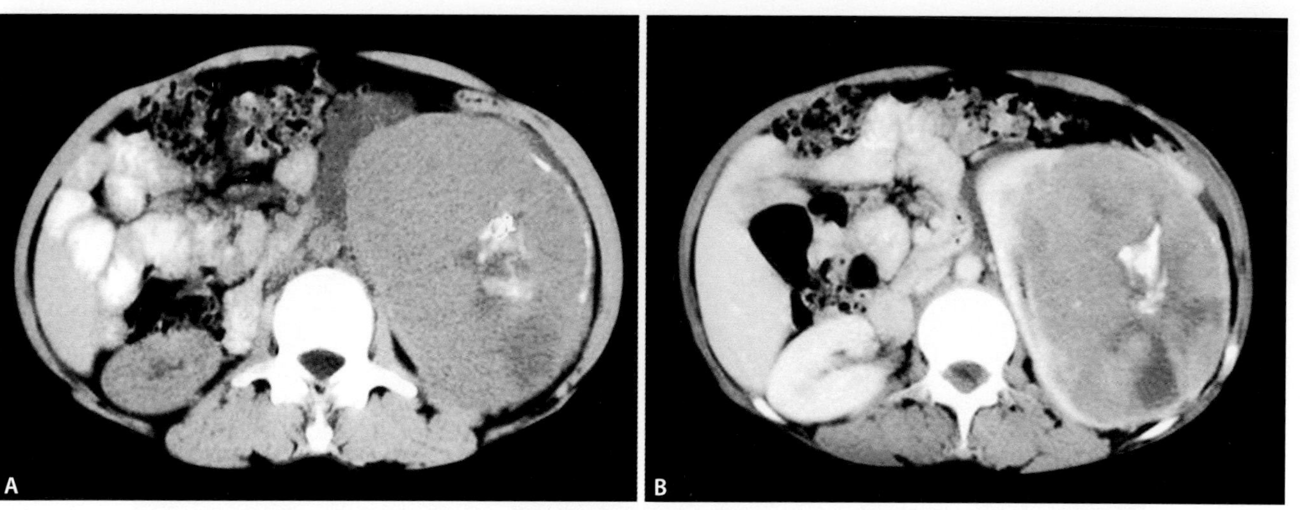

Figs. 7A and B: (A) Noncontrast CT; (B) Contrast-enhanced CT showing a large enhancing mass with peripheral and central coarse calcification in the left kidney.

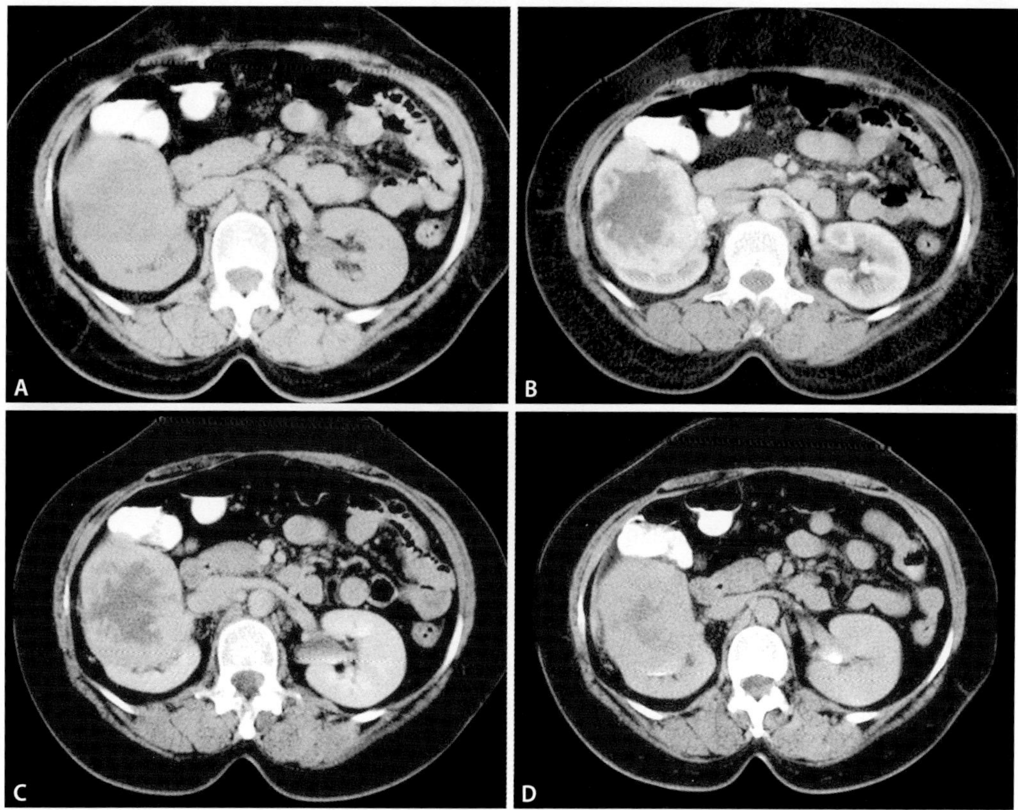

Figs. 8A to D: CT features of renal cell carcinomas in four phases: (A) Noncontrast; (B) Corticomedullary; (C) Nephrographic; (D) Excretory phases. Shows a right renal mass with mixed enhancement pattern containing enhancing soft tissue and low attenuation areas representing necrosis or cystic change arising from the anterior renal cortex. The mass is best demarcated on nephrographic phase and shows "de-enhancement" in the later phase.

A zone of relative radiolucency surrounding the tumor or "Halo sign" may be noted. This represents the compressed ischemic renal parenchyma around the tumor—"pseudocapsule".

Most renal carcinomas are solid with an attenuation of at least 20 HU on precontrast scans. An increase of attenuation of more than 20 HU, post administration of IV contrast indicates a possible malignant etiology **(Figs. 8 and 9)**.

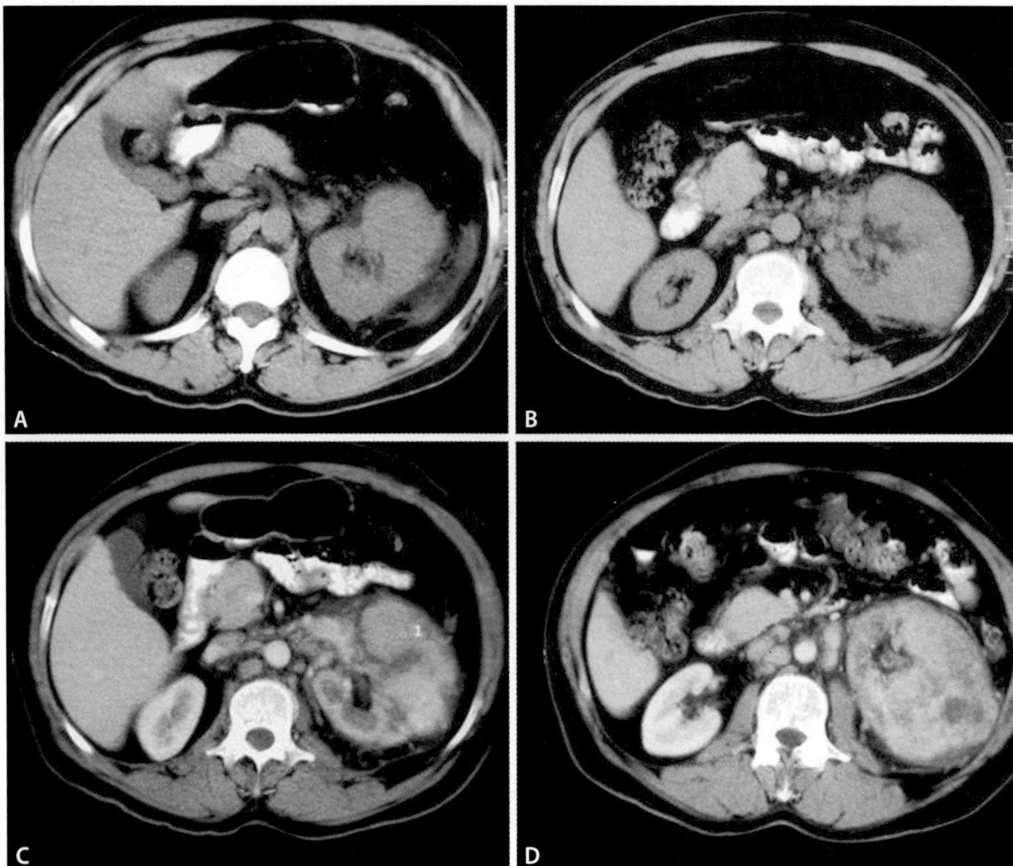

Figs. 9A to D: (A and B) CT precontrast; and (C and D) CT postcontrast—solid left renal mass with increase in attenuation of 20 HU—malignant etiology—renal cell carcinoma.

Heterogeneous enhancement correlates with the presence of cellular regions within the tumor, but does not correlate with grade. Cystic and necrotic change is seen in clear cell type, whereas papillary and chromophobe are more homogeneous. Clear cell carcinomas enhance to a greater degree than other subtypes of malignant lesions, especially papillary carcinoma. A low tumor to aorta enhancement or tumor to normal renal parenchyma enhancement ratio is indicative of papillary RCC.[21,22]

The RCC shows a propensity for renal vein invasion and the thrombus may extend into the IVC, seen in almost 30% of cases. CT is specific for renal vein invasion by tumor thrombus with specificity of 98% **(Fig. 10)**. A hypodense filling defect outlined by contrast in the renal vein on a CT on CM or nephrographic phase is diagnostic for thrombus. Tumor thrombus may extend into IVC, often enlarging the caliber of the IVC. There may be bland thrombus inferior to the tumor thrombus in the IVC, as a result of occlusion of the lumen. Inadequate contrast bolus, motion and flow artefacts may cause a technically inadequate CT scan. On the right side, it may be difficult to distinguish between intraluminal tumor thrombus and extrinsic caval compression caused by a large primary tumor or enlarged lymph nodes.

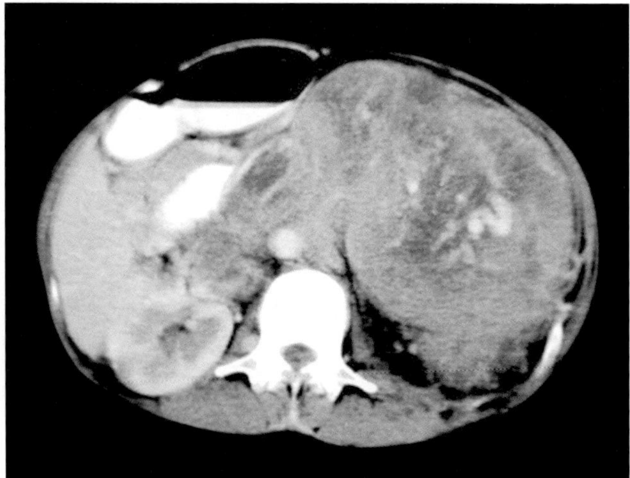

Fig. 10: Contrast-enhanced CT abdomen shows a large mass in the left kidney with neovascularity, definite extension into perinephric space, left renal vein and inferior vena cava—renal cell carcinoma.

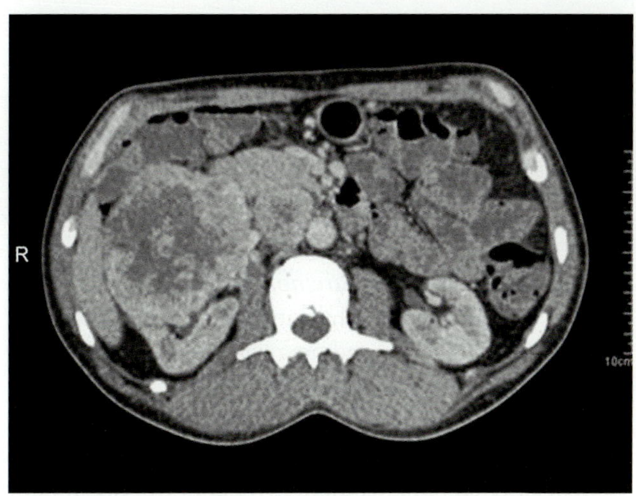

Fig. 11: Contrast-enhanced CT abdomen—right renal mass with retroperitoneal adenopathy.

Metastatic adenopathy in the retroperitoneum, associated with RCC has poor prognostic significance **(Fig. 11)**. The criterion of 1 cm threshold has proved to be unsuccessful in differentiating reactive nodes from metastatic adenopathy. Lymph nodes greater than 2 cm are always malignant. Nodes, less than 1 cm, may contain metastasis.

Dual-energy computed tomography: Dual-energy computed tomography (DECT) plays an important role in the characterization of renal masses, especially in the incidentally discovered mass. Virtual unenhanced and the water density images substitute for conventional noncontrast images, where acquisition in precontrast phase has not been done. In patients who are imaged for a multiphase renal CT, omitting noncontrast phase can lead to decrease in radiation dose. Color-coded iodine maps or iodine density maps demonstrate enhancement and can help in diagnosing nonenhancing cysts.[23]

Estimating the iodine content from a region of interest may help in the diagnosis of hyperdense cyst, complex cysts, and hypovascular renal tumor. An iodine density threshold of 0.5 mg/mL has a reported sensitivity of 100% and a specificity of 97.7% for distinguishing enhancing from nonenhancing lesions. Similarly, tumor iodine concentration of 0.9 mg/mL may serve as a threshold to differentiate between clear cell from papillary subtypes of RCC. DECT also provides virtual monochromatic data sets can help to overcome the problem of pseudoenhancement in small lesions. A recent advance of atomic number mapping can help to differentiate nonenhancing lesions from enhancing masses. DECT has a role in posttreatment imaging of renal tumors. Color-coded iodine maps can help to differentiate postoperative changes such as hyperdense foci and nodular appearance seen after ablative therapy that mimic residual changes from residual/recurrent tumor.[24,25]

Magnetic resonance imaging of renal masses: Functional imaging [diffusion-weighted imaging (DWI) and dynamic contrast-enhancement (DCE)] techniques combined with T2-weighted (T2W) and chemical-shift imaging (CSI), with or without urography, constitutes a comprehensive multiparametric (MP) MRI protocol of the kidneys.

MR imaging allows detection and characterization of renal masses. MR also helps in differentiating benign from malignant renal mass, suggests various subtypes of RCC **(Tables 4 and 5)** and possible histological grade leading to a role in management decisions. With the advent of newer treatment options and adjuvant therapies like immunotherapy with interleukin-2, interferon-α, and autolymphocytes, antiangiogenic therapy, cytotoxic chemotherapy, predicting the subtype of RCC is important in the management. Clear cell and chromophobe RCC may show response to immunotherapy, which is not

Table 4: MR features of various renal cell carcinoma subtypes.

Clear cell RCC	*Papillary RCC*	*Chromophobe RCC*
Hypervascular	Hypovascular	Hypovascular
Heterogeneous	Homogeneous	Homogeneous
Renal vein and IVC involvement common	Rare	Rare
Lymph nodal involvement is less	More common	Least common
Metastasis common	Less common	Least common
Hyperintense on T2WI	Hypointense on T1W1	

Table 5: Multiparametric MRI of renal masses.

Renal mass	*MRI feature*
Clear cell RCC	High SI on T2WI, microscopic fat, hypervascular
Papillary RCC	Low SI on T2WI, hypovascular, may contain hemosiderin
Chromophobe RCC	No definitive features—biopsy
Classic AML	Macroscopic fat suppresion on frequency-selective Fat Sat sequence, artefact on CSI
Lipid-poor AML	Low SI on T2WI, avid early enhancement, may contain microscopic fat
Oncocytoma	No definitive features-biopsy

useful in papillary RCC. Various studies have correlated MRI appearance of renal masses with pathology.[26-27] An MRI classification system has been proposed to predict the histological subtype and nuclear grade. This is based on certain characteristics like lesion size, peripheral vs central location, T2 signal intensity and degree of enhancement of the lesion, the presence of subvoxel fat on CSI, intratumoral necrosis, retroperitoneal vascular collaterals, and vascular thrombosis.[28]

Clear cell RCC, which demonstrates high T2 signal with heterogeneity due to associated cystic change and necrosis, are hypointense to isointense to normal renal parenchyma on T1W images. The presence of necrosis in a renal mass has been shown to correlate with tumor size and grade. Presence of intralesional microscopic fat in 60% of cases leads to a drop of signal on opposed phase imaging compared to in-phase images. A signal loss of 25% or more has predictive value. Clear cell RCC are hypervascular tumors, enhancing avidly (more than other subtypes of RCCs). A tumor pseudocapsule, representing compressed renal parenchyma, which is hypointense on both T1 and T2 may be seen. Clear cell RCCs tend to extend into the renal vein and inferior vena cava. Presence of intralesional necrosis, retroperitoneal collaterals, renal vein thrombosis interruption of pseudocapsule, large size correlate with an aggressive tumor grade[29,30] **(Figs. 12 and 13)**.

Papillary renal cell carcinoma: Papillary RCC are usually well-circumscribed, peripherally located small tumors less than 3 cm. Papillary tumors are characteristically hypointense on T2W images and are hypovascular. As the tumor increases in size, internal hemorrhage may cause heterogeneous appearance **(Figs. 14A to D)**. Presence of hemosiderin due to hemorrhage leads to signal drop on in-phase images. Cystic papillary RCCs show internal papillary projections, mural nodules, and hemorrhagic fluid.

Chromophobe renal cell carcinoma: No specific features are seen on MR, they may show intermediate-to-low signal on T2WI; cystic change and necrosis are uncommon. The enhancement is intermediate, more than pRCC, and less than ccRCC. In some cases, a central stellate scar and spoke wheel pattern (similar to oncocytoma) may be seen. Segmental enhancement inversion, wherby initially enhancing components of a renal mass subsequently become lower in attenuation than the initially hypo-enhancing ones is another shared feature with oncocytoma.

Diffusion-weighted Imaging[31-37]

Diffusion-weighted MR imaging adds to the diagnostic ability of MRI. It is a valuable tool in evaluating pathology in patients with renal impairment in whom contrast administration is contraindicated. ADC value of renal tumor is less than normal parenchyma, a fact of utility in ruling out malignancy in pseudotumors. Solid lesions have higher cellular density, which restrict Brownian motion of water and have low ADC values whereas benign lesions lose signal with increasing b-values and have high ADC values **(Figs. 15A to E)**. In a few studies, RCCs show

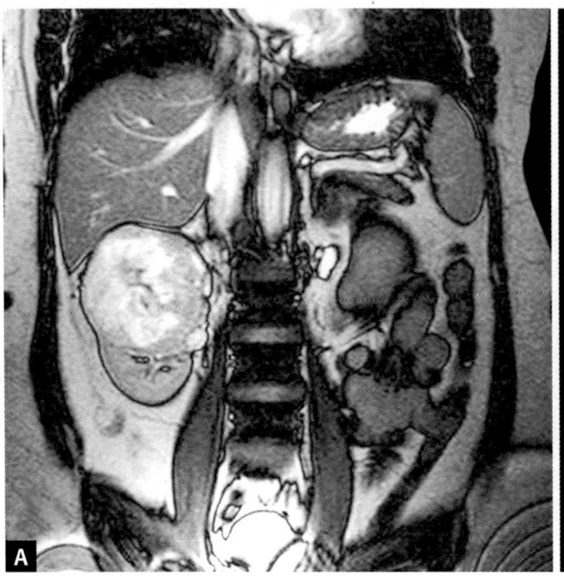

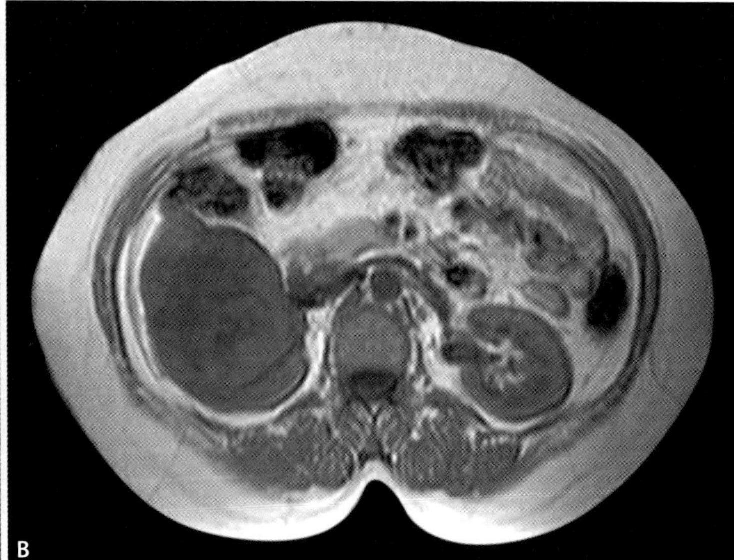

Figs. 12A and B: Renal cell carcinoma—(A) MRI; (B) TRUEFISP coronal T1W1 axial showing a well-circumscribed mass with necrotic change hypointense on T1 and hyperintense on T2 arising from upper pole of right kidney. Inferior vena cava appears normal. Clear cell renal cell carcinoma.

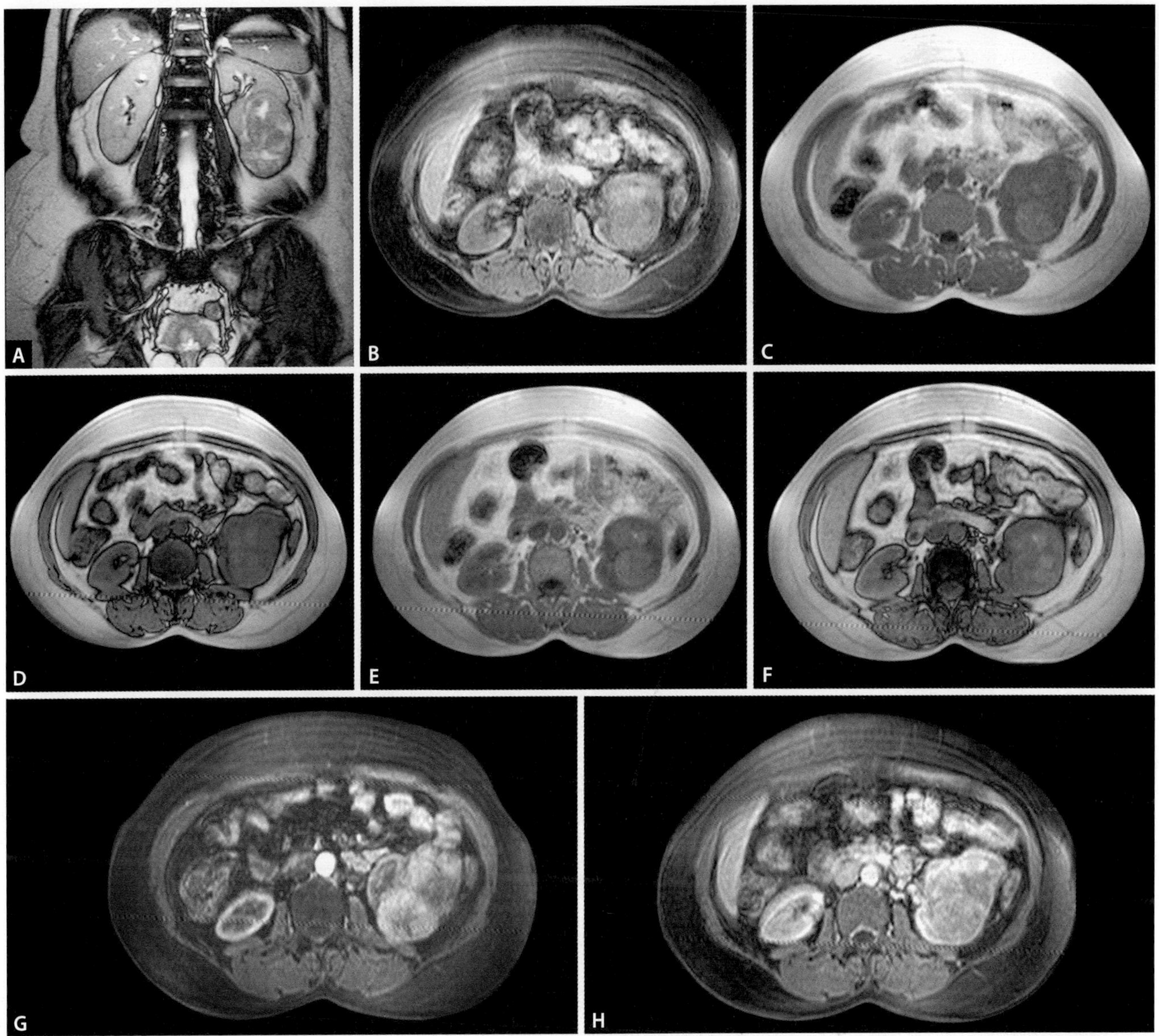

Figs. 13A to H: (A) MRI T2 TRUE FISP coronal; (B) TI VIBE axial; (C and E) TI in phase; and (D and F) opposed phase; (G and H) TI axial postgadolinium—a solid-enhancing mass is seen in left kidney, hypointense on T1, hyperintense on T2, with a drop in signal intensity on opposed phase images compared to in phase images. Note lack of "India ink" effect on opposed phase—clear cell renal cell carcinoma.

significantly lower ADC than benign lesions ($1.61 \pm 0.08 \times 10^{-3}mm^2/s$ vs $2.10 \pm 0.09 \times 10^{-3}mm^2/s$). Cysts have highest ADC values followed by normal renal tissue ($2.26 \pm 0.10 \times 10^{-3}mm^2/s$).

There is a difference in the reported ADC value between oncocytoma ($2.01 \pm 0.08 \times 10^{-3}mm^2/s$) and RCC, a point that can potentially help in differentiating the two. DWI helps to differentiate various subtypes of RCCs. Clear cell RCCs have significantly higher ADC values than papillary and chromophobe subtypes. ADC values are lower for high-grade clear cell RCCs compared with those of low-grade clear cell RCCs. There is a considerable overlap in ADC values between benign and malignant lesions and it cannot be used to differentiate between them. Research is going on to evaluate role of DWI as a predictor for treatment response postchemotherapy (Sorafenib in metastatic RCC).[38]

Renal Cell Carcinoma Staging

The overall accuracy of MR staging is comparable to CT. It has certain advantages over CT in the evaluation of tumor vascular extension, differentiation of perihilar vessels from nodes and the assessment of direct tumor extension into other organs. MRI is an excellent staging modality when the CT findings are equivocal.[39,40]

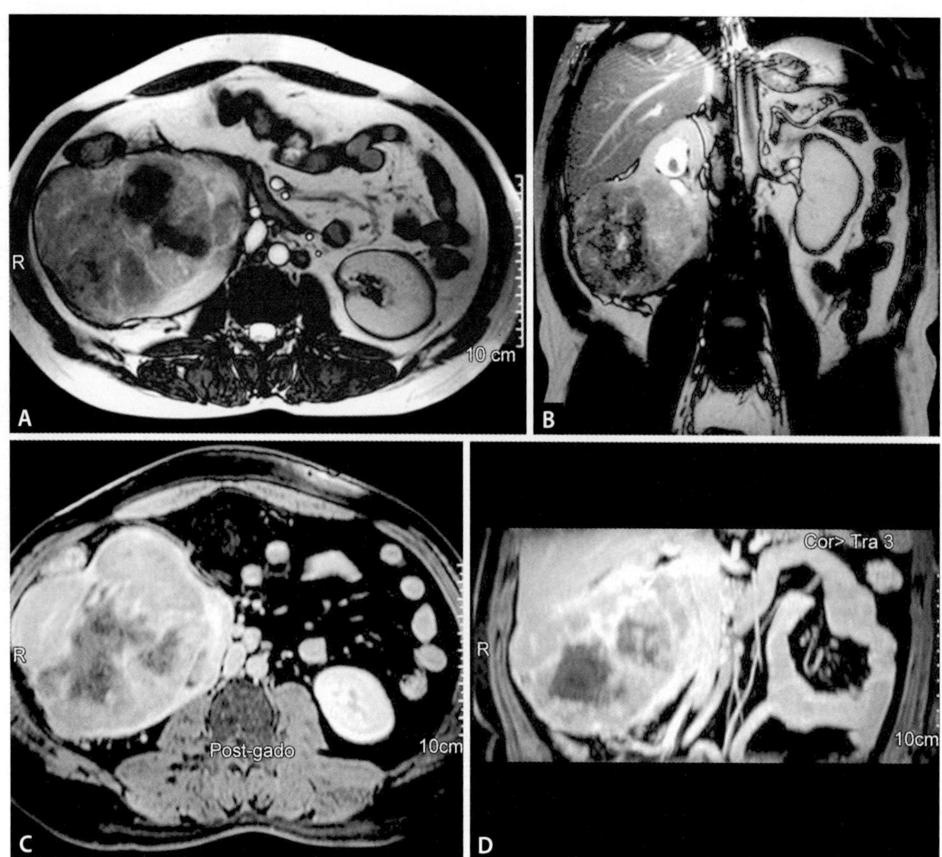

Figs. 14A to D: MRI TRU FISP (A) Axial; and (B) Coronal—mixed intensity right lower polar mass with areas of hemorrhage; (C) TI postgadolinium axial; and (D) Coronal maximum intensity projection (MIP) shows enhancing soft-tissue component of the mass—papillary renal cell carcinoma.

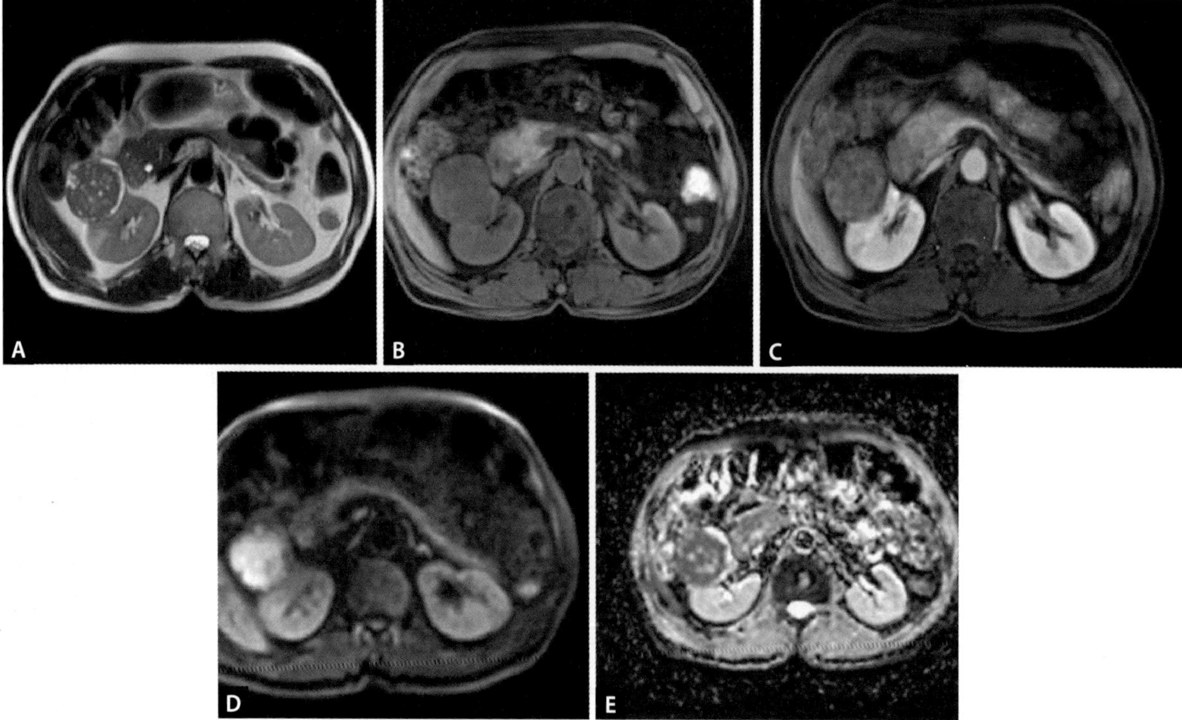

Figs. 15A to E: (A) T2 axial; (B) T1 axial pre; (C) Postcontrast; (D) Diffusion-weighted; and (E) Apparent diffusion coefficient (ADC) maps—well-circumscribed, peripherally located T2 hypointense, hypovascular mass with restricted diffusion—renal cell carcinoma.

Currently the most commonly used staging system is the TNM system of the American Joint Committee on Cancer **(Box 2)**. The patient's overall stage is determined by the American Joint Committee on Cancer stage groupings **(Box 3)**.

Box 2: TNM staging for renal cell cancer.

TNM staging (7th edition)

T
- T1
  - *T1a:* Tumor confined to kidney, <4 cm
  - *T1b:* Tumor confined to kidney, >4 cm but <7 cm
- *T2:* Limited to kidney >7 cm
  - *T2a:* Tumor confined to kidney, >7 cm but not >10 cm
  - *T2b:* Tumor confined to kidney, >10 cm
- *T3:* Tumor extension into major veins or perinephric tissues, but not into ipsilateral adrenal gland or beyond Gerota's fascia
  - *T3a:* Tumor grossly extends into the renal vein or its segmental (muscle-containing) branches, or tumor invades perirenal and/or renal sinus fat but not beyond the Gerota fascia
  - *T3b:* Spread to infradiaphragmatic IVC
  - *T3c:* Spread to supradiaphragmatic IVC or invades the wall of the IVC
- *T4:* Involves ipsilateral adrenal gland or invades beyond Gerota's fascia

N
- *N0:* No nodal involvement
- *N1:* Metastatic involvement of regional lymph node(s)

M
- *M0:* No distant metastases
- *M1:* Distant metastases

Box 3: Stage grouping for renal cancer.

- *Stage I:* T1 N0 M0
- *Stage II:* T2 N0 M0
- *Stage III:* T3 or N1 with M0
- *Stage IV:* T4 or M1

The staging and histological grading affects the survival and the therapeutic approach. 5-year survival rates vary from 95% for T1 to 20% for T4.

Tumor stage: Size of the tumor and extent of local extension determine the T stage. Tumor size is critical for staging cancer confined to the kidney **(Figs. 16A and B)**. Tumors limited to the kidney are staged T1 or T2 depending on the size. Tumors are staged T1 when they are <7 cm in size with a further subclassification into *T1a* and *T1b* at a cutoff of 4 cm. Improved survival of patients is seen with tumors measuring <4 cm compared to patients with a tumor size of 4–7 cm. Tumors confined to the kidney, measuring >7 cm are staged as *T2* **(Figs. 17A and B)**.

Stage T3, characterized by extrarenal extension of tumor, an important prognostic factor, is marked by infiltration into perinephric or renal sinus fat and venous infiltration.

Some signs like stranding of perinephric fat, fascial thickening (>3 cm), obliteration/blurring of fat, adrenal involvement, and visible collaterals are considered suggestive for extracapsular spread.

Perinephric stranding and obliteration of fat planes alone cannot be taken as a sign for extrarenal extension as it may result from edema, congestion, and mass effect. The most reliable imaging sign of RCC spread is presence of discrete perinephric mass > 1 cm in diameter **(Figs. 18 and 19)**. Presence of an intact pseudocapsule on MRI has a high accuracy in differentiating T1/T2 from T3a tumor.

Renal cancers can be staged with more than 90% accuracy; however, identification of stage T3a disease can be problematic.[21] Renal sinus fat invasion *(T3a)*, considered the most common site for extrarenal extension

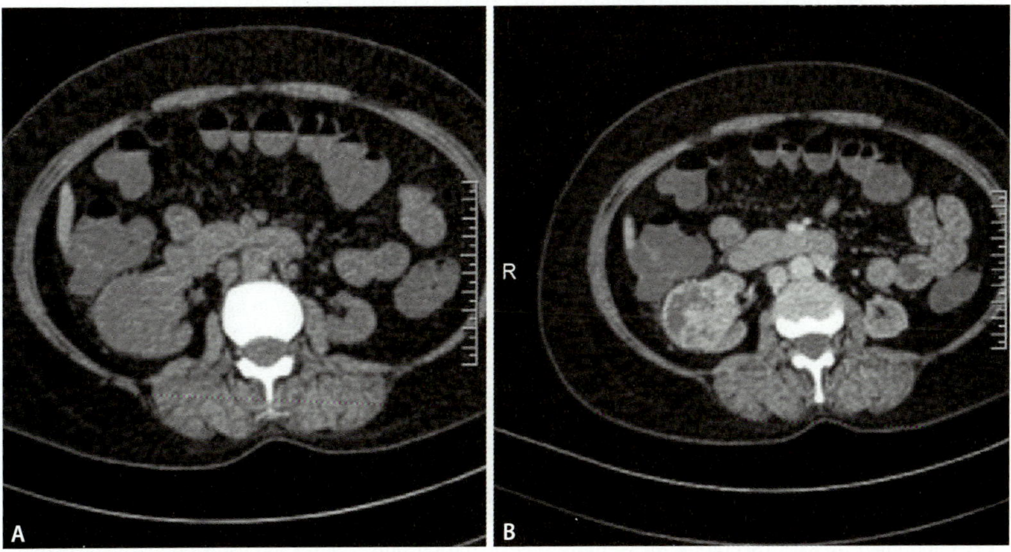

Figs. 16A and B: CT abdomen: (A) Precontrast; and (B) Postcontrast—an enhancing mass limited to the kidney—T1A.

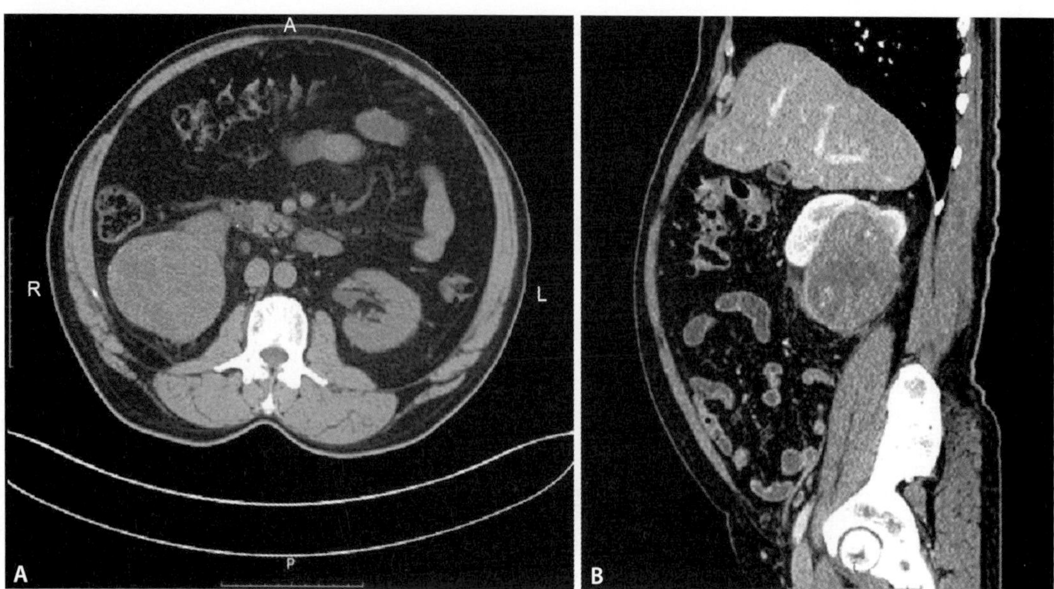

Figs. 17A and B: (A) Noncontrast CT axial; (B) Contrast-enhanced CT sagittal multiplanar reconstruction (MPR)—right renal solid enhancing mass measuring >7 cm, confined within Gerota's fascia. Stage T2.

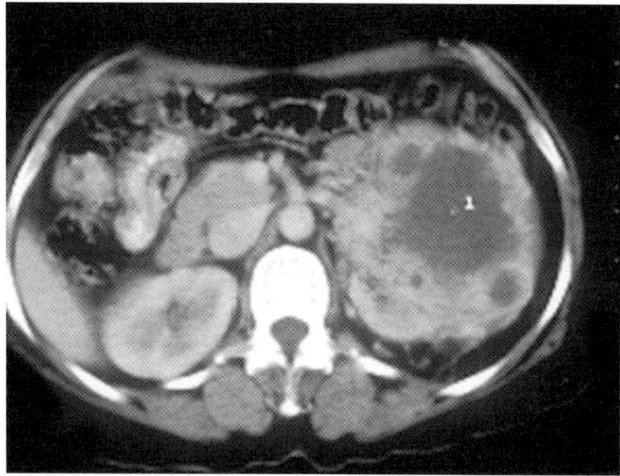

Fig. 18: CT—a large left renal mass with extension into the perinephric space.

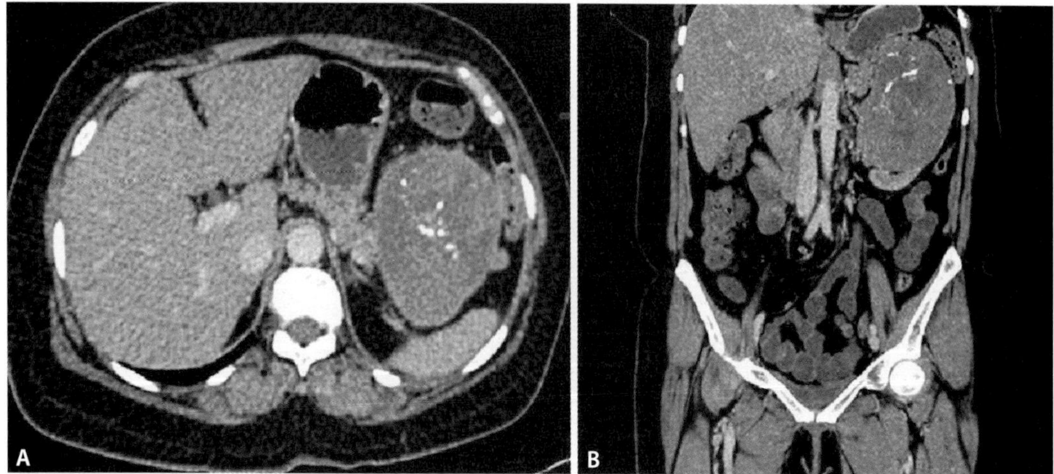

Figs. 19A and B: CECT abdomen: (A) Axial; (B) Coronal MPR—mass >7 cm in the left kidney with a soft tissue nodule in the perinephric region—T3.

of RCC, is also difficult to accurately assess on CT. Presence of renal sinus fat invasion makes nephron-sparing surgery a challenge.

Tumor extension into segmental renal vein or the main renal vein is stage *T3a*. Extension of tumor thrombus into IVC must be looked for, including the cephalad extent of the thrombus **(Figs. 20A to C)**. This has management and prognostic significance with a poorer prognosis associated with supradiaphragmatic extension of IVC thrombus (T3c). Surgical planning for these patients depends on accurate preoperative staging. If tumor extends only into subdiaphragmatic cava, then a flank approach is sufficient. If it extends beyond this, then thoracoabdominal approach has to be followed.

Thrombus can be identified on the venous phase of CT. In cases, where the findings are indeterminate, MRI may be done. Noncontrast MRI has a higher sensitivity and specificity for detecting venous extension than noncontrast CT. It is more sensitive, for IVC wall invasion and to confirm tumor thrombus **(Figs. 21A and B)**. Gradient echo images may detect a low-signal defect within the high signal lumen of IVC. Bland thrombus on MRI shows a uniform signal intensity and lack of enhancement, whereas a tumor thrombus shows intermediate-to-high signal intensity, is heterogeneous and has small vessels, which enhance similar to the renal mass. Artefacts can hamper detection of venous thrombus on MRI. Contrast-enhanced MR venography is highly accurate for the detection of venous thrombus.

Contiguous invasion into adrenal, liver, diaphragm, psoas muscle, pancreas, and bowel denotes advanced *T4* stage. CT has a 100% negative predictive value in detecting contiguous spread into the adrenal gland, positive predictive value is less as it is difficult to differentiate abutment from invasion **(Figs. 22 and 23)**. It has been suggested that only when the adrenal gland is not identified, not displaced or enlarged on CT, adrenal is said to be involved.

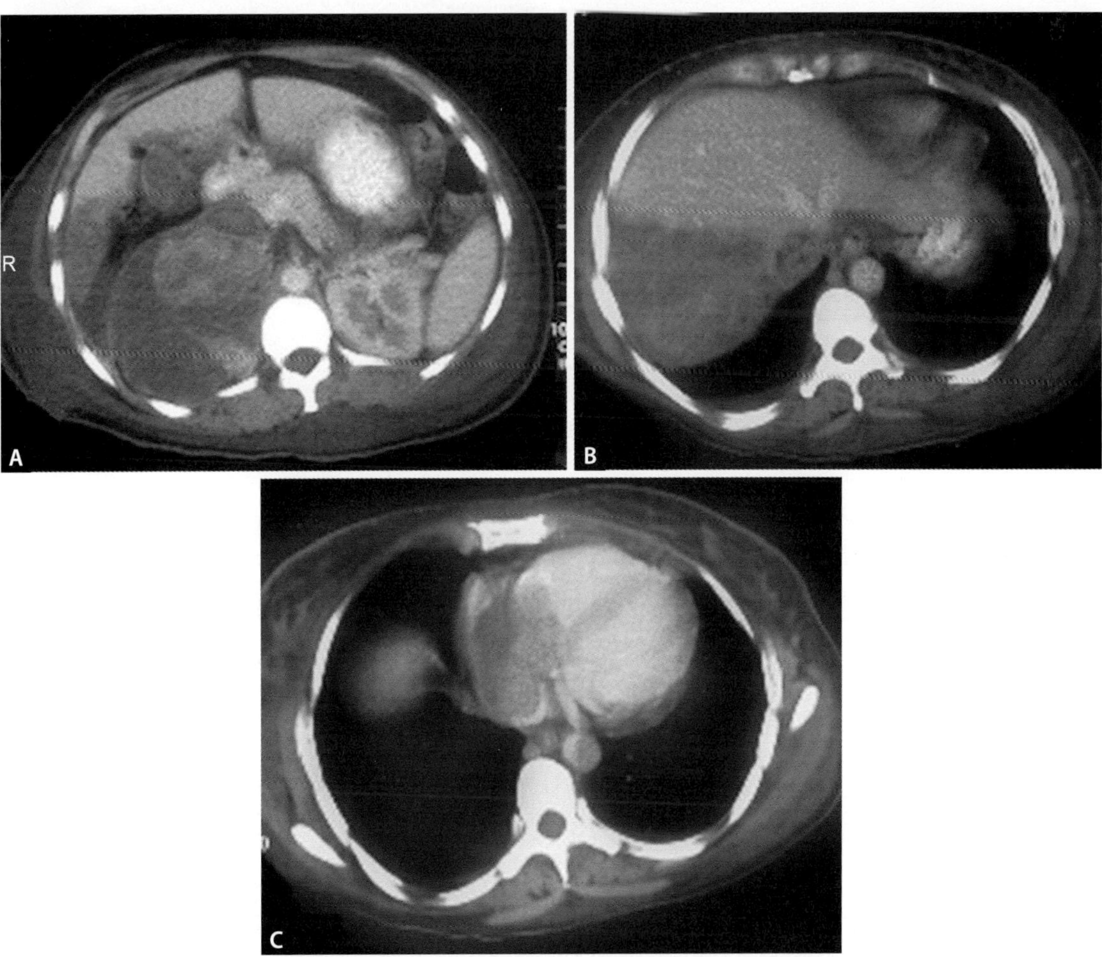

Figs. 20A to C: Renal cell carcinoma—CT shows (A) A complex solid cystic mass with intraluminal filling defect seen in renal vein which is enlarged; (B) A more cephlad section shows the enhancing thrombus within the inferior vena cava and a consequent to this, a perfusion deficit in liver; (C) The thrombus is seen to extend into the right atrium.

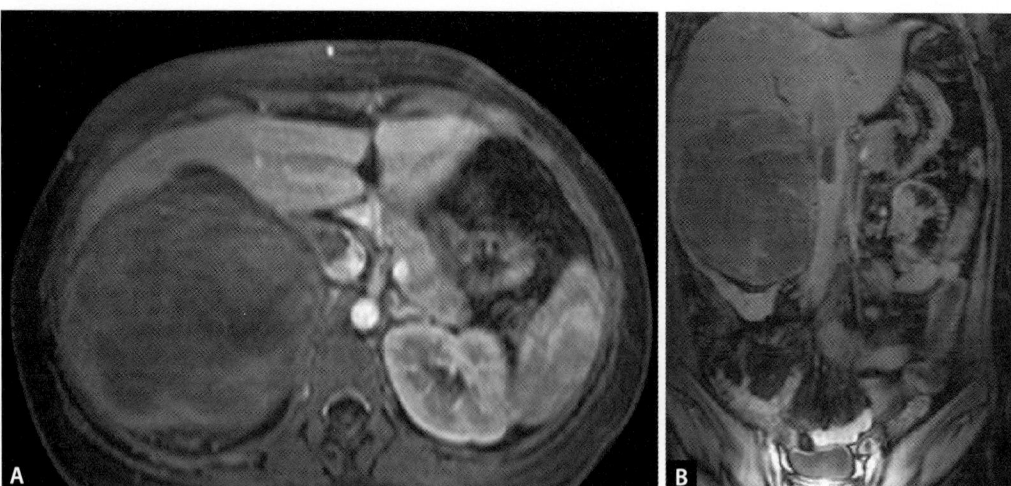

Figs. 21A and B: MRI abdomen postcontrast—right renal mass with venous extension into renal vein and inferior vena cava. The tumor and the thrombus are showing similar enhancement.

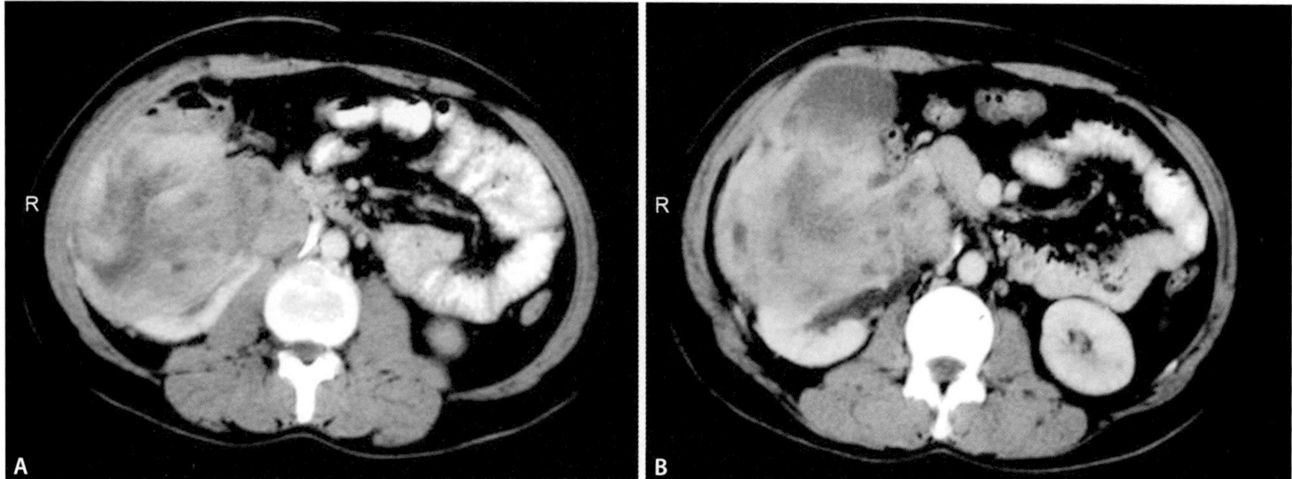

Figs. 22A and B: Contrast-enhanced CT abdomen: Axial—direct infiltration from right renal mass into liver, gallbladder fossa, duodeneum, and colon—stage IV.

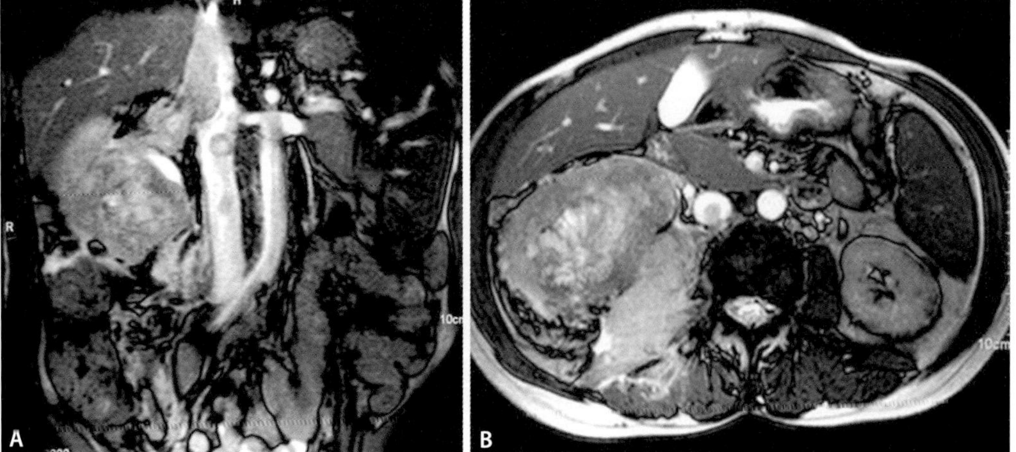

Figs. 23A and B: T2 TRUE FISP: (A) Coronal; (B) Axial—extension of the renal mass into right renal vein which is enlarged and into the IVC. Direct infiltration into the psoas is also noted.

Nodal staging: Lymph node size of >1 cm and disruption of lymph node architecture are criteria for diagnosing nodal metastasis. Based on nodal size criteria alone, MRI and CT are similar in sensitivity and specificity for metastatic adenopathy. False-positive rates of 58% have been reported, however, a size criterion of 1 cm is used, owing to reactive or other benign nodal disease. These false positives are more frequent in patients with tumor involvement of the renal vein and tumor necrosis. Similar to other tumors, nodal staging for RCC by imaging is suboptimal, as up to 50% of enlarged nodes are benign and metastasis in smaller nodes is not detected.

Distant metastases: Stage-IV renal cancer denotes distant metastases or spread to other organs, except the adrenal. Metastatic disease involves lung, liver, bone or brain. RCC <3 cm rarely metastasize. A renal mass may appear to invade the liver or spleen, when it is actually distorting the margin without direct invasion.

Chest radiograph: A *chest radiograph* is essential for the workup of RCC. A *chest CT* can be done if the radiograph is abnormal or the local disease is advanced. RCC is associated with hypervascular liver metastasis; particularly from clear cell RCC. Portal venous phase imaging of *abdominal CT* detects 90% of metastases. Bone metastases are usually lytic. Bone scan is performed only in patients with bone pain or raised alkaline phosphatase. *Bone scan* may be negative as the lytic metastasis produces little osteoblastic reaction. MRI may be more sensitive to CT in detection of unsuspected bony metastasis, because of bone marrow imaging capability.

Positron emission tomography-computed tomography in staging of RCC: There is no established role of PET CT in the initial staging of renal cancer. Due to high background activity of the tracer in kidney, it is difficult to detect primary renal tumor by PET scan alone. PET combined with CT has a sensitivity of 90%. 18F-fluoro-2-deoxy-2-D-glucose (FDG) uptake within a renal mass confirms that solid elements are present. False-positive diagnosis is a problem as benign solid renal masses such as oncocytoma can be FDG avid. PET may be useful in detecting activity in metastatic lesions detected by CT and MRI bone scan.[41] The recommendations for the expert group for staging of renal malignancy is given in **Box 4**.

Box 4: Recommendations for staging renal tumor.

- Contrast-enhanced multiphasic abdomen CT is the modality of choice for staging primary renal tumor. MRI is a suitable substitute when patient cannot undergo CECT abdomen
- If status of renal vein and IVC cannot be determined on CT, then contrast-enhanced multiphasic 3D MR venography can be done
- Computed tomography chest to be done in large or locally advanced tumor to look for pulmonary metastasis. Chest X-ray is sufficient for patients with small tumors
- Brain MRI and bone scan should be done in patients with suspicion of metastatic disease, based on symptoms, laboratory findings or metastasis elsewhere

Treatment of Renal Cell Carcinoma

Renal cell carcinoma is managed surgically. The operative management can be radical nephrectomy or nephron-sparing surgery (partial nephrectomy). The preferred treatment of renal masses measuring 4 cm or less in maximal diameter is now *partial nephrectomy*, and *thermal ablation* in patients who are poor surgical candidates.[42] Imaging assists in planning these treatments with the least possible complications.

There is an alternative management strategy called *"active surveillance"*. This is used in biopsy proven small renal cancers (≤4 cm in size) in elderly patients who are more likely to die with, rather than of their cancer and who have a favorable histological prognosis (low-grade papillary and chromophobe) as assessed by percutaneous biopsy. Active surveillance consists of periodic imaging with no intervention till the size increases or there is rapid growth (>5 mm in 12 months).[43,44]

Renal Mass Scoring

The decision to perform partial nephrectomy was often subjective and required a standardized method to score renal mass complexity. The scoring systems, now most commonly used are nephrometry score and the Padua score.

R.E.N.A.L nephrometry score[45] **(Table 6)** was developed to categorize renal masses into low, intermediate, and high complexity, based on cross-sectional imaging findings. The score helps in decision making, patient counseling, surgical planning, and patient follow-up, as well as for academic reporting. R.E.N.A.L is an acronym for the five components of this system

1. Renal size
2. Exophyticity
3. Nearness to the collecting system or renal sinus
4. Anterior or posterior location
5. Location with respect to the renal poles. This is determined by polar lines drawn on coronal images, at the level where the medial lip of the kidney is interrupted by renal sinus fat **(Figs. 24A to C)**.

Table 6: R.E.N.A.L. nephrometry score.

	1 point	*2 point*	*3 point*
Radius (maximal diameter in cm)	<4	4–7	>7
Exophytic/endophytic properties	≥50%	<50%	Entirely endophytic
Nearness of the tumor to the collecting system or sinus (mm)	≥7	>4 but <7	≤4
Anterior or posterior	No points given. Mass assigned a descriptor of a, p or x		
Location relative to polar lines*	Entirely above the upper line or below the lower line	Lesion crosses polar line	>50% of mass is across polar line (a) or mass crosses the axial renal midline (b) or the mass is entirely between polar lines (c)

*Suffix "h" if mass touches the main renal artery/vein.

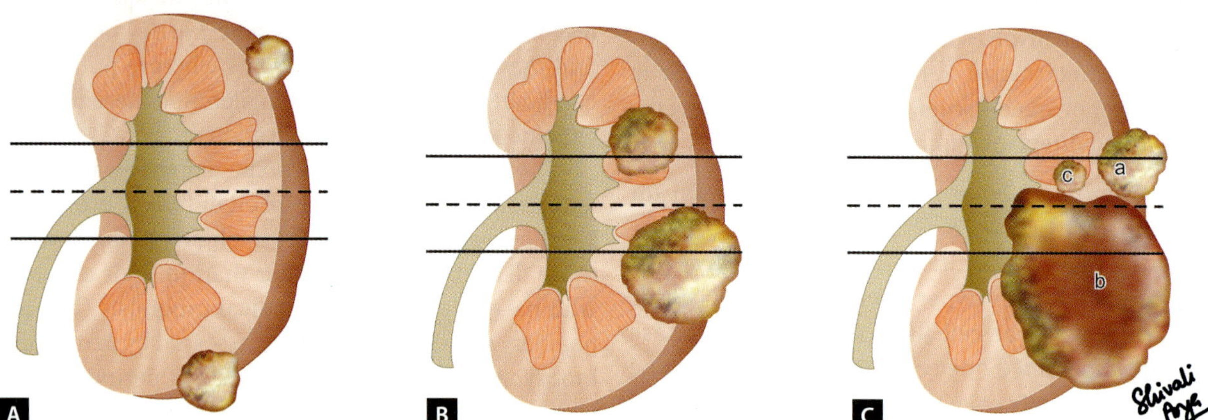

Figs. 24A to C: Polar lines (solid lines) and axial renal midline (dashed lines) are depicted on each coronal view of the kidney. Polar lines are determined in the coronal plane and run through the axial plane. They pass through the point where the medial renal parenchyma touches the renal sinus. Assigning location (L) score. In image (A), L = 1 because masses are above or below polar lines. In image (B), L = 2 because masses cross polar lines. In image (C), L = 3 because mass "a" crosses polar line > 50%; "b" is located between polar lines; and "c" crosses axial midline.

Each component, except location is graded on a scale of 1-3. All scores are summed to give a final nephrometry score.

- Score of 4-6: Low complexity
- Score of 7-9: Moderate complexity
- Score of 10-12: High complexity.

A low score of 4-6 is associated with fewer complications such as postoperative bleed or urinary fistula after partial nephrectomy. In addition to greater postsurgical complications, a higher nephrometry score of 12-14 has been shown to correlate with pathological stage and grade.

Another system to assess renal masses prior to surgery is the *PADUA classification,*[46] which is also an acronym for Preoperative Aspects and Dimensions Used for Anatomical classification. In this system, nearness to the collecting system and to renal sinus is assessed separately. The polar location of the mass is determined by drawing a renal sinus line at the first (upper pole) and the last (lower pole) axial level where pericollecting system fat is seen entirely within the kidney.

Box 5: Imaging protocol for follow-up of treated RCC.

- *For low-risk/T1 tumors*:
  - Chest imaging: Every 12 to 24 months for 3–5 years
  - Abdominal imaging: Baseline between 3 months and 12 months, especially after partial nephrectomy, then yearly for 3–5 years
- *For intermediate-risk/T2 primary tumors*:
  - Chest and abdominal imaging-baseline study at 3 months, then at 6 and 12 months, followed by every 6–24 months for 5 years
- *For high-risk/T3 tumors*:
  - Chest and abdominal imaging: Baseline study at 3 months, then at 6 and 12 months, followed by every 6–12 months for 5 years

Imaging Post-treatment

The imaging protocol for follow up of treated RCCs is given in **Box 5**.

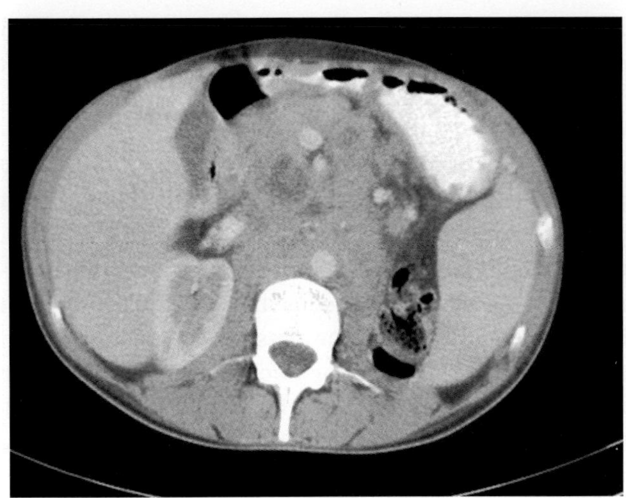

Fig. 25: CT abdomen in a postoperative case of renal cell carcinoma, presenting 1 year later with metastatic retroperitoneal lymphadenopathy.

Post-total/partial nephrectomy: In the imaging follow-up of patients after surgical excision of RCC, CT abdomen with IV contrast, CT abdomen without and with IV contrast are recommended as equivalent alternatives for imaging. The use of MRI of abdomen and pelvis with and without IV contrast as alternative in this scenario may be appropriate, but is controversial. There is a renal parenchymal defect along with some soft tissue changes and surgical staples postpartial nephrectomy. Hemostatic packing material may look like fluid collection or residual masses gradual decrease in size will be noted, if it is normal postoperative appearance. Recurrent tumor is identified as an enhancing soft tissue nodule/mass[47] **(Fig. 25)**.

Post-thermal ablation: In the imaging follow-up of patients after localized RCC ablation, CT abdomen with IV contrast/CT abdomen without and with IV contrast/MRI of abdomen, and pelvis without and with IV contrast are recommended as equivalent alternatives (i.e. only one of the above procedures to be ordered).

The ablation bed may initially be significantly larger in size than the initial mass. It may take 1–2 years to decrease in size. Increased perinephric stranding with invagination of perinephric fat into the defect may be seen normally. The appearance may mimic an angiomyolipoma. A thin-enhancing rim may be seen 2–6 weeks following ablation. An enlarging ablation bed should be considered as a sign of recurrent disease.[48] Persistent areas of enhancement, especially nodular or crescentic in appearance, seen at the interface with normal renal parenchyma signifies residual/recurrent tumor. Certain procedural complications, though rare, may be seen on follow-up imaging such as hematomas, pseudoaneurysms and chyluria.

Postchemotherapy: Patients with metastasis are treated with chemotherapeutic agents like multikinase inhibitors. These produce tumor necrosis as a marker of response without decrease in size. These patients have to be evaluated for changes in enhancement along with change in size on follow-up imaging.

Active surveillance: Active surveillance is reserved for patients with these small renal masses who are poor surgical candidates due to comorbidities or are not willing for surgery. The American Urological Association (AUA) and National Comprehensive Cancer Network (NCCN) recommend CT/MR of the abdomen CT/MR within 6 months of start of surveillance followed by imaging annually till patient is on watch.[49] In the imaging follow-up of patients who are on active surveillance of localized RCC, CT abdomen with IV contrast/CT abdomen without and with IV contrast/MRI of abdomen and pelvis without and with IV contrast/ultrasound abdomen with IV contrast are recommended as equivalent alternatives. Size has to be carefully monitored with an average growth of 0.3 cm/year. A higher growth rate is associated with unfavorable outcome.

Screening for Kidney Cancer

There are no guidelines for RCC screening in general population due to lack of a large randomized controlled trial for renal cancer screening.[50] Patients with genetic predisposition to RCC require surveillance, starting at an early age based on the syndrome. Certain syndromes like hereditary leiomyomatosis and RCC (HLRCC) require surveillance to begin at an early age, as tumors are aggressive with metastatic potential. Patients with Birt–Hogg–Dubé syndrome and von Hippel–Lindau syndrome are recommended to undergo annual or biannual surveillance, starting at 20 years of age with tumors more than 3 cm being treated. In hereditary papillary RCC, tumors develop in sixth decades onward and are slow growing, hence there is no screening protocol for these patients.

Oncocytoma

Renal oncocytoma is the most common benign, solid, nonfat-containing renal mass. It is a benign renal epithelial tumor, arising from intercalated cells of proximal tubule with many characteristics of RCCs. Oncocytomas are histologically composed of large cells (oncocytes) with mitochondria rich cytoplasm. The appearance of a typical oncocytoma cannot be reliably differentiated from RCC.[51]

Most oncocytomas are asymptomatic (80%), but few may present with hematuria, pain, or mass. The peak age of incidence is in the seventh decade with a male preponderance. The incidence of oncocytomas is higher in incidentally discovered renal masses, as compared with patients who have urinary symptoms. They may be quite large at time of presentation. Oncocytoma appears as a well demarcated, unencapsulated, fairly homogeneous renal cortical tumors.

In 10% of oncocytomas, there can be a coexistent RCC, as an incidental microscopic finding or as a hybrid tumor. Oncocytomas are multifocal in 2.5–16% and bilateral in 4–12% of cases. Multifocality can be sporadic or syndromic in Birt–Hogg–Dubé syndrome and renal oncocytosis (renal parenchyma is replaced by multiple oncocytomas, hybrid tumors, and chromophobe RCCs).[52,53]

On *ultrasound*, renal oncocytomas appear as solitary hypoechoic or isoechoic masses originating from the renal cortex with a well-defined margin. On *color Doppler imaging* blood flow signals are seen in the periphery and strip-like flow signals within the mass. Contrast-enhanced sonography, shows early enhancement, hyperenhancement, and fast washout compared to the adjacent renal cortex. Irregular nonenhanced areas may be seen within the central area corresponding to area of central fibrous scar, which may be echogenic.

On *CT*, they are solid, well-marginated tumors, slightly hypodense to renal parenchyma on unenhanced images. Some may exhibit a central low attenuation scar with a branched appearance **(Fig. 26)**. However, central necrosis with RCC may mimic this. Invasion into perinephric fat occurs is 11%. There is usually no adenopathy or vascular invasion. Various patterns of enhancement have been described for oncocytomas. Segmental enhancement inversion is considered a hallmark of small (<4 cm) oncocytomas. There are two distinct zones of enhancement, which show different pattern on CM and excretory phase (EP). The zone that is hyperenhancing on CM phase becomes hypoenhancing on EP and vice versa[54-56]. Other authors found that an early heterogeneous enhancement becoming homogeneous in delayed phase is seen in small oncocytomas. The presence of a central scar, absence of calcification or necrosis and hemorrhage suggests the diagnosis, though there is no specific CT finding to differentiate oncocytoma from RCC. Surgery is usually performed for these. The MRI appearance is of a hypo- to isointense (22%) mass on T1W images with high signal on T2WI, enhancing homogeneously after IV gadolinium. It may exhibit spoke-wheel pattern of enhancement. The central scar is T1 hypointense and T2 hyperintense with delayed enhancement. A spoke-wheel pattern of feeding arteries associated with a homogeneous nephrogram is a characteristic finding on catheter angiography.

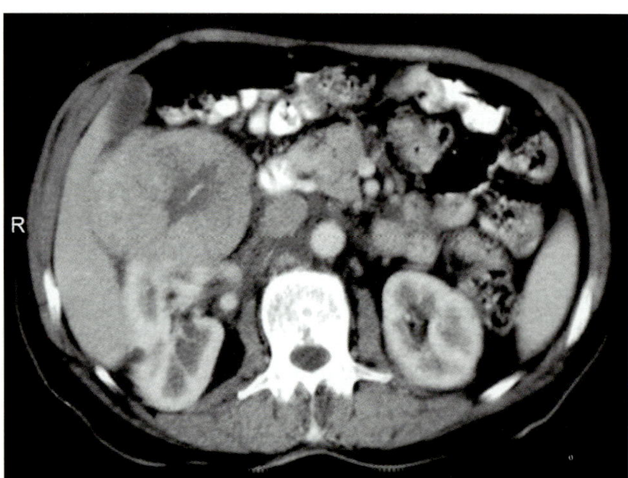

Fig. 26: CT—well-defined, homogeneously enhancing mass right renal with a central scar—oncocytoma.

METANEPHRIC TUMORS

Renal Adenomas

Papillary adenomas are the most common renal epithelial neoplasm. According to some authors, renal adenoma is an earlier stage of evolution of renal cell carcinoma. By definition, papillary adenomas measure 5 mm or less. According to an autopsy series, approximately 40% of patients above the age of 70 harbor a renal adenoma. Papillary adenomas are also found in patients with acquired renal cystic disease and in those undergoing long-term hemodialysis. They usually occur as cortical subcapsular tumors less than 1 cm and are indistinguishable from RCCs. *Metanephric adenoma* is a benign neoplasm with a peak age in 5–6th decade. Polycythemia, a characteristic finding, is seen in 10% and disappears after surgery. Metanephric adenoma typically occurs as a well-defined, unencapsulated, solitary solid mass. Metanephric adenomas display hypovascularity and delayed, minimal enhancement.

MIXED EPITHELIAL AND STROMAL TUMORS

Cystic nephroma, mixed epithelial and stromal tumors belong to this subgroup of tumors.[57] They are seen almost exclusively in perimenopausal women, most patients receiving estrogen therapy. They usually present incidentally and are believed to be a hormonally dependent tumor. Mixed epithelial and stromal tumors (MESTs) are characterized by variegated imaging patterns including complex cysts and mixed solid cystic masses that show delayed and heterogeneous enhancement. On MR imaging, the degree of delayed enhancement and T2 hypointense signal is dependent on the amount of stromal component.

MESENCHYMAL TUMORS

Mesenchymal tumors constitute a wide spectrum of tumors with variable histology and imaging findings. Benign mesenchymal tumors include angiomyolipoma (AML), leiomyoma, lymphangioma, hemangioma, lipoma, etc. Malignant mesenchymal tumors include leiomyosarcoma, rhabdomyosarcoma, angiosarcoma, and osteosarcoma. Some mesenchymal tumors like AML, lipoma, and hemangioma may be diagnosed on imaging. Percutaneous biopsy is usually required for the diagnosis of mesenchymal tumors and to rule out RCC.

Mesenchymal renal tumors can be classified, based on the predominant tissue type **(Box 6)** or on the pattern of distribution[58] **(Box 7)**.

Box 6: Mesenchymal tumors based on tissue type.

- *Soft tissue mass:*
  - Fat-poor AML
  - Leiomyoma
  - Hemangioma
  - Schwannoma
  - Juxtaglomerular cell tumor
  - Medullary fibroma
  - Solitary fibrous renal tumor
  - Leiomyosarcoma
  - Synovial sarcoma
  - Osteosarcoma
- *Fat-containing:*
  - Classic angiomyolipoma
  - Lipoma
- *Cystic mass:*
  - Lymphangioma
- *Calcified mass:*
  - Hemangioma
  - Osteosarcoma

Box 7: Distribution of mesenchymal tumors.

- *Capsular distribution:*
  - Leiomyoma
  - Lymphangioma
  - Solitary fibrous tumor
  - Leiomyosarcoma
  - Angiosarcoma
- *Cortical distribution:*
  - Angiomyolipoma
  - Schwannoma
  - Synovial sarcoma
- *Medullary distribution:*
  - Angiomyolipoma
  - Hemangioma
- *Renal sinus distribution:*
  - Leiomyoma
  - Hemangioma
  - Lymphangioma

Angiomyolipoma

Angiomyolipoma is the most common solid benign tumor. These lesions are mesenchymal neoplasms (previously considered as hamartomas), representing excess growth of mature fat, smooth muscle and thick-walled blood vessels, the amount of each component being variable.

Angiomyolipomas are now considered to be a heterogeneous group of tumors with different imaging features, histology, and are grouped under a family of tumors characterized by the proliferation of perivascular epithelioid cells (PEComas).[59] Usually benign, a rare potentially malignant variant called epithelioid angiomyolipoma is listed separately in the WHO classification of renal tumors.

They are usually seen in women between 40 and 60 years of age. The majority being sporadic, 20% are associated with tuberous sclerosis (TS). Angiomyolipomas may rarely be associated with NF-I, Von Hippel-Lindau disease or ADPKD. TS-associated AMLs are seen in asymptomatic, young patients without sex predilection. AMLs associated with TS are often multiple, bilateral, and larger at the time of presentation. These are also likely to grow and be symptomatic. As the tumor grows, there is vessel dilatation and pseudoaneurysm formation. Tumors greater than 4 cm have an increased risk of hemorrhage (Wunderlich syndrome), potentially life-threatening and need to be prophylactically managed.

Angiomyolipoma may originate from the cortex or the medulla. The tumor is usually well defined and appears as large, heterogeneous mass with varying amount of macroscopic fat, intralesional aneurysms, and hypervascular soft tissue. As angiomyolipomas are composed of thick-walled inelastic blood vessels, the risk of intratumoral and perinephric hemorrhage is higher in lesions > 4 cm diameter.

Classification of AML: There are two classifications of AML. One is based on clinical and imaging features, histological grade, and genetic features, while the second is based purely on CT and MRI features. Jinzaki et al.[60] classified AML on the basis of clinical and imaging features, histological grade, and genetic features.

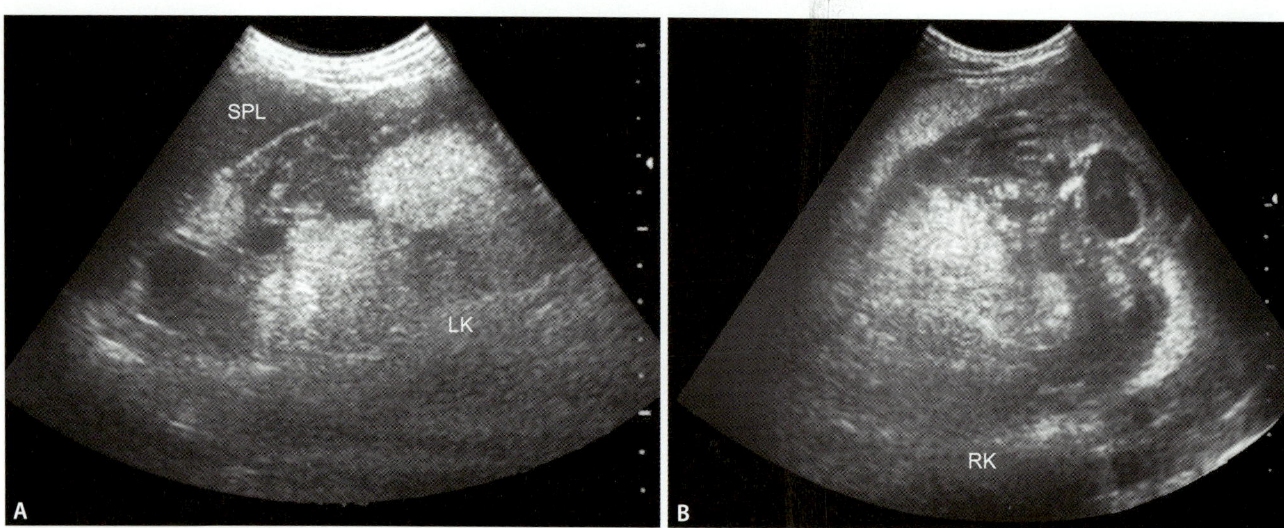

Figs. 27A and B: Ultrasound of the upper abdomen depicts multiple well-defined homogeneously hyperechoic lesions with no perilesional halo in both kidneys, suggestive of angiomyolipomas (AML).

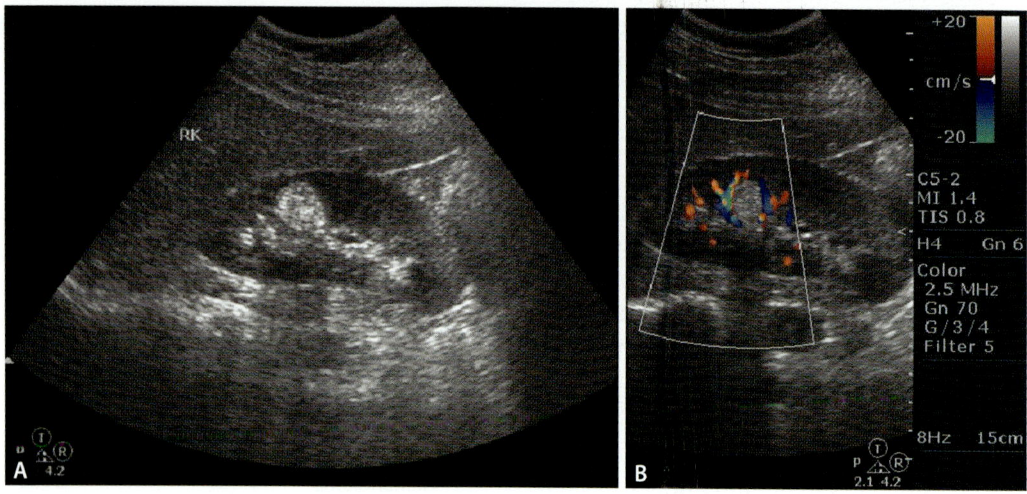

Figs. 28A and B: Ultrasound of the upper abdomen shows: (A) Well-defined rounded hyperechoic lesion; (B) In the right kidney with peripheral vascularity on color Doppler.

Triphasic AML is a benign mesenchymal tumor consisting of three components in varying proportion—dysmorphic blood vessels, smooth muscle, and mature fat.

This is further subdivided radiologically into classic and fat-poor varieties.

Classic Angiomyolipomas

They are characterized by abundant fat and are easily diagnosed by imaging. Classical AML appears as a hyperechoic circumscribed mass (more echogenic than central fat) on ultrasound **(Figs. 27 and 28)**. 32% of renal carcinomas are also highly reflective, although there are other pointers toward RCC such as hyporeflective rim or focal small spotty areas (intratumoural cysts) of reduced central reflectivity. Another feature that helps in distinguishing an AML from a small RCC, is posterior shadowing, seen in approximately 30% of AML, but is not seen in small hyperreflective renal carcinomas.

Computed tomography is the most accurate imaging technique for detection and characterization of classic angiomyolipomas. The lesions show low attenuation, typically less than 10 HU and presence of gross fat being a typical finding[61] **(Figs. 29 to 31)**. Thin slices are necessary to demonstrate fat in small AMLs because of volume averaging. Higher specificity may be obtained with threshold measurements of –15 to –30 HU. The fat may be interposed with solid components. A subset of lesions will not meet fat attenuation criteria due to volume averaging or hemorrhage, others are fat-poor, and rarely, a well-differentiated RCC can mimic this appearance.

Computed tomography pixel mapping, over a region of interest within the tumor may be useful to detect small quantities of fat. With pixel mapping, three to six contiguous pixels with negative Hounsfield units averaging below -20 HU indicates intratumoral fat.[62] AMLs are usually well-marginated, but do not have a true capsule, the lesion is usually at the margin of the kidney and may expand beyond as a small hypodense wedge-shaped defect in the renal parenchyma. This wedge-shaped defect is diagnostic of angiomyolipoma. These lesions are vascular, large vessels may be identified. Intratumoral aneurysms may be present and AMLs exhibit moderate enhancement after IV contrast. Homogeneous and prolonged enhancement is a valuable predictor for differentiating AML with minimal fat from RCC.

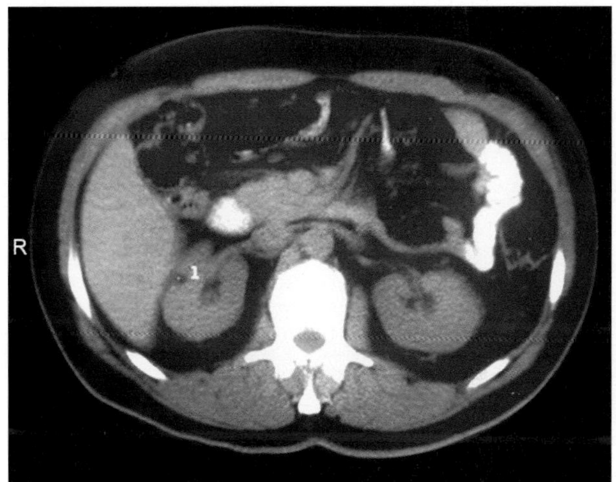

Fig. 29: CT shows a small pinhead lesion in right kidney with fat attenuation S/o angiomyolipomas (AML).

Angiomyolipomas may have to be differentiated from a perirenal/capsular liposarcoma. Pathological differentiation between a well-differentiated liposarcoma from an angiomyolipoma may be difficult, unless radiological appearance is considered. Liposarcomas are rare, seen in older patients, are large at time of diagnosis, and are centered at perinephric space or capsule rather than intraparenchymal like AML. A renal origin of the mass seen as beak sign, presence of enlarged vessels, aneurysms, and perinephric hematoma favor a diagnosis of AML. Liposarcomas are hypovascular, without enlarged vessels and aneurysms. The renal parenchyma defect in AML as stated earlier is not seen in well-differentiated liposarcomas, which will displace, compress, and distorts the kidney, but will not invade renal parenchyma **(Figs. 32 and 33)**. Rarely RCC also contains fat, either engulfing the sinus or perinephric fat or due to metaplasia. In the latter case, presence of calcification, which is not seen in AML favors the diagnosis of RCC.[63,64]

On *MRI,* fat component of an angiomyolipoma can be detected by *Frequency-selective (FS) fat suppression technique* and *chemical shift imaging.*

Classical AMLs have a characteristic high T1 signal and fat-saturated images exhibit a drop in signal. Chemical shift imaging helps to detect small quantities of bulk fat. In classic AML, a characteristic *India ink artefact* is seen at the interface between the mass and the normal renal parenchyma on opposed phase T1 images, whereas the central part of the lesion does not demonstrate changes in signal intensity compared with in-phase images **(Figs. 34A to F)**. This

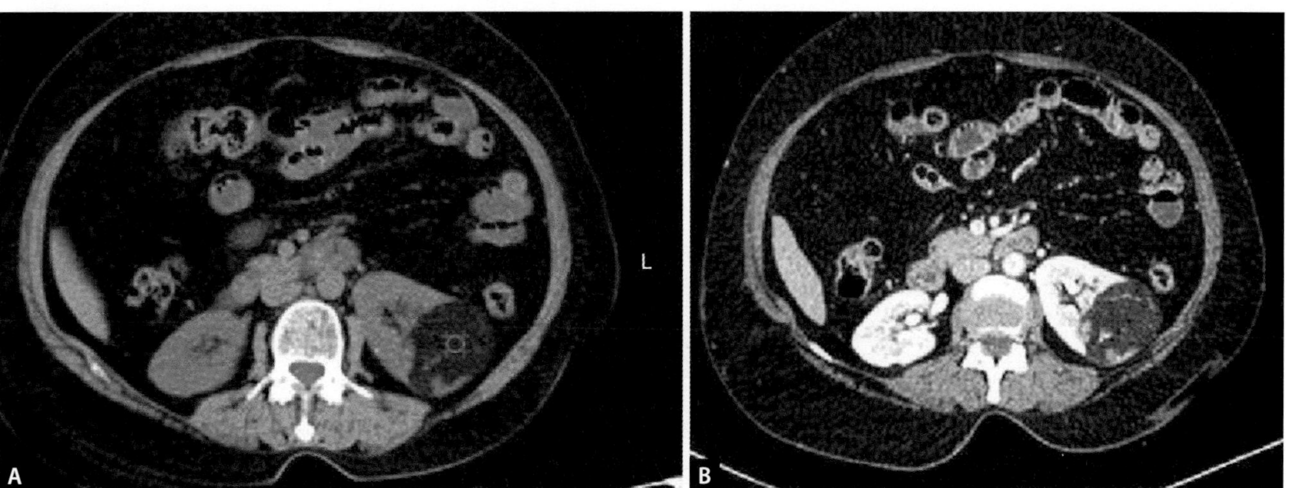

Figs. 30A and B: (A) Noncontrast CT; (B) Contrast-enhanced CT—mass with macroscopic fat and enhancing vessels in the left kidney—angiomyolipoma.

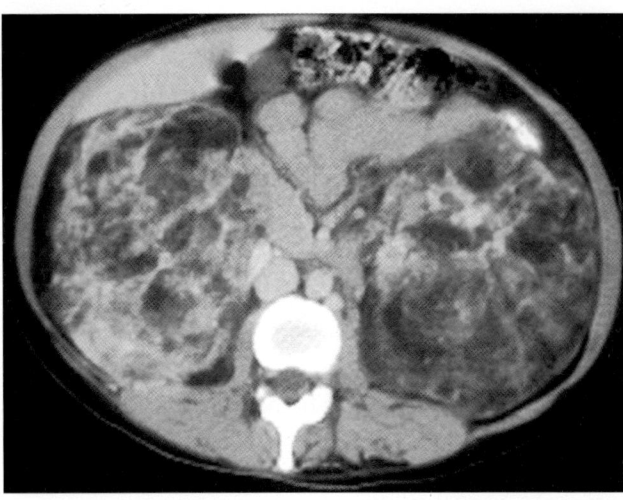

Fig. 31: CT showing bilateral large fat attenuation lesions with enhancing soft tissues —angiomyolipoma.

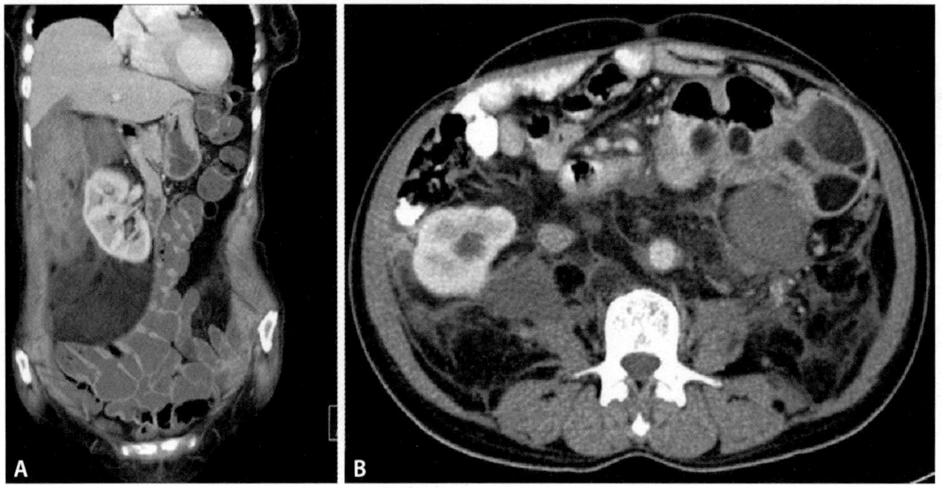

Figs. 32A and B: Contrast-enhanced CT abdomen: (A) Coronal MPR; (B) Axial shows a large fat-containing mass surrounding and displacing the right kidney and extending into left renal fossa—perirenal liposarcoma.

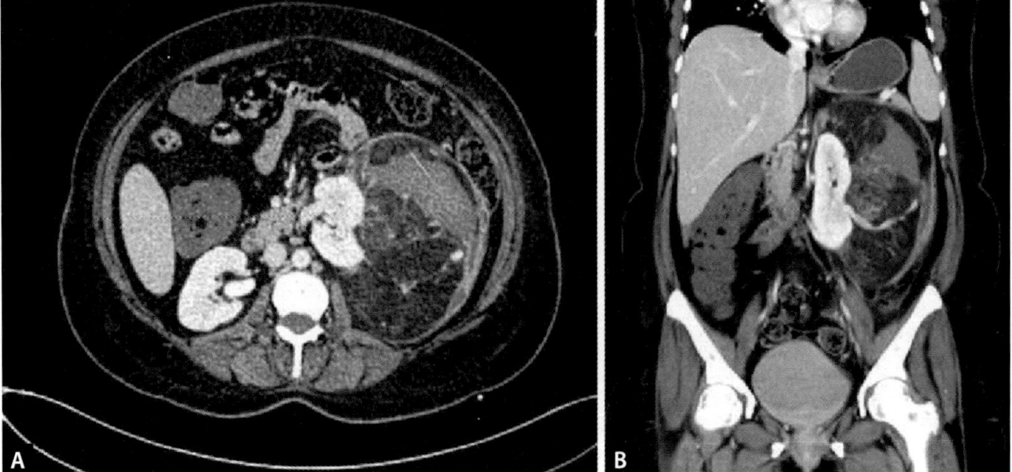

Figs. 33A and B: Contrast-enhanced CT abdomen: (A) Axial; (B) Coronal reformat—shows a large fat-containing mass in relation to the left kidney with a wedge-shaped defect and a vessel seen within the mass—renal angiomyolipoma.

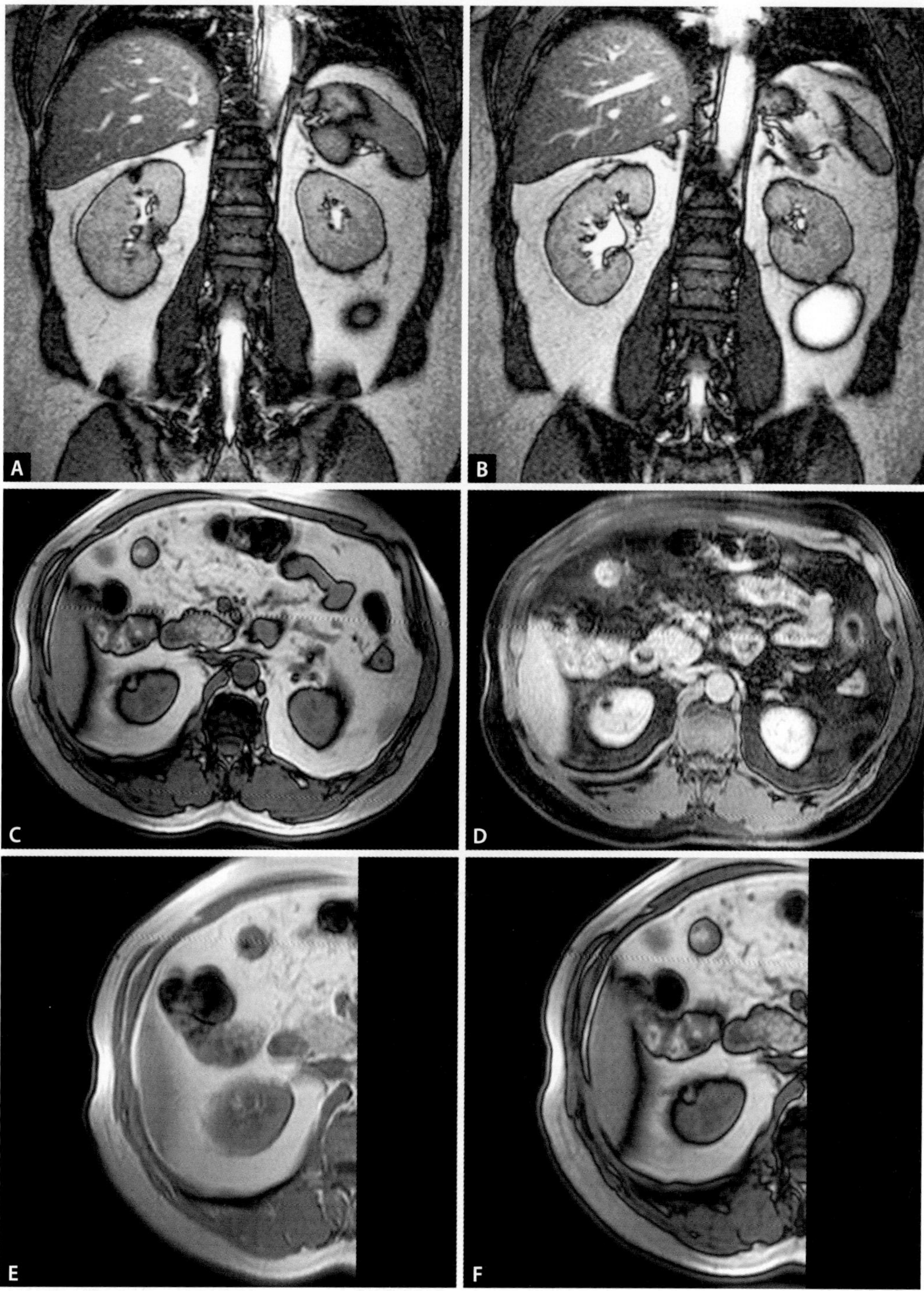

Figs. 34A to F: (A and B) MRI coronal TRUFISP; (C) T1 axial; (D) T1 axial fat suppressed; (E) T1 axial in phase; (F)T1 axial opposed phase. A small hyperintense lesion in right kidney with signal suppression on fat-saturated image. On opposed phase image, there is a signal drop when compared with in-phase image. An India ink artifact is also noted at lesion parenchyma interface—angiomyolipoma.

is useful in very small lesions, where direct comparison with T1 images, with and without fat suppression may be difficult. The appearance of AML on T2-weighted images is variable and depends on bulk fat present in the lesion. An AML composed of predominantly fat would demonstrate homogeneous high signal at T2 images.

Angiography may demonstrate multiple aneurysms and onion layer appearances.

Fat-poor Angiomyolipoma (Minimal-fat AML and Lipid-poor AML)

These lesions, by definition, do not reveal fat on unenhanced CT, even on thin sections. Pathologically they are defined as containing no more than 25% fat cells per high-power field. Fat-poor AML are further divided into three subtypes based on the amount of fat cells and the distribution of the same in the mass:

1. Hyperattenuating
2. Isoattenuating
3. Epithelial cysts.

Hyperattenuating angiomyolipoma: Usually small, they contain only 3-10% fat cells.[65] The predominant component is smooth muscle making them appear hyperdense to renal parenchyma on CT and isoechoic on ultrasound. Homogeneous enhancement is seen. On MRI, they are T1 hypointense and show no bulk fat. When a voxel contains cells with no fat or only intracytoplasmic fat, frequency-selective fat suppression will not detect fat.

Isoattenuating angiomyolipoma: These have CT attenuation between –10 and 45 HU, with diffuse scattered fat cells and appear isodense on noncontrast CT and mildly hyperechoic on ultrasound. They are typically T2 hypointense and show suppression on chemical shift imaging. There is no specific feature to differentiate them from RCC.

Fat-poor angiomyolipoma or renal cell cancer?

This continues to be a diagnostic challenge. Fat-poor AMLs are usually T2 hypointense, a feature that is not seen in clear cell RCC, but seen in papillary subtype of RCC. Chemical suppression cannot be used to differentiate small amounts of fat in AML from cells containing intracytoplasmic fat in ccRCC. AMLs have similar ADC as RCCs and this cannot be used as a point of differentiation. It has been suggested that T2 hypointensity and early enhancement with subsequent washout can be used as a marker for fat-poor AML, though in clinical practice, biopsy is indicated.[66] Certain points of differentiation are enumerated in **Table 7**.

Angiomyolipoma with epithelial cysts: This is an extremely rare subtype of AML, which contains epithelial-lined cysts.[67] These are benign lesions and are more common in women. Imaging features include a cystic component and noncystic-enhancing component. The differential diagnoses are other multilocular cystic masses such as multilocular RCC, cystic nephroma, and mixed epithelial and stromal tumor-MEST. Percutaneous biopsy may be helpful, as AML with epithelial cells and MEST stain positive for Desmin or Actin, while RCC does not.

Table 7: Minimal-fat AML vs RCC.

Minimal-fat AML	*RCC*
Lower attenuation	Higher CT number
Calcification, necrosis rare	Calcification and necrosis common
Well-defined margins	Ill-defined margins
Renal vein/IVC invasion rare	Venous involvement common
Arterial/delay enhancement ratio*>1.5	<1.5
Arterial/delay enhancement ratio* = SI (arterial-precontrast)/SI (delayed-precontrast)	

Table 8: Differences between sporadic and syndromic AML.

Sporadic AML	*Syndromic AML*
Solitary	Multiple
Unilateral	Bilateral
Female predominance (4:1)	M = F
Older	Younger
Smaller lesions	Larger lesion

Epithelioid angiomyolipoma: First described in 1997, this is an extremely rare tumor, which is potentially malignant, locally aggressive, and can metastasize.[68,69] Pathologically, these are composed of numerous atypical epithelioid muscle cells and few or no fat cells. These are large masses with intratumoral hemorrhage and necrosis, with small foci of fat. Hyperattenuating on CT and T2 hypointense, they may present as enhancing solid or multilocular cystic masses.

Angiomyolipoma in tuberous sclerosis complex: There is a strong association between angiomyolipoma and tuberous sclerosis. Most are the classical variety, though fat-poor AMLs are also seen. AMLs associated with TSC are usually bilateral, large with an increased rate of growth (1.25 cm/year), compared to the sporadic variety (0.19 cm/year).[70] Treatment is required in patients of angiomyolipomas with TSC. Recurrent bleeding in syndromic AML is also a notable feature. Transcatheter embolization is the preferred treatment. Patients with bilateral AMLs should be evaluated for TSC. The differences between sporadic and syndromic AML are listed in **Table 8**.

Angiomyolipoma in lymphangioleiomyomatosis: A disease seen predominantly in young females, rarely in males and children, *angiomyolipoma in lymphangioleiomyomatosis (LAM)* is characterized by cystic changes in lung and

Table 9: Differentiating features of subtypes of AML.

Imaging features	*Fat-rich AML*	*Fat-poor AML*	*Fat-invisible AML*
Ultrasound appearance	Hyperechoic	Intermediate	Isoechoic
CT attenuation ≤ 10 HU	Present	Absent	Absent
MRI tumor to spleen ratio <0.71/ Signal intensity index >16.5%	Present	Present	Absent
Lesion management	Observation	Undetermined	Biopsy

other multisystem manifestations like renal AMLs, abdominal lymphadenopathy, chylous ascites, and cystic lymphatic masses. This disease occurs sporadically or in association with TSC. In sporadic LAM, the incidence of AML is almost 50%. The European Respiratory Society recommends screening of patients with unilateral AML, no clinical features of TSC or respiratory system to be screened for LAM.[71]

In the second *classification* based purely on CT and MRI features, Song et al. have classified AML into *fat-rich, fat-poor, and fat-invisible AML* using quantitative values.[72] Fat-rich AML is a lesion with CT attenuation of ≤–10 HU. Fat-poor AML has CT attenuation >–10 HU, tumor to spleen ratio < 0.71, or a signal intensity index > 16.5%. Fat-invisible AML is defined as a lesion with CT attenuation >–10 HU, tumor to spleen ratio ≥ 0.71 and a signal intensity index of 16.5% or less **(Table 9)**.

Management of Angiomyolipoma

Conservative management is indicated for classic AMLs. Annual follow-up is recommended for asymptomatic lesions < 4 cm. For larger lesions, due to risk of hemorrhage, semiannual evaluation is suggested. Approximately 58–75% of these lesions grow with time, though a slow growth rate is seen. Growth of an isolated AML without TS is less than of those with TS and multiple lesions. For patients with larger tumors, treatment is recommended due to potential of bleeding, an intralesional aneurysm >5 mm is likely to bleed.[73] Renal artery embolization and partial nephrectomy are the treatment options available **(Box 8)**.

Box 8: Management of AML.

Indications for treatment of AML:
- Hemorrhage/pain/mass effect
- Most important predictor for hemorrhage—tumor size

Treatment of symptomatic AML:
(Irrespective of size)
- Angiogram
- Selective TCE/enucleation/partial nephrectomy

Management of asymptomatic AML:
≥4 cm—6 monthly CT/USG
<4 cm—12 monthly CT/USG.

Leiomyosarcoma

It is an aggressive and rapidly growing tumor, which accounts for 50–60% of all renal sarcomas. Leiomyosarcoma may arise from the renal capsule, renal parenchyma, smooth muscle of the renal pelvis, or the renal vein. On CT, it appears as a large expansile heterogeneous solid mass with areas of necrosis and enhancement. It may rarely appear as a multilocular cystic mass. Leiomyosarcoma that arises from the renal capsule may envelop the entire kidney, whereas that with a parenchymal origin may replace a large part of the parenchyma and extend into perinephric fat or renal sinus. Venous extension of the tumor like RCC is also seen. On MRI, it appears T1 and T2 hypointense due to the fibrous component.

UROTHELIAL TUMOR

Transitional Cell Carcinoma

Urothelial tumors are less common in the upper urinary tract than renal cell carcinoma. However, transitional cell carcinoma (TCC) is the second most common renal neoplasm in adults. It is most common in urinary bladder, followed in frequency by ureter and the renal pelvis. They may be bilateral in 10% and multicentric in 20–44% of cases. This known multifocality warrants that the entire collecting system must be evaluated in patients with upper tract TCC because of high prevalence of an associated tumor in the lower tract.

The risk factors for TCC include nonsteroidal anti-inflammatory drug (NSAID) abuse, tobacco use or some occupational exposure. The incidence of TCC is more common is males, in the seventh decade. They commonly present with hematuria and flank pain. Hematogenous spread is less common than RCC, but lymphatic spread occurs earlier. High-grade tumors are more common in upper tract than the urinary bladder. It has been suggested that the stage rather than tumor grade is the main prognostic factor for urothelial tumor of the upper tract.

Intravenous Urography

Intravenous urography (IVU) has traditionally been used for imaging a suspected TCC before the advent of CT urography. The findings include a filling defect outlined by excreted contrast. The filling defect may be in pelvis (35%) or calyces (26%). "Stipple sign" may be seen due to trapping of contrast in the interstices of a papillary growth. There may be obstruction of kidney with nonopacification of the collecting system (phantom calyces) due to extensive areas of parenchymal infiltration. Calyces may be amputated or obliterated due to malignant infundibular stricturing. Calyces may be distended with tumor called as "oncocalcyces".

None of the signs on IVU are pathognomonic and can be simulated by a blood clot, radiolucent stone, or granuloma. Retrograde or percutaneous antegrade pyelography may be useful in such situations to delineate the site of obstruction and to obtain brush biopsy.

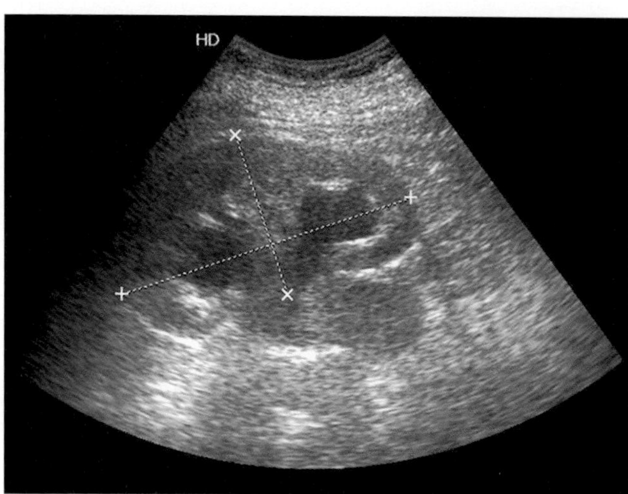

Fig. 35: Longitudinal sonogram of the left kidney shows a solid lesion in the renal pelvis and upper, a case of transitional cell carcinoma.

Ultrasonography

A large TCC is seen as an iso- to hypoechoic solid mass separating the central sinus echoes. A small TCC may not be detected on USG. Focal enlargement of renal cortex suggests infiltration of renal parenchyma. Other non-specific findings include hydronephrosis, and pyelo-calyceal wall thickening. USG can help to differentiate a radiolucent calculus from a tumor. It cannot differentiate from a blood clot unless followed up to show interval change **(Fig. 35)**.

Computed Tomography and Magnetic Resonance Imaging

Computed tomography and MRI urography have increased the diagnostic confidence; however, mucosal detail is still best seen on IVP and RGP.[74] For CT or MRI evaluation, imaging should include excretory phase (3–5 minutes after injection) to show low attenuation mass involving the collecting system or ureter, outlined by the concentrated dense contrast.

There are three appearances on CT of a small TCC, the most common is of a small hypodense lesion in the renal collecting system, the lesion has a soft tissue attenuation (<40 HU), less than most renal calculi, slightly lower than a blood clot, but higher than urine. TCC will enhance approximately 10–50 HU, with the enhancement being less than renal parenchyma, this mild enhancement helps to differentiate it from blood clot and calculi. In the kidney, TCC is usually more central than RCC, owing to the origin in the urothelium.[75-77] TCC does not commonly involve renal vein, through rare cases of IVC involvement have been reported.[78] The central mass expands the kidney symmetrically and with centrifugal extension preserves the shape. The soft tissue component in the renal sinus obliterates and displaces intervening fat to merge with the renal parenchyma, an appearance described as "faceless" kidney **(Figs. 36A and B)**.[79]

The TCC may present as a locally aggressive infiltrative renal mass, margins being ill defined. Involvement of renal parenchyma may be seen as a hypoenhancing mass involving parenchyma or heterogeneous abnormal hypoenhancement disrupting the normal parenchyma. A different appearance is thickening of collecting system urothelium or ureteral wall, the thickening may be asymmetric or eccentric. Focal infiltrative renal lesion may mimic RCC or tuberculosis. TCC tends to be more centrally located and is more likely to expand the kidney centrifugally, while preserving the shape, the coexistence of a stone is a pointer toward squamous cell carcinoma. A small area of parenchymal infiltration with papillary necrosis, is a major clue suggesting TB.

The appearance of TCC is of a small focal lesion involving renal pelvis or calyceal system. TCCs are typically isointense relative to renal medulla on T1WI, making the detection of small tumors virtually impossible. Larger infiltrative tumors may obliterate the fat in the renal sinus, this may be appreciated on T1WI. TCC is best seen on T2-weighted images due to excellent soft tissue contrast between tumor and bright signal intensity due to urine in the collecting system. Infiltrative TCCs may be seen on single shot T2WI as intermediate signal intensity mass infiltrating the renal parenchyma. A cup-shaped dilatation of the ureter just distal to a focus of TCC in the ureter may be seen called the "chalice/goblet" sign. [80] Enhancement

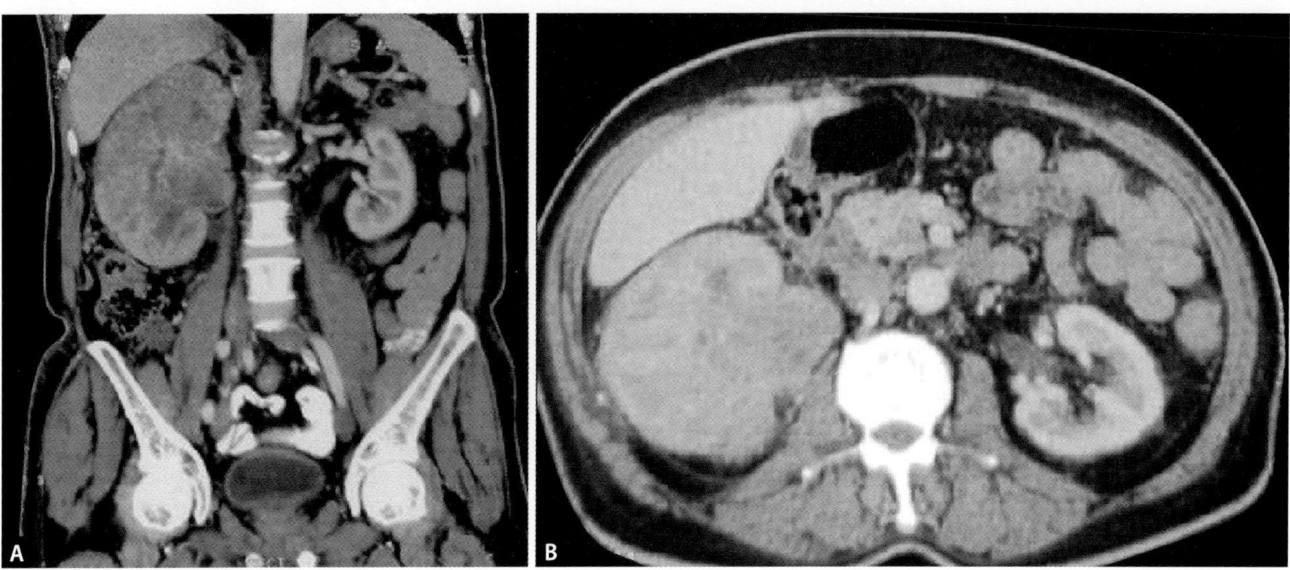

Figs. 36A and B: Contrast-enhanced CT abdomen—large centrally located mass in the right kidney with preserved renal shape. Renal sinus fat is obliterated giving the "faceless kidney" sign—a case of transitional cell carcinoma.

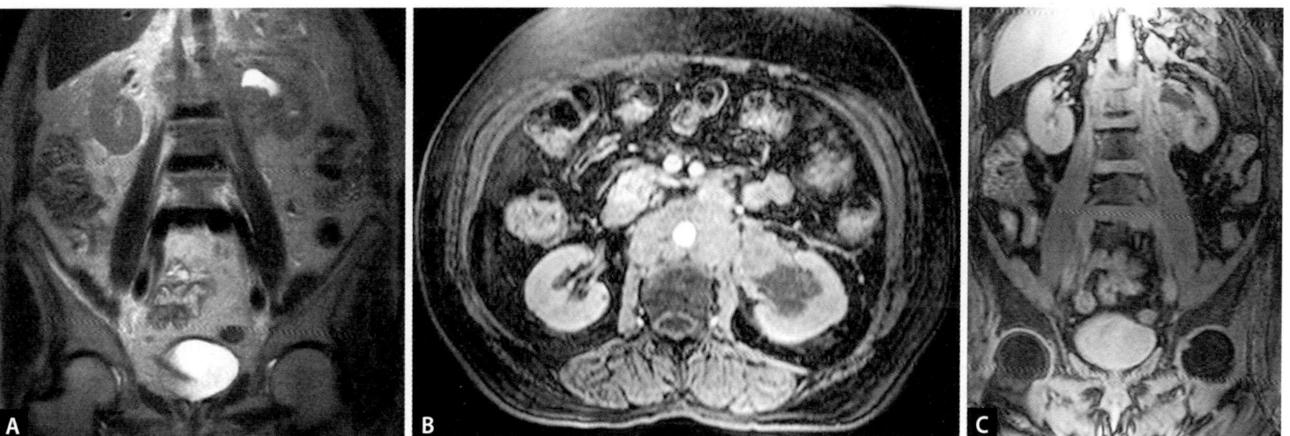

Figs. 37A to C: MRI T2 TRUE FISP: (A) Coronal; (B) T1 VIBE, postgadolinium axial; and (C) Coronal—enhancing mass in the renal pelvis with hydronephrosis and retroperitoneal adenopathy— transitional cell carcinoma.

of a focal filling defect in the collecting system is strongly suggestive of TCC **(Figs. 37A to C)**.

Staging

The TNM classification of malignant tumors (TNM) staging of TCC in upper urinary tract has different prognostic indications from bladder tumors **(Boxes 9 and 10)**. Carcinoma in situ and tumors limited to submucosa have best prognosis, tumors beyond subepithelial tissue (Stage II) and muscularis (Stage III) have worse prognosis. CT cannot accurately distinguish T1 (limited to uroepithelium and lamina propria) from T2 (extending into muscularis propria). Indications of Stage III disease are parenchymal involvement or peripelvic and periureteral fat involvement.

Squamous Cell Carcinoma

Squamous cell carcinoma (SCC) of the renal pelvis is a relatively rare tumor. It is highly aggressive, with a poor clinical prognosis. Chronic infection and renal calculi are implicated in its etiology. It often involves the renal parenchyma and perinephric tissue and may present with metastasis. Intravenous urography may reveal nonfunctioning kidney, hydronephrosis, a central mass, or a pelvicalyceal filling defect seen in 83% of patients. On cross-sectional imaging, this cannot be differentiated

Box 9: TNM Staging of transitional cell carcinoma of the renal pelvis.

T
- *Ta:* Noninvasive papillary tumor
- *Tis:* In situ (noninvasive flat)
- *T1:* Through lamina propria into subepithelial connective tissues
- *T2:* Into muscularis propria
- *T3:* Invasion into peripelvic fat or renal parenchyma
- *T4:* Direct invasion into adjacent structures or beyond renal capsule

N

Nodal staging is the same for TCC of any part of the urinary tract
- *N0:* No nodal involvement
- *N1:* Single node involved <2 cm
- N2
  - Single node 2–5 cm or
  - Multiple nodes all <5 cm
- *N3:* One or more nodes >5 cm

M
- *M0:* No metastases
- *M1:* Metastases identified

Box 10: Staging groups for transitional cell CA of renal pelvis.

- *Stage 0:* Ta or Tis, N0, M0
- *Stage I:* T1, N0, M0
- *Stage II:* T2(a or b), N0, M0
- *Stage III:* T3(a or b) or T4a, N0, M0
- *Stage IV:*
  - T4b, any N, any M
  - N1-3, any T, any M

from transitional cell carcinomas. Pointers toward the diagnosis of SCC include the fact that SCC grows fast, and rapid progression on sequential studies favors SCC. As SCC develops following metaplasia due to chronic inflammation, associated calculi are seen in 50% of cases.

LYMPHOMA

Renal lymphoma is usually *secondary* to systemic disease and associated with adenopathy or involvement of other organs such as liver and gastrointestinal tract (GIT). Contiguous involvement of retroperitoneal disease often affects the genitourinary system with the kidneys, being the most commonly involved organ. Renal involvement is more commonly seen in non-Hodgkin lymphoma than in Hodgkin lymphoma.

Renal lymphoma is often asymptomatic, with detection incidentally at imaging studies. The incidence at autopsy being as high as 41.6%. Despite the high prevalence, imaging studies demonstrate involvement in only 3–8% of patients.[81]

Malignant lymphocytes reach the renal parenchyma by means of hematogenous spread and proliferate within the interstitium, using nephrons, tubules, and blood vessels as scaffolding for further growth. If it follows this infiltrative pattern, kidneys enlarge, maintaining the reniform shape. In many cases, there is focal proliferation giving rise to single or more commonly bilateral renal expansile masses. Some tumors spread by means of contiguous extension from the retroperitoneal disease, penetrating the renal capsule. Renal involvement is usually bilateral, in form of nodules or diffuse infiltration, bulky single tumor, invasion from perirenal disease or microscopic invasion.

Primary renal lymphoma (PRL) is extremely rare, due to lack of lymphatic tissue within the kidney. It should be suspected, if the disease affects only the kidney, or the patient presents with renal impairment in absence of any other cause of renal impairment; rapid improvement and decrease in renal size is noted following the initiation of chemotherapy. The tumor is aggressive and shows bilateral renal involvement in majority of cases. PRL is usually a B cell non-Hodgkin lymphoma and affects patients who are middle-aged or older. In chronic lymphatic leukemia, kidney may be involved in 90% of cases and is associated with membranous glomerulonephritis.

Imaging of Renal Lymphoma

Renal lymphoma has a variety of imaging appearances depending on the pattern of tumor spread **(Box 11)**.[81,82]

Lymphoma masses consist of large number of uniform cells. On *ultrasonography*, this results in a homogeneous, nearly anechoic appearance which may mimic renal cysts, but there is no thorough transmission and subtle low-level echoes may be seen **(Figs. 38A and B)**. The sinus fat surrounding the central pelvicalyceal echoes may completely disappear. This sonographic pattern is

Box 11: Renal lymphoma—patterns.

- *Multiple masses*—most common pattern (50–60%)
  - Usually 1–3 cm in size
  - Associated with enlarged retroperitoneal nodes (≥50%)
- *Single mass* (10–25%)
  - Homogeneous, hypodense without cystic change
- *Invasion from retroperitoneal nodal mass* (25–30% of cases)
  - Usually >10 cm
  - Encasement of vessels without thrombosis, +/–hydronephrosis
- *Diffuse infiltration* (up to 20% of cases)
  - No discrete mass
  - Usually bilateral
  - Seen with Burkitt lymphoma
- *Perirenal mass* (less than 10% of cases)
  - Perirenal stranding
  - Thickening of Gerota's fascia
  - Perirenal nodules.

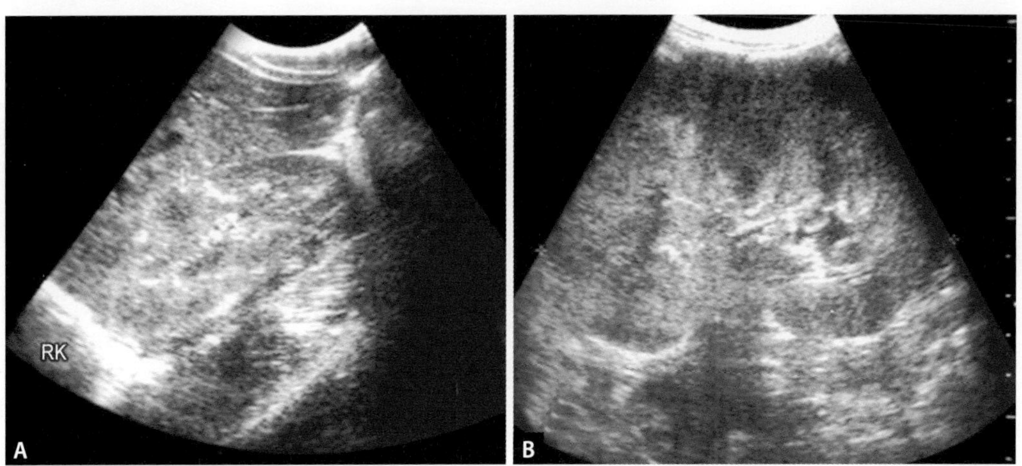

Figs. 38A and B: USG bilateral renal enlargement with poorly defined hypo/anechoic nodules giving a homogeneous appearance—lymphoma.

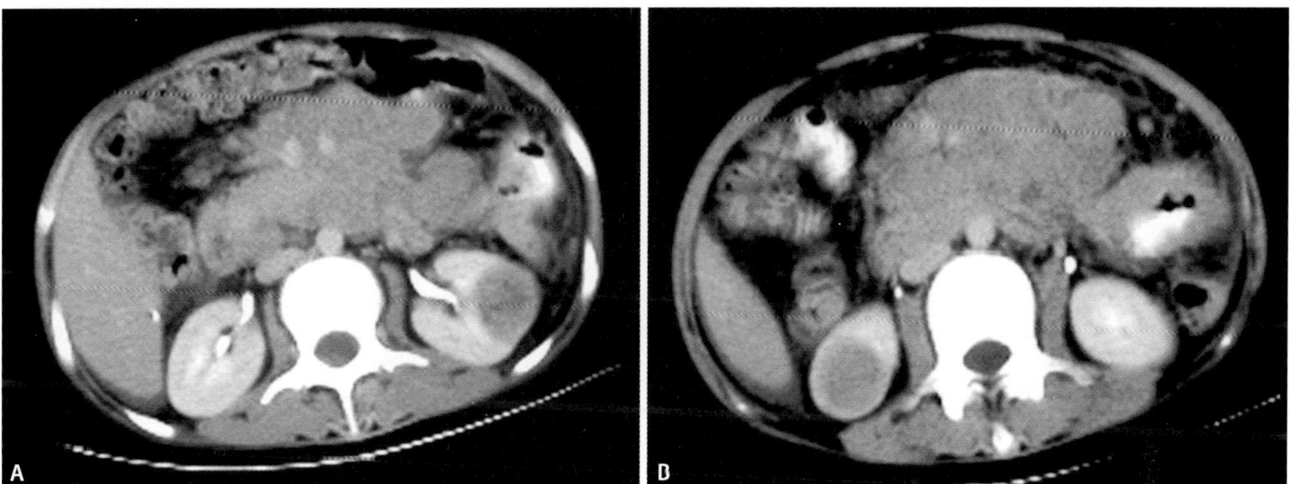

Figs. 39A and B: Contrast-enhanced CT showing well-defined focal hypodense masses in both kidneys with significant retroperitoneal adenopathy and bowel thickening—a case of lymphoma.

unique to renal lymphoma. Ultrasound may also detect hydroureteronephrosis, adenopathy and other foci in liver and spleen. Large retroperitoneal nodes may be seen encasing the vessels.[83]

Computed tomography is more sensitive than ultrasound in detection of renal lymphoma. The most common appearance, which is seen in 50–60% of cases is of multiple focal masses which have attenuation similar or only slightly less than renal parenchyma on unenhanced images (nephrographic phase-contrast CT is essential, as many lesions are small and affect the medullary part of the kidney and may be missed on CM phase). Lymphoma enhances less than normal parenchyma.[82,83] Heterogeneity and necrosis may be seen with larger lesions. Calcification is usually not seen, unless there has been therapy. Invasion into renal vein and IVC is rare.[84]

Renal lymphoma can also manifest as a solitary mass in 10–25% of patients **(Figs. 39A and B)**. It characteristically demonstrates homogeneous attenuation and low-grade enhancement, providing a point of differentiation from clear cell RCC. Biopsy may be required to differentiate from other subtypes of RCC.

Contiguous involvement to kidneys or perinephric space from large retroperitoneal nodal masses is the second most common pattern (25–30%).[85] Perinephric involvement is noted in approximately one-third of patients, most of whom also have parenchymal involvement **(Fig. 40)**.

Another appearance of renal lymphoma is a perinephric ring of soft tissue noted around the kidney without a focal parenchymal lesion; the soft tissue is of low attenuation, compresses the renal parenchyma without

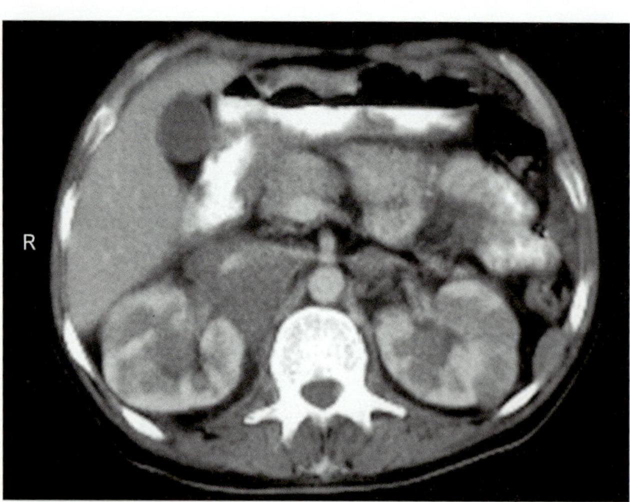

Fig. 40: Renal lymphoma—contrast-enhanced CT shows multiple nodules in both kidneys with perirenal disease on the right side.

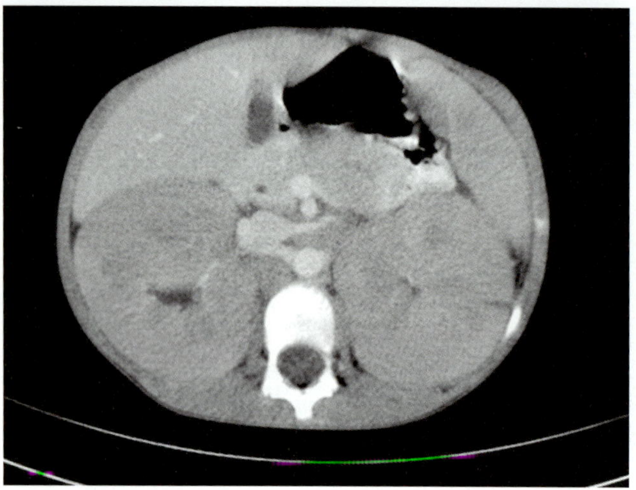

Fig. 41: CT abdomen—bilateral kidneys are enlarged with loss of corticomedullary differentiation—a case of Burkitt's lymphoma.

significant impairment of renal function. Extramedullary hematopoiesis, metastasis, and retroperitoneal sarcoma are differentials for perinephric soft tissue masses.

Diffuse renal enlargement may be seen in the infiltrative form in up to 20% of cases. It is seen as a low-attenuation mass expanding the kidney with predominant, involvement of the renal medulla, with relative sparing of cortical margins. This is more common in Burkitt lymphoma, either disseminated or limited to the kidneys **(Fig. 41)**. Heterogeneous enhancement of the kidneys, with loss of normal differential enhancement is seen. Lymphoma can affect the renal sinus preferentially, the normal sinus fat is replaced by homogeneous soft tissue mass. The mass usually causes encasement of the renal vessels leading to poor enhancement.

The morphological appearance of lymphoma on MRI is similar to that on CT. Renal lymphoma is iso- to slightly hypointense relative to the renal cortex on T1 and iso- to mildly hyperintense on T2-weighted images. There is minimal heterogeneous enhancement on postgadolinium images, the enhancement being less than that of the normal parenchyma.

In suspected cases of lymphoma, biopsy is indicated for differentiating from other tumors. The distinction is important as lymphoma is usually treated medically.

PRIMITIVE NEUROECTODERMAL TUMOR/ EXTRASKELETAL EWING'S TUMOR

This is a highly aggressive renal neoplasm, which comprises only less than 1% of all adult renal tumors, patient is usually a young adult with a median age of 27. Primitive neuroectodermal tumor (PNET) of the kidney belongs to small round cell tumors of the kidney, which include lymphoma, clear cell sarcoma, carcinoid, monophasic Wilms' tumor, synovial sarcoma, desmoplastic small round cell tumor and extraskeletal Ewing's sarcoma (EES)/ PNET. It appears as solitary, large, ill-defined, irregular heterogeneous mass. Invasion of the renal cortex and renal pelvis as well as perirenal fat and adjacent organs, presence of tumor thrombus, at the time of the initial diagnosis is seen in most cases. Early metastases to liver and bone are noted. Diagnosis is based on histology and immunocytohistochemisty.[86,87]

RENAL METASTASES

The prevalence of metastatic disease to the kidney varies from 20% in autopsy series to less than 1% in clinicopathological series. The most common sites of primary tumor are lung, colon, breast, melanoma, and reproductive organs. Melanoma, when present, frequently metastasizes to the kidney. Most renal metastases are hematogenous, although a few may be due to direct invasion (adrenal, colonic, and pancreas). Usually the primary tumor is known and there is metastasis to other organs. Metastases to the kidney are usually asymptomatic, but may rarely present with hematuria.

The appearance of metastases is usually of small bilateral, multiple renal masses, an appearance not commonly seen in RCC, though solitary renal metastasis are not uncommon **(Figs. 42A and B)**. Metastases are usually at the junction of the renal cortex and medulla with ill-defined borders with poor enhancement, except those from hypervascular tumors. Direct involvement of perinephric space by metastasis, representing lymphatic

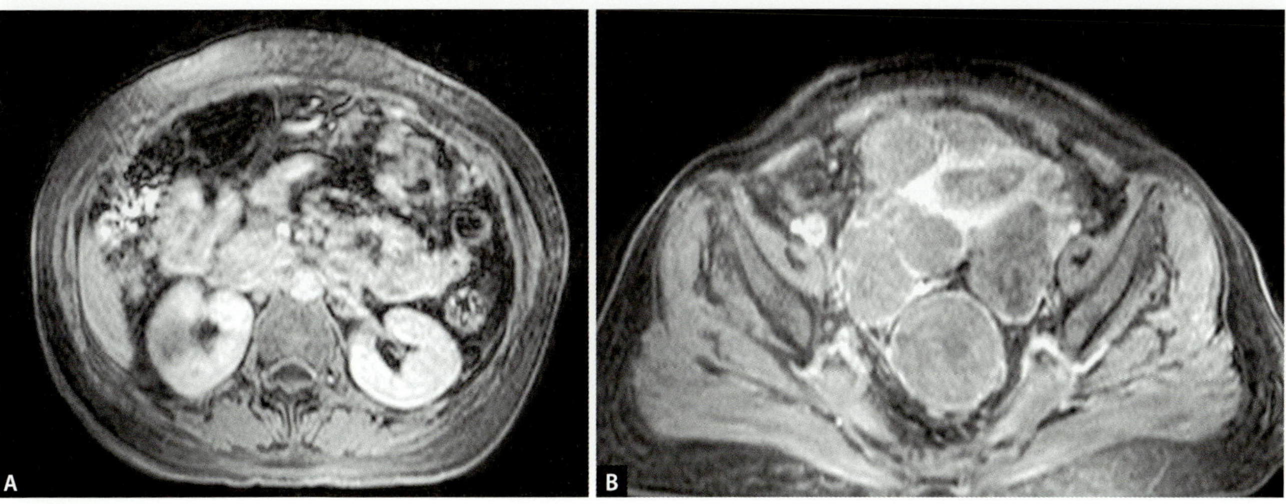

Figs. 42A and B: MRI T1 vibe postcontrast: (A) A focal poorly enhancing mass in the right kidney; (B) Renal metastasis from disseminated ovarian malignancy.

spread is noted in metastasis from melanoma and lung carcinoma. Hemorrhagic renal metastases are seen in melanoma and pheochromocytomas.[88,89]

In the presence of an extrarenal malignancy that is known to metastasize to the kidney, the renal mass may represent a primary renal malignancy or metastatic disease. In patients with a history of extrarenal malignancy, 50–85% of solitary solid renal masses are metastatic. Large solitary renal metastasis that disrupt the renal cortical margins may be associated with breast, lung, or colon carcinomas. Solitary metastasis may resemble RCC, which however, has no necrosis. Hyperenhancement and renal vein involvement favors RCC. The margination of metastasis is often less well defined than RCC. Biopsy of the renal mass is indicated in the clinical dilemma of a solitary metastasis versus RCC.

RENAL MASS BIOPSY

Traditionally, percutaneous biopsy played a limited role in evaluation of all solid renal tumors. However, renal biopsy has become an accepted part of diagnostic algorithm of an indeterminate renal and in a small renal mass (<4 cm), to decide treatment options. The American Urological Association has postulated guidelines for performing renal mass biopsy. It should be offered if an alternate diagnosis is suspected such as hematological, metastatic, inflammatory or infectious etiology. Biopsy is also done for confirming RCC in certain circumstances, including prior to ablative therapies, when a solid mass is present in a solitary or transplant kidney, or when disease is either locally advanced or metastatic, when the surgical risk is high, and when the disease is locally advanced and metastatic, in the setting of a solitary/transplant kidney, and prior to ablative therapy.[90]

Renal biopsy is gaining acceptance and is increasingly used in characterizing and managing renal masses. Accepted indications include confirming an infected cyst, identifying lymphoma or a metastasis as the cause of the indeterminate renal mass, and renal mass biopsy may not be done in the older patients, who will be treated conservatively irrespective of the result, and in the young or healthy patients who may be unwilling to accept uncertainties associated with biopsy. Biopsy may underestimate aggressive features in a renal tumor.

The guidelines state that multiple core needle biopsy sampling should be done rather than fine needle aspirations. Renal mass biopsy may help predict the biological behavior of a renal tumor, its aggressive nature, and thus guide management decisions. Renal mass biopsy, done under image guidance is considered safe with a 92% diagnostic rate and a complication rate of less than 5%. No case of needle tract seeding has been reported with use of the coaxial technique.[91]

INDETERMINATE RENAL MASS

An indeterminate renal mass is one that cannot be diagnosed confidently as benign or malignant at the time it is discovered. MDCT is the most utilized imaging technique for evaluating the indeterminate renal mass, playing an important role in the characterization of both solid and cystic lesions. Presence of macroscopic fat in a renal mass marks it as benign. Enhancing solid renal masses or enhancing components in cystic masses indicate a possible malignant etiology. The small (≤1.5 cm

Flowchart 1: Diagnostic algorithm for characterization of renal mass on CT.

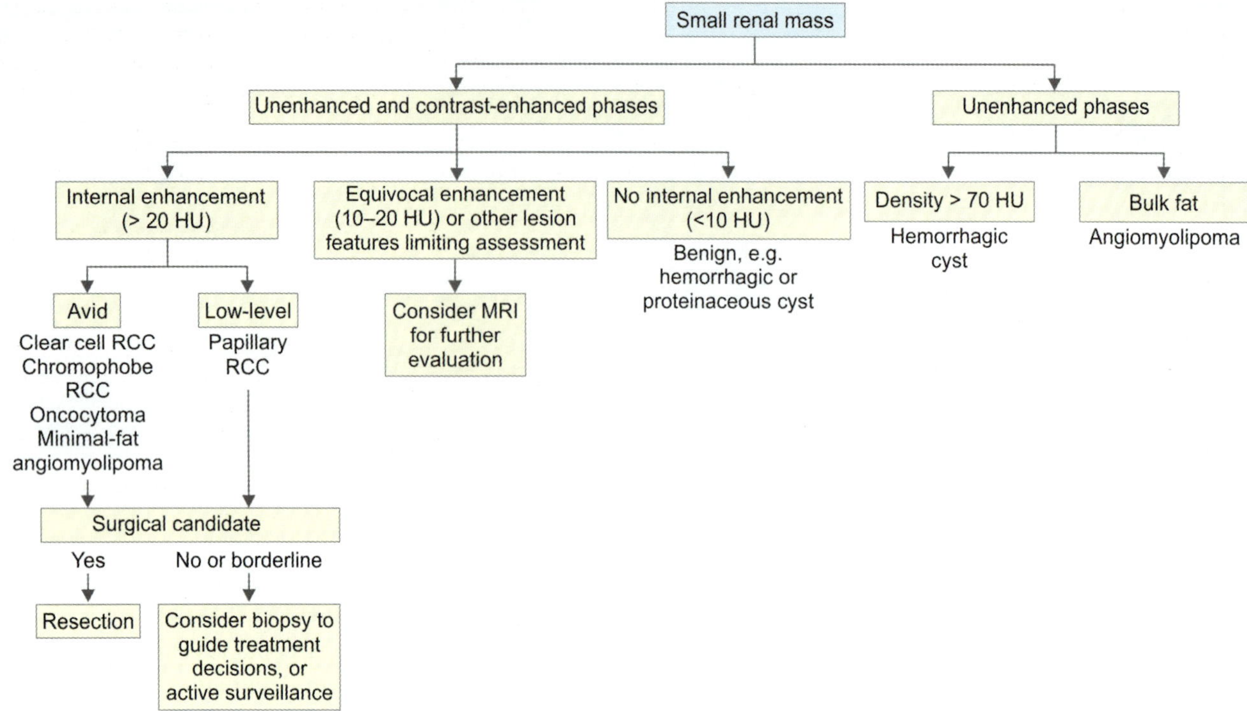

(RCC: renal cell carcinoma; HU: Hounsfield units)

in diameter) renal mass poses a more complex problem for CT imaging, in that volume averaging effects occur, making it difficult to assess accurately the density on noncontrast images and to evaluate for enhancement after IV-contrast administration.[92]

Magnetic resonance imaging is a rapidly evolving modality, currently valuable as a problem solving tool.[93] The addition of diffusion-weighted imaging provides additional inputs in workup of indeterminate lesions, especially in pseudotumors or in cases where IV contrast is contraindicated. The diagnostic dilemma of fat-poor AML vs RCC remains.

A diagnostic algorithm for characterization of renal masses has been suggested **(Flowchart 1)**.

Newer advances such as texture analysis may further refine the pre operative characterization of renal neoplasms.

ACKNOWLEDGMENT

Thanks to Dr Shivali Arya, MD student in the department of Radiodiagnosis, MAMC for the illustrations.

REFERENCES

1. Moch H, Cubilla A, Humphrey PA, et al. The 2016 WHO Classification of Tumours of the Urinary System and Male Genital Organs—Part A: Renal, Penile, and Testicular Tumours. Eur Urol. 2016;70(1):93-105.
2. Burgan CM, Sanyal R, Lockhart ME. Ultrasound of renal masses. Radiol Clin North Am. 2019;57(3):585-600.
3. Kay FU, Pedrosa I. Imaging of solid renal masses. Radiol Clin North Am. 2017;55(2):243-58.
4. Dyer R, DiSantis DJ, McClennan BL. Simplified imaging approach for evaluation of the solid renal mass in adults. Radiology. 2008;247(2):331-43.
5. Hartman DS, Davidson AJ, Davis CJ Jr, et al. Infiltrative renal lesions: CT-sonographic-pathologic correlation. AJR Am J Roentgenol. 1988;150(5):1061-4.
6. Pickhardt PJ, Lonergan GJ, Davis CJ Jr, et al. Infiltrative renal lesions: radiologic-pathologic correlation. Radiographics. 2000;20(1):215-43.
7. Bhatt S, MacLennan G, Dogra V. Renal pseudotumors. AJR Am J Roentgenol. 2007;188:1380-7
8. Maki DD, Birhbaum BA, Chakraborty DP, et al. Renal cyst pseudoenhancement: beam hardening effects on CT numbers. Radiology. 1999;213(2):468-72.
9. Isreal GM, Bosniak MA. Pitfalls in renal mass evaluation and how to avoid them. Radiographics. 2008;28(5):1325-38.
10. Atkins MB, Choueiri TK, Richie JP, et al. (2019). Epidemiology, pathology and pathogenesis of renal cell carcinoma. [Online]. Available from: https://www.uptodate.com/contents/epidemiology-pathology-and-pathogenesis-of-renal-cell-carcinoma. [Last accessed from October, 2019]
11. Cheville JC, Lohse CM, Zincke H, et al. Comparisons of outcome and prognostic features among histological subtypes of renal cell carcinoma. Am J Surg Pathol. 2003;27(5):612-24.
12. Zhang J, Lefkowitz RA, Bach A. Imaging of kidney cancer. Radiol clin North Am. 2007;45(1):119-47.

13. Raman SP, Johnson PT, Allaf ME, et al. Chromophobe renal cell carcinoma: multiphase MDCT enhancement patterns and morphological features. AJR Am J Roentgenol. 2013;201(6):1268-76.
14. Wahal SP, Mardi K. Multilocular cystic renal cell carcinoma: a rare entity with review of literature. J Lab Physicians. 2014;6(1):50-2
15. Peyromaure M, Thiounn N, Scotte F, et al. Collecting duct carcinoma of the kidney: a clinicopathological study of 9 cases. J Urol. 2003;170(4 Pt 1):1138-40.
16. Allappan N, Marak CP, Chopra A, et al. Renal medullary cancer in a patient with sickle cell trait. Case Rep Oncol Med. 2013;2013:129813.
17. Blitman NM, Berkenblit RG, Rozenblit AM, et al. Renal medullary carcinoma: CT and MRI features. AJR Am J Roentgenol. 2005;185(1):268-72.
18. Woo S, Kim SY, Lee MS, et al. MDCT findings of renal cell carcinoma associated with Xp11.2 translocation and TFE3 gene fusion and papillary renal cell carcinoma. AJR Am J Roentgenol. 2015;204(3):542-9.
19. Sureka B, Bansal K, Arora A. Imaging hallmark of Xp 11.2 translocation renal cell carcinoma. Can Urol Assoc J. 2015;9(7-8):E572.
20. Malhi H, Grant EG, Duddalwar V. Contrast-enhanced ultrasound of the liver and kidney. Radiol Clin North Am. 2014;52(6):1177-90.
21. Cohan RH, Ellis J. Renal masses: imaging evaluation. Radiol Clin N Am. 2015;53(5):985-1003.
22. Mittal MK, Sureka B. Solid renal masses in adults. Indian J Radiol Imaging. 2016;26:429-42.
23. Kaza RK, Platt JF. Renal applications of dual energy CT. Abdom Radiol. 2016;41:1122-32.
24. Mileto A, Marin D, Ramirez-Giraldo JC, et al. Accuracy of contrast-enhanced dual-energy MDCT for the assessment of iodine uptake in renal lesions. AJR Am J Roentgenol. 2014;202(5):W466-74.
25. Mileto A, Nelson RC, Paulson EK, et al. Dual-energy MDCT for imaging the renal mass. AJR Am J Roentgenol. 2015;204(6):W640-7.
26. Vendrami CL, Villavicencio CP, DeJulio TJ, et al. Differentiation of solid renal tumors with multiparametric MR imaging. Radiographics. 2017;37(7):2026-42.
27. Pedrosa I, Chou MT, Ngo L, et al. MR classification of renal masses with pathological correlation. Eur Radiol. 2008;18(2):365-75.
28. Pedrosa I, Sun MR, Spencer M, et al. MR imaging of renal masses:correlation with findings at surgery and pathological analysis. Radiographics. 2008;28(4):985-1003.
29. Cornelis F, Tricaud E, Lasserre AS, et al. Multiparametric magnetic resonance imaging for the differentiation of low and high grade clear cell renal carcinoma. Eur Radiol. 2015;25(1):24-31.
30. Kaelo CA, Donati OF, Burger IA, et al. MR imaging of renal cortical tumours: qualitative and quantitative chemical shift imaging parameters. Eur Radiol. 2013;23(6):1738-44.
31. Choi YA, Kim CK, Park SY, et al. Subtype differentiation of renal cell carcinoma using diffusion weighted and blood oxygenation level dependent MRI. Am J Roentgenol. 2014;203(1):W78-84.
32. Rosenkrantz AB, Niver BE, Fitzgerald EF, et al. Utility of the apparent diffusion coefficent for distinguishing clear cell renal cell carcinoma of low and high nuclear grade. AJR Am J Roentgenol. 2010;195(5):W244-51.
33. Goyal A, Sharma R, Bhalla AS, et al. Diffusion weighted MRI in renal cell carcinoma: a surrogate marker for predicting nuclear grade and histological subtype. Acta Radiol. 2012:53(3):349-58.
34. Lassel EA, Rao R, Schwenke C, et al. Diffusion weighted imaging of focal renal lesions: a meta-analysis. Eur Radiol. 2014;24(1):241-9.
35. Maurer MH, Harma KH, Thoney H. Diffusion-weighted genitourinary imaging. Radiol Clin North Am. 2017;55(2):393-411.
36. Goyal A, Sharma R, Bhalla AS, et al. Diffusion-weighted MRI in inflammatory renal lesions: all that glitters is not RCC! Eur Radiol. 2013;23(1):272-9.
37. Goyal A, Sharma R, Bhalla AS, et al. Comparison of MDCT, MRI and MRI with diffusion-weighted imaging in evaluation of focal renal lesions: the defender, challenger, and winner! Indian J Radiol Imaging. 2018;28(1):27-36.
38. Jeon TY, Kim CK, Kim JH, et al. Assesment of early therapeutic response to sorafenib in renal cell carcinoma xenografts by dynamic contrast enhanced and diffusion weighted MR imaging. Br J Radiol. 2015;88(1053):20150163.
39. Johnson CD, Dunnick NR, Lohan RH, et al. Renal adenocarcinoma: CT staging of 100 tumors. AJR Am J Roentgenal. 1987;148(1):59-63.
40. Hallscheidt PJ, Bock M, Riedasch G, et al. Diagnostic accuracy of staging renal cell carcinomas using multidetector row computed tomography and magnetic resonance imaging: a prospective study with histopathological correlation. J comput Assist Tomogr. 2004;28(3):333-9.
41. Montravers F,Grahek D, Kerrou K, et al. Evaluation of FDG uptake by renal malignancies (primary tumor or metastases) using a coincidence detection gamma camera. J Nucl Med. 2000;41(1):78-84.
42. Boss A, Clasen S, Kuczyk M, et al. Image guided radiofrequency ablation of renal cell carcinoma. Eur Radiol. 2007;17(3):725-33.
43. Silverman SG, Israel GM, Herts BR, et al. Management of the incidental renal mass. Radiology. 2008;249(1):16-31.
44. Heilbrun ME, Remer EM, Casilino DD, et al. ACR Appropriateness Criteria indeterminate renal mass. J Am Coll Radiol. 2015;12(4):333-41.
45. Kutikov A, Uzzo RG. The R.E.N.A.L. nephrometry score: a comprehensive standardized system for quantitating renal tumor size, location and depth. J Urol. 2009;182(3):844-53.
46. Ficarra V, Novara G, Secco S, et al. Preoperative aspects and dimensions used for an anatomical (PADUA) classification of renal tumors in patients who are candidates for nephron-sparing surgery. Eur Urol. 2009;56(5):786-93.
47. Lall CG, Patel HP, Fujimoto S, et al. Making sense of post-operative CT imaging following laparoscopic partial nephrectomy. Clin Radiol. 2012;67(7):675-86.
48. Rutherford EE, Cast JEI, Breen DJ. Immediate and long-term CT appearances following radiofrequency ablation of renal tumours. Clin Radiol. 2008;63(32):220-30.
49. Donat SM, Diaz M, Bishoff JT, et al. Follow-up for clinically localized renal neoplasms: AUA guideline. J Urol. 2013;190(2):407-16.
50. Leon AD, Pedrosa I. Imaging and screening of kidney cancer. Radiol Clin North Am. 2017;55(6):1235-50.
51. Prasad SR, Surabhi VR, Menias CO, et al. Benign renal neoplasms in adults: cross-sectional imaging findings. AJR AM J Roentgenol. 2008;190(1):158-64.

52. Ishigami K, Jones AR, Dahmoush L, et al. Imaging spectrum of renal oncocytomas: a pictorial review with pathological correlation. Insights Imaging. 2015;6(1):53-64.
53. Dechet CB, Bostwick DG, Blute ML, et al. Renal oncocytoma: multifocality, bilateralism, metachronus tumor development and coexistent renal cell carcinoma. J Urol . 1999;162(1):40-2.
54. Woo S, Cho JY, Kim SH, et al. Segmental enhancement inversion of small renal oncocytom: differences in prevalence according to tumor size. AJR Am J Roentgenol. 2013;200(5):1054-9.
55. Kim JI, Cho JY, Moon KC, et al. Segmental enhancement inversion at biphasic multidetector CT: characteristic finding of small renal oncocytoma. Radiology. 2009;252(2):441-8.
56. McGahan JP, Lamba R, Fisher J, et al. Is segmental enhancement inversion on enhanced biphasic MDCT a reliable sign for the non invasive diagnosis of renal oncocytomas? AJR Am J Roentgenol. 2011;197(4):W674-9.
57. Wilkinson C, Palit V, Bardapure M, et al. Adult multilocular cystic nephroma: report of six cases with clinical, radio-pathologic correlation and review of literature. Urol Ann. 2013;5(1):13-7.
58. Katabathina VS,Vikram R, Nagar AM, et al. Mesenchymal Neoplasms of the kidney in adults.Imaging spectrum with radiological and pathological correlation. Radiographics. 2010;30(6):1525-40.
59. Prasad SR, Mino Kneudson M, Narra VR, et al. Neoplasms of the perivascular epithelioid cell including the abdomen and pelvis: cross sectional imaging findings. J Comput Assist Tomogr. 2007;31(5):688-96.
60. Jinzaki M, Silverman SG, Akita H, et al. Renal angiomyolipoma: a radiological classification and update on recent developments in diagnosis and management. Abdom Imaging. 2014; 39(3):588-604.
61. Bosniak MA, Meigbow AJ, Hulnick DH, et al. CT diagnosis of renal angiomyolipomas: the importance of detecting small amounts of fat. AJR Am J Roentgenol. 1988;151(3):497-501.
62. Takahashi K, Honda M, Okubo RS, et al. CT pixel mapping in the diagnosis of small angiomyolipomas of the kidneys. J Comput Assist Tomogr. 1993;17(1):98-101.
63. Israel GM, Bosniak MA, Slywotzky CM, et al. CT differentiation of large expophytic renal angiomyolipomas and perirenal liposarcomas. AJR Am J Roentgenal. 2002;179(3):769-73.
64. Ellingson JJ, Coakley FV, Joe BN,et al. Computed tomographic distinction of perirenal liposarcoma from exophytic angiomyolipoma: a feature analysis study. J Comput Assist Tomgr. 2008;32:548-52.
65. Silverman SG, Mortele KJ, Tuncali MD, et al. Hyperattenuating Renal Masses: etiologies, pathogenesis and imaging evaluation. Radiographics. 2007;27:1131-43.
66. Choi HJ, Kim JK, Ahn H, et al. Value of T2-weighted MR imaging in differentiating low-fat renal angiomyolipomas from other renal tumors. Acta Radiol. 2011;52(3):349-53.
67. Mikami S, Oya M, Mukai M. Angiomyolipoma with epithelial cysts of the kidney in a man. Pathol Int. 2008;58(10):664-7.
68. Froemming AT, Boland J, Cheville J, et al. Renal epithelioid angiomyolipoma: imaging characteristics in nine cases with radiologic-pathologic correlation and review of the literature. AJR Am J Roentgenol. 2013;200(2):W178-86.
69. Tsukada J, Jinzaki M, Yao M, et al. Epithelioid angiomyolipoma of the kidney: radiological imaging. Int J Urol. 2013;20(11): 1105-11.
70. Crino PB, Nathanson KL, Henske EP. The tuberous sclerosis complex. N Engl J Med 2006;355(13):1345-56.
71. Johnson SR, Cordier JF, Lazor R, et al. European Respiratory Society guidelines for the diagnosis and management of lymphangioleiomyomatosis. Eur Respir J. 2010;35(1):14-26.
72. Song S, Park BK, Park JJ. New radiologic classification of renal angiomyolipomas. Eur J Radiol. 2016;85:1835-42.
73. Yamakado K, Tanaka N, Nakagawa T, et al. Renal angiomyolipoma: relationships between tumor size, aneurysm formation and rupture. 2002;225(1):78-82.
74. Caoili EM, Cohan RH, Inampudi P, et al. MDCT urography of upper tract urothelial neoplasms. AJR Am J Roentgenol. 2005;184(6):1873-81.
75. Raza SA, Sohaib SA, Sahdev A, et al. Centrally infiltrating renal masses on CT:differentiating intrarenal transistional cell carcinoma from centrally located renal cell carcinoma. AJR Am J Roentgenol. 2012;198(4):846-53.
76. Gatewood OM, Goldman SM, Marshall FF, et al. Computerized tomography in the diagnosis of transitional cell carcinoma of the kidney. J Urol. 1982;127(5):876-87.
77. Parienty RA, Ducellier R, Pradel J, et al. Diagnostic valve of CT number in pelvicalcyeal filling defects. Radiology. 1982;145(3):743-7.
78. Leo ME, Petrou SP, Barrett DM. Transitional cell carcinoma of the kidney with vena caval involvement: report of 3 cases and a review of the literature. J Urol. 1992;148(2 Pt 1):398-400.
79. Hulnick DH, Bosniak MA. 'Faceless kidney' CT sign of renal duplicity. J Comput Assit Tomogr. 1986;10(5):771-2.
80. Daniels RE 3rd. The Goblet sign. Radiology. 1999;210(3):737-8.
81. Sheth S, Ali S, Fishman E. Imaging of renal lymphoma: patterns of disease with pathological correlation. Radiographics. 2006; 26(4):1151-68.
82. Ganeshan D, Iyer R, Devine C, et al. Imaging of primary and secondary renal lymphoma. Am J Roentgenol. 2013;201: W712-9
83. Ruchman RB, Yeh H-C, Mitty HA, Cohen BA, et al. Ultrasonographic and computed tomographic features of renal sinus lymphoma. J Clin Ultrasound. 1988;16(1):35-40.
84. Reznek RH, Mootoosamy I, Webb JA, et al. CT in renal and perirenal lymphoma: a further look. Clin Radiol. 1990;42(4):233-8.
85. Urban BA Fishman EK. Renal Lymphoma: CT patterns with emphasis on Helical CT. Radiographics. 2000;20(1):197-212.
86. Lee H, Cho JY, Kim SH, et al. Imaging findings of primitive neuroectodermal tumors of the kidney. J Comput Assist Tomogr. 2009;33(6):882-6.
87. Akkaya Z, Peker E, Gulpinar B, et al. CT and MRI findings in a rare case of renal primitive neuroectodermal tumor. Pol J Radiol. 2016;81:401-6.
88. Choyke PL, White EM, Zemen RK, et al. Renal metastasis: clinicopathological and radiological correlation. Radiology. 1992;159(6):1229-34.
89. Zhou C, Urbauer DL, Fellman BM, et al. Metastases to the kidney: a comprehensive analysis of 151 patients from a tertiary referral center. BJU Int. 2016;117(5):775-82.
90. Marconi L, Dabestani S, Lam TB, et al. Systematic review and meta-analysis of diagnostic accuracy of percutaneous renal tumour biopsy. Eur Urol. 2016;69(4):660-73.
91. Jason Abel E. Percutaneous biopsy facilitates modern treatment of renal masses. Abdom Radiol (NY). 2016;41(4):617-9.
92. Pahernik S, Ziegler S, Roos F, et al. Small renal tumors: correlation of clinical and pathological features with tumor size. J Urol. 2007;178(2):414-7.
93. Kang SK, Huang WC, Pandharipande PV, et al. Solid renal masses: what the numbers tell us. AJR Am J Roentgenol. 2014;202(6):1196-206.

Chapter 9

Renovascular Hypertension

Sanjeev Kumar, Vineeta Ojha, Sanjiv Sharma

HYPERTENSION

Conventionally hypertension is defined as blood pressure (BP) more than or equal to 140/90 mm Hg. However, according to the latest American College of Cardiology (ACC) guidelines,[1] hypertension is defined as a blood pressures of more than or equal 130/80, measured while following proper techniques. Stage 1 hypertension is systolic BP of 130–139 mm Hg and diastolic BP of 80–89 mm Hg. Stage 2 hypertension is BP of at least 140/80 mm Hg.[1] Hypertension is a common cause of cardiovascular and neurological morbidity and mortality by the virtue of causing complications like left ventricular hypertrophy, heart failure, ischemic heart disease, chronic kidney disease (CKD), ischemic stroke, intracerebral hemorrhage. The overall prevalence of hypertension is 29.8% in India.[2] In adults, mostly (~90%) hypertension is idiopathic and is called as essential hypertension. Rest 10% have hypertension attributable to a particular cause (secondary hypertension). The incidence of hypertension in children is 1–5% and up to 10% in adolescents. Unlike adults, secondary hypertension is more prevalent (70–80%). Risk factors are age, obesity, family history, high sodium diet, alcohol, etc. In a minority of patients, a specific etiology can be identified and such patients are said to have secondary hypertension. The major etiologies implicated in this category include drugs, renovascular, renal parenchymal, obstructive sleep apnea, endocrine, and neurologic.

CAUSES OF HYPERTENSION

The major causes are:

- Primary
- Secondary
    - Renal—parenchymal, vascular
    - Other vascular—coarctation, steno-occlusive lesion of the aorta
    - Endocrine—primary aldosteronism, Cushing's syndrome, pheochromocytoma, hypothyroidism, and primary hyperparathyroidism
    - Drugs—oral contraceptives, nonsteroidal anti-inflammatory drugs (NSAIDs), and antidepressants
    - CNS disease.

RENOVASCULAR HYPERTENSION

Renovascular hypertension (RVH) is a potentially correctable form of secondary hypertension. It denotes the cause and effect relationship between a renal artery stenosis (RAS) and its clinical sequelae, namely: (1) hypertension or (2) chronic ischemic nephropathy. It is also defined as hypertension that improves or resolves after correction of renal artery stenosis.[3]

Epidemiology

The prevalence of RAS in general population is unknown. It is more prevalent in people younger than 30 years and those older than 60 years of age. The prevalence of RVH among adult hypertensive patients is 1–5%.[4] Approximately 20% have bilateral disease or many a times, a single functional kidney may be affected.[5] About 70–80% of hypertension in children is secondary, out of which 5–25% is attributable to renovascular cause. The incidence of surgically correctable hypertension in children less than 5 years of age is approximately 80%, 40–45% in 6–20 years of age, and 20% in 11–18 years of age.

The prevalence of coronary artery disease, cerebrovascular disease, and peripheral vascular disease in patients with RAS is 67%, 37%, and 56%, respectively. In patients with CAD, the angiographic prevalence of RAS is 30%, of which nearly half of the cases have a stenosis greater than 50%. About 50% of patients with RAS do not have hypertension.[6,7]

Renovascular hypertension is mostly seen in younger women and older men. In young women, Takayasu's arteritis (proximal and distal renal arteries) and fibromuscular dysplasia (FMD) (distal and segmental renal artery) are common etiologies. In older men, atherosclerotic RAS affecting the ostia is common. There is no sex predilection in children.

Flowchart 1: Mechanism of renovascular hypertension.

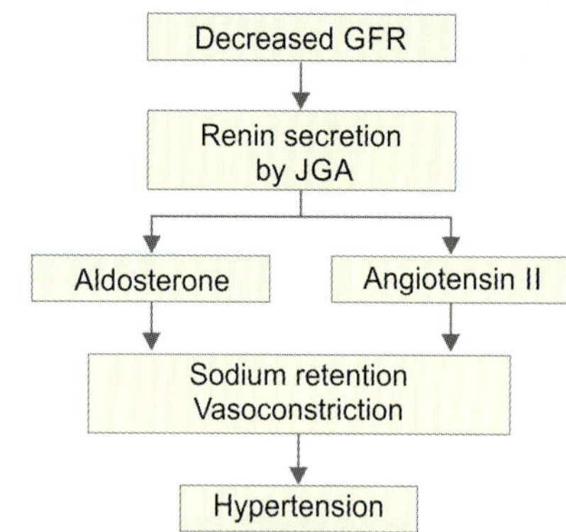

(JGA: juxtaglomerular apparatus; GFR: glomerular filtration rate)

Natural History

Atherosclerotic RAS is progressive. Risk of progression is highest with high-grade stenosis, severe hypertension, and diabetes. Less than 10% of patients with RAS progress to high-grade stenosis or occlusion within 5 years.[8] RVH in the setting of renal dysfunction is associated with the greatest mortality.

Diagnosing RVH is important because treatment of RAS may cure patient's hypertension. Renal artery stenosis is also an important cause of ischemic nephropathy and end-stage renal disease (ESRD) which can be prevented by early and appropriate intervention.[9] Also in view of the widespread use of angiotensin-converting enzyme (ACE) inhibitors, it is important to exclude the presence of RAS as these agents may precipitate renal failure in the presence of bilateral RAS or stenosis of renal artery in a solitary functioning kidney.

Pathophysiology

Renal artery stenosis causes a decrease in perfusion pressure and glomerular filtration rate (GFR) by decreasing the hydrostatic pressure in the afferent arterioles. The reduction in intrarenal arterial pressure is sensed by the juxtaglomerular apparatus of the afferent arterioles. The renin-angiotensin-aldosterone system is triggered in an attempt to maintain glomerular filtration pressure. Renin secreted by juxtaglomerular apparatus of the kidney, converts plasma angiotensinogen to angiotensin I. This is converted by ACE in the lungs to angiotensin II. Angiotensin II is a potent vasoconstrictor and increases blood pressure by direct effect on arterioles and by stimulating aldosterone secretion leading to salt and water retention. Angiotensin II also causes vasoconstriction of the efferent arterioles in an attempt to restore glomerular filtration to normal. It also leads to vascular and myocardial remodeling.

Flowchart 1 is a schematic diagram of the mechanism of RVH.

In significant unilateral RAS increased levels of angiotensin II causes not only vasoconstriction of afferent arterioles of the affected kidney but also a decrease in GFR and sodium excretion by the contralateral kidney. The normal kidney also demonstrates marked decrease in renin secretion. It is called "angiotensin-dependent hypertension". Increased blood pressure ultimately results in pressure natriuresis from the contralateral kidney resulting in the classic "high renin-normal volume" pattern of unilateral RAS.[10]

In patients with bilateral stenosis or a solitary kidney with RAS the entire mass of nephrons is ischemic, resulting in increased renin, excess angiotensin II and aldosterone, which by counter regulatory mechanisms, decrease renin production. Since pressure natriuresis cannot occur from either kidney, there is volume retention. The overall picture in bilateral RAS is a mixed one with both renin and volume factors typically being involved. Because of volume overload these patients are prone to recurrent sudden "flash" pulmonary edema.[10]

Clinical Manifestations of Renovascular Disease

Flowchart 2 shows various clinical manifestations of renovascular disease. The following criteria have been proposed, in the presence of which prevalence of RVH is 20–30% **(Box 1)**:[3,11]

Laboratory tests that may indicate renovascular disease include blood urea nitrogen > 20 mg/dL, serum potassium < 3.4 mEq/L, proteinuria, etc.

Flowchart 2: Clinical manifestations of renal artery stenosis (RAS).

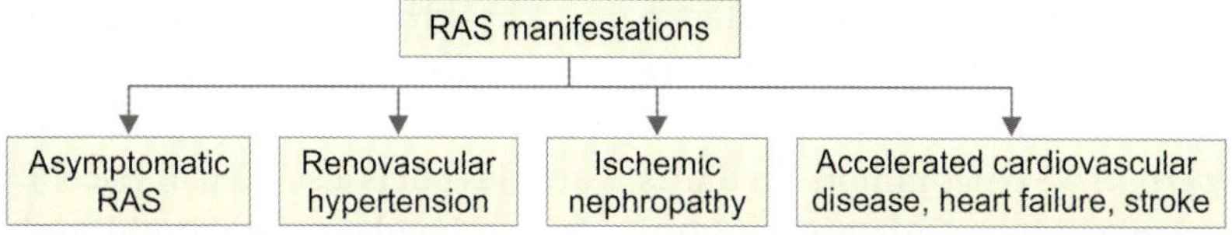

Box 1: The various clinical criteria for suspecting RAS.

- Abdominal or flank bruit (systolic or diastolic)
- Patients presenting with accelerated/malignant hypertension
- Unilateral small kidney
- Onset of hypertension less than 20 years or more than 50 years of age
- Sudden worsening of renal function in a hypertensive patient
- Impairment of renal function after treatment with an angiotensin-converting enzyme (ACE) inhibitor
- Hypertension uncontrolled by triple-drug therapy
- Patients with hypertension and extensive arterial occlusive disease

Box 2: Causes of renovascular hypertension.

Renal artery stenosis

- Atherosclerosis
- Nonspecific aortoarteritis/Takayasu's arteritis
- Fibromuscular dysplasia
- Vasculitis
- Dissection
- Thromboembolism
- Coarctation syndrome
- Neurofibromatosis
- Congenital RAS, supravalvular aortic stenosis
- Congenital rubella
- Syphilitic arteritis
- Tuberous sclerosis
- *Extrinsic compression*: Tumor, median arcuate ligament
- Middle aortic syndrome
- Williams syndrome

Other causes of renovascular hypertension

- Aneurysm of renal artery
- Renal artery embolus
- AVM/AVF
- Irradiation
- Renal transplant
- Trauma

(AVM/AVF: arteriovenous malformation/arteriovenous fistula; RAS: renal artery stenosis)

MAJOR CAUSES OF RENOVASCULAR HYPERTENSION

In the western literature, FMD and midaortic syndrome are the most common causes of RVH, however, in India, Takayasu (61%), FMD (26%), atherosclerosis (8%), polyarteritis nodosa (2.5%), etc. account for most of the cases, as pointed out by Chugh et al.[12]

The various causes of RVH are listed in **Box 2**.

Table 1 depicts most common causes of secondary hypertension by age.

Atherosclerotic Renal Arterial Disease

Atherosclerosis accounts for approximately two-thirds of patients of RAS in the western world. It occurs more commonly in men over the age of 50 years. Obstruction usually results from aortic plaque engulfing the renal ostium (i.e. within 4 mm of aortic lumen). Less frequently plaque develops independently in the proximal third of the renal artery. The stenosis is often circumferential but may be eccentric and is commonly associated with calcification **(Fig. 1)**. Differentiation between proximal and ostial lesions is important because of their different response to angioplasty. Because atherosclerosis is a generalized process both renal arteries are frequently affected. If atheromatous lesions are left untreated there is a high probability of progression to complete occlusion.[13]

Fibromuscular Dysplasia

Fibromuscular dysplasia has only been recognized for the past 30 years or so but accounts for almost a third of the patients with of RVH according to western literature. It typically occurs in young women. It comprises 10–25% of all etiologies of RAS. It may involve any layer of the artery and is classified as intimal, medial or adventitial.

- *Intimal fibroplasia*: There is concentric accumulation of collagen beneath the internal elastic membrane which causes focal smooth stenosis usually in the midportion of renal artery. It is more common in children and is progressive.
- *Medial dysplasia*: This is the most common type of dysplasia and accounts for approximately 95% cases.
    - *Medial fibroplasia*: This is the most common type of medial dysplasia in which there is replacement of smooth muscle by collagen. These alternate with small areas of dilatation due to aneurysm formation and result in the classic "string of beads" appearance. It is more common in women between 20 years and 50 years of age and is progressive. It usually responds to angioplasty **(Figs. 2A and B)**.

- *Perimedial fibroplasia*: Collagen infiltrates outer layer of media. A beaded appearance similar to medial fibroplasia is seen but the "beads" are smaller as aneurysms do not develop.
- *True medial hyperplasia:* Uncommon media is replaced by hyperplastic smooth muscle and fibrous tissue. A tubular smooth narrowing of the vessels is seen on angiography.
- *Medial dissection*: Also uncommon. A new channel is formed in the outer one-third of the media with visualization of a false channel in media on angiography.

Table 1: Common causes of secondary hypertension by age.

Age group	*Common etiologies*
Children (<12 years)	Coarctation of aorta, renovascular hypertension (including congenital renal artery stenosis), midaortic syndrome
Adolescents (12–20 years)	Renal parenchymal disease, renal artery stenosis
Young adults (20–40 years)	Vasculitis causing aortic stenosis (Takayasu's arteritis), renal artery stenosis [Takayasu's arteritis in India, fibromuscular dysplasia (FMD) worldwide], hypothyroidism, coarctation of aorta, renal parenchymal disease
Middle age (40–65 years)	Medication, vasculitis, extrinsic band, aldosteronism, obstructive sleep apnea, renal trauma, dissection, thromboembolism, thyroid dysfunction, pheochromocytoma, Cushing's syndrome
Old age (>65 years)	Atherosclerotic renal artery stenosis, chronic kidney disease (CKD), thromboembolism, dissection, radiation fibrosis, hypothyroidism

- *Adventitial dysplasia*: Collagenous infiltrate surrounds the adventitia, producing a tubular smooth narrowing on the angiogram.

Fibromuscular dysplasia is not confined to renal arteries but is also seen in visceral and peripheral arteries. It also involves the carotid and vertebral arteries, but tends to spare the intracranial vessels. Approximately 30% progressively worsen but total occlusion is rare.

Nonspecific Aortoarteritis/Takayasu's Arteritis[14,15]

Nonspecific aortoarteritis, also known as Takayasu's disease is a chronic, idiopathic, granulomatous arteritis

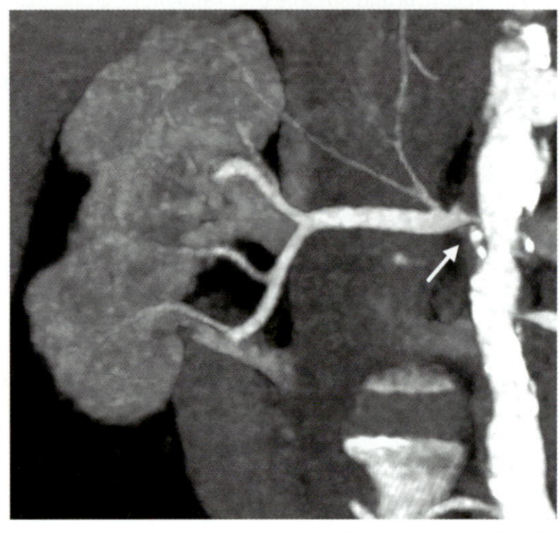

Fig. 1: Computed tomography angiography (CTA) coronal multiplanar reconstruction reveals atherosclerotic renal artery stenosis with calcific plaque at the ostium of the right renal artery (arrow).

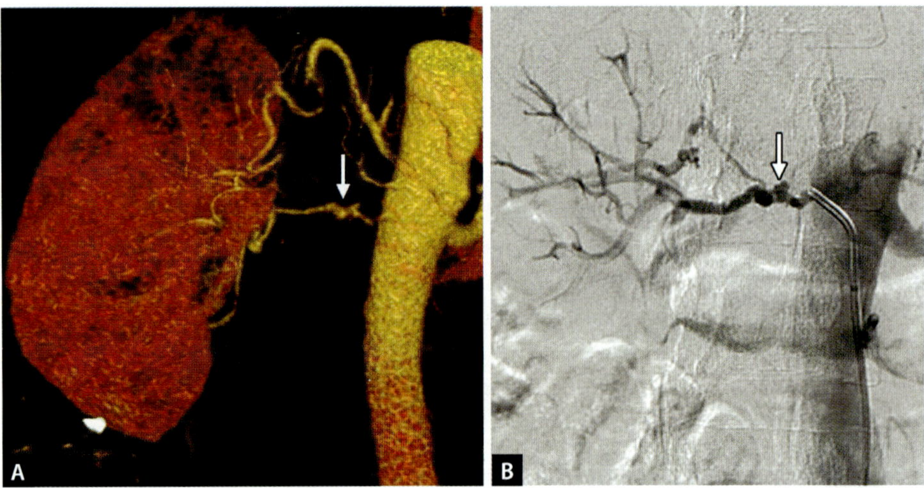

Figs. 2A and B: (A) Volume-rendered CTA and (B) DSA reveal multiple tandem stenoses and dilatations (string of beads appearance) in a patient with medial fibroplasia type of FMD (CTA: computed tomography angiography; DSA: digital subtraction angiography; FMD: fibromuscular dysplasia).

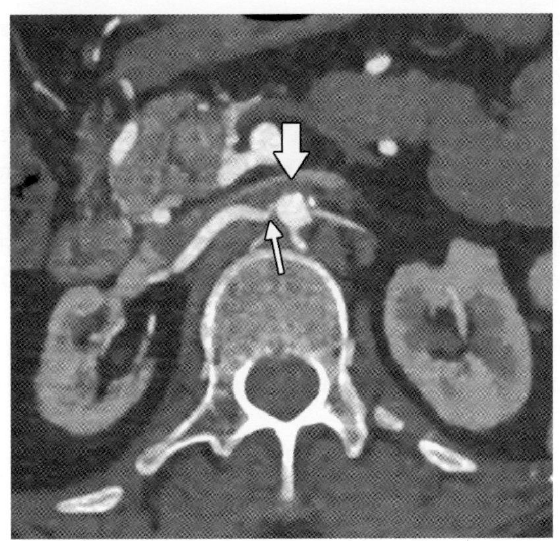

Fig. 3: Axial CTA image shows ostial stenosis of the main renal artery in a patient with Takayasu's arteritis (thin arrow). There is circumferential thickening of the aorta (thick arrow).

that commonly involves the aorta and its major branches and the pulmonary and coronary arteries. The disease tends to affect young females (in second and third) particularly from Southeast Asia and India. Histopathology has shown Takayasu's arteritis to be a granulomatous panarteritis characterized by infiltration of lymphocytes, macrophages and giant cells in the vessel wall. Nonspecific inflammation of the vascular wall leads to progressive adventitial fibrosis, which leads to luminal narrowing and occlusions. In the active stage, the disease is associated with clinical features like fever, carotid tenderness and increased sedimentation rate. Hypertension in Takayasu's disease may be caused by coarctation of aorta or main renal artery stenosis **(Fig. 3)**.

According to a recent classification, it can be classified into six types: [16]

1. *Type I* involves only the aortic arch branches.
2. *Type IIa* involves the ascending aorta, aortic arch, and its branches.
3. *Type IIb* affects ascending aorta, aortic arch, its branches, and descending thoracic aorta.
4. *Type III* involves the descending aorta, abdominal aorta and/or the renal arteries.
5. *Type IV* involves only the abdominal aorta and/or renal arteries.
6. *Type V* has combined features of type IIb and IV.

Type V is the most common pattern. Involvement of the coronary and pulmonary arteries is indicated as C (+) or P (+), respectively.

The morphological pattern of involvement in aortoarteritis shows racial and geographical differences.[17] In Japan, thoracic aortic involvement is more common and neck vessels are most often involved. In most other Asian countries abdominal aorta is most often affected particularly renal and subclavian arteries. Pulmonary artery involvement is less frequently seen in Indian patients. Steno-occlusive lesions of aorta and renal arteries are the most common type of lesions found in the north Indian population, dilatative lesions are more common in Northeastern parts of India. South Indian population has mainly abdominal vessel involvement.

Other Vasculitis

Polyarteritis nodosa is a necrotizing systemic vasculitis involving medium and small sized arteries. Most cases are idiopathic. It causes approximately 2.5% of the RVH in India. Renal involvement often leads to hypertension and renal insufficiency. Imaging reveals patchy parenchymal infarcts with stenoses, microaneurysms, and post-stenotic dilatations, which can rupture and cause hematomas.

Other vasculitis that can cause RAS are systemic arterial mediolysis, scleroderma, etc.

Congenital Renal Artery Stenosis

Congenital RVH may remain asymptomatic for a long time. The RAS in neurofibromatosis usually involves the ostia and bilateral kidneys. Because of fibrotic nature, they are tough to dilate. Surgery usually shows better results than endovascular management.

Transplant Renal Artery Stenosis

It occurs in the first 6 months after renal transplant and cause graft failure or premature death in transplant recipients **(Fig. 4)**. It accounts for 1–5% cases of post-transplant hypertension. Flash pulmonary edemas can develop and is called pickering syndrome. It usually occurs at the ostium/anastomotic site as well at the external iliac artery where RA is anastomosed. It is a potentially treatable condition, usually respond to balloon dilatation. Contralateral femoral access is preferred.

Aortorenal Dissection

Dissection in renal artery, either isolated **(Fig. 5)** or that extending form concomitant aortic dissection can also cause RVH. Spontaneous RA dissection can be seen in connective tissue disorders. Therapeutic options include

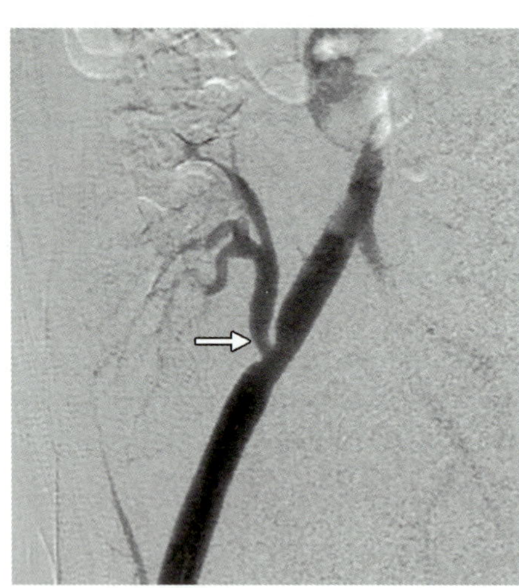

Fig. 4: Transplant renal artery stenosis: Digital subtraction angiography shows narrowing of the ostioproximal segment (arrow) of the renal artery from right external iliac artery.

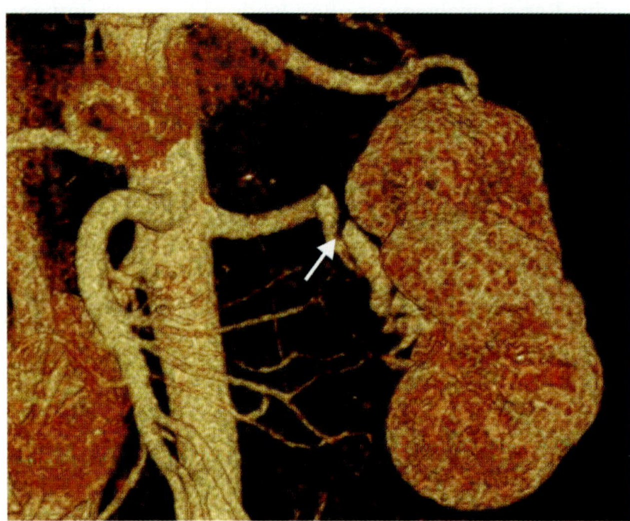

Fig. 5: Volume rendered CTA image shows isolated renal artery dissection in left main renal artery (arrow).

conservative management and revascularization. It is more frequent in middle-aged male patients.

SCREENING FOR RENOVASCULAR HYPERTENSION

Hypertension is common but RVH is not, therefore, screening should be reserved for patients at moderate-to-high risk for RVH.

Indications for Testing for Renovascular Hypertension[11,18,19]

The 2013 American College of Cardiology/American Heart Association (ACC/AHA) and 2017 European Society of Cardiology (ESC) guidelines recommend performing diagnostic studies to identify RAS in patients with any of the following (They have high likelihood of benefitting from the procedure):

1. Onset of hypertension before the age of 30 years or after age of 55 years (level of evidence, LOE-B).
2. Accelerated hypertension (sudden and persistent worsening of previously controlled hypertension) (LOE-C).
3. Resistant hypertension (failure to achieve goal BP in patients adhering to full doses of a 3-drug regimen that includes a diuretic).
4. Malignant hypertension (hypertension with coexistent end-organ damage, i.e. acute kidney injury (AKI), flash pulmonary edema, LVF, aortic dissection, new visual or neurological disturbance, and/or advanced retinopathy).
5. New azotemia or worsening renal function (>30% creatinine) after the administration of an ACE inhibitor or an ARB (LOE-B).
6. Unexplained atrophic kidney or size discrepancy of >1.5 cm between the kidneys (LOE-B).
7. Unexplained congestive heart failure or refractory angina (LOE-C).

The above clinical features suggest a cause of secondary hypertension rather than primary hypertension. Additionally, testing for renovascular disease is prudent if:

- Other causes of secondary hypertension such as primary kidney disease, primary aldosteronism, or pheochromocytoma, have been excluded.
- An intervention can be planned if a significant stenotic lesion is found.

Testing should not be performed if there is:

- Moderate or low likelihood of having clinically significant renovascular disease (This is because the RCTs comparing percutaneous revascularization with medical therapy primarily consisted of patients with moderate and low likelihood of clinically important renovascular disease; during 3–5 years of follow-up, they showed no evidence of benefit from adding revascularization to optimal medical therapy), or
- In those who respond well to medical therapy.

There is no perfect screening test for the detection of RVH. The situation is further complicated by the fact that the presence of RAS may not always indicate a causal relationship. Not every RAS leads to RVH and patients with essential hypertension may also develop RAS. The degree of stenosis that causes RVH has not been established although most investigators treat stenosis measuring 50%

or greater.[20] Also, there are potential risks in testing for RVH, especially in patients with impaired renal function, which include contrast-induced nephropathy and nephrogenic systemic fibrosis.

Physiologically, RAS is defined as inadequate renal blood flow leading to reduction in GFR and loss of renal parenchyma, hence it becomes prudent to establish the functional significance of RAS before proceeding to revascularization.[21]

DIAGNOSTIC MODALITIES

Clinical and Biochemical Tests

Clinical/nonradiological tests that have been used for the diagnosis of RVH include: Plasma renin activity, ACE inhibitor challenge test, aspirin challenge test and 24 hours ambulatory blood pressure monitoring.

Imaging Modalities for Assessment of Renal Artery Stenosis

In patients with clinical suspicion of RAS, noninvasive screening is required to select patients for conventional angiography and renal revascularization.[22]

An ideal renal artery imaging study should answer the following questions:[23]

- Localization and number of arteries
- Characterization of renal stenosis, including etiology of stenosis, localization, and post-stenotic dilatation
- Hemodynamic and functional significance of the stenosis
- Further pathologies or variants that might have an influence on treatment planning.

The useful diagnostic tools are:

Noninvasive:

- Ultrasound/Doppler/contrast US
- Computed tomography (CT)
- Magnetic resonance imaging (MRI)
- Intravascular ultrasound (IVUS)
- Any other [nuclear imaging, optical coherence tomography (OCT)]

Invasive: Arteriography

Table 2 shows the strength of recommendations for using these tests for detection of RAS.[19]

Table 2: Tests for detection of RAS.

Recommendation	*Class*	*Level*
Duplex ultrasonography, computed tomography angiography (CTA) [in patients with estimated glomerular filtration rate (eGFR) > 60 mL/min] and magnetic resonance angiography (MRA) (in patients with eGFR > 30 mL/min) are recommended as screening tests	I	B
When the clinical index of suspicion is high and the results of the noninvasive tests are inconclusive, catheter angiography is recommended as a diagnostic test	IIB	C
Captopril renal scintigraphy, selective renal vein renin measurements and plasma renin activity are not recommended as a useful screening test	III	C

Ultrasound and Color Doppler

A normal appearance of the kidneys on ultrasound does not exclude a significant unilateral or bilateral renal artery stenosis. Renal size and shape may be normal unless the stenosis is greater than 60% when a small decrease in size may be found.[24]

Brief anatomy of renal arteries: Renal arteries arise from aorta just below the level of superior mesenteric artery, usually at L1-L2 level. There can be one or more accessory renal arteries. Stenoses in accessory renal arteries can also cause RVH. Anterior to each renal artery runs the renal vein on each side. The right renal artery has a longer course due to downward location of the right kidney. Double main renal arteries and accessory renal arteries occur in nearly 12–22% of patients.

Doppler USG is first-line imaging modality for assessment of RAS.

Advantages of Doppler ultrasound:

- Widely available
- Inexpensive
- Good sensitivity and specificity for detection of RAS
- It can be repeated to assess stenosis progression
- To exclude an obvious structural abnormality or coexistent condition.

Disadvantages of Doppler ultrasound:

- It remains operator dependent and time consuming
- It can overestimate the degree of stenosis.

Information provided by a duplex USG for assessment of severity and suitability for revascularization are:

- *Size of kidneys*: Shrunken kidneys with size < 7 cm have lower chance of improvement with revascularization as kidney sizes decrease after setting in of CKD **(Figs. 6A and B)**.
- *Parenchymal cortical thickness*: Cortical thickness of at least 1 cm is necessary for considering revascularization.
- *Echogenicity*: Increased echogenicity and loss of corticomedullary differentiation are findings of CKD,

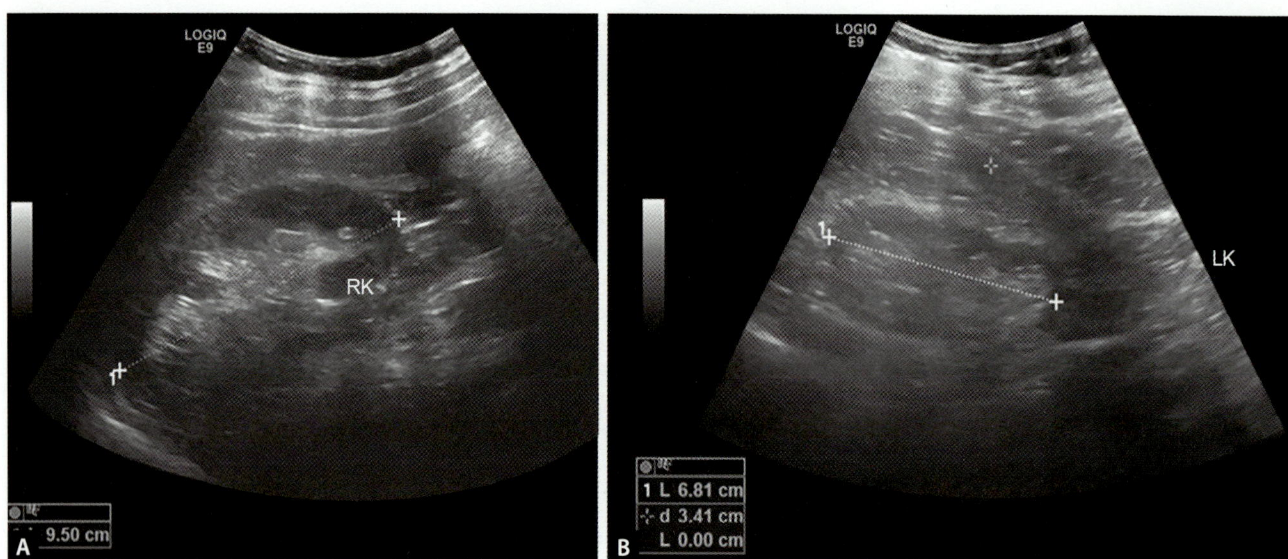

Figs. 6A and B: Grayscale ultrasound images show (A) a normal-sized kidney, and (B) a shrunken kidney.

and such kidneys should not be revascularized as there are minimal chances of improvement.

- Direct evaluation of the renal arteries as well as transrenal Doppler waveform analysis (as discussed below)

Two approaches are used with Doppler ultrasound. The first is the direct visualization and interrogation of the stenotic segment of the renal artery. The second is an assessment of the arterial waveform distal to the stenosis within segmental renal vessels **(Fig. 7)**.

Direct approach: This requires evaluation of the entire main renal artery, spectral traces are then obtained from areas of stenosis identified on color Doppler. The aorta is also interrogated and peak systolic velocity (PSV) obtained at the level of renal origins. An anterior or anterolateral approach usually allows insonation of both the arteries. A coronal approach can be used when bowel gas is present. The criteria used to diagnose significant stenosis or occlusion of a renal artery is as follows:[3,25]

- An increase in PSV (thresholds commonly applied in current literature to diagnose RAS include PSV (max) in the renal artery >180 cm/ sec **(Figs. 8A and B)**.
- Renal artery/aortic ratio (RAR ratio) > 3.5 calculated as:

$$\frac{\text{PSV (max) renal arteries}}{\text{PSV aorta at the origin of renal arteries}}$$

- Turbulent flow in the post-stenotic area
- Visualization of the renal artery without detectable Doppler signal, a finding that indicates occlusion.

As main renal arteries may not be visualized in up to 42% cases, in practice, these measurements often cannot

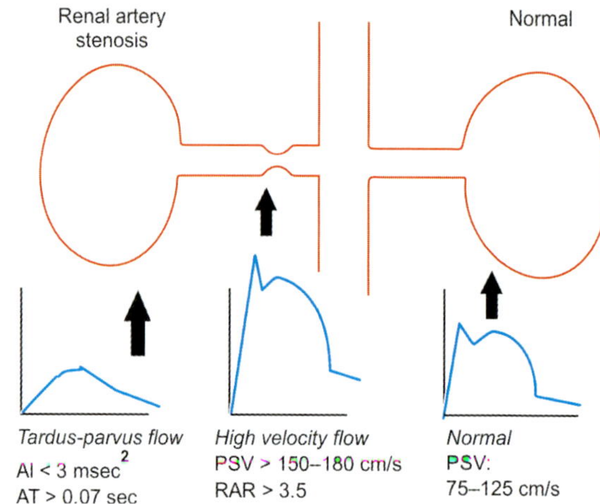

Fig. 7: Schematic diagram of the renal artery Doppler tracings showing the normal renal artery trace on the left side. On the right side high velocity at the site of stenosis and "tardus-parvus" waveform is seen distal to the stenosis (PSV: peak systolic velocity; RAR: renal-aortic ratio; AI: acceleration index; AT: acceleration time).

be obtained. The procedure is time consuming and operator dependent. Accessory renal arteries and branch artery stenosis cannot be diagnosed. In cases of renal artery occlusion collaterals may be sampled.

Indirect approach: Arterial waveforms from the segmental renal arteries from the upper, mid, and lower poles are evaluated. The normal waveform from these vessels shows a steep systolic upstroke with a peak in early systole referred to as early systolic peak (ESP). The early systolic acceleration seems to be the best predictor of RAS and should be measures along the initial portion of the systolic

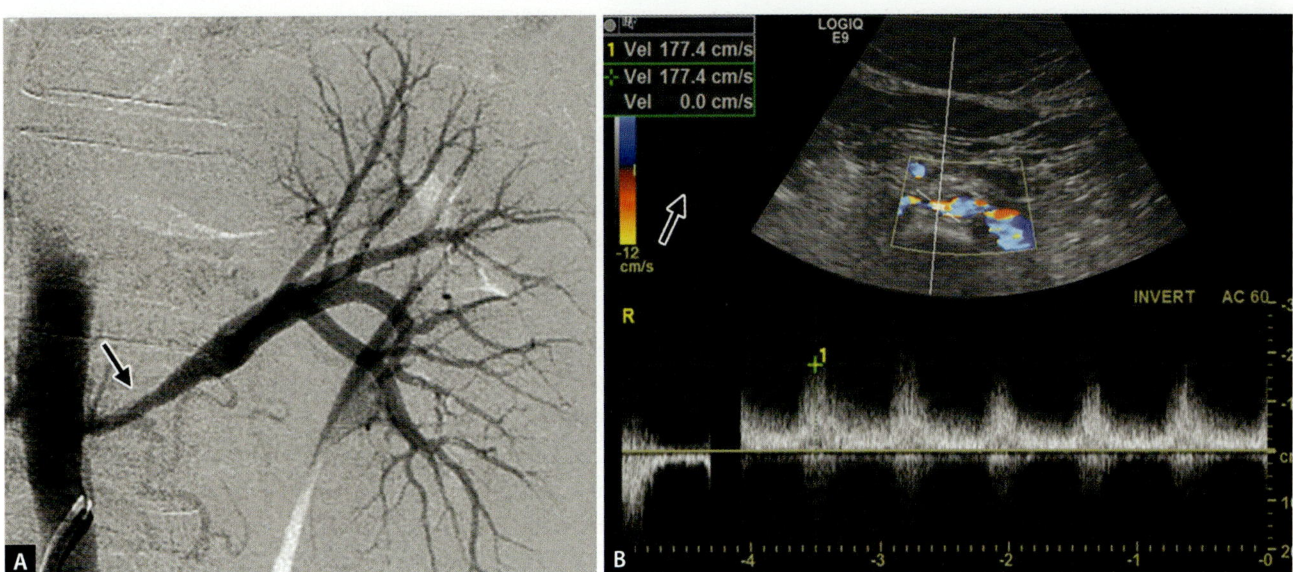

Figs. 8A and B: Digital subtraction angiography: (A) Frame reveals stenosis in proximal left renal artery (arrow); (B) Spectral trace with high peak systolic velocity (PSV >180 cm/s) at the site of stenosis.

rise and should not include the late compliance peak.[26] The waveform in patients with RAS lacks both these features and is known as "tardus-parvus" waveform. Tardus refers to the slowed systolic acceleration and parvus refers to the low amplitude of the systolic peak **(Fig. 9)**.

There are two quantitative measurements that are used: (1) the acceleration time (AT) and (2) the acceleration index (AI). AT is the time from start of systole to peak systole. AI is the slope of the systolic upstroke.

Findings suggestive of significant RAS are:

- Parvus-tardus waveform
- Acceleration time greater than 0.07 sec
- Acceleration index reduced to less than 3 m/s^2.
- Change in resistive index (RI) of greater than 5% between the right and left kidneys (RI and pulsatility index decrease).

Some authors have shown that simple pattern recognition of "tardus-parvus" waveform is more accurate than calculation of "AT" and "AI".[27] The waveform may also demonstrate a decrease in RI and pulsatility index.[28] Administration of captopril in individuals with significant RAS produces measurable changes in Doppler waveform which increases the degree of pulsus tardus and decreases the RI.[29]

These criteria only detect stenosis of greater than 70–90% reliably. A positive test is more informative than a negative test. The shape of the waveform is not simply related to the pressure drop across the stenosis but also compliance of renal arteries.[37] Coexisting parenchymal disease may also affect the waveform due to changes

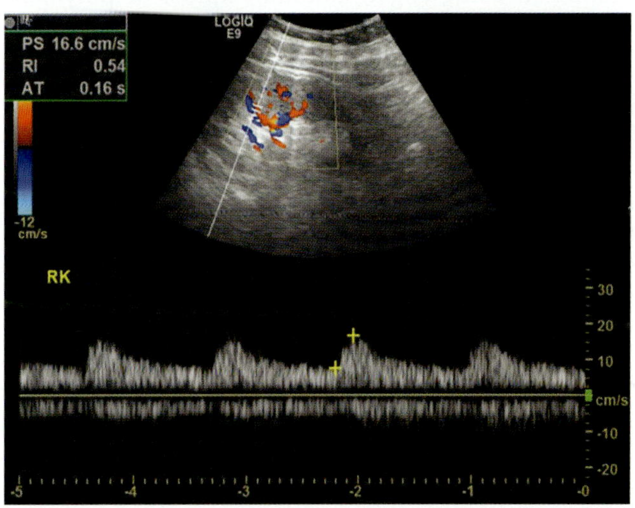

Fig. 9: Color Doppler image showing tardus-parvus waveform in intralobar artery due to main renal artery stenosis.

in peripheral resistance. The technique also cannot distinguish between high-grade stenosis and complete occlusion with collateral flow. Tardus-parvus waveform may also be produced by abdominal coarctation.[30]

A meta-analysis of 88 studies including 9,974 arteries assessed the accuracy of each of these parameters and found that PSV, with a sensitivity and specificity of 85% and 92%, respectively, was more accurate than the renal aortic ratio and acceleration index.[31]

Use of resistive index [Ratio of (PSV–EDV) to PSV]: Normal values are 0.6–0.7. RI may also be used to predict the outcome of therapy for RAS.[32] A "RI" of more than 80 probably identifies patient with RAS in whom angioplasty or surgery will not improve renal function or blood pressure because of greater intrinsic renal damage. Other than parenchyma, RI can also be regarded as a marker of systemic vascular properties. A low (<6) RRI can reflect (in addition to RAS greater than 70%), valvular aortic stenosis, thoracic or suprarenal abdominal aortic stenosis, hypervolemia, tachycardia, and parasympathetic activation (extrarenal determinants). High RRI (>7) can reflect arteriolosclerosis, vasoconstriction, increased interstitial, and venous pressure (intrarenal determinants) or increased systemic pulse pressure, adrenergic hyperactivity, and bradycardia (extrarenal determinants).

Contrast-enhanced ultrasound: Renal contrast-enhanced ultrasound (CEUS) is a newer method for detecting RAS noninvasively and some studies have shown it to be superior than routine duplex sonography for the same.[33] The common ultrasound contrast agents are microbubbles stabilized using sugar, albumin, lipids, or polymers. Microbubbles are smaller than 10 μm in diameter and are effective and safe agents. The most widely used agent is Levovist. It has been found to enhance the visualization of main renal vessels resulting in higher technical success rates.[34] It can be used in cases in which usual duplex Doppler is nondiagnostic or suboptimal.[35]

Computed Tomography Angiography

Computed tomography angiography (CTA) offers a noninvasive technique for obtaining angiographic images. The advent of spiral CT and more recently multidetector computed tomography (MDCT) has revolutionized CT and CTA. MDCT has made possible the acquisition of isotropic data with high spatial and temporal resolution in shorter scan times. With current generation scanners, the data can be acquired within a few seconds. We, at our institute, use a 384 slice dual source CT scanner. The protocol that we follow is as follows:

- *Arterial phase scan (including diaphragm to iliac arteries to cover potential accessory renal arteries):* The thinnest collimation is used (0.75 mm). A contrast volume of 1 mL/kg (350 mg I/mL) is injected IV at 4–6 mL/sec followed by a 20–30 mL saline chase. No oral contrast is given. Bolus tracking techniques is used to trigger the scan with ROI in the region of abdominal aorta, with trigger threshold of 100 HU.
- *Parenchymal phase scan:* Three minutes after contrast injection, only kidneys are included in scan, low-dose protocol. This scan helps in identifying the areas of hypoperfusion/infarcts and corticomedullary thicknesses.

The axial images are reconstructed in multiple planes using multiplanar reconstruction (MPR), maximum intensity projection (MIP) or real-time volume rendering techniques (VRTs) for morphological evaluation of kidneys and main renal arteries **(Figs. 10A to C)**.

The sensitivity of CTA in identifying main renal arteries has been 100%; accessory arteries are also almost always detected with any area of narrowing. The sensitivity and specificity for diagnosis of RAS has ranged between 90% and 95%.[36]

CTA is highly accurate for imaging renovascular disease due to atherosclerosis but less so for fibromuscular disease (as it involves distal arteries difficult to image).

Advantages of CTA:

- CTA can demonstrate the wall of the aorta unlike angiography which only visualizes the lumen of the vessel, important in cases of atherosclerosis and also aortoarteritis **(*see* Fig. 3)**, where the lumen may appear angiographically normal in places but may show vessel wall involvement in cross-sectional studies.
- It demonstrates the extent of plaque projecting into the vessel lumen, aiding in determining the form of intervention planned such as angioplasty versus primary stent placement.
- It has high efficacy for diagnosis of ostial stenosis.
- MDCT/CTA can also detect collaterals as well as stenoses in accessory renal arteries with great accuracy **(Figs. 11A and B)**.
- Unlike magnetic resonance angiography (MRA), CTA can also be used to examine the patency of vessels that have been dilated by intravascular stents.

Disadvantages of CTA:

- Relatively high cost
- Use of large amount of iodinated contrast medium precluding its use in renal insufficiency
- Mural calcification in the aorta or renal artery may result in overestimation of stenosis.

Magnetic Resonance Angiography

After published reports of nephrogenic systemic fibrosis (NSF) following gadolinium-based contrast agent in patients with deranged renal functions, contrast-enhanced MRI as a screening test is being avoided.[37] It is of great importance that radiologists be aware of this serious disease and exercise caution when considering the use of gadolinium-based contrast media in patients with

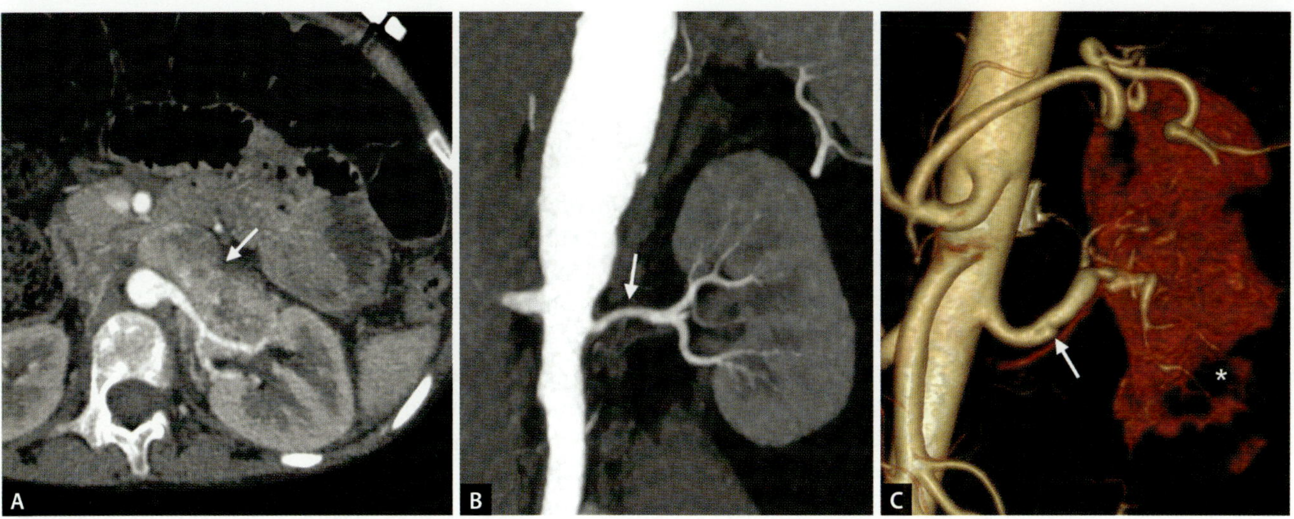

Figs. 10A to C: Applications of different CTA postprocessing in identifying etiologies of RVH: (A) Axial MPR shows narrowing of the main renal artery due to mass (arrow) at the perihilar region (RVH due to extrinsic compression); (B) MIP coronal image in a patient with Takayasu's arteritis shows mild stenosis (arrow) in mid left renal artery; (C) VRT image reveals left renal artery dissection (arrow) with resultant parenchymal infarcts (star) (CTA: computed tomography angiography; MIP: maximum intensity projection; MPR: multiplanar reconstruction; RVH: renovascular hypertension; VRT: volume rendering technique).

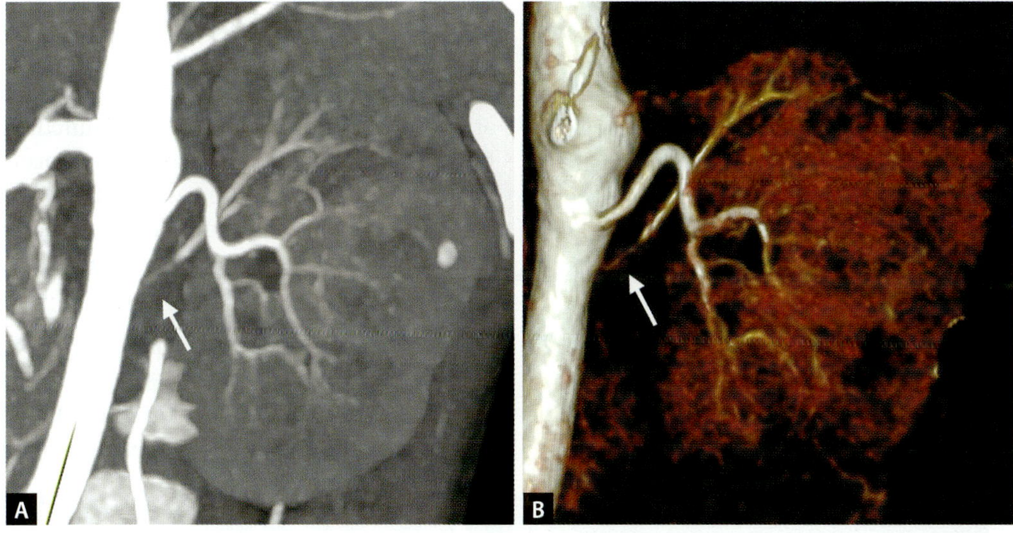

Figs. 11A and B: CTA MIP: (A) MPR and (B) VRT image reveal tight stenosis (arrow) of the lower accessory renal artery supplying upper pole of the left kidney.

moderate (GFR < 60 mL/min/1.73 m^2) to severe (GFR < 15 mL/min/1.73 m^2) renal disease. In this situation various other MR techniques which can assess renal arterial morphology, perform functional measurements of arterial flow and parenchyma perfusion without the administration of gadolinium are being investigated and found useful in patients with deranged renal functions. These techniques are noncontrast studies such as time-of-flight (TOF), phase contrast (PC), steady-state free precession (SSFP), and arterial spin labeling (ASL).[37] These advancements explain why renal MRI is evolving as the first-line imaging modality for the evaluation of renovascular disease.

Most series have shown excellent correlation between conventional angiography and MRA (sensitivity > 99% and specificity > 96%) for detection of RAS 50% or greater in diameter.

Contrast-enhanced MRA: Recent advances in the magnetic resonance gradient hardware with availability of 3.0 T, acquisition of isotropic data with submillimeter resolution is allowing the detection of renal artery narrowing with high sensitivities (94–97%) and specificities (85–93%). Moreover, it is now possible to demonstrate the functional consequences of RAS, such as a decline in renal perfusion and glomerular filtration.[38]

Intravenous gadolinium is used in a dose of 0.1–0.3 mmol/kg with bolus tracking. With the advent of 3.0 T, the amount of contrast can be reduced because of increase in T1 of tissue. Entire acquisition is performed during a single-breath hold. In patients unable to withhold breath for long-time parallel imaging technology provides high-resolution images with shorter acquisition times. Three-dimensional (3D) contrast MRA overcomes the limitations of noncontrast MRA. As a result, renal arteries are assessed in their entirety, including the major segmental branch vessels, as well as small accessory renal arteries **(Figs. 12A and B)**. In addition, speed, operator independence, high spatial and contrast resolution, and lack of side effects have contributed to making 3D contrast MRA a well-suited screening alterative for detection of renovascular disease. The technique has sensitivities of 93–100% and a specificity of 90–100%.

In several centers, contrast-enhanced MRA is complemented by 3D-PC acquisition. Areas of hemodynamically significant stenosis are detected by their associated turbulence seen as a signal void on 3D-PC images. The presence of a signal void at or immediately downstream from a stenosis suggests pressure drop across the stenosis. For 3D-PC MRA to be optimally sensitive to turbulent flow echo time should be approximately 8 ms and velocity encoded value (VENC) should be kept at 25–50 cm/sec.

Advantages of MRA:
- Absence of ionizing radiation
- Production of 3D arteriogram not affected by calcific plaques
- Phase contrast studies can provide information about blood flow velocity also (as phase is related to time)
- Multiplanar reconstructions
- Evaluation of renal masses and renal excretion function.

Drawbacks of MRA:
- High cost
- Limited availability
- Artifacts due to bowel peristalsis
- Evaluation of branch vessels and detection of accessory arteries are a challenge
- Tendency toward overestimation of stenosis.
- The presence of a metallic stent also hampers evaluation.

The MRI is also being evaluated in acquiring the functional data that can provide comprehensive assessment of renal morphology and renal function prior to any intervention.[39]

Dynamic contrast-enhanced (DCE) MRI is a technique in which fast repetitious imaging of the kidney is performed using first pass of the contrast agent. In a series, significant correlations between raising serum creatinine levels and decreasing renal perfusion parameters are found indicating that renal first pass perfusion may reflect, at least to a certain degree of renal function.[40] The DCE-MRI can evaluate the kidneys after the placement of stents which otherwise cannot be assessed due to susceptibility artifacts. In such situations, demonstration of normal perfusion parameters proves the patency of stent.

Noncontrast-enhanced MRI of the renal arteries:[37] Various noncontrast MRA techniques have evaluated such as TOF, PC, SSFP, and ASL **(Fig. 13)**.
- *Time-of-flight MRA:* Signal in TOF MRA is produced by unsaturated blood flowing into the plane of imaging

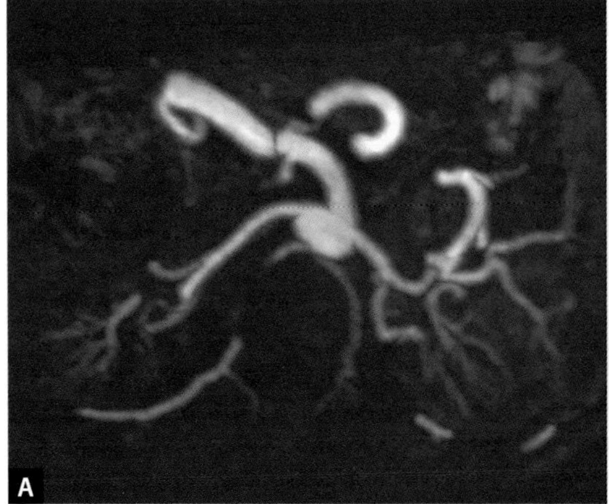

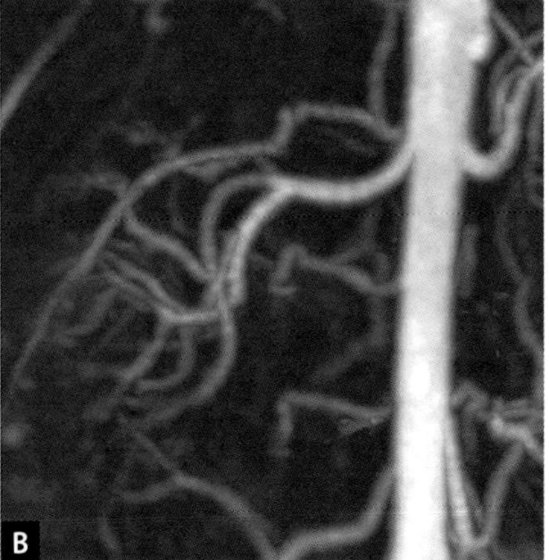

Figs. 12A and B: (A) 3D CE-MRA axial and (B) coronal section reveal the anatomy of main renal artery as well as segmental branches in great details (3D CE-MRA: three-dimensional contrast-enhanced magnetic resonance angiography).

(flow related enhancement). TOF MRA is not an useful technique for the evaluation of renal arteries because of the following reasons:

- It tends to overestimate the degree of stenosis, in particular 2D techniques do not compensate for vessel tortuosity and therefore, tend to overestimate vessels stenosis
- Loss of signal in slow flow when vessel is oriented in axial plane (in-plane saturation)
- Inherently a slow technique requiring several minutes, causing breathing related degradation or extremely long scan times for signal averaging
- Poor visualization of the distal arterial segment where flow is slow.

- *Phase-contrast MRA*: It depicts not only the morphologic nature of a stenosis, but also provides quantitative analysis of flow dynamics in RAS. Combining PC with cardiac gating, a 2D velocity map can be obtained, which is termed as "quantitative" or "q" flow. With this flow maps similar to Doppler ultrasound can be generated and analyzed.
- *Steady-state free precession MRA*: 3D SSFP with short echo and repetition times is the most promising noncontrast bright blood technique for evaluation of renal arteries as it is intrinsically fast, high in signal-to-noise ratio (SNR), and flow compensated in all the three axis. SSFP, either breath-hold or navigator-gated can be performed as a first-line MRA technique to rule out RAS especially in patients in risk of NSF. If SSFP is negative for high-grade RAS (>50%), RAS can be excluded without using any gadolinium-based contrast agents, vice-a-versa if SSFP is positive, then further studies [contrast-enhanced MRI, digital subtraction angiography (DSA), CTA] can be done for better delineation of stenosis.
- *Arterial spin labeling*: Arterial spin labeling uses blood as an endogenous contrast agent to obtain angiograms with an advantage to obtain tissue perfusion as well. The perfusion parameters are being investigated and initial reports suggest a good correlation with scintigraphy.

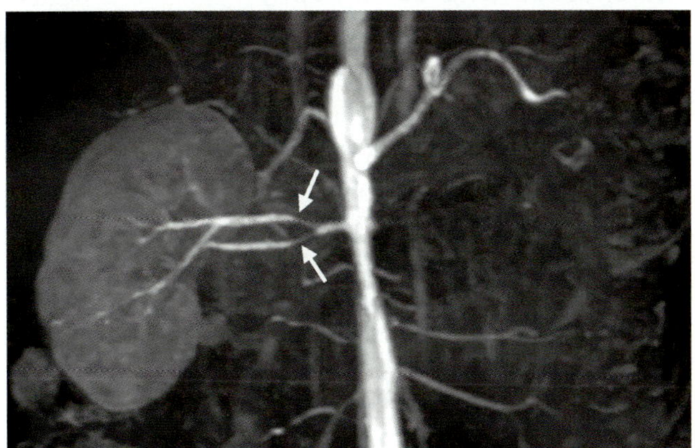

Fig. 13: Noncontrast MRA (SSFP) reveals stenosis (arrows) in both upper and lower division of the right renal artery in a patient with Takayasu's arteritis (MRA: magnetic resonance angiography; SSFP: steady-state free precession).

Renal Angiography

Conventional angiography (or DSA) is the gold standard for diagnosis of RAS. However, its invasiveness prevents it from becoming a screening test. All patients proceeding to percutaneous treatment of RAS initially undergo diagnostic angiography as part of the procedure.

Angiographic evaluation should include aortography and bilateral selective renal arteriography. The initial aortogram is necessary to evaluate the renal artery ostia, identifying accessory renal arteries, and avoid mistaking guidewire-induced arterial spasm for fixed disease.

Flush aortography is usually adequate to demonstrate main renal arteries and any proximal renal stenosis **(Fig. 14)**. When intrarenal or branch artery stenosis are suspected selective injections are necessary. Because the origin of right renal artery is anterolateral and left renal artery is posterolateral, an ostial lesion may be missed on an AP aortogram due to overlap by the opacified aorta, superimposition of intrarenal vessels may also mask stenosis. Depending on the site of stenosis oblique/lateral view, cranial/caudal angulation or magnification views may be required to optimally delineate stenosis.[41]

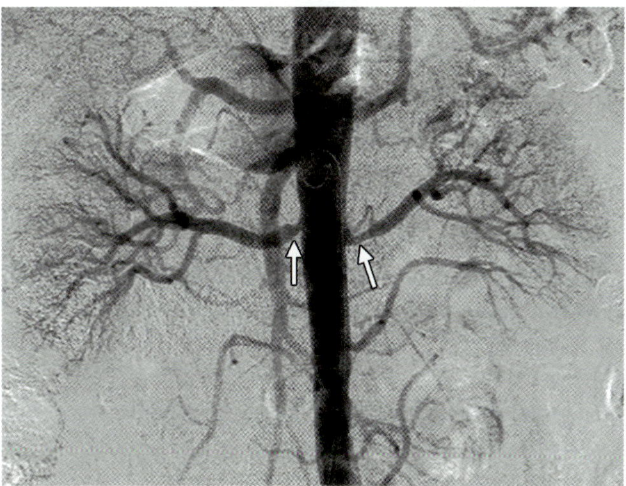

Fig. 14: Digital subtraction angiography flush aortography demonstrates bilateral proximal renal artery stenoses (RAS) in a patient with atherosclerotic RAS.

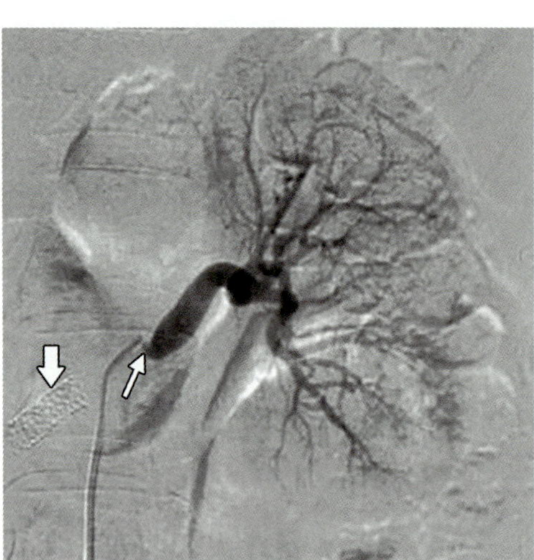

Fig. 15: Selective angiogram of left renal artery shows approximately 90% ostioproximal stenosis (thin arrow) of the left renal artery and poststenotic dilatation in a patient with atherosclerosis. Stenting (thick arrow) had previously been done for contralateral renal artery.

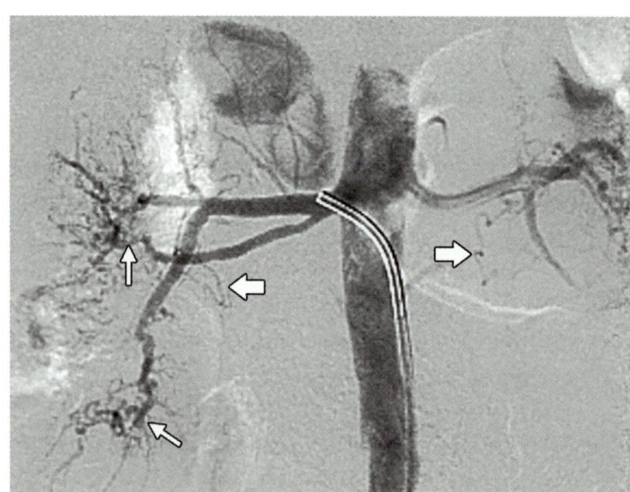

Fig. 16: Digital subtraction angiography reveals diffuse irregularities and stenoses (thin arrow) in the intrarenal vessels with multiple collaterals (thick arrows) in a patient with vasculitis.

Society for Cardiovascular Angiography and Interventions (SCAI) recommends DSA as the gold standard for invasive assessment of hemodynamically significant RAS and categorizes stenosis severity as follows:

- *Mild*: <50%
- *Moderate*: 50–70%
- *Severe*: >70%—hemodynamically significant **(Fig. 15)**

Other criteria for hemodynamic significance are:

- Systolic pressure gradient >20 mm Hg across the stenosis
- Evidence of collateral circulation into distal vessel
- Poststenotic dilatation
- Renal fractional flow reserve (FFR) ≤ 0.8.

Pressure gradients are the most accurate indicator of hemodynamic significance.

Advantages of conventional angiography/DSA:

- High resolution of the technique
- Visualizing branch renal artery stenosis
- Pressure gradients can be measured to assess hemodynamic significance
- Selective renal catheterization may be followed by appropriate intervention in the same sitting
- Allows for evaluation of collaterals and intrarenal vasculature with high accuracy **(Fig. 16)**.

Limitations of arteriography:

- Expensive
- Invasive
- Use of iodinated contrast
- Angiography only provides intraluminal information; no intramural information is gained about the vessel wall or plaques
- Transient decrease in renal function may occur in up to 5% patients
- Access site complications, RA dissection, thromboembolism.

Flowchart 3 demonstrates the diagnostic algorithm commonly followed for RVH.

Table 3 demonstrates the imaging findings in various common etiologies of RVH.

Radionuclide Renal Scintigraphy

Radionuclide renal scintigraphy especially with ACE inhibitors is highly sensitive and accurate in detection of unilateral RAS but its accuracy decreases in patients suffering from bilateral RAS or azotemia and in patients with single functioning kidney.[42]

Radionuclide imaging of the kidney is the most widely performed screening test for the diagnosis of RVH I-131 orthoiodohippurate (OIH) was used in the past. Currently technetium 99m (99mTc) die-thylenetriaminepentaacetic acid (DTPA) (marker of GFR) and mercaptoacetic triglyceride (MAG 3) (secreted by proximal tubule) are commonly used for isotope renography.

The standard renogram reflects the salt and water retention on the ischemic side by demonstrating slow transit and excretion of radiotracer. The classic

Flowchart 3: Diagnostic algorithm for RVH.

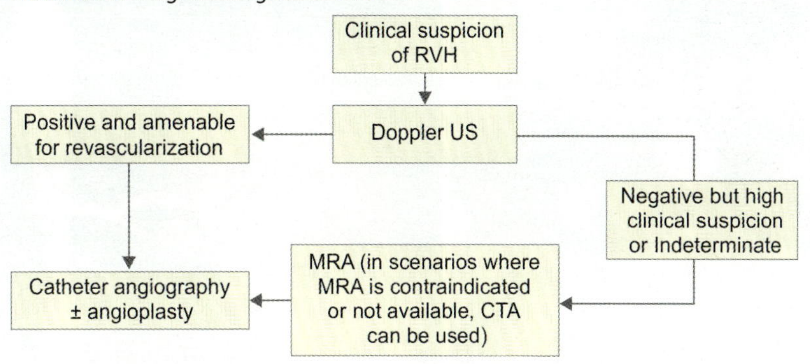

Table 3: Imaging findings in various common etiologies of renovascular hypertension (RVH).

Etiology	*CTA*	*MRA*	*DSA*
Atherosclerosis **(Figs. 1, 14, and 16)**	• Focal/segmental, eccentric stenosis • *Location*: Ostium or proximal 2 cm of RA • Bilateral disease is common • Calcifications • Infrarenal aortic involvement usually exist • Coronary, carotid involvement seen	• Limited role as calcification may cause artifacts • Same findings as CTA except that calcifications not well seen	• Irregular circumferential or eccentric narrowing of the ostium or proximal third of the renal arteries • Calcification visible • Intrarenal vessels usually not involved • Collaterals can be seen
Aortoarteritis **(Figs. 17 and 18)**	• Mural thickening of aorta, aortic arch branches and other involved vessels • Better for ostial ostioproximal involvement • Steno-occlusive or dilatative lesions depending on the type • Delayed enhancement of the vessel wall suggests active disease • Calcification sets in when there is accelerated atherosclerosis	• Useful tool • Whole body 3D MRA can reveal other vascular involvement • 3D space—can reveal wall thickening • T2 hyperintensity in wall—sensitive marker for active disease	• Involves aorta, its major branches and PAs—mainly ostioproximal segments • Intrarenal vessels may be involved • Midsegment involvement better seen
FMD **(Fig. 2)**	• Focal concentric narrowing of distal two-thirds main RA and intrarenal branches • The right kidney is affected more commonly than the left • Bilateral disease may be seen in about two-thirds of cases • Aorta is usually disease free • Calcification uncommon	• MR usually less useful as it is not an optimal modality for evaluation of distal vessels. Intrarenal stenoses can be missed • Sensitivities of only 22–28% have been noted with MRA and CTA in this setting	• Middle to distal renal arteries • Less commonly intrarenal branches • Often, poststenotic dilatation • The classic appearance of the medial fibroplasia type—String of beads. • Aneurysms can be seen
PAN **(Figs. 19A and B)**	• Vessel stenoses (renal, mesenteric, peripheral arteries) • Microaneurysms • Intra-abdominal organ infarcts, and/or bowel thickening	Not much helpful due to artifacts due to peristalsis	• Stenoses • Microaneurysms • Infarcts • In abdominal aortic branches

(CTA: computed tomography angiography; DSA: digital subtraction angiography; FMD: fibromuscular dysplasia; MRA: magnetic resonance angiography; PAN: polyarteritis nodosa RA: renal artery)

appearance is that of a small kidney with decreased uptake and delayed tracer transit and excretion. Captopril renal scintigraphy can be used as a screening test, to establish the hemodynamic significance of RAS, to predict the outcome of revascularization and in the follow-up after successful revascularization.

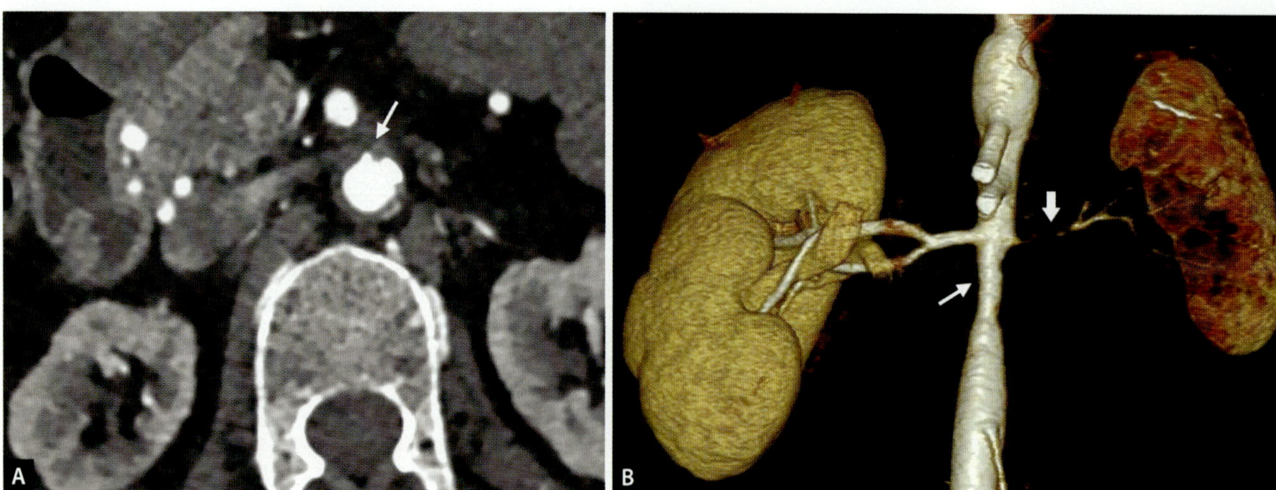

Figs. 17A and B: Takayasu's arteritis: (A) Axial CTA image reveals circumferential wall thickening of aorta (arrow) in a patient with Takayasu's arteritis; (B) VRT in a different patient reveals diffuse tight 99% stenosis of the left renal artery (thick arrow). Additionally, narrowing of the juxtarenal aorta (thin arrow) can also be seen in (B) (CTA: computed tomography angiography; VRT: volume-rendering technique).

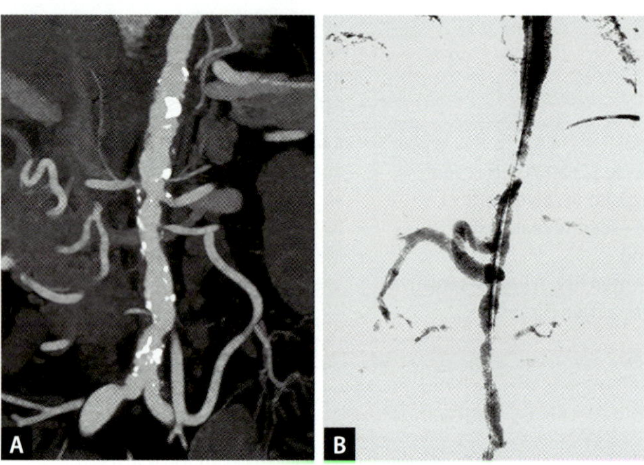

Figs. 18A and B: Takayasu's arteritis: (A) MIP coronal CT and (B) DSA reveal tight ostioproximal RRA stenosis approximately 50% LRA stenosis with accelerated atherosclerosis (calcifications) and diffuse involvement of abdominal aorta (DSA: digital subtraction angiography; LRA: left renal artery; MIP: maximum intensity projection).

Principles of ACE inhibitor (captopril) scintigraphy: In a patient with a significant RAS the efferent arterioles of the glomeruli are constricted by angiotensin II to maintain glomerular filtration pressure in the face of diminished afferent arteriolar pressure.

Administration of ACE inhibitor decreases this angiotensin related constriction of efferent arterioles which reduces glomerular filtration and hence urine flow. ACE inhibitor does not affect GFR in patients with normal renal arteries or those with essential hypertension.

Protocol: ACE inhibitor scintigraphy is performed 1 hour after the oral dose of 25 mg of captopril or 15 minutes after an intravenous dose of 0.04 mg/kg of enalapril maleate. Patients are well-hydrated, are taken off antihypertensive medication 2–5 days prior to the study according to the half-life. Resting blood pressure is monitored. After a baseline study, the scan is repeated 30 minutes after administration of ACE inhibitor. Time-activity curves are generated from renal cortex and pelvis.

Results: A positive result is said to be present if there is a decrease in uptake and delayed clearance by the affected kidney on the post-captopril study compared to the baseline study or if there is exaggeration of the baseline asymmetry between the normal and abnormal kidney in patients with unilateral RAS.

The overall sensitivity and specificity of the test exceeds 90% in most series with a few exceptions.[43] Advantages include low cost, relative reliability, and noninvasive nature. A positive captopril renography may suggest a cure or improvement in blood pressure after intervention. It may also be used in the follow-up of patients after intervention. Disadvantages and pitfalls include low sensitivity in patients with azotemia or underlying renal dysfunction and in patients with bilateral RAS. Branch artery stenosis cannot be diagnosed. It has a low spatial resolution and provides functional nonanatomic data. In patients who develop severe hypotension in response to captopril, bilateral symmetric parenchymal retention may be seen (false positive). Symmetrical retention even in the absence of hypotension is usually a false positive finding. Presence of pelvic retention may complicate interpretation of cortical retention and scintigraphy must be interpreted with caution in the presence of pelvic retention.[44]

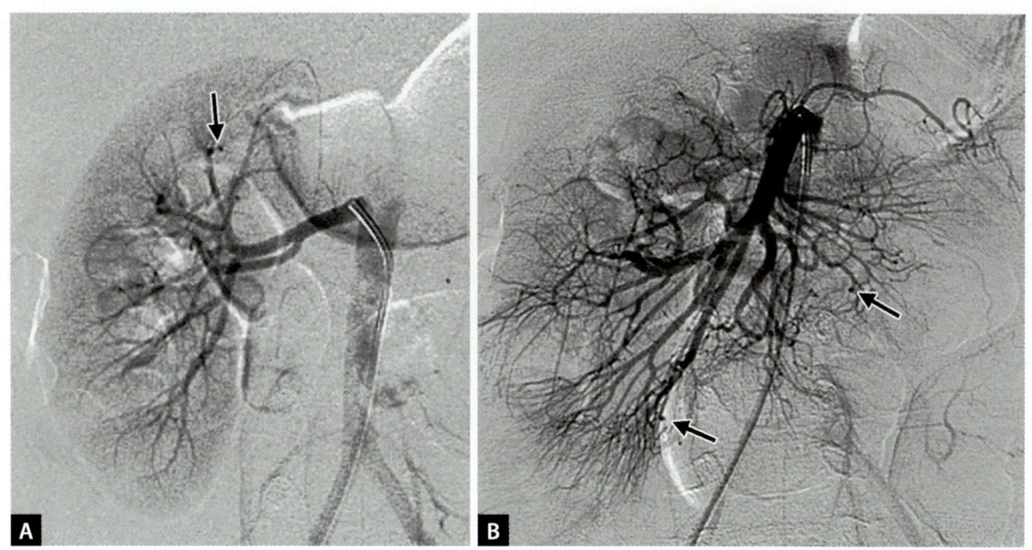

Figs. 19A and B: (A) Renal and (B) SMA arteriograms (DSA) reveal multiple microaneurysms in both vascular territories in a patient with PAN (DSA: digital subtraction angiography; PAN: polyarteritis nodosa; SMA: superior mesenteric artery).

Plasma renin activity (PRA): Peripheral venous PRA is elevated in only 50–80% of patients with RVH. The predictive value of the PRA can be increased by measuring the rise in PRA 1 hour after the administration of 25–50 mg of captopril. A positive test is when postcaptopril renin level is above 12 ng/mL, increases by 10 ng/mL/h or more, and is at least 150% above the baseline value. Patients with RAS have an exaggerated increase in the PRA as perhaps due to removal of the normal suppressive effect of high angiotensin II levels.

Renal vein renin measurements: It more precise estimation of "pressor kidney" renin that is ≥1.5 times the value from the contralateral kidney which is suppressed in RVH. It can be helpful in bilateral RAS in whom RV renin measurements can be used to determine which side contributes most to the hypertension or in patients considered for nephrectomy of a pressor kidney.

Newer Modalities

Intravascular ultrasound is the best modality for the correct evaluation of stenosis and plaque morphology, but it being invasive and expensive it is unlikely to become a screening modality.[35]

It allows for characterization of vessel wall layers and hence can help in identification of disease etiology.

Optical Coherence Tomography

The advantages of OCT include demonstration of the layers of arterial wall, pathological findings of the disease, and to guide percutaneous interventions. The major limitation of OCT is its lower penetration, which may cause imaging of large vessels difficult.

INDICATIONS OF REVASCULARIZATION AND TREATMENT OPTIONS

The ACC/AHA guidelines recommend percutaneous revascularization in patients with hemodynamically significant RAS and any of the following:[18]

- Recurrent congestive heart failure or sudden unexplained pulmonary edema (class I)
- Accelerated, resistant, or malignant hypertension or hypertension with unexplained unilateral small kidney and intolerance to medication (class IIa)
- Unstable angina (class IIa)
- Asymptomatic bilateral or single functioning kidney (class IIb)
- In addition, percutaneous revascularization is reasonable for patients with progressive CKD and bilateral RAS or a RAS to a single functioning kidney and can be considered for unilateral RAS with chronic renal insufficiency.

Before percutaneous transluminal renal angioplasty (PTRA) is performed the salvage ability of the procedure must be established. The commonly used criteria are:

- Residual function-single kidney GFR by radionuclide studies
- Kidney size of 8–9 cm
- Renal biopsy showing preservation of glomeruli and tubule

- Presence of collateral circulation to intrarenal vessels confirmed by arteriography. Revascularization is usually not beneficial in patients with severe renal failure (serum creatinine > 4.0 mg/dL).

The SCAI concluded that patients with any of the following are typically not good candidates for renal artery stenting: mild or moderate blockages (less than 70%), long-standing loss of blood flow or complete blockage of the renal artery.

Atherosclerotic Renal Artery Stenosis

There are three primary modes of treatment for renovascular hypertension: (1) Medical therapy, (2) surgery, and (3) angioplasty. First-line treatment is optimal medical therapy.

Percutaneous Transluminal Renal Angioplasty and Stenting

Percutaneous transluminal renal angioplasty and stenting are justified in selected patients who have both normal renal function and normal blood pressure because of the natural history of RAS to progress and ultimately result in impaired renal function.

The ACA/AHA and ESC recommend renal stent placement for ostial atherosclerotic renal artery stenosis (ARAS) (class I). If untreated, there is high probability of progression to complete occlusion. PTRA is best suited to discrete tight concentric, short segment stenosis located away from ostium and branches of renal arteries. Eccentric, long segment and calcified lesions, occlusion in tortuous vessels, stenosis adjacent to an aneurysm and occlusion or stenosis with a thrombus increase the risk of complications and reduce the likelihood of success **(Figs. 20A and B)**.[13]

Renal Artery Stenting

Angioplasty failure is an absolute indication for stenting. The criteria for angioplasty failure include: residual stenosis of more than 30%, residual aortorenal pressure gradient of > 20 mm Hg, acute occlusive, flow limiting dissection flap and late restenosis (recurrent stenosis > 50%) **(Figs. 20A and B)**.[45]

In selected patients in whom the risk of intervention or anatomic considerations make a repeat procedure in the future unlikely primary stenting is justifiable. It should be the technique of choice for ostial atherosclerotic RAS.

Outcome: Success in renal revascularization can be judged by the technical success of angioplasty and by the clinical response. Criteria for technical and clinical success are given later in this chapter. The results of PTRA depend on the type of lesion, indication for treatment, and factors such as age, coexistent essential hypertension, and nephrosclerosis.

For atherosclerotic lesions both angiographic and clinical results for nonostial stenosis are superior to those for ostial stenosis (within 2–10 mm of aortic lumen). Technical success occurs in 75–95% cases, although some authors have reported lower rates of 43% for nonostial lesions and 29% for ostial lesions. Long-term clinical

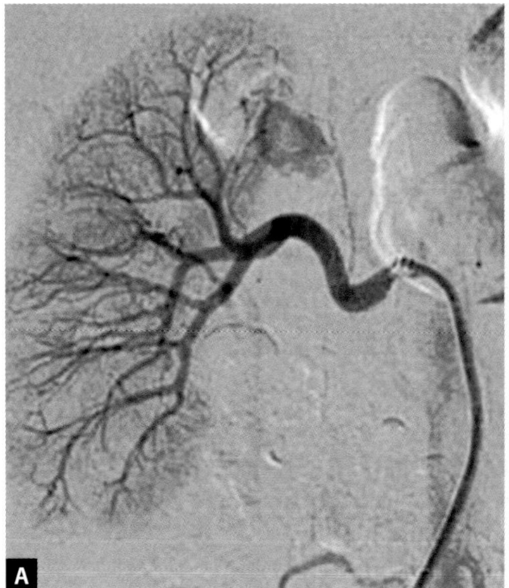

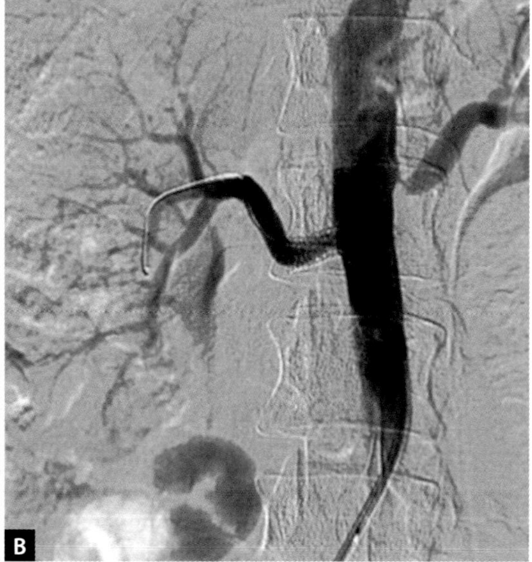

Figs. 20A and B: In-stent restenosis is seen on (A) DSA in a previously treated patient of atherosclerotic RAS and (B) reveals luminal opening after angioplasty within the stent (DSA: digital subtraction angiography; RAS: renal artery stenosis).

benefit is seen in 76% patients with ostial lesions and 83% patients with nonostial lesions.[46]

Lesser success can be expected in patients with bilateral RAS, generalized atherosclerosis, with heavily calcified or segmental artery lesion. For renal salvage the results are less favorable and improvement is seen in 40–60% cases.

Surgical revascularization can be considered if multiple small renal arteries are present or there is a primary early branching of renal artery (class 1 ACC)

Takayasu's Arteritis/Nonspecific Aortoarteritis

The diffuse nature of the disease and complexity of pathological changes in the vessel wall make surgical revascularization difficult. Graft occlusion is also common. Hence, current guidelines recommend endovascular as the initial treatment.

Since chances of dissection or restenosis are more in active disease, endovascular treatment is not recommended unless there are absolute indications indications like:

- Refractory hypertension
- "Flash" pulmonary edema or severe left ventricular dysfunction
- Hypertensive retinopathy, cerebropathy.

Specific technical difficulties may be encountered during PTRA for aortoarteritis because of the tough noncompliant nature of the stenosis which is difficult to cross and resists repeated prolonged balloon dilatation. Patients may also develop hypotension and backache during the procedure **(Figs. 21A to C)**.[47]

However, reports have shown high rate of technical success and frequently good clinical response. One large series including 193 patients reported technical success rate of 96%, clinical benefit of 91%, complication rate of 5.8%, restenosis rate of 17% and 5-year patency rate of 67%. Factors predicting restenosis included ostial stenosis, residual stenosis of more than 30%, residual gradient of more than 10 mm Hg after angioplasty, juxtadiaphragmatic aortic stenosis, and active disease.[48]

Following angioplasty for any cause at least 3–6 months of follow-up is required to assess durability of clinical response.

Primary stenting of renal artery stenoses is not recommended in Takayasu's arteritis as:

- Patients are young and the vessel can outgrow the stent.
- The anatomy is often complex with diffuse disease involving the aorto-ostial region and extending to the renal artery bifurcation
- The risk of in-stent restenosis is higher.

Stenting is usually reserved as a bailout procedure for complications like obstructive dissection, arising out of angioplasty. Balloon mounted stents are preferred. If there is significant residual stenosis, cutting balloons are an option.

Surgical Therapy

Surgical revascularization is now indicated only in situations where PTRA fails or is contraindicated.

Techniques include aortorenal, lienorenal, ileorenal arterial bypass, nephrectomy, and autorenal transplantation.

Fibromuscular Dysplasia

If technically feasible, PTRA should be attempted on all patients with FMD. The ACC/AHA gives a class I recommendation for balloon angioplasty with ballout stent placement if necessary for fibromuscular dysplasia lesions. The results in FMD are uniformly good. Technical

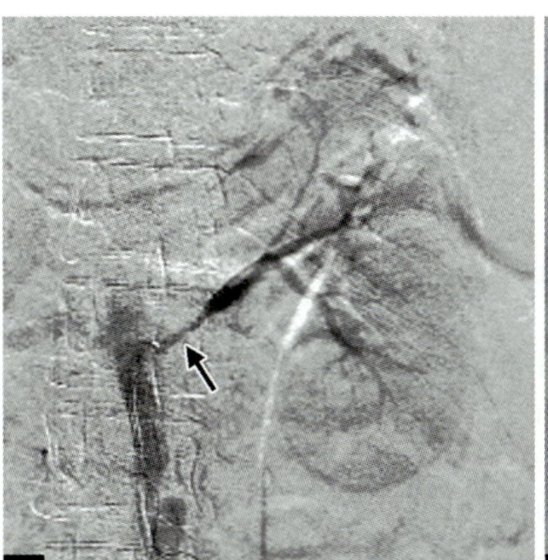

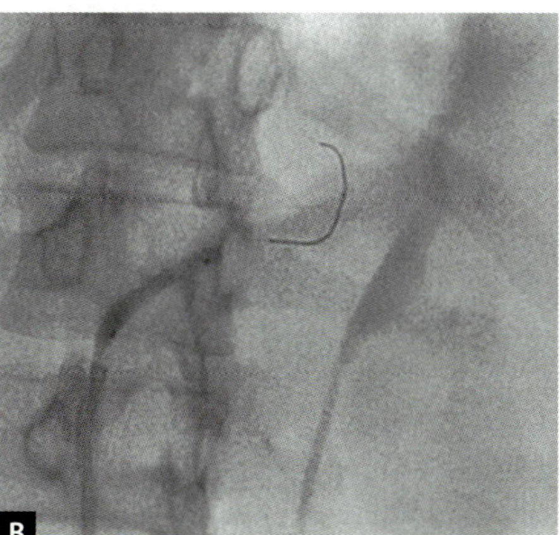

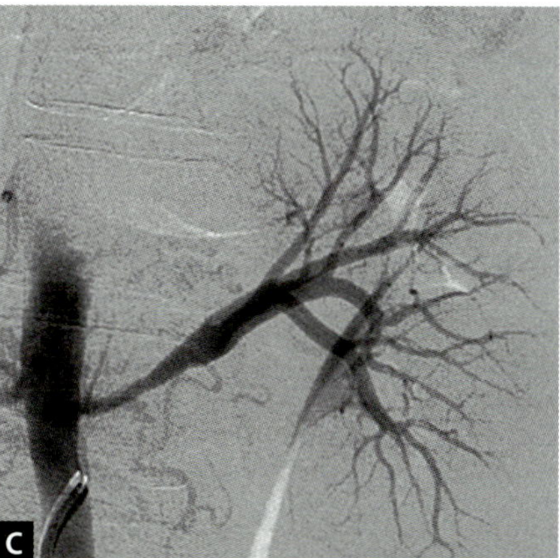

Figs. 21A to C: Percutaneous transluminal angioplasty for Takayasu's arteritis: (A) Initial angiogram which reveals approximately 95–99% stenosis of left renal artery (arrow); (B) Figure B shows balloon inflation at the site of stenosis; (C) Postangioplasty angiogram shows significant improvement in luminal caliber.

success is achieved in 90–100% patients. Hypertension is cured or improved in 98% patients. Intimal FMD may require much greater pressures than medial fibroplasia type of FMD. Restenosis is uncommon in these patients and primary patency at 15 months is 92%.

Spasm more likely during angioplasty. Liberal use of NTG is recommended. Cutting balloons can be used for intimal fibroplasia type. Stenting is only done as a bailout procedure.

Surgical revascularization is a class 1 indication for complex FMD extending into bifurcation or those with aneurysms.

Renal Artery Stenosis in Children[49]

Although RAS is uncommon in children the incidence is much higher in children with hypertension than in adults. About 4–20% of children with hypertension have RAS.

Causes

Fibromuscular dysplasia: The classical string of beads appearance is rarely seen with intimal fibroplasia being the most common type of lesion. The lesions are more often found in boys unlike adults. Branch artery stenosis is also more common.

Neurofibromatosis: Stenosis of bilateral proximal renal arteries is the main finding in RAS associated with neurofibromatosis. This may be associated with hypoplasia of abdominal aorta.

Nonspecific aortoarteritis and middle aortic syndrome are other important causes.

Because of the higher incidence of RAS in children with hypertension patients with a strong clinical suspicion often undergo DSA.

Percutaneous transluminal renal angioplasty is being used with increasing frequency in children, however, the success rate is lower than adults for two reasons—smaller size of vessels and more frequent vasospasm make children more difficult to angiogram and dilate. Adult FMD and atherosclerosis respond well to PTRA while children have a more fibrotic process that cannot be adequately dilated.

TRIAL EVIDENCE

Numerous studies have looked into the outcomes of different therapies for renal artery stenoses.

The major studies comparing initial angioplasty without stenting with optimal medical therapy are EMMA (Essai Multicentrique Medicaments vs Angioplastie),[50] the Scottish and Newcastle Renal Artery Stenosis trial,[51] and the DRASTIC (the Dutch Renal Artery Stenosis Intervention Cooperative).[52] A meta-analysis of these trials suggested that there was a small but significant decrease in the blood pressures (mean change in systolic/diastolic pressures = 6.3/3.3 mm Hg, $p = 0.02/0.03$) in the angioplasty group when compared to those receiving only optimal medical therapy. Also, there was some decrease in serum creatinine levels as well, but it was not significant ($p = 0.06$).

Many studies have also compared the results of optimal medical therapy with angioplasty and stenting. The ASTRAL study was a randomized trial to evaluate if renal revascularization delays the decline of renal function when compared to optimal medical therapy. The study did not show any additional advantage of revascularization for rate of decline of renal function. However, this study did not include patients in whom revascularization is often required and performed, that is patients with flash pulmonary edema, critical RAS or uncontrolled hypertension. Also, it did not study the effect of revascularization in BP control.[53] Similar results were obtained from STAR trial (revascularization versus medical therapy for renal artery stenosis).[54] CORAL (Cardiovascular Outcomes in Renal Atherosclerotic Lesions) study is the most recent study which included 947 patients with RAS of at least 60% diameter, (ASTRAL and STAR studies used 40% as cutoff) and significant hypertension. These patients were randomized to receive either optimal medical therapy alone or medical therapy with renal arterial stenting. Stenting did not offer any additional benefit to prevent death from MACE, hospitalization, heart failure, progression of renal failure or need for renal replacement therapy.[55]

ENDOVASCULAR TREATMENT: TECHNICAL CONSIDERATIONS

Endovascular management of RAS includes angioplasty of the stenosed segment with or without stent placement, the procedure is known as PTRA. The procedure includes taking a vascular access, usually the common femoral route or may be brachial artery approach depending on ease of renal artery cannulation. A flush aortogram is done by a pigtail catheter which has multiple side holes, to delineate the origin of the renal arteries, any accessory renal arteries and also to rule out any other abdominal vascular involvement. Further, a double curve catheter is used to hook the ostium of each of the renal arteries and a selective angiogram is done. After establishing the diagnosis and identifying the stenosed segment, a balloon angioplasty is planned if the lesion is significantly stenosed. Significant stenosis is defined as a stenosis more than 50% for renal arteries, or that causing post-stenotic dilatation or any lesion that has a pressure gradient of 20 mm Hg across it.

For PTRA, a renal guiding catheter (usually 7Fr) is taken to provide a route for exchange of balloons and wires and also to do angiograms. Usually the balloons which are selected are compatible with 0.014" or 0.018 guidewires and are a monorail system (common lumen for wire and balloon). Size of the balloon is decided by using distal vessel diameter as reference. The balloon is advanced via the guide catheter over the wire and put across the lesion. The position of the balloon is checked by doing a check angiogram with the guiding catheter. Balloons are inflated for 1–2 minutes at their nominal pressures. Postangioplasty, a repeat angiogram is done to look for technical success or any complications. Primary stenting is usually done in case of atherosclerotic ostial RAS.

Technical success is defined as either of:

- Increase in the luminal diameter by 50%
- Residual stenosis of less than 30%, or
- Residual gradient of less than 20 mm Hg.

For clinical success:

- Patients are considered cured if normal BP is obtained without antihypertensive regimen.
- Improved if there is at least a 15% reduction in diastolic pressure or the diastolic pressure is less than 90 mm Hg with the patient taking less medication than before the procedure
- Failed if there is no change in BP after the procedure
- In patients treated for renal salvage a reduction in serum creatinine levels of >20% may be considered successful treatment.

Complications: Complication rate in PTRA varies from 3% to 6%. Complications include those related to the arteriographic procedure and those due to angioplasty and stenting. These include renal artery injury, guidewire perforation of kidney, flow limiting renal artery dissection **(Fig. 22)**, renal artery thrombosis, renal artery rupture. There may be puncture site complications such as hematoma, pseudoaneurysm or at the level of renal arteries because of selective catheterization. Stent-related complications include stent malposition, misdeployment of stent, endovascular infection, and cholesterol embolization.

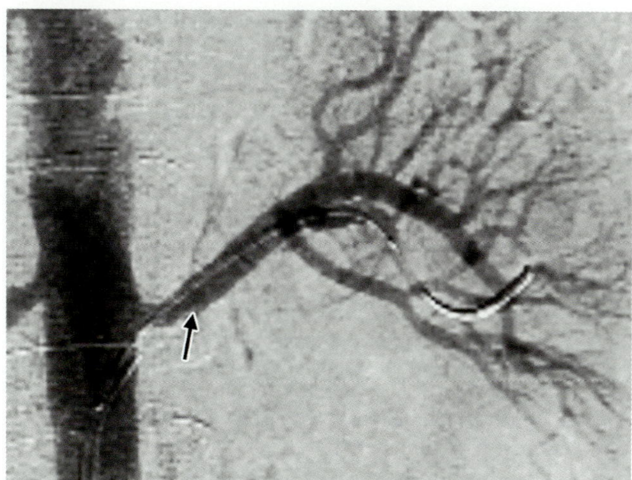

Fig. 22: Complication: Post-PTRA, small nonobstructive dissection flap is seen in LRA (arrow). (LRA: left renal artery; PTRA: percutaneous transluminal renal angioplasty).

CONCLUSION

The prevalence of RVH is 1–5%. Atherosclerotic renal artery disease (RAD) is the most common cause of "renovascular hypertension". Renal artery stenosis should be considered in any patient with refractory or severe hypertension, or those with declining renal function or those who have atherosclerosis in other vessels. ACC/ESC suggests test only those patients who are thought to have a high likelihood of benefiting from the procedure. Initial workup includes renal function tests, ultrasound with Doppler, etc. If Doppler is positive, patients may proceed directly to noninvasive angiography. If Doppler is inconclusive or not available MRA, preferred over CTA can be used. Arteriography is gold standard for diagnosing RAS and should be done in all patients who are planned for intervention or if all other modalities are inconclusive/negative and clinical suspicion is high. Optimal medical therapy, balloon angioplasty with or without stenting or surgical revascularization can be considered in suitable patients depending on the characteristics of the lesion.

REFERENCES

1. Whelton PK, Carey RM, Aronow WS, et al. 2017 ACC/AHA/AAPA/ABC/ACPM/AGS/APhA/ASH/ASPC/NMA/PCNA Guideline for the Prevention, Detection, Evaluation, and Management of High Blood Pressure in Adults: Executive Summary: A Report of the American College of Cardiology/American Heart Association Task Force on Clinical Practice Guidelines. Hypertension. 2018;71(6):1269-324.
2. Anchala R, Kannuri NK, Pant H, et al. Hypertension in India: a systematic review and meta-analysis of prevalence, awareness, and control of hypertension. J Hypertens. 2014;32(6):1170-7.
3. Soulez G, Oliva VL, Turpin S, et al. Imaging of renovascular hypertension: respective values of renal scintigraphy, renal Doppler US, and MR angiography. Radiographics. 2000;20(5):1355-68.

4. Circulation (2005). ACC/AHA 2005 Practice Guidelines for the Management of Patients With Peripheral Arterial Disease (Lower Extremity, Renal, Mesenteric, and Abdominal Aortic). [online] Available from https://ahajournals.org/doi/10.1161/circulationaha.106.174526. [Last accessed October, 2019].
5. Mann SJ, Pickering TG. Detection of renovascular hypertension. State of the art: 1992. Ann Intern Med. 1992;117(10):845-53.
6. Olin JW, Melia M, Young JR, et al. Prevalence of atherosclerotic renal artery stenosis in patients with atherosclerosis elsewhere. Am J Med. 1990;88(1N):46N-51N.
7. American College of Physicians (1993). Annals of Internal Medicine. Atherosclerotic renovascular disease and progressive renal failure. [online] Available from https://annals.org/aim/article-abstract/706341/atherosclerotic-renovascular-disease-progressive-renal-failure. [Last accessed October, 2019].
8. Jennings CG, Houston JG, Severn A, et al. Renal artery stenosis-when to screen, what to stent? Curr Atheroscler Rep. 2014;16(6):416.
9. 1995 update of the working group reports on chronic renal failure and renovascular hypertension. National High Blood Pressure Education Program Working Group. Arch Intern Med. 1996;156(17):1938-47.
10. Brunner HR, Kirshman JD, Sealey JE, et al. Hypertension of renal origin: evidence for two different mechanisms. Science. 1971;174(4016):1344-6.
11. Textor SC, Lerman L. Renovascular hypertension and ischemic nephropathy. Am J Hypertens. 2010;23(11):1159-69.
12. Chugh KS, Jain S, Sakhuja V, et al. Renovascular hypertension due to Takayasu's arteritis among Indian patients. Q J Med. 1992;85(307-308):833-43.
13. Lao D, Parasher PS, Cho KC, Yeghiazarians Y. Atherosclerotic renal artery stenosis—diagnosis and treatment. Mayo Clin Proc. 2011;86(7):649-57.
14. Matsunaga N, Hayashi K, Sakamoto I, et al. Takayasu arteritis: protean radiologic manifestations and diagnosis. Radiogr Rev Publ Radiol Soc N Am Inc. 1997;17(3):579-94.
15. Zhu FP, Luo S, Wang ZJ, et al. Takayasu arteritis: imaging spectrum at multidetector CT angiography. Br J Radiol. 2012;85(1020):e1282-92.
16. Hata A, Noda M, Moriwaki R, et al. Angiographic findings of Takayasu arteritis: new classification. Int J Cardiol. 1996;54 Suppl:S155-63.
17. Sharma S, Rajani M, Talwar KK. Angiographic morphology in nonspecific aortoarteritis (Takayasu's arteritis): a study of 126 patients from north India. Cardiovasc Intervent Radiol. 1992;15(3):160-5.
18. Anderson JL, Halperin JL, Albert NM, et al. Management of patients with peripheral artery disease (compilation of 2005 and 2011 ACCF/AHA guideline recommendations): a report of the American College of Cardiology Foundation/American Heart Association Task Force on Practice Guidelines. Circulation. 2013;127(13):1425-43.
19. Aboyans V, Ricco JB, Bartelink MLEL, et al. 2017 ESC Guidelines on the Diagnosis and Treatment of Peripheral Arterial Diseases, in collaboration with the European Society for Vascular Surgery (ESVS). Document covering atherosclerotic disease of extracranial carotid and vertebral, mesenteric, renal, upper and lower extremity arteriesEndorsed by: the European Stroke Organization (ESO)The Task Force for the Diagnosis and Treatment of Peripheral Arterial Diseases of the European Society of Cardiology (ESC) and of the European Society for Vascular Surgery (ESVS). Eur Heart J. 2018;39(9):763-816.
20. Harden PN, MacLeod MJ, Rodger RS, et al. Effect of renal-artery stenting on progression of renovascular renal failure. Lancet Lond Engl. 1997;349(9059):1133-6.
21. Preston RA, Epstein M. Ischemic renal disease: an emerging cause of chronic renal failure and end-stage renal disease. J Hypertens. 1997;15(12 Pt 1):1365-77.
22. Watson PS, Hadjipetrou P, Cox SV, et al. Effect of renal artery stenting on renal function and size in patients with atherosclerotic renovascular disease. Circulation. 2000;102(14):1671-7.
23. Dellegrottaglie S, Sanz J, Rajagopalan S. Technology insight: Clinical role of magnetic resonance angiography in the diagnosis and management of renal artery stenosis. Nat Clin Pract Cardiovasc Med. 2006;3(6):329-38.
24. Guzman RP, Zierler RE, Isaacson JA, et al. Renal atrophy and arterial stenosis. A prospective study with duplex ultrasound. Hypertens Dallas Tex 1979. 1994;23(3):346-350. doi:10.1161/01.hyp.23.3.346.
25. Haan MW de, Kroon AA, Flobbe K, et al. Renovascular disease in patients with hypertension: detection with duplex ultrasound. J Hum Hypertens. 2002;16(7):501-507. doi:10.1038/sj.jhh.1001429.
26. Kliewer MA, Tupler RH, Carroll BA, et al. Renal artery stenosis: analysis of Doppler waveform parameters and tardus-parvus pattern. Radiology. 1993;189(3):779-87.
27. Stavros AT, Parker SH, Yakes WF, et al. Segmental stenosis of the renal artery: pattern recognition of tardus and parvus abnormalities with duplex sonography. Radiology. 1992;184(2):487-92.
28. Schwerk WB, Restrepo IK, Stellwaag M, et al. Renal artery stenosis: grading with image-directed Doppler US evaluation of renal resistive index. Radiology. 1994;190(3):785-90.
29. Oliva VL, Soulez G, Lesage D, et al. Detection of renal artery stenosis with Doppler sonography before and after administration of captopril: value of early systolic rise. Am J Roentgenol. 1998;170(1):169-75.
30. Bude RO, Rubin JM. Detection of renal artery stenosis with Doppler sonography: it is more complicated than originally thought. Radiology. 1995;196(3):612-3.
31. Williams GJ, Macaskill P, Chan SF, et al. Comparative accuracy of renal duplex sonographic parameters in the diagnosis of renal artery stenosis: paired and unpaired analysis. Am J Roentgenol. 2007;188(3):798-811.
32. Radermacher J, Chavan A, Bleck J, et al. Use of Doppler ultrasonography to predict the outcome of therapy for renal-artery stenosis. N Engl J Med. 2001;344(6):410-17.
33. Ciccone MM, Cortese F, Fiorella A, et al. The clinical role of contrast-enhanced ultrasound in the evaluation of renal artery stenosis and diagnostic superiority as compared to traditional echo-color-Doppler flow imaging. Int Angiol J Int Union Angiol. 2011;30(2):135-9.
34. Dowling RJ, House MK, King PM, et al. Contrast-enhanced Doppler ultrasound for renal artery stenosis. Australas Radiol. 1999;43(2):206-9.
35. Drelich-Zbroja A, Jargiello T, Drelich G, et al. Renal artery stenosis: value of contrast-enhanced ultrasonography. Abdom Imaging. 2004;29(4):518-24.
36. Kaatee R, Beek FJ, de Lange EE, et al. Renal artery stenosis: detection and quantification with spiral CT angiography

versus optimized digital subtraction angiography. Radiology. 1997;205(1):121-7.
37. Potthast S, Maki JH. Non-contrast-enhanced MR imaging of the renal arteries. Magn Reson Imaging Clin N Am. 2008;16(4):573-84, vii.
38. Mostardi PM, Glockner JF, Young PM, et al. Contrast-enhanced MR angiography of the abdomen with highly accelerated acquisition techniques. Radiology. 2011;261(2):587-97.
39. Leiner T, Michaely H. Advances in contrast-enhanced MR angiography of the renal arteries. Magn Reson Imaging Clin N Am. 2008;16(4):561-572, vii.
40. Michoux N, Montet X, Pechère A, et al. Parametric and quantitative analysis of MR renographic curves for assessing the functional behaviour of the kidney. Eur J Radiol. 2005;54(1):124-35.
41. Verschuyl EJ, Kaatee R, Beek FJ, et al. Renal artery origins: best angiographic projection angles. Radiology. 1997;205(1):115-20.
42. Huot SJ, Hansson JH, Dey H, et al. Utility of captopril renal scans for detecting renal artery stenosis. Arch Intern Med. 2002;162(17):1981-4.
43. Jaarsveld BC van, Krijnen P, Derkx FHM, et al. The place of renal scintigraphy in the diagnosis of renal artery stenosis. Fifteen years of clinical experience. Arch Intern Med. 1997;157(11):1226-34.
44. Krijnen P, Oei HY, Claessens RA, et al. Interobserver agreement on captopril renography for assessing renal vascular disease. J Nucl Med Off Publ Soc Nucl Med. 2002;43(3):330-7.
45. Burket MW, Cooper CJ, Kennedy DJ, et al. Renal artery angioplasty and stent placement: predictors of a favorable outcome. Am Heart J. 2000;139(1 Pt 1):64-71.
46. Eldrup-Jorgensen J, Harvey HR, Sampson LN, et al. Should percutaneous transluminal renal artery angioplasty be applied to ostial renal artery atherosclerosis? J Vasc Surg. 1995;21(6):909-14; discussion 914-915.
47. Martin LG, Cork RD, Kaufman SL. Long-term results of angioplasty in 110 patients with renal artery stenosis. J Vasc Interv Radiol. 1992;3(4):619-26.
48. Sharma S, Gupta A. Visceral artery interventions in Takayasu's arteritis. Semin Interv Radiol. 2009;26(3):233-44.
49. Robinson L, Gedroyc W, Reidy J, et al. Renal artery stenosis in children. Clin Radiol. 1991;44(6):376-82.
50. Plouin PF, Chatellier G, Darné B, et al. Blood pressure outcome of angioplasty in atherosclerotic renal artery stenosis: a randomized trial. Essai Multicentrique Medicaments vs Angioplastie (EMMA) Study Group. Hypertens Dallas Tex 1979. 1998;31(3):823-9.
51. Webster J, Marshall F, Abdalla M, et al. Randomised comparison of percutaneous angioplasty vs continued medical therapy for hypertensive patients with atheromatous renal artery stenosis. Scottish and Newcastle Renal Artery Stenosis Collaborative Group. J Hum Hypertens. 1998;12(5):329-35.
52. van Jaarsveld B, Krijnen P, Bartelink A, et al. The Dutch Renal Artery Stenosis Intervention Cooperative (DRASTIC) Study: rationale, design and inclusion data. J Hypertens Suppl. 1998;16(6):S21-7.
53. ASTRAL Investigators, Wheatley K, Ives N, et al. Revascularization versus medical therapy for renal-artery stenosis. N Engl J Med. 2009;361(20):1953-62.
54. Bax L, Woittiez AJ, Kouwenberg HJ, et al. Stent placement in patients with atherosclerotic renal artery stenosis and impaired renal function: a randomized trial. Ann Intern Med. 2009;150(12):840-8, W150-1.
55. Cooper CJ, Murphy TP, Cutlip DE, et al. Stenting and medical therapy for atherosclerotic renal-artery stenosis. N Engl J Med. 2014;370(1):13-22.

Chapter 10

Imaging of Renal Transplant

Ajay Gulati, Manavjit Singh Sandhu, Tulika Singh

INTRODUCTION

Renal transplantation is currently the established standard treatment in patients of end-stage renal disease (ESRD), which leads to improvement of renal function, alleviation of the uremic syndrome with complete rehabilitation from the renal dysfunction. This has been made possible by advancements in the surgical techniques and availability of newer potent immune-suppressive medications and better donor-recipient matching.

Renal function impairment of the transplant kidney can be secondary to parenchymal abnormality, renal vascular causes, or due to collecting system abnormality. Depending upon the clinical findings, appropriate diagnostic studies are carried out. Renal biopsy remains the definitive way to diagnose the parenchymal abnormalities.

TECHNIQUE

The graft kidney is generally positioned extraperitoneally in patient's right lower quadrant with the pelvis lying anteriorly. In cadaveric renal transplants, an aortic patch (Carrel patch) is commonly removed with main renal artery. With live donors, the renal artery is harvested with anastomosis done commonly in end-to-side manner with recipient's external iliac artery. The donor renal vein is always anastomosed end-to-side with external iliac vein. The standard preferred method of reestablishing continuity of urinary tract is by formation of ureteroneocystostomy (commonly by using a submucosal tunnel to decrease the incidence of vesicoureteric reflux).[1,2]

Post-transplantation complications may be characterized in time frame as early or delayed. Early complications develop in the first few weeks and happen generally due to technical surgical challenges. Delayed complications manifest after few weeks and are normally due to medical causes (usually due to immunosuppression or due to drug toxicity).

Early complications include acute tubular necrosis (ATN), pyelonephritis, acute rejection, urinoma, hematoma, abscess, acute ureteral obstruction, and vascular complications. Late complications include chronic rejection, lymphocele, cyst formation, malignancies, and opportunistic infections of the transplant kidney.[3]

The greatest risk in the early post-transplant period is of early graft failure, which presents with oliguria. To diagnose this early, there is a routine policy of clinical surveillance complimented with laboratory tests and imaging.[4]

COMPLICATIONS

Various complications seen in post-transplant recipients may be broadly categorized as described here.

Vascular Complications

Renal Artery Stenosis

Well-recognized complication occurs in 0.9–8%[5] of cases, which is usually seen in the first 3 months.[5,6] It typically presents clinically as hypertension with or without deterioration of renal function. Auscultation may reveal bruit over the graft site. This is generally secondary to atherosclerotic vascular disease involving either the donor or recipient vessels and improper suture technique or iatrogenic vascular injury during graft harvesting. Color Doppler sonography is a commonly used technique, which reveals areas of focal color aliasing secondary to turbulent flow across the stenotic segments. Raised peak systolic velocity (PSV) (>200 cm/sec) is a sensitive and specific finding. Velocity gradient of >2:1 between stenotic and prestenotic segments also suggests the diagnosis. Tardus parvus waveform in distal segmental branches of the transplant kidney may be observed.[6] Computed tomography angiogram or magnetic resonance angiogram are complimentary imaging techniques which may be required in cases of technical difficulties in sonography due to vascular tortuosity or limited acoustic window.

Renal Artery Thrombosis

It is a rare complication seen in 0.4–3.5% of recipients.[5] The clinical features include oliguria and increased serum creatinine levels. Causes include vessel kinking, arterial dissection, acute rejection, and hypercoagulable states. Lack of flow with contents within the main renal artery with extension into its distal branches is seen on ultrasound (US), contrast-enhanced computed tomography, and contrast-enhanced magnetic resonance.

Renal Vein Thrombosis

It is also an uncommon complication encountered in 0.5–4% of the graft recipients.[5] Clinical presentation includes fever, pain, swelling over the transplant kidney, and or ipsilateral lower limb. It may be due to twisting or kinking at the time of surgery causing venous torsion and extrinsic compression over the vein. US shows lack of flow in main renal vein of the graft kidney.

Pseudoaneurysm

These are generally iatrogenic due to biopsy of graft kidney. These are well seen on color Doppler imaging typically showing yin yang sign and may be managed by graded compression technique. Interventional techniques such as percutaneous injection of thrombin or endovascular coils may be required in selected cases.

Arteriovenous Fistula

These also occur mainly due to iatrogenic reasons secondary to renal biopsies. They are formed when the biopsy needle accidentally hits both arterial as well as venous walls. Color Doppler along with spectral waveform analysis helps in the diagnosis. These usually follow self-limiting course and may close spontaneously. Some large fistulae may require endovascular embolization.

Nonvascular Complications

Medical Complications

Acute tubular necrosis: ATN occurs due to renal ischemia during transplantation and reperfusion injury. It clinically presents with anuria immediately or within first few days after an initial diuresis. The patients remain constitutionally well and urine sodium levels (Na^+) are high. It is usually self-limiting with renal parameters returning to normal in few days to weeks. It is almost exclusively seen in cadaveric transplants.[4]

Graft rejection: Acute rejection is the most commonly encountered complication, which may be potentially serious if not managed appropriately. Currently, invasive core needle biopsy is still regarded as the gold standard for confirming the suspected acute rejection, however, carries the risk of graft injury or other vascular complications.[7]

Clinically, there are three distinct types of rejections: (1) hyperacute, (2) acute, and (3) chronic. Hyperacute rejection (due to circulating antibodies) usually occurs within hours to 1 or 2 days after the transplantation. It is characterized by the presence of fibrin thrombi in small arteries with cortical necrosis. The treatment is only the graft removal.

Acute rejection (mediated through cell-mediated immunity) is seen most frequently in first 1–3 weeks. It is characterized clinically by oliguria with flu-like symptoms, pyrexia, hypertension, graft tenderness, and swelling. The urine Na^+ is usually low (c.f. ATN in which urine Na^+ is high). If early diagnosis is made, this may be potentially reversed either by administering steroids or in some cases by antibody therapy.[4]

Chronic rejection is the most common reason for delayed graft dysfunction and usually manifests 3 months after transplant.[6] It does not respond to increased immunosuppressive therapy. Removal of the graft is required in majority of the patients.

Drug toxicity: Calcineurin inhibitors such as cyclosporine and tacrolimus are main immunosuppressive agents given to avoid acute rejection. These drugs are potentially nephrotoxic and cause interstitial fibrosis with long-term usage.[6] Serum drug levels need to be monitored and dosage reduced if features of drug toxicity develop.

Infections: Early diagnosis is pivotal to improve patient outcome although the clinical features and early imaging features are generally variable and nonspecific. The involvement may be focal or diffuse pyelonephritis, which may progress on to abscess formation and/or pyonephrosis.

US may reveal focal areas of hypo- or hyperechogenicity.[8] Abscess may have complex cystic appearance and may be treated by percutaneous drainage along with systemic antibiotics. Nuclear imaging using Gallium 67 citrate and Indium 111 tagged leukocyte may aid as a complimentary technique in diagnosing infection in equivocal cases.[9]

Neoplasms and post-transplantation lymphoproliferative disorder: Immunosuppressive medications predispose the patients receiving graft kidney to increased risk of subsequently developing cancers particularly of the cervix, rectum, skin, Kaposi's sarcoma, and lymphoma (non-Hodgkin lymphoma).[8,10,11]

This risk has been estimated to be 100 times more as compared to the general population. Post-transplantation lymphoproliferative disorder (PTLD) is another uncommon malignancy, which may be seen in approximately 1% of graft recipients this is commonly secondary to Epstein-Barr virus infection, which usually involves the B cells. The frequently seen radiological manifestations are extrarenal with generalized lymphadenopathy.[7] In addition, extra nodal involvement may be seen, which can be solitary or multifocal lesions affecting the lung, liver, spleen, central nervous system (CNS), and gastrointestinal tract (GIT).[3,11,12]

Involvement of the graft kidney is not common but when present, it may present as nodular renal masses, perihilar, or perinephric soft tissue masses.

Renal cell carcinoma also shows increased prevalence in kidney graft recipients with 90% occurring in the native kidneys and 10% in the transplant kidney.[11]

Surgical Complications

Peritransplant Fluid Collections

Hematoma: They commonly occur due to inadequate surgical hemostasis, anticoagulation, coagulopathy, or after biopsy. They may be subcapsular or peritransplant in location. Significant subcapsular hematomas produce mass effect, which can alter the renal perfusion. On US, they may appear as complex hypoechoic masses with internal echoes and septation. Computed tomography (CT) and magnetic resonance (MR) are adjunct imaging techniques, which may add more confidence to the diagnosis.[8]

Urinoma: They occur from urine leaks, commonly found between kidney and the bladder. The clinical presentations may include oliguria with fullness, swelling, and tenderness over the graft. On US, they appear as well-defined hypoechoic to anechoic fluid collections making it difficult to differentiate from seroma or lymphocele.[8] Aspiration of fluid with raised creatinine levels helps to confirm the diagnosis. Percutaneous nephrostomy may be required for urinary diversion.

Abscess: They are an uncommon complication, which may present during first few weeks. The clinical features include pain, fever, tenderness over the graft kidney, and features of sepsis. On US, they appear as complex fluid collection with internal echoes and occasionally may be multiloculated. The treatment includes intravenous antibiotics, aspiration or drainage based upon the size.[8]

Lymphocele: Surgical disruption of adjacent lymphatic vessels leads to development of lymphoceles. They generally occur later (4–8 weeks after surgery).[8,13] On US, they appear as variable-sized anechoic to hypoechoic fluid collections with thin septations. Most patients are asymptomatic; symptoms may develop when they produce hydronephrosis secondary to mass effect.

Urinary obstruction: Most commonly ureteral stenosis occurs in the distal third due to relatively less blood supply or by compression from fluid collections.[8] It manifests by increasing serum creatinine levels. US shows dilated renal pelvis and calyceal system and fluid collections, if present. CT also helps in detecting the level of and cause of obstruction. Balloon ureteroplasty or stent placement may be done for management.

IMAGING TECHNIQUES

Impaired renal allograft function during the post-transplant period warrants an immediate and thorough evaluation to distinguish between the parenchymal and surgical complications.

The various imaging techniques and their indications are as follows.

Radiography

Plain Radiography

Plain radiographs are useful in demonstrating radio-paque calculi and air within the collecting system or renal parenchyma in rare cases of emphysematous pyelonephritis.

Intravenous Urography

Intravenous urography was a useful study when ureteral obstruction or extravasation was suspected in a transplant recipient with adequate renal function. Presently, it is not indicated due to the newer advancements in various imaging technologies, which offer more comprehensive evaluation within acceptable radiation limits.

Cystography

Cystography is indicated to rule out vesicoureteral reflux in patients with persistent or recurrent urinary tract infection.

Nuclear Imaging

Radioimmunoassay is the most useful imaging technique for evaluating the renal function both qualitatively and quantitatively while screening for common complications. Obtaining a baseline scan in the immediate postoperative period is extremely important.[5] Serial radionuclide scans allow early detection of rejection and can be used to monitor the recovery from ATN. The most common technique used is dynamic renal imaging using ^{99}Tc DTPA (diethylenetriaminepentaacetic acid), which helps in assessing the renal perfusion and dimercaptosuccinic acid (DMSA) scan, which detects any morphological abnormalities.

Ultrasonography

Ultrasonography (USG) is most commonly employed imaging technique for evaluation of transplant recipients owing to its wider availability and lack of ionizing radiation. High-frequency transducers (5 MHz or higher) provide excellent details of the transplant kidney because of the superficial location. Several sonographic findings including enlargement of kidney, poor corticomedullary differentiation, reduced amplitude of sinus echoes, and enlarged pyramids may be seen in graft dysfunction, which can be due to early rejection, ATN, or infection. Real-time USG combined with duplex Doppler or color and power flow imaging techniques is the most frequently used examination to evaluate worsening renal function in the post-transplantation period[5,6,14-16] **(Figs. 1A to C)**. Vascular complications of transplantation, i.e. infarction, arteriovenous fistulae, pseudoaneurysms, arterial or venous thrombosis, and stenosis are readily identified by color and duplex Doppler sonography[5,6] **(Figs. 2A and B)**.

American College of Radiology appropriateness criteria for renal transplant dysfunction also recommend US duplex Doppler as a first-line imaging modality. Color Doppler is used to evaluate the status of graft vessels and to detect any areas of focal stenosis or thrombosis. Studies

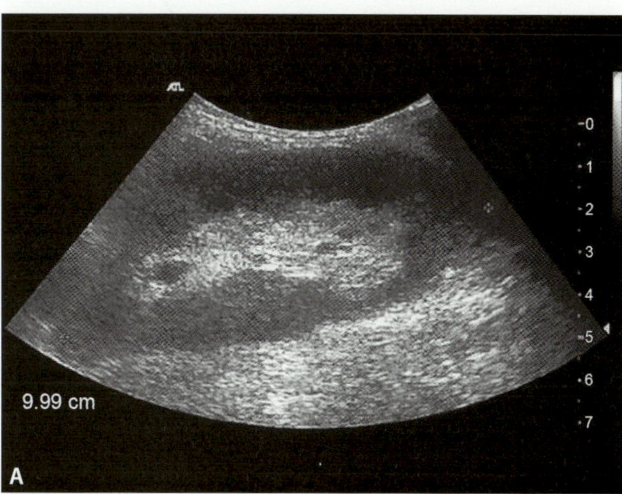

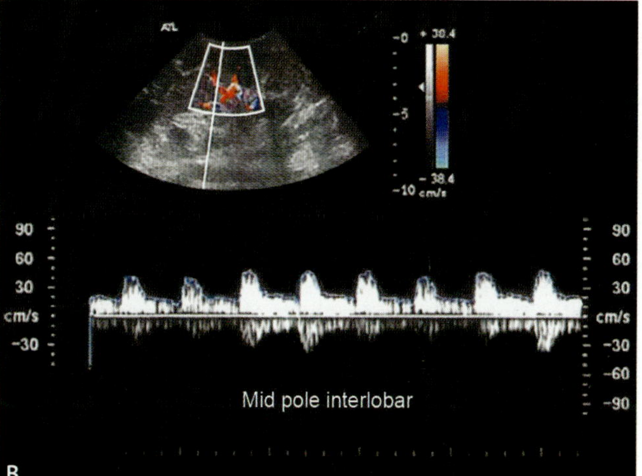

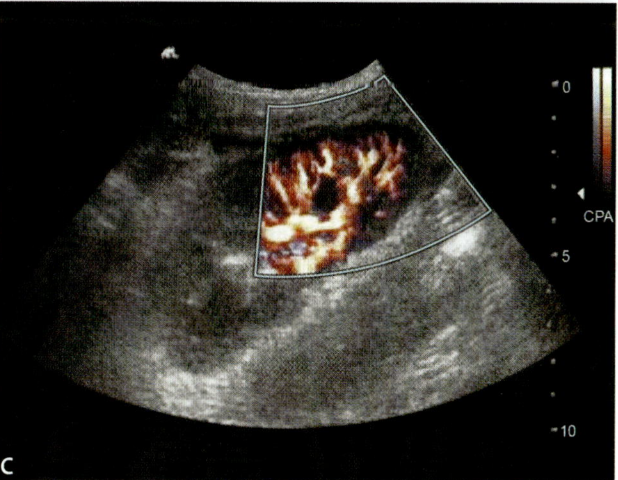

Figs. 1A to C: Ultrasonography and Doppler images of the normal transplant kidney. (A) Gray-scale sonogram showing normal size, outline, echogenicity, corticomedullary differentiation, and pelvicalyceal system. (B) Duplex Doppler from interlobar artery shows normal low resistance flow with resistive index of 0.69 (<0.8) and pulsatility index of 1.23 (<1.5). (C) Power Doppler image shows normal cortical perfusion showing reaching up to the periphery of the renal cortex.

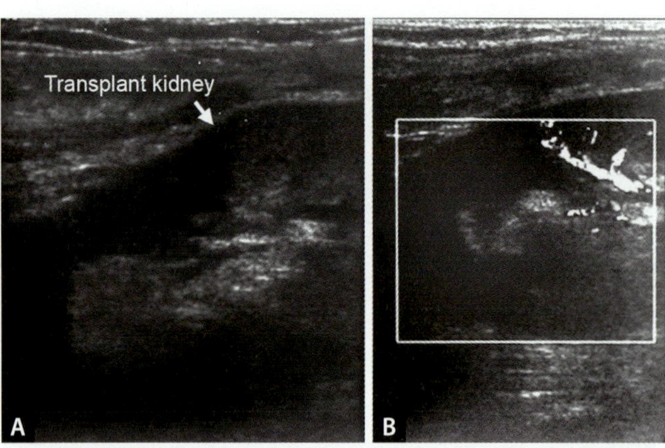

Figs. 2A and B: Renal infarction. (A) Ultrasound images show well-demarcated hypoechoic areas involving the renal parenchyma. (B) Power Doppler shows absence of flow in the involved renal parenchyma.

have shown that power Doppler sonography is superior to duplex Doppler sonography in screening patients with acute rejection. On spectral analysis, PSV, acceleration time, pulsatility index, and resistive index (RI) are assessed. The upper limit of normal PSV in renal artery is 200 cm/sec. The RI is considered to be normal if it is lesser than 0.8 **(Figs. 3A to C)**.[5,6]

Color Doppler sonography is also primary diagnostic modality for identifying various vascular complications. Focal stenotic segment may reveal color aliasing with velocities more than 200 cm/sec. Absent or reversed end diastolic flow is seen in severe rejection, ATN, and thrombosis in graft renal vein. Raised RI (>0.8) may also be present in acute rejection and ATN.[5,6]

Minimal dilatation of the collecting system in the immediate postoperative period is acceptable and is usually due to edema at the ureteroneocystostomy site.

Hydronephrosis may be secondary to the ureteral stricture or peritransplant fluid collections. USG is sensitive for identifying the fluid collections such as urinoma, hematoma, and abscess around the graft kidney but it is not specific for fluid type, and aspiration of the fluid collection with US guidance is helpful in the management. US guidance minimizes the risk and discomfort of the percutaneous renal transplant biopsy **(Figs. 4 and 5)**.

Recent advances in the form of contrast-enhanced ultrasound (CEUS), US elastography, and ARFI (acoustic radiation force impulse imaging) are being used to improve the diagnostic performance for early detection of graft dysfunction.

Contrast-enhanced ultrasound provides more precise information about the status of vessels and parenchymal flow; it also provides quantitative analysis of the renal

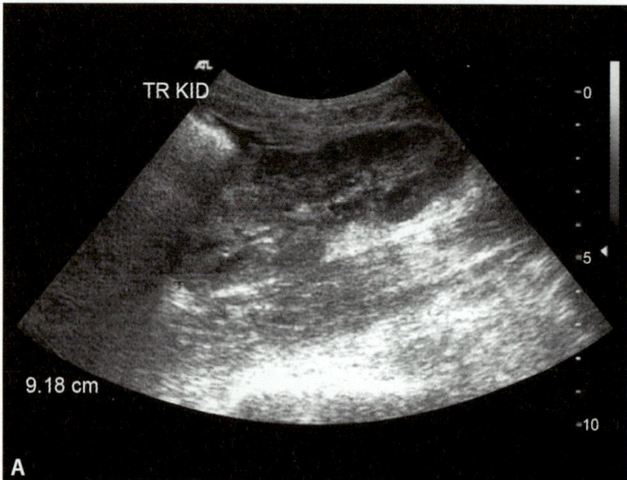

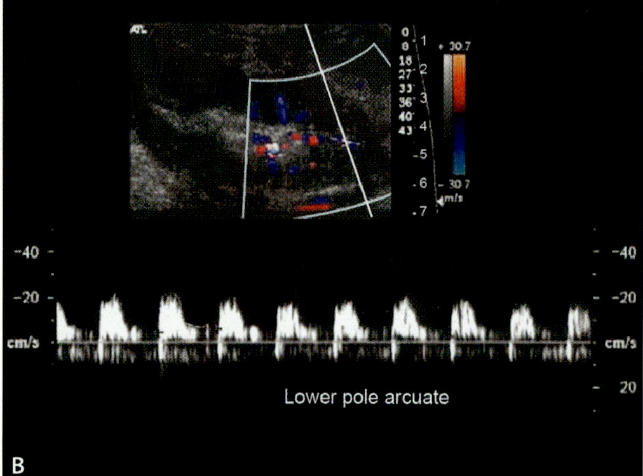

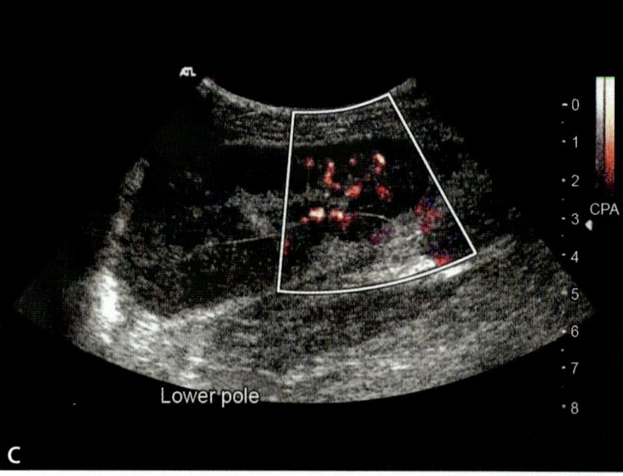

Figs. 3A to C: Ultrasonography and Doppler images of the transplant kidney with acute rejection (confirmed on renal biopsy). (A) Gray-scale sonogram shows normal renal length and echogenicity with indistinct corticomedullary differentiation and reduced renal sinus echoes. (B) Duplex Doppler from interlobar artery shows raised resistive index of 0.81 and pulsatility index of 1.67. (C) Power Doppler image shows reduced cortical perfusion.

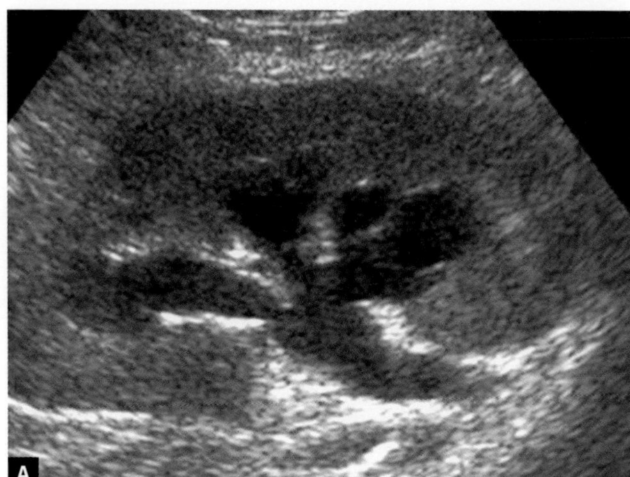

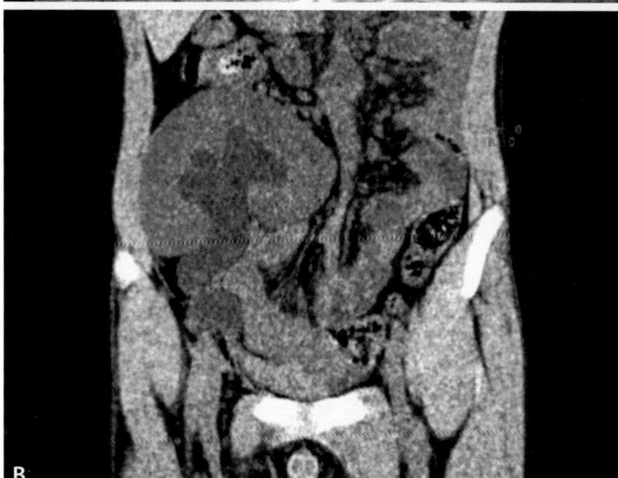

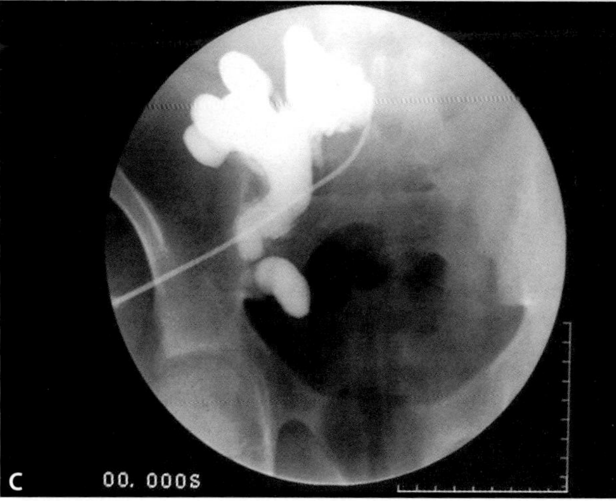

Figs. 4A to C: Hydroureteronephrosis with ureteric stricture. (A) Sonogram of transplant kidney shows hydronephrosis. (B) Coronal reformatted computed tomography images show hydroureteronephrosis with ureteric stricture. (C) Antegrade urogram shows hydroureteronephrosis with ureteric stricture.

perfusion thereby adding more information for identifying various causes of graft dysfunction.[17]

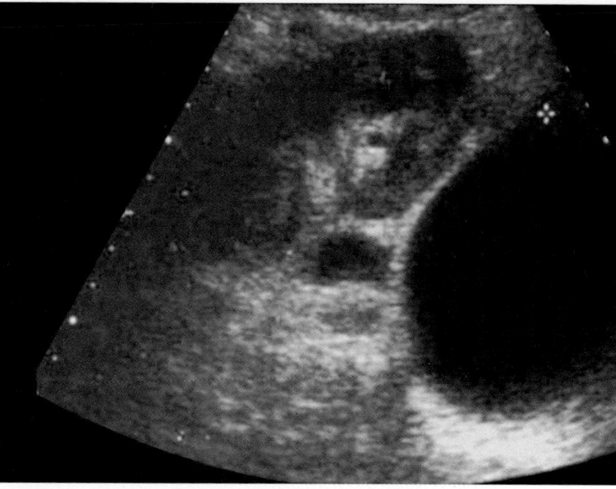

Fig. 5: Urinoma. Sagittal ultrasound image shows a large anechoic fluid collection seen posterior to the kidney. Note the dilatation of the ureter is attributable to the compression by the urinoma.

Another recent advancement is US elastography and ARFI for assessing early graft dysfunction. These techniques noninvasively assess the tissue's stiffness, which may help in early detection of parenchymal abnormalities, however, lack specificity for identification of precise underling disease.[7]

A novel technique for objective quantification of vascularity has been described by Gruenewald et al. This technique involves assessment of vascularity from the information obtained from Doppler cine loops, which are transferred to a computer for analysis. The vascularity is assessed by percentage color pixel density and mean flow velocity in mid kidney regions of interest. This technique can reliably detect allograft nephropathies.[18]

Computed Tomography

Helical CT is an accurate, noninvasive technique, which can comprehensively delineate the renal parenchyma, vasculature, pyeloureteric system, and perirenal region **(Figs. 6A to F)**. It helps to differentiate acute rejection from obstructive uropathy, urinary fistula, perinephric fluid collections, mass lesions, etc. In assessing the complex problems such as detection of malignancy such as PTLD and lymphoma or identifying sites of infection or sepsis, CT is the most useful modality **(Figs. 7 and 8)**. PTLD may present with focal lesions involving various visceral organs such as lungs, liver, spleen, CNS, and GIT **(Figs. 9 and 10)**. Dynamic CT has been used in the evaluation of physiological status of the renal transplants. It often delineates fluid collections and their anatomic relationship to adjacent structures better than USG. It can

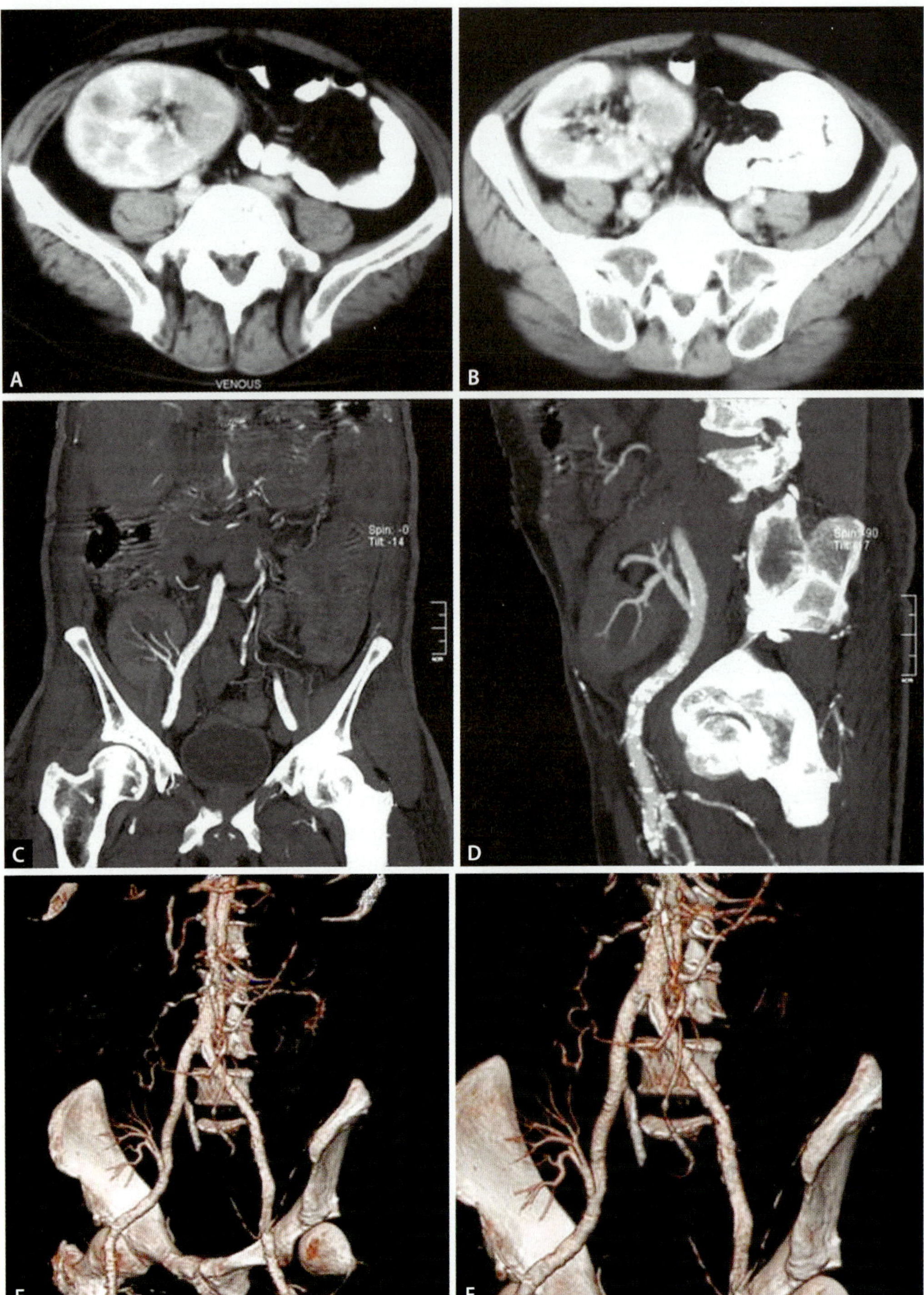

Figs. 6A to F: Normal transplant kidney. (A and B) Contrast-enhanced venous phase show uniformly enhanced parenchyma of the transplant kidney. Note made of a simple cyst. (C and D) Vascular myocardial infarction preformatted images depict the transplant renal artery anastomosed to the external iliac artery. (E and F) Volume-rendered images show the end-to-side anastomoses of the graft artery and the external iliac artery.

also distinguish the nature of fluid collections **(Fig. 11)**. Fresh blood in the form of hematoma has the highest attenuation value (55–66 HU), lymphoceles are between 10 HU and 20 HU, and the abscesses between 20 HU and 30 HU. In addition, drainage procedures may be performed with CT guidance when USG cannot clearly define the relationship to the collections to adjacent bowel loops. CT can reliably diagnose various infective conditions including focal or diffuse pyelonephritis or areas of abscess formation[8] **(Figs. 12A and B)**.

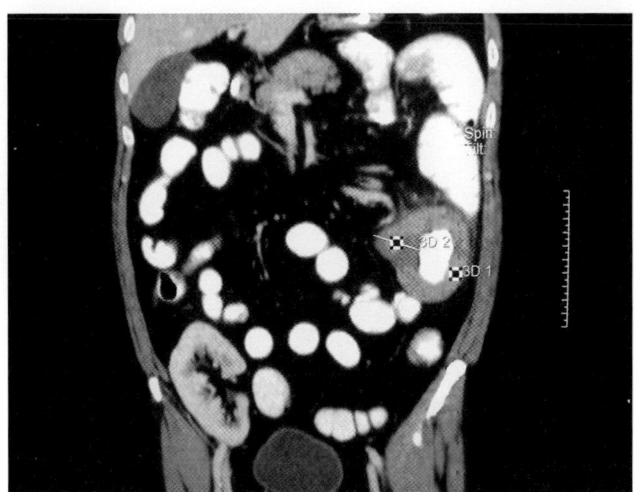

Fig. 7: Post-transplantation lymphoma. Coronal reformatted computed tomography image shows homogeneous circumferential mural thickening involving the jejunum.

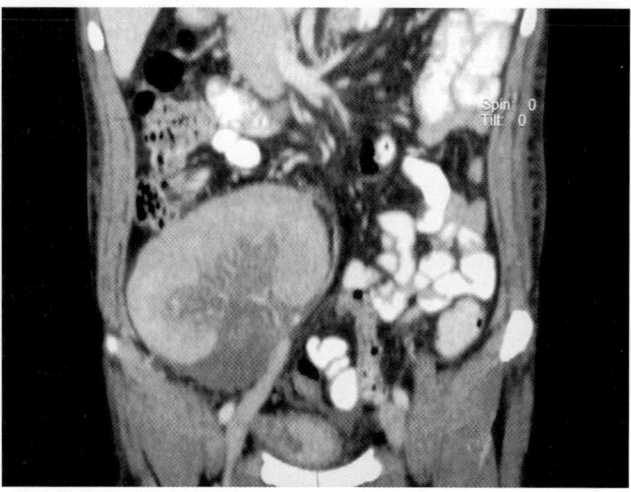

Fig. 8: Post-transplantation lymphoproliferative disorder involving renal transplant. Coronal reformatted computed tomography image shows infiltrating mass in the renal hilum surrounding the graft pedicle.

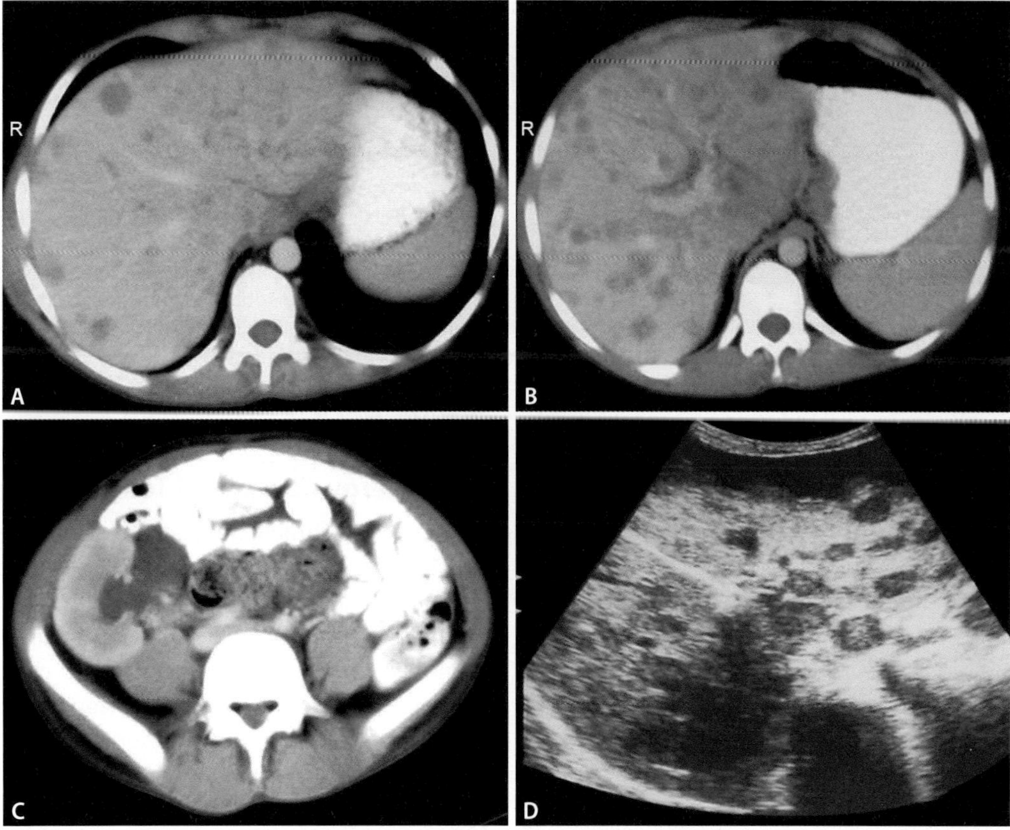

Figs. 9A to D: Hepatic post-transplantation lymphoproliferative disorder. (A and B) Contrast-enhanced computed tomography scan shows multiple hypodense lesions involving both the lobes. (C) Computed tomography scan at lower level shows hydronephrosis in renal transplant secondary to narrowing at ureterovesical anastomoses. (D) Ultrasound image shows multiple well-defined hypoechoic lesions in the liver parenchyma.

Computed tomography angiography with three-dimensional (3D) reformatted images allows accurate imaging of the vascular diseases such as stenosis, thrombosis, pseudoaneurysms, and arteriovenous fistulae when US studies are inconclusive. Associated parenchymal abnormalities such as infarction may be well seen with CT imaging **(Figs. 13A to C)**.

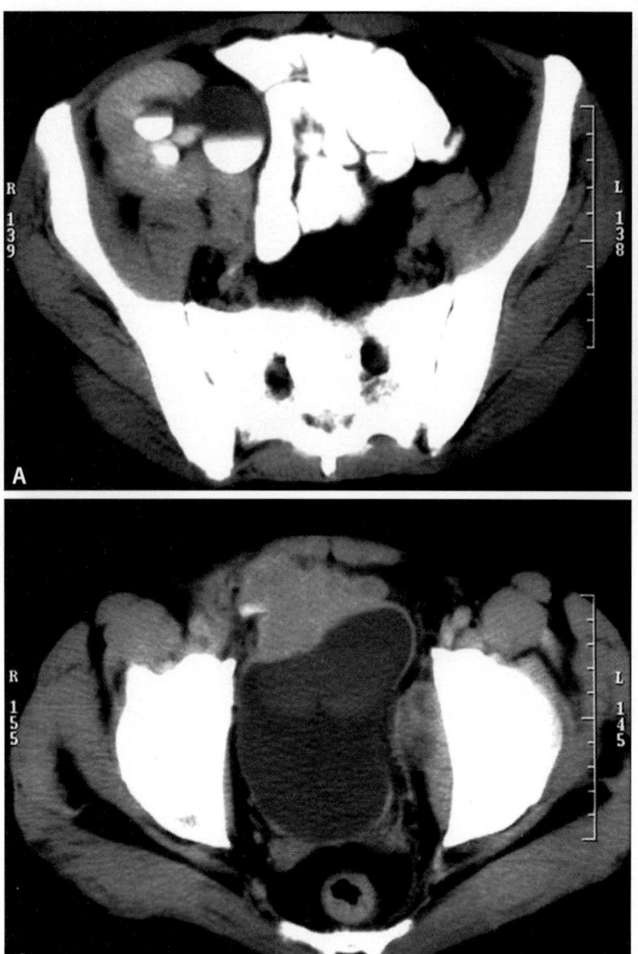

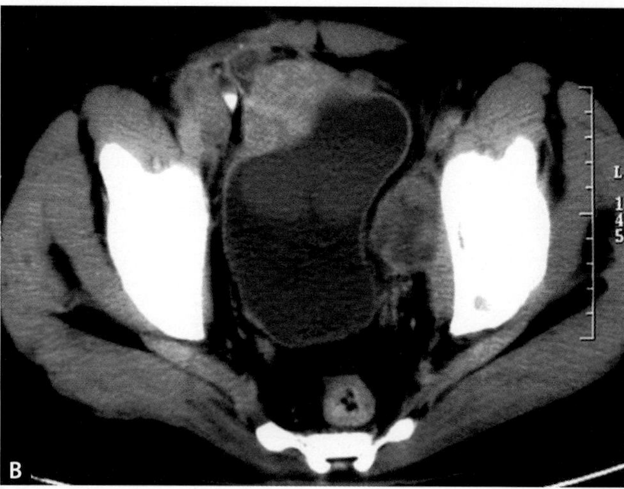

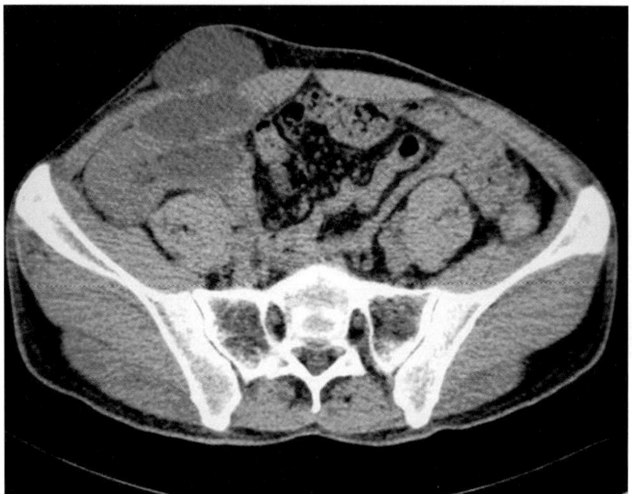

Figs.10A to C: Lymphoma in renal allograft recipient involving ureterovesical anastomoses. (A) Contrast-enhanced computed tomography scan demonstrates hydroureteronephrosis. (B and C) Contrast-enhanced scans obtained at lower levels show homogeneous soft-tissue mass lesion at the ureterovesical anastomoses.

Fig. 11: Urinoma. Noncontrast computed tomography of KUB region shows hydronephrosis with perinephric urinoma extending into the anterior abdominal wall.

Dual Energy Computed Tomography

It is a novel technical advancement in CT technology in which acquisition is performed at two different energy levels generating two data sets, which aids in better lesion detection and characterization over traditional single-energy CT. In kidney transplant cases, it helps in differentiating hyperdense cystic lesion from an enhancing renal mass and also in characterization (differentiating uric acid stones from stones of other composition).

Magnetic Resonance Imaging

Magnetic resonance imaging (MRI) is employed as second-line modality for evaluation of the graft kidney as it also gives comprehensive information on the status of the renal vasculature, renal parenchyma, and peritransplant region. It can also identify or exclude various causes of renal graft dysfunction (e.g. occlusion of transplant vessels,

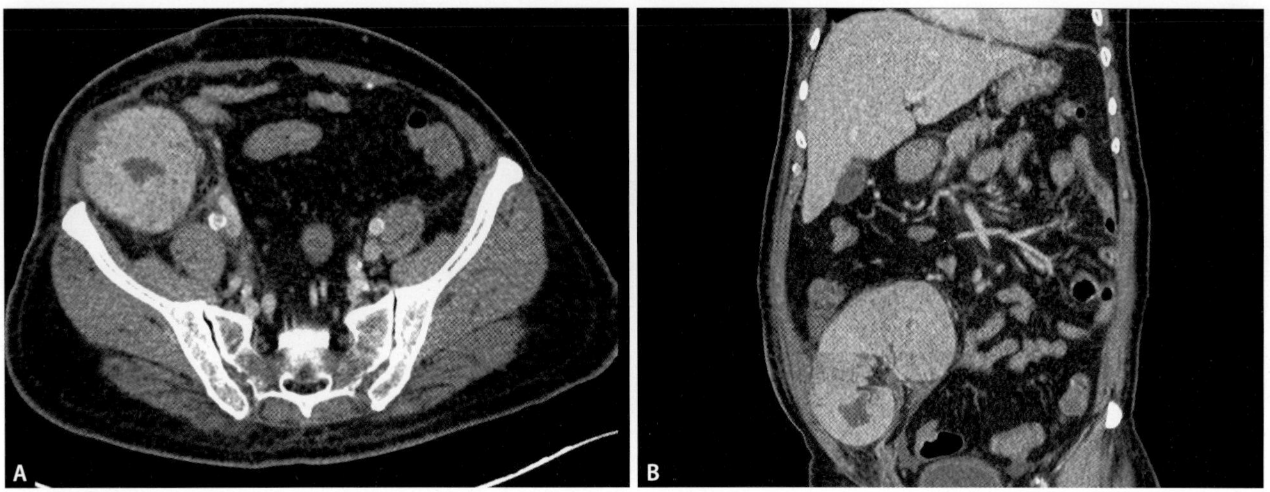

Figs. 12A and B: Computed tomography (axial and coronal reformatted images) showing diffuse pyelonephritis in graft kidney with focal hypodense areas of abscess formation in the lower part.

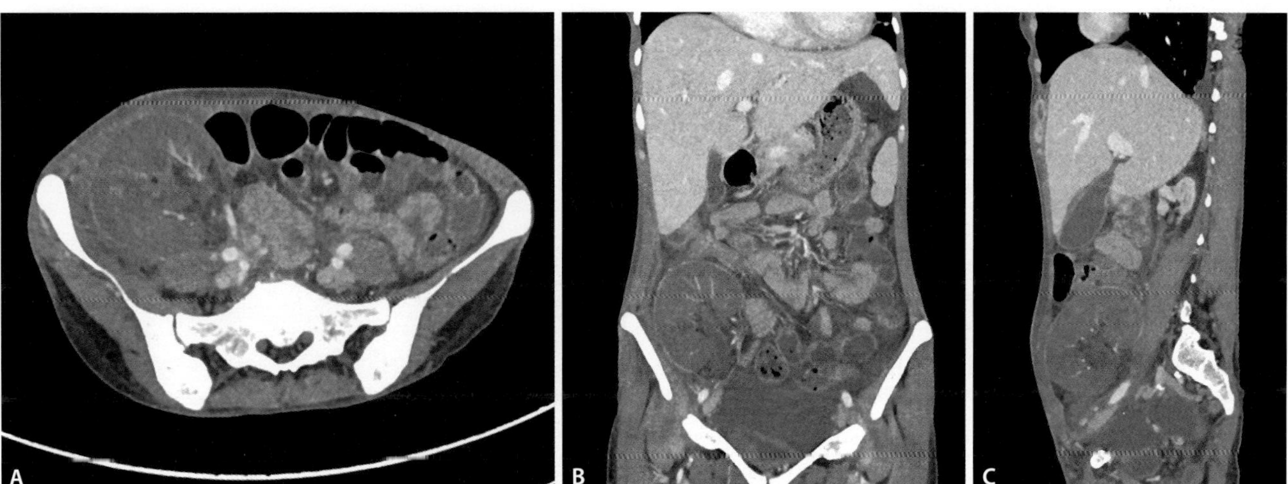

Figs. 13A to C: Computed tomography (axial, coronal, and sagittal reformatted images) showing globular nonenhancing graft kidney consistent with global infarction.

fluid collections around the graft kidney, and ureteral obstruction).[19]

From the renal safety perspective, although the risk of renal toxicity after gadolinium injection is debatable,[20] there is added risk of nephrogenic systemic fibrosis in recipients with already compromised renal parameters.[21]

Due to high spatial resolution, nonenhanced pulse sequences may provide good details in graft recipients with compromised renal function.

A dynamic MR performed with 3D fat saturated gradient echo T1-weighted sequence provides adequate information regarding the vessels and functional status of the transplant. Half-Fourier single-shot turbo spin-echo T2-weighted acquisition also provides rapid assessment of the anatomy along with the detection of hydronephrosis, perirenal collections, and malignancy, if present **(Figs. 14A and B)**.

The usefulness of MRI in renal transplant dysfunction is rapidly evolving. Decreased or absent corticomedullary differentiation on T1-weighted image is seen in majority of patients with acute rejection; however, this is nonspecific for etiology and may also be seen in allograft infection, immunosuppressant drug toxicity, and infiltrative or diffuse parenchymal diseases. On dynamic gadolinium-enhanced imaging, there is a blunted-up rise and delayed peak in the cortical signal intensity curves. The medulla also shows decreased enhancement in acute rejection.[22]

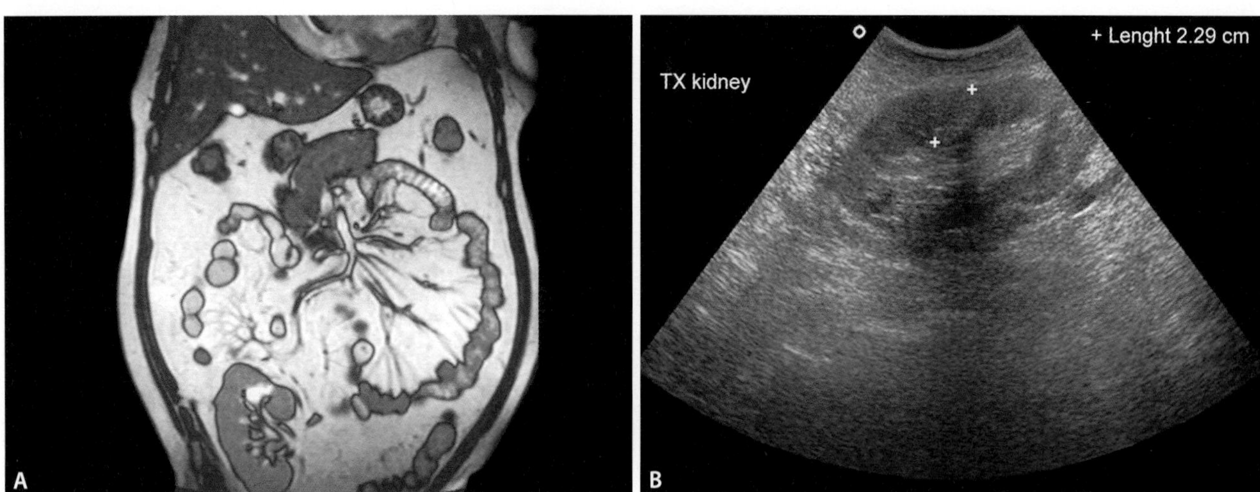

Figs. 14A and B: Renal cell carcinoma in renal graft. (A) Coronal MR T2WI shows focal hyperintense lesion in the transplant kidney. (B) Ultrasound image shows the lesion is iso-to-hypoechoic to the renal parenchyma.

Preliminary published data indicate that ^{31}P-MR spectroscopy may be useful in differentiating the rejection from other causes of the renal transplant failure. The use of MR spectroscopy for evaluating the phosphorus metabolism of allografts is still under development and has been reported to be useful. The long-term assessment of post-transplant renal prognosis with ^{31}P-MR spectroscopy has been recently evaluated and a beta-adenosine triphosphate/inorganic phosphate ratio more than 1.2 will favor increased probability of 3-year renal survival, whereas a value more than 2.5 may suggest that graft kidney may survive over 5 years.[23]

Recent advanced MRI techniques such as diffusion-weighted imaging (DWI) and blood oxygen level-dependent imaging has also shown promising role in detecting functional changes in kidney without intravenous contrast.[24]

By DWI, the Brownian motion can be detected, which is the random movement of the water molecule in the tissue. DWI along with quantitative apparent diffusion coefficient can detect renal allograft dysfunction wit high specificity.[25]

Blood oxygen level-dependent imaging sequence is technically obtained by altering levels of paramagnetic deoxyhemoglobin and can detect intrarenal oxygenation. This may be of benefit in differentiating between acute rejection from ATN from hypoxia caused by renal artery stenosis.[26]

Magnetic resonance is an excellent modality for screening of renal artery stenosis and other vascular complications **(Fig. 15)**. MR angiographic examination can help in avoiding unnecessary catheter angiographies in majority of cases. Noncontrast magnetic imaging angiography (NCMRA) with steady-state free procession imaging can help avoiding use of MR contrast and risk of developing nephrogenic systemic fibrosis.[27]

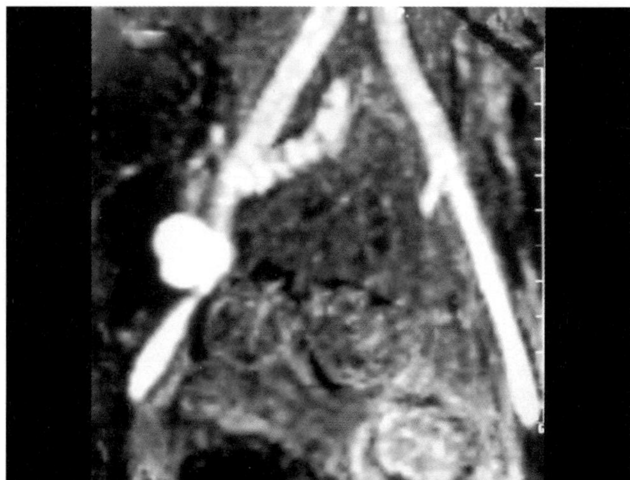

Fig. 15: Pseudoaneurysm. Maximum intensity projection reformatted magnetic resonance angiogram depicts stenosis involving the external iliac artery with a pseudoaneurysm at the anastomotic site.

Few studies showed that NCMRA was capable of detecting renin-angiotensin system in graft kidney with accuracy comparable to contrast-enhanced MRA.[28]

Angiography

Some important indications of renal transplant angiography are acute anuria, hypertension not responding to medication, and graft dysfunction, in which definitive diagnosis of rejection or renal artery stenosis is required order to plan subsequent appropriate management.[29,30]

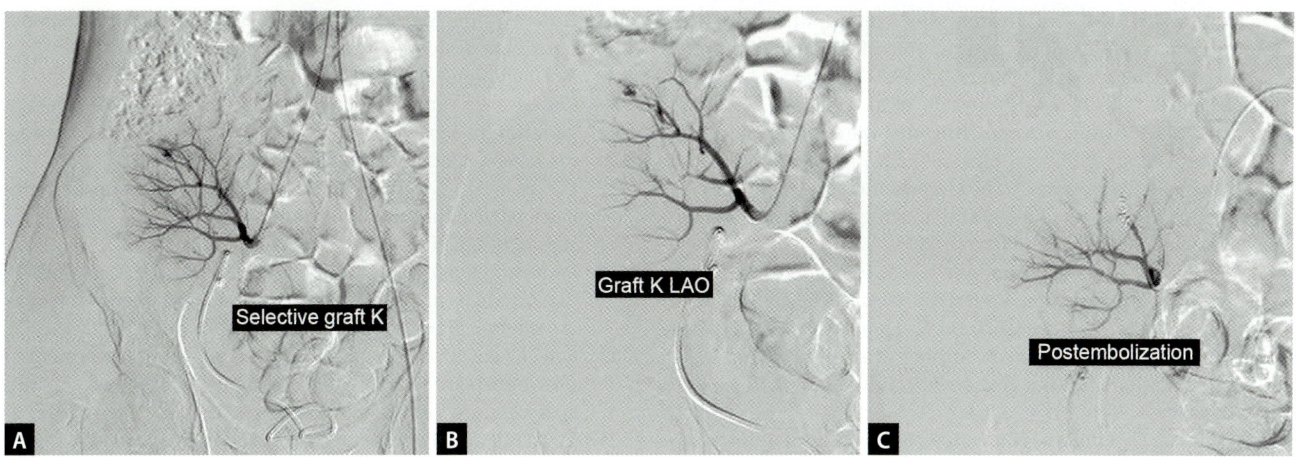

Figs. 16A to C: Transcatheter embolization of pseudoaneurysm. (A and B) Angiogram of transplant renal artery [anterior-posterior and left anterior oblique (LAO) projection] shows a pseudoaneurysm in upper segmental artery. (C) Angiogram obtained after coil embolization shows successful obliteration of the aneurysm with preservation of the flow in the rest of the parenchyma.

In acute rejection, there is a pruned-tree appearance secondary to the loss of second- and third-order branches. The arteriogram is essentially normal in ATN. In chronic rejection, arteriography demonstrates small graft size with irregularity, attenuation, and occlusion of interlobar arteries and a patchy nephrogram secondary to the areas of cortical infarction.

Angiography is indicated in patients with hypertension not responding to the medical therapy. Angiography in such situation may demonstrate degree of renal artery stenosis. Hemodynamically significant (>50%) stenosis can be simultaneously treated with percutaneous transluminal angioplasty with covered metal stents or drug eluting stents.[31] Arteriovenous fistula (AVF) and pseudoaneurysm formation are generally iatrogenic secondary to percutaneous needle biopsy. Interventional techniques such as transcatheter embolization are the treatment of choice for both enlarging pseudoaneurysms and symptomatic AVFs. Super-selective embolization performed with metallic coils or stent grafts minimizes the loss of functioning allograft tissue and ensures long-term graft survival **(Figs. 16A to C)**. It allows selective occlusion of targeted vessels more precisely unlike particle embolization where particles may reflux into nontargeted vessels. Surgery is regarded as the treatment of last resort, with partial or total nephrectomy being two options.

Percutaneous Interventional Techniques

Percutaneous interventional radiological techniques play a pivotal role in management of the complications in the graft kidney recipients and the timely use of these techniques may obviate surgery in some cases.

Complication such as urinary obstruction or leak can occurs up to 3–10% in graft kidney patients.[32] Antegrade pyelography is the most accurate and informative examination for the demonstration of ureteral stricture as well as the site of ureteral leak **(*see* Fig. 4C)**. Nephrostomy drainage catheter is placed in patients with urine leak and ureteral obstruction.

Ureteral strictures can be dilated percutaneously by using angioplasty catheter, and indwelling ureteral stents left in place. Renal calculi removal through a percutaneous nephrostomy in a graft kidney recipient can also be successfully accomplished. Peri graft fluid collections such as urinoma or lymphocele are managed definitively by percutaneous drainage procedures with or without adjunct sclerosis. The commonly used sclerosing agent is dehydrated ethanol. The other agents which may be used for sclerotherapy are povidone iodine, doxycycline, bleomycin, and fibrin glue.[33] Percutaneous management of postoperative hematoma is controversial and is generally avoided, however, may be helpful in subacute and chronic stages of hematoma with significant liquefied component or in case of superadded infection.

ACKNOWLEDGMENTS

Sincere thanks to Dr Hema HK, Junior Resident, Department of Radiodiagnosis, PGIMER, Chandigarh.

REFERENCES

1. Rankin S. Renal parenchymal disease, including renal failure, renovascular disease and transplantation. In: Grainger RG, Allison DJ (Eds). Diagnostic Radiology, 5th edition. London: Churchill Livingstone; 2009. pp. 851-5.

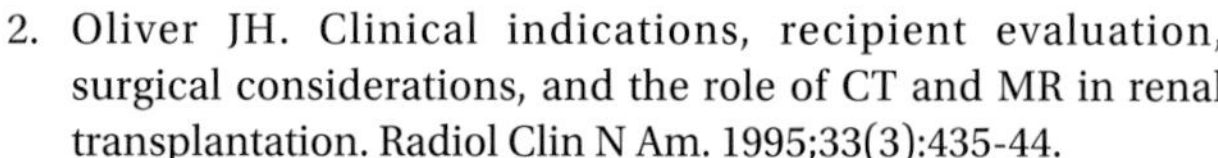

2. Oliver JH. Clinical indications, recipient evaluation, surgical considerations, and the role of CT and MR in renal transplantation. Radiol Clin N Am. 1995;33(3):435-44.
3. Sebastria C, Quiroga S, Boye R, et al. Helical CT in renal transplantation: normal findings and early and late complications. Radiographics. 2001;21(5):1103-17.
4. Kabala JE, Roobottom C. The kidneys and ureters. In: Sutton D (Ed). Textbook of Radiology and Imaging, 7th edition. London: Churchill Livingstone; 2002. pp. 982-6.
5. Moreno CC, Mittal PK, Ghonge NP, et al. Imaging complications of renal transplantation. Radiol Clin N Am. 2016;54(2):235-49.
6. Chrysafoula K, Konstantinos S, Demosthenes D. Ultrasonographic features of kidney transplants and their complications: an imaging review. ISRN Radiol. 2013;2013: 480862.
7. Thölking G, Schuette-Nuetgen K, Kentrup D, et al. Imaging-based diagnosis of acute renal allograft rejection. World J Transplant. 2016;6(1):174-82.
8. Kim N, Juarez R, Levy AD. Imaging non-vascular complications of renal transplantation. Abdom Radiol. 2018;43(10):2555.
9. Akbar SA, Jafri ZH, Amendola MA, et al. Complications of renal transplantation. Radiographics. 2005;25(5):1335-56.
10. Kumar R, Wilson DD, Santa Cruz FR. Postoperative urological complications of renal transplantation. Radiographics. 1984;3 (4):531-47.
11. Langer JE, Jones LP. Sonographic evaluation of the renal transplant. Ultrasound Clinics North Am. 2007;2:73-88.
12. Sandhu MS, Kalra N, Sidhu R. Post-transplant lymphoproliferative disorder (PTLD) localised near the allograft mimicking a collection. Indian J Radiol Imaging. 2002;12: 132-33.
13. Brown ED, Chen YM, Wolfman NT, et al. Complication of renal transplantation: evaluation with US and radionuclide imaging. Radiographics. 2000;20(3):607-22.
14. O'neill WC, Baumgarten DA. Ultrasonography in renal transplantation. Am J Kidney Dis. 2002;39:663-78.
15. Tublin ME, Dodd GD. Sonography of renal transplantation. Radiol Clin N Am. 1995;33:447-59.
16. Datta R, Sandhu M, Saxena AK, et al. Role of duplex Doppler and power Doppler sonography with acute renal parenchymal dysfunction. Australasian Radiol. 2005;49(1):15-20.
17. Álvarez RS, Hevia PV, Sanz ME, et al. The usefulness of contrast-enhanced ultrasound in the assessment of early kidney transplant function and complications. Diagnostics (Basel) 2017;7(3):pii: E53.
18. Gruenewald S, Skerrett D, Dolimier D, et al. Technique of colour Doppler quantification of vascularity in transplanted kidneys. J Clin Ultrasound. 2002;30(3):151-7.
19. Hohenwalter MD, Skowlund CJ, Erickson SJ, et al. Renal transplant evaluation with MR angiography and MR imaging. Radiographics. 2001;21(6):1505.
20. Ledneva E, Karie S, Launay-Vacher V, et al. Renal safety of gadolinium-based contrast media in patients with chronic renal insufficiency. Radiology. 2009;250(3):618-28.
21. Broome DR, Girguis MS, Baron PW, et al. Gadodiamide-associated nephrogenic systemic fibrosis: why radiologists should be concerned. Am J Roentgenol. 2007;188(2):586-92.
22. Pedrosa I, Rofsky NM, Kidneys. In; Edelman RR, Hesselink JR, Zlatkin MB, et al. (Eds). Clinical Magnetic Resonance Imaging, 3rd edition. Philadelphia: Saunders; 2007. pp. 2851-2.
23. Seto K, Ikechira H, Obata T, et al. Long-term assessment of post-transplant renal prognosis with 31 P magnetic resonance spectroscopy. Transplantation. 2001;72(4):627-30.
24. Vermathen P, Binser T, Boesch C, et al. Three-year follow-up of human transplanted kidneys by diffusion-weighted MRI and blood oxygenation level-dependent imaging. J Magn Reson Imaging. 2012;35(5):1133-8.
25. Eisenberger U, Binser T, Thoeny HC, et al. Living renal allograft transplantation: diffusion-weighted MR imaging in longitudinal follow-up of the donated and the remaining kidney. Radiology. 2014;270(3):800-8.
26. Juillard L, Lerman LO, Kruger DG, et al. Blood oxygen level dependent measurement of acute intra-renal ischemia. Kidney Int. 2004;65(3):944-50.
27. Liu X, Berg N, Sheehan J, et al. Renal transplant: nonenhanced renal MR angiography with magnetization-prepared steady-state free precession. Radiology. 2009;251(2):535-42.
28. Lanzman RS, Voiculescu A, Walther C, et al. ECG-gated nonenhanced 3D steady-state free precession MR angiography in assessment of transplant renal arteries: comparison with DSA. Radiology. 2009;252(3):914-21.
29. Orons PD, Zajko AB. Angiography and interventional aspects of renal transplantation. Radiol Clin N Am. 1995;33(3):461-71.
30. Kobayashi K, Censullo ML, Rossman LL, et al. Interventional radiologic management of renal transplant dysfunction: indications, limitations, and technical considerations. Radiographics. 2007;27(4):1109-30.
31. Beecroft JR, Rajan DK, Clark TWI, et al. Transplant renal artery stenosis: out come after percutaneous intervention. J Vasc Interv Radiol. 2004;15(12):1407-13.
32. Pollak R, Veremis SA, Maddux MS, et al. The natural history of and therapy for perirenal fluid collections following renal transplantation. J Urol. 1988; 140(4):716-20.
33. Karcaaltincaba M, Akhan O. Radiologic imaging and percutaneous treatment of pelvic lymphocele. Eur J Radiol. 2005;55(3):340-54.

SECTION

2

Lower Urinary Tract

Chapter 11

Imaging Techniques and Radiological Anatomy of Lower Urinary Tract

Gaurav Shanker Pradhan, Satyam, Jyoti Kumar

INTRODUCTION

Radiological evaluation of the lower urinary tract was attempted in early twentieth century. John Cunningham had done urethrography for the first time in 1910 using highly dilute solution of mercuric iodide as contrast. Many contrast agents were subsequently tried to improve radiological visualization. Presently, nonionic iodinated contrast media are in widespread use because of their good radiopaque opacification and relatively less toxicity compared to other agents.

Micturating cystography is a useful technique for evaluation of bladder. Retrograde Urethrography (RGU) and Voiding Cystourethrography (VCUG) have become the gold standard for imaging of urethra. Cross-sectional imaging modalities including ultrasonography, computed tomography and magnetic resonance (MR) imaging are now frequently being used for detailed evaluation of bladder, urethral and periurethral abnormalities.

ANATOMY

Urinary Bladder

The urinary bladder is a subperitoneal musculomembranous sac which act as reservoir of urine. The size, shape, position and relation depend on the amount of fluid it contains. The empty bladder is flattened tetrahedron in shape while full bladder is round or oval in shape. The normal capacity of bladder is between 500 mL and 600 mL in adults. The empty bladder lies in the lesser pelvis and extend into the abdomen when full.

The bladder is situated posterior to symphysis pubis separated by fatty Retzius' space. Superiorly the bladder is covered by peritoneum, which continues posteriorly and is reflected on anterior surface of rectum. It is surrounded by perivesical fat and laterally bordered by obturator internus muscles and inferiorly by prostate gland. The bladder is connected to lateral pelvic wall by endopelvic fascia, which is strengthened by pubovesical and rectovesical ligaments.

It has four anatomical parts: apex, fundus, base and neck. The apex of the bladder is attached to the anterior abdominal wall by median umbilical ligament. The base of the bladder is continuous with bladder neck.

The wall of urinary bladder is smooth, regular with uniform thickness, not exceeding 6 mm in adult. The layers of the wall from inside out are serosa, smooth muscle, lamina propria, submucosa, and mucosa. The detrusor muscle has three layers: inner longitudinal, middle circular, and an outer longitudinal. Bladder is lined with a mucosal membrane consisting of the urothelium (a form of transitional epithelium), a basement membrane, and the lamina propria **(Fig. 1)**. The mucous membrane is

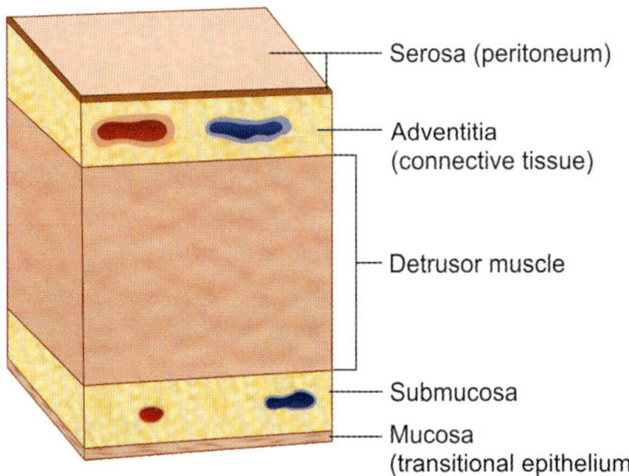

Fig. 1: Schematic diagram of constituents of wall of urinary bladder—The layers of the wall from inside out are serosa, smooth muscle, laminar propria, submucosa, and mucosa.

loosely attached to the muscular layer, except in triangular area just above and behind the internal orifice of urethra, termed as trigone, where it is firmly attached. The anterior angle is formed by internal orifice and its posterolateral orifice is formed by ureters. The interureteric ridge extending between two ureteric orifices, forms the posterior aspect of trigone. The distance between two orifices is same as the distance from internal urethral orifices, 2.5 cm in contracted state and 5 cm in distended state.

The arteries supplying bladder are superior, middle and inferior vesical arteries derived from anterior trunk of internal iliac artery. The inferior gluteal and obturator arteries gives a small visceral branch to the bladder and in females, additional supply is from uterine and vaginal arteries. The veins form a complicated plexus and drain into the hypogastric vein. The lymphatic drainage of bladder is primarily to external iliac lymph nodes.

Urethra

Male Urethra

The male urethra extends from the bladder to the external urethral meatus and is approximately 18 to 20 cm long. It has four parts and is divided into posterior and anterior portions **(Fig. 2)**, each of which is further divided into two parts.

The *posterior urethra* extends from the internal urethral orifice at bladder neck passing through anterior part of prostate distally to the inferior urogenital diaphragm. The posterior urethra consists of a prostatic segment and a membranous segment and is lined by transitional epithelium.

The *prostatic urethra* is surrounded by the prostate gland and measures 3 to 3.5 cm in length. It is the widest and most dilatable part of male urethra, being widest in the middle part and narrowest where it joins membranous urethra. The posterior wall of prostatic urethra has a median longitudinal ridge of smooth muscle (urethral crest) extending from bladder neck to membranous urethra. The longitudinal ridge continues into an ovoid mound known as verumontanum (15–17 mm in length and 3 mm in height). The prostatic utricle is a small saccular depression in the center of verumontanum. The ejaculatory ducts open distal and lateral to the utricle. The prostatic gland opens into prostatic urethra via prostatic sinuses.

The *membranous urethra* measures 1.5–2 cm in length and is surrounded by sphincter urethrae. It is the narrowest and least dilatable part of male urethra with the exception of external orifice. It extends from the distal end of verumontanum to the tip of cone of bulbous urethra. It runs downward and forward through the deep perineal space piercing the urogenital diaphragm about 2.5 cm below and behind the pubic symphysis. The urogenital diaphragm contains the external urethral sphincter with a Cowper gland on either side.

The *anterior urethra* extends from inferior edge of urogenital diaphragm distally to the external meatus and measures 15 cm in length. The anterior urethra consists of a bulbous segment and a penile or pendulous segment and is lined by stratified columnar epithelium.

The *bulbous urethra* is located between the inferior margin of the urogenital diaphragm and the penoscrotal junction. The bulbous urethra courses within the root of the penis and is tubular structure in the midline within the bulb of the corpus spongiosum. The proximal portion of bulbar urethra is dilated and called "sump" of bulbar

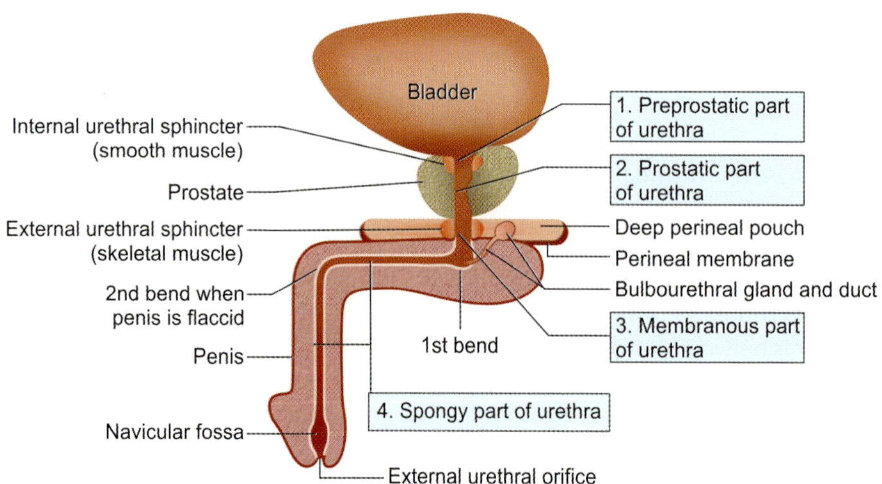

Fig. 2: Schematic diagram of male urethra.

urethra. It assumes a conical shape at bulbomembranous junction. The duct of Cowper glands are 2 cm long and empty into the bulbar urethral sump in midline. The periurethral Littre gland are present in anterior urethra.

The *penile urethra* extends from the penoscrotal junction to the external meatus with the distal 2 cm of dilated portion urethra known as *fossa navicularis.*

Urethral Sphincters

There are two sphincters which maintain continence of urine.

The *internal urethral sphincter* (sphincter vesicae) extends from the bladder neck through the prostatic urethra above the verumontanum and is composed of smooth muscle. It is the primary sphincter of urinary continence and involuntary in nature.

The *external sphincter* (sphincter urethrae) has both intrinsic and extrinsic components and is voluntary in nature. The *intrinsic urethral sphincter* is a concentric muscular structure that lies below the mound of the verumontanum in the distal third of the prostatic urethra and surrounds the membranous urethra. The intrinsic sphincter is composed of smooth muscle and also functions as muscle that maintains passive incontinence, along with internal sphincter. The intrinsic sphincter functions as the secondary continence sphincter. The *extrinsic sphincter* is paraurethral, composed of striated muscle with contributions from the levator ani complex and is voluntary in nature.

Female Urethra

The female urethra is a 4 cm long tubular structure, extending from the internal urethral meatus at bladder neck, 5 cm behind pubic symphysis, to external urethral meatus in the vestibule traversing through urogenital diaphragm. The external meatus opens directly in front of vaginal opening and about 2.5 cm behind glans clitoris. In the undilated stage, it is 6 mm in diameter. Numerous small submucosal paraurethral and periurethral glands opens into the urethra. The paraurethral glands of Skene secrete mucous material into either side of the distal urethra at the external meatus.

The proximal third of the urethra is lined by transitional cell epithelium and distal two-third of urethra is lined by stratified squamous epithelium. The urethropelvic and pubourethral ligaments help in maintaining urinary continence and urethral stability. The lower portion of the urethra is intimately situated next to the anterior vaginal wall and enveloped by common musculature (the urethrovaginal sphincter), which extends to the inferior pubic ramus above urogenital diaphragm.

IMAGING MODALITIES

Radiological evaluations of the urinary bladder and urethra are done by various imaging modalities such as:

- Plain radiograph
- Voiding cystourethrography
- Retrograde urethrography
- Cystography
- Retrograde pyelography
- Conduitogram
- Ultrasonography
- Computed tomography (CT)
- Magnetic resonance imaging (MRI)
- Urodynamic studies
- Radionuclide imaging.

Plain Radiographs

The plain radiograph is the primary modality for detection of radiopaque calculi in patients presenting with hematuria or foreign bodies, calcification, abnormal gas pattern and in identification of soft tissue and the bony abnormalities. **(Fig. 3)**. It is referred to as *scout film* prior to contrast studies to identify any radiopacity that may be obscured with contrast subsequently.

The plain radiograph done for evaluation of kidneys, ureters and bladder (KUB) is known by term X-ray KUB in which X-ray beam is centered in midline at level of iliac

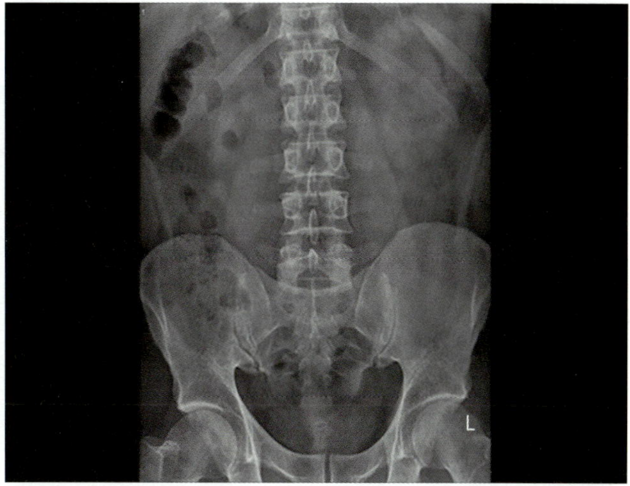

Fig. 3: X-ray Abdomen KUB- Bowel preparation is necessary. Patient micturates before examination (to see the bladder outline) and the radiograph is taken in full inspiration to include area of abdomen from adrenals to a point 2 cm below the inferior margin of pubic symphysis, with beam centering in midline at level of iliac crests.

crest and exposure factors generally used are low Kvp (65–75 Kvp) and high mA (60–100 mA).

Calcification of the bladder wall may be seen in tuberculosis, hydatid disease, tumors, radiation cystitis, cyclophosphamide induced cystitis, alkaline incrustation cystitis, amyloidosis and schistosomiasis. Radiolucent foreign bodies may get encrusted with calcium.

The plain radiograph typically shows gas within the bladder lumen and wall in emphysematous cystitis. Presence of gas is seen within the ureter wall in the emphysematous pyeloureteritis or emphysematous pyelonephritis.

It is also helpful for the detection of bony abnormalities such as metastases, spinal abnormalities in cases of neurogenic bladder and diastasis of the pubic symphysis in patients with exstrophy/epispadias anomaly.

Voiding Cystourethrography

Voiding cystourethrography is the standard technique in the evaluation of the posterior urethra of male, female urethra and bladder. It allows detection of bladder neck pathology, postsurgical stenosis and urethral stricture. The main indications of VCUG include evaluation of vesicoureteric reflux (VUR), urinary leak (post-trauma, surgery) and for urodynamic study. This study is particularly useful in evaluation of posterior urethral valves and for evaluation of diverticula, false tracts and strictures in the urethra.

Technique and Normal Appearance

Voiding cystourethrography is usually performed after filling the bladder with contrast material via a transurethral or suprapubic catheter. Patient is asked to empty bladder prior to the procedure. The patient is then catheterized and Foley's bulb is inflated in bladder followed by instillation of contrast, till patient can tolerate. Once the bladder is distended, urethral catheter is withdrawn, and patient is asked to void under fluoroscopic monitoring. The spot radiographs of the bladder and urethra are then obtained after positioning the patient in right and left anterior oblique positions to avoid super imposition of the urethra on the pubic symphysis. Full KUB radiograph is taken to assess bladder anatomy and presence of any undetected VUR. This is followed by a postvoid film to evaluate residual volume of bladder (PVR). In case clinical suspicion of vesicovaginal fistula (VVF) or rectovaginal fistula (RVF), a lateral view must also be taken.

During active voiding, the bladder neck opens widely and becomes funnel shaped in both male and female patients by means of the internal sphincter mechanism. In males, the verumontanum appears elongated and the proximal bulbar urethra has a less conical appearance. The membranous urethra remains the narrowest segment between these parts of the urethra **(Figs. 4A and B)**. During voiding, it may dilate up to 6 or 7 mm in diameter.

Voiding cystourethrography may not demonstrate certain abnormalities of the male anterior urethra because the normal anterior urethra is not fully distended. It is an invasive study and does not provide information regarding the periurethral tissues.

Retrograde Urethrography

Retrograde urethrography is considered the standard imaging technique for evaluation of *anterior urethra.*

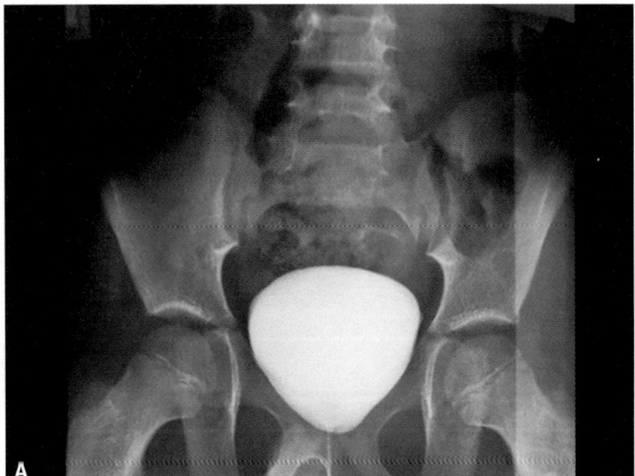

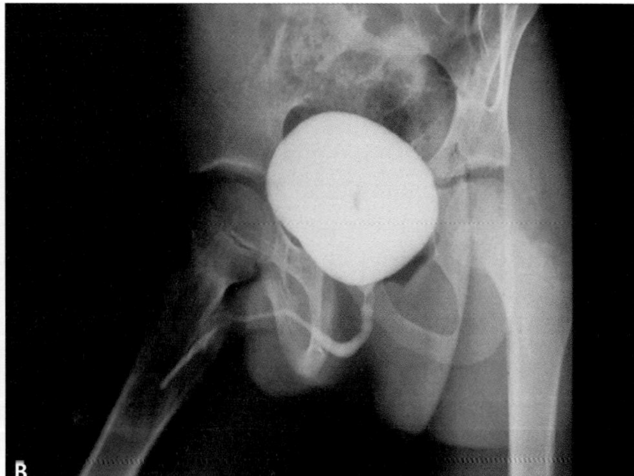

Figs. 4A and B: Micturating cystography involves the introduction of contrast into the urinary bladder followed by micturition urinary bladder for the evaluation of the urinary bladder and urethra.

It is the primary modality indicated in the evaluation of urethral injuries, inflammatory disease, strictures and fistulas. Assessment of the location, length and severity of urethral pathologies can be done based on RGU studies.

Technique and Normal Appearance

The patient is placed in a supine 45 oblique position. The penis should be placed laterally over the proximal thigh with moderate traction. The patient should be reassured about the discomfort that is experienced during balloon inflation. A 16-F or 18-F Foley's catheter is inserted into urethra so that the balloon lies in fossa navicularis and is inflated with 2 to 3 mL of water to anchor catheter and occlude the meatus. Then, 20–30 mL of iodinated contrast material is injected in the anterior urethra under fluoroscopic guidance through the Foley's catheter till it is adequately distended **(Fig. 5)**.

After the visual confirmation of contrast material flowing into the bladder, spot radiographs are obtained. Sometimes, normal structures such as prostatic duct, Littre's gland and Cowper duct are also opacified due to intravasation of contrast.

The external urethral sphincter spasm encountered during injection can be overcome by slow and gentle pressure. Sometimes, lidocaine gel or normal saline may be used to obtain urethral distention in such cases. Sometimes, there is disruption of urethral mucosa due to increased pressure during injection, which causes opacification of corpora and draining vein due to intravasation of contrast.

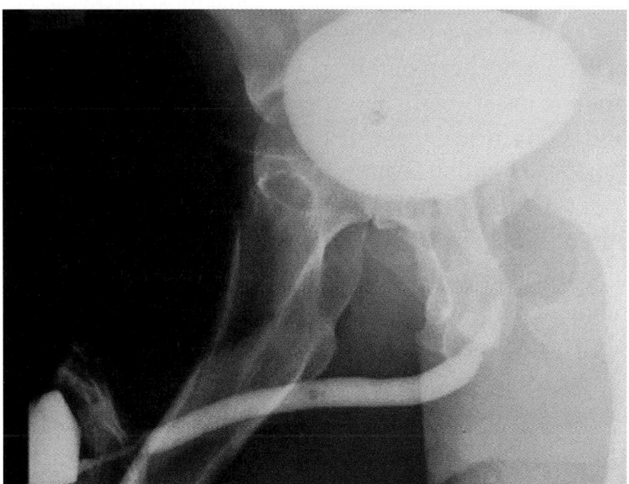

Fig. 5: For retrograde urethrography, the patient is placed in a supine 45 oblique position. 20–30 mL of iodinated contrast is injected under fluoroscopic guidance through the catheter with tip in fossa navicularis, so that the anterior urethra is filled. Spot radiographs are obtained when there is visual confirmation of contrast material flowing into the bladder.

Acute urinary tract infection (UTI), urethral trauma and intravasation of contrast are few *complications* of the procedure. Recent instrumentation and acute UTI are two *contraindications* of this procedure.

Cystography

Cystography (retrograde, excretory or suprapubic) is a contrast study of bladder to evaluate its position, morphology, integrity and distensibility. It allows evaluation of both intraluminal and intramural lesions and functional abnormalities. Contrast cystogram can clearly depict wall irregularities, tumors, intraluminal calculi and hematomas. It also demonstrates the type of bladder rupture (extraperitoneal or intraperitoneal) along with pelvic fractures in traumatic injury. Extrinsic compression of the bladder produced by pelvic hematoma or lipomatosis results in "teardrop bladder" and is better evaluated on cross-sectional imaging.

Conventional retrograde cystography is considered as gold standard in suspected bladder injury and plays an important role in patients with renal failure having lesions in the bladder.

In the *excretory cystogram,* bladder is evaluated simultaneously along with upper urinary tracts in intravenous pyelography (IVP), but it is difficult to recognize reflux.

Cystography of bladder and Voiding cystourethrography are indicated for demonstration of anatomic abnormalities of the bladder neck and urethra.

About 300 to 400 mL appropriately diluted nonionic contrast is instilled in bladder using Foley's catheter. Images are then obtained under fluoroscopic guidance in various projections (AP, oblique, lateral, during rest and strain/or voiding) appropriate to the indications for the study.

Pregnancy, UTI and allergy to iodinated contrast are contraindications to the procedure.

Retrograde Pyelography

This investigation is infrequently used for evaluation of lower ureters when pathology like lower ureteric stones, mitotic process or strictures are not demonstrated by other imaging modalities. It is an invasive procedure where ureteral orifice is cannulated cystoscopically and catheter is advanced into renal pelvis and contrast is injected. The examination is performed with graded withdrawal of catheter under fluoroscopic monitoring and appropriate spot films are taken.

Conduitogram

An ileal conduit is constructed for urinary diversion after partial or complete cystectomy. One end of the ileum is brought to skin as an ileocutaneous stoma and ureters are implanted in the opposite end of the loop. Contrast material is instilled into the ileal loop through stoma. It demonstrates ureters and renal collecting system. The study is also called loopogram or an ideal conduit study. The study is useful in patient with impaired renal function and serves to exclude ureteral obstruction. It also helps to evaluate stricture or leak at the site of anastomosis of ureter and ileal conduit.

Ultrasonography

Urinary Bladder

Real-time ultrasonography (US) is the primary modality in the evaluation of bladder lesions.

Bladder US indications include:

- Evaluation of bladder wall, its base, distal ureter and urethral orifice anatomy.
- For evaluation of thickening, diverticula and trabeculations.
- Pre and post-void residual volume.
- Bladder calculi including radiolucent calculi, which may be missed on plain radiographs.
- Blood clots and sediments within the lumen.
- Intraluminal filling defects and extraluminal masses causing bladder compression.
- For guiding diagnostic and therapeutic interventions.

Technique: The urinary bladder must be examined when it is comfortably distended either by oral intake of fluid and voiding restrictions. In anuric patient, it can be retrogradely filled with normal saline through a catheter. The bladder sonography is done by transabdominal, perineal, endorectal or endovaginal approaches.

Transabdominal approach is the most common. In this approach, a 3.5–5 MHz sector scanning transducer is placed in suprapubic region and angled appropriately for longitudinal and transverse views of bladder.

Transrectal/Transvaginal transducer (frequency range from 3.5–7 MHz) is used to image bladder base, its neck and for evaluation of posterior wall masses. It is useful in defining the plane between the bladder, prostate and seminal vesicles.

Transurethral US scan provides better details of urinary bladder wall and is used to visualize and stage bladder tumor.

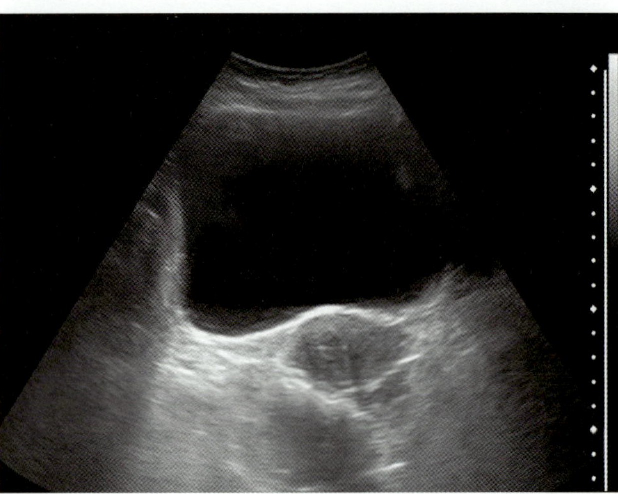

Fig. 6: Examination of the urinary bladder requires well filled bladder for its detailed evaluation for the adjoining structures and tissues.

Normal sonographic appearance: The bladder is present in midline in true pelvis and appears as a sonolucent structure with smooth thin wall. Its shape is oval in the trans-axial plane and triangular in sagittal plane **(Fig. 6)**. Reverberation artefact seen during bladder scanning can be avoided by slightly changing the angle of transducer.

Bladder wall measures 3–6 mm, is comprised hyperechoic outer serosa and mucosa with hypoechoic detrusor muscle in between.

The formula used to calculate full bladder volume and postmicturition residual volume is 0.523 × length × width × height.

The ureteric orifice is seen as small focal thickening in the bladder base on either side, through which low level of echoes are seen entering bladder which are known as ureteric jets. Ureteric jets are best evaluated on Doppler and their presence rules out complete obstruction **(Fig. 7)**. In normal healthy person, ureteric jet frequency is of two or more per minute on either side. If ureteric jets are absent during steady diuresis phase for 10 more minutes of observation, it represent complete obstruction and frequency of less than two per minute may indicate partial obstruction.

Male Urethra

Urethral ultrasound plays an important role in the evaluation of urethra, periurethral tissue and for diagnosis, assessment of thickness and length of urethral strictures. It is equally efficacious as RGU in detection and characterization of anterior urethral strictures and false

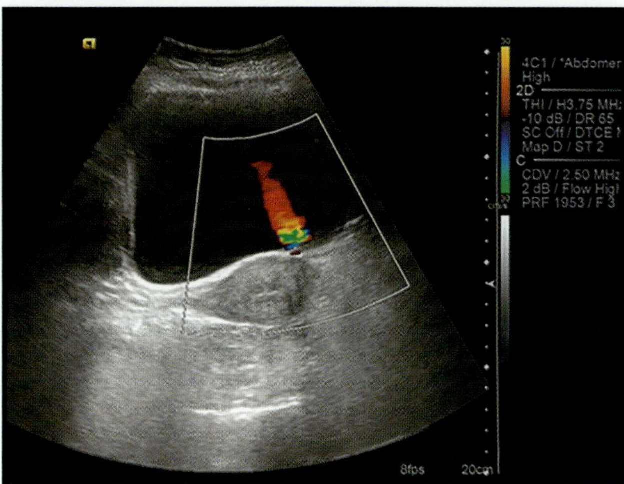

Fig. 7: For routine, transabdominal urinary bladder imaging, bladder must be full. UV junction obstruction can also be inferred by evaluation of lower ureteric jets on color Doppler.

tracts with the added advantage of lower incidence of complications.

Voiding urethral sonography detects the bladder neck and posterior urethra pathology (anatomical and functional), postsurgical stenosis and neoplasm.

Technique and normal appearance: Sonography of the urethra is usually performed using a broadband 5–10 MHz linear array for transpenile or transperineal scanning and a broadband 5–9 MHz curved array for transrectal scanning. The *posterior male urethra* can be evaluated by TRUS. Endourethral sonography is performed with a catheter (6.2-F) based transducer (12.5 MHz) on a dedicated intravascular US machine.

Penile urethra can be seen through penile shaft using the linear probe after filling the penile urethra with fluid or gel. The normal urethra is seen as an anechoic tubular structure. It is also called *ascending urethral sonography.* Subscrotal and perineal views delineate anterior urethra clearly in longitudinal and transverse scanning planes.

A modification of this technique is *descending urethral ultrasound* technique in which urethral distension is achieved during voiding, which is interrupted by gently clamping 2 cm proximal to the tip of penis. Under distension of urethra can lead to false diagnosis of stricture. This technique is useful in evaluating strictures in region of navicular fossa, pre- and postoperative patients of hypospadias repair, trauma and in planning reconstructive anterior urethroplasty.

Advances in imaging technology like extended field of view imaging have enhanced the use of this modality in clinical practice.

Female Urethra

Ultrasound allows detailed evaluation of female urethra and periurethral disease by using transabdominal, transvaginal, transperineal, and transurethral US approaches.

Technique and normal appearance: In transvaginal US, a 5–9 MHz curved-array transducer is used and is inserted approximately 1–2 cm into the vagina and in transperineal US, a 5–10 MHz linear-array transducer is placed on the perineum between the labia for obtaining sagittal and transverse images. For transurethral US, a catheter (6.2 F) based transducer (12.5 MHz) on an intravascular US machine is used. Axial images are obtained as catheter is withdrawn. Patients lie in the lithotomy position with partially filled bladder. The urethra is evaluated from the bladder neck to the distal urethral opening, with subsequent attention given to the periurethral area. It is used for diagnosis of urethral diverticula and strictures.

The female urethra is visualized on transabdominal scan as short anechoic channel with anteroposterior diameters just inferior to the bladder measuring 1–1.5 cm. It appears less echogenic than the surrounding connective tissue or the bladder wall.

There is an important role of dynamic US in the diagnosis and classification of pelvic floor dysfunction and pelvic organ prolapse. Dynamic US with endoluminal transducers is an emerging technique in the evaluation of pelvic floor dysfunction. It allows real-time evaluation of the displacement of pelvic floor muscles and pelvic organs during provocative maneuvers such as coughing and the Valsalva maneuver.

In women with symptoms of stress incontinence, hypermobility of the urethra or a "funnel" appearance of the proximal urethra may be noted during coughing due to laxity of connective tissues. After surgical correction of pelvic organ prolapse, endoluminal US is valuable in assessing achievement of normal genitourinary anatomy and the absence of urethral funneling and recurrent cystourethrocele.

Computed Tomography

Computed tomography urography (CTU) has emerged as a promising tool in the evaluation of urologic conditions over IVU. CT cystography is an accurate and safe means for identification of bladder injury and urine leakage following bladder or posterior urethra rupture in abdominal trauma patient.

The important indications of CTU in lower urinary tract (LUT) are:

- Evaluation of hematuria
- Identification of size and number of distal ureteric, vesicle or urethral calculi and calcification
- Staging of bladder and urethral malignancy
- Pelvic trauma and bladder rupture
- Postoperative complications
- Congenital anomalies.

Technique

Computed tomography urography is mainly done to evaluate upper tract collecting system, ureters and urinary bladder in excretory phase. The three techniques used are single bolus, split bolus and triple bolus protocols.

Single bolus technique is the most common and routinely used. In this, first noncontrast image is acquired. After full bolus of contrast injection, images are acquired in the nephrographic phase (80 to 120s), corticomedullary phase (30 to 40s) and delayed excretory phase (5 to 15 min), however, corticomedullary phase is optional for evaluation in case of bladder pathologies. The bladder tumor can be best evaluated in nephrographic or excretory phase.

In split bolus technique, the contrast is given into separate injections. After taking noncontrast scan, a part of contrast is given and corticomedullary images are obtained. The second portion of contrast is given 5 to 8 minutes after the first injection and combined nephrographic and excretory phase images are acquired. The images acquired from entire abdomen and pelvis. It is done in younger patients to reduce radiation dose.

Computed tomography cystography consists of imaging of bladder following retrograde filling of bladder with contrast up to patient tolerance (200–300 mL) followed by a CT of the pelvis. It should be followed by intravenous contrast administration and acquisition of abdomen and pelvis after that. Postdrainage scan are not required. It should be done in all patients with pelvic fracture or with gross hematuria.

Normal Computed Tomography Appearance

The urinary bladder is seen as a homogeneous midline structure of water density. The outer margin of the bladder wall is smooth and has soft tissue attenuation. It is well-delineated by the perivesical fat. The urine shows water density attenuation. The size and configuration depends on the amount of urine present **(Figs. 8A to C)**.

Noncontrast scans are useful for detection of vesicle calculi, intravesical hemorrhage, bladder wall calcification and gas in bladder wall and lumen.

In contrast enhanced CT scan, opacified urine usually occupies the dependent portion of the bladder and unopacified urine layers above it. However, this relationship may be reversed in patients with glycosuria or infectious debris in the bladder. Contrast-enhanced CT (CECT) is essential in tumor staging especially for evaluation of bladder wall and transmural extent and distinction of lymph node from vascular structures and adjacent masses compressing or displacing the bladder. CT can also reveal elevation and narrowing of the bladder (pear shaped bladder) in retroperitoneal fibrosis, pelvic lipomatosis, hematoma and lymphoceles. It also helps in the evaluation of lower ureter if thickened or inflamed as evidenced by its wall thickening and periureteral fat stranding.

Virtual Cystoscopy

Virtual cystoscopy is a diagnostic tool for evaluation of bladder pathology. It is dedicated for evaluating the mucosal surface of the bladder and therefore, can detect superficial lesion greater than 5 mm. It allows the operator to navigate the mucosal surface in various projections. The technique of virtual cystoscopy/endoscopy has been refined and clinically improved over the last few years.

It can either be done as part of the routine CTU protocol using contrast-filled bladder, or using an air-filled bladder. The contrast filled bladder protocol are more commonly used over air-filled technique as latter requires catheterization and there is possibility of leakage of air with change in position. The most commonly used multidetector computed tomography (MDCT) protocol include unenhanced scan in supine and prone and postcontrast scan as per CT urography protocol. Volumetric data set is acquired and are computer rendered to generate 3D images. Special software then allows navigation through the bladder. Virtual endoscopy techniques may provide ureteral "flythrough" allowing to have an ureteroscopic viewpoint of the urinary tract.

The main complications of air-filled technique are infection due to the use of room air and CT must be acquired in both prone and supine position and that of contrast filled technique are contrast allergy and inability to be done in renal insufficiency.

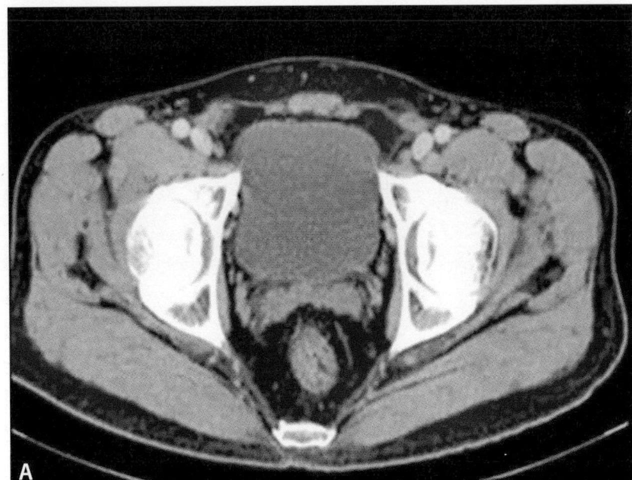

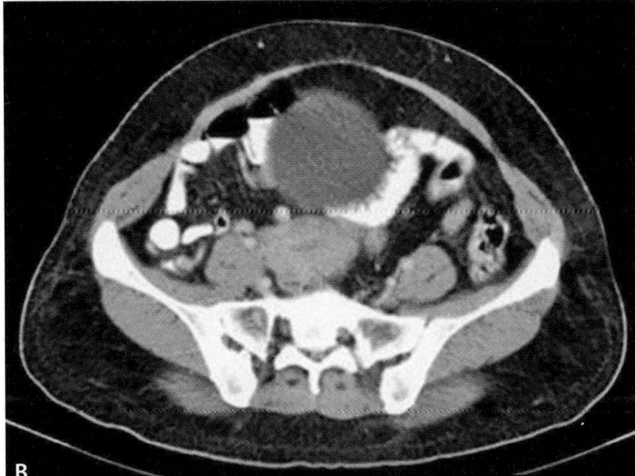

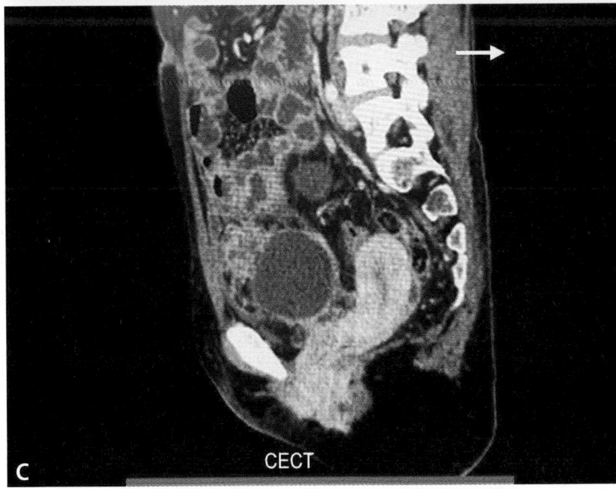

Figs. 8A to C: (A) On CT scan, the urinary bladder is seen as a homogeneous midline structure of water density. Outer margin of the bladder wall is smooth and usually well delineated by the perivesical fat; (B) Scans obtained before and after administration of contrast medium can detect subtle vesical and perivesical abnormalities; (C) Contrast-enhanced CT depicting very well the relation of enhancing bladder wall with adjacent structures (uterus and cervix) in a female patient of carcinoma cervix.

Its advantages are noninvasive nature and no risk for local infection, bladder perforation, strictures and scarring. The disadvantages include failure to detect flat lesions and to distinguish mucosal thickening due to fibrosis from neoplasm.

Magnetic Resonance Imaging

Recent technological advances in MR imaging allows more detailed evaluation of urinary bladder, urethral and periurethral abnormalities. Advances in MR imaging hardware and pulse sequences allow high-resolution, high-contrast static and dynamic imaging of the urinary bladder, urethral and periurethral region in the context of the entire pelvic floor.

Magnetic resonance images provide an excellent insight into the anatomy and pathology of the urinary bladder due to its exquisite contrast resolution and multiplanar ability. It clearly differentiates the three layers of the bladder wall and enables accurate assessment of the depth of tumor invasion and extravesical extension in patients with bladder tumors. Multiparametric MRI techniques enables better evaluation and staging of bladder cancer. It also offers functional information through pulse sequences such as diffusion weighted MRI (DW MRI) and dynamic contrast MRI (DCE MRI).

Magnetic resonance cystography is used for bladder tumor detection, complication of tumor, trauma such as leak, fistulae, or sinus tract formation and VUR. It is mainly used in a patient who have iodine allergy or contraindication to CT.

Technique and Recommended Sequence

The standard MRI sequences used in the bladder imaging are T1 and T2 weighted in all three axial, coronal and sagittal planes, diffusion-weighted MRI (DWI) and T1-weighted with fat saturation pre and post IV administration of gadolinium. Dedicated phased array multi coils and endorectal coils significantly improve image resolution.

Dynamic contrast-enhanced T1-weighted MRI is used for tumor staging and prognostication.

Lymphotropic nanoparticle-enhanced MRI can be used for differentiating bowel loops from lymph nodes and thus prove to be helpful in nodal staging in bladder cancer patients using MR oral intestinal contrast agents such as ferrite particles.

In MR cystogram, initially a precontrast image is taken and then imaging is done after installation of gadolinium in 1:100 concentration (5 mL in 500 mL of saline). In patients with contrast allergies gadolinium is replaced by saline solution.

Normal Magnetic Resonance Appearance

The urinary bladder is clearly demonstrated on MRI regardless of distension. Urine has low signal intensity on T1W and high on T2W. Muscle layer has low signal intensity on T2-weighted image and low to intermediate signal intensity on T1-weighted images. Both mucosa and lamina propria have higher signal intensity as compared to muscle on proton density sequences **(Figs. 9A to C)**. Lateral wall are best evaluated on axial section. Dome, base, anterior and posterior wall of the bladder are primarily evaluated on sagittal images, however, coronal images do play complimentary role. T1W Fat-Sat spin echo is helpful in evaluation of lymph node and bone.

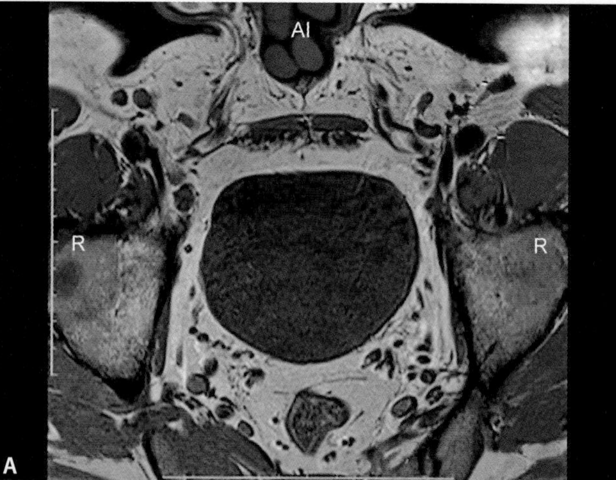

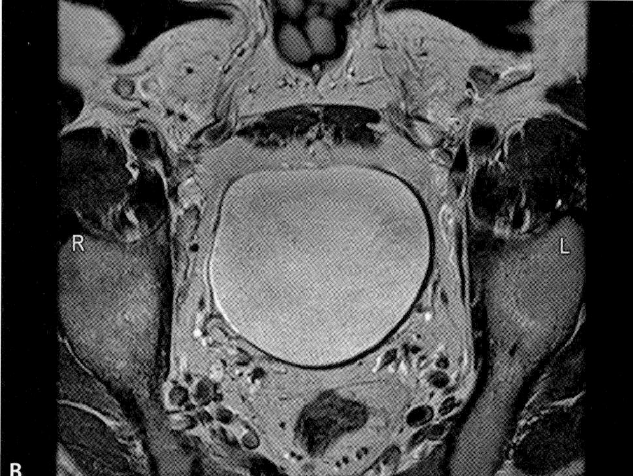

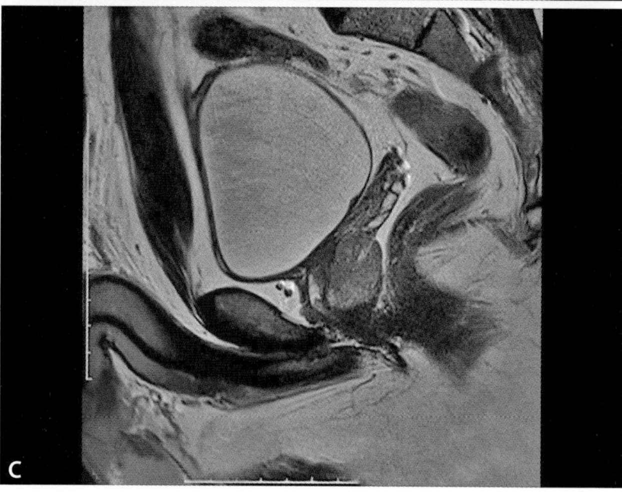

Figs. 9A to C: MR-T1 and T2-weighted fast spin-echo axial sections (A and B) with phased array coil showing normal distended urinary bladder. The urine appears hypointense on T1 with intermediate signal bladder wall. The urine appears bright on T2 with low-signal wall. The perivesical fat appears bright on T1 and intermediate signal on T2. The pelvic side walls, rectum and fat planes are well seen; (C) Dome, base, anterior and posterior wall of the bladder are primarily evaluated on sagittal images.

Urethra

Magnetic resonance imaging provides detailed multi-planar evaluation of urethra and periurethral tissues. Both T1- and T2 weighted imaging are used to evaluate the male and female urethra. Dedicated phased array or endocavitary coils can be used for detailed evaluation.

Male urethra: T2-weighted images show the course of the anterior and posterior urethras in sagittal and coronal planes. The proximal portion of the prostatic urethra and distal penile urethra is properly visualized on MR images only if an indwelling catheter is placed. Initial evaluation of the membranous urethra is done in the axial plane and images in sagittal and coronal planes are useful to assess relationship with adjoining structures, especially in cases of trauma. Contrast enhanced MR imaging can be performed in patients with mitotic or inflammatory processes involving the urethra and periurethral tissues.

Female urethra: Magnetic resonance imaging because of its superior temporal resolution is suitable for anatomic evaluation of various urethral and periurethral abnormalities. It is useful in local staging of urethral tumors. It can also be of help in evaluating congenital anomalies, diverticulum, inflammation, trauma, and fistula of the urethra in female patients. On MR imaging, a fistula can be seen as a direct communication channel with an adjacent organ.

Virtual Cystoscopy Magnetic Resonance

Magnetic resonance based virtual cystoscopy newer technique being increasingly used as an adjunct to conventional cystoscopy to assess bladder noninvasively. It is better than conventional cystoscopy as, it is impervious to hematuria, and anterior bladder wall lesion and urethral stricture. It has certain limitations such as time consuming, costly and require expertise. It is not possible to do biopsy with MR cystoscopy (MRC) or detect flat lesions.

Magnetic resonance cystoscopy is done by two ways: (1) 3D T1W MRI is acquired after filling the bladder with gadolinium retrogradely by catheter or intravenously, (2) 3D T2W MRI is acquired after luminal distension with urine. The 3D data sets obtained from both methods can be evaluated by multiplanar, 3D or virtual cystoscopic "fly through" reconstruction method.

Urodynamic Studies

Urodynamic studies are functional studies of urinary bladder and are considered to be the most definitive tests for determining the source of symptoms involving the lower urinary tract, including the bladder and the urethra for storing and releasing urine. These tests can help to pinpoint the anatomic or neurologic source of symptoms such as leakage, frequent urination, problem in initiating stream, dribbling, painful urination, difficulty in completely emptying the bladder and recurrent UTI.

The types of tests that are administered depend on the patient's symptoms and may include one or more of the tests like uroflowmetry, cystometry, pressure studies for stress incontinence, VCUG, video urodynamics and assessment of postvoid residual urine, etc.

Nuclear Imaging

Radionuclide cystography has been accepted as the technique of choice for evaluation and follow-up of children with UTI and reflux.

Positron emission tomography-CT (PET-CT) and PET -MR are hybrid imaging modalities that have combined both morphologic and functional imaging simultaneously for providing better information for guiding therapy.

The most commonly used PET radiotracer is 2-deoxy-2-(18F)-fluorodeoxyglucose (18F-FDG).

FDG-PET is useful in monitoring response to therapy and management urinary bladder cancer. It also helps in identification of distant metastasis. FDG PET has limited role in urologic cancer because of high urinary activity of radiotracer.

PET-CT has established its role in metastatic work up for bladder cancer. It helps in detection of primary tumor and nodal metastasis.

PET-MR due to its better soft tissue resolution and with simultaneous use of DW-MRI and DCE MRI detects local tumor, nodal and distant metastasis.

Recent advances in PET-CT/PET MR techniques and with few new radiotracer such as C11-choline and C11-acetate have increased the role of this technique in urinary bladder cancer.

CONCLUSION

The imaging techniques for evaluation of lower urinary tract have advanced seemingly in past decades. VCU and RGU remains the mainstay of conventional imaging procedures for evaluation of lower urinary tract, while ultrasound remains a promising a screening tool. Cross-sectional imaging like CT and MRI are the modality of choice for staging and follow up of urothelial malignancy. With the advent of the multiparametric MRI incorporating anatomic and functional sequences such as DWI, DCE-MRI, and lymphotropic nanoparticle-enhanced MRI, MR has become the mainstay in the diagnosis, staging, and follow-up of bladder cancer.

SUGGESTED READING

1. Arif SH, Mohammed AA. Primary hydatid cyst of the urinary bladder. BMJ Case Rep. 2018. pii: bcr-2018-226341. doi: 10.1136/bcr-2018-226341.
2. Berná-Mestre JD, Berná-Serna JD. Anterior urethral trauma: role of sonourethrography. Emerg Radiol. 2009;16(5):391-4.
3. Bernhardt TM, Rapp Bernhardt U. Virtual cystoscopy of the bladder based on CT and MRI data. Abdom Imaging. 2001;26(3):325-32.
4. Bernhardt TM, Schmidl H, Philipp C, et al. Diagnostic potential of virtual cystoscopy of the bladder. MRI vs CT preliminary report. Eur Radiol. 2003;13(2):305-12.
5. Buckley JC, Wu AK, McAninch JW. Impact of urethral ultrasonography on decision-making in anterior urethroplasty. BJU Int. 2012;109(3):438-42.
6. Chan DP, Abujudeh HH, Cushing GL Ir Novelline RACl cystography with multiplanar reformation for suspected bladder rupture: experience in 234 cases. AJR Am J Roentgenol. 2006;187(5):1296-302.
7. Choudhary S, Singh P, Sundar E, et al. A comparison of sonourethrography and retrograde urethrography in evaluation of anterior urethral strictures. Clin Radiol. 2004;59(8):736-42.
8. Choyke PL, Bluth EI, Bush WH Jr, et al. Radiological investigation of patients with hematuria. American College of Radiology, ACR Appropriateness Criteria, 2005.
9. Clinical Magnetic Resonance Imaging. Vol 3 2006,Elsevier Inc. Page 2889-2905.
10. Cruz J, Figueiredo F, Matos AP, et al. Infectious and inflammatory diseases of the urinary tract: role of MR imaging. Magn Reson Imaging Clin N Am. 2019;27(1):59-75.
11. David S. A Textbook of Radiology. 1993;2:1079-97.
12. Ferguson GG, Bullock TL, Anderson RE, et al. Minimally invasive methods for bulbar urethral strictures: a survey of members of the American Urological Association. Urology. 2011;78(3):701-6.

13. Gupta N, Dubey D, Mandhani A, et al. Urethral stricture assessment: a prospective study evaluating urethral ultrasonography and conventional radiological studies. BJU Int. 2006;98(1):149-53.
14. Johnin K1, Kobayashi K1, Tsuru T1, et al. Pediatric voiding cystourethrography: An essential examination for urologists but a terrible experience for children. Int J Urol. 2019;26(2): 160-71.
15. Karavaş E, Gürel S, Kıyan A, et al. Effect of Prone and Supine Positioning on Computed Tomography Urography Examination. Urol Int. 2018;101(2):167-74.
16. Kawashima Ã, Glockner JF, King BF Jr. CT urography and MR urography. Radiol Clin North Am. 2003;41(5):945-61.
17. Kim JK, Park SY, Kim HS, et al. Comparison of virtual cystoscopy, multiplanar reformation and source CT images with contrast material filled bladder for detecting lesions. AJR Am J Roentgenol. 2005;185(3):689-96.
18. Kim JY, Harisinghani MG. MR imaging staging of pelvic lymph nodes. Magn Reson Imaging Clin N Am. 2004;12(3):581-6.
19. Kim SU, Han MC. Reversed contrast-urine levels in urinary bladder: CT findings. Urol Radiol. 1992;13(14):249.52.
20. Maher MM, Kalra MK, Rizzo S, et al. Multidetector CT urography in imaging of the urinary tract in patients with hematuria. Korean J Radiol. 2004;5(1):1-10.
21. Mallampati GK, Siegelman ES. MR imaging of the bladder. Magn Reson Imaging Clin N Am. 2004:12(3):545-55.
22. McCallum RW. The adult male urethra normal anatomy, pathology, and method of urethrography. Radiol Clin North Am. 1979;17(2):227-44.
23. Mitterberger M, Christian G, Pinggera GM, et al. Gray scale and color Doppler sonography with extended field of view technique for the diagnostic evaluation of anterior urethral strictures. J Urol. 2007;177(3):992-6.
24. Morgan DE, Nallamala LK, Kenney PJ, et al. CT cystography: Radiographic and clinical predictors of bladder rupture. AJR Am J Roentgenol. 2000;174(1):89-95.
25. Pollack HM, Banner MP Martinez LO, et al. Diagnostic considerations in urinary bladder wall calcification. AJR. 1981;136(4):791-7.
26. Price CI, Adler RS, Rubin JM. Ultrasound depiction of differences in density: Explanation of ureteral jet phenomenon and implications for new ultrasound applications. Invest Radiol. 1989;24(11):876-83.
27. Raman SP, Fishman EK. Upper and Lower Tract Urothelial Imaging Using Computed Tomography Urography. Urol Clin North Am. 2018;45(3):389-405.
28. Rickards D, Hare C. The lower urinary tract. In Meire HB, Cosgrove D, Dewbury KC, Farrant P (Eds). Abdominal and General Ultrasound. Edinburgh, Churchill Livingstone; 585-611,200
29. Silverman SG, Leyendecker JR, Amis SE Jr. What is the current role of CT urography and MR urography in the evaluation of the urinary tract? Radiology. 2009;250(2):309-23.
30. Taveras N, Demas BE, Hricak H. MR Imaging of bladder neoplasms: correlation with pathologic staging. Urol Radiol. 1990;12(1):27-33.
31. The Journal of Urology. 1932;28(4):461-76.
32. Thurston W, Wilson SR. The Urinary Tract in Rumack CM, Wilson SR, Charboneau JW (Eds) Diagnostic ultrasound. 3rd edition. Elsevier Mosby; 2005. pp. 321-93.
33. Vaccaro JP, Brody JM. CT Cystography in the Evaluation of Major Bladder Trauma. RadioGraphics. 2000;20(5):1373-81.

Chapter 12

Urinary Bladder and Urethral Diseases

Anupam Lal, Paramjeet Singh, Harish Bhujade

ANATOMY

Urinary Bladder

The urinary bladder is a musculomembranous sac which acts as a reservoir for the urine. Its size, shape, position, and relations vary according to the amount of fluid it contains. The empty bladder takes a form of flattened tetrahedron and when it is distended with urine, it becomes round or oval in shape. In adults, the normal bladder capacity is highly variable but is usually between 500 mL and 600 mL. The normal wall of the bladder is smooth, regular, and uniform in thickness (typically 2–3 mm in fully distended bladder) not exceeding 6 mm in adults.

The bladder lies in the anterosuperior portion of the pelvic cavity, behind the pubic ramus, with "space of Retzius" in between, which contains fat and obliterated urachus. Superiorly, the bladder is enveloped by peritoneum which continues posteriorly and is then reflected onto the anterior surface of the rectum (anterior surface of uterus in females). The bladder is surrounded by perivesical fat; and is connected to pelvic wall by the endopelvic fascia which is strengthened by the pubovesical and rectovesical ligaments. It is bordered laterally by the obturator internus muscles and inferiorly by the prostate gland. The superoanterior portion of the bladder, the apex, is attached to the anterior abdominal wall by the median umbilical ligament, a remnant of the urachus. The posteroinferior wall, referred to as the base, is continuous with the bladder neck. The urinary bladder wall consists of mucosa, lamina propria, submucosa, and smooth muscle layer.

The mucous membrane consists of multilayered transitional epithelium, which is loosely attached to the muscular coat over greater part of the viscus and appears folded/wrinkled when the bladder is contracted. Over a small triangular area, termed the "trigone," immediately behind and above the internal orifice of the urethra, the mucous membrane is firmly bounded to the muscular coat and is always smooth. The internal orifice of urethra forms the anterior angle of the trigone and its posterolateral angles are formed by the orifices of the ureters. A ridge of muscle, "the interureteric ridge," extends between the ureteral orifices and forms the posterior aspect of the trigone. In the contracted bladder the ureteric orifices are ~2.5 cm apart and at same distance from the internal urethral orifice. These measurements may be increased to about 5 cm in the distended bladder. The muscular component of the bladder wall is composed of longitudinal and circular smooth muscle bundles that form distinct layers near the bladder neck.

The arterial supply of the bladder consists of the superior, middle, and inferior vesical arteries, which are derived from the anterior trunk of the internal iliac artery. The obturator and inferior gluteal arteries also supply smaller visceral branches to the bladder; and in the female additional branches are derived from the uterine and vaginal arteries. The veins form a complex plexus on the inferior surface, and fundus near the prostate, and end in the hypogastric veins. Lymphatic drainage of the bladder is primarily to the external iliac chain of lymph nodes.

Urethra

The urethra is made up of mucous membrane, which is supported by a submucous tissue connecting it with the various other structures through which it passes.

The Male Urethra

The male urethra measures between ~17.5 cm and 20 cm in length. It is represented by a double curve in the ordinary relaxed state of penile shaft. It has anterior and posterior parts, which are further subdivided into two parts. The anterior urethra extends from the external meatus to the inferior margin of the urogenital diaphragm, courses through the corpus spongiosum. The anterior urethra is traditionally divided into the pendulous (or penile) and bulbar parts at the penoscrotal junction based on anatomical and imaging appearance. The penile segment ends in the glans penis forming a *"fossa navicularis"*, which measures ~1–1.5 cm long. The proximal part of the bulbar urethra appears dilated and termed the "sump" of bulbar urethra. The bulbar urethra has a conical shape at the bulbomembranous junction just proximal to the sump. This portion of the bulb is called as the "cone." The anterior urethra has periurethral "Littre glands," which are more in number in the bulbar urethral sump and at the dorsal side of the penile urethra. Two pea-sized glands, namely "Cowper's glands", are present within the urogenital diaphragm on either side of the membranous part of the posterior urethra. The Cowper's gland's ducts are ~2 cm long and drain into the bulbar urethral sump on each side of midline.

The posterior urethra consists of prostatic and membranous urethras. The prostatic urethra, the widest and most dilatable part of the canal, is ~3–3.5 cm long. It courses almost vertically through the prostate from its base up to apex and lies nearer to anterior surface than posterior surface. It forms spindle-shaped canal, which is wider in the middle than at either ends and narrowest where it joins the membranous part. A longitudinal ridge of smooth muscle on the posterior wall of the posterior urethra, known as "urethral crest," extends from the bladder neck to the membranous urethra. This ridge continues into "verumontanum," an ovoid mound (about ~15–17 mm in length and 3 mm in width), present in the posterior wall of the prostatic urethra.

A small saccular depression lies in the center of the verumontanum, known as "prostatic utricle." It is a vestigial remnant of the müllerian duct. The orifices of the paired ejaculatory ducts lie distally and laterally to the utricle. Prostatic glands via multiple small openings drain into the prostatic urethra which surround the verumontanum. The prostatic urethra continues into the membranous urethra, which is about ~1–1.5 cm in length, distal and it ends at lower margin of the urogenital diaphragm.

The membranous urethra, which is the shortest and least distensible, (except for external meatus), is the narrowest part of the urethra. It courses forward and downward, between the prostatic apex and the bulb of the urethra, with a slight anterior concavity. It perforates the urogenital diaphragm approximately ~2.5 cm inferior and posterior to the pubic-symphysis.

The internal (proximal) urethral sphincter is extending between neck of bladder and the verumontanum, through the prostatic urethra. It is having different neurogenic innervation in spite of being similar to the detrusor muscle. The external (distal) sphincter has two components—intrinsic and extrinsic. The "intrinsic" urethral sphincter is a concentric muscular ring which is present in the distal one-third of the prostatic urethra that surrounds the membranous urethra and below the verumontanum. The internal sphincter and intrinsic component of external sphincter are made up of smooth muscle and maintain passive continence. The primary continence is the function of internal sphincter while secondary continence is function of intrinsic sphincter. The extrinsic component of external sphincter is a paraurethral, voluntary, striated muscle which has muscle fibers from the levator ani. Active continence is a function of sphincter surrounding membranous urethra.

The Female Urethra

The female urethra has ~4 cm length and lies from the neck of bladder at the urethrovesical junction up to the vestibule, where it forms the external urethral meatus between labia minus. It lies posterior to the pubis symphysis, confined in the anterior vaginal wall. It courses obliquely forward and downward. It is slightly curved with forward concavity. When undilated, its diameter measures ~6 mm. It penetrates the fascia of the urogenital diaphragm and its external opening is situated directly in front of the vaginal opening and 2.5 cm inferior to the clitoris. A number of small periurethral glands empty into the urethra. These glands group together on each side of the urethra ("Skene glands") distally and has two small ducts on each side of the external meatus. The proximal segment of the urethral wall consists of two layers of smooth muscle (inner longitudinal and outer circular) which are in continuation with the smooth muscle of the neck of bladder. The outer layer of the urethra is made up of striated muscle which is primarily circular in the upper two-thirds of the urethra and extends superiorly to mingle with the bladder base.

The lower portion of the urethra lies closely to the vaginal wall anteriorly and is surrounded by same musculature (the urethrovaginal sphincter), above the urogenital diaphragm and extends to the inferior pubic ramus.

IMAGING MODALITIES

Various imaging modalities available for the urinary bladder and urethra include the following:

- Plain films
- Retrograde urethrography (RGU)
- Voiding cystourethrography (VCUG)
- Cystography
- Urodynamic studies
- Ultrasonography (US)
- Computed tomography (CT)
- Magnetic resonance imaging (MRI)
- Radionuclide imaging.

Plain Films

The main role of plain films is in the detection of radio-paque calculi or foreign bodies, calcification, abnormal gas pattern, and in identification of soft tissue and the bony abnormalities. A plain radiograph or fluoroscopic examination is mandatory before starting the contrast studies to identify any radiopacity (calculi, calcification or foreign body) that may be obscured with contrast subsequently. Radiolucent foreign bodies can be seen if these get encrusted with calcium. Causes of bladder wall calcification include tuberculosis, tumors, radiation cystitis, cyclophosphamide-induced cystitis, alkaline incrustation cystitis, amyloidosis and schistosomiasis.[1] Bladder neoplasms may be suggested on detection of stippled calcification.

In emphysematous cystitis, the plain film typically shows gas within the lumen of bladder and streaky irregular radiolucencies within the wall of bladder. The presence of gas within the ureter may be seen in the setting of emphysematous pyeloureteritis or emphysematous pyelonephritis. Plain films may occasionally be helpful for the detection of bony metastases, spinal abnormalities in cases of neurogenic bladder and diastasis of the pubic symphysis in patients with exstrophy/epispadias anomaly.

Retrograde Urethrography

Retrograde urethrography is an initial best imaging technique for urethral and periurethral assessment in men and is useful in evaluating urethral injuries, fistulas, and strictures. The patient needs to be placed in 45° supine-oblique position. With moderate traction, the penile shaft should be pulled laterally over toward thigh. Reassurance should be given to patient regarding discomfort which may be experienced on balloon inflation. Then, under fluoroscopic guidance, ~20–30 mL of 60% iodinated-contrast material is pushed through the 16F or 18F Foley catheter (having Foley's bulb gently inflated in fossa navicularis) to fill anterior urethra with diluted contrast. Gentle, slow, gradual injection of contrast is usually required to overcome the resistance occurred due spasm of the external urethral sphincter which may prevent filling of the entire extend of urethra including posterior urethra. On fluoroscopy, when the contrast material is seen filling the bladder, the spot radiographs are obtained. During RGU, there can be the opacification of various ducts and periurethral glands (like prostatic or Cowper's ducts or periurethral Littre glands), however, this is not always associated with urethral disease.[2] Sometimes, an increased pressure due to contrast material injection may result in disruption of lining of urethral mucosa leading to intravasation of contrast medium causing opacification of the corpora and draining vein **(Fig. 1)**.

Voiding Cystourethrography

Voiding cystourethrography is radiographic study often used to evaluate the female urethra and male posterior urethra. In VCUG, urinary bladder is filled with diluted contrast through a suprapubic or transurethral catheter. After which, the transurethral catheter is removed and the patient is asked to void under fluoroscopic monitoring and spot X-rays are acquired. On active voiding, due to

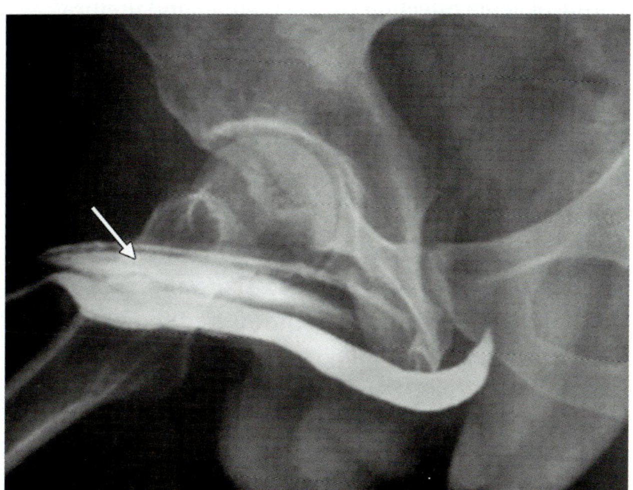

Fig. 1: Retrograde urethrography (RGU) image showing opacification of the corpora (arrow) and draining veins due to increased pressure of injection.

wide opening of neck of the bladder, funneling of urethra is seen in both male and female cases due to presence of the internal sphincteric mechanism. The verumontanum is seen elongated in male patients and the proximal bulbous urethra is less conical. The membranous urethra still appears to be the narrowest segment between these parts of the urethra, although it can regain up to ~6–7 mm diameter while voiding.[2] Voiding cystourethrography cannot be able to visualize some pathologies of the anterior urethra in male due to the fact that the distension of anterior urethra is less compared to as seen in RGU. For anterior urethra evaluation, RGU is the most appropriate and for evaluation of the posterior urethra, VCUG is the most appropriate study.

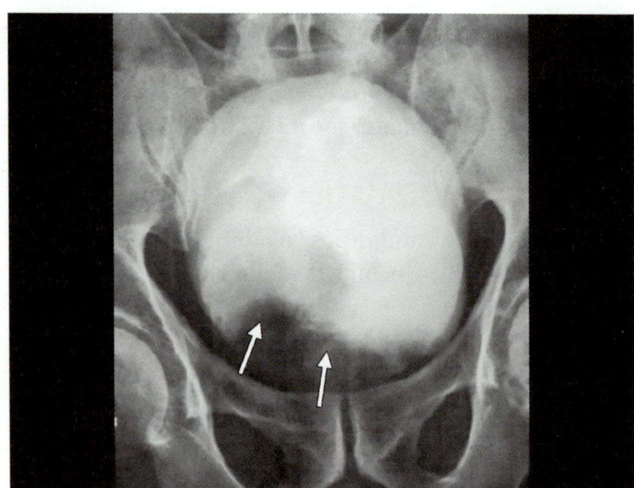

Fig. 2: Excretory cystogram showing irregular lobulated filling defect (arrows) at bladder base due to malignant growth.

Cystography

Cystography (excretory, retrograde, and suprapubic) is a well-established modality for urinary bladder evaluation. The best cystogram is obtained by the retrograde method. Meglumine salts of diatrizoate and iothalamate are now universally used for cystography. Solution of 15% is generally adequate for cystography. In the excretory cystogram, bladder can be evaluated simultaneously along with upper urinary tracts, but it is not possible to recognize the presence of reflux.

In patients with renal failure having lesions in the bladder, retrograde cystography has a role. Cystography and micturating cystography is indicated for demonstration of the ability of the bladder to contract and control the micturition, with assessment of vesical diverticula and anatomic abnormalities of the urinary bladder neck and urethra. However, the examination is contraindicated in setting of acute infections of the bladder and urethra.

Contrast cystogram can distinctly demonstrate intraluminal calculi, hematomas, tumors **(Fig. 2)**, and wall irregularities. In traumatic injury of the bladder, cystogram depicts the type of bladder rupture (extraperitoneal or intraperitoneal), in addition to detection of pelvic fractures.

Extrinsic compression of the bladder can be produced by pelvic hematoma or lipomatosis resulting in appearance of bladder that has been referred to as "teardrop bladder". In such pathologies, ultrasound and CT play an important role in evaluating the cause of extrinsic compression.

Urodynamic Studies of the Lower Urinary Tract

Urodynamic studies are among the most appropriate tests to determine the source of symptoms in the lower urinary tract. A number of urodynamic tests can be useful in evaluation of the bladder and urethra and can evaluate their functioning like storing and releasing urine. These studies may be helpful to pinpoint the neurologic cause or anatomic site for source of symptoms like frequency, urgency, problems initiating a stream, dribbling, painful micturition, problems in completely emptying the bladder and recurrent urinary tract infections. Depending on the patient's symptoms, the types of tests can be done and may include one or more of the tests like uroflowmetry, cystometry, electromyelogram, pressure studies for stress incontinence, VCUG, video urodynamics, and assessment of postvoid residual urine, etc.

Ultrasonography

Real-time ultrasonography (US) is a versatile modality in the detection of bladder lesions, and is frequently employed as the first imaging tool for its assessment. US of urinary bladder can be carried out by transabdominal, endorectal or endovaginal approach. However, transabdominal approach is the simplest and the easiest. Urinary bladder should be evaluated when it is properly distended. In the majority of patients this means a volume of about ~350 mL. The bladder is seen as a smooth thin-walled anechoic structure rectangular to round in configuration on transverse scanning with no intravesical filling defects.

Ultrasonography of urinary bladder is used to evaluate the following:

- Urinary bladder wall anatomy:
  - Thickening of the wall and focal abnormalities
  - Presence of trabeculation
  - Diverticula

- Capacity of the bladder and postmicturition residual volume
- Anatomy of bladder base and urethral opening
- Distal ureteric anatomy
- Intravesical filling defects and extraluminal masses causing bladder compression.

Radiolucent calculi, which may be missed on plain radiographs, are easily picked up on US. Blood clots and sediments are usually freely mobile within the lumen. In obese patients and those with peritonitis in whom palpation of the bladder is difficult, ultrasound is very useful in determining whether the bladder is full enough to allow safe suprapubic catheterization. Transrectal US (TRUS) is useful in defining the plane between the prostate, seminal vesicle, and urinary bladder, in posterior wall masses. Ultrasound cystodynamogram can be performed in patients with symptoms of voiding disorders.

Sonography of the urethra mostly been used for diagnosis of urethral diverticula and strictures, is generally done by broad-band linear probe (5–10 MHz) for trans penile or transperineal scanning and a broad-band curved probe (5–9 MHz) for transvaginal or transrectal scanning. Endourethral USG is done with a 12.5MHz, 6.2F, transducer based on catheter on the intravascular USG machine. However, the need for a costly intravascular USG machine is disadvantageous. A disposable urethral catheter and restricted field of view are other disadvantages for this technique.

Sonourethrography has shown good sensitivity and specificity in evaluation and diagnosis of anterior (penile and bulbous) urethral strictures. RGU and sonourethrography are equally effective in detection of penile and bulbar urethral strictures **(Fig. 3)**. Further characterization and evaluation of strictures in forms of diameter, length and periurethral pathologies, like spongiofibrosis or false tracts, is performed with more sensitivity using sonourethrography as compared to RGU, with the added benefit of radiation free modality and lower incidence of complications.[3]

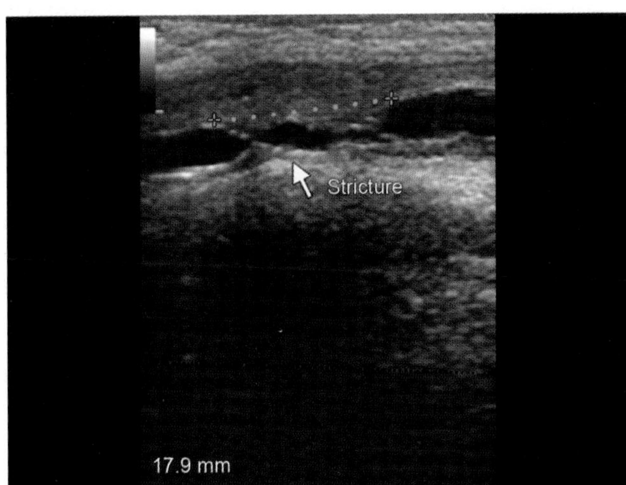

Fig. 3: Sonourethrogram showing a stricture (arrows) of penile urethra.

Computed Tomography

The role of CT is in identification of size and number of distal ureteric, vesical or urethral calculi, pelvic trauma, and in staging of vesicle or urethral malignancy.

On CT scan, the urinary bladder appears as a homogeneous midline structure of water density. The size and configuration varies greatly which depends on the amount of urine present. The outer margin of the bladder wall is smooth and usually well-delineated by the perivesical fat. Although urine is of near water density, the bladder wall has soft tissue attenuation. In contrast-enhanced CT scan, contrast opacified urine usually gets the dependent portion of the bladder with layer of unopacified urine above it. However, this relationship may be reversed in patients with glycosuria or infectious debris in the bladder, where the unopacified urine may have higher specific gravity than the excreted opacified urine.[4] Scans obtained before and after administration of contrast medium can detect subtle vesical and perivesical abnormalities. Dense opacification of the lumen may obscure small tumors or calculi and can produce scan artifacts which degrade the image **(Figs. 4A and B)**. In the male pelvis, the seminal vesicles are seen posterior to bladder and anterior to the rectum. They are oval to tear shaped structures. A small amount of fat is usually present between posterior aspect of the bladder and the seminal vesicles. This relationship may be distorted by a distended rectum or when the patient is prone. The prostate gland is located anteriorly to the rectum and just posteriorly to the symphysis pubis. Masses seen on intravenous urography compressing or displacing the bladder are readily evaluated by CT. True masses are easily distinguished from bladder impression produced by the bowel loops present in the pelvis, if the loops are adequately filled with contrast material. Alteration in the shape of the bladder can be produced by retroperitoneal fibrosis, pelvic lipomatosis, hematoma, and lymphoceles, etc. In these benign conditions, CT reveals elevation and narrowing of the bladder (pear-shaped bladder).

Contrast-enhanced CT with delayed imaging or retrograde bladder filling (CT cystography) has been shown to be highly accurate and equivalent to conventional cystography in the detection of bladder rupture.[5]

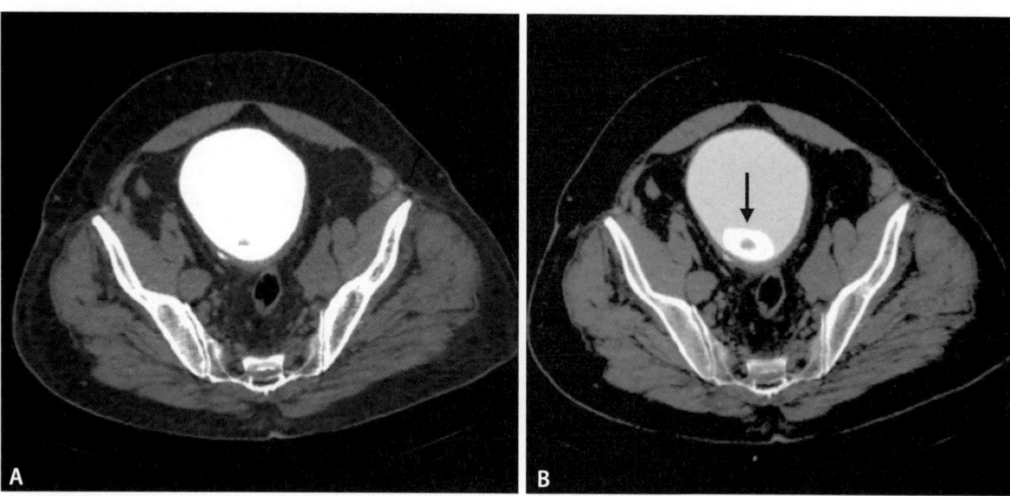

Figs. 4A and B: Bladder calculus: Dense opacification of bladder in CT axial image completely obscuring the calculus (A), which is visualized (arrow) in wide window setting (B).

Magnetic Resonance Imaging

Magnetic resonance imaging is commonly done for cases of intersex and complex genitourinary abnormalities in patients with congenital anomalies, in which assessment of pelvic organs is very important. MRI can show diverticulum or periurethral inflammation, periurethral abscess or sinus, which are not seen on conventional radiographic modalities. In trauma cases, MRI is useful in evaluating the injuries of anterior and posterior urethra, thereby predicting the associated complications. On MRI, a fistula is seen as communicating tract with an adjacent organ. There is also important role of MRI in local staging of urethral tumors.[6]

Magnetic resonance images act as an excellent tool to delineate the anatomic structure and various pathologic conditions of the urinary bladder. Both T1-weighted and T2-weighted spin echo (SE) sequences are useful in imaging of the bladder. The muscle layer shows a T1 intermediate and T2 low signal-intensity same as of skeletal muscle **(Fig. 5)**. The mucosa and lamina propria may occasionally be differentiated from the muscle layer on proton density images, due to higher signal-intensity of the mucosa and lamina propria.

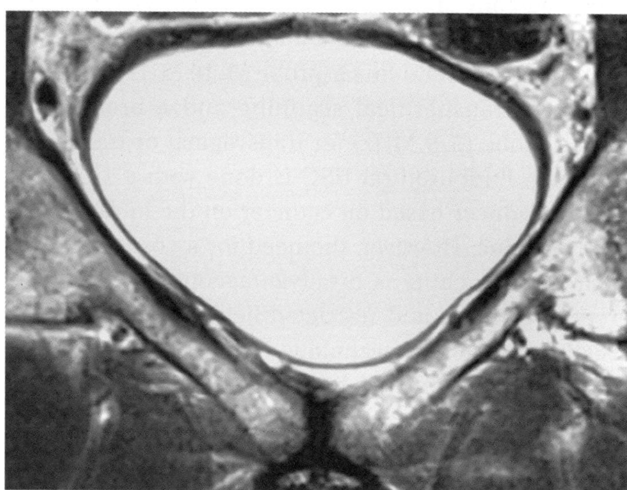

Fig. 5: MR Coronal T2 image of urinary bladder. Note low signal intensity of detrusor muscle.

Fast SE sequences provide superior quality in T2-weighted MR images with 3–5 fold less study time compared to conventional spin-echo sequences. At present, fast SE is pioneering to obtain T2W images of the pelvis. Three-dimensional (3D) techniques with offline reconstruction of high resolution images in any arbitrary plane are also very useful. The introduction of short TR (<10 msec) gradient echo sequences that use a preparation pulse, such as turbo FLASH (fast low angle shot), snapshot FLASH and MP-RAGE (magnetization prepared rapid gradient echo) and fast spin-echo (FSE) sequences significantly reduce imaging time without compromising signal to noise ratio. For T1-weighted 3D imaging, the use of an MP-RAGE sequence has been described. Also, use of phased-array multicoils and endorectal coils improves resolution. Dynamic contrast-enhanced MR provides the best information to help differentiate malignant from benign lesions.

Development of oral intestinal MR contrast agents such as ferrite particles has improved the delineation of small bowel loops and para-aortic region.

Images of the urethra may be acquired in three orthogonal planes (axial, coronal, sagittal). Alternatively, oblique images along the course of urethra can be

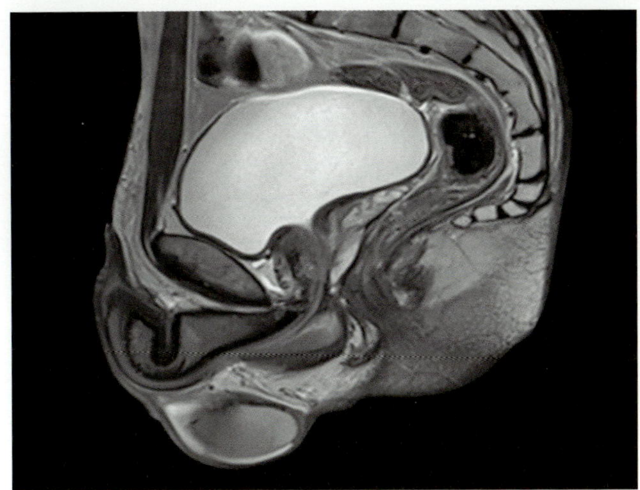

Fig. 6: MR sagittal T2 image showing the entire extent of urethra.

obtained. Both T1W and T2W imaging are necessary for evaluation of the male and female urethra. In male patients, axial plane is the best for evaluation of the membranous urethra and the coronal or sagittal plane are useful for the course of the membranous and bulbous urethra (especially in traumatic cases). To obtain images of the anterior urethra, the penile shaft should be taped to the abdominal wall and positioned anteriorly in supine position under the surface coil **(Fig. 6)**. In female patients, axial images are essential.[7] A combination of imaging planes or sequences may be useful to evaluate a urethral diverticulum or local extension of urethral malignancy.

A thin slice thickness (~3–5 mm) and smaller inter-slice gap (~1–2 mm) are appropriate for imaging the urethra. The signal-to-noise ratio (SNR) may be improved by use of surface coils, endovaginal or endorectal coils. The endocavitary coils can give better spatial resolution; however, small field of view may be disadvantageous. Also, the high signal intensity in the near field can cause degradation of image quality. Use of intravenous contrast media is helpful in selected cases, especially in patients with extensive spread of tumor or inflammation.

Radionuclide Imaging

Radionuclide cystography has been a technique of choice for assessment and follow-up of children with urinary tract infections and reflux. The advantages being simplicity, lower radiation dose, and no catheterization needed. The sensitivity of radionuclide cystography is more than VCUG in diagnosing vesicoureteric reflux; however, this has poor anatomical resolution than the conventional VCUG. Direct and indirect radionuclide cystography can be substitute to the radiographic technique and can be incorporated into the process of diagnosis and follow-up of vesicoureteral reflux.[8]

SPECIFIC DISEASES OF THE URINARY BLADDER

Bladder Diverticula

Bladder diverticulum refers to out-pouching of the bladder wall. These may be congenital, but are more commonly acquired as a result of bladder outlet obstruction or neurogenic bladder. Congenital bladder diverticula develop as a result of herniation or protrusion of bladder mucosa through the detrusor muscle, usually at a location slightly above and lateral to the ureteric orifice (Hutch diverticulum). These can vary from small to quite large and can cause either obstruction of, or reflux into the ipsilateral ureter. Diverticula are sites of urinary stasis and thus lead to infection, stone formation, and lower urinary tract symptoms.

On cystogram, bladder diverticula are seen as out-pouchings from the bladder which may show persistence of contrast in the postmicturition phase. On US these appear as well-defined, thin-walled fluid-containing structures communicating with the bladder lumen. The most important use of US is to detect the complications, i.e. stone or tumor in the diverticulum, which is not always possible to assess on cystography or endoscopy.

Urachal Anomalies

The urachus is developed from the superior part of the urogenital sinus and joins the allantoic duct and the dome of bladder during fetal life. It lies posterior to abdominal wall (behind transverse fascia) and anterior to parietal peritoneum, in the extraperitoneal "space of Retzius". Normally, it obliterates before birth forming a fibrous median umbilical ligament. The various congenital anomalies of urachus arise from failure to develop urachus to completely obliterate its lumen leading to the various entities given in **Table 1**.

Urachal anomalies can be delineated on US, CT, and MRI. USG is the first line and most commonly used modality with high sensitivity and diagnostic accuracy. CT and MRI are very helpful as they permit multiplanar imaging especially in the sagittal plane and are usually employed when USG fails to allow diagnosis of anomaly.

Patent urachus is often suspected in a newborn when there is leakage of urine from the umbilicus. It can be directly identified by retrograde injection of contrast into umbilical opening. It may also fill up during voiding

Table 1: Urachal anomalies.

Urachal anomalies	*Entity*
Completely patent urachus	Vesicocutaneous fistula between bladder and umbilicus
Patent caudal portion opening into the bladder	Vesicourachal diverticulum
Patent cephalic portion opening into the umbilicus	Urachal sinus
Mid-portion is patent, both cephalic and caudal ends closed	Urachal cyst

cystourethrogram, best demonstrated in the lateral projection. Urachal cyst is not delineated on conventional urography studies. An urachal diverticulum is seen as urine filled anterosuperior protrusion of the dome of bladder on cystography. US reveals a tubular, anechoic structure in the lower, mid anterior abdominal wall, communicating with bladder in case of urachal fistula. Urachal cyst appears as midline homogenous fluid-filled structure in path of urachus. Urachal sinus appear as blind fusiform dilatation of urachus toward umbilical end without any communication to bladder. Urachal diverticulum is identified as a focal midline protrusion arising from dome of bladder. They can be detected incidentally or when symptomatic and suspected complications are associated with them [such as infections, stone formation, malignancy (adenocarcinoma)] **(Figs. 7 and 8)**.

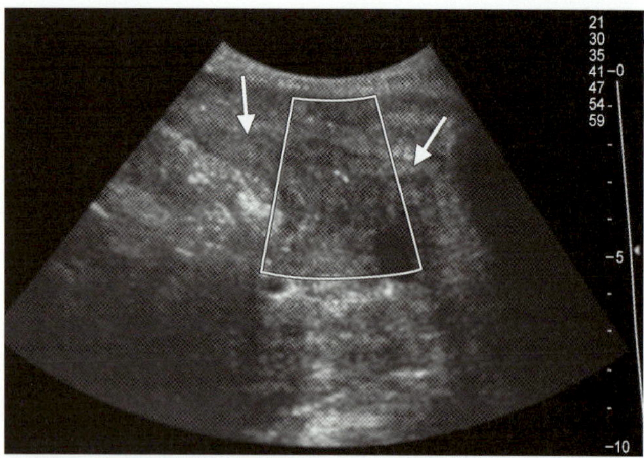

Fig. 7: Urachal diverticulum (arrows) complicated with infection: US image showing thickening of diverticular wall with increased vascularity.

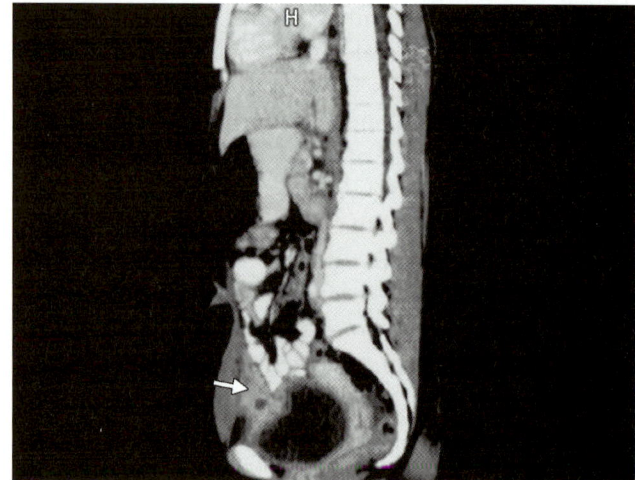

Fig. 8: Sagittal 3D reformatted CT image of the same patient as in Figure 7 showing thickening and enhancement of urachus.

Exstrophy

Exstrophy of the bladder is a spectrum of defects resulting from varying degree of failure of fusion of midline mesodermal tissue below the umbilicus with resultant defect in the formation of the anterior abdominal wall. Classical exstrophy includes epispadias, separation of pubic bones (>10 mm), and communication of bladder with the anterior skin surface **(Fig. 9)**. On excretory urography, there is a wide lateral curve of the pelvic portion of the distal ureters, which then turn upward and medially, in the shape of a hook, passing through the bladder wall in a perpendicular direction. Cystogram is performed in postoperative follow-up of these patients.

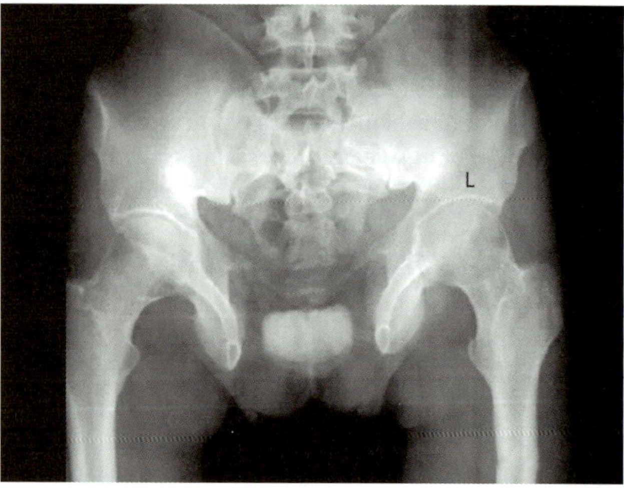

Fig. 9: Exstrophy of bladder: Radiograph showing diastasis of pubic symphysis.

Other Anomalies

Other major anomalies include bladder agenesis and hypoplasia which are associated with other congenital anomalies, which when severe may even be incompatible with life. Duplication of bladder may be partial or complete with two separate urinary bladders, present side by side separated by a peritoneal fold (sagittal duplication). Coronal duplication of bladder is very unusual and rare. Each bladder receives the corresponding ureter and drains into a separate urethra. This can be associated with anomalies of the gastrointestinal tract, genital system, external genitalia, and lower spine. Anatomy of duplication can be well-demonstrated on US and MRI.

Neurogenic Bladder

Neurogenic bladder dysfunction may be caused by CNS abnormalities, spinal dysraphism, cord compression or cord injury. Cystography is very helpful in diagnosis of neurogenic bladder. US is also useful to assess bladder size, shape, volume, post void residue, renal parenchymal changes, and secondary calculi.

In the condition called as detrusor-external sphincter dyssynergia (DSED), contraction of the external sphincter occurs involuntarily at the same time as detrusor contraction thus impeding urinary flow and resulting in bladder outlet obstruction. In this condition bladder is often vertically oriented, with an irregular contour with trabeculation; frequently with multiple diverticula and is referred to as "Christmas tree" or "pine tree" bladder. On voiding cystourethrography, there may or may not be vesicoureteral reflux. In detrusor areflexia voiding cystourethrography often reveals a smooth, thin-walled bladder with increased capacity, occasionally up to several liters and extending high into the abdomen. Significant post void residue is seen in both these conditions.

Infections

Acute Cystitis

Acute cystitis due to bacterial infection is most commonly the result of transurethral infection, and is common in females due to short urethral length and proximity to anus. *Escherichia coli* is the most common pathogen. Imaging is usually advocated in complicated cystitis, recurrent infection and to diagnose upper urinary tract infection. Cystography is contraindicated in acute infection. US is the most useful modality allowing evaluation of the upper tracts as well as the bladder. On US, cystitis show thickened and less distinct bladder wall with internal echoes or debris. Cobble-stone appearance of bladder wall can be seen in severe bladder edema due to acute cystitis. Contour irregularity due to bladder mucosal edema can also be seen in radiation cystitis, cyclophosphamide cystitis, and eosinophilic cystitis, and these can be associated with hemorrhage.

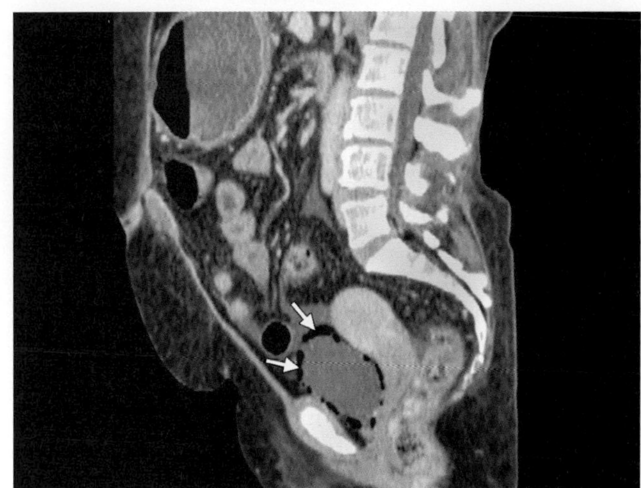

Fig. 10: Emphysematous cystitis: Sagittal reformatted CT image showing air pockets (arrows) within the bladder wall.

Emphysematous cystitis is almost always seen in diabetic or immunocompromised patients and *E. coli* is the most common pathogen **(Fig. 10)**.

Chronic Cystitis

The hallmark of chronic cystitis is thickening, calcification, and irregularity of the bladder wall associated with trabeculation and often diminished bladder capacity. Biopsy should be done in focal mural thickening to rule out underlying malignancy. Tuberculosis of the bladder has been discussed in detail in a chapter on "Tubercular Infection of the Urinary Tract."

Cystitis Cystica and Cystitis Glandularis

Cystitis cystica and cystitis glandularis are benign inflammatory conditions commonly seen in females with recurrent or chronic cystitis, or in chronically irritated bladders such as those catheterized for long periods or with calculus disease of the bladder. Metaplasia of urothelium, with proliferation and downward extension into the connective tissue of lamina propria is seen pathologically. Cystitis glandularis is commonly associated with pelvic lipomatosis, bladder exstrophy, and bladder obstruction. On cystogram, multiple round contour defects at the bladder base can be seen in both conditions. Masses from both the conditions may vary in number and size. A hypervascular polypoidal mass has been observed on CT and MR imaging. These show low signal on T1 and T2 with central high signal on T2 with intense contrast enhancement (corresponding to vascular stalk). It is important to demonstrate intact muscular layer which differentiate these masses from malignancy.

Malakoplakia

Malakoplakia is an uncommon granulomatous response to an infection of the urinary tract, predominantly with *E. coli, especially in immunocompromised patients with female: male ratio of 4:1*. Submucosal granulomas containing macrophages with inclusion bodies known as "Michaelis-Gutmann bodies" are characteristic. It may affect any part of the urinary tract. Radiographically, these are seen as single or multiple mural filling defects due to polypoidal, vascular masses especially in the trigone and bladder base. Accompanying bladder wall thickening may also be seen, with or without perivesical extension simulating carcinoma.

Schistosomiasis

Schistosomiasis or bilharziasis is a parasitic infection caused by Schistosoma haematobium, producing polypoidal bladder wall thickening, which is nonspecific in appearance. In late stages, fibrosis leads to a small capacity bladder with focal or curvilinear dense wall calcification. Distal ureteric dilatation with calcification can also been seen.

Extravesical Processes

Appendicitis, diverticulitis, and pelvic abscesses may produce reactive thickening of bladder wall with mucosal irregularities. Endometriosis and inflammatory pseudotumor can also present with focal bladder lesions.

Bladder Tumors

Primary bladder tumors have mostly epithelial origin and less than 10% arises from a nonepithelial source. Almost all epithelial tumors are malignant, majority being transitional cell type with squamous cell carcinoma and adenocarcinoma being relatively uncommon. The bladder carcinoma can also be classified by growth pattern apart from histology into superficial (papillary or flat) and muscle invasive. Nonepithelial tumors may be benign (such as leiomyoma, fibroma) or malignant (such as leiomyosarcoma and rhabdomyosarcoma). The other primary tumors or masses may occur including pheochromocytoma, hemangioma, leukoplakia, and lymphoma. Metastases can be rarely seen in bladder. The staging system most often used for bladder cancer is the TNM system given in **Table 2** [The American Joint Committee on Cancer (AJCC) Staging System, 8th edition, 2017].

Table 2: TNM staging.

Primary tumor (T)		
Ta	Noninvasive papillary carcinoma	
Tis	Carcinoma in situ	
T1	Invades subepithelial connective tissue	
T2	Muscular invasion	T2a: Inner half
		T2b: Outer half
T3	Invades perivesical tissues	T3a: Microscopic disease
		T3b: Macroscopic disease
T4	Invades adjacent organs, pelvic–abdominal wall	T4a: Prostate, uterus or vagina
		T4b: Pelvic or abdominal wall
Regional lymph nodes (N)		
N0	No nodal metastasis	
N1	Single regional lymph node metastasis in the true pelvis (perivesical, obturator, internal and external iliac, or sacral lymph node)	
N2	Multiple regional lymph node metastasis in the true pelvis (perivesical, obturator, internal and external iliac or sacral lymph node metastasis)	
N3	Common iliac lymph node metastasis	
Distant metastasis		
M0	No distant metastasis	
M1	Distant metastasis	M1a: Distant metastasis limited to nodes beyond the common iliac lymph nodes
		M1b: Nonlymph nodal distant metastases

The clinical staging (with deep fractioned transurethral resection) is much less accurate in staging invasive (stages T2-T4) tumors. Cystogram cannot detect an early growth, extent of extravesical spread or status of the adjacent organs **(Fig. 11)**.

Although the intravesical position of many tumors can be visualized on US, an exact evaluation of depth of penetration of bladder wall cannot be done with US **(Fig. 12)**. The diagnostic accuracy of the transabdominal US for depth of infiltration ranges from 55% to 95%. Perivesical invasion cannot be frequently determined; however, extravesical spread may be recognized by the asymmetry due to infiltration.

Tumors involving the posterior bladder wall and neck, prostate and seminal vesicles may be better visualized with transrectal approach. Finally, none of the ultrasound methods optimally assesses the regional nodal status.

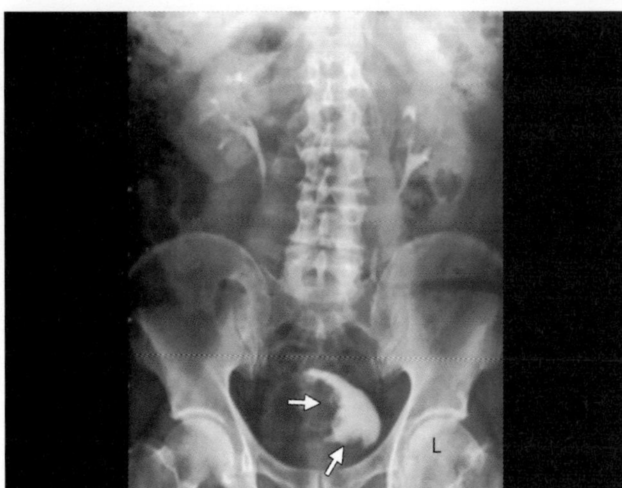

Fig. 11: Transitional cell carcinoma (TCC) of bladder: Intravenous urogram (IVU) image showing large polypoidal filling defects (arrows) within the bladder.

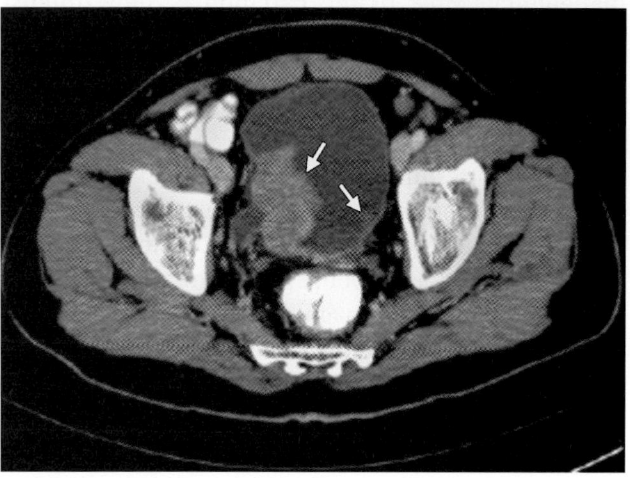

Fig. 13: Transitional cell carcinoma (TCC) of bladder: CT axial image showing a large polypoidal growth (arrow) along right lateral wall and base of bladder causing ureteric obstruction. A small tumor is also seen along left lateral wall (arrow).

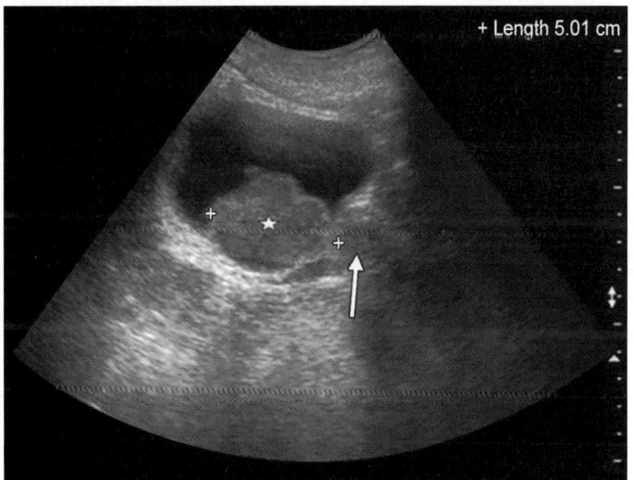

Fig. 12: Transitional cell carcinoma (TCC) of bladder: US image showing intraluminal polypoidal mass within the bladder with invasion of left ureter (arrow).

The important role of CT in the bladder carcinoma is to stage than detection of the primary neoplasm. However, CT is not accurate for the early stages and it is more reliable with advanced disease **(Fig. 13)**. CT cannot distinguish the different layers of urinary bladder wall; therefore, it cannot differentiate the lesions limited to the lamina propria (T1) from other lesions invading the superficial (T2) and deep (T3a) muscles. CT is useful for detecting extravesical extension which is seen by an increased density/stranding of the perivesical fat with poor definition of the outer margin of the bladder wall. Tumor involvement of the pelvic side wall is characterized by a soft tissue mass extending into the obturator internus muscle or by strands of soft tissue extending from main tumor mass to pelvic wall.

Tumor invasion of seminal vesicles should be suspected if the seminal vesicle angle gets obliterated by a soft tissue mass. However, this should be evaluated cautiously because the seminal vesicle angle may be lost if rectum is overdistended or if prone position is used for the scanning. CT is useful in detecting lymph nodal metastases; involvement being interpreted by the size of the node. Node greater than 10 mm in short axis is considered malignant. The obturator and external iliac lymph nodes are first to involve. CT has limited accuracy compared to MRI in detecting perivesical infiltration and lymph nodal metastasis in invasive bladder carcinoma[9,10] (accuracy of CT varies from 40% to 90% for staging, 65–85% for detection of perivesical extension and 65–97% for lymph node detection).

On MR, T1W imaging is the best for assessing tumor spread into adjacent hyperintense fat, to detect lymph node enlargement and bone marrow evaluation.[11] There is better delineation of bladder malignancy from urine with T2W imaging. Compared to 2-dimensional T1-weighted spin echo (SE) imaging, 3-dimensional MP-RAGE imaging has improved bladder carcinoma staging by 15%.[12] When compared with conventional SE, fast SE sequences significantly have reduced acquisition time by 3-fold to 5-fold without decrease in quality of T2-weighted image.[13] Presently, fast spin-echo is pioneering for acquiring T2W images of pelvis. Contrast-enhanced study and fast dynamic imaging can improve the capability of MRI in detection and staging bladder malignancy. Most of the carcinomas show intense enhancement following intravenous contrast material administration. Tumor tissue generally enhances earlier (average ~6.5 s) than postbiopsy granulation tissue (~13.5 s).[14]

Magnetic resonance imaging is the most accurate technique in staging the invasive tumors. T2W or postcontrast T1W sequences are required to evaluate the infiltrating component of the tumor. Presence of the low intensity line on T2W images represents the uninvolved wall of bladder between tumor and perivesical fat, which is an important feature in MRI staging in differentiating stage T3a from stage T3b. Any interruption of the low signal intensity muscular layer of the urinary bladder or irregularity of the outer bladder wall and perivesical stranding suggest stage T3b **(Figs. 14 to 16)**.

The demonstration of direct tumor invasion into surrounding organs is facilitated by multiplanar imaging. A sagittal image is helpful for assessment of uterine or vaginal invasion. Assessment of invasion of the seminal vesicles is also assisted by use of sagittal image, invasion being indicated by an enlargement of vesicle, drop in signal intensity on T2W images, and loss of the angle between seminal vesicle and the posterior wall of bladder.

Infiltration of the prostate and rectum is depicted as direct tumor spread with an increase in signal intensity on T2W images. Due to multiplanar imaging capability, MR is especially useful for evaluation of tumors at dome or base of bladder.

T1W images are more suitable for assessing lymph nodes due to lower signal intensity than the adjacent fat. MRI with ultra-small super paramagnetic iron oxide agents has potential to detect metastases in normal sized node and in differentiating reactive enlargement of node from metastases.[15]

All modalities have limitation in determining extension of tumor growth in the muscular layer of the bladder wall, i.e. distinguishing between stages T2 and T3a. The imaging with endorectal surface coils or phased array

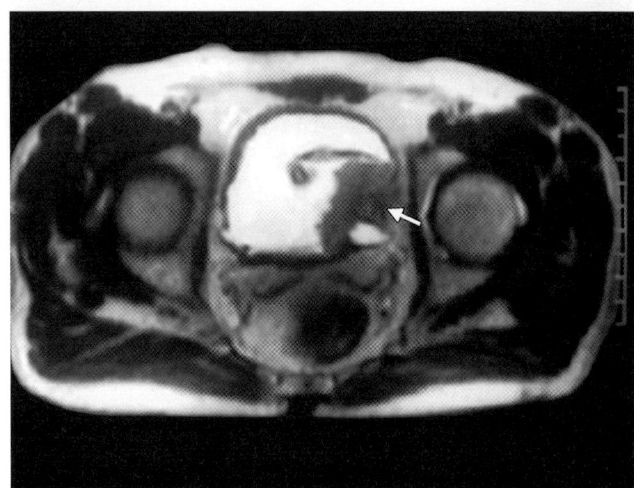

Fig. 15: Transitional cell carcinoma (TCC) of bladder: T2 axial section showing left posterolateral wall tumor (TCC) with deep muscle infiltration leading to ureteric obstruction. Early perivesical spread is seen as stranding of fat along left posterolateral aspect (arrow).

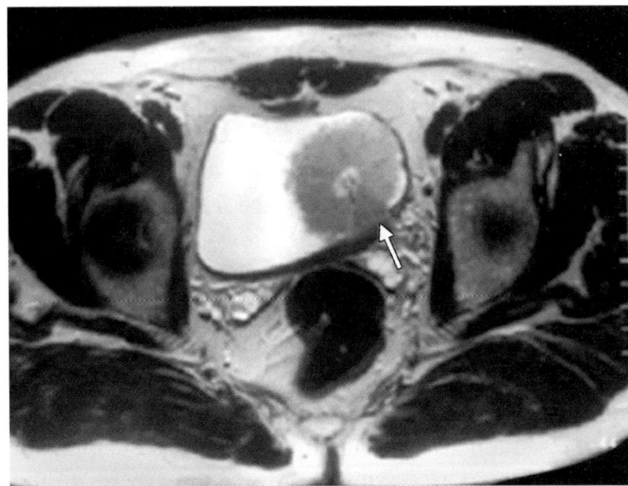

Fig. 14: Transitional cell carcinoma (TCC) of bladder: Axial T2-weighted image of a papillary transitional cell carcinoma shows an intraluminal mass which is intermediate in signal intensity. The pedicle is clearly seen (arrow). The muscle wall is not infiltrated. Perivesical enlarged vessels are noted adjacent to the tumor on left side.

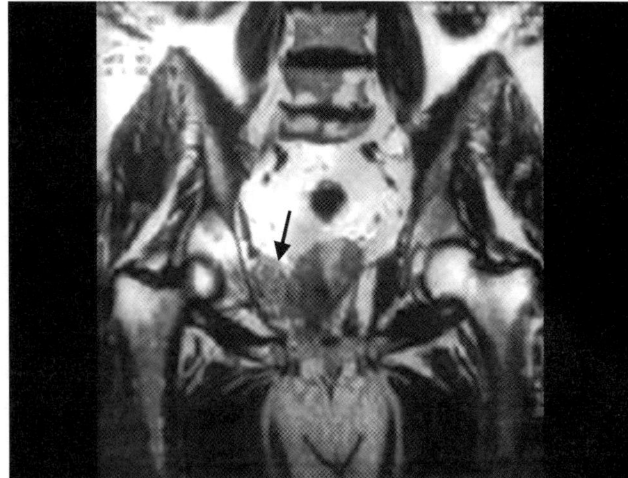

Fig. 16: Transitional cell carcinoma (TCC) of bladder: Stage T4 disease with infiltration of the right pelvic sidewall muscles (arrow) by bladder cancer. Note normal marrow signal of the pelvic bones on this T1 image.

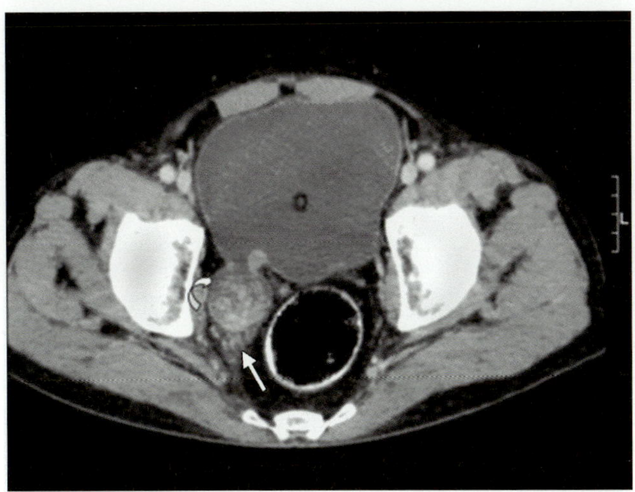

Fig. 17: Transitional cell carcinoma (TCC) of bladder diverticulum: Axial CT image shows an enhancing mass almost completely filling the bladder diverticulum (curved arrow) along right posterolateral wall. Note extravesical extension of the tumor (arrow).

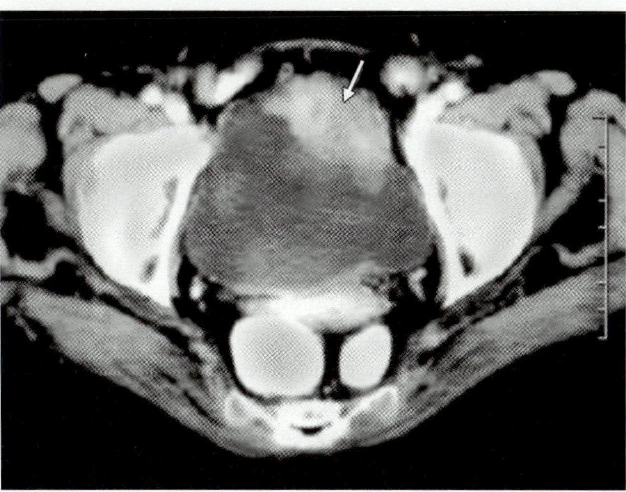

Fig. 18: Urachal carcinoma: Axial CT image showing a polypoid tumor mass (arrow) along the anterosuperior aspect of bladder.

multicoils in combination with IV contrast agents or T2W fast spin-echo sequences may resolve problem of distinguishing stage T2 from stage T3 tumors.

CT or MR urography (15 minute delayed image) is usually obtained with rest of the phases and sequences to increase the sensitivity or tumor detection.

Other newer imaging modalities like fluorescence cystoscopy, optical coherence tomography, and narrow-band imaging are under evaluation and may be proven useful in staging of early bladder cancer.[16] Virtual cystoscopy can help in noninvasive diagnosis, treatment planning, and surveillance. There is a promising role of diffusion weighted imaging (DWI) for evaluation of bladder tumors, differentiating benign and malignant tumor and lymph node assessment.

Because of high incidence of synchronous upper tract malignancy, kidney and ureters should also be carefully scrutinized.

Because of urinary stasis and chronic inflammation, there is ~2–10% increased incidence of carcinoma that develops within urinary bladder diverticulum.[17] Most of the neoplasms arising from bladder diverticulum are urothelial in origin. As the detrusor muscle is not present in diverticulum, tumors generally invade the perivesical fat **(Fig. 17)**. A narrow neck of diverticulum or unusual location can preclude adequate visualization at cystoscopy; therefore, cross-sectional imaging has an important role in detecting such occult neoplasm.

Most urachal carcinoma are mucin-producing adenocarcinomas of the juxta vesical segment of the urachus.[18] The diagnosis is commonly made by the characteristic midline location of tumor anterosuperior to the bladder, which is optimally delineated in the sagittal and coronal planes **(Fig. 18)**.

Chronic stasis and inflammation predispose to squamous cell carcinoma. Schistosomiasis (bilharziasis) is associated with an increase in incidence of vesical squamous cell carcinoma.

Benign Bladder Tumors

Epithelial (papilloma), nonepithelial (leiomyoma, fibroma, hemangioma, paraganglioma, neurofibroma), and inflammatory (nephrogenic adenoma, inflammatory myofibroblastic tumor) are common benign vesical lesions, of which leiomyoma is most common. There can be varied appearance and differentiation from malignancy can be difficult on imaging. Leiomyoma is commonly encountered in women, which is subepithelial in location, smoothly marginated and characteristically demonstrates low signal intensity on T2W image. Paraganglioma should be suspected in patient with episodic hypertension during micturition with intensely enhancing lesion in bladder.

SPECIFIC DISEASES OF URETHRA

Gonococcal and Nongonococcal Urethritis

Gonococcal urethritis is caused by Gram negative *Diplococcus, Neisseria gonorrhea. Chlamydia trachomatis* is the most commonly associated with nongonococcal urethritis, which accounts for ~30–50% of cases. Patients having gonococcal urethritis commonly manifest with purulent discharge per urethra. Nongonococcal urethritis has usually scanty urethral discharge. Acute gonococcal and nongonococcal urethritis are usually diagnosed clinically and by laboratory findings. Imaging is generally not needed in cases of noncomplicated urethritis. Urethral stricture, periurethral abscess, and periurethral fistula are complications seen with gonococcal urethritis which are more common and severe than those seen in nongonococcal urethritis.

The gonococcal urethral stricture appears as a long segment irregular narrowing of urethra **(Fig. 19)**. About ~15% of male having gonococcal urethritis develop stricture, with an interval of 2–30 years between infection and the onset of obstructive symptoms.[19] In 70% of cases, there will be hard fibrous scars at the distal part of the bulbar urethra. These scars are formed because of uneffective flushing by micturition and the preponderance of Littre glands in this area. On urethrography, there may be associated dilatation of Littre glands. When the cone shape of bulbous urethra is narrowed, elongated, asymmetric, irregular, or absent, the stricture extends into the membranous urethra in >90% of cases.[20] This imaging finding is very important to the urologist because surgical intervention may involve resection of scar tissue and, subsequently, the distal sphincter, which might lead to iatrogenic incontinence.

Periurethral abscess is developed when there is Littre gland obstruction by inspissated pus or fibrosis **(Fig. 20)**. Gram-negative rods, *Enterococci*, and anaerobes are the most common infecting organisms. Periurethral abscess can be a life-threatening infection of the urethra and periurethral tissue in male patients. These are frequently sequelae of gonococcal infection, urethral stricture disease or urethral catheterization. The urethral communication with a periurethral abscess leads to pseudodiverticulum formation. As the tunica albuginea of the penis restricts the dorsal spreading of infection, the abscess courses ventrally along the corpus spongiosum, where it is limited by the "Buck fascia". However, when there is disruption of Buck fascia, extensive subcutaneous tissue and fascia necrosis can occur. Early and quick diagnosis and treatment is necessary in such cases. Imaging technique can be needed, if diagnosis cannot be made out clinically. Urethrography may show an abscess that drains into the urethra. Ultrasonography can evaluate the presence of periurethral abscess. Cross-sectional imaging such as CT or MR is helpful for demonstrating the spread of the periurethral abscess and also complications like fasciitis and Fournier gangrene.

Urethroperineal fistulas are often seen as sequelae of a periurethral abscess. The initial abscess cavity contracts

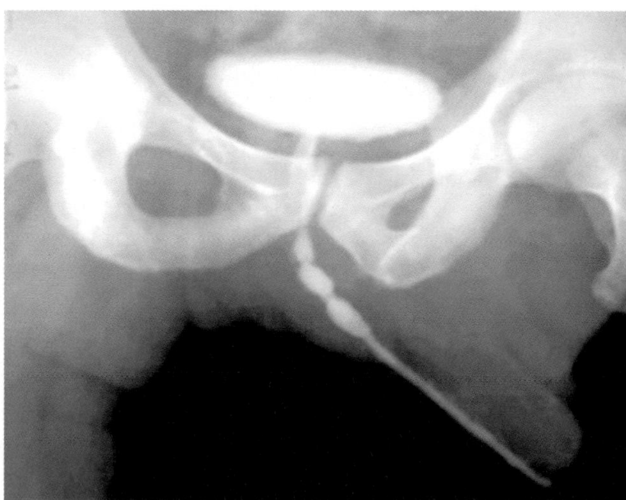

Fig. 19: Gonococcal urethral stricture: Retrograde urethrography (RGU) image showing a panurethral stricture.

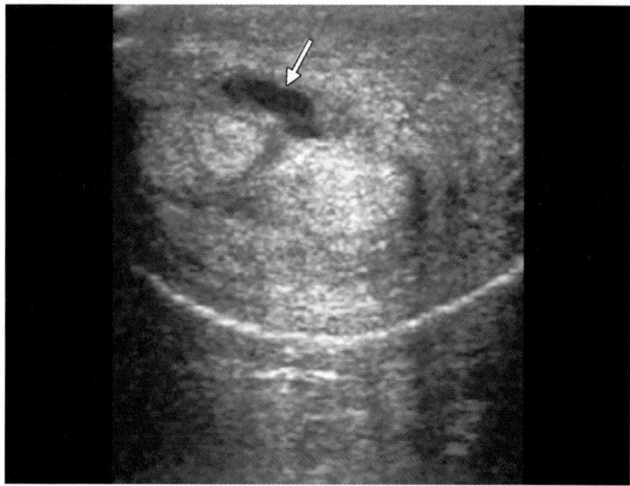

Fig. 20: Periurethral abscess: US image shows an abscess cavity (arrow) in relation to the penile urethra.

by healing fibrosis, which leads to the narrow fistulous tract from the urethra to the perineum. Consequently, micturition usually occurs through the perineal fistulas, which results in so called "watering can perineum".[21] Urethroperineal fistulas are generally the result of tuberculosis and schistosomiasis infections.

Condyloma Acuminata (Venereal Warts)

Condyloma acuminata produce soft, sessile, squamous papillomas on the glans, shaft and prepuce, are caused by viral infection. Urethral involvement occurs in 0.5–5% of male cases. Sometimes, condyloma acuminata can extend to prostatic urethra and urinary bladder. Voiding cystourethrography can help in diagnosis and is modality of choice. However, suspicion of the diagnosis is often not suspected until retrograde urethrography has been performed. On urethrography, anterior urethra shows typical multiple papillary filling defects.

Tuberculosis

Usually, urogenital tuberculosis is a descending infection and often present with renal tuberculosis. The prostate is involved in 70% of cases with genital tuberculosis. Abscess in prostate can rupture into surrounding structure, which may lead to prostatorectal and prostatoperineal or prostatourethral fistulas **(Fig. 21)**. In the acute phase, there is discharge perurethra with involvement of the epididymis, prostate, and other parts of the urinary system. In the chronic phase, patients have obstructive symptoms secondary to urethral strictures, therefore the diagnosis becomes difficult. Tuberculous strictures of urethra result in periurethral abscesses, which, unless treated, can lead to numerous perineal and scrotal fistulas resulting in "watering can perineum." RGU typically shows a stricture of anterior urethra associated with multiple prostatocutaneous and urethrocutaneous fistulas. In addition, fistulagraphy can be helpful for evaluating the entire urethra.

Urethral Strictures

The causes of most urethral strictures are infections, instrumentation or trauma. The anterior urethral strictures can be inflammatory (for example-infectious urethritis, balanitis xerotica obliterans), traumatic (straddle injury, iatrogenic instrumentation) or congenital. Straddle injury is the most common external cause of traumatic stricture. Iatrogenic trauma to the urethra may occur from pressure necrosis in the urethra from indwelling catheters **(Fig. 22)**. Instrumentation related strictures generally occur in the bulbomembranous part and rarely at the penoscrotal junction.

The stricture of posterior urethra is mostly an obliterative process which occurs due to disruption of urethra by trauma or surgery **(Fig. 23)**. Post-traumatic stricture of posterior urethra is generally associated with displacement of the axis of urethra from intervening fibrosis. Iatrogenic prostatic urethral stricture

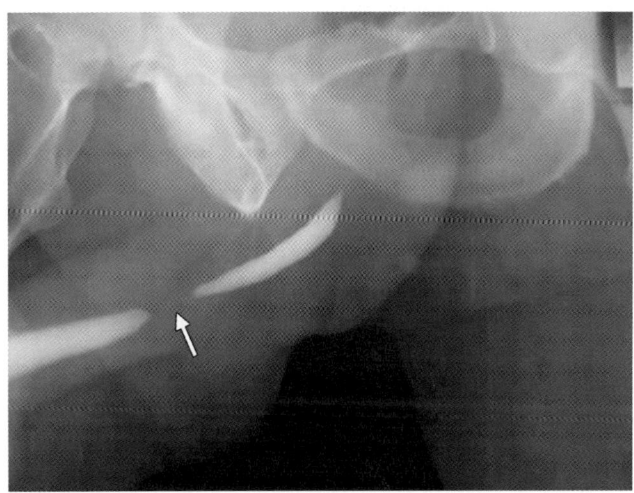

Fig. 22: Post-traumatic anterior urethral stricture: Retrograde urethrography (RGU) image showing a penile urethral stricture due to instrumentation for transurethral resection of prostate

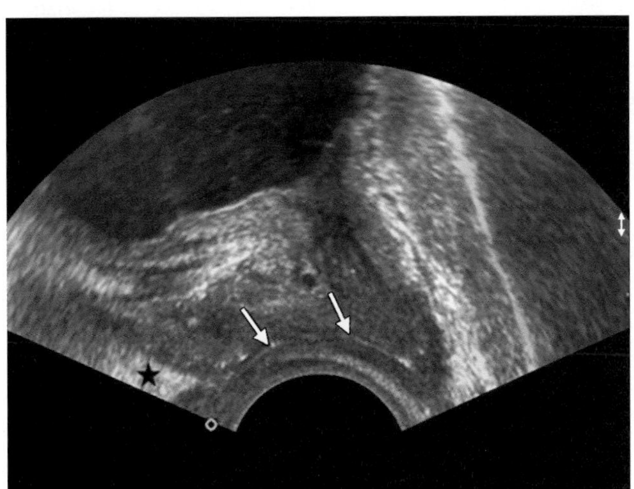

Fig. 21: Rectourethral fistula in a young male who had tuberculous prostatic abscesses and presented with pneumaturia: Transrectal US image shows the echogenic fistulous tract (arrows) between the rectum (star) and the prostatic urethra.

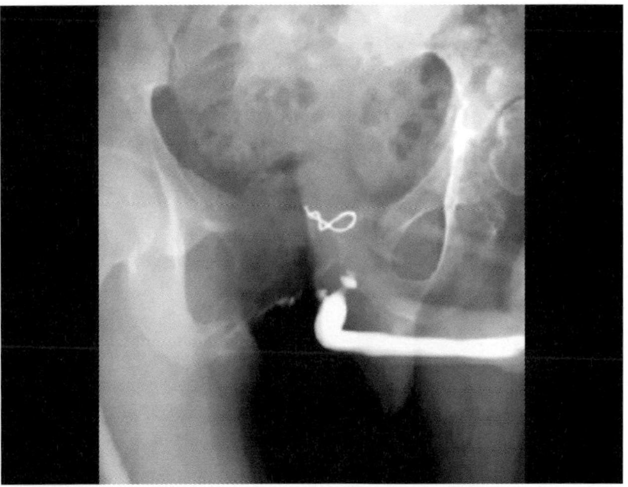

Fig. 23: Post-traumatic posterior urethral stricture: Retrograde urethrography (RGU) image showing a tight posterior urethral stricture at membranous urethra due to pelvic trauma.

("bladder neck contracture") is usually seen after transurethral resection of the prostate or open radical prostatectomy.[22]

Urethral Diverticulum

Acquired urethral diverticulum are seen more commonly in females and rarely in males. Most of the times, it involves midurethra and posterolateral wall. It is likely due to inflammation and trauma of the periurethral Skene glands and ducts, resulting in local glandular enlargement and subsequent rupture into urethra. It may be seen associated with a congenital anomaly, such as cloacal epithelium or wolffian or müllerian duct remnant. Urethral diverticulum are seen in ~1.4% of female with stress urinary incontinence.[23] Other commonly seen etiology is breach of the periurethral fascia during bladder neck suspension surgery for stress incontinence, which may lead to focal posterior urethral prolapse. The diagnosis is usually based on VCUG or cross-sectional imaging **(Fig. 24A)**. VCUG has an overall accuracy of ~65%.[24]

Ultrasonography can show a relatively echo-free cavitary structure adjacent to the urethra and may also show intracavitary debris or surrounding edema. MRI has more sensitivity than VCUG and double-balloon urethrography in the detecting urethral diverticulum, especially in the cases of narrow neck noncommunicating urethral diverticulum.[25] The differential diagnosis of a urethral diverticula are vaginal cyst (Gartner duct cyst, paramesonephric or müllerian duct cyst, epithelial inclusion cyst), ectopic ureterocele, endometrioma, and urethral tumors.[26]

Urethral diverticulum is often complicated by infection, stone formation, and malignant changes. Adenocarcinoma is the most commonly seen tumor in female urethral diverticulum.

Urethral diverticula in male anterior urethra, though rare, are the second most common etiology of congenital urethral obstruction in male. It typically occurs along the anterior aspect of penile urethra and on VCUG, the diverticulum of anterior urethra gets opacified with contrast media and can be seen as an oval outpouching on the ventral aspect of anterior urethra. Sonourethrogram is also useful in detecting anterior urethral diverticulum and delineating communication with urethral lumen **(Fig. 24B)**.

Megalourethra and Urethral Fistula

Megalourethra is a congenital abnormality with dilation of urethra which can be scaphoid type or fusiform type.

Urethral fistulas are commonly associated with imperforate anus and High Anorectal malformations (ARM).

Urethral Calculi

The most of urethral calculi are the small calculi coming out from the urinary bladder into the urethra during micturition (migrant calculi). Occasionally, primary (native) formation of a calculus is seen in the urethra when there is stricture or diverticulum. On a preprocedural low abdominal X-ray film, the calculus can be visualized before contrast media is injected. RGU will demonstrate a rounded filling defect in the urethra **(Figs. 25A and B)**. On sonography, the urethral calculus

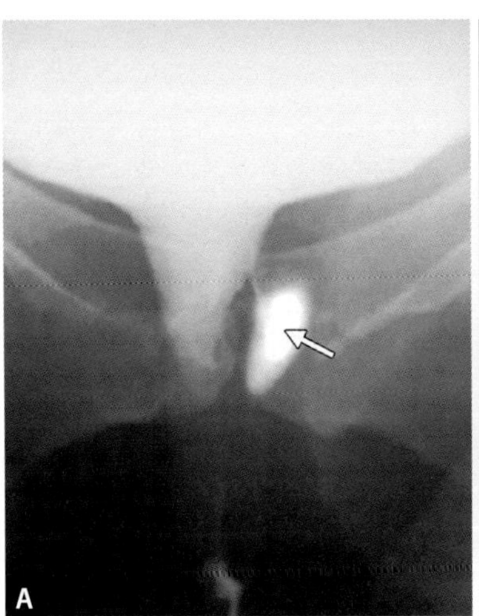

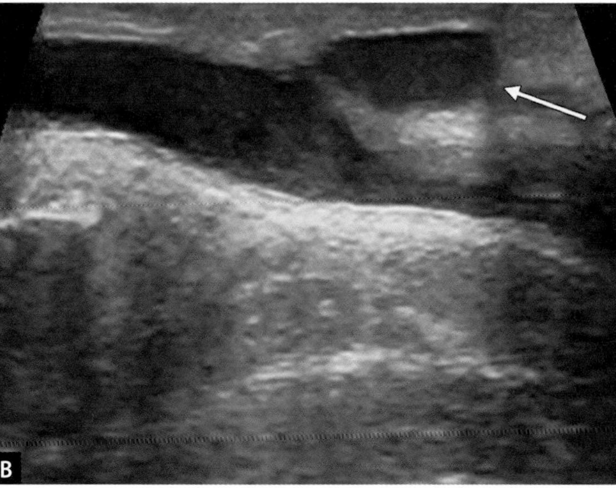

Figs. 24A and B: Urethral diverticulum in an elderly female: (A) Voiding cystourethrography (VCUG) image showing the urethral diverticulum (arrow). (B) Anterior urethral diverticulum in a male: Sonourethrogram showing the urethral diverticulum (arrow).

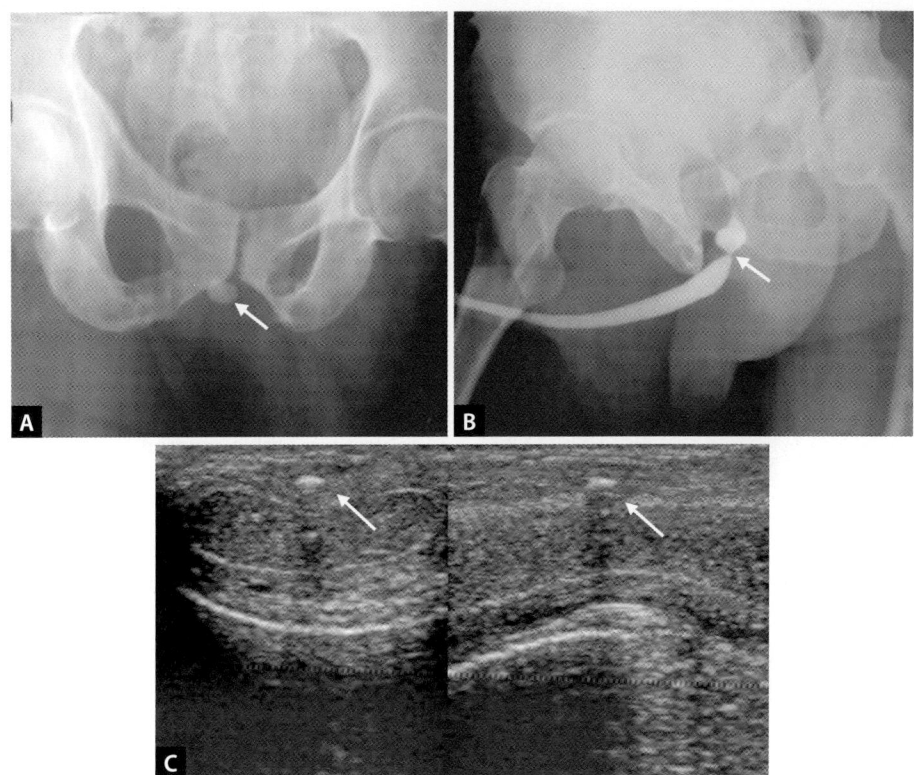

Figs. 25 A to C: Urethral calculus: Radiograph showing a calculus (arrow) in expected location of prostatic urethra, (A). Retrograde urethrography (RGU) image showing the stricture (arrow) at bulbar urethra distal to the impacted calculus, (B) Note the calculus is obscured by injected contrast, and (C) Urethral calculus: US showing the urethral calculus (arrow) as echogenic focus with distal shadowing within the urethral lumen.

may be seen and appears as echogenic focus with distal shadowing within the urethral lumen **(Fig. 25 C)**.

Tumors of the Male Urethra

Benign urethral tumors are very uncommon. They can be of epithelial or mesenchymal origin with biopsy often required to establish the correct diagnosis. Malignant tumors comprise of <1% of all urologic malignancy and are generally seen after age of 50 years. At presentation, the most frequent symptom appears a palpable mass along course of the urethra or in perineum or in penile shaft with or without obstructive voiding problems. Urethral stricture or bleeding per urethra, obstructive symptoms, serosanguinous discharge, urethral fistula, periurethral abscess in an elderly man likely suggest of carcinoma of urethra.

The bulbomembranous urethra is the most common site (~60% of cases), followed by the penile urethra (~30%) and the prostatic urethra (~10%).[27] Overall, ~80% of carcinomas in male urethra are squamous cell carcinoma, ~15% are transitional cell carcinoma, and ~5% being adenocarcinoma or undifferentiated carcinoma. The histologic subtype of urethral malignancy also varies as per anatomic sites. The involvement of prostatic urethra by transitional cell carcinomas is seen in ~90% of cases and by squamous cell carcinomas in ~10%. The involvement of bulbomembranous urethra by squamous cell carcinomas is seen in ~80% of cases, by transitional cell carcinomas is seen in ~10%, and by adenocarcinomas or undifferentiated carcinomas is seen in ~10%. The penile urethral squamous cell carcinomas are seen in ~90% of cases and that of transitional cell carcinomas are seen in ~10% **(Figs. 26 and 27)**. Adenocarcinoma may originate from the Littre's or Cowper's glands. More than 50% of cases with a carcinoma of the urethra have a history of urethral stricture disease and about one-fourth have a history of sexually transmitted disease.

The carcinoma of male urethra may spread by direct extension to surrounding structures or metastasize to regional lymph nodes. Stage I is confined to the sub-epithelial connective tissue. Stage II tumor involves the corpus spongiosum, prostate, or periurethral muscle. Stage III tumor involves the corpus cavernosum and neck of bladder or extends beyond the prostatic capsule. Stage IV tumor invades other adjacent organs. The lymphatic drainage from the anterior urethra occurs to

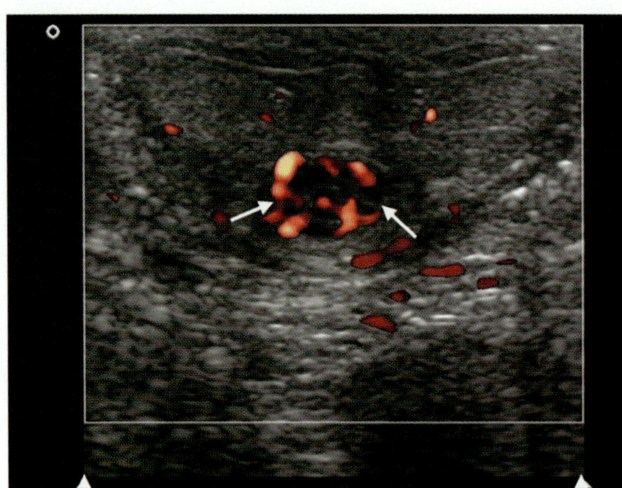

Fig. 26: Urethral transitional cell carcinoma (TCC) in an elderly male: US power Doppler image shows a hypoechoic hypervascular mass (arrows) at penile urethra.

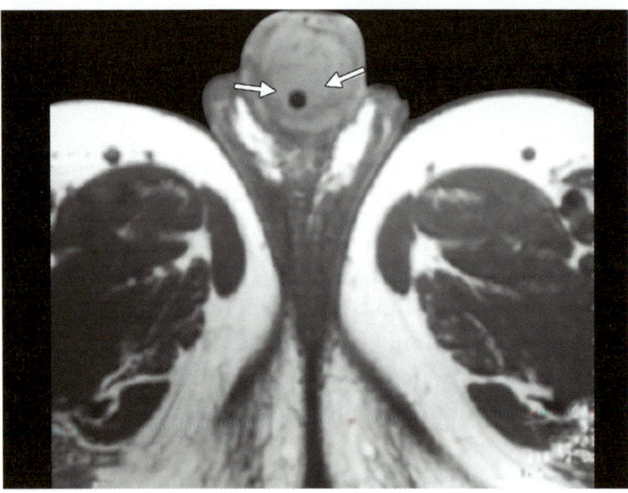

Fig. 27: Urethral squamous cell carcinoma (SCC): Contrast-enhanced magnetic resonance (CEMR) axial image showing a hypoenhancing periurethral mass (arrows) of penile urethra. Note, the urethral outline can be clearly made due to presence of urinary catheter.

the superficial and deep inguinal lymph nodes and sometimes, into the external iliac lymph nodes. Tumors of posterior urethra most frequently metastasize to pelvic lymph nodes. Carcinomas of bulbomembranous urethra can involve the urogenital diaphragm, prostate, perineum, and scrotal skin. Hematogenous spread is rare, seen in advanced local disease or with primary transitional cell carcinoma of the prostatic urethra. Generally, carcinoma of anterior urethra is more likely to have surgical control and has a better prognosis than carcinoma of posterior urethra, which commonly results in extensive local invasion and distant metastasis.

The diagnosis of urethral tumors is generally made by physical examination. Urethrography may be helpful in detecting urethral carcinoma, which can show an irregular focal narrowing of urethra. The MRI shows a soft tissue mass with less signal intensity compared to the normal corpora at both T1W and T2W sequences. MRI can depict invasion of the corpora cavernosa and is helpful for depicting tumor location, size, and local staging.[28]

Tumors of the Female Urethra

Urethral carcinoma in women is frequently seen than men urethra, with a women to men ratio of 4:1, however, it accounts for <0.01% of all malignancies in women. Most of these patients are >50 years of age. The various factors in association with female urethral malignancy are urinary tract infection, chronic irritation, and proliferative lesions such as adenomas, polyps, caruncles, papillomas, and leukoplakia of the urethra. Initial presentations in urethral malignancy are urethral bleeding, urinary frequency, obstructive symptoms, and at times may present as palpable mass or induration. Tumors of female urethra are divided as either "anterior" urethral or "entire" urethral tumors.[27] Anterior female urethral tumors are located exclusively in the distal one-third of the urethra and responsible for ~46% of urethral tumors. The entire urethral carcinomas are generally locally advanced and high grade in nature, most commonly with squamous cell carcinoma (60% of cases), followed by transitional cell carcinoma (20%), adenocarcinoma (10%), undifferentiated tumor and sarcoma (8%), and melanoma (2%). Local spread of primary tumors into the neck of bladder, vagina or vulva is commonly seen; hence, differentiation of the primary urethral tumors from the vulva or vagina can be troublesome.

The diagnosis of female urethral tumors are usually made clinically. Urethrography shows irregular narrowing of urethra. MRI is very accurate in assessing local urethral tumors in ~90% of patients. Tumors of urethral typically appear hypointense on T1W images and relatively hyperintense on T2W images. Tumor extent is best evaluated on sagittal T2W sections.

Metastatic Tumors of Urethra

Metastatic tumors of the male urethra are rarely seen. Bladder transitional cell carcinomas may disseminate to anterior urethra by seeding while doing urethral instrumentation or at cystectomy; these lesions are usually identified as multiple small mucosal nodules on urethrography. Contiguous extension of carcinoma from adjacent structure (prostate, rectum, spermatic cord, and testis) can involve the corpus spongiosum, which leads to extensive urethral narrowing and irregularity. Hematogenous secondaries to the corpora cavernosa and corpus spongiosum are uncommonly seen in cases of malignant melanoma, primary prostate, bladder, colonic, testicular, and renal malignancies.

Role of Contrast-enhanced Ultrasound and Recent Advances in Lower Urinary Tract Imaging

Contrast-enhanced ultrasound involves administration of ultrasound contrast agent combined with gray scale imaging. Intravenous use is very reliable to study the dynamics of organ and lesion perfusion, demonstrating the microvascularity.[29] It is a good investigation technique for preoperative characterization of urothelial carcinoma with easy availability and being safe and noninvasive especially advantageous in patients with deranged RFT.[30] It has very good sensitivity and specificity to detect bladder malignancy (due to its hypervascular status) especially when >1 cm in size, to differentiate superficial and muscle invasive bladder malignancies.[31] By studying the contrast dynamics, high grade and low grade lesions can also be differentiated pre operatively.

Contrast-enhanced voiding urosonography is a dynamic imaging technique that enables both morphological and functional evaluation of entire urinary tract by introducing contrast into the bladder and has a major advantage of being radiation free. After emptying the bladder with Foleys or infant feeding tube, CEUS contrast (SonoVue) is instilled intravesically mixed with saline at a dose of 0.2–1% of bladder volume. Transpelvic or suprapubic placement of USG probe is used with preferable interscrotal transperineal approach in boys. It can be used to study normal variants, congenital abnormalities (megaureter, urethral diverticulum, ureteroceles), VUR, and urethral strictures.

Advances in Imaging of Lower Urinary Tract

3D ultrasound can be employed to reconstruct the tumor with visualization of bladder walls with improved rate of tumor diagnosis and staging with USG.[32]

Dual energy CT can be useful tool for CT evaluation of bladder to look calcifications, increased conspicuity of hypervascular lesions, and differentiating small posterior wall bladder carcinomas from benign prostatic hyperplasia (BPH).

Diffusion weighted imaging is a functional imaging modality and has a potential to give with qualitative and quantitative information to aid tumor detection and characterization as well as follow-up for response to chemoradiotherapy.[33]

Positron emission tomography (PET) CT/PET MRI combines both anatomical and functional imaging modalities and can improve detection accuracy of bladder cancer as well as response assessment.[32,33]

Molecular imaging with targeted agents like antibodies, peptides or small molecules thus hold a potential for real time endoscopic cancer detection.

REFERENCES

1. Pollack HM, Banner MP, Martinez LO, et al. Diagnostic considerations in urinary bladder wall calcification. AJR. 1981;136(4):791-7.
2. McCallum RW. The adult male urethra: normal anatomy, pathology, and method of urethrography. Radiol Clin North Am. 1979;17(2):227-44.
3. Choudhary S, Singh P, Sundar E, et al. A comparison of sonourethrography and retrograde urethrography in evaluation of anterior urethral strictures. Clin Radiol. 2004;59(8):736-42.
4. Kim SH, Han MC. Reversed contrast-urine levels in urinary bladder: CT findings. Urol Radiol. 1992;13(4):249-52.
5. Chan DP, Abujudeh HH, Cushing GL Jr, et al. CT cystography with multiplanar reformation for suspected bladder rupture: experience in 234 cases. Am J Roentgenol. 2006;187(5):1296-302.
6. Ryu J, Kim B. MR imaging of male and female urethra. Radiographics. 2001;21(5):1169-85.
7. Tan IL, Stoker J, Zwamborn AW, et al. Female pelvic floor: endovaginal MR imaging of normal anatomy. Radiology. 1998;206(3):777-83.
8. Piepsz A, Ham HR. Pediatric applications of renal nuclear medicine. Semin Nucl Med. 2006;36(1):16-35.
9. M Jinzaki, A Tanimoto, H Shinmoto, et al. Detection of bladder tumors with dynamic contrast-enhanced MDCT. Am J Roentgenol. 2007;188(4):913-8.
10. Baltaci S, Resorlu B, Yagci C, et al. Computerized tomography for detecting perivesical infiltration and lymph node metastasis in invasive bladder carcinoma. Urol Int. 2008;81(4):399-402.
11. Lee JK, Rholl KS. MRI of the bladder and prostate. AJR. 1986;147:732-6.
12. Barentsz JO, Jager G, Mugler JP 3rd. Staging urinary bladder cancer: value of T1-weighted three-dimensional magnetization prepared- rapid gradient echo and two dimensional spinecho sequences. Am J Roentgenol. 1995;164(1):109-15.
13. Barentsz JO, Ruijs SH, Strijk SP. The role of MR imaging in carcinoma of the urinary bladder. Am J Roentgenol. 1993;160(5):937-74.
14. Barentsz JO, Jager GJ, van Vierzen PB. Staging urinary bladder cancer after transurethral biopsy: value of fast dynamic contrast-enhanced MR imaging. Radiology. 1996;201(1):185-93.

15. Deserno WM, Harisinghani MG, Taupitz M, et al. Urinary bladder cancer: preoperative nodal staging with ferumoxtran-10-enhanced MR imaging. Radiology. 2004;233(2):449-56.
16. Goh AC, Lerner SP. Application of new technology in bladder cancer diagnosis and treatment. World J Urol. 2009;27(3):301-7.
17. Dondalski M, White EM, Ghahremani GG, et al. Carcinoma arising in urinary bladder diverticula: imaging findings in six patients. Am J Roentgenol. 1993;161(4):817-20.
18. Sheldon CA, Clayman RV, Gonzalez R, et al. Malignant urachal lesions. J Urol. 1984;131(1):1-8.
19. DiSantis DJ. Inflammatory conditions of the urethra. In: Pollack AH, McClennon BL (Eds). Clinical Urography, 2nd edition. Philadelphia: Saunders; 2000. pp. 1041-57.
20. Gallentine ML, Morey AF. Imaging of the male urethra for stricture disease. Urol Clin North Am. 2002;29(2):361-72.
21. Sharfi AR, Elarabi YE. The 'watering-can' perineum: presentation and management. Br J Urol. 1997;80(6):933-6.
22. Pansadoro V, Emiliozzi P. Iatrogenic prostatic urethral strictures: classification and endoscopic treatment. Urology. 1999;53(4):784-9.
23. Fortunato P, Schettini M, Gallucci M. Diverticula of the female urethra. Br J Urol. 1997;80(4):628-32.
24. Keefe B, Warshauer DM, Tucker MS, et al. Diverticula of the female urethra: diagnosis by endovaginal and transperineal sonography. J Roentgenol. 1991;156(6):1195-7.
25. Daneshgari F, Zimmern PE, Jacomides L. Magnetic resonance imaging detection of symptomatic noncommunicating intraurethral wall diverticula in women. J Urol. 1999;161(4):1259-61.
26. Hahn WY, Israel GM, Lee VS. MRI of female urethral and periurethral disorders. Am J Roentgenol. 2004;182(3):677-82.
27. Donat SM, Cozzi PJ, Herr HW. Surgery of penile and urethral carcinoma. In: Walsh PC, Reitik AB, Vaughan ED Jr, Wein AJ (Eds). Campbell's Urology, 8th edition. Philadelphia: Saunders; 2002. pp. 2983-99.
28. Vapnek JM, Hricak H, Carroll PR. Recent advances in imaging studies for staging of penile and urethral carcinoma. Urol Clin North Am. 1992;19(2):257-66.
29. Nicolau C, Bunesch L, Sebastia C, et al. Diagnosis of bladder cancer: contrast-enhanced ultrasound. Abdom Imaging. 2010;35(4):494-503.
30. Gupta VG, Kumar S, Singh SK, et al. Contrast enhanced ultrasound in urothelial carcinoma of urinary bladder: an underutilized staging and grading modality. Cent Eur J Urol. 2016;69(4):360-5.
31. Caruso G, Salvaggio G, Campisi A, et al. Bladder tumor staging: comparison of contrast-enhanced and gray-scale ultrasound. Am J Roentgenol. 2010;194(1):151-6.
32. Hafeez, Huddart. Advances in bladder cancer imaging. BMC medicine. 2013;11(1):104.
33. Srivastava A, Douglass LM, Chernyak V, et al. Advances in imaging in prostate and bladder cancer. Curr Urol Rep. 2017;18(9):69.

SECTION 3

Female Genital Tract

Chapter 13

Imaging Techniques and Radiological Anatomy of Female Genital Tract

Swati Gupta, Sapna Singh, Anju Garg, Satyam

INTRODUCTION

The imaging appearance of female genital tract is dynamic and changes dramatically during the lifespan of a woman.[1] Imaging plays a significant role and ultrasonography (USG) is currently the imaging modality of choice for assessing the female genital organs. Its safety has been established, and it provides excellent depiction of normal and pathologic findings in gynecologic diseases. Magnetic resonance imaging (MRI) is used to complement sonography and to answer specific pretreatment questions about malignant and benign conditions of the female pelvis. MRI allows acquisition of multiplanar images with excellent soft tissue contrast and a large field of view. Computed tomography (CT) is commonly performed in patients with acute symptoms and generally not the primary imaging modality of choice for the evaluation of suspected gynecologic disease due to low contrast of soft tissues. There has been significant advancement in nuclear imaging studies with the advent of hybrid scanners like positron emission tomography-computed tomography (PET-CT) and PET-MRI that are capable of providing both anatomical and functional information.

PLAIN FILM RADIOGRAPHY

The role of plain radiographs in the field of gynecological imaging is limited. One condition where a plain radiograph may be performed includes a radiograph to locate an intrauterine contraceptive device (IUCD) that is not visualized on ultrasound **(Figs. 1A and B)**. Pelvic calcification can be seen on an abdominal radiograph and can be due to various causes. One of the common causes is fibroids; popcorn calcification is seen in few of them. Calcification is seen in about 12% of ovarian cystadenocarcinomas.[2] Dermoid cysts may show tooth-like structure and/or a fat fluid level. Close scrutiny of pelvic bones should always be done to look for areas of erosion in suspected pelvic masses.[3]

HYSTEROSALPINGOGRAPHY

Hysterosalpingography (HSG) is an important diagnostic tool in determining anatomical contour of uterine cavity, tubal anatomy, and patency. It is indicated in cases of infertility and recurrent pregnancy loss. Rare indications include checking the completion of tubal sterilization and evaluation of tubes prior to attempted reversal of sterilization. HSG is contraindicated in patients having comorbidities such as endometriosis and pelvic inflammatory disease (PID).

Technique

Hysterosalpingography is done in the preovulatory phase of the menstrual cycle in order to ensure that the patient is not pregnant at the time when the procedure is performed, preferably between 6th day and 10th day of the cycle. Examination in the postovulatory phase of cycle is avoided also because the chances of venous intravasation and probability of false positive diagnosis of cornual occlusion are increased by thickened secretory endometrium. Routine administration of antibiotics is not recommended and decisions regarding prophylactic use of antibiotics in patients with a history of PID are left to the referring clinicians. One such specific regimen for prophylaxis is doxycycline 100 mg twice a day for 5 days, beginning 2 days prior to the procedure. It is advisable to administer a

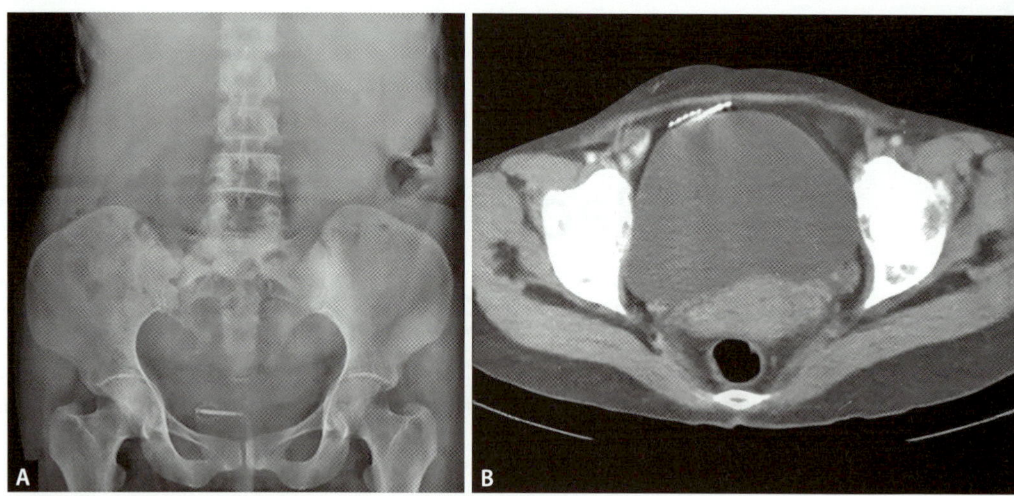

Figs. 1A and B: (A) Plain radiograph showing displaced intrauterine contraceptive device (IUCD); (B) Contrast-enhanced axial CT scan image of the same patient with IUCD visualized anterior to urinary bladder.

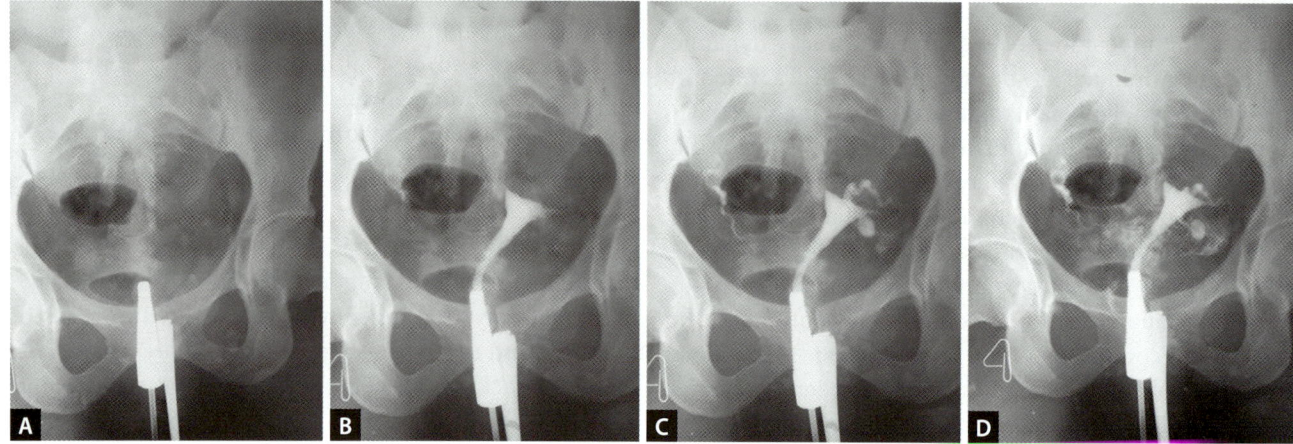

Figs. 2A to D: Normal hysterosalpingogram comprising scout, early uterine, early tubal and late filling phase.

dose of nonsteroidal anti-inflammatory drug (NSAID) half an hour before the study to alleviate pain. The procedure should be explained to the patient before obtaining informed consent. Urinary bladder should be empty before the patient is positioned in lithotomy position. The perineum is prepared with povidone-iodine solution and draped with sterile towels. Cervix and vagina are exposed using speculum and cleansed with antiseptic solution. Tenaculum is used to grasp the anterior cervical lip. Leech Wilkinson cannula or a 5F HSG catheter is introduced, stabilized into the cervix and uterus retracted. A catheter is preferred as it causes less pain, is easier to perform and requires less fluoroscopic time. Nonionic water soluble contrast media in a dilution ratio of 1:1 is introduced into uterus. The first film is a scout radiograph in supine position. Spot film is taken during early filling phase after instillation of 5 mL of contrast to ensure that contrast does not obliterate the small filling defects and during early tubal filling before contrast obscures the isthmic portions. In the next step, additional 5 mL is instilled to completely fill the tube and to demonstrate free spill **(Figs. 2A to D)**. Delayed films help to study the pattern of peritoneal spillage. Additional oblique views may be taken if needed.[4]

Complications of HSG include pain, infection, vasovagal reactions, venous intravasation and allergic reaction to contrast media.

Though HSG has been used for tubal assessment since several years, meta-analysis has shown a sensitivity and specificity of 0.65 [95% confidence interval (CI): 0.50–0.78] and 0.83 (95% CI: 0.77–0.88), respectively for HSG as a test for tubal obstruction. When the HSG suggests that the tubes are patent, this can be confirmed by laparoscopy in 94% of the women. A tubal block seen on HSG will be confirmed by laparoscopy in only 38% of the women.[5]

Thus, HSG is a reliable indicator of tubal patency but not of tubal block.

ULTRASOUND

Ultrasound remains the first line of investigation while evaluating the female genital tract. It gives an excellent visualization of the organs of the genital tract. With the addition of Color Doppler USG, the vascular dynamics can also be very well-evaluated. The introduction of USG contrast agents has made it possible to interrogate even the slow flow areas. Multiplanar and surface rendered images are possible with three-dimensional (3D) technology. However, it is essential to recognize that operator's skill; regardless of the equipment used, ultimately determines the final benefit of ultrasound in patient care.

Indications for Evaluation of Uterus and Adnexa

The indications for sonographic evaluation include:

- Menstrual disorders
- Postmenopausal bleeding
- Pelvic inflammatory disease
- Pelvic mass
- Infertility
- Recurrent pregnancy loss
- Lower abdominal pain
- Guided procedures.

Technique

Sonographic evaluation of the uterus and the adnexa can be done by the transabdominal and transvaginal routes. These are complementary techniques and are used extensively in evaluation of the female pelvis. The *transabdominal scan (TAS)* is performed with a 3.5–5 MHz sector transducer, with a distended bladder as an essential prerequisite. The urinary bladder is considered adequately distended when it covers the entire fundus of the uterus. Overdistension is to be avoided as it may distort the anatomy and may push the pelvic organs beyond the focal zone of the transducer. Imaging of the uterus is performed in both sagittal and axial planes. The adnexa are imaged by scanning obliquely from the contralateral side, although in many cases good visualization may be achieved by scanning directly over the adnexa.

The limitations of transabdominal scan are as follows:

- The patient may not be able to fill the bladder adequately.
- In patients with retroverted uterus, fundus may be beyond the focal zone of the transducer.
- Limited resolution.

Transvaginal scanning (TVS) affords improved resolution of the pelvic organs. Specially designed probes of 4–9 MHz frequency are used for this procedure. The urinary bladder should be empty. However, a minimal distension may be required if the uterus is severely anteflexed. The patient is positioned supine in lithotomy position with the knees flexed and hips slightly elevated. The probe is covered with a latex barrier and inserted gently into the vagina till the uterus is identified. The uterus is imaged in its longitudinal axis, first sweeping from left to right. Short-axis images are then obtained sweeping from anterior to posterior. The relative position of the uterus can be inferred by the orientation of the probe that best images the uterus, e.g. if the uterus is best imaged with a posterior inclination, the uterus is retroflexed and vice versa. For imaging the cervix, the transducer should be withdrawn to the mid-vaginal level.

The ovaries are imaged by tilting the transducer to either side of the midline in the transverse section. The internal iliac vessels can be identified as anechoic tubular structures along the pelvic side walls. The ovaries usually lie anterior and medial to these vessels; however, their position can vary.

Limitations of this technique are:

- Limited field of view
- Examination may not be possible in vaginal atrophy or when the woman is virgo intacta.

Transrectal ultrasound can be performed in patients with a contraindication to transvaginal scan. *Transperineal* scans also help in determining the origin and extent of some tumors.

DOPPLER EVALUATION

The gynecological Doppler ultrasound examination can be used to study pathological and physiological circulatory changes in the female pelvis noninvasively.

Indications

The indications for Doppler examination include:

- Characterization of uterine/ovarian masses
- Infertility and assisted reproduction.

After simultaneous evaluation of morphology and color flow, pulsed gate is placed to obtain flow information. The course of the uterine artery is suited for transvaginal assessment with ideal geometry for Doppler signal recording. It is also possible to record Doppler signals transabdominally when the uterus is anteverted.

The branches of the uterine artery extending towards the ovary can be identified in the broad ligament and the superior aspect of the ovary, respectively. Because of their tortuosity, only short segments of the arteries are usually identified in any scan plane. The lowest possible filter (<50–60 Hz), with a high color gain should be used to detect slow flow. Endometrial vascularity can also be evaluated by Doppler sonography. The extent of vascular penetration into the endometrium correlates well with successful conception. Variations in the depth of vascular penetration before, during, and after the mid-cycle can be seen.

The ovarian artery is a branch of the abdominal aorta and reaches the ovary through the infundibulopelvic ligament. Signals from the ovary are identified as low Doppler shifts of a small vessel with low velocity. The waveform shape varies with state of activity of ovary.[6] Guerriero et al. demonstrated that specificity in diagnosing adnexal malignancies can be increased by association of color flow localization and the B-mode analysis of internal architectural appearance.[7]

Three-dimensional displays enable visualization of multiple overlapping vessels and their relation to other vessels, tumor, and surrounding tissues. A variation of Doppler imaging which uses the amplitude termed power Doppler imaging or color Doppler energy (CDE) is also used. The greatest advantage of CDE includes the relative angle independence and absolute lack of aliasing. It has a higher detection rate of vascularity in malignant and benign adnexal masses. The disadvantages of power imaging are high motion sensitivity and the absence of information about direction and speed of flow.

GEL SONOVAGINOGRAPHY

Regular transvaginal sonography is known to have limitations in assessing local cervical and vaginal lesions. This is due the close proximity of the vaginal and cervix walls to the transducer. In such cases, a recently described technique called gel sonovaginography is helpful. This technique involves instillation of 20 mL of ultrasound gel into the vagina followed by examination with a transvaginal transducer. The instilled gel causes a partial distension of vaginal walls and standoff resulting in increased clarity on gel sonovaginography. Disorders such as vaginal and cervical cancer, vaginal septa, deep infiltrating endometriosis, and cervical polyps can be visualized better with gel sonovaginography.[8]

THREE-DIMENSIONAL AND FOUR-DIMENSIONAL SONOGRAPHY

Three-dimensional ultrasound or volume sonography is an imaging advancement that involves acquisition of a series of two-dimensional (2D) images from a volume of the patient. They are then displayed in different planes after the acquisition **(Figs. 3A to C)**.

Indications

Three-dimensional ultrasound may be useful in following conditions:

- Diagnosing congenital uterine malformations **(Fig. 4)**
- Accurate volume measurement, e.g. endometrial, ovarian cysts, follicles and tumor masses
- Exact localization of pathology—intrauterine fibroid, IUCD etc

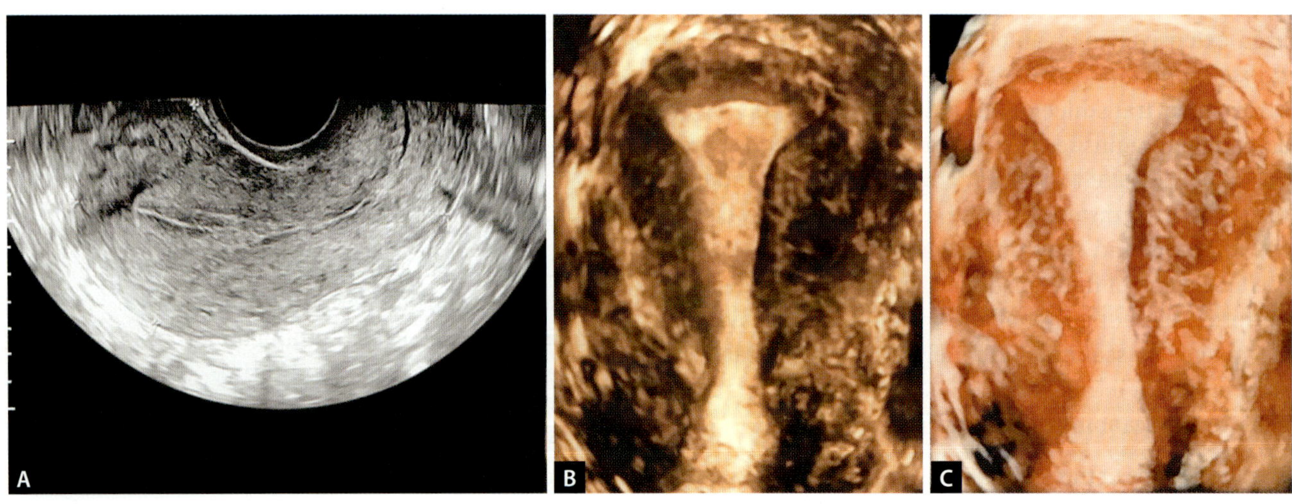

Figs. 3A to C: 3D ultrasound with data obtained from a volume of tissue and visualization of the third or coronal plane of the uterus with rendering techniques.

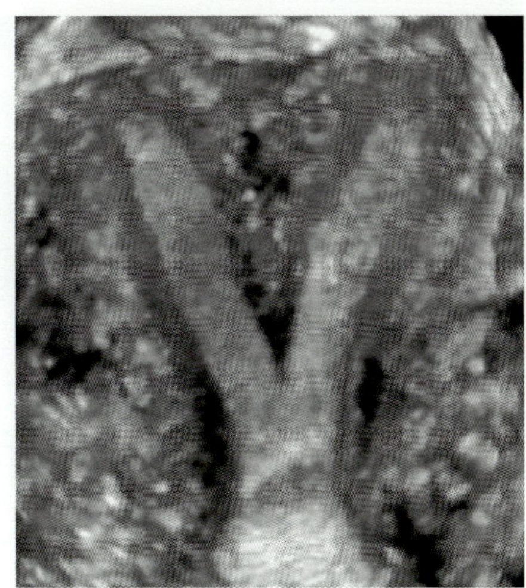

Fig. 4: 3D reconstructed coronal view showing a subseptate uterus.

- Mapping of myomata
- Characterization of adnexal masses
- Extent of tumor infiltration into adjacent tissues/organs
- 3D power Doppler can aid in characterization of vessel morphology.

Technical Considerations

When used in conjunction with 2D ultrasound, 3D ultrasound has added clinical and diagnostic value for selected indications and circumstances in gynecologic ultrasound. 3D imaging has several obvious benefits that relate to demonstration of multiplanar views and an improved spatial orientation, of which the coronal plane is particularly useful in gynecological practice.[9] It offers a more reproducible and objective measurement of vascularity and volume of the region of interest through further postprocessing modalities. It also has the added advantages of teleconsultation, reduced scanning time, and storage of images for reevaluation. There are different types of 3D acquisitions—manual, sensor-based, and automatic. Demonstration of 3D images in real time is variously known as 4D ultrasound, real-time 3D ultrasound and live 3D ultrasound.

SALINE INFUSION SONOHYSTERO-SALPINGOGRAPHY

Saline infusion sonohysterosalpingography (SIS) involves the instillation of sterile saline into the endometrial cavity under ultrasound guidance. The saline distends the cavity, separating the walls of the endometrium. Saline infusion sonohysterosalpingography (SIS) has several advantages over HSG including simplicity, reduced cost, lack of ionizing radiation, a high level of diagnostic accuracy, and minimal invasiveness with an ability to characterize masses within the endometrial cavity. Assessment of tubes and uterine cavity is possible in presence of fluid within them. The procedure of SIS for testing tubal patency was first reported by Richman.[10]

Technique

Saline infusion sonohysterosalpingography is done in proliferative phase just like HSG, however, it can be done anytime in postmenopausal women. Patient's preparation is similar to that described under HSG. Initial screening using TVS probe is done to look for any pathology that may hinder successful completion of procedure.[4]

The endometrial cavity is distended with 20–40 mL normal saline introduced via a self-retaining catheter, prior to transvaginal sonography. The fluid within the cavity gives an excellent visualization of any pathology within the cavity and also differentiates between intracavitary versus extracavitary pathology **(Figs. 5A and B)**. Sonosalpingography can be done to establish the patency of the fallopian tubes by instilling fluid into the uterus and then visualizing passage of fluid through the tubes or presence of fluid in the pouch of Douglas on USG.[11] While intracavitary lesions are clearly delineated by anechoic media, very small hollow cavities, such as normal tubes are not always easily visualized using SIS.

HYSTEROSALPINGO-CONTRAST SONOGRAPHY

Deichert et al. were the first to evaluate tubal patency using injection of contrast agent and transvaginal sonography.[12] Demonstration of the lumen of tubes requires visualization of movement of fluid using highly echogenic medium. A cost-effective alternative is the use of saline mixed with air. It produces high contrast due to the presence of air bubbles; these bubbles, however, stand only for a very short period and tubal patency assessment may become difficult practically. Therefore, commercially available contrast media were launched with microbubbles that can stand longer. On ultrasound evaluation, this contrast appears echogenic. The scanning technique is the same as that for SIS. It is possible to delineate the uterine cavity along with the tubes using contrast. Total amount of contrast needed is as little as 2–3 mL/tube. The findings appreciated by conventional 2D-HyCoSy (hysterosalpingo-contrast sonography) are, however, sometimes difficult to interpret. Due to the tortuosity of the tube, the whole fallopian tube

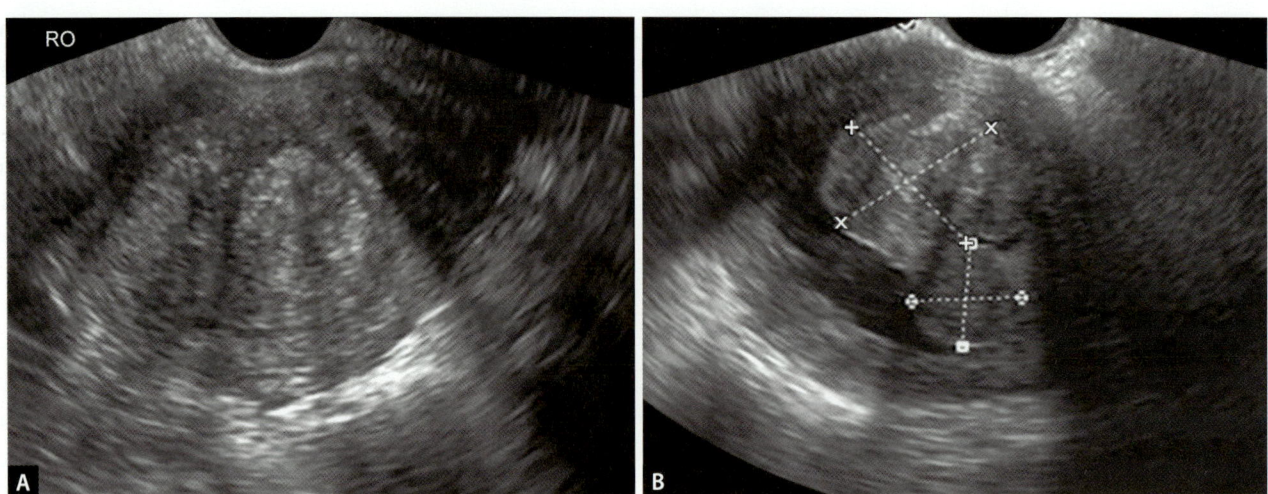

Figs. 5A and B: Sonohysterography. (A) Transvaginal scan shows hyperechoic masses within the uterus; it is not possible to determine their relation with the endometrium; (B) On instillation of intracavitary saline, two well-defined masses (within callipers) are seen projecting into the endometrial cavity—submucous fibroids.

cannot be visualized in the majority of scanning planes. Furthermore, differentiation of echogenic tube from bowel becomes difficult due to the spill of the echo-positive contrast medium. This has been overcome by use of 3D and 4D imaging in conjunction with HyCoSy.[13]

A comprehensive meta-analysis was published in 2016 to assess the diagnostic value of 4D and 3D HyCoSy for detecting tubal patency and it included 23 studies. This systematic review showed a high diagnostic accuracy of 3D/4D HyCoSy for tubal patency with an overall specificity of 0.91 (95% CI: 0.89–0.93) and sensitivity of 0.92 (95% CI: 0.90–0.94). The results had a good stability among the included studies.[14]

EXTENDED FIELD-OF-VIEW IMAGING[15]

Extended field-of-view (EFOV) overcomes the drawback of limited field of view of sonography, enabling the visualization of large fields of view in a single image. This technology is now available in most of the modern equipment. The technique is relatively simple and requires only a steady sweep of the transducer over the concerned area to acquire the data. The EFOV image is then reconstructed automatically by the computer. Doppler EFOV allows a panoramic visualization of vascularity in mass lesions, helping in their characterization. Transvaginal EFOV is also possible to illustrate the relation of smaller pelvic masses with the uterus and ovaries in a single image. EFOV images are comparable to CT/MRI images as they provide a panoramic view.

ELASTOGRAPHY[16]

Elastography is an imaging method that evaluates the elasticity of tissue. All available ultrasound elastography methods employ ultrasound to measure the mechanical response resulting from an applied force. The mechanical response measured may be displacement, strain or amplitude and phase of vibration.

There are three main techniques used in sonoelastography: (1) shear wave elastography (SWE), (2) strain elastography (SE), and (3) transient elastography (TE). Both SE and SWE can be used in evaluation of uterus and cervix; however, the application in the field of gynecology has mostly been experimental and further validation requires extensive research. Stoelinga et al. and Frank et al. have investigated the use of transvaginal elastography in uterine evaluation.[17,18] Both studies concluded that transvaginal elastography could help differentiate uterine fibroids from adenomyosis. Elastography can also be used in the diagnosis of cervical malignancies. Thomas et al. have reported use of cervical elastography in 113 patients, among whom 24 had cervical malignancies. The study showed that elastography was able to differentiate malignant from normal cervical tissue.[19]

CONTRAST-ENHANCED ULTRASONOGRAPHY

Ultrasonography contrast agents can help delineate vascular structures and enhanced Doppler signals from small volumes of blood make it possible to image organ and lesion perfusion in real time.[20] These contrast agents are gas-filled microbubbles of size 2–5 μm. They are stabilized by a shell and are injected intravenously. They are capable of passing through the smallest capillaries. Microbubbles oscillate particularly at frequencies used for diagnostic imaging (1–10 MHz), reflecting a unique nonlinear echo.

The use of contrast-enhanced ultrasonography (CEUSG) in the assessment of liver lesions, renal carcinoma, and cardiac imaging is already quite established, the use of this technique is still limited in the field of gynecology. Contrast uptake and wash out can be studied subjectively or objectively by time intensity curves. These curves have a role in characterization of ovarian mass lesions. It is also possible to distinguish between endometrial hyperplasia and endometrial malignancy by analysis of intensity and time parameters recorded after contrast administration. Ultrasound contrast agents can be extremely useful in differentiating uterine fibroids from focal adenomyosis as their uptake patterns are very different.[21]

MAGNETIC RESONANCE IMAGING

Magnetic resonance imaging is now recognized as an important problem solving tool in the evaluation of female pelvis due to its multiplanar capability, lack of significant motion degradation of images, and higher soft tissue contrast resolution.

Indications

Indications for MRI include the following:

- Evaluation of congenital anomalies
- Evaluation of cervical and uterine malignancy
- Selected cases of leiomyoma, like cases that require differentiation from adnexal masses and leiomyosarcoma, treatment planning and monitoring after therapy etc.
- Assessing response to medical therapy
- Pelvic floor assessment
- Search of submucosal lesions in infertile patients
- Diagnosis of adenomyosis and endometriosis
- Problem solving modality in characterization of ovarian lesions, especially ovarian dermoid.

Patient Preparation

Imaging is performed in the supine position with a moderately full bladder after fasting for at least 4 hours to limit bowel motion. In the absence of glaucoma, 20 mg of butyl scopolamine (Buscopan) is injected intramuscularly to reduce bowel peristalsis. A variety of receiver coil (body coil allowing better coverage and endoluminal coil for better anatomical depiction) have been used for pelvic imaging but phased array coils have been found to provide the best results. Ideally, the coil position should allow imaging from mid-symphysis pubis to renal hilum. Rectal and vaginal gel contrast media can be used for specific indications.[22] Vaginal opacification has shown to be beneficial in conditions like cervical cancer, endometrial cancer, and vaginal developmental anomalies. Both rectal and vaginal opacification are recommended when imaging patients of deep pelvic endometriosis. Vaginal injection involves an average of 60 mL of sterile ultrasound gel. Rectal opacification is performed with 100–120 mL of nonsterile ultrasound gel.

Sequences

After the localizer sequence, anterior and upper saturation bands are placed to cover the subcutaneous fat for each sequence. The standard protocol for pelvic imaging comprises unenhanced T1- and T2-weighted sequences. Spoiled gradient recalled echo (GRE) and spin-echo (SE) sequences form the basis of most of the protocols. Standard sequences include the following:

- Sagittal T2-weighted sequence of the pelvis.
- One or two additional T2-weighted sequences with slice orientation based on the clinical indication and findings of the sagittal sequence (one T2 fat saturation sequence may also be acquired based on the area of interest).
- One to three T1-weighted images (the optional orientation of this native T1-weighted image depends on the slice orientation that best demonstrates the pathology and its extent).
- Fat suppressed T1 sequence whenever the lesion demonstrates hyperintensity on the T1-weighted images.
- Contrast-enhanced T1-weighted images with fat suppression—mandatory for staging of malignancies, evaluation of deep endometriosis, and characterization of adnexal masses.

Technique of MRI for Uterine and Cervical Pathologies

For uterine indications, short-axis MR images are acquired perpendicular to the hyperintense stripe of the endometrium in the uterine body. This will usually be paraxial, but in patients with extreme anteversion of the uterus, this may be closer to a true coronal plane. Long-axis MR images are acquired parallel to the stripe.

Occasionally, the uterus may be anteflexed, i.e. there may be a considerable angle between the body of the uterus and cervix. In these circumstances, the main clinical question should be answered; for example, if the procedure is being done for the assessment of a cervical carcinoma, the orientation of axial oblique T2-weighted images should be perpendicular to the hyperintense stripe of endocervical channel, permitting complete visualization of the T2 hypointense stromal ring. If this is equivocal, a fat-suppression sequence, such as short-TI inversion-recovery (STIR), may be helpful. Fat suppressed T1-weighted images should be acquired before and after gadolinium enhancement. Coronal plane imaging is occasionally helpful, particularly if disease spread to the vagina is suspected on the initial imaging sequences. Investigation of benign conditions of the uterus, such as adenomyosis and leiomyoma, will usually require a briefer protocol than imaging for preoperative staging in cases of malignancy.

Technique of MRI for Pathologies of Ovary

The axial plane is most important. Coronal imaging is often useful in clarifying the relationship of masses to vessels and the uterus. The sagittal plane is found to be of limited use.

Technique of MRI for Imaging of Vagina

T2-weighted images once again form the mainstay of the imaging technique. Layers of the vaginal can sometimes be differentiated using small field-of-view, high-resolution images. Axial, sagittal, and coronal planes are all useful in demonstrating the relationship of vagina to adjacent organs. Axial and sagittal images demonstrate the relationship to rectum and bladder while coronal images demonstrate the relationship to the levator ani muscle to its best advantage.

Nodal Survey

A common indication for pelvic MRI is staging gynecological or urological malignancy. An essential part of this investigation is surveying the retroperitoneum and pelvis for enlarged nodes. It is prudent to complete this part of the investigation first, as gut relaxation is maximum in the beginning of the procedure. Images of the pelvis are obtained using T1-weighted spoiled GRE (breath-hold) and T2-weighted sequences, in the axial plane, from the aortic bifurcation to the inguinal region just below the femoral canal. Slice thickness should be 8–10 mm using a 0–4-mm gap. This may be varied to cater to patients of varying heights. Subsequently, an evaluation of the retroperitoneum should be carried out.

Special Techniques

Various special techniques that can be added to standard protocol include the following:

- The characterization of adnexal masses may require additional in phase and out of phase sequences to allow a diagnosis of teratoma with minimal fat.
- Dynamic contrast-enhanced (DCE)-MRI involves intravenous injection of standard low-molecular weight paramagnetic intravascular contrast agents (typically gadolinium diethylenetriamine penta-acetic acid), either as a constant infusion or fast bolus injection. Serial image acquisitions are performed every few seconds over a length of few minutes, the region of interest and exact protocols depend on the tumor type being imaged. DCE-MR is useful in characterization of adnexal lesions and cases of recurrence of malignancies.[23]
- Diffusion-weighted imaging (DWI)-MRI is a robust tool for evaluation of functional status of gynecological malignancies. It has shown to have high accuracy and sensitivity for detection of nodal metastases in cervical cancer patients according to a recent meta-analysis involving 67 studies.[24] DWI-MRI is especially capable of accurate determination of the depth of myometrial invasion in patients with endometrial cancer.[25] It has also been proposed to be a potential response biomarker in cervical cancer.[26] DWI is highly sensitive for picking up peritoneal spread in gynecological malignancies and plays an important role in their management especially ovarian cancer.[27]
- Blood oxygenation level-dependent (BOLD) hypoxia imaging is an MR tool to analyze vascular functionality associated with angiogenesis. It uses deoxyhemoglobin as a natural paramagnetic contrast agent and is found to be sensitive to changes in blood flow, blood volume, and blood oxygenation. Combined physiologic and anatomic information obtained from multiparametric MRI (MPMRI) with BOLD hypoxia imaging helps in detection and grading of tumors.[28]
- Diffusion tensor imaging (DTI) has been used to quantify defects and determine direction of muscle fibers during pelvic floor assessment.[29]
- Multiphase dynamic MR defecography can be performed following intrarectal instillation of contrast to evaluate pelvic floor and defecatory dysfunction.[30]
- Magnetic resonance lymphography is performed to assess the lymph nodes. It involves intravenous

injection of ultrasmall superparamagnetic particles of iron oxide (USPIO) and can detect presence of metastases in the nodes with high sensitivity and specificity.[31]

- Proton MR spectroscopy also has a role in differentiating malignant from borderline epithelial ovarian tumors (EOTs). A high Choline (CHO) peak suggests a malignant EOT and a significantly elevated N-Acetyl Aspartate (NAA) peak is highly suggestive of a borderline EOT. The NAA/Cho ratio is a reliable biomarker for differentiating malignant from borderline EOTs.[32]

COMPUTED TOMOGRAPHY

The role of CT in the evaluation of gynecologic disorders has declined due to endovaginal scanning and MRI. MRI is better than CT for staging uterine and cervical carcinoma, particularly with respect to local extent. But CT has a role in evaluation of ovarian carcinoma due to its potential to detect peritoneal deposits.[33] CT is frequently added as an imaging modality in patients with nonspecific lower abdominal symptoms such as pain.

Technique

A standard pelvic CT scan consists of continuous sections from the level of the symphysis pubis cephalad to the iliac crest. In cancer staging or abdominopelvic mass evaluation, sections are then taken from the symphysis pubis to the diaphragm. Bowel opacification achieved orally with 1,000 mL of diluted contrast medium is generally recommended. Patients are requested to drink 450 mL of water soluble contrast medium 10–12 hours before the examination to opacify the large bowel, and 450 mL 45 minutes preceding the study to opacify small bowel. In patients with suspected ovarian cancer, PID, endometriosis, 200 mL water soluble contrast enema is preferred to delineate the disease extent. Intravenous opacification is pivotal for assessing adnexal lesions, staging uterine and ovarian cancers, and assessing vascular or inflammatory diseases. A dose of 90–120 mL contrast medium with a concentration of 300–370 mg iodine/mL administered at a rate of 2–3 mL/sec is sufficient. In multidetector computed tomography (MDCT), images are obtained in transaxial planes and reformatted in coronal and sagittal planes.

CT also plays an important role in the aspiration or drainage of fluid collections such as blood or pus.

Evaluation of the pelvic vasculature is indicated in MDCT of pelvic arteriovenous malformations after embolization and fibroids after uterine artery embolization. It is recommended to determine individual circulation time by using a bolus-tracking program for CT angiography of the pelvic arteries. The pelvis is scanned during the arterial phase after a faster injection rate (3–5 mL/sec).

PET-CT AND PET-MR

There is an increase in evidence advocating the use of PET-CT in evaluation of gynecologic malignancies. These are typically identified with increased glucose metabolism and therefore present with increased fluorodeoxyglucose (FDG) uptake, whereas benign tumors are usually negative on PET. However, common pitfalls include normal physiologic activity in bowel, endometrium, blood vessels, increased FDG uptake in normal ovaries during ovulation and focal retained activity in pelvic kidneys, ureters, bladder diverticula, and urinary diversions.

Indications

Positron emission tomography-computed tomography has been used widely in patients with advanced disease or in cases of recurrence. It is indicated in patients of ovarian and cervical carcinoma with suspected relapse. In patients of carcinoma cervix stage 2A and above, PET-CT is indicated for prognostication and treatment planning. It is also used in assessing response to therapy in patients of carcinoma cervix.[34] MRI and PET individually play important and supporting roles in assessing gynecologic malignancy. MRI is the imaging procedure of choice for assessing local extension of tumors, and PET aids in detection of distant metastases.[35]

Technical Considerations

Ideally, the bladder should be empty to avoid artifacts on PET images from high radioactivity concentration in the bladder. It is advised that the patient is scanned in a caudal to cranial direction, thereby imaging the pelvis in the beginning of the study. The CT portion of PET/CT is often important to identify focal retained activity in ureters and bladder diverticula. Pelvic imaging can be made better by intravenous injection of a diuretic agent to lessen tracer retention in the urinary system. A technique of hydration, diuretic administration, and preimaging voiding obviates the need for invasive procedures like bladder drainage in most patients.

ANATOMY

Uterus

The uterus lies between the bladder anteriorly and rectosigmoid posteriorly **(Fig. 6)**. Its size and shape vary

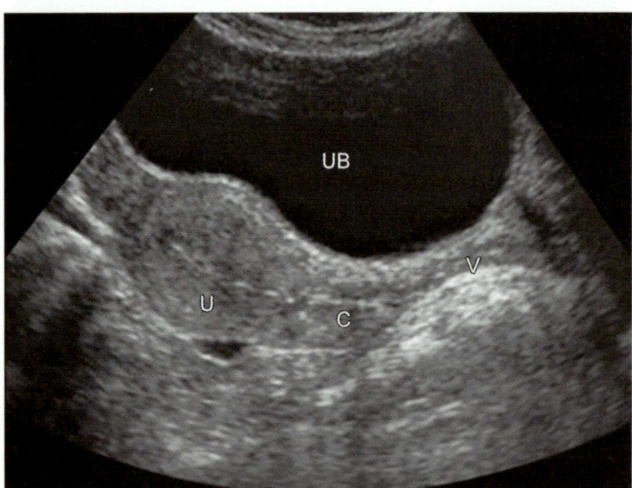

Fig. 6: Normal uterus (U), cervix (C), and vagina (V) on a transabdominal sagittal scan.

Fig. 7: Normal neonatal uterus—sagittal scans. Inverse pear shape with cervix (C) having greater width than body (B) of uterus.

Table 1: Normal uterine size and shape by life stage.[1]

Stage	*Uterine Length (cm)*	*Uterine body to cervix ratio*
Neonatal	3.5	2:1
Pediatric	1–3	1:1
Prepubertal	3–4.5	1–1.5:1
Pubertal	5–8	1.5–2:1
Reproductive	8–9	2:1
Postmenopausal	3.5–7.5	1.5:1

throughout life-related to age, hormonal status, and parity **(Table 1)**. The infantile or prepubertal uterus has an inverse pear-shaped appearance with a disproportionately larger cervix occupying up to one-half to two-thirds the size of the uterus **(Fig. 7)**. In the immediate neonatal period, the uterus is slightly larger and shows an echogenic endometrium, because of residual maternal hormonal stimulation. A small amount of endometrial fluid may also be seen in 25% of neonatal uteri.[36] There is little growth of the prepubertal uterus from infancy till about 8 years of age. The uterus gradually increases in size till puberty; when it attains a pear-shaped appearance with the body of the uterus becoming approximately double the cervix.

The normal postpubertal or adult uterus varies considerably in size. The maximal dimensions of the nulliparous uterus are approximately 8 cm in length, 4 cm in anteroposterior (AP) diameter and 5 cm in width. Parity increases the normal dimensions by more than 1 cm in each dimension.[37] After menopause, atrophy of uterus occurs, with the most rapid decrease in size occurring in the first 10 years following the cessation of menstruation. The uterus

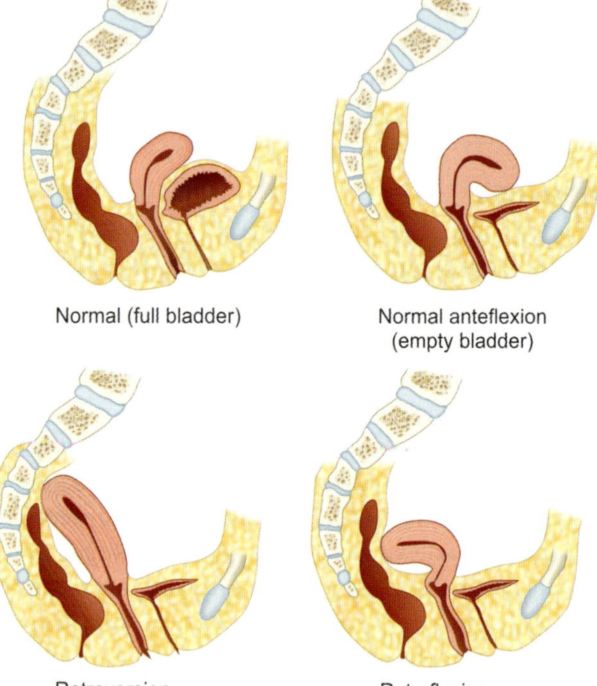

Fig. 8: Alterations in uterine position. The normal position of uterus in most women is anteverted with a mild degree of anteflexion. In retroversion, the long axis of the uterus and cervix point more posteriorly than the long axis of the vagina. In retroflexion, the body of the uterus is angled posteriorly relative to the cervix.

usually assumes a position that is both anteverted and anteflexed **(Fig. 8)**. The degree of bladder filling alters the lie of the uterus; with an empty bladder the uterus is angled forward from the lie of the vagina, whereas a full bladder straightens the uterus. In case of retroverted or retroflexed uterus, the fundus lies posteriorly. It is often not possible to distinguish between retroversion and retroflexion on sonography so the general term retroposition is used. On transabdominal scanning, the deeper portions of the fundus may be difficult to delineate and may even appear abnormal because of shadowing from the intervening body and cervix. Transvaginal scanning gives an excellent visualization of the retropositioned uterus as the probe can be directed posteriorly.[38]

Uterus consists of an external serosa (*perimetrium*), a middle muscle layer (*myometrium*) and the internal mucosa (*endometrium*). The perimetrium is not visible on ultrasound examination, although subserosal veins may be seen as a normal variant. *On sonography*, the myometrium has three layers: the inner myometrium (or the subendometrial halo) appears as a thin hypoechoic area surrounding the echogenic endometrium. The intermediate layer is the thickest and has a uniformly homogeneous low-to-moderate echogenicity. The thin outer layer is less echogenic and separated from the intermediate layer by the arcuate vessels, which can be visualized on ultrasound as small anechoic foci in the periphery of the uterus. Calcification may be seen in the arteries in postmenopausal women. Sometimes small highly echogenic foci may be seen in the inner layer of myometrium. These small, single or multiple, nonshadowing foci are thought to represent dystrophic calcification related to previous instrumentation like dilatation and curettage or endocervical biopsy.[39]

The endometrium is best measured on the midline sagittal scan of the uterus. The measurement is taken as the distance between the two interfaces formed by junction of subendometrial halo and the more echogenic endometrium. This is the double layer thickness **(Fig. 9)**.

The normal endometrial cavity is seen as a central echogenic line as a result of specular reflection from the interface between apposing surfaces of the endometrium. It should be straight or smoothly curved.

The cervix is better visualized by transvaginal sonography as a tubular structure of homogeneous echogenicity **(Fig. 10)**. The mucus within the endocervical canal usually appears as an echogenic interface which may become hypoechoic during the periovulatory period as the fluid content increases. Retention (nabothian) cysts of the cervix are commonly seen during routine sonography. They may vary in size from a few mm to 4 cm. They may be single or multiple and usually diagnosed incidentally, although they may be associated with chronic cervicitis.

On MRI, three distinct uterine zones can be differentiated in women of reproductive age on T2-weighted imaging. The endometrium represents the

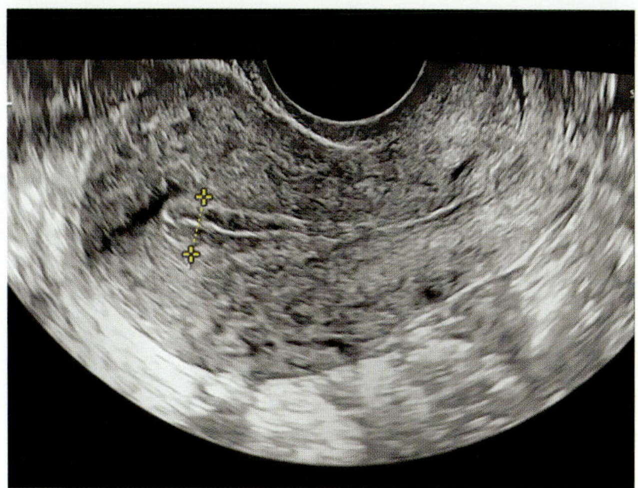

Fig. 9: Measurement of endometrial thickness on ultrasound.

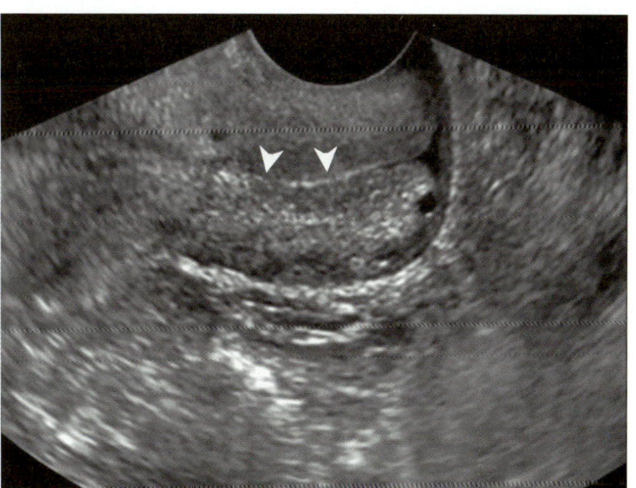

Fig. 10: The normal cervix as seen on sagittal transvaginal scan, with a central echogenic line (arrowheads) representing the cervical canal. Two small nabothian cysts are seen.

central high signal intensity portion of the uterus. The middle low signal intensity layer is the junctional zone and represents the inner myometrium. The thickness of normal junctional zone is less than 8 mm. The outer medium signal intensity represents the outer myometrium. Its signal intensity depends on the phase of menstrual cycle, but it usually exhibits intermediate signal intensity on T2-weighted image **(Fig. 11)**. The zonal anatomy is important to assess the depth of myometrial invasion of endometrial carcinoma. On T1-weighted images, uterus is seen as an organ with medium to low signal intensity.[40] Uterus also undergoes subtle wave-like peristalsis caused by contractions of the inner myometrium. The direction, height, and frequency of the wave vary throughout the phase of menstrual cycle, with an average of 2–3 cycles

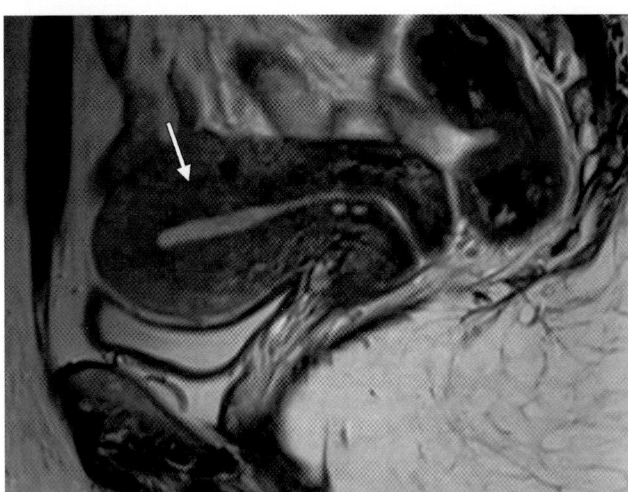

Fig. 11: T2-weighted sagittal magnetic resonance image. Outer limit of junctional zone is marked by arrow.

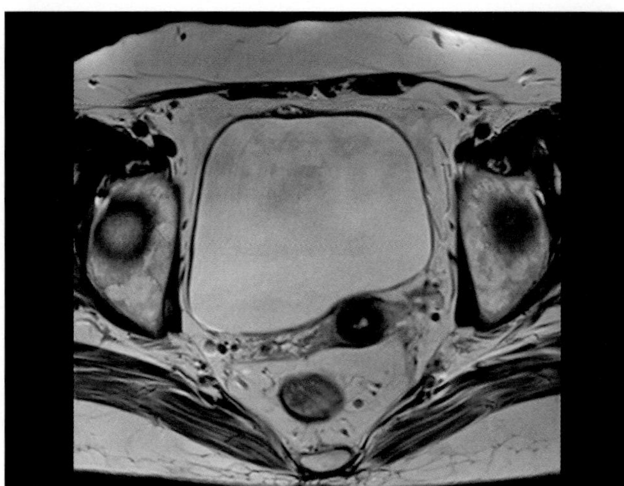

Fig. 12: Magnetic resonance appearance of cervix with T2 hypointense stroma surrounding the hyperintense endocervix.

per minute. The direction is generally antegrade during menstruation and retrograde (cervicofundal) in mid-cycle. On cine mode display, wavy and subtle movement of this area can be seen, with occasional stripping movement of the endometrium. The appearance of the uterus on the DCE-MRI study is variable and depends on the time interval after intravenous contrast administration. Usually, the myometrium is homogeneous and hyperintense in the arterial and venous phase, while the endometrium enhances later and slowly, showing hypointensity when compared to myometrium. On delayed evaluation, endometrium and outer myometrium show pronounced contrast enhancement while the junctional zone is of low signal intensity, thus displaying the zonal anatomy.

The cervix shows four layers on T2-weighted MR images. The central high signal layer represents mucus, which is surrounded by high signal intensity endocervix. The hypointense stroma surrounds the endocervix and is continuous with the junctional zone of uterus. The outer intermediate signal intensity is from smooth muscle and is continuous with outer myometrium **(Fig. 12)**. Strong contrast enhancement of the endocervix and parametrium is seen on postcontrast images, whereas stroma shows initial faint enhancement with progression on delayed images.

On *CT*, the cervix and body of uterus appear as soft tissue masses, only identifiable from each other by their shape, i.e. cervix is round and uterus oval or triangular in cross section. In women of reproductive age, the endometrium exhibits hypodensity relative to the inner myometrium during most phases of contrast enhancement, a finding that might be mistaken as fluid within the uterine cavity **(Fig. 13)**.

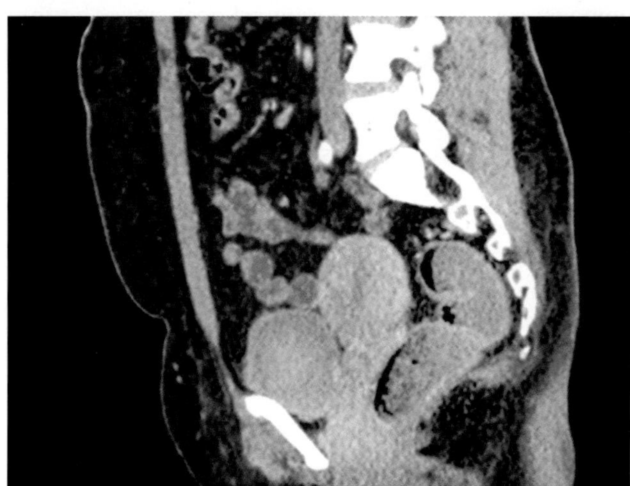

Fig. 13: Sagittal reformat of contrast-enhanced CT scan showing the normal uterus posterior to the bladder with reduced enhancement of the endometrium.

Vagina

The vagina runs anteriorly and caudally from the cervix between the bladder and rectum. On *USG*, it is best seen on the mid-sagittal transabdominal scans as a collapsed hypoechoic tubular structure with a central hyperechoic line due to the apposed surfaces of the vaginal mucosa. A vaginal tampon can be visualized as a highly reflective structure with a strong acoustic shadow. On TVS, examining the vaginal walls is possible during slow withdrawal of the probe as they collapse around the end of probe. In patients who have had hysterectomy, the vaginal cuff should not be mistaken for a mass. The normal upper limit of the AP diameter of the vaginal cuff is 2.1 cm.[41] The vagina has three layers on T2-weighted MR images. The central high-signal intensity represents mucus; middle low-signal intensity represents submucosa and muscularis; and outer high-signal intensity representing vaginal venous plexus. On *CT axial scans*, the vagina is identified as a thin rectangular structure with an enhancing mucosa. The vulva includes the mons pubis, labia majora and minora, prepuce, frenulum, clitoris, and vestibule. A complex system of anastomoses accounts for variations in arterial, venous, and lymphatic supply.

Upper corpus and uterine fundus are drained by the common iliac and para-aortic lymph nodes. Lower and middle parts of the uterus are drained by parametrial, paracervical, and obturator nodes. In general, lymphatic drainage from the distal vagina and vulva passes along inguinal and femoral nodes. The upper two-thirds of the vagina drains to the external iliac and obturator nodes. The posterior vagina may also drain to the gluteal and anorectal lymph nodes.

Adnexae

The adnexae consist of the ovaries, the fallopian tubes, ligaments, and vessels. The *ovaries* most commonly lie lateral to the uterus (usually within a few centimeters) at about the level of the cornua. Variations are common and insignificant. A relatively constant relationship of the ovaries is their location anterior to internal iliac vessels, which serves as a useful landmark for the ovaries particularly during *TVS*.

The ovaries are typically seen as oblong structures with a relatively homogeneous echotexture. Well-defined small anechoic follicles may be seen peripherally in the cortex. The variable appearances of ovaries during different stages of life are described in **Table 2**.

Because of the variability in shape, ovarian volume is considered the best method for evaluating the ovarian size (0.523 × length × width × AP diameter). For this measurement, any cyst larger than 1 cm in diameter is excluded. The two ovaries should be approximately equal in volume; and neither should be more than twice the volume of the other. Small echogenic, nonshadowing foci may sometimes be seen in a normal ovary, which are thought to be due to specular reflection from tiny unresolved cysts below the spatial resolution of the ultrasound machine.

On *MRI*, normal ovaries can be visualized in 85% of women of reproductive age. They are identified by following the course of the round ligament or gonadal vessels. On T1-weighted images, the ovaries are seen as low- or medium-signal intensity structures, and on T2-weighted images, they show low signal intensity in the central stroma and high signal intensity follicles and functional cysts of varying sizes **(Fig. 14)**. A low signal intensity rim around ovaries represents the fibrous capsule. On *CT images*, the ovaries are usually seen in adult premenopausal patients as soft tissue masses posterolateral to uterus; however, their position is variable **(Fig. 15)**. The normal ovary displays intense early enhancement with a secondary washout.

The nondistended fallopian tubes are difficult to see on ultrasound. Delineation of the tubes is possible if intraperitoneal fluid is present in the peritoneal cavity or if they are distended by saline/contrast agent.

The posterior cul-de-sac (pouch of Douglas) is the most posterior and inferior reflection of the peritoneal cavity located between the rectum and vagina. Small quantities of fluid (1–3 mL) in the cul-de-sac is a normal finding in asymptomatic women, and can be seen in all phases of the menstrual cycle.

Table 2: Normal ovarian volume and appearance by life stage.[1]

Stage	*Ovarian volume (cm^3)*	*Ovarian appearance*
Neonatal	1–3.5	Follicles and cysts common
Pediatric	0.5–1.5	Fewer than six follicles; cysts uncommon
Prepubertal	1–4	Follicles and cysts common
Pubertal	2–6	Follicles and cysts common
Reproductive	4–16	Follicles and cysts common
Postmenopausal	1.3–5.8	Follicles and cysts in approximately 15–20%

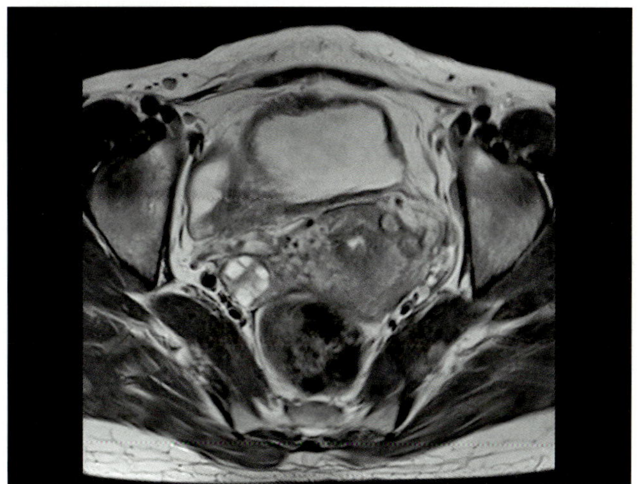

Fig. 14: Magnetic resonance appearance of ovaries. T2-weighted axial image showing multiple hyperintense follicles in ovary on the right side.

The pelvic side walls are lined by psoas and iliacus muscles. Iliacus muscle arises from the iliac wings and progresses posterolateral to the psoas into the pelvis. These muscles run obliquely passing posterior to inguinal ligament and form a joint tendon to insert on greater trochanter. These muscles are visualized on ultrasound as paired hypoechoic structures separated by echogenic fascial plane. The iliac vessels lie on the psoas muscle.

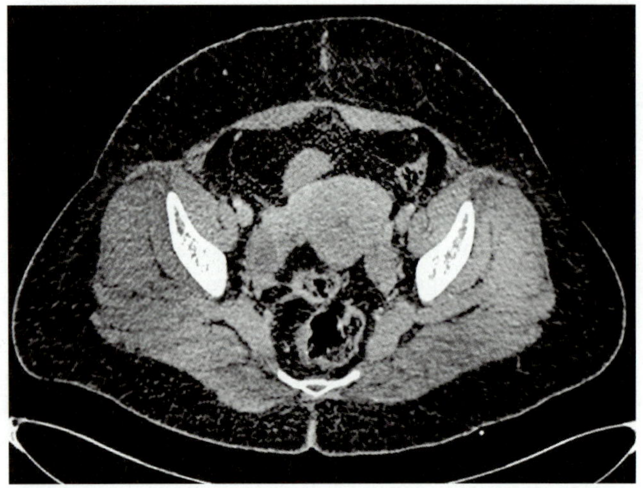

Fig. 15: Axial contrast-enhanced CT scan image showing the uterus and bilateral ovaries located posterolateral to it.

Pelvic floor muscles including iliococcygeus, coccygeus, puborectalis, and pubococcygeus muscles, as well as the external and internal anal sphincter are clearly shown on MRI. Pelvic diaphragm are displayed as two layers of low signal intensity at the level of lower vagina. In addition to a precise demonstration of anatomy, dynamic MRI also helps in imaging the kinematics of pelvic organs.

The Menstrual Cycle

The appearance of the endometrium and ovaries varies during the menstrual cycle.[42] Their appearance during the various phases of the menstrual cycle has been described in **Table 3 (Figs. 16 and 17)**.

Table 3: Appearance of endometrium and ovaries in a normal menstrual cycle.

Day of cycle	*Phase*	*Endometrial thickness (mm)*	*Ultrasound appearance of endometrium*	*Ultrasound appearance of ovaries*	*MR appearance of uterus*
1–4	Menstrual phase	1–4	Small amounts of fluid may be seen endovaginally. Thin interrupted central echo	Development of a small number of follicles.	Loss of zonal appearance. Blood clot may be present in the endometrial cavity
5–14	Proliferative phase	4–8	Central hyperechoic line with surrounding thin hypoechoic band	By Day 8 or 9 of the menstrual cycle, one follicle becomes dominant, and the others become atretic. Nondominant follicles are usually less than 14 mm in diameter	Internal myometrial enhancement occurs earlier and is more intense in the proliferative than in the luteal phase of the cycle
	Periovulatory	6–10	Trilayered appearance; the hypoechoic band becomes more prominent with thin echogenic lines on either side	About Day 14, when the dominant follicle measures 18–25 mm, ovulation occurs	
15–28	Secretory phase	8–16	Thick Echogenic with through transmission.	Following ovulation, a corpus luteum develops which can commonly be seen as a hypoechoic or isoechoic structure peripherally within the ovary, but may show a very varied sonographic appearance. Sometimes, it may form a cyst and become very large. **(Fig. 18)**. A repeat scan 2–6 weeks later will usually resolve the dilemma	Signal intensity of outer myometrium increases. Increased thickness of junctional zone

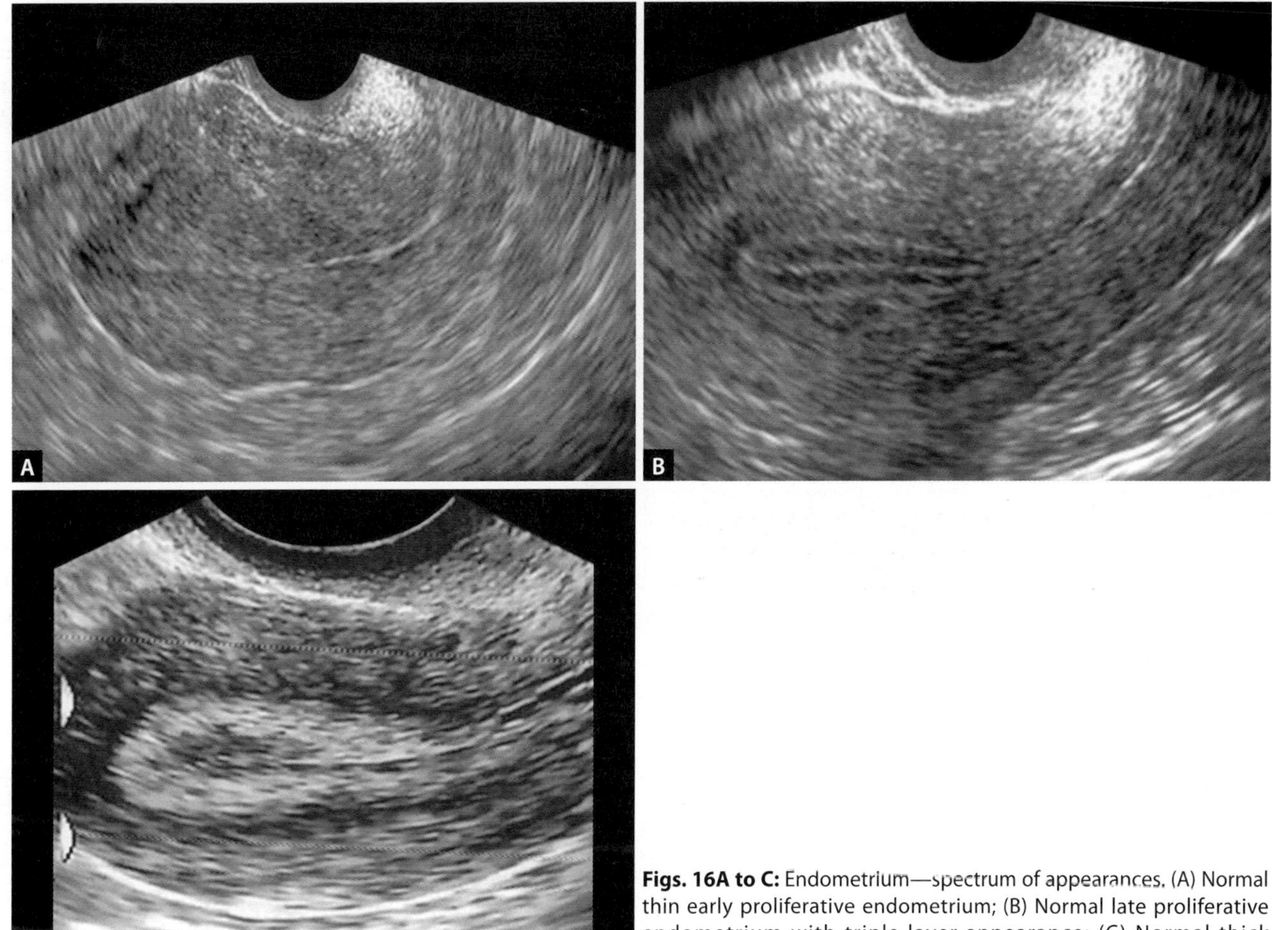

Figs. 16A to C: Endometrium—spectrum of appearances. (A) Normal thin early proliferative endometrium; (B) Normal late proliferative endometrium with triple layer appearance; (C) Normal thick hyperechoic secretory phase endometrium.

Imaging in Postmenopausal Period

In postmenopausal women, the outer myometrium displays lower signal intensity and the junctional zone is often missing or indistinctly visualized. The normal sonographic endometrial appearance varies according to absence or presence of hormonal replacement therapy (HRT). Additionally, the type of HRT (i.e. combined, sequential or continuous) is important.[43] In postmenopausal asymptomatic women not receiving HRT, several reports suggest that endometrial thickness should not exceed 4 mm, whereas others use 8 mm as the upper limit of normal value.[1] For women receiving HRT, the ultrasound appearance of the endometrium depends on whether the patient takes a combination of estrogen and progesterone (either continuously or sequentially) or continuous estrogen. Sequential HRT results in monthly cyclic endometrial thickening and withdrawal bleeding. At mid-cycle, the upper limit of maximal endometrial thickness frequently goes beyond 8 mm, and in some cases may reach up to 15 mm. In these women, it is essential to do a follow-up scan. In women taking either continuous estrogen or continuous estrogen and progesterone, the maximum endometrial thickness is 8 mm, and cyclic endometrial changes should not occur. Postmenopausal women may often have a trace of fluid (approximately 1 mm in thickness) in the endometrial cavity due to cervical stenosis.[43] The postmenopausal patients have similar internal and external myometrial enhancement which is significantly less intense than in the premenopausal patients.

The postmenopausal ovaries may be difficult to recognize sonographically as they are relatively small and do not contain follicles **(Fig. 19)**. Mean postmenopausal ovarian volume ranges between 1.2 cc and 5.8 cc with the volume decreasing in size with increasing age. An ovarian volume of more than 8 cc is definitely abnormal. Small anechoic cysts (less than 3 cm) may be seen in up to 15%

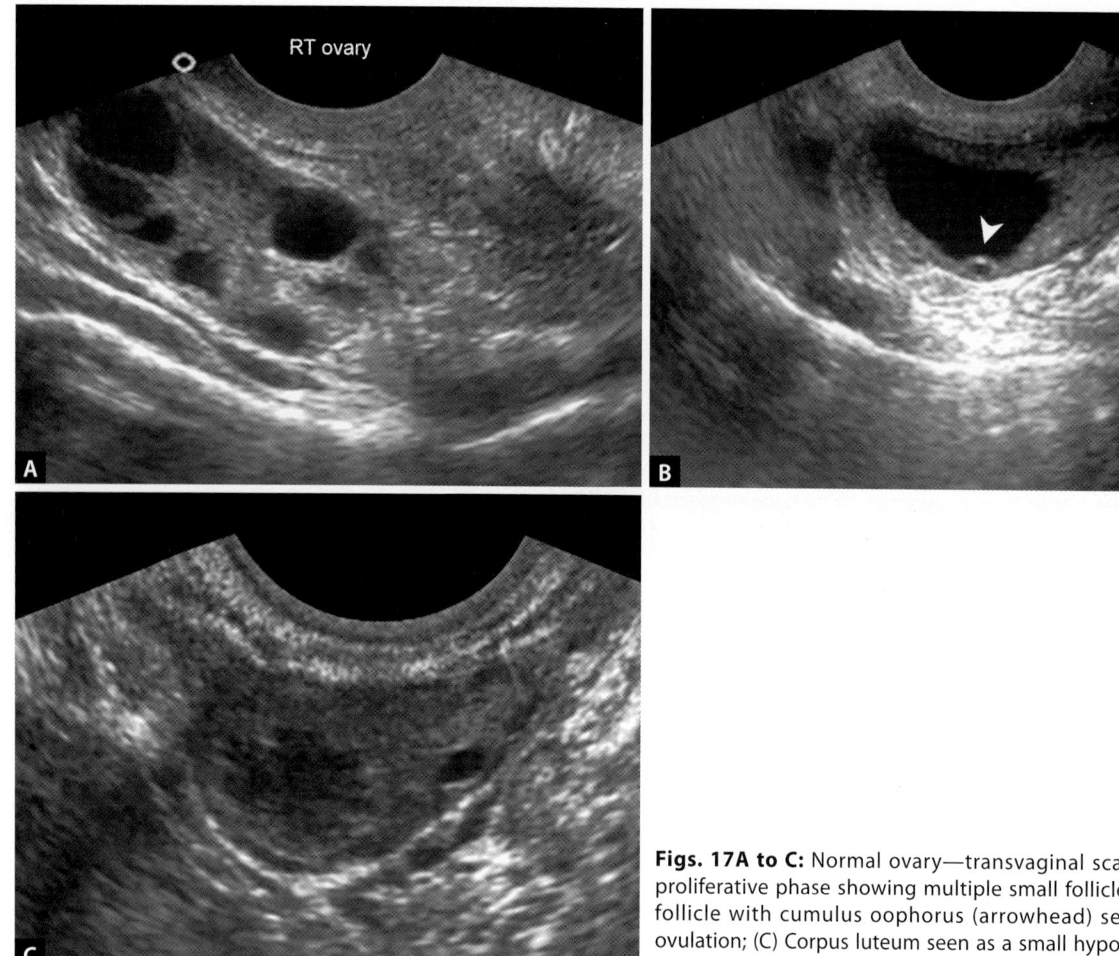

Figs. 17A to C: Normal ovary—transvaginal scans. (A) Ovary in proliferative phase showing multiple small follicles; (B) Dominant follicle with cumulus oophorus (arrowhead) seen just prior to ovulation; (C) Corpus luteum seen as a small hypoechoic area with crenated margins within the ovary.

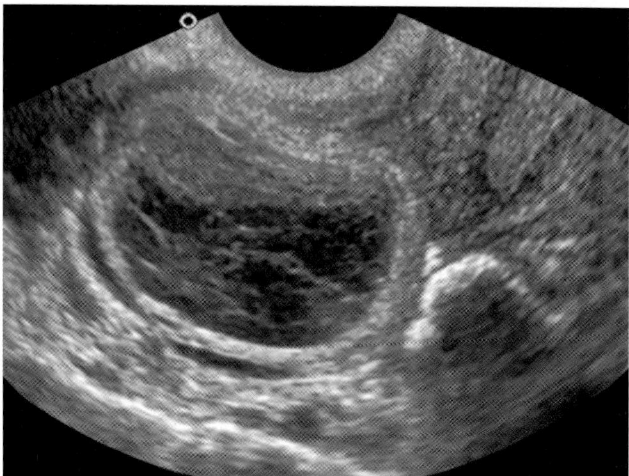

Fig. 18: Hemorrhagic corpus luteum cyst. Characteristic reticular pattern of internal echoes seen within the cyst.

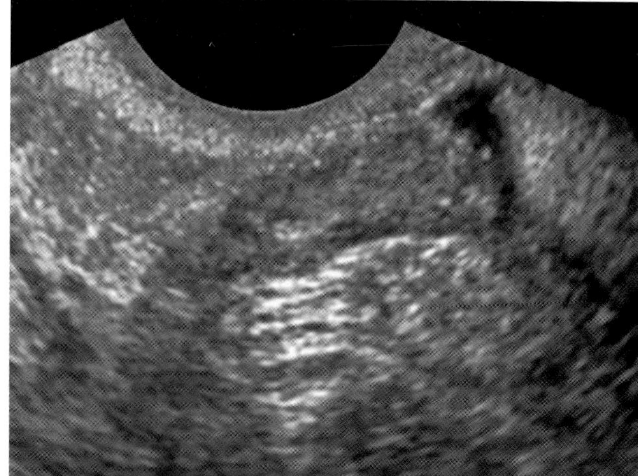

Fig. 19: Postmenopausal ovary. Small in size with no follicles, often difficult to identify.

of postmenopausal ovaries and are not related to age, length of time since menopause or hormone use. These cysts can disappear or change in size over time.[44] The atrophic ovaries of postmenopausal women are frequently indistinguishable from surrounding structures on CT images.

Vascular Anatomy

The blood supply to the uterus is via the *uterine artery*, a branch of the internal iliac artery. The uterine artery enters the uterus at the cervico-corporal junction and ascends along the lateral aspect of the uterine body to the cornua. At the cornua, an adnexal branch originates that supplies the ipsilateral ovary and anastomoses with the ipsilateral ovarian artery. The uterine arteries anastomose through the anterior and posterior arcuate arteries which are located in the outer one-third of the myometrium. Radial arteries arise from the arcuate vessels and extend through the myometrium up to the endometrium where they form: (1) the basal arteries which supply the basalis layer of endometrium and (2) the spiral arteries which supply the functional layer of endometrium. The spiral arteries are responsive to hormonal changes. During the reproductive years, both color and duplex Doppler patterns change concomitantly with grayscale changes.[45] The general pattern of uterine blood flow throughout the menstrual cycle is that perfusion increases in response to rising plasma estrogen and progesterone and decreases with periovulatory fall in estrogen. The typical spectral waveform shows a high resistance pattern characterized by high flow velocity with an early diastolic notch **(Figs. 20A to C)**.

The *ovarian arteries* arise from the abdominal aorta and enter the pelvis through the infundibulopelvic ligament. They reach the ovaries through the hila via the mesovarium. After supplying the ovary, terminal branches anastomose with branches of the uterine artery. The ovarian arteries are more difficult to assess as they run a transverse course through the pelvis. The ovarian arterial supply also exhibits different flow characteristics during different phases of a normal menstrual cycle. In general, the index value is high during the early follicular phase which progressively decreases till the early luteal phase and then rises again in the late luteal phase **(Table 4)**.[46] Differences in flow characteristics may also be seen between the dominant and nondominant ovaries. In the ovary containing the dominant follicle, continuous

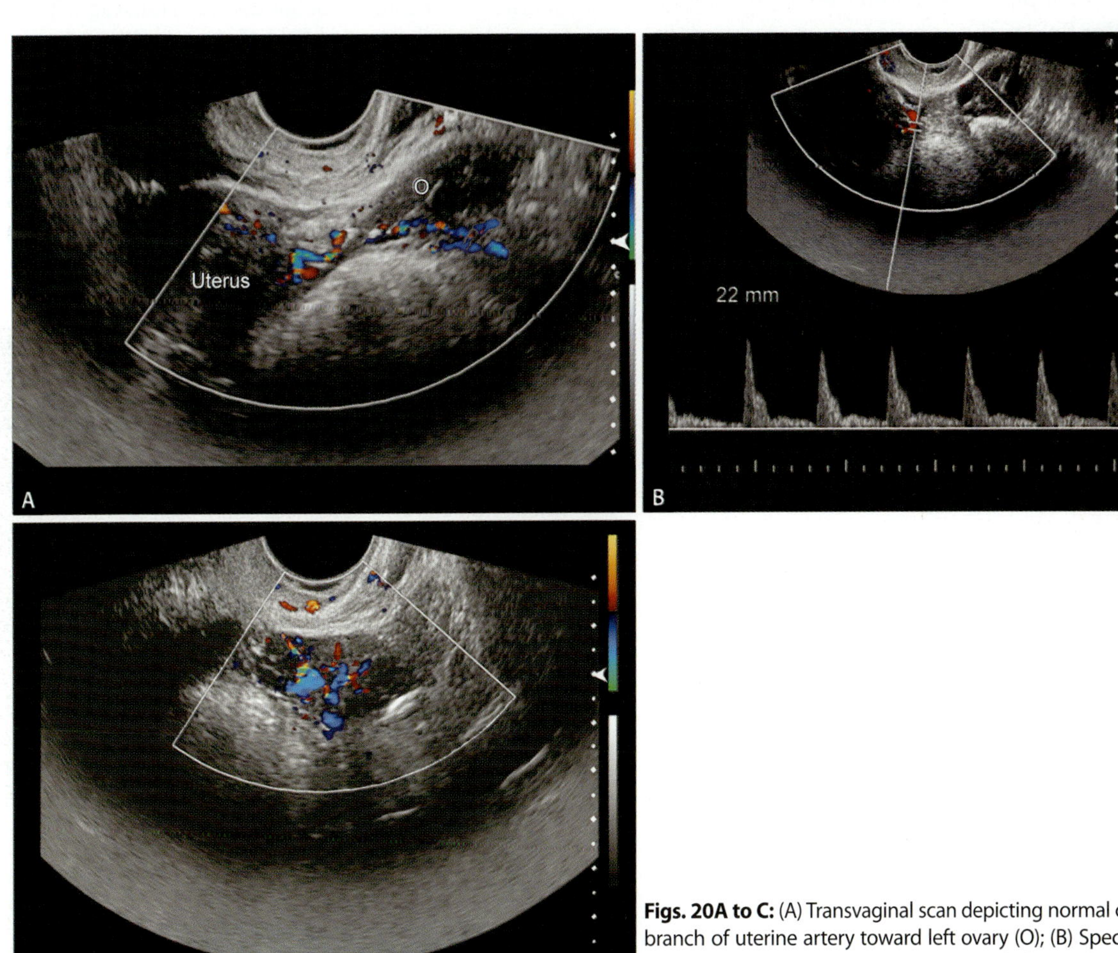

Figs. 20A to C: (A) Transvaginal scan depicting normal course of adnexal branch of uterine artery toward left ovary (O); (B) Spectral waveform of the uterine artery characterized by a high flow velocity, a postsystolic notch and low diastolic flow; (C) Scan showing vascularity in the ovary.

Table 4: Variation in Doppler indices in the uterine and ovarian arteries.

Phase	*RI OVA*	*PI OVA*	*PI UTA*
Early proliferative	0.65–0.7	1.8–2.2	1.67 ± 0.22
Late proliferative	0.55–0.6	1.0–1.3	1.89 ± 0.4
Luteal	0.6–0.65	1.3–1.8	1.23 ± 0.67
Postmenopausal	0.6–1.0	1.3–4.0	1.8–3.8

(RI: resistance index; PI: pulsatility index; OVA: ovarian artery; UTA: uterine artery)

diastolic flow may be seen by the early luteal phase. In contrast, both diastolic flow and cyclical changes may be absent in the nondominant ovary.

Doppler ultrasound can demonstrate neovascularity within the wall of the corpus luteum. Demonstrable color flow surrounding the developing dominant follicle becomes more apparent as the midcycle approaches and continues around the corpus luteum until the late luteal phase. In the event of pregnancy, both the low resistance flow and the color flow to the corpus luteum may remain until the 11th week of amenorrhea.[45]

The normal values are given in **Table 4**.

CONCLUSION

Rapid advancements have been made in the radiologic evaluation of patients with gynecological disorders. Ultrasound forms the first line imaging modality. CT and MRI techniques have become essential tools for problem solving and in guiding presurgical treatment planning. Imaging techniques providing insights into the molecular processes in the tumor environment are gaining importance and their use is likely to expand in future.

REFERENCES

1. Langer JE, Oliver ER, Lev-Toaff AS, et al. Imaging of the female pelvis throughout the life cycle. Radiographics. 2012;32:636-9.
2. Lingley JR. The significance of psammoma body calcification in the roentgen diagnosis of papillary tumors of the ovary. Am J Roentgenol. 1942;47:563-70.
3. Sutton D. Textbook of Radiology and Imaging. 7th edition, Volume 2. Churchill Livingstone; 2003. pp. 1069-107.
4. Simpson WL Jr, Beitia LG, Mester J. Hysterosalpingography: a reemerging study. Radiographics. 2006;26(2):419-31.
5. Panchal S, Nagori C. Imaging techniques for assessment of tubal status. J Hum Reprod Sci 2014;7:2-12.
6. Kurjak A, Kupesic-Urek S, Schulman H, et al. Transvaginal color Doppler in the assessment of ovarian and uterine blood flow in infertile women. Fertil Steril. 1991;56:870-3.
7. Guerriero S, Ajossa S, Risalvato A, et al. Diagnosis of adnexal malignancies by using color Doppler energy imaging as a secondary test in persistent masses. Ultrasound Obstet Gynecol. 1998;11:277-82.
8. Sibal M. Gel sonovaginography: a new way of evaluating a variety of local vaginal and cervical disorders. J Ultrasound Med. 2016;35(12):2699-715.
9. Pretorirus DH, Borok NN, Coffler MS, et al. Three dimensional sonography in obstetrics and gynaecology, RCNA. 2001;39(3):499-521.
10. Richman TS, Viscomi GN, deCherney A, et al. Fallopian tube patency as assessed by ultrasonogram following fluid injection. Radiology. 1984;152:507-10.
11. Lindheim SR, Sprague C, Winter TC 3rd. Hysterosalpingography and sonohysterography: lessons in technique. AJR Am J Roentgenol. 2006;186(1):24-9.
12. Deichert U, Schlief R, van de Sandt M, et al. Transvaginal hysterosalpino-contrast-sonography (Hy-Co-Sy) compared with conventional tubal diagnostics. Hum Reprod. 1989;4:418-24.
13. Zhou L, Zhang X, Chen X, et al. Value of three-dimensional hysterosalpingocontrast sonography with SonoVue in the assessment of tubal patency. Ultrasound Obstet Gynecol. 2012;40:93-9.
14. Wang Y, Qian L. Three- or four-dimensional hysterosalpingocontrast sonography for diagnosing tubal patency in infertile females: A systematic review with meta-analysis. Br J Radiol. 2016;89:20151013.
15. Henrich W, Fuchs I, Schmider A. Transvaginal and transabdominal extended field of view (EFOV) and power Doppler EFOV sonography in gynecology: advantages and applications. J Ultrasound Med. 2002;21:1137-44.
16. Ophir J, Céspedes I, Ponnekanti H, et al. Elastography: A quantitative method for imaging the elasticity of biological tissues. Ultrason Imaging. 1991;13(2):111-34.
17. Stoelinga B, Hehenkamp WJK, Nieuwenhuis LL, et al. Accuracy and reproducibility of sonoelastography for the assessment of fibroids and adenomyosis, with magnetic resonance imaging as reference standard. Ultrasound Med Biol. 2018;44:1654-63.
18. Frank ML, Schafer SD, Mollers M, et al. Importance of transvaginal elastography in the diagnosis of uterine fibroids and adenomyosis. Ultraschall Med. 2016;37:373-8.
19. Thomas A, Kümmel S, Gemeinhardt O, et al. Real-time sonoelastography of the cervix: tissue elasticity of the normal and abnormal cervix. Acad Radiol. 2007;14:193-200.
20. Burns PN. Microbubble Contrast for Ultrasound Imaging: Where, How and Why in Rumack CM, Wilson SR, Charboneau JW (Eds). Diagnostic ultrasound, 3rd edition. Maryland Heights: Elseiver Mosby; 2001. pp. 55-76.
21. Stoelinga B, Dooper AMC, Juffermans LJM, et al. Use of contrast-enhanced ultrasound in the assessment of uterine fibroids: a feasibility study. Ultrasound in Medicine and Biology. 2018;44(8):1901-9.
22. Haaga JR, Boll DT. CT and MRI of the Whole Body. 6th edition. Philadelphia, PA: Elsevier, 2017.
23. Thomassin-Naggara I, Balvay D, Rockall A, et al. Added value of assessing adnexal masses with advanced MRI techniques. Biomed Res Int. 2015;2015:785206.
24. Liu B, Gao S, Li S. A comprehensive comparison of CT, MRI, positron emission tomography or positron emission tomography/CT, and diffusion weighted imaging-MRI for detecting the lymph nodes metastases in patients with cervical cancer: a meta-analysis based on 67 studies. Gynecol Obstet Invest. 2017;82:209Y222.

25. Manoharan D, Das CJ, Aggarwal A, et al. Diffusion weighted imaging in gynecological malignancies—present and future. World J Radiol. 2016;8:288-97.
26. Makino H, Kato H, Furui T, et al. Predictive value of diffusion-weighted magnetic resonance imaging during chemoradiotherapy for uterine cervical cancer. J Obstet Gynaecol Res. 2014;40:1098-104.
27. Fujii S, Matsusue E, Kanasaki Y, et al. Detection of peritoneal dissemination in gynecological malignancy: evaluation by diffusion- weighted MR imaging. Eur Radiol. 2008;18:18-23.
28. Hallac RR, Ding Y, Yuan Q, et al. Oxygenation in cervical cancer and normal uterine cervix assessed using blood oxygenation level-dependent (BOLD) MRI at 3T. NMR Biomed. 2012;25:1321-30.
29. Zijta FM, Lakeman MME, Froeling M, et al. Evaluation of the female pelvic floor in pelvic organ prolapse using 3.0-Tesla diffusion tensor imaging and fibre tractography. Eur Radiol. 2012;22:2806-13.
30. Colaiacomo MC, Masselli G, Polettini E, et al. Dynamic MR imaging of the pelvic floor: a pictorial review. Radiographics. 2009;29:e35.
31. Narayanan P, Iyngkaran T, Sohaib SA, et al. Pearls and pitfalls of MR lymphography in gynecologic malignancy. Radiographics. 2009;29:1057-69.
32. Ma FH, Qiang JW, Cai SQ, et al. MR spectroscopy for differentiating benign from malignant solid adnexal tumors. Am J Roentgenol. 2015;204;W724-30.
33. Iyer VR, Lee SI. MRI, CT, and PET/CT for ovarian cancer detection and adnexal lesion characterization. Am J Roentgenol. 2010;194(2):311-21.
34. Rockall AG, Cross S, Flanagan S, et al. The role of FDG-PET/CT in gynaecological cancers. Cancer Imaging. 2012;12:49-65.
35. Ohliger MA, Hope TA, Chapman JS, et al. PET/MR imaging in gynecologic oncology. Magn Reson Imaging Clin N Am. 2017;25(3):667-84.
36. Siegel MJ. Pediatric gynaecologic sonography. Radiology. 1991;170:593-600.
37. Salem S, Wilson SR. Gynaecologic ultrasound. In: Rumack CM, Wilson SR, Charboneau JW (Eds). Diagnostic Ultrasound, 3rd edition. Maryland Heights: Elsevier Mosby; 2001. pp. 527-87.
38. Coleman BG, Arger PH, Grumbach K, et al. Transvaginal and transabdominal sonography: prospective comparison. Radiology. 1988;168:639-43.
39. Burks DD, Stainken BF, Burkhard TK, et al. Uterine inner myometrial echogenic foci: relationship to prior dilatation and curettage and endocervical biopsy. J Ultrasound Med. 1991;10:487-92.
40. Aubel S, Wozney P, Edward RP. MRI of female uterine and juxta-uterine masses: clinical application in 25 patients. Magn Reson Imaging. 1991;9:485-91.
41. Schoenfield A, Levavi H, Hirsch M, et al. Transvaginal sonography in postmenopausal women. J Clin Ultrasound. 1990;18:350-58.
42. Forrest TS, Elyaderani MK, Muilenburg MI, et al. Cyclic endometrial changes: US assessment with histologic correlation. Radiology. 1988;167:233-7.
43. Laing FC, Brown DL, DiSalvo DN, et al. Gynecologic ultrasound. RCNA. 2001;39(3):523-40.
44. Wolf SI, Gosink BB, Feldesman MR, et al. Prevalence of simple adnexal cysts in postmenopausal women. Radiology. 1991;180:65-71.
45. Applebaum M. in The menstrual cycle, menopause, ovulation induction, and in vitro fertilization. In: Copel JA, Reed KL (Eds). Doppler Ultrasound in Obstetrics and Gynecology. New York: Raven Press; 1994.pp. 71-86.
46. Dubbins PA. The female pelvis. In: Allan PL, Dubbins PA, Pozniak MA, et al. (Eds). Clinical Doppler Ultrasound. London: Churchill Livingstone; 2000. pp. 237-58.

Chapter 14

Benign Adnexal Disease

Anju Garg, Alpana Manchanda, Radhika Batra

INTRODUCTION

The adnexa is the region adjacent to the uterus that includes the ovary, fallopian tube, and associated structures. Pathology in this region can arise from the ovary, the fallopian tube, from adjacent organs like the uterus and less commonly from other nongynecological structures like bowel, connective tissues, etc. Benign adnexal lesions are far more common than malignant lesions and thus an accurate characterization of adnexal disease is essential for management. Imaging is an essential part of the diagnostic workup to establish the presence, identify the organ of origin, and characterize the nature of lesions in the adnexal region. This chapter deals with imaging of adnexal disease from gynecological causes.

OVARIAN DISEASE

As most of the pathological conditions of the ovary present in the form of masses, the first step after detection of a mass lesion in the adnexal region is to identify if it arises from the ovary. This can be achieved by identifying both the ovaries, seeing whether they look normal and then looking at their relation to the pathological findings. A mass arising from the ovary will deform the ovary and alter its normal shape. A positive "*beak sign*" can be identified when a mass deforms the edge of the ovary into a "beak" shape, suggesting that the mass arises from it; while an adjacent ovary with dull edges suggests that the mass compresses it but does not arise from the ovary **(Fig. 1)**. The "crescent sign" or "embedded organ sign" shows the ovarian tissue splayed around a mass which arises from the ovary. Another sign which can be used to identify a mass as of ovarian origin is to trace the ovarian vessels, especially the ovarian vein. The ovarian vein is easily identified as it lies anterior to the psoas muscle and can be followed up to the pelvic mass—the *"vascular pedicle sign"*. In a study by Lee et al., this CT finding was found to indicate that a mass was of ovarian origin, with a 91% diagnostic accuracy, 97% positive predictive value, and 69% negative predictive value.[1] The direction of displacement of other pelvic structures by the mass can also give a clue to the origin of the mass. The ureter is often displaced posteriorly or posterolaterally by an ovarian mass, whereas the iliac vessels are pushed laterally.

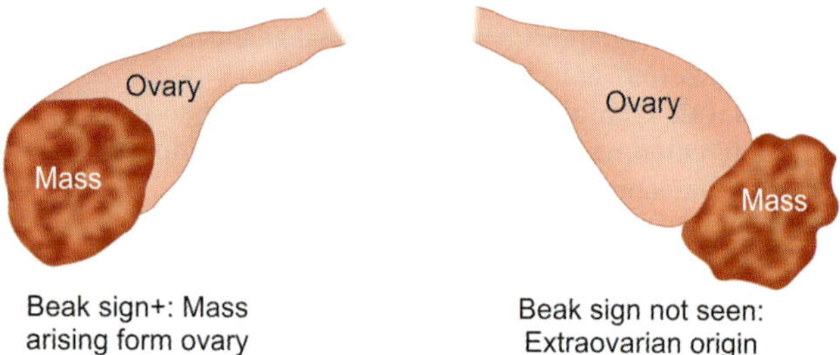

Fig. 1: Ovarian versus extraovarian origin—look at the ovary-mass interface.

FUNCTIONAL CYSTS OF THE OVARY

Functional cysts comprise the most common benign cystic lesions of the ovary. They are formed when Graafian follicles or corpora lutea grow too large or bleed internally. They can be of three types—follicular cysts, corpus luteum cysts, and hemorrhagic cysts. Majority of these cysts are seen during the premenopausal reproductive age, however, sporadic ovulatory cycles may still occur in the postmenopausal women with occasional formation of functional cysts. Even in late menopause, 20% of women may have small simple cysts. In a study by Modesitt et al., in 3529 simple ovarian cysts of less than 10 cm, no cancers were detected in postmenopausal women. The authors estimated the risk of malignancy in simple cysts as less than 0.1%.[2]

Follicular Cyst

A follicular cyst occurs when a dominant Graafian follicle does not ovulate or fails to involute. When it becomes larger than 3 cm, it is called a follicular cyst. Most follicle cysts lose the ability to produce estrogen, however, sometimes the granulosa cells remain productive, with prolonged secretion of estrogen.

Clinical Features

Most cysts are asymptomatic and discovered incidentally. However, some patients may develop pain because of rapid enlargement of the cyst, rupture, or hemorrhage.

Imaging Features

On ultrasound (US), follicular cysts are seen as unilateral, unilocular, anechoic cysts with thin (<3 mm), smooth walls, often measuring between 3 cm and 8 cm in size. Occasionally, they may become larger.[3] A compressed rim of ovarian tissue can often be visualized around the periphery of the cyst **(Figs. 2A and B)**. They generally do not show any septations or solid components. On CT, they appear as well-defined round simple fluid collections with thin nonenhancing walls, with an attenuation generally less than 15 HU.[4] On magnetic resonance imaging (MRI), these cysts are typically homogeneously hypointense on T1-weighted image (T1WI), very high signal intensity (SI) on T2W images. Follicular cysts usually resolve spontaneously after 1–2 menstrual cycles. A follow-up US should be done on days 5–10 of a subsequent menstrual cycle to look for resolution.

Differential Diagnosis

The differential diagnosis of follicular cysts include nonfunctional cysts and cystic neoplasms like benign teratoma and simple benign epithelial neoplasms which are seen in an older age group, are larger and persistent, atypical endometrioma, and hydrosalpinx. Nonfunctional cysts include surface epithelial inclusion cysts, rete cysts, and paraovarian or paratubal cysts. Paraovarian cysts are indistinguishable from functional cysts by imaging criteria except by location. A diagnosis of paraovarian cyst can be made when the ipsilateral ovary is seen close to but separate from the cyst.

Corpus Luteum Cyst

Corpus luteum cysts form when a corpus luteum fails to regress following the release of an ovum, filling up with fluid or blood. They occur in the postovulatory phase of the menstrual cycle and grow under the influence of the luteinizing hormone. They are usually less than 2 cm in size and resolve within 1–2 menstrual cycles. Corpus luteum cysts can also occur in pregnancy, which grow under the influence of beta-human chorionic gonadotropin (β-hCG), are much larger (3–4 cm, can reach up to 15 cm), usually resolve by 12–16 weeks but may fail to involute and persist after the first trimester.

Clinical Features

These cysts are also most commonly seen in the reproductive age group. Women on birth control pills

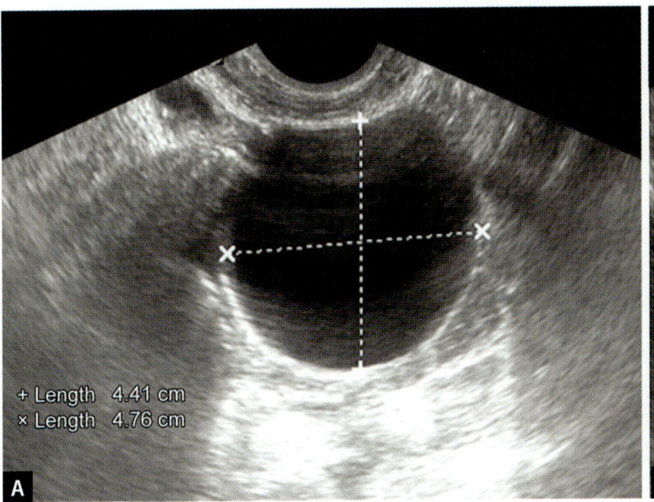

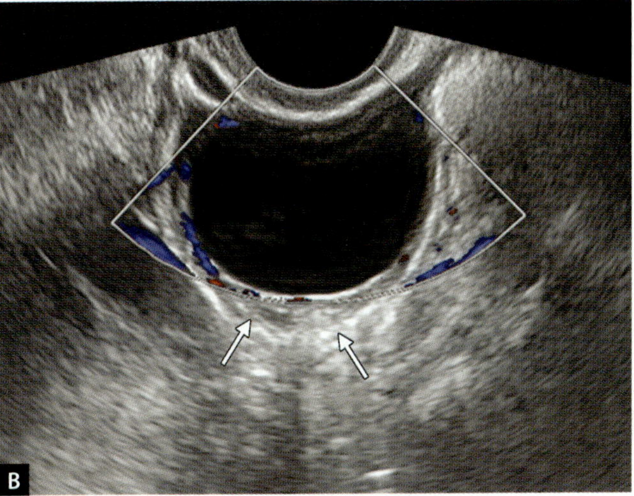

Figs. 2A and B: Simple follicular cyst. (A) Transvaginal scan shows a unilocular, rounded, thin-walled, anechoic cyst in the right ovary; (B) Color Doppler shows mild perifollicular color flow. Compressed ovarian rim—"crescent sign" (arrows) seen in posterior aspect of the cyst.

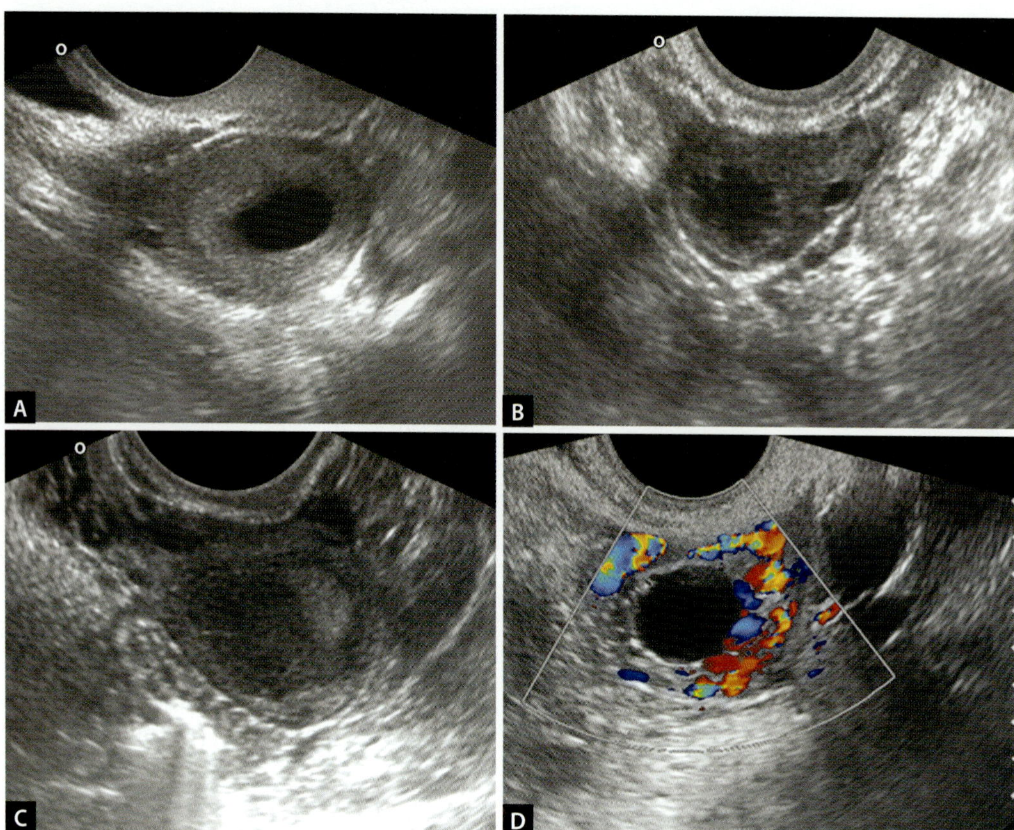

Figs. 3A to D: Varied appearances of corpus luteum cysts. (A) Transvaginal scan shows an anechoic corpus luteum cyst with thick echogenic walls. Ovarian tissue with follicles seen surrounding the cyst; (B) Transvaginal scan in another case shows the crenulated margins in a corpus luteum cyst with low level internal echoes; (C) Large corpus luteal cyst with differential internal echoes; (D) Peripheral vascularity seen around the corpus luteum cyst.

usually do not form a corpus luteum, as birth control pills prevent ovulation, and so will not have corpus luteum cysts; whereas women who are on ovulation stimulating drugs, like clomifene, have an increased incidence of corpus luteum cysts. They constitute the most common pelvic mass encountered within the first trimester of pregnancy and large cysts may present with pain.

Imaging Features

On US, they are seen as small, <3 cm sized cysts with thick, crenated margins, internal echoes, and good through transmission **(Figs. 3A to C)**. The contents are usually hyperechoic and represent some bleeding into the follicle that has ovulated. A higher fat content of the cyst wall is a likely cause for the hyperechogenic wall of the corpus luteal cyst.[3] Doppler shows peripheral vascularity—the characteristic "ring of fire" sign **(Fig. 3D)**. They need to be differentiated from a tubal ring in an ectopic pregnancy in some situations, and correct clinical interpretation is required. CT will show an irregular, low-attenuating cyst (<25 HU), with enhancing walls.[4] On MRI, these cysts are typically homogeneously hypointense on T1WI, very high SI on T2W images, and show intense wall enhancement on postcontrast scans **(Fig. 4)**. A small amount of free fluid is often seen to be associated with these cysts.

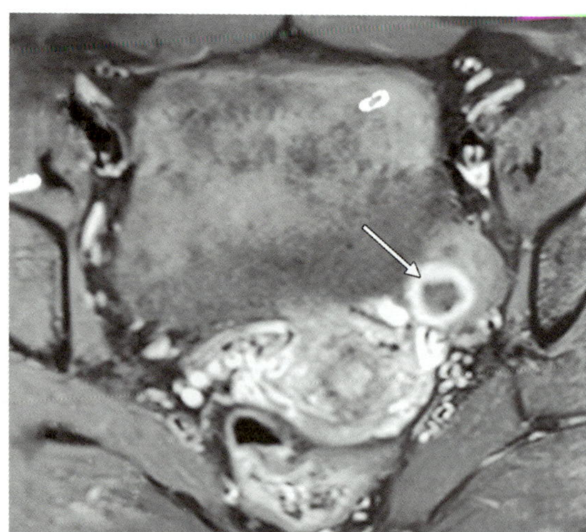

Fig. 4: Contrast-enhanced axial T1-weighted fat-suppressed MR image shows a corpus luteum cyst in the left ovary with an intensely enhancing ring (arrow).

Complications

Functional cysts may bleed leading to the formation of a hemorrhagic cyst, may rupture or cause the ovary to undergo torsion.

Hemorrhagic Ovarian Cysts

Hemorrhagic ovarian cysts (HOCs) occur due to hemorrhage into a follicle or a corpus luteum cyst. As the Graafian follicle matures, the granulosa cell layer becomes very vascular. These vessels are very fragile and rupture easily, causing bleeding into the cyst, giving rise to a hemorrhagic cyst.

Clinical Features

Patients present with sudden-onset pelvic pain, pelvic mass, or they may be asymptomatic.[5] A hemorrhagic or a ruptured ovarian cyst is the most common cause of acute pelvic pain in an afebrile, premenopausal woman presenting to the emergency room.

Imaging Features

The imaging features vary depending on the time of the radiologic evaluation, as the hemorrhagic cysts evolve through various stages of acute hemorrhage, clot formation, and clot retraction. The HOC is seen as a thin-walled cyst with an average diameter of 3.0–3.5 cm (range 2.5–8.5 cm). In the early stages, the HOC may show diffuse, low level, internal echoes (ground-glass pattern). The echogenicity decreases with time as the red cells undergo hemolysis. A whirled, spongy pattern of mixed echogenicity can be seen. A fine reticular pattern also known variously as the "fishnet", "cobweb", "spider web" or "lacy" pattern occurs due to the fibrin strands **(Fig. 5A)**. Retracting blood clot can be seen as solid appearing, nonvascular mass within the cyst **(Fig. 5B)**. This mass may be seen to jiggle when probe pressure is applied on transvaginal scan (TVS). Sometimes a fluid-debris level may be seen within the cyst **(Fig. 5C)**. Doppler sonography helps in establishing the diagnosis as no vascularity is seen in the septae or solid nodule. On CT, HOCs are seen as unilocular cysts with a high internal attenuation of about 25–100 HU.[6] On MRI, HOCs have a characteristic appearance of blood products and the SI will vary depending on age of bleed. They are seen as intermediate or relatively high SI on T1W and intermediate to high SI on T2W images. Layering may be seen on T2W images and only mild heterogeneous signal loss will be seen as compared to T1WI, not the characteristic T2 shading of endometriomas **(Figs. 6A to E)**. On diffusion-weighted imaging (DWI), hemorrhagic cysts may display restricted diffusion because of their blood content. HOCs can be seen to resolve spontaneously in 6–8 weeks, with follow-up US showing either complete resolution or a marked decrease in size and change in morphologic appearance **(Figs. 7A to C)**.

A hemorrhagic cyst may rupture, leading to hemoperitoneum. Patients present with acute pelvic pain. On US, the HOC can often be seen in the adnexal region along with hemoperitoneum **(Figs. 8A to E)** seen as peritoneal fluid with low-level echoes in the pouch of Douglas, Morison's pouch, or in the left upper quadrant. A close differential diagnosis is ruptured ectopic pregnancy as the clinical presentation and US imaging may be similar. A clinical history (cyst rupture occurs more often in the luteal phase, whereas ectopic pregnancy is associated with a history of delayed menstrual periods) and β-HCG levels help in differentiation.

Differential Diagnosis

The most important differential diagnosis of a hemorrhagic cyst is an endometrioma, especially in the early stage. The differentiating features are discussed later in the chapter.

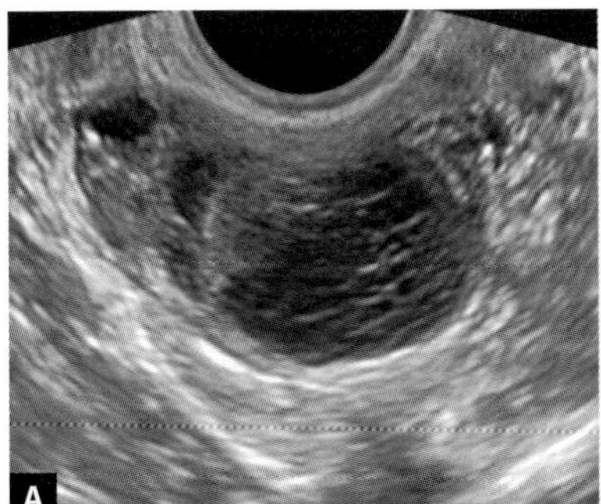

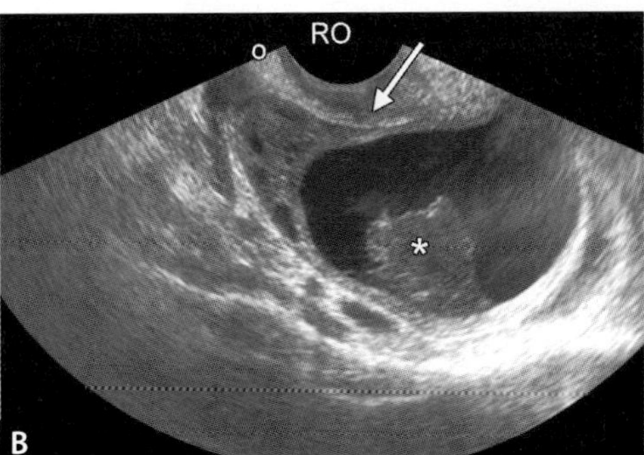

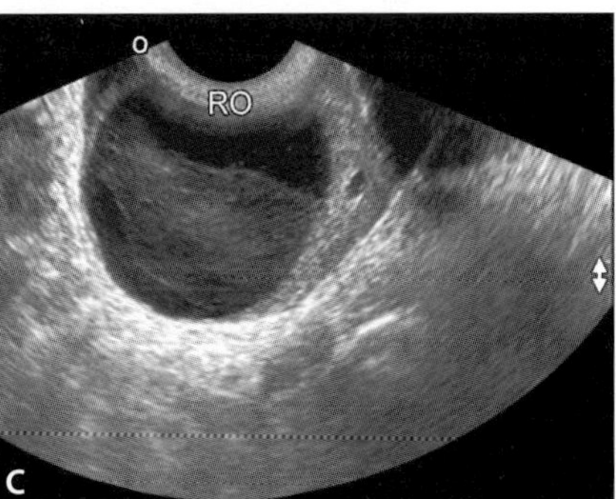

Figs. 5A to C: Spectrum of hemorrhagic cysts on transvaginal scan. (A) Fine reticular strands seen within the cyst—"fish net" appearance; (B) Echogenic, solid-appearing, retracted clot along dependant margin (*), did not show any vascularity on Doppler. "Beak sign" of ovarian parenchyma well seen (arrow); (C) Blood-fluid level seen in a right ovarian hemorrhagic cyst.

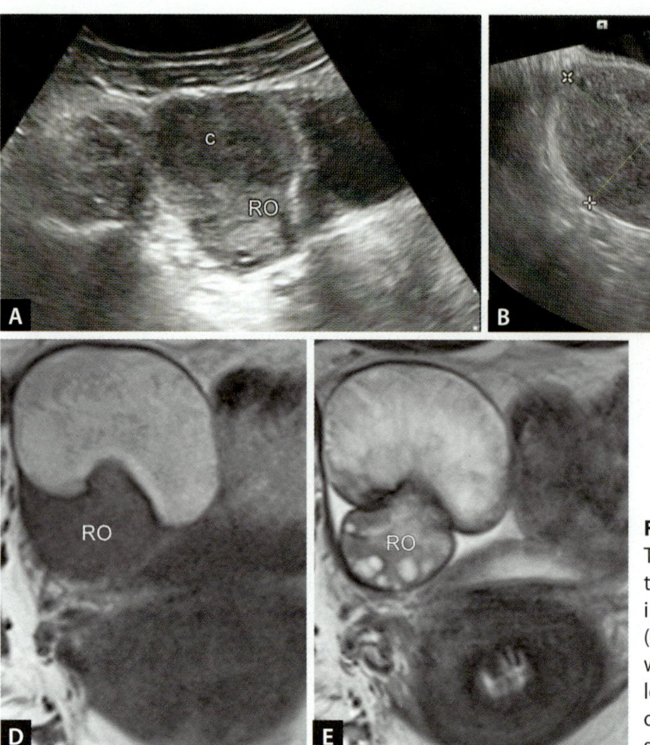

Figs. 6A to E: Hemorrhagic cyst in a 20-year-old female. (A) Transabdominal scan shows a hypoechoic mass lesion (c) in close relation to the right ovary (RO); (B) It appears as a well-defined, homogeneous, intermediate echogenicity, solid-looking mass on transvaginal scan; (C) However, there is no internal vascularity on Doppler; (D) Axial T1-weighted and (E) T2-weighted magnetic resonance images show the lesion arising exophytically from the right ovary appearing hyperintense on T1-weighted and iso- to-hyperintense on T2-weighted images (not showing T2 shading). Small amount of adjacent free fluid is seen.

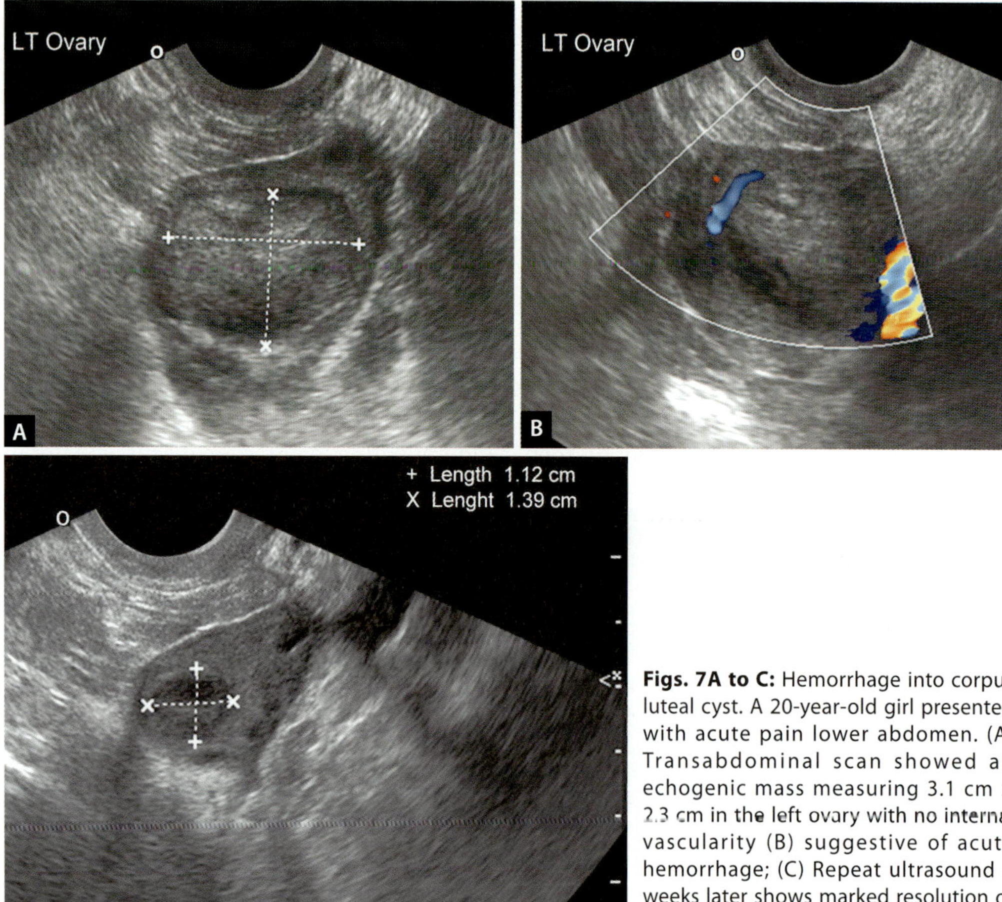

Figs. 7A to C: Hemorrhage into corpus luteal cyst. A 20-year-old girl presented with acute pain lower abdomen. (A) Transabdominal scan showed an echogenic mass measuring 3.1 cm × 2.3 cm in the left ovary with no internal vascularity (B) suggestive of acute hemorrhage; (C) Repeat ultrasound 4 weeks later shows marked resolution of the hemorrhagic corpus luteum cyst.

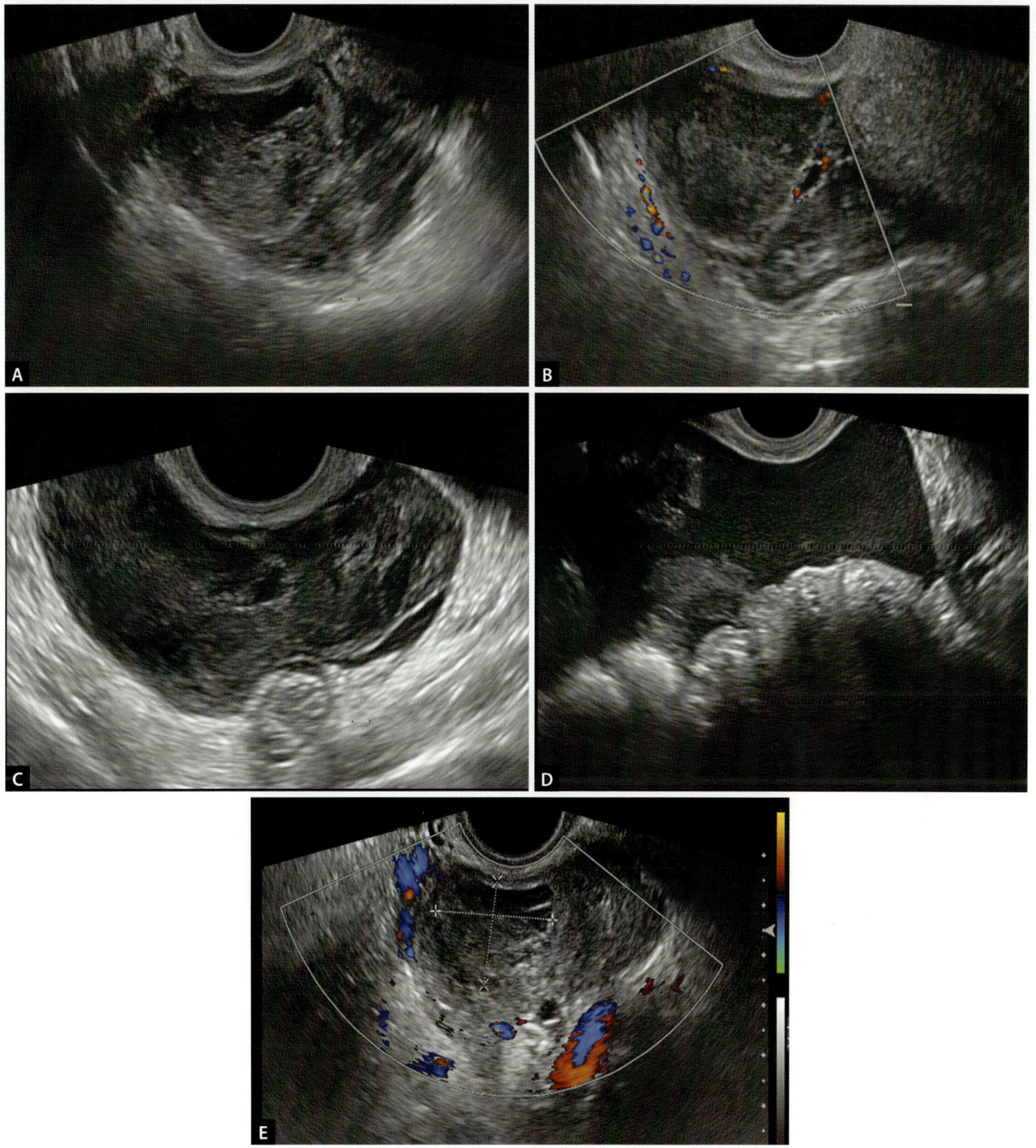

Figs. 8A to E: Hemorrhagic cyst in a 29-year-old female with rheumatic heart disease with mitral valve replacement and on anticoagulants. Patient presented with complaints of abdominal pain and distension since 8 days. She was premenstrual and pregnancy test was negative. Transvaginal ultrasonography (USG) reveals a well-defined heterogeneously hypoechoic lesion with hyperechoic contents within, in the right ovary (A) showing no significant vascularity on addition of color Doppler (B). Associated pelvic hematoma (showing similar characteristics as that of hemorrhagic cyst) was also noted adjacent to the right ovary (C). Additionally, there was moderate fluid in pelvis with internal echoes within—hemoperitoneum (D). In view of above findings, a diagnosis of ruptured hemorrhagic corpus luteal cyst was suggested and patient was managed conservatively. (E) On subsequent follow-up with USG after 6 weeks, there is reduction in size of hemorrhagic cyst within the right ovary (RO) and hematoma (H) with complete resolution of hemoperitoneum. Also, note the change in morphology of hemorrhagic cyst due to evolution of the blood products within the cyst.

They may also need to be differentiated from a tubo-ovarian abscess (TOA), ectopic pregnancy, and even a malignant neoplasm when a retracted solid-appearing clot resembles a malignant mural nodule. A detailed clinical history and follow-up scans which show a changing appearance, can help in clinching the diagnosis.

Follow-up Guidelines for Functional Ovarian Cysts

The most widely used guidelines for management of functional ovarian cysts imaged sonographically in asymptomatic women, are the consensus statement by the Society of Radiologists in Ultrasound 2010.[7] For simple ovarian cysts with no suspicious features on US, current follow-up guidelines are based on menopausal status, presence of any risk factors and the cyst size **(Flowchart 1)**. HOCs have a different follow-up schedule than simple cysts **(Flowchart 2)**. Patients who are symptomatic need to be managed accordingly.

Polycystic ovary syndrome (PCOS) and hyperstimulated ovarian disease have been dealt with elsewhere in this book.

ENDOMETRIOMA

Endometriomas are blood containing cysts within the ovaries formed due to endometriosis. Endometriosis is defined as presence of functional endometrial tissue (consisting of glands and stroma) outside the uterus. The common sites of involvement include ovaries (most common), uterosacral ligaments, serosal surfaces, pouch of Douglas, fallopian tubes, rectosigmoid, and urinary bladder. It is a leading cause of chronic pelvic pain and infertility in reproductive age group.

Pathophysiology

The exact etiology and pathogenesis of endometriosis is unclear and remains controversial. Three theories of pathogenesis have been proposed: (1) the *metastatic theory*, i.e. metastatic implantation of endometrial tissue from retrograde menstruation, (2) the *metaplastic theory* which is related to metaplastic differentiation of the serosal surfaces (coelomic epithelium) and remnants of Müllerian tissue, and (3) the *induction theory* which combines the first two proposed mechanisms and suggests

Flowchart 1: Algorithmic approach for reporting, follow-up, and management of asymptomatic ovarian cysts (Society of Radiologists in Ultrasound, 2010).[7]

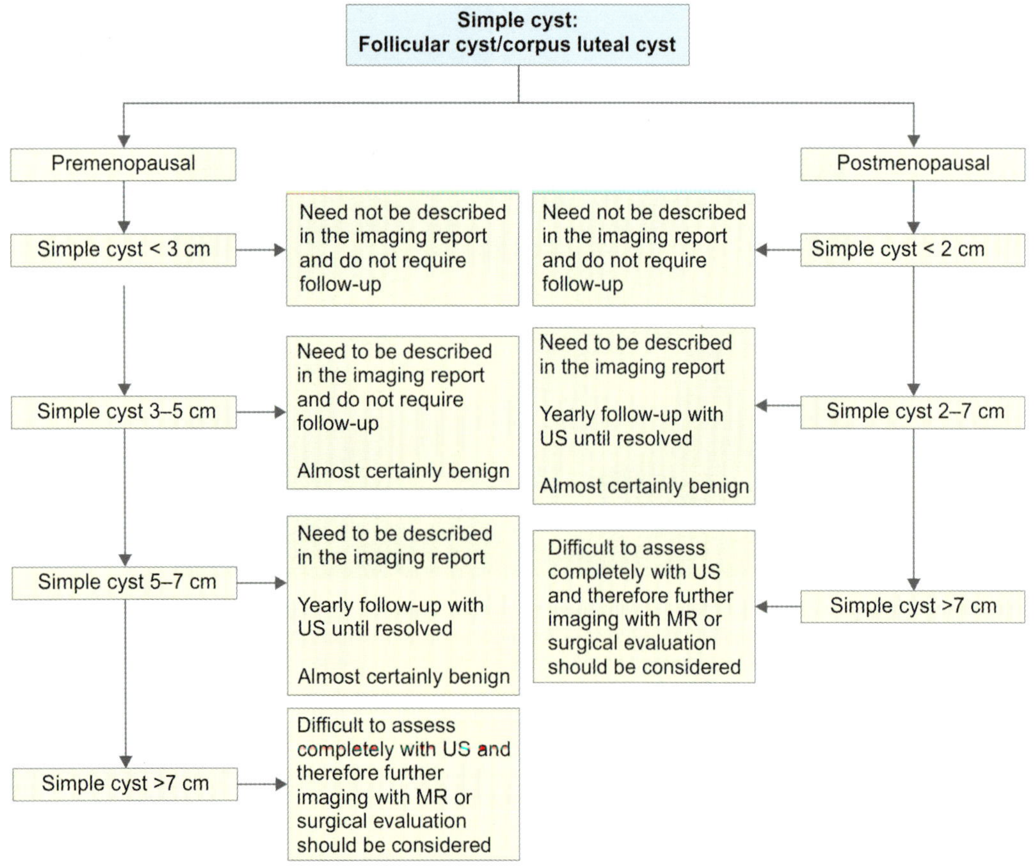

Flowchart 2: Algorithmic approach for reporting, follow-up, and management of asymptomatic hemorrhagic cysts (Society of Radiologists in Ultrasound, 2010).[7]

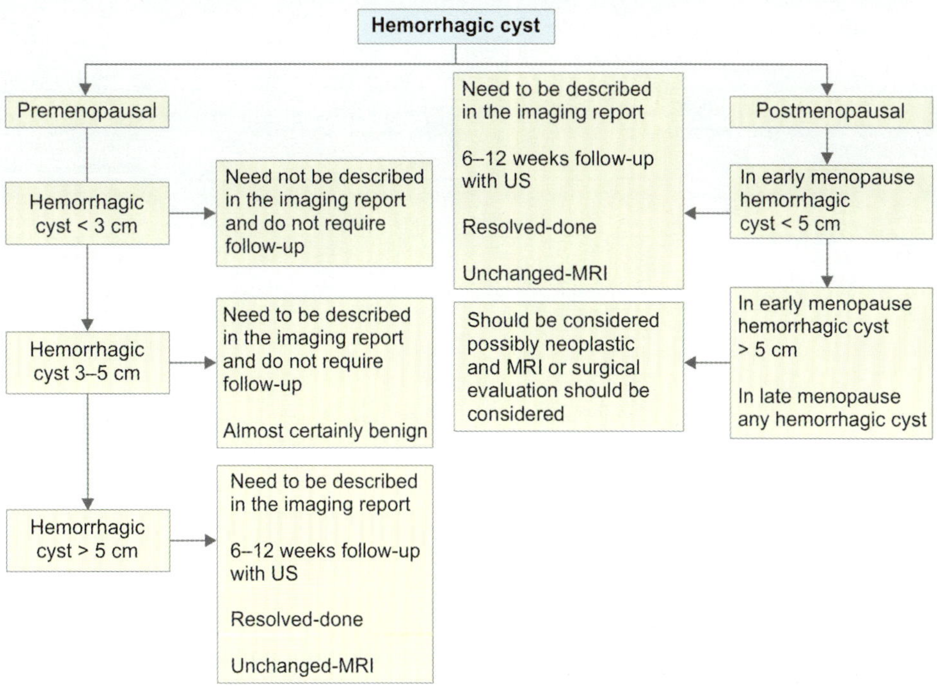

that shed endometrium releases substances that induce undifferentiated mesenchyme to form endometrium. Circulating estradiol and estrone, which stimulate ectopic and eutopic endometrial tissue have been linked in propagation of this condition.

Endometriosis may present in various forms which includes endometrial nodules or plaques on the peritoneal surface, endometriotic cysts in ovaries (endometriomas), and deep infiltrative endometriosis (DIE).

Endometriomas are formed when endometrial tissue deposited in the ovaries undergoes cyclical bleeding during menstruation. With time, such repeated episodes lead to accumulation of fluid and blood products within the involved ovary with compression and peripheral displacement of rest of ovarian tissue giving rise to formation of benign chronic retention cysts or endometriomas (also known as chocolate cysts). Besides being the most common presenting form of endometriosis, they are also a marker of severity of deep infiltrating endometriosis, with the risk for multifocal and intestinal involvement in patients with endometrioma being two to three times more than those without endometrioma.[8]

Clinical Features

Patients usually present with the complaints of dysmenorrhea, dyspareunia, and chronic pelvic pain. Endometriomas are also associated with decreased ovarian function and inhibition of ovulation thus leading to infertility. In addition they can interfere with assisted reproductive technologies which are often utilized in management of infertility. In association with deep pelvic endometriosis, patients can also present with symptoms of dyschezia and dysuria. CA-125 levels (normal levels being 0–35 units/mL) are also found to be raised in patients with endometriosis but they are highly nonspecific and hence are unable to aid in diagnosis.

Imaging Features

On USG, typical endometriomas appear as well-defined, rounded, unilocular cystic lesions with regular margins which characteristically exhibit homogeneous, low level internal echoes **(Figs. 9A and B)**, and occasional fluid-fluid levels within.[9] When endometriomas are bilateral, they may be found adherent to each other above or behind the uterus, being termed as "kissing ovaries" **(Fig. 10)**. The positive predictive value of sonography in diagnosis of surgical proven typical endometriomas has been estimated to be about 97%.[10]

Endometriomas usually do not exhibit any internal vascularity on color Doppler (even if present, it is usually peripheral). As such the role of Doppler in diagnosis of endometriotic cysts has been found to be limited. A study by Alcázar et al.[11] demonstrated that the use of color or pulsed Doppler sonography did not improve the diagnostic accuracy of diagnosis of endometriomas.

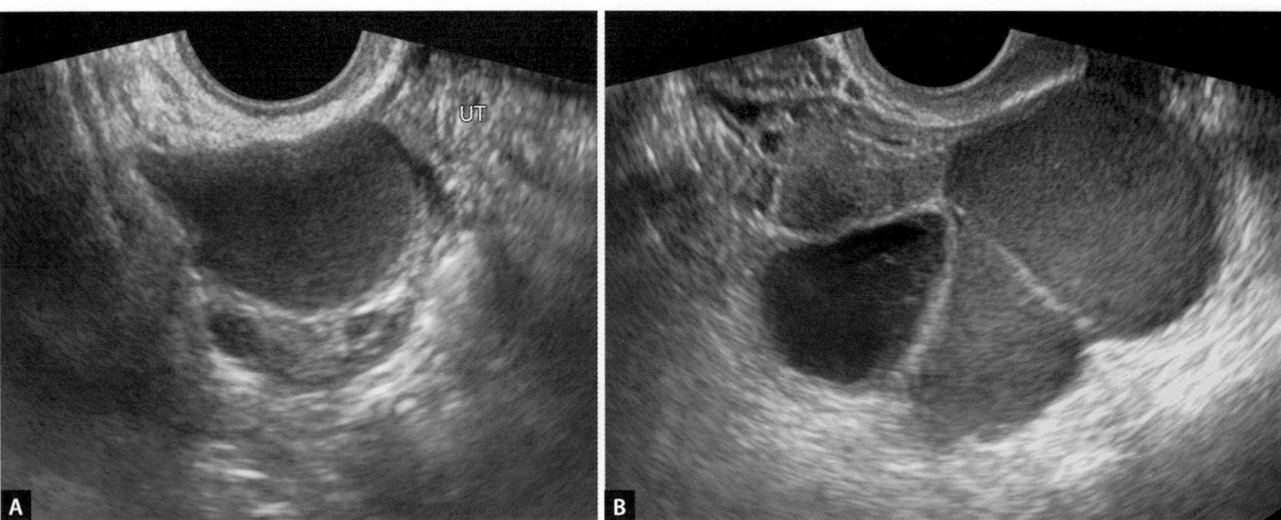

Figs. 9A and B: Endometriotic cysts in a 25-year-old woman with chronic pelvic pain. (A) Transvaginal scan showing the typical appearance of an endometrioma as a unilocular cyst with diffuse, low level internal echoes—"ground-glass" appearance, with a rim of normal right ovarian tissue, adherent to the uterus (UT); (B) Multiple endometriomas in the left ovary.

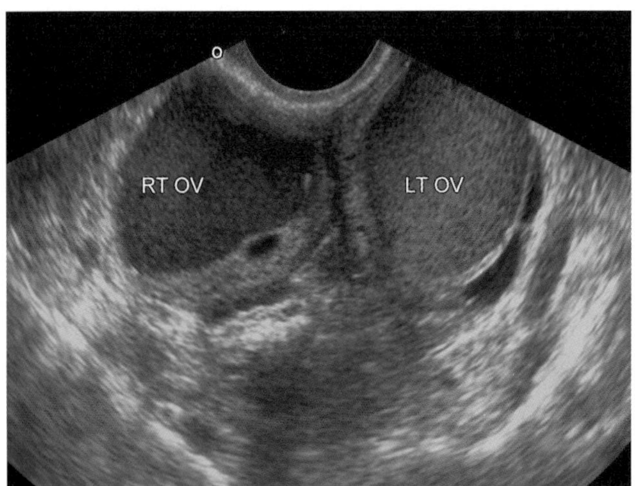

Fig. 10: Endometriomas in bilateral ovaries adherent to each other—"kissing ovaries" sign.

Atypical forms of endometriomas, on the other hand, can have a variety of characteristics attributed to other adnexal masses thus posing a challenge for diagnosis. They may have anechoic appearance and may show irregular margins. Thin or thick septae, giving a multilocular appearance **(Figs. 11A and B)** and echogenic peripheral foci (representing cholesterol deposits), may also be seen. Punctate calcifications, also seen as echogenic foci, have been described in walls of endometriomas **(Figs. 12A to C)**, they may show central calcifications which make the differentiation from teratomas difficult.

In addition, multiple solid components and papillary excrescences may be seen within thereby mimicking malignancy, however, these usually do not show vascularity on color Doppler **(Figs. 12A to C)**.

Magnetic resonance imaging is widely accepted as a highly specific imaging modality for diagnosing endometriomas due to the ability to detect aged blood. Endometriomas are characterized by blood and blood products of different ages, being particularly rich in methemoglobin. This extra- and intracellular concentration of methemoglobin results in marked T1 shortening with resultant high SI on T1W images **(Figs. 13A and B)**.[12] Additionally, this T1 shortening due to blood products persists even after addition of fat saturation and becomes much more conspicuous. Hence, use of fat-saturated T1 sequences has been recommended in imaging of endometriomas **(Fig. 13C)**. It has been found to increase the specificity and sensitivity in diagnosis especially increasing the detection rate of small endometriomas.[13]

On T2W images, endometriomas typically exhibit the characteristic "*shading sign*", being described as focal or diffuse reduction in SI due to old blood products having rich concentration of iron and proteins **(Fig. 13D)**. The wall of the endometriotic cyst is hypointense on both, T2W and T1W images, caused by hemosiderin deposition. Recently, "*T2 dark spot sign*" has been shown to be more specific than T2 shading in detecting endometriomas and differentiating them from hemorrhagic cysts.[14] These

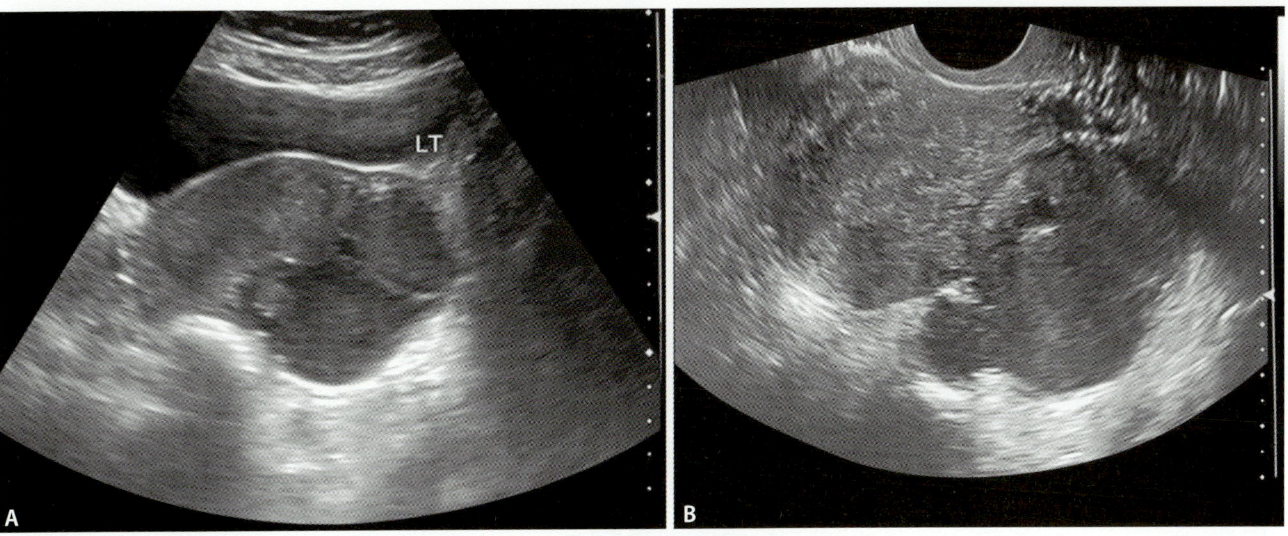

Figs. 11A and B: Multiloculated endometriotic cyst in a 36-year-old female. Transabdominal (A) and transvaginal (B) ultrasound images show presence of a multiloculated cystic lesion in left ovary with typical ground-glass texture.

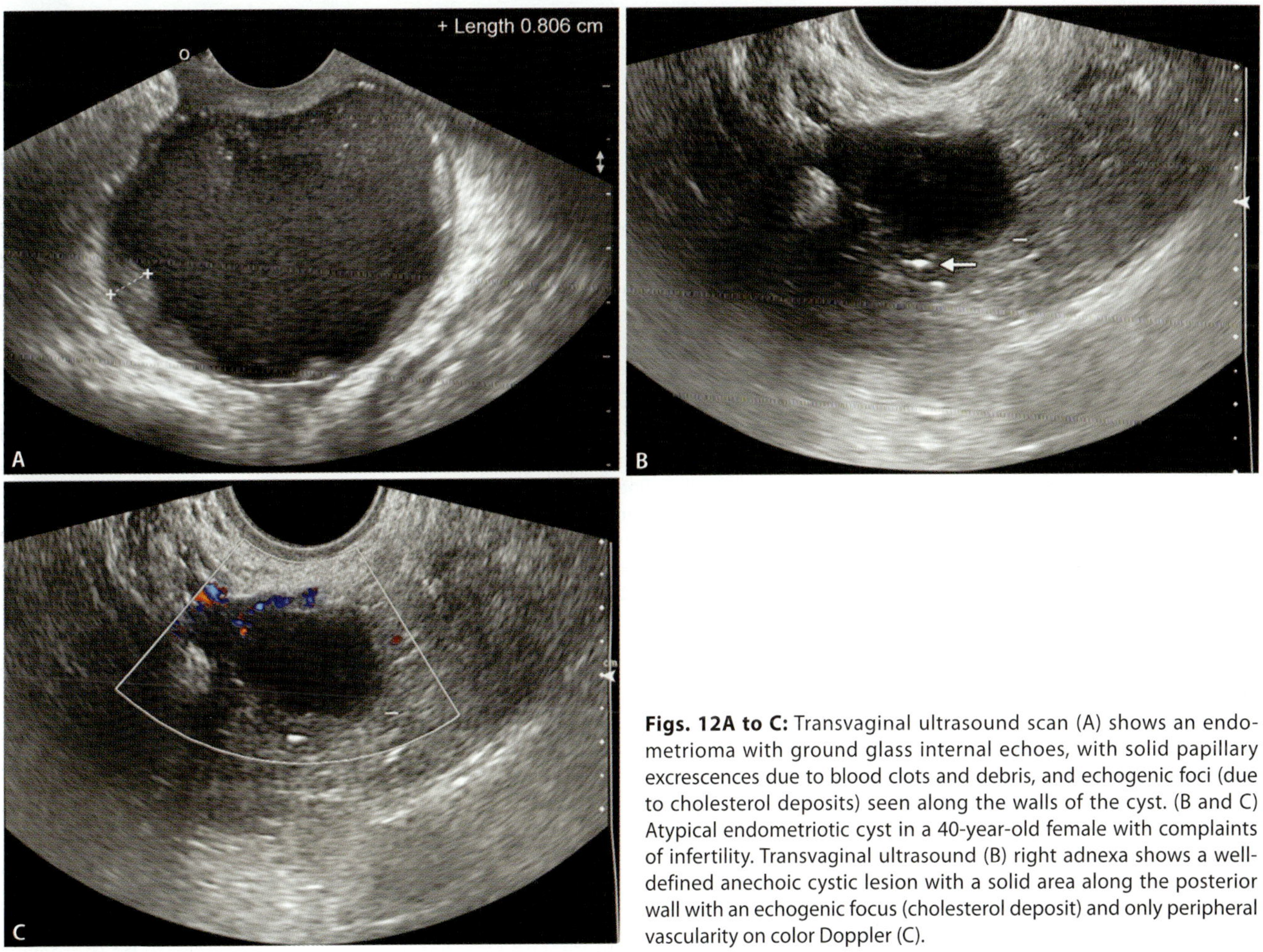

Figs. 12A to C: Transvaginal ultrasound scan (A) shows an endometrioma with ground glass internal echoes, with solid papillary excrescences due to blood clots and debris, and echogenic foci (due to cholesterol deposits) seen along the walls of the cyst. (B and C) Atypical endometriotic cyst in a 40-year-old female with complaints of infertility. Transvaginal ultrasound (B) right adnexa shows a well-defined anechoic cystic lesion with a solid area along the posterior wall with an echogenic focus (cholesterol deposit) and only peripheral vascularity on color Doppler (C).

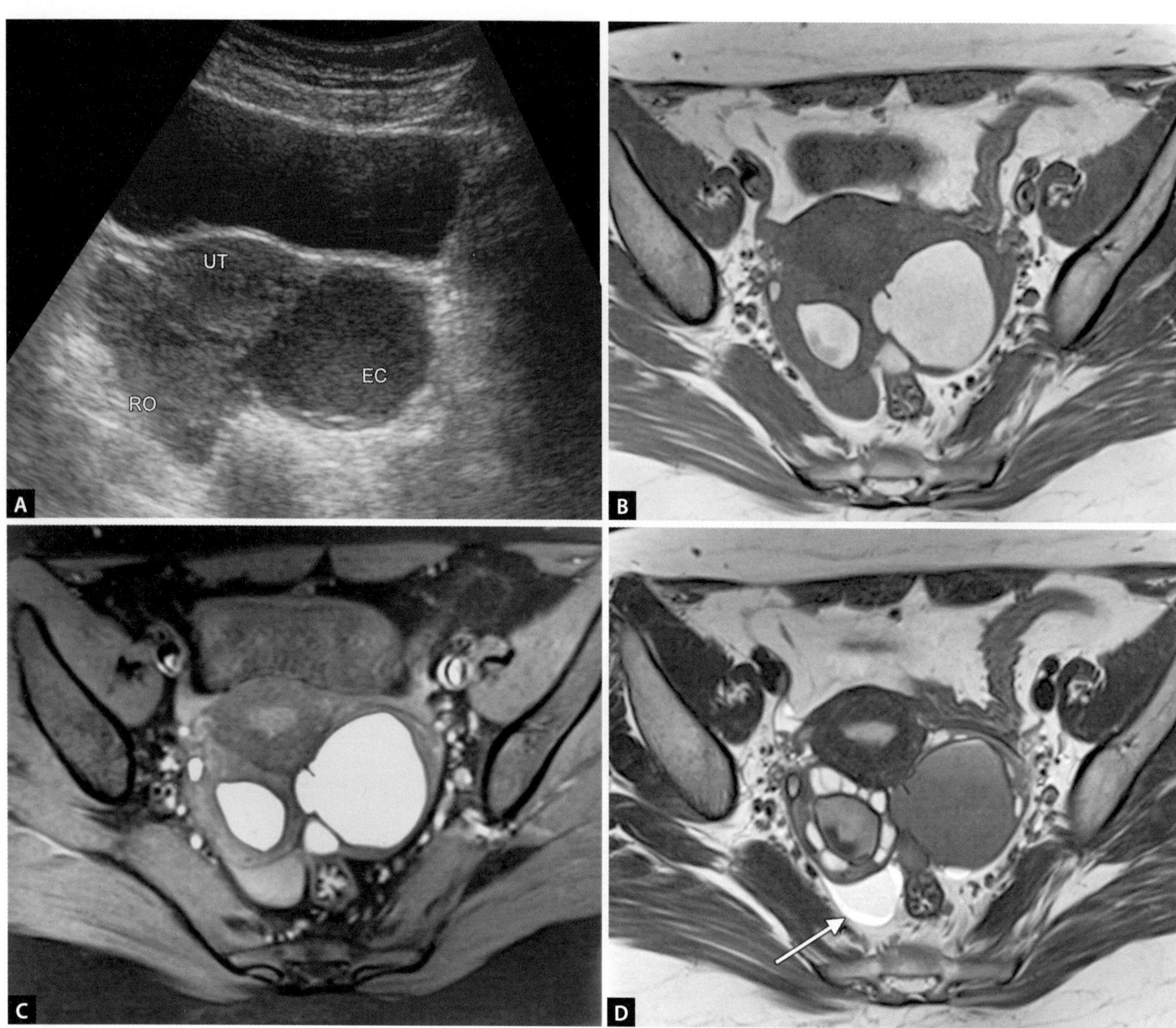

Figs. 13A to D: Endometriomas in a 20-year-old unmarried girl with complaints of long-standing chronic pelvic pain. (A) Transabdominal ultrasound scan shows an endometriotic cyst (EC) in the left ovary with an enlarged right ovary (RO). Both the ovaries are adherent to the uterus and to each other in the POD. Axial T1W (B) MR image shows well-defined hyperintense cystic lesions involving bilateral ovaries, which appear more hyperintense in the T1 fat-saturated image (C). They characteristically show signal drop on the axial T2W image—"shading sign" (D). In addition, both the lesions are situated in rectouterine pouch and closely abut each other in midline—"kissing ovaries". Multiple hyperintense follicles are seen in both the ovaries around the endometriomas on T2W image "embedded organ sign". The presence of loculated fluid collection is seen (arrow in D) around the right ovary appearing hyperintense on T2W image.

are discrete, well-defined, markedly hypointense foci seen on T2W images which can be located anywhere within the endometriotic cyst with the exception of wall of cyst **(Fig. 14)**. They are thought to occur due to long-standing accumulation of iron and protein within the lesions. Contrast-enhanced scans do not add any value to the noncontrast scans in the imaging of endometriomas **(*see* Fig. 12C)** Due to their thick proteinaceous and hemoglobin degradation products, endometriomas show a restricted diffusion pattern, exhibiting high SI on DWI at b = 1000 sec/mm^2 and low SI on apparent diffusion coefficient (ADC) maps **(Figs. 15A and B)**.[15,16]

Associations

Deep pelvic endometriosis, adenomyosis, and fibroids are found to be associated with endometriosis probably due to increased estrogen levels which are found to be increased in endometriosis.

Deep infiltrative endometriosis, which is defined as the presence of invasive endometriotic lesions that extend into the retroperitoneal space or involving the pelvic organ wall to a depth of at least 5 mm, often coexist with endometriotic cysts. These are commonly found in patients who have a long-term history of endometriosis (which may remain undiagnosed) and is responsible for symptoms like deep seated chronic pelvic pain, dysmenorrhea, dysuria, and dyschezia. Diagnosis of coexistent deep endometriotic deposits by USG/MRI is necessary for complete diagnosis and treatment. The common sites of DIE include the uterosacral ligaments, the rectosigmoid colon, the vagina, and the bladder.

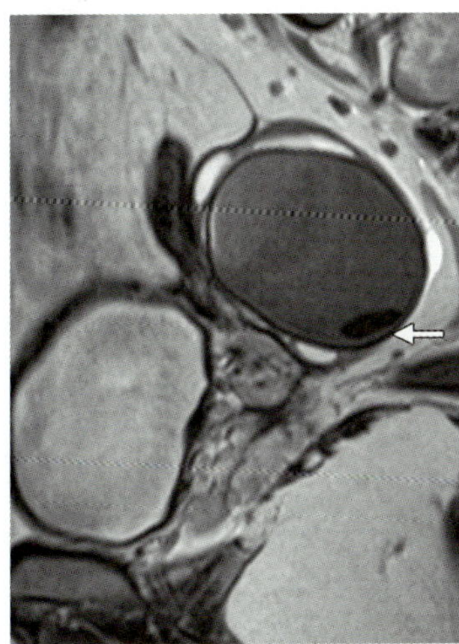

Fig. 14: Sagittal T2-weighted MR image shows the presence of a dependent hypointense focus (arrow) in left sided endometriotic cyst—*"T2 dark spot"*. This sign (although less sensitive than T2 shading sign) is highly specific for endometriotic cyst.

Recently, transvaginal sonography has been used to detect DIE of specific regions especially rectosigmoid region **(Fig. 16A)**. Sonographically, these lesions appear as solid hypoechoic masses with irregular margins involving the bowel wall which show lack of peristalsis and absent color flow. In addition, fixity of uterus and cervix with rectal wall can also be assessed with the help of sliding sign, which involves the demonstration of relative mobility of the uterus to the adjacent organs.[17]

On MRI, the diagnosis of DIE is made on a constellation of morphological and signal abnormalities. These lesions are due to fibromuscular hyperplasia surrounding ectopic endometrial glands. The regions of fibrous and smooth muscle tissue show intermediate to low SI on T1W and low SI on T2W images **(Figs. 16B and C)**. DIE may also present as soft tissue thickening involving ligaments and organ walls. Hyperintense foci on T2W images may be present representing the dilated ectopic endometrial glands. In addition, hemorrhagic foci appearing as hyperintense foci on T1W and fat-suppressed T1W images can be seen.

On CT, endometriomas have a nonspecific appearance appearing as high density cystic, or solid appearing masses with no enhancement after contrast administration. Varying degrees of adherence can be seen with the uterus, adjacent organs, and between the ovaries.

Complications

Adhesions: Endometriomas are associated with extensive adhesions leading to distortion of anatomical structures and symptoms in patients. Indirect signs of adhesions include elevation of the posterior vaginal fornix, posterior and lateral displacement of the uterus or ovaries, or

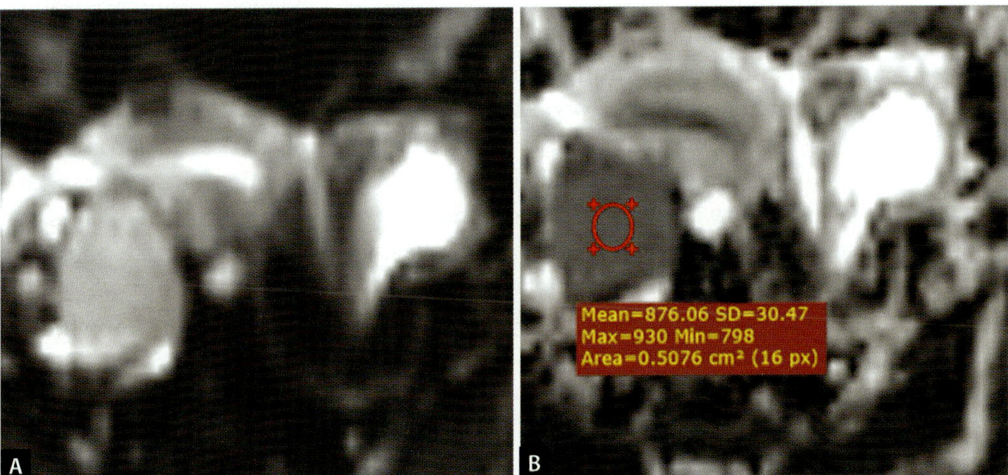

Figs. 15A and B: Diffusion-weighted imaging (DWI) in endometriomas. DWI (A) and corresponding apparent diffusion coefficient (ADC) map (B) demonstrating diffusion restriction (ADC value = $0.87 \times 10^{-3} \pm 0.03$ /mm^2).

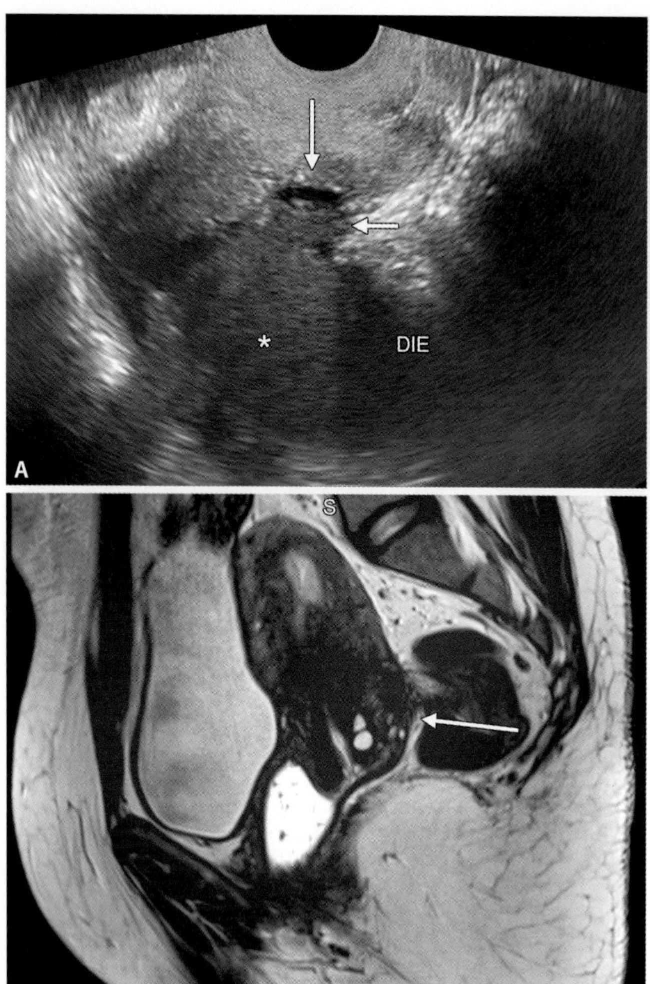

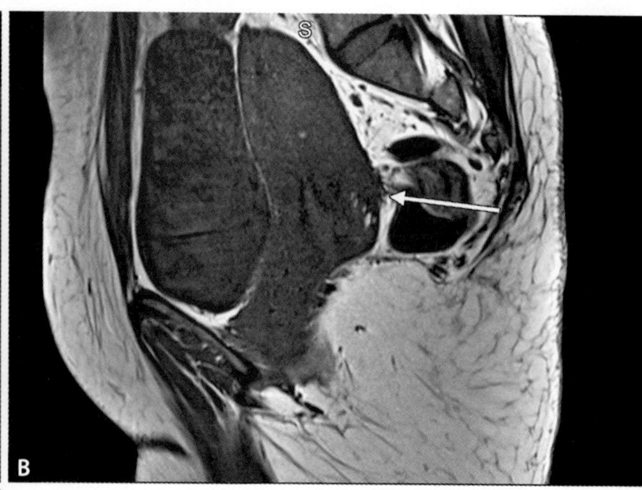

Figs. 16A to C: Deep infiltrating endometriosis (DIE) located in rectouterine pouch. Transvaginal scan (A) reveals an ill-defined hypoechoic lesion (arrow) adherent to the posterior wall of uterus and endometriotic cyst (*). DIE involving cervix and vagina in 36-year-old patient with dyspareunia and dyschezia—an ill-defined stellate-shaped lesion (arrow) is seen involving the upper portion of posterior cervical region, posterior vaginal wall with resultant obliteration of posterior vaginal fornix appearing hypointense on sagittal T1W (B) and T2W (C) images. It also shows few hyperintense foci on T1W images suggestive of hemorrhagic foci.

both, loss of fat planes between the structures without a clear interface, hydrosalpinx or hematosalpinx, hydroureteronephrosis, angulation of bowel loops, transition points in bowel diameter, and loculated fluid collections. On MRI, adhesions may be identified as spiculated low SI strands extending between the organs on both T1W and T2W images **(Figs. 17A and B)**.

Malignant transformation of endometrioma, although rare (about 1%), is well known.[18] It may arise from within the endometriotic cyst itself or from the normal ovary. The most common histological subtypes include clear cell and endometrioid carcinoma. They are mostly seen in women older than 40 years, after several years of latency and in endometriomas larger than 9 cm. Malignant transformation is uncommon in endometriomas <6 cm.[19] Any endometrioma-exhibiting features like mural nodules or papillary components showing vascularity on Doppler should be evaluated further in view of malignancy. Other features include ascites, septal thickness >3 mm and peritoneal metastasis. Loss of T2 shading has also been described as a magnetic resonance feature of coexisting neoplasm which is attributed to dilution of hemorrhagic fluid by tumor.

Ovarian torsion and rupture: Due to formation of extensive adhesions, risk of torsion is rare in endometriotic cysts. Rupture of endometriotic cysts usually occurs in pregnancy due to rapid growth of endometriomas under the effects of estrogen. Endometrioma rupture is clinically indistinguishable from rupture of a hemorrhagic cyst. There may be hemoperitoneum, which becomes a surgical emergency if the patient is unstable.

Decidualization: During pregnancy, endometriomas can undergo decidual changes in the endometrial tissue lining the cysts, which can be seen as solid papillary projections with a rounded contour and increased vascularity within the ground-glass background.

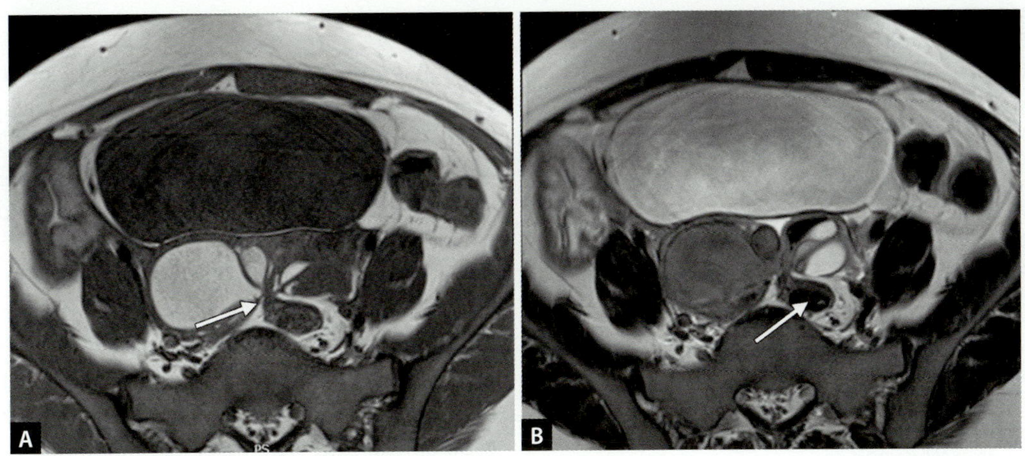

Figs. 17A and B: Axial T1-weighted (A) and T2-weighted (B) images reveal endometriotic cyst in right ovary with both ovaries adherent to each other in the midline—"kissing ovaries". There is tenting of the anterior wall of sigmoid colon with focal adherence to posterior aspect of ovaries (arrows).

On MRI, the nodules may show SI and texture similar to the decidualized uterine endometrium. They can resemble malignant neoplasms. These changes generally subside in the third trimester and regress completely following pregnancy.

Differential Diagnosis

The differential diagnosis of endometriomas includes mature cystic teratomas (MCTs), hemorrhagic cysts, TOA, cystadenomas, and other ovarian neoplasms with most of the lesions being differentiated on basis of USG and MR findings.

On USG, a MCT of the ovary presents as a unilocular cystic lesion with echogenic components (representing calcification or tooth components) within. Associated posterior acoustic shadowing may also be present. Like endometriomas, dermoid cysts can also depict fluid-fluid levels. However, the two may be distinguished by assessing the pattern of distribution of fluid within the cyst. In a dermoid, supernatant layer is echogenic representing fat while in endometriomas, the supernatant layer appears hypoechoic with blood and its components in the dependent hyperechoic layer.[20] MR evaluation even though reserved for doubtful cases, has a high sensitivity owing to its ability to detect presence of fat. Although both lesions may appear hyperintense on T1-weighted images, T1 fat-saturated (T1FS) MRI can easily help in distinction. Endometriotic cysts appear hyperintense on T1FS images while dermoid cysts (containing fat) appear hypointense on T1FS images, thereby aiding in differentiation between the two.

On USG, HOCs are seen as thinned-walled, cystic lesions with fine reticular network within. Echogenic foci are specific to endometriomas. On MRI, they show high signal on T1- and T2W images and show lack of T2 shading sign. However, hemorrhagic cysts of longer duration may show T2 shading like features thereby mimicking endometriomas. T2 dark spots have a higher specificity for diagnosis of endometriomas than shading sign and can help to differentiate between them. Since hemorrhagic cysts are relatively short-lived, they do not show such spots. It has been suggested that addition of DWI can help to differentiate between endometriomas and hemorrhagic cysts. However, both show restricted diffusion due to the presence of blood products, and the ADC values have not shown a consistent pattern to allow a confident differentiation.[21,22]

However, there have been variable reports on the ADC values management.

Medical treatment of endometriomas is aimed for alleviation of symptoms and reduction in size. These include the use of nonsteroidal anti-inflammatory drugs (NSAIDs) and hormonal therapy to temper estrogen levels. These include oral contraceptive pills, progesterone analogs, and gonadotropin-releasing hormone (GnRH) agonists.[21] Despite medical management, most endometriotic cysts require surgery for definitive treatment, especially in cases of infertility. However, even after complete resection, these cysts are known for recurrence.

BENIGN OVARIAN NEOPLASMS

Ovarian neoplasms can be broadly classified into epithelial tumors, germ cell tumors, sex-cord stromal tumors, and metastatic tumors **(Box 1 and Fig. 18)**.

Box 1: Broad classification of ovarian tumors.

1. **Epithelial tumors—arise from surface epithelium**
   - *Serous epithelial tumors:*
     - Benign (serous cystadenoma/cystadenofibroma), borderline, and malignant
   - *Mucinous tumors:*
     - Benign (mucinous cystadenoma/cystadenofibroma), borderline, and malignant
   - *Endometroid tumors:*
     - Benign, borderline, and malignant
   - *Clear cell tumors:*
     - Benign, borderline, and malignant
   - *Transitional cell tumors:*
     - Brenner (benign, borderline, and malignant)
     - Transitional cell carcinoma (non-Brenner type)
   - *Epithelial-stromal tumors:*
     - Adenosarcoma
     - Carcinosarcoma
2. **Germ cell tumors—arise from the primordial germ cells**
   - *Teratoma:*
     - Mature teratoma (dermoid)
     - Immature teratoma
   - Yolk sac tumor (endodermal sinus tumor)
   - Dysgerminoma
   - Embryonal cell carcinoma
   - Choriocarcinoma
   - *Monodermal tumors:*
     - Struma ovarii
     - Carcinoid
3. **Sex cord–stromal tumors—arise from ovarian stroma and/or sex cord cells**
   - Thecoma
   - Fibroma
   - Fibrothecoma
   - Granulosa cell tumors
   - Sertoli-Leydig cell tumors
   - Steroid (lipid) cell tumors
4. **Metastatic tumors**

Surface epithelium-stroma
Serous
Mucinous
Clear cell
Endometrioid
Transitional cell

Sex cord-stroma
Granulosa cell
Sertoli cell
Sertoli-Leydig cell
Thecoma
Fibroma
Steroid

Germ cells
Dysgerminoma
Yolk sac tumor
Teratoma
Choriocarcinoma
Embryonal cell carcinoma

Fig. 18: Diagram to show the origin of ovarian tumors from the various cells within the ovary.

EPITHELIAL TUMORS

Benign epithelial ovarian tumors are mainly cystic in appearance. They are seen in a younger age group as compared to their malignant counterparts. The two most common types of benign epithelial neoplasms are the serous cystadenoma and the mucinous cystadenoma.

Serous Cystadenoma

Serous cystadenomas are a commonly occurring neoplasm accounting for approximately 25% of all benign ovarian neoplasms. They are thought to arise from ovarian epithelial inclusions, which itself is derived from fallopian tube epithelium. The peak age incidence is 30–50 years with bilateral tumors seen in 12–23% cases.[22]

Pathology

Serous cystadenomas are usually unilocular (sometimes multilocular) cysts measuring 10 cm in average diameter (sometimes may be extremely large), containing thin and straw-colored fluid. Microscopically, the cyst wall is composed of a solitary layer of simple epithelium with cilia that may be columnar or flat. Psammomatous calcifications can be seen.

Clinical Features

Patients may be asymptomatic and the tumor is often discovered incidentally. In case of large tumors, patients can present with pain, abdominal fullness or distension.

Imaging Features

On US, they are often seen as unilocular cystic lesions with thin walls and anechoic internal contents **(Fig. 19)**.

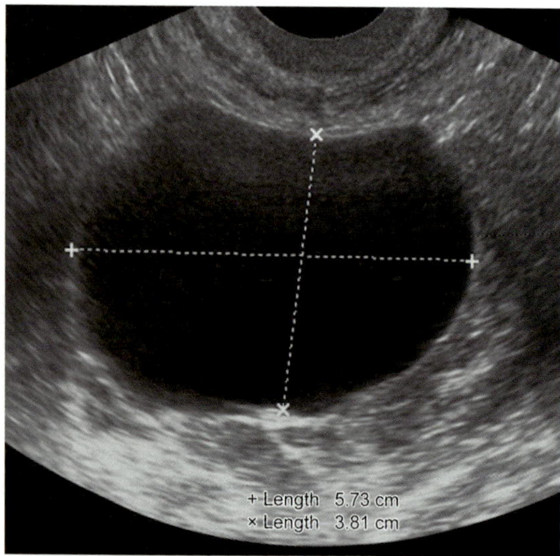

Fig. 19: Serous cystadenoma in a 70-year-old postmenopausal woman seen as a unilocular, anechoic cyst on transvaginal ultrasound.

Some lesions may be multilocular, with thin internal septations **(Fig. 20A)**. On Doppler evaluation, mild peripheral or septal vascularity may be seen **(Fig. 20B)**, which shows higher resistive and pulsatility indices on pulsed Doppler as compared to malignant neoplasms. On CT, a unilocular (typically) or multilocular cystic mass is seen with homogeneous attenuation, with thin regular walls or septae and no solid component **(Figs. 21A and B)**. On MRI, the lesions show T1W hypointense and T2W hyperintense contents on images with enhancement of the cyst wall on contrast administration. When large, these cysts can be seen to fill most of the lower pelvis and extend into the upper abdomen.

Differential Diagnosis

The common differentials are from other benign looking cystic masses in the adnexal region like functional ovarian cysts, paraovarian cysts, peritoneal inclusion cysts (PICs), and large hydrosalpinx. Presence of a solid component, even small, especially if showing internal vascularity, needs to be evaluated for malignant etiology.

Management

As these are benign lesions, they usually have a good prognosis. However, ovarian cystadenomas may evolve into cystadenocarcinomas, and thus are usually removed

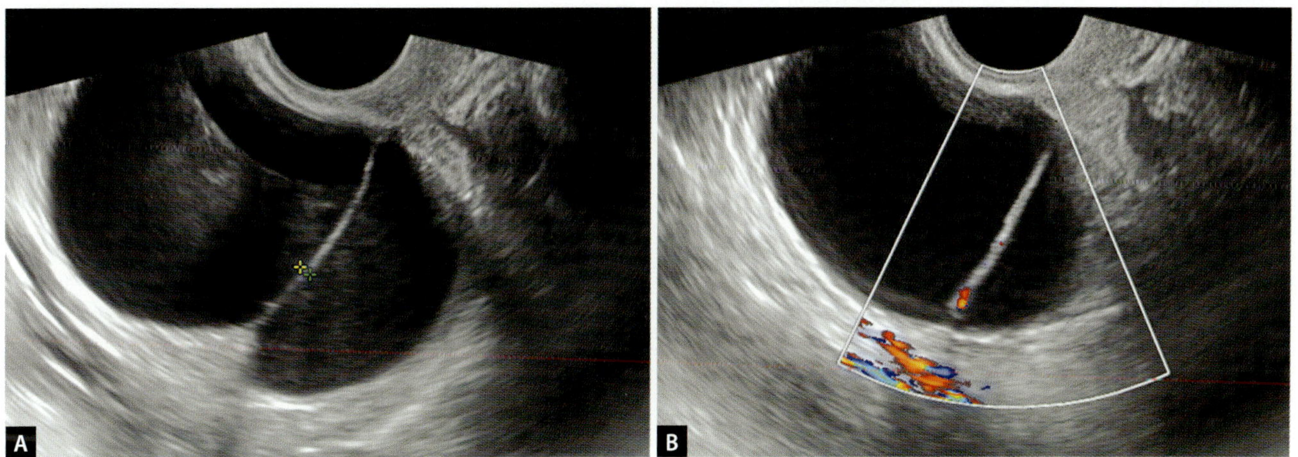

Figs. 20A and B: Serous cystadenoma in a 55-year-old woman. Transvaginal scan (A) shows a thin septum within a large, anechoic, cystic mass. The septum shows mild vascularity on color Doppler (B).

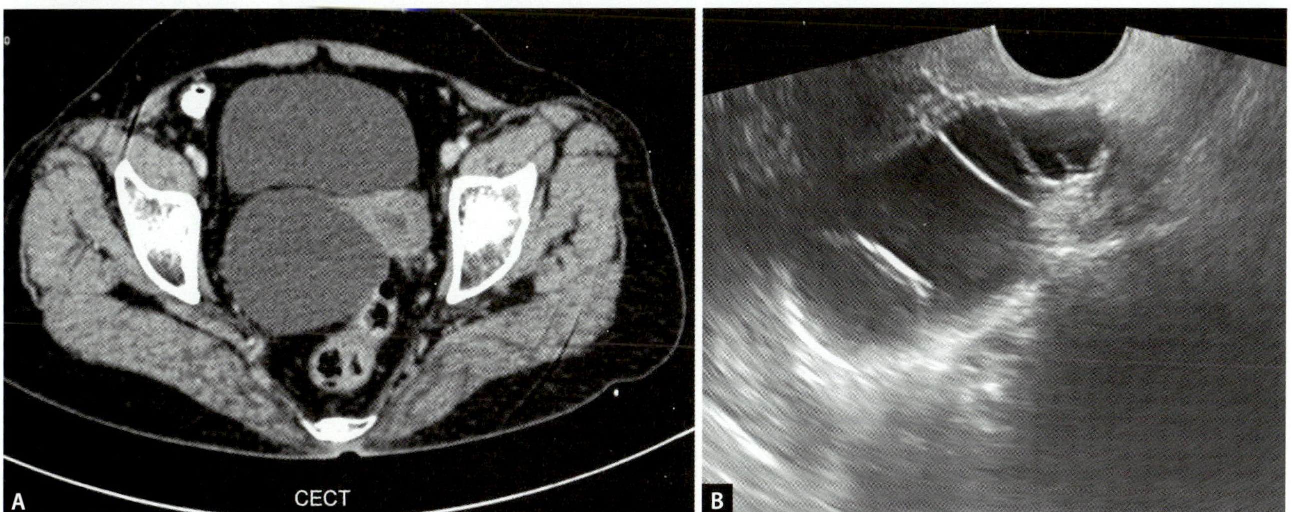

Figs. 21A and B: Serous cystadenoma in a 60-year-old woman. Contrast-enhanced CT scan (A) shows a unilocular, thin-walled cystic lesion in right adnexal region. On transvaginal ultrasound (B) a few, thin septae were seen within the cyst.

either by cystectomy or oophorectomy. They can also form a lead point for ovarian torsion. Cystadenomas do not recur following oophorectomy.

Mucinous Cystadenoma

Mucinous cystadenomas account for approximately 15–20% of benign ovarian neoplasms and 80% of mucinous ovarian tumors.[23] They are less common than their serous counterparts.

Pathology

They are usually multilocular cystic masses (rarely they can be unilocular), larger than their serous counterparts. Only 2–5% are bilateral. Microscopically, they are lined by columnar epithelial cells which secrete thick, gelatinous mucin which fills the locules. In 5% cases, mucinous cystadenomas may occur in association with other tumors of the ovary like Brenner tumors or dermoid cysts.

Clinical Features

Patients present with abdominal distension, pain and/or pelvic mass. In rare cases, hormonal manifestations can occur due to stromal luteinization. They commonly occur between 30 years and 50 years of age.

Imaging Features

On imaging, mucinous cystadenomas are seen as large, multilocular cystic masses with numerous thin septations which are smooth and regular **(Figs. 22A and B)**. The locules show low-level internal echogenicity on US. As the locules contain fluid of various viscosity, they often show variable density on CT and signal intensities on both T1 and T2 sequences on MRI giving a "stained glass" or "honeycomb" appearance. On T1W images, loculi with watery mucin have a lower SI than the loculi which have thicker mucin. On T2-weighted images, the loculi with watery mucin have high SI and loculi with thicker mucin appear slightly hypointense **(Figs. 23A to C)**. Lack of solid components and presence of regular smooth septa confirm the benign nature of the lesion. Small papillary projections may be present but are often difficult to visualize on imaging.[24] Mural calcification occurs more commonly than in serous tumors.[25]

Differential Diagnosis

Large cystic masses can be confused with omental or mesenteric cysts, PICs, and large serous cystadenomas. Although the "stained glass" appearance has been said to be pathognomonic for mucinous ovarian tumors, it may rarely be seen in MCT, fibrothecoma, endometrioma, Brenner tumor of the ovary, and degenerated leiomyoma of the uterus.[26]

Management

Mucinous cystadenomas are benign masses with excellent prognosis, however, often need to be surgically removed to confirm benign histology, due to the mass effect of large tumors and potential for ovarian torsion.

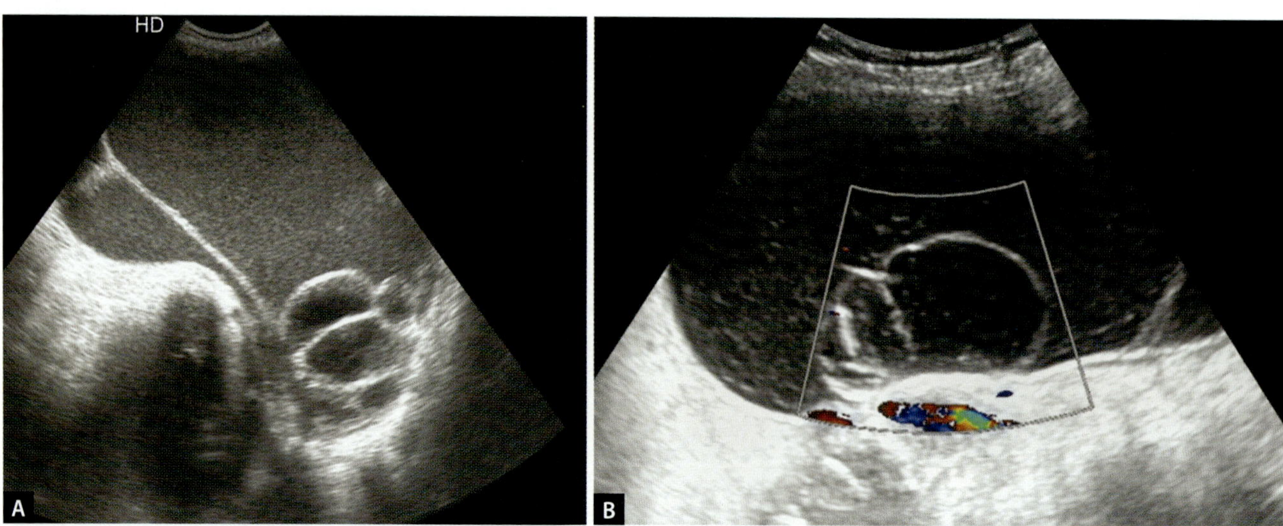

Figs. 22A and B: Mucinous cystadenoma in a 45-year-old woman presenting with abdominal fullness and pain. (A) Transvaginal ultrasound image shows a multiloculated cystic mass with multiple thin septae, differential internal echoes and no solid component; (B) No vascularity was seen in the septae or adjacent wall on transabdominal color Doppler scan.

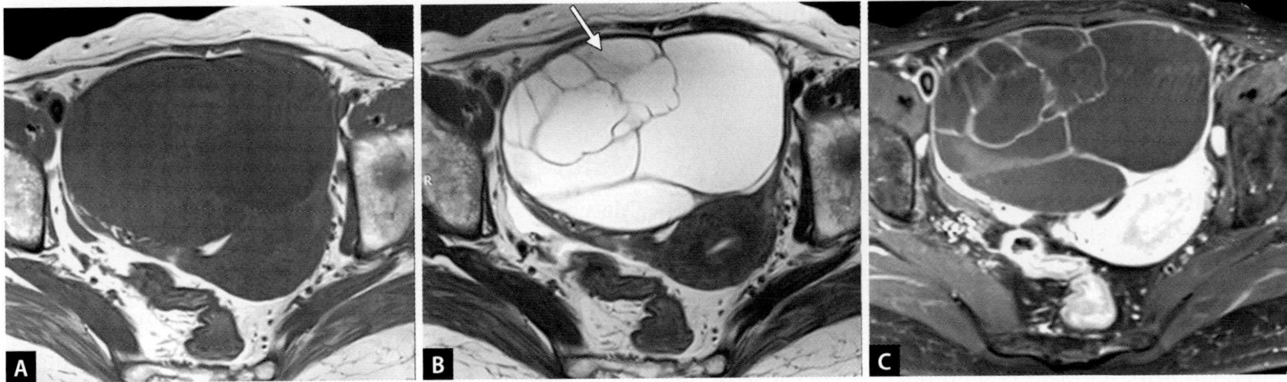

Figs. 23A to C: Mucinous cystadenoma. T1-weighted (A) and T2-weighted (B) axial MR images show a large multiloculated cystic mass with multiple thin, smooth septae within appearing hypointense on T1W, hyperintense on T2W images with thin, regular, hypointense septae, and cyst wall. Variable signal intensities are seen in some of the locules on T2W image (arrow). On contrast-enhanced T1W image (C) the cyst wall and septae are seen to enhance.

Ovarian Cystadenofibroma

Cystadenofibromas of the ovary are uncommon benign neoplasms which contain both epithelial and fibrous stromal components, and account for 1.7% of all benign ovarian tumors.[27] They occur in females in the reproductive age group. Cystadenofibromas may be predominantly cystic, predominantly solid or complex cystic with variable amount of solid components and may have a serous or mucinous cystic component. Due to the presence of irregular thick septae or solid components within the lesion, they are often mistaken for malignant lesions not only on imaging, but even at surgery. A frozen section at time of surgery is necessary to make an accurate diagnosis to avoid unnecessary extensive surgery.

Imaging Features

On US, a cystadenofibroma may be seen as a solitary cyst or a multiloculated cystic mass, with solid nodules or papillary projections with some of them showing increased vascularity on Doppler evaluation. The fibrous component in the solid part may show acoustic shadowing which can give a clue to the diagnosis. On CT, a nonspecific complex cystic mass with enhancing solid component, mimics a malignant lesion.[28]

On MRI, the presence of low-SI on T2W images in the solid part of the tumor, due to its fibrous tissue component, helps in characterizing this neoplasm. A sponge-like appearance may also be seen due to multiple tiny hyperintense T2W cysts alongwith a low SI solid fibrous component. Diffuse or focal thickening of the cyst wall may be seen with low SI on T2W images. There is mild enhancement of the solid component on postcontrast images. In a study by Cho et al., 16 cases of cystadenofibromas of the ovary, presenting as complex cystic masses with solid components, were misdiagnosed as malignant ovarian neoplasms on CT scan or MRI.[27]

Differential Diagnosis

The differential diagnosis will depend on the appearance of the cystadenofibroma—whether predominantly cystic, solid or complex cystic-solid. Thus, it can vary from a serous or mucinous neoplasm to other T2W hypointense masses like fibroma, fibrothecoma, Brenner tumor, and even leiomyomas.

Brenner Tumor

Brenner tumors are surface epithelial-stromal tumors of the ovary comprising approximately 2% of all ovarian neoplasms, so-called as they were first described by Fritz Brenner in 1907.[29] They are also called "transitional cell tumors" because of their histological similarity to the urothelium. They usually occur in women between the ages of 45 years and 65 years. There may be an associated second tumor in the same ovary in about 30% of cases, which is most often a serous or a mucinous cystadenoma.

Clinical Features

Brenner tumors are unilateral masses often discovered incidentally. Symptomatic patients present with vaginal bleeding (due to excess estrogenic activity), pelvic pain or pelvic mass. Large tumors may give rise to urinary retention, ascites or even Meigs' syndrome. Histological examination shows epithelial cell nests growing in a fibrous stroma. Although 99% of Brenner tumors are benign, malignant Brenner tumors may arise from their benign counterparts, so careful histopathological examination of all Brenner tumors is essential.

Imaging Features

On US, these tumors are seen as predominantly solid masses, small in size, with few, if any, cystic areas in the benign lesions. Extensive amorphous calcification may be present. On Doppler examination, they are either avascular or show minimal vascularity. *CT* shows the calcifications better. On *MRI*, a low SI is seen on T2WI because of the solid fibrous content **(Figs. 24A and B)**. In cases where an associated cystic tumor, like mucinous or serous cystadenoma, is present along with the Brenner tumor, a lesion with both cystic (cystadenomas) and solid (Brenner) component is seen on imaging. Borderline or invasive Brenner tumors are characterized by the presence of solid-cystic or cystic appearance, with papillary structures, and mild or moderate enhancement in the solid mass.[30]

Differential Diagnosis

The important differentials include ovarian fibromas, fibrothecomas, and a pedunculated leiomyoma all of which can be seen as hypoechoic masses on US and T2 hypointense masses on MRI. Absence of a normal ipsilateral ovary helps distinguish from pedunculated leiomyomas. The presence of small follicles surrounding the mass helps identify the ovarian origin. Abundant calcification, if present, goes in favor of Brenner tumor.

GERM CELL TUMORS

Ovarian germ cell tumors arise from primordial germ cells of the ovary. The only benign germ cell tumor is the MCT.

Mature Cystic Teratoma

Mature cystic teratomas are the most common germ cell neoplasms, accounting for about 15–20% of all ovarian neoplasms.[31] These tumors arise from a single germ cell after its first meiotic division and contain mature tissue from all three germ cell layers (ectoderm, mesoderm, and endoderm) with predominance of ectodermal component. When ectodermal tissues predominate, these teratomas are called as dermoid cysts.

Pathology

Mature teratomas are usually seen as unilocular cystic masses at macroscopic examination. However, they may be multilocular at times. Fat is present in more than 90% of cases,[32] either as sebum or macroscopic fat, and is the most specific finding of a mature teratoma. The cyst cavity is filled with sebaceous and keratinized material secreted by the squamous epithelial lining. Sebaceous material contains most of the lipid content whereas adipose tissue is less common. Sebum is an oily, waxy material produced by sebaceous glands in the epidermis and is primarily composed of fatty acids and triglycerides. There is usually a raised protuberance, projecting into the cyst cavity, known as the *Rokitansky protuberance or dermoid plug*. Bone and teeth tend to be located in this protuberance and most of

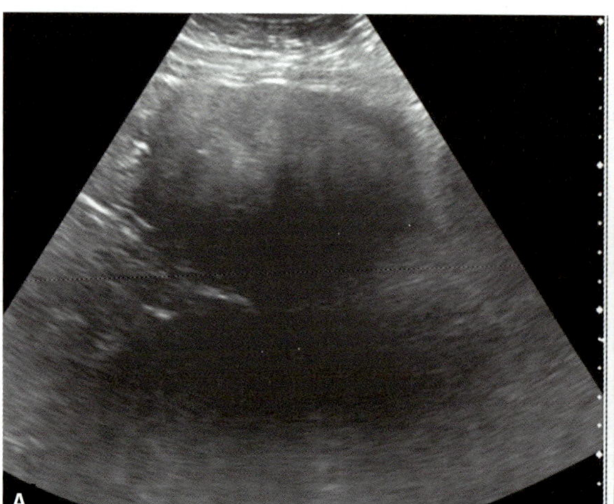

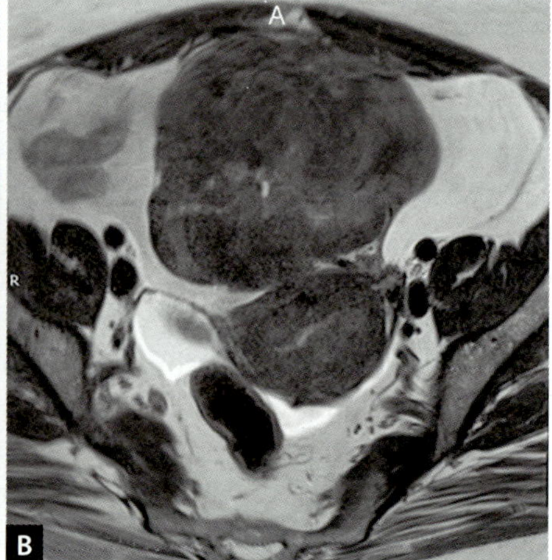

Figs. 24A and B: Brenner tumor in a 50-year-old patient with abdominal distension and abnormal uterine bleeding. (A) Transabdominal ultrasound image shows a hypoechoic solid mass with lobulated outer margins and some acoustic shadowing; (B) T2-weighted axial MR image shows lobulated hypointense mass anterior to the uterus with small amount of ascites.

the hair arises from it. The rare malignant transformation also occurs at this site.

Histologically, mature tissues from different cell lines are seen within the wall. Walls of the cyst are frequently lined by squamous epithelium. In an MCT, ectodermal elements are almost always present. Endodermal tissues (mucinous or ciliated epithelium) can also be seen in the majority of cases and mesodermal tissues are present in over 90% of cases.

Clinical Features

Mature cystic teratomas occur in a younger age group with mean age of 30 years, but can range between 4 months and 70 years.[33] They are the most common ovarian mass lesion found in children. The tumors are bilateral in about 10–12% of cases.[34]

They are slow growing tumors and are often discovered incidentally. Pain in the lower abdomen or other nonspecific symptoms may occur in a few cases. Complicated dermoid cysts can present with acute symptoms, the most common complication being torsion of the ovary.

Imaging Features

On *plain radiographs*, around 40% of ovarian teratomas show diagnostic characteristics with presence of teeth or fat in the pelvis.

A variety of appearances can be seen on cross-sectional imaging due to the multiple tissues within these teratomas. The classic *US* appearance is a complex cystic mass with solid mural component called *"dermoid plug"* or *"Rokitansky nodule"*. This is seen in almost 90% of cystic teratomas **(Figs. 25A and B)**. The dermoid plug contains hair, teeth or fat and is usually echogenic and frequently casts an acoustic shadow. Rarely, the Rokitansky nodule may appear entirely cystic.[35] The dermoid cyst may show focal or diffuse, homogeneous or heterogeneous, *hyperechogenecity* which may be associated with areas of acoustic shadowing which is due to presence of mixed sebaceous material and hair **(Fig. 26A)**.

"Tip of the iceberg" sign can be seen, on both transabdominal and transvaginal US scans, as an amorphous echogenic mass which causes posterior shadowing that obscures the posterior portion of the lesion and any structures behind it **(Fig. 26B)**.[36] This is produced by a mixture of matted hair, fatty fluid, and cellular debris which is highly echogenic because of the multiple tissue interfaces. This sign is seen. It may mimic a fecal/air-filled bowel segment and may be missed on US.

"Dot-dash" sign or *"dermoid mesh"* seen as hyperechoic lines and dots within the cyst. It occurs due to strands of hair in different orientations **(Fig. 26C)**.[37]

Fat-fluid/fluid-fluid levels can be seen when anechoic sebum layers above the hyperechoic aqueous/debris-containing layer **(Fig. 26D)**. Sometimes the supernatant

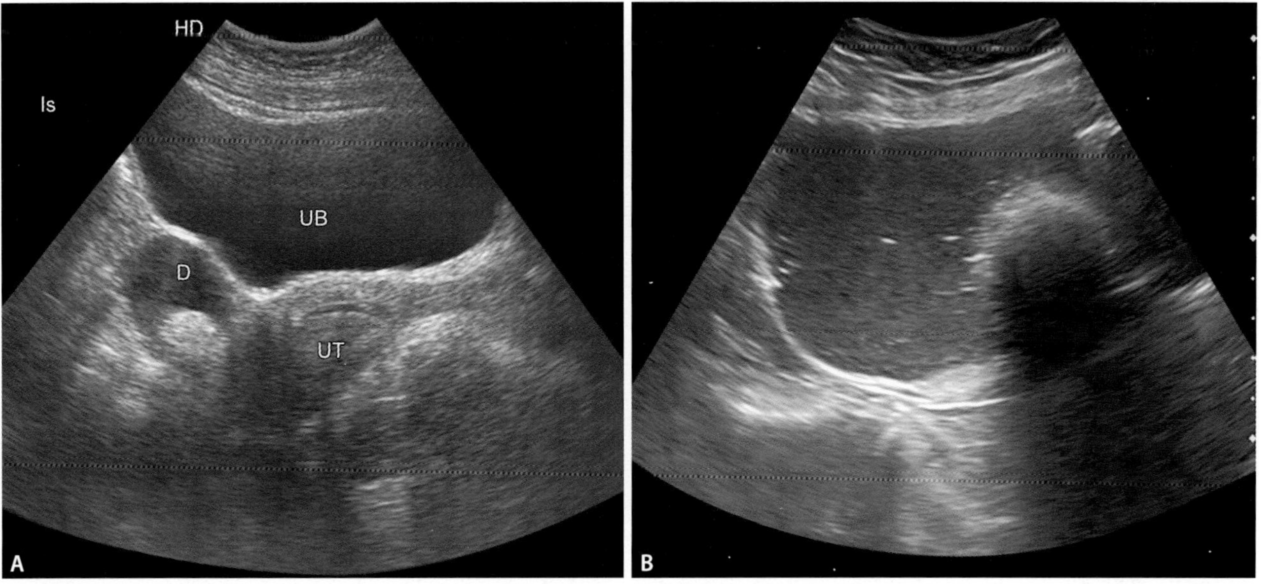

Figs. 25A and B: (A) Right ovarian dermoid. Transabdominal ultrasound image showing right ovarian cystic mass (D) with an echogenic nodule—Rokitansky nodule; (B) Transvaginal scan. Typical mature cystic teratoma showing a Rokitansky nodule as an echogenic nodule with marked acoustic shadowing within a cystic mass. The cyst shows low level ground-glass echoes within. Multiple hyperechoic dots and dashes seen along surface of the nodule and within the cyst represent hair. (UB: urinary bladder; UT: uterus).

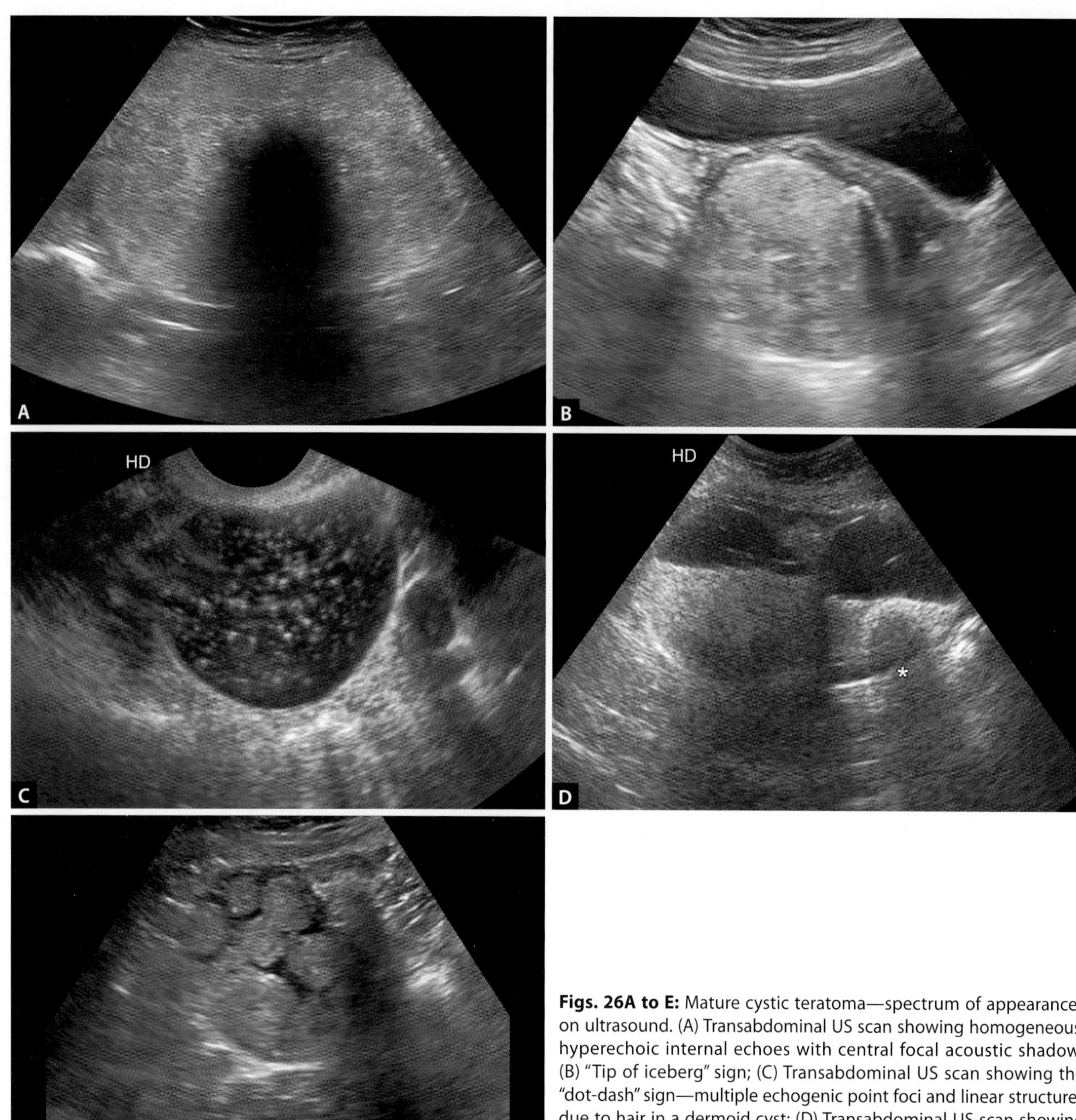

Figs. 26A to E: Mature cystic teratoma—spectrum of appearances on ultrasound. (A) Transabdominal US scan showing homogeneous, hyperechoic internal echoes with central focal acoustic shadow; (B) "Tip of iceberg" sign; (C) Transabdominal US scan showing the "dot-dash" sign—multiple echogenic point foci and linear structures due to hair in a dermoid cyst; (D) Transabdominal US scan showing bilateral dermoids lying next to each other, with fat fluid levels, hyperechoic linear dashes representing hair and acoustic shadowing (*) in left dermoid; (E) "Floating ball" sign.

hyperechoic sebum layers above the hypoechoic aqueous fluid.

"Floating balls" sign is seen as intracystic floating hyperechoic globules or nodules within a cystic mass **(Fig. 26E)**. This is another pathognomonic sign, but is uncommonly seen.[38]

The US appearance may vary from a very specific (when the characteristic signs can be identified), to a totally nonspecific appearance requiring further CT or MRI to confirm the nature of the mass.

Computed tomography can provide a definitive diagnosis in majority of cases due to its high sensitivity in detecting fat. The characteristic CT features include detection of fat (density <–20 HU), hair, teeth, and fat-fluid level. Rokitansky nodule is also best seen on CT, as a rounded or oval structure, generally <5 cm in diameter,

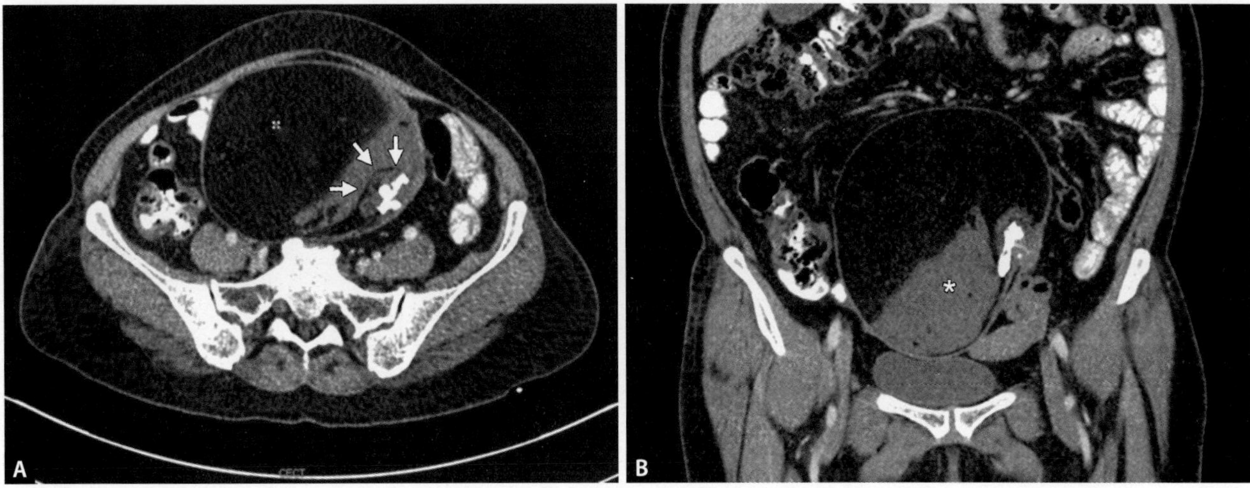

Figs. 27A and B: Typical mature cystic teratoma in a 45-year-old woman. (A) Axial contrast-enhanced CT shows a large, thinly encapsulated, fat containing (–113 HU) cystic mass with a rounded Rokitansky nodule (arrows) which has teeth-like structures within it. A fat fluid level is seen; (B) On the coronal CECT, the Rokitansky nodule can be seen to be arising from the soft tissue along the cyst wall. Fluid density content (*) can also be seen adjacent to the nodule within the predominantly fat-containing mature cystic teratoma.

protruding into the cyst. It frequently contains tooth, calcification, hair or adipose tissue **(Figs. 27A and B)**. Rarely, a Rokitansky protuberance may be seen as a mural thickening or a bridge across the cyst.[39] Curvilinear or globular calcification can be seen in the Rokitansky protuberance or in the wall of the dermoid cyst. Fat-fluid level and floating balls sign can also be well seen on CT. When a dermoid cyst does not have fat or calcification, CT may not be helpful in the differential diagnosis.[40] It may have shown only water density content, due to excess watery fluid or gelatinous fluid **(Fig. 28)**. Sometimes a large amount of hair maybe mixed with the fat density, resulting in a cystic density of >–20 HU. Dermoids which have undergone torsion may show a high internal density due to hemorrhage or necrosis.

Contrast administration is not really helpful in diagnosis of dermoids as most of the characteristic features are well seen on noncontrast scans. Slight enhancement may be seen in the wall, septae and the Rokitansky protuberance on delayed contrast-enhanced scans.

On *MRI*, fat within the MCT shows high intensity on T1W images with a signal drop on fat-saturated T1W images **(Figs. 29 and 30)**. This drop in signal allows a definitive diagnosis of a MCT ruling out a hemorrhagic cyst or an endometrioma which remain hyperintense on the fat saturation images. Small areas of fat maybe identified on chemical shift imaging **(Fig. 29C)**. However, MRI may fail to pick up very small fatty areas (about 1 mm) when compared with CT.[41] On T2W images the intensity can be intermediate or higher than the subcutaneous adipose tissue. Reversed chemical shift artifact (boundary artifact

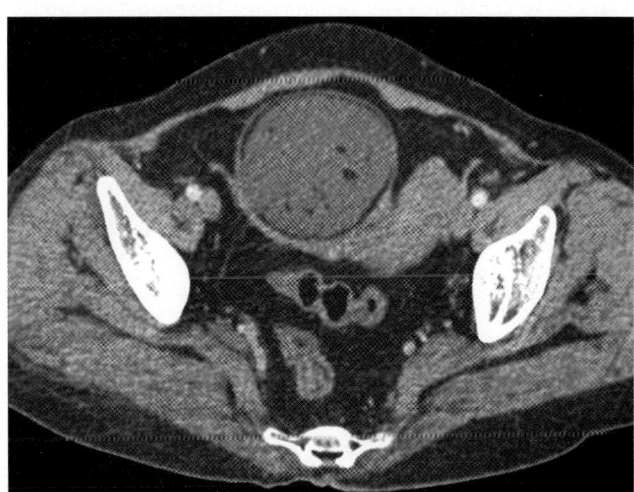

Fig. 28: Atypical mature cystic teratoma. Contrast-enhanced CT shows a well-defined, fluid density cystic lesion with a few floating fat density foci within the cystic fluid. It also shows a fatty rim along the inner margin of the wall.

perpendicular to the direction of the frequency encoding gradient) may also be seen on T2W images as foci or areas of very high SI at the interface of fatty tissue and nonfatty tissue, with a low-intensity band on the opposite side **(Fig. 30D)**.[34]

The size, number, shape, and content of the Rokitansky nodule can be easily evaluated with MRI, along with its relationship to the cyst wall **(Figs. 29A to D)**.

Fat-fluid level maybe seen as layering with high SI of supernatant fatty layer on T1W images and low SI on fat suppressed TWI **(Figs. 31A and B)**. On T2WI, variable signal intensities can be seen in the supernatant and dependent layers. A ball of debris, fat, and hair may be seen floating at the interface of the fat-fluid level or layering along the dependent wall. Matted hair can layer as dependent debris and large amounts of hair lead to lower SI on T2W images.[34] Floating globules or spherules can be seen in the cyst **(Figs. 32A and B)**. These globules may also contain macroscopic or microscopic fat, which can be detected by fat-suppression techniques or in outpatient imaging.[42]

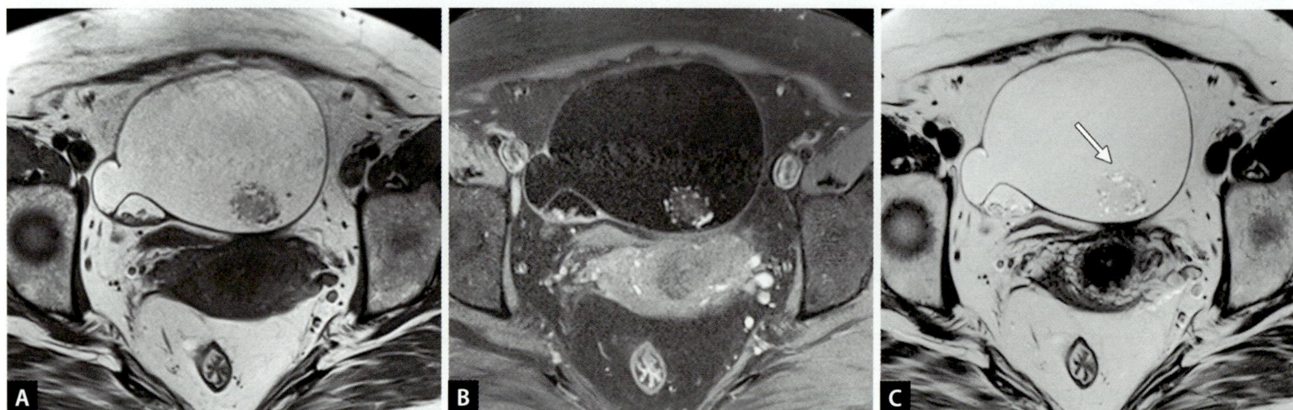

Figs. 29A to C: Mature cystic teratoma in a 16-year-old girl. (A) Large, thin-walled, multiloculated cystic mass, seen anterior to the uterus, homogeneously hyperintense on T1-weighted image, which is totally suppressed on the fat suppressed T1W image; (B) A Rokitansky nodule is seen on the posterior wall; (C) Axial T2-weighted image shows chemical shift artifact (arrow) at the interface of the Rokitansky nodule with the cyst fluid. It was consistent with matted hair and keratinoid material in the macroscopic specimen.

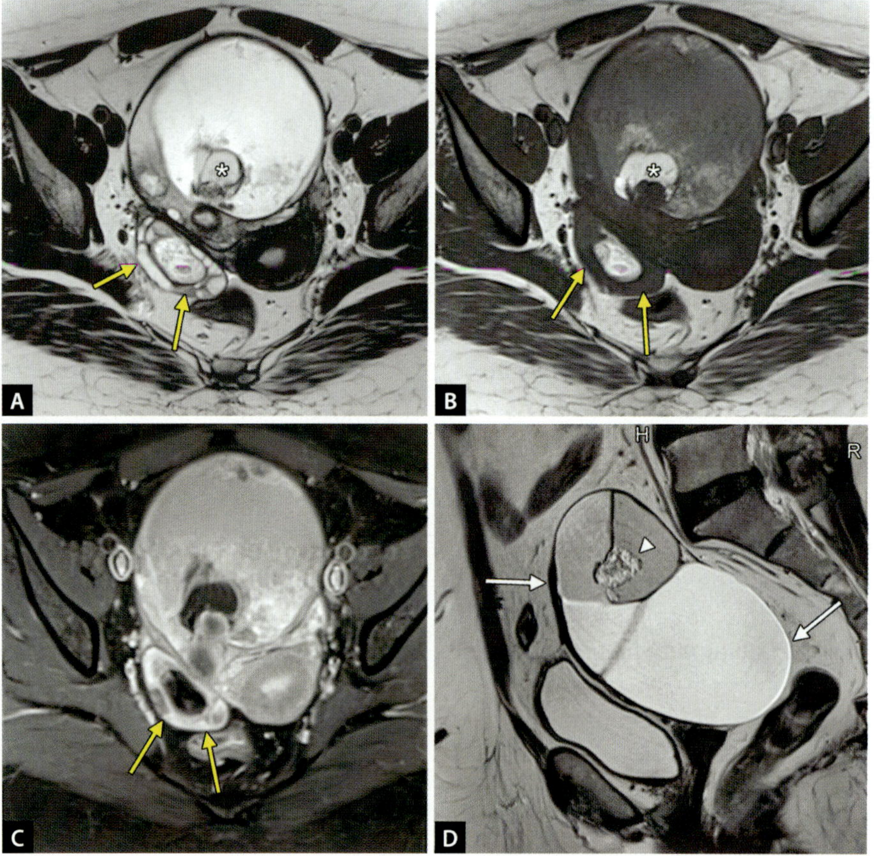

Figs. 30A to D

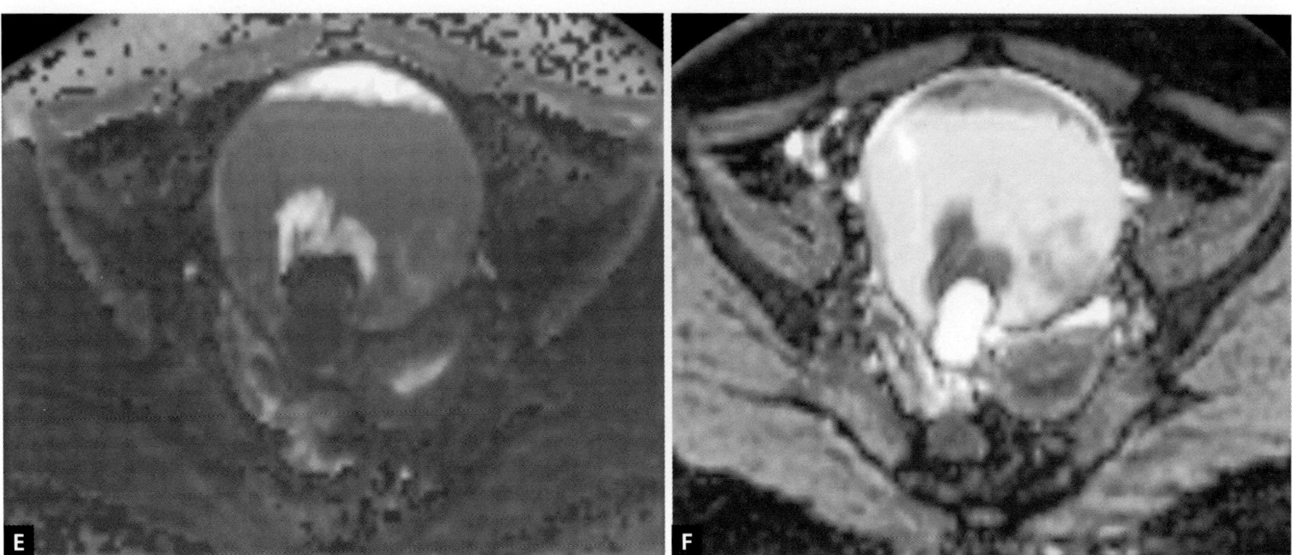

Figs. 30E and F

Figs. 30A to F: Bilateral mature cystic teratomas in a 24-year-old woman. T2-weighted (A), T1-weighted (B), and contrast-enhanced T1WFS axial MR images show a large, well-defined, hyperintense, cystic left ovarian teratoma, with a Rokitansky protuberance (*). A smaller similar mass in the right ovary (yellow arrows). Few hypointense elements seen in the protuberence on both T2- and T1-weighted images correspond to tooth/bony elements. T1-weighted image shows few scattered hyperintense foci and hyperintensity in the Rokitansky protuberance which show signal suppression on the fat-suppressed image (C). (D) On the sagittal T2W image, chemical shift artifact can be seen as a low signal intensity band (straight arrow) on the anterior border of the cyst with a high intensity band on the opposite wall (oblique arrow). The floating hair ball is also well seen in this image (arrowhead). Axial diffusion-weighted image at b = 800 sec/mm^2 (E) shows hyperintensity in few areas in the left ovarian teratoma, which appear dark on the corresponding ADC map (F) suggesting diffusion restriction in the keratin component of the teratoma.

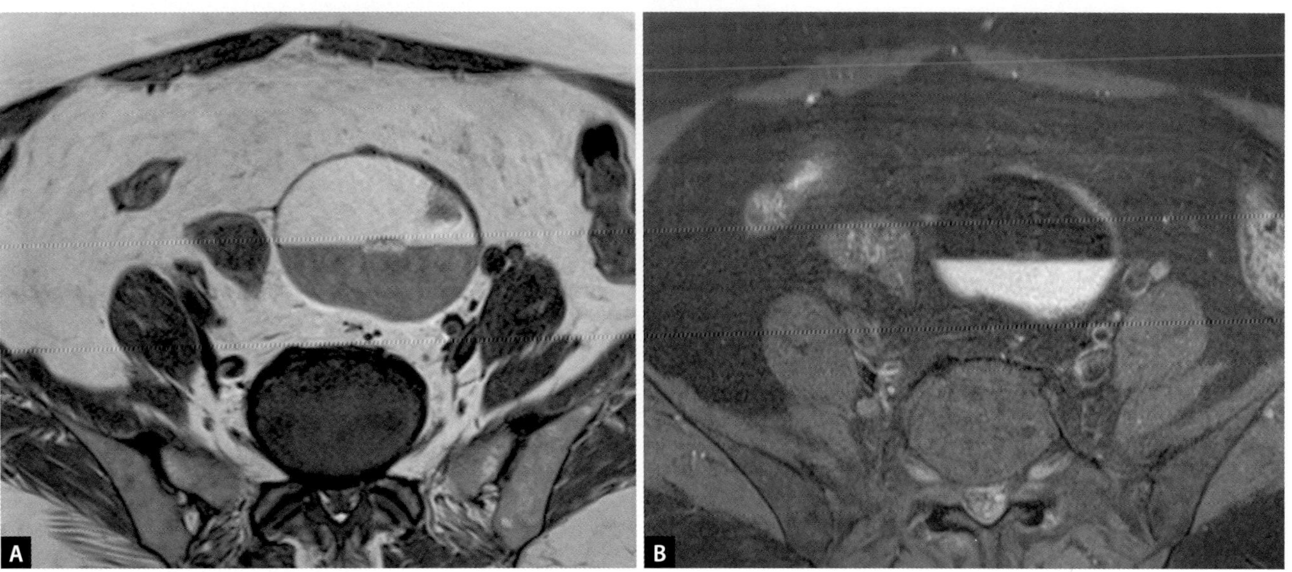

Figs. 31A and B: Axial T1-weighted MR image of a 60-year-old woman with mature cystic teratoma (A) shows high signal intensity of the supernatant fatty layer creating an interface with a low signal intensity aqueous layer. Fat-suppressed T1-weighted image (B) shows decreased signal intensity in the supernatant fatty layer. A free-floating ball is seen at the interface between the fat and fluid.

Polypoid palm tree-like protrusions maybe seen projecting into the cyst cavity **(Figs. 33A and B)**. They consist of desquamated, degenerated epithelial cells mixed with hair and the signal intensity varies according to the proportion of hair and cheese-like material.

Diffusion-weighted imaging has been used in an attempt to identify MCTs. MCTs contain a keratinoid substance, a scleroprotein, that originates from the cytoskeletal structure of the epidermis, and is a major component of skin, hair, and nails. Keratinoid is seen

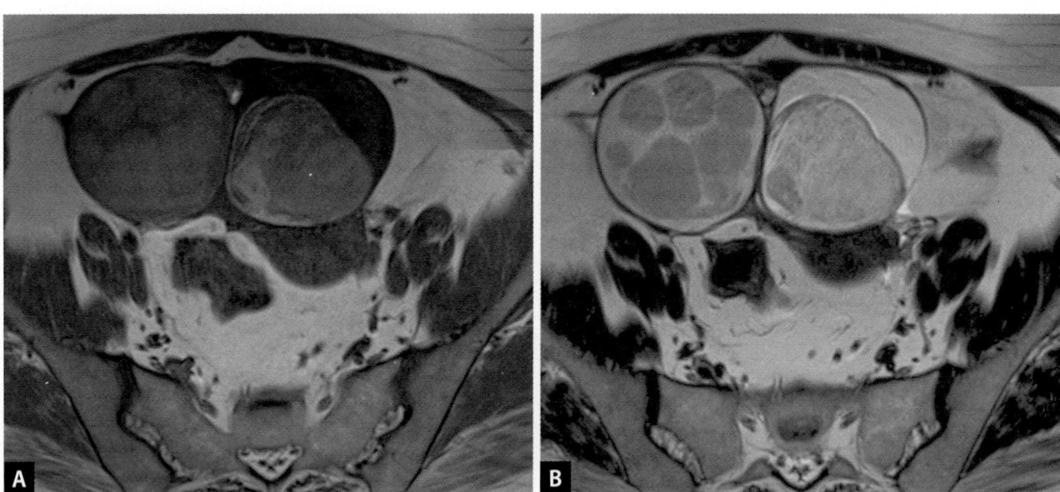

Figs. 32A and B: Mature cystic teratoma (MCT) in a 16-year-old girl. (A) T1-weighted and (B) T2-weighted axial magnetic resonance images. Biloculated MCT of right ovary with "floating ball sign" in the right locule and a large single heterogeneous ball within the left locule which appear hyperintense on the T1-weighted image. Normal left ovary was seen separately.

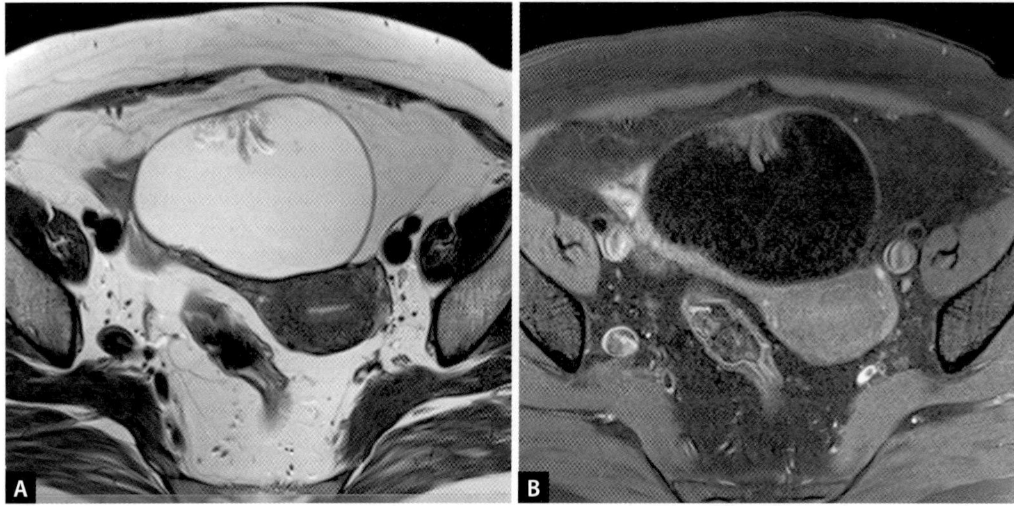

Figs. 33A and B: Palm tree protrusions in mature cystic teratoma (MCT). (A) Axial T2-weighted and (B) T1-weighted fat-suppressed magnetic resonance images showing the characteristic palm tree protrusions seen arising from the wall of the MCT.

as low SI on T1- and high SI on T2-weighted images resembling serous fluid. However, it shows a restricted diffusion pattern on DWI, i.e. a high signal on DWI and a low ADC value (***see* Figs. 30E and F**). Thus, in some MCTs, particularly when fat is not obvious, DWI may serve as an accessory sequence for the correct diagnosis.[43]

Complications

The most common complication associated with MCTs is torsion. Almost 16% of ovarian teratomas will undergo torsion, and MCTs are also considered to be the most common cause of ovarian torsion. Other complications which can occur are leak or rupture (1–4%), in which the sebaceous contents enter into the peritoneal cavity and can result in a granulomatous peritonitis; malignant transformation can occur in 1–2% cases, of which squamous cell carcinoma is the most common (>80%) but other cancers such as adenocarcinomas, sarcomas, and even carcinoids may occur. The Rokitansky's nodule is the common site for malignant transformation. Malignant transformation can be suspected, if there is irregular wall thickening, enhancing solid mass within the cystic cavity, or invasion of adjacent structures.[44] Superadded infection may be seen in few cases. Autoimmune hemolytic anemia has been reported as a rare complication, occurring in <1% cases.[45] Collision tumors have been reported with MCTs, most commonly with mucinous tumors and other germ cell tumors.

Differential Diagnosis

As MCTs have a very variable appearance on imaging due to the numerous constituents, there are a large number of conditions which can mimic them. On US, endometriomas, ovarian abscesses, and mucinous cystadenomas can be confused with MCTs having homogeneous low-level internal echoes. On CT and MRI, the typical MCT with fat and calcification do not constitute a problem, however, atypical MCTs with small or no fat content may pose a diagnostic problem.

Management

Mature cystic teratomas grow slowly at an average rate of <2 mm each year, prompting a nonsurgical management of smaller tumors (<6 cm). However, due to the high rate complications, especially torsion, most clinicians advise surgical removal. MCTs requiring removal can be treated with simple cystectomy. In case a conservative approach is adopted, then a 6-monthly to annual follow-up by US is recommended, to ensure that the lesion is not changing in size or internal architecture. In case of complicated MCTs, the management will depend on nature and severity of the complication.

SEX CORD-STROMAL TUMORS

These are a subgroup of tumors derived from the *stromal* component of the ovary, i.e. from the theca cells, fibroblasts, and Leydig cells or the *gonadal primitive sex cord cells* which include granulosa cells and Sertoli cells. They form approximately 7% of all primary ovarian tumors.[46] In the recently revised WHO classification (2014) of ovarian neoplasms, these sex cord-stromal tumors were regrouped into the following clinicopathologic entities: pure stromal tumors, pure sex cord tumors, and mixed sex cord-stromal tumors.[47] As some of the cells of these types of tumors secrete ovarian steroid hormones (e.g. estrogens, androgens, and corticosteroids), sex cord-stromal tumors are often associated with various hormone-mediated syndromes and may exhibit a wide spectrum of clinical features, e.g. precocious puberty in a child, abnormal uterine bleeding, endometrial hyperplasia or carcinoma, which are signs of increased estrogen, or signs of virilization, i.e. androgen excess in association with adnexal mass.

Ovarian fibromas, thecomas, and fibrothecomas are pure stromal tumors and are thought to be variants of a single entity. They are the most common benign solid lesions of the ovaries and usually occur in middle-aged women. They are usually asymptomatic; sometimes they may be associated with ascites and pleural effusion and this condition is called Meigs' syndrome.

Fibromas contain spindle-shaped cells and secrete collagen. They do not contain thecal cells and so do not have any estrogenic activity. On US, fibromas are commonly seen as solid, hypoechoic masses. On CT, a solid homogeneous mass with delayed contrast enhancement is seen. Sometimes diffuse intratumoral calcification maybe present. MRI shows an ovarian mass which is hypointense on both T1- and T2W images **(Figs. 34A and B)**. Hyperintense areas may be seen in the T2W images due to edema and cystic degeneration. On contrast administration, a weak and delayed enhancement pattern is seen. Majority of the ovarian fibromas do

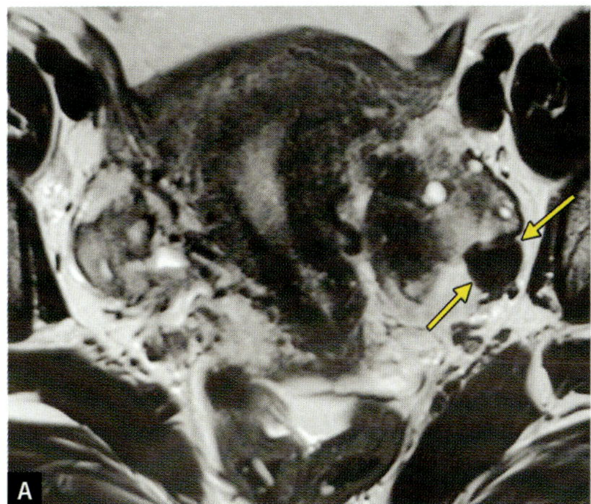

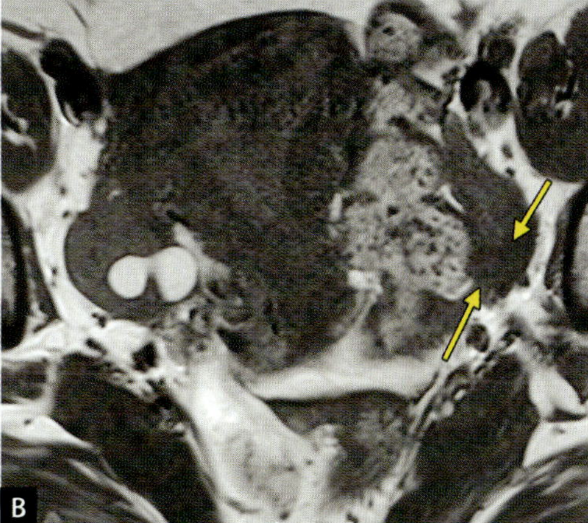

Figs. 34A and B: Ovarian fibroma. T2-weighted (T2W) (A) and T1-weighted (T1W) (B) axial magnetic resonance images show a small well-defined mass arising from the left ovary (yellow arrows), which is hypointense on both T2- and T1W images. Two small endometriotic cysts are also seen in the right ovary which show fluid-fluid levels on T2W image and are hyperintense on the T1W image.

not show any evidence of restricted diffusion on DWI, however, cellular fibromas may show some restriction. However, ADC measurements in the solid component may be low, possibly due to the lower mean ADCs in benign fibrous tumors associated with dense fibrous stromal proliferation. No signal increase is observed on DWI, despite their low ADCs, probably as a consequence of the T2 blackout effect. Ovarian torsion can occur with fibromas leading to infarction and necrosis. Typically fibromas are benign tumors and can be surgically excised.[2] Nevertheless, some fibromas and thecomas in this group may show restricted diffusion. For instance, functioning thecomas and cellular fibromas may show high SI on DWI and relatively low ADCs (***see* Fig. 4**), due to their relatively high cellularity.[35-37]

Thecomas contain lipid rich thecal cells. *Fibrothecomas*, as the name suggests, contain both thecal cells and fibrous tissue. These tumors are much rarer than fibromas and can present with hormonal features of excess estrogen. They do not have distinct US or CT features but as compared to fibromas, may be more hyperintense on T2W images and may show a greater degree of enhancement.

The differential diagnosis of these tumors is similar to that of Brenner tumors as discussed above.

Sclerosing stromal tumor is a rare benign tumor, which is more commonly seen in young adolescent girls, who present with pelvic pain and menstrual irregularity. On US, this neoplasm may mimic a malignant ovarian tumor, as it may be seen as a unilateral solid mass with multiple small hypoechoic cleft-like areas, or a multilocular mass with irregular septae may be seen with intratumoral vascularity. On MRI, it is seen as a solid heterogeneous tumor which is iso- to hyperintense on T2WI, with a spoke-wheel pattern. Dynamic contrast-enhanced (DCE) MRI shows early and avid peripheral contrast uptake, with centripetal progression on late images.[48]

Steroid cell tumors and Leydig cell tumors are other pure stromal tumors which are very rare and often manifest as virilizing tumors of the ovary.

OVARIAN TORSION

Ovarian torsion is the twisting of an ovary on its ligamentous supports resulting in a compromised blood supply. *Adnexal torsion* is a term that is inclusive of torsion of the ovary, the fallopian tube or both. Simultaneously, ovarian and tubal torsion has been shown to occur in upto 60% of cases of adnexal torsion.

Pathophysiology

Ovarian torsion proceeds in a stepwise manner. In the *early phase*, twisting of the vascular pedicle leads to the compromise of the low pressure venous system and lymphatic system first, which causes edema and enlargement of the ovary. In the *later phase*, the arterial circulation also gets compromised causing ischemia and hemorrhagic necrosis.

In more than 50% cases, an underlying mass acts as a lead point for the torsion. The mass can be a functional ovarian cyst (most common—17% of torsed ovaries), benign ovarian neoplasms (of which most common is dermoid cyst, others can be a fibroma or cystadenoma) or a malignant ovarian neoplasm—both primary and metastatic.[49] Even extraovarian masses like a paraovarian cyst or hydrosalpinx can lead to adnexal torsion.

A normal ovary may also undergo torsion, and this is seen more frequently in the younger, adolescent age group, and has been attributed to developmental anomalies like long pelvic ligaments, mobile fallopian tube or mesosalpinx. The right ovary is more likely to torse as compared to the left, which has been attributed to the protective effect of the sigmoid colon on the left.

Clinical Features

Although torsion can occur at any age, it is seen to occur commonly in women of reproductive age, with approximately 20% cases occurring in pregnant women.[48] This could be due to the fact that both, physiological and pathologic ovarian masses, occur more commonly in this age group. Clinically, the patients present with nonspecific acute lower abdominal pain, with associated nausea, vomiting, low grade fever, and moderate leukocytosis. There may be a palpable, tender mass in the lower abdomen.

The clinical differential diagnoses include acute appendicitis, renal colic, diverticulitis, pelvic inflammatory disease (PID), rupture of corpus luteum or hemorrhagic cyst, etc.[50] Sometimes patients may present with repeated attacks of abrupt onset pain with intervening asymptomatic intervals, which occurs due to episodic torsion and detorsion.

Imaging Features

On imaging, the findings will vary depending on the phase in which the patient presents. US is often the first line imaging modality in a case of suspected ovarian torsion. In the early phase, the ovary is seen to be enlarged (>20 cc in volume, or a single maximum diameter >4 cm in premenopausal women), often lying in unusual locations—in the midline, in the pouch of Douglas or anteriorly **(Fig. 35A)**. The enlarged ovary shows hyperechoic stroma, with peripherally placed follicles (due to the follicles being pushed to the periphery by the edematous stroma). The follicles show 1–2 mm thick, hyperechoic margins—the *"follicular ring sign"* which has been described as a specific feature for torsion, and occurs due to edema and hemorrhage in the walls of the follicles. It is better visualized on transvaginal than transabdominal scans **(Fig. 35B)**.[51] When present, an associated mass, the cause of the torsion, can also be identified **(Figs. 36 and 37)**. In later stages, an infarcted or necrotic ovary may be seen as a heterogeneous mass with complete loss of architecture **(Figs. 38A and B)** real-time transvaginal probe tenderness can be elicited.

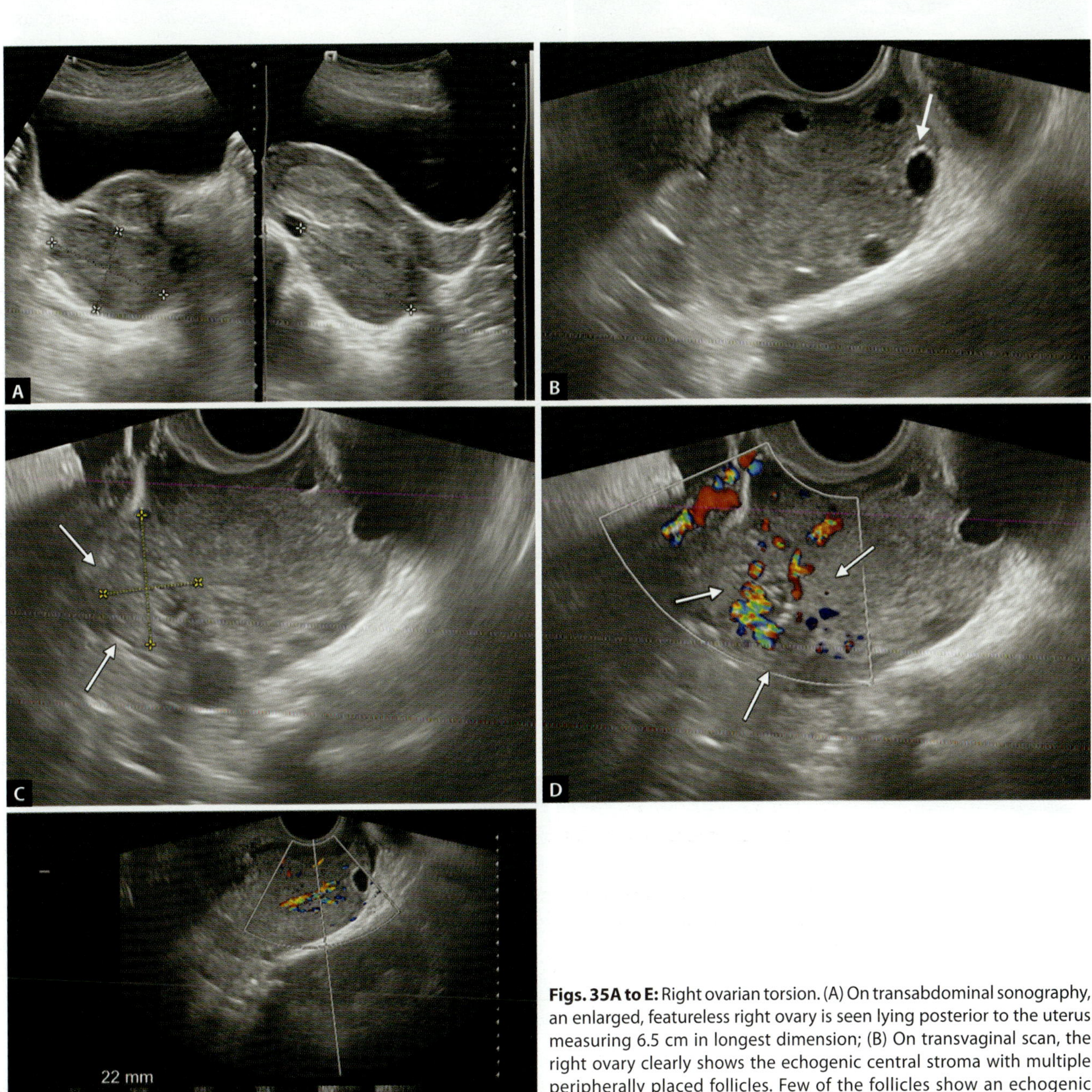

Figs. 35A to E: Right ovarian torsion. (A) On transabdominal sonography, an enlarged, featureless right ovary is seen lying posterior to the uterus measuring 6.5 cm in longest dimension; (B) On transvaginal scan, the right ovary clearly shows the echogenic central stroma with multiple peripherally placed follicles. Few of the follicles show an echogenic rim—"the follicular ring sign" (arrow). Small amount of adjacent fluid is seen. The twisted pedicle seen on gray scale (C) and Doppler (D) as a soft tissue density mass adjacent to the torsed ovary with swirling color flow within—"whirlpool sign" (arrows); (E) Color Doppler in the torsed ovary shows only arterial signal.

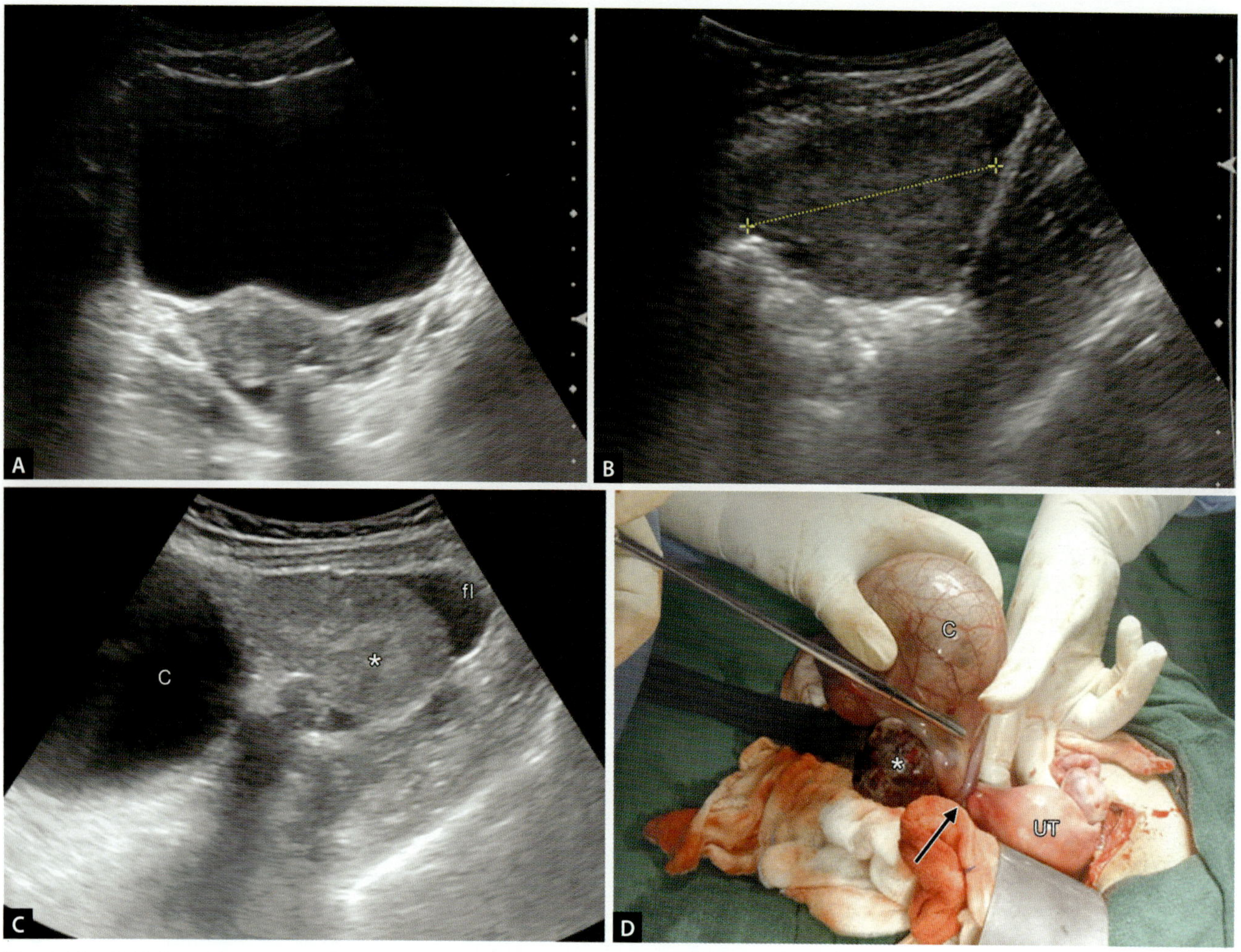

Figs. 36A to D: Right ovarian torsion with adjacent paraovaian cyst. A 19-year-old girl presenting with pain in right iliac fossa (RIF). Transabdominal ultrasound of pelvis (A) shows the normal uterus and left ovary. An enlarged superficially placed right ovary is seen in the RIF (B) measuring 5 cm in maximum diameter, with an echogenic groundglass stroma with few peripherally placed follicles. Longitudinal scan in the RIF shows the torsed ovary (*) with a clear, cystic mass superiorly (C); On surgery (D) the discolored, enlarged ovary is seen with its twisted pedicle (arrow) and the paraovarian cyst (C). (UT: uterus; fl; free fluid).

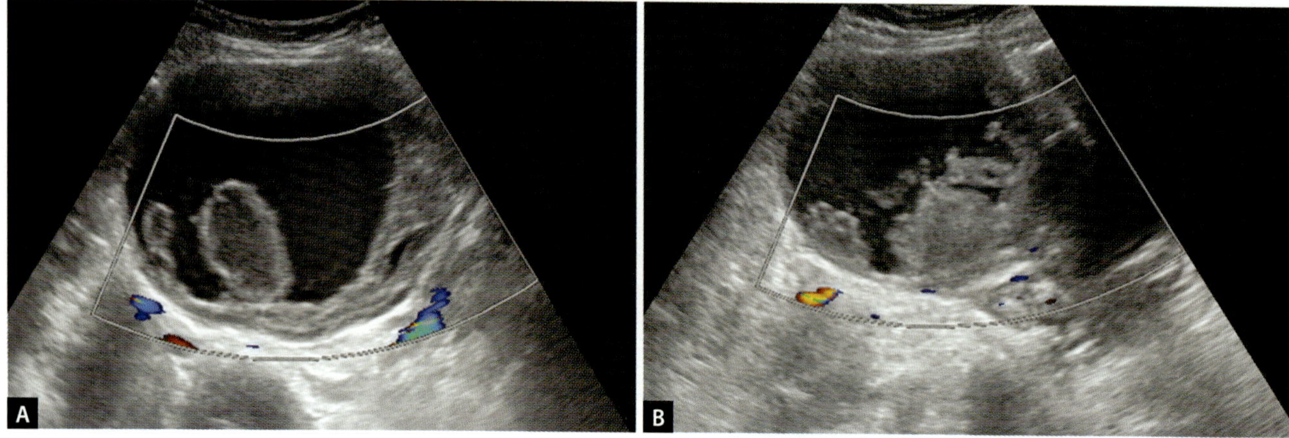

Figs. 37A and B: Transabdominal ultrasound scans show torsed hemorrhagic cyst of right ovary with thick walls and no color flow. Retracted clots and debris seen within the cyst.

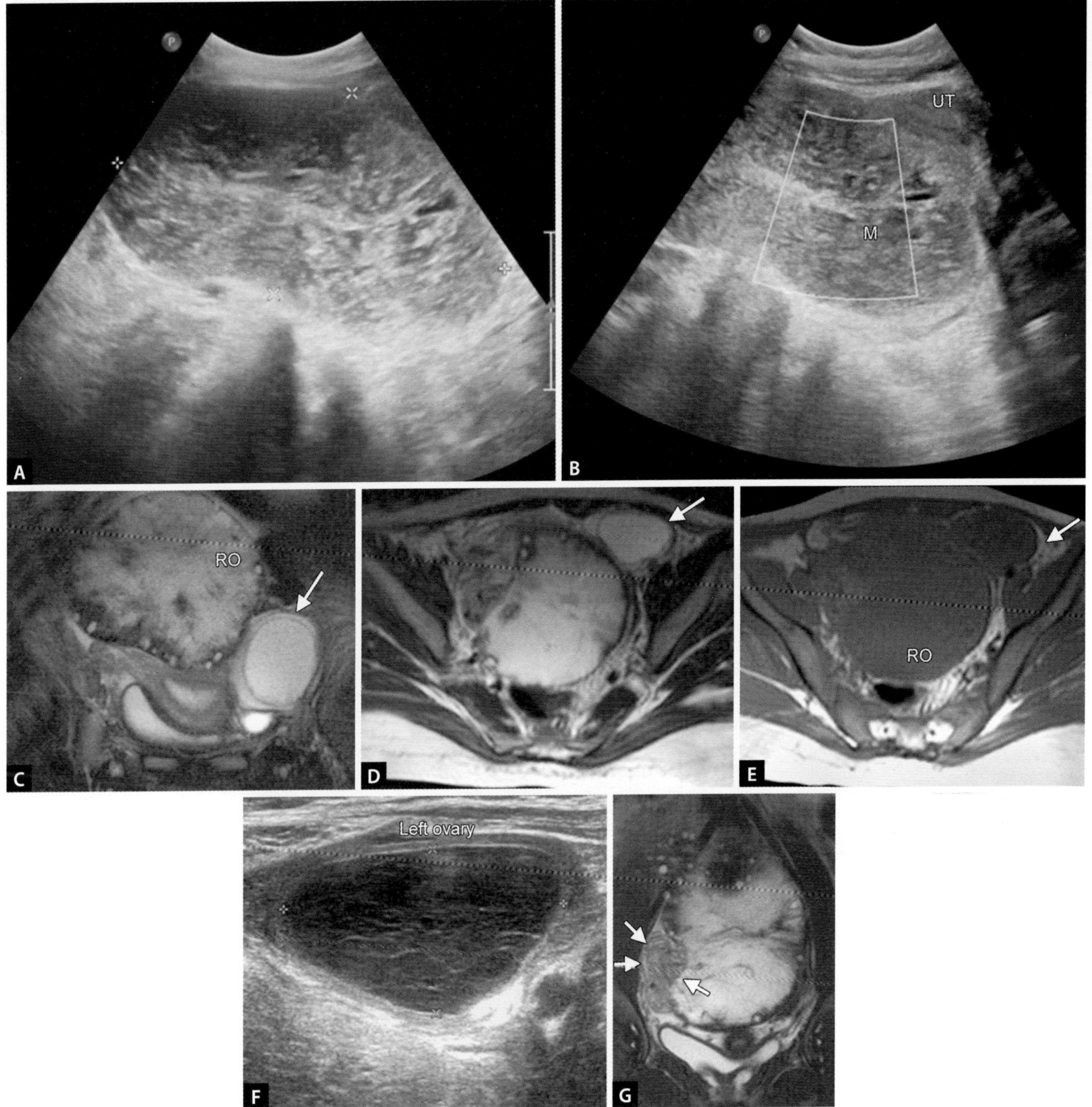

Figs. 38A to G: Right ovarian torsion—late stage with a left hemorrhagic cyst. Transabdominal ultrasound (A) in a 17-year-old girl with acute pain lower abdomen shows a markedly enlarged right ovary (measures 14 cm maximum dimension) with a heterogeneous internal echotexture and no flow on color Doppler (B) T2-weighted (T2W) coronal (C) and axial (D) MR images show a markedly enlarged, centrally placed right ovary with hyperintense stroma and multiple peripheral follicles (RO). The left ovary shows a hemorrhagic cyst appearing homogeneously hyperintense on the T2W images (arrows). Both appear hypointense on T1W image; (E) The characteristic internal "fish-net" appearance is better seen on a high frequency, transabdominal ultrasound (F) as the haemorrhagic cyst is superficially placed; (G) T2W coronal MR image taken more posteriorly shows the adjacent twisted pedicle (arrows) (RO = torsed right ovary; UT = uterus).

Identification of the twisted pedicle adjacent to the torsed ovary, although difficult to identify, is a specific sign for torsion. It is seen as a "*target sign*" with a central hyperechoic area with multiple concentric rings around it on cross-section, and an ellipsoid or tubular mass with heterogeneous echotexture in the longitudinal section. The "*whirlpool sign*" is seen on Doppler, when swirling vessels are seen within the twisted pedicle **(Figs. 35C and D)**.[52]

On Doppler, flow in the ovary is variable depending on the degree of vascular obstruction, intermittent torsion and presence of dual blood supply of ovary (from the ovarian and uterine artery). Abnormal Doppler flow has been reported in 35–93% of patients in many studies **(Fig. 35E)**, who have pathologically proven torsion.[50] As the flow patterns are assessed qualitatively, rather than quantitatively, it is difficult to generalize results.[53] However, it is important to remember that the presence of arterial or venous flow, does not exclude the diagnosis of ovarian torsion. Additionally, the lack of color can also be due to technical factors (especially in a transabdominal scan), and does not necessarily mean that the ovary is nonviable.

Ultrasound has a reported sensitivity of almost 100% and specificity of 97%, if there is an enlarged ovary with absent blood flow.[54]

As the clinical picture is one of nonspecific acute abdomen, a CT may often be done as first imaging investigation. MRI is not a primary imaging modality in a suspected case of torsion, but it can be helpful if sonographic findings of torsion are indeterminate. On both, CT and MRI, ovarian torsion can be seen as an enlarged ovary with or without an underlying mass and a twisted pedicle. The uterus is often deviated to the side of the torsion. The enlarged edematous ovary with peripheral follicles is best seen on contrast-enhanced CT or on fast spin-echo T2-weighted MRI **(Figs. 38A to F)**. On noncontrast CT, hemorrhagic infarction is seen as a high-density ovarian hematoma with an HU value ranging between 50 HU and 100 HU, and on T1W fat suppressed MRI, a hyperintense rim of the hematoma can be seen within an enlarged ovary **(Figs. 39A and B)**.[50] Associated free fluid and fat stranding is often seen. An underlying lead point can be identified.

Multiplanar CT reformations or MRI acquisitions can depict the twisted pedicle better as the helical configuration

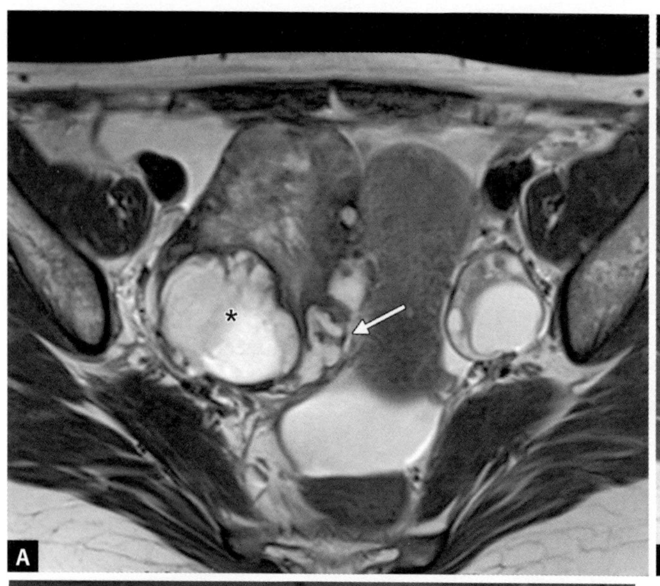

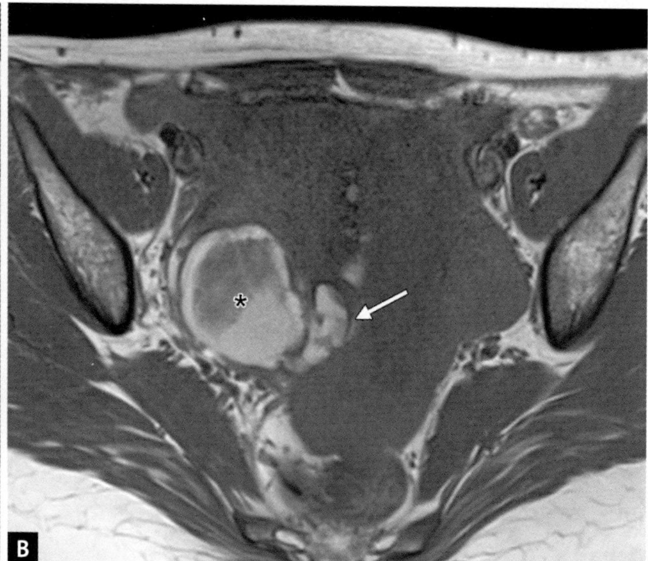

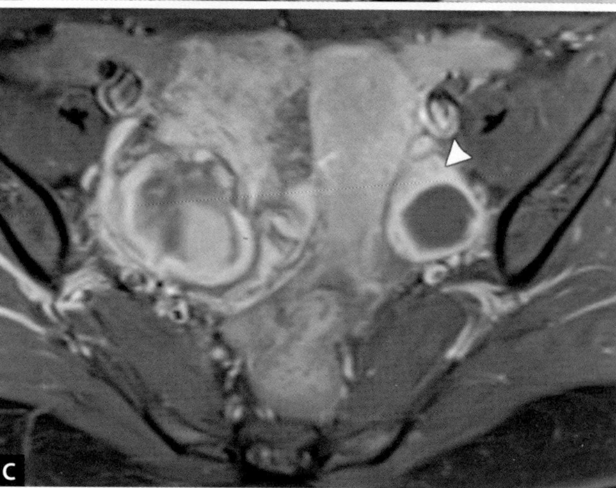

Figs. 39A to C: T2W axial (A) MR image shows a markedly enlarged right ovary with few peripheral follicles and a hyperintense central stroma. An ovarian hematoma is seen as an irregular, well-defined mass within the ovary appearing hyperintense on T2W and T1W MR image (B). Associated hematosalpinx seen medially as a tubular structure hyperintense on T2- and T1W images (arrow); (C) Gadolinium-enhanced T1W MRI with fat saturation shows patchy irregular enhancement of the afollicular stroma in the torsed right ovary. Left ovary (arrowhead) shows normal enhancement with a follicular cyst within.

of the broad ligament containing the vascular pedicle and fallopian tube can be better seen on the sagittal or coronal planes **(Fig. 38G)**.

On contrast-enhanced CT and MRI, the torsed ovary may show an abnormal enhancement pattern **(Fig. 39C)**. As the ovarian ischemia progresses to infarction, there may be minimal or absent enhancement. However, as mentioned before, the presence of enhancement does not exclude torsion.

Differential Diagnosis

The differential diagnosis for ovarian torsion is long and includes ectopic pregnancy, hemorrhagic corpus luteum cyst, massive ovarian edema, hyperstimulated ovaries, oophoritis, PID, necrotic metastases, and nonepithelial primary ovarian tumors. Absence of a twisted pedicle and/or presence of a normal enhancement decreases the possibility of ovarian torsion. Sometimes torsion of a pedunculated subserosal or broad ligament fibroid may mimic ovarian torsion. Identification of both the ovaries separate from the torsed, infarcted fibroid can rule out ovarian torsion.

Management

The treatment of choice for ovarian torsion is laparoscopic untwisting of the adnexa with resection of any underlying cystic lesion. It has been found that ovaries can remain viable up to 36 hours after twisting. Multiple studies have suggested that even nonviable looking ovaries may retain ovarian function following detorsion and so oophorectomy can be avoided in majority of women. Postoperative follow-up with US has shown that over 80% of patients had a normal follicular development after detorsion.[55,56]

MASSIVE OVARIAN EDEMA

It is rare condition in which there is a marked, tumor-like enlargement of one (or rarely both) ovaries due to accumulation of edema fluid in the ovarian stroma. The right ovary is more commonly involved than the left. The etiology could be due to a partial or intermittent torsion with obstruction of venous and lymphatic supply, sparing the arterial supply, or there may be an underlying stromal proliferation complicated by torsion. It is seen in preadolescent girls, women undergoing ovulation induction or during pregnancy. Patients present with acute or intermittent lower abdominal pain of long duration. Sometimes abnormal uterine bleeding and features of masculinization may be seen due to elevated levels of androgens.

Imaging Features

On imaging, the ovary is markedly enlarged with a mean maximum diameter of 11.5 cm (range 5–40 cm) with a multicystic appearance. On US, the ovary is seen as a hypoechoic, hypovascular solid mass-like lesion. There is presence of central increased ovarian stroma, and multiple follicles arranged in the peripheral cortex with internal vascularity on color Doppler.[57] MRI shows a hypo- to isointense signal on T1W and markedly hyperintense signal on T2W images, with enhancement on postcontrast scans.[58] Long-standing ovarian edema may lead to *ovarian fibromatosis* in which case US will show a markedly hypoechoic mass, with hypointense mass on both T1 and T2W MR images.[59]

PELVIC INFLAMMATORY DISEASE

Pelvic inflammatory disease includes all upper genital tract infections including cervicitis, endometritis, salpingitis, pyosalpinx, oophoritis, TOA, and peritonitis.

Etiopathogenesis

The most frequent cause of PID is an ascending lower genital tract infection, by direct upward extension from the vagina to the cervix, uterine cavity, followed by the fallopian tubes and ovaries, and, finally, to the peritoneal cavity. Less commonly, it may occur by hematogenous spread or extension from adjacent organs. The common causative organisms are the sexually transmitted microorganisms such as *Chlamydia trachomatis, Neisseria gonorrhoeae, Mycoplasma genitalium,* and gram-negative bacteria. Mixed infections are seen in a large number of cases. Tuberculosis and actinomycosis are more often associated with chronic PID.

Acute PID of the adnexal region may manifest as isolated inflammation of one or both fallopian tubes—*salpingitis*, obstructed tube filled with pus; *pyosalpinx*, isolated inflammation of one or both ovaries; *oophoritis*, or more commonly a combined inflammation of the tube and ovary, forming a *tubo-ovarian mass*. Associated *endometritis* and *peritonitis* is often seen. Further progression of infection and inflammation results in the formation of a complex cystic and solid mass with complete destruction of the normal adnexal architecture—the *TOA*.

Clinical Features

Pelvic inflammatory disease is commonly seen in young women with a history of a prior uterine procedure, presence of intrauterine contraceptive device (IUCD) or history of multiple sexual partners.[60] Clinically, patients present with lower abdominal pain, fever, vaginal discharge, dyspareunia, leukocytosis, and other vague constitutional symptoms.

Imaging Features

In *salpingitis*, the inflamed tubes may be seen as thickened (more than 10 mm), tortuous structures with increased color flow due to hyperemia on US and marked enhancement on CT and MRI. *Pyosalpinx* is seen as a tortuous, thick-walled, tubular structure with low level internal echoes representing pus **(Fig. 40)**, with incomplete septae on longitudinal section or a "cog-wheel" appearance on cross-section due to protrusion of mucosa into the lumen. Doppler evaluation shows increased vascularity in the thickened walls and septae. On MRI, the internal contents of a pyosalpinx show an intermediate SI on T1WI and high SI on T2WI. MRI can help in the differentiation of pyosalpinx from hematosalpinx, as hematosalpinx will not show wall thickening and will show high or variable SI on T1W MR images because of the presence of blood products. On CT, the internal contents are usually higher than water density. Adjacent inflammatory fat stranding and free or loculated fluid in the peritubal region and/or the cul-de-sac are often present.

It is rare for *oophoritis* to occur in isolation, but if so, it is seen as enlarged unilateral or bilateral ovaries with hyperemia, and associated adjacent inflammatory changes.

A *tubo-ovarian mass* is seen as a lobulated, solid or complex cystic-solid mass with increased color flow signals on Doppler interrogation. It is not possible to identify the tubes or ovaries separately **(Figs. 41A and B)**. A *TOA* has a variable appearance on sonography. Typically, it is seen as a unilocular or multilocular complex cystic-solid mass with irregular borders and thickened wall, with internal debris or fluid-debris level within the cystic component. Color Doppler shows peripheral vascularity and allows distinction of fluid from solid areas **(Figs. 42 and 43)**. Probe tenderness on US is often elicited. On CT, a complex cystic solid mass with marked enhancement of walls and septae can be seen. Presence of air within the cystic component is

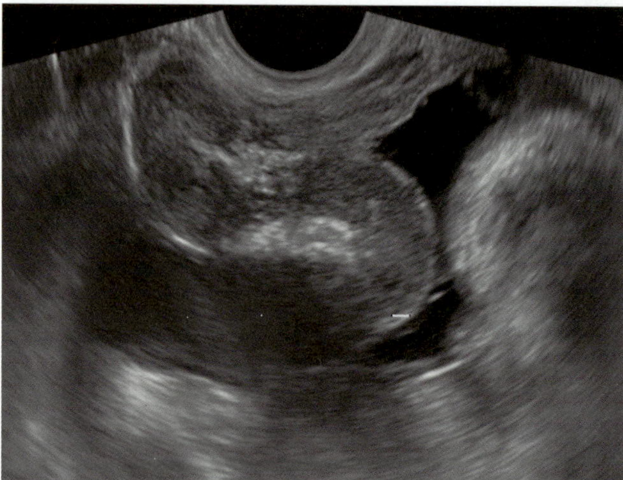

Fig. 40: Pyosalpinx. Transvaginal US shows a convoluted, tubular structure with low level internal echoes and thick walls seen in right adnexal region, with adjacent free fluid.

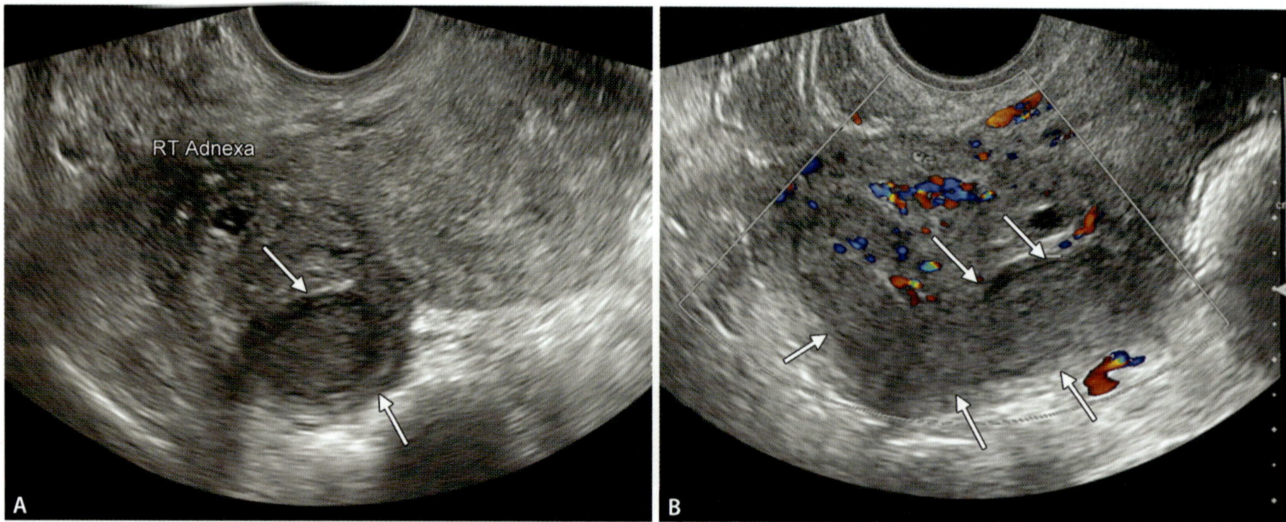

Figs. 41A and B: Tubo-ovarian mass. Transvaginal ultrasound transverse (A) and longitudinal Doppler (B) scans show an ill-defined hypoechoic solid mass in the right adnexal region, adherent to the uterus. A focal area of low level echoes represents the pus-filled fallopian tube (arrows). Scattered color signals are seen in the inflammatory solid mass and walls of the pyosalpinx.

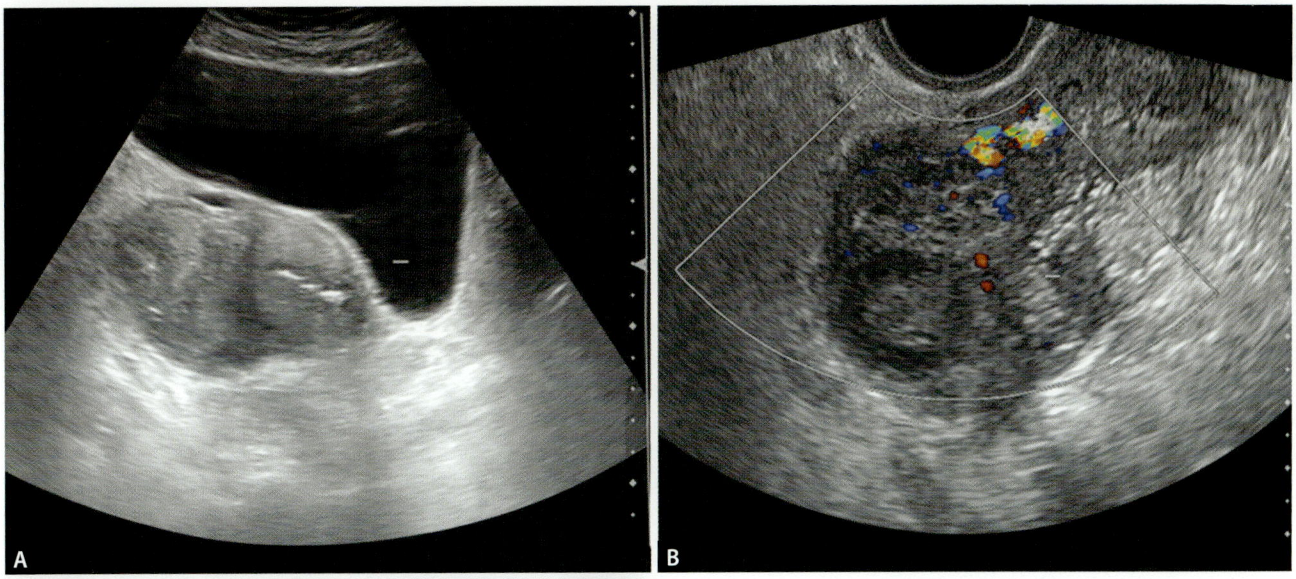

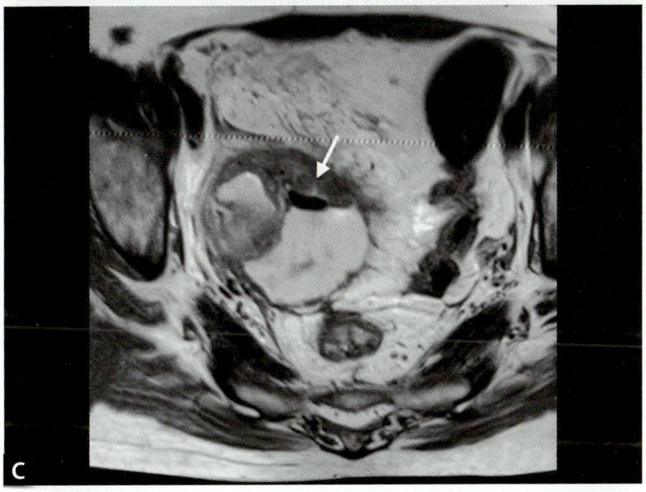

Figs. 42A to C: Tubo-ovarian abscess (TOA). US scan: transabdominal sonography (A) and transvaginal scan (B). A predominantly solid right adnexal mass adherent to the uterus (with IUCD *in situ*) and scattered vascularity. (C) T2W axial MR image shows the heterogeneous intensity of the adnexal mass with hyperintense abscess. Adjacent inflammatory stranding is seen. Presence of air-fluid level (arrow) confirms the diagnosis of a TOA.

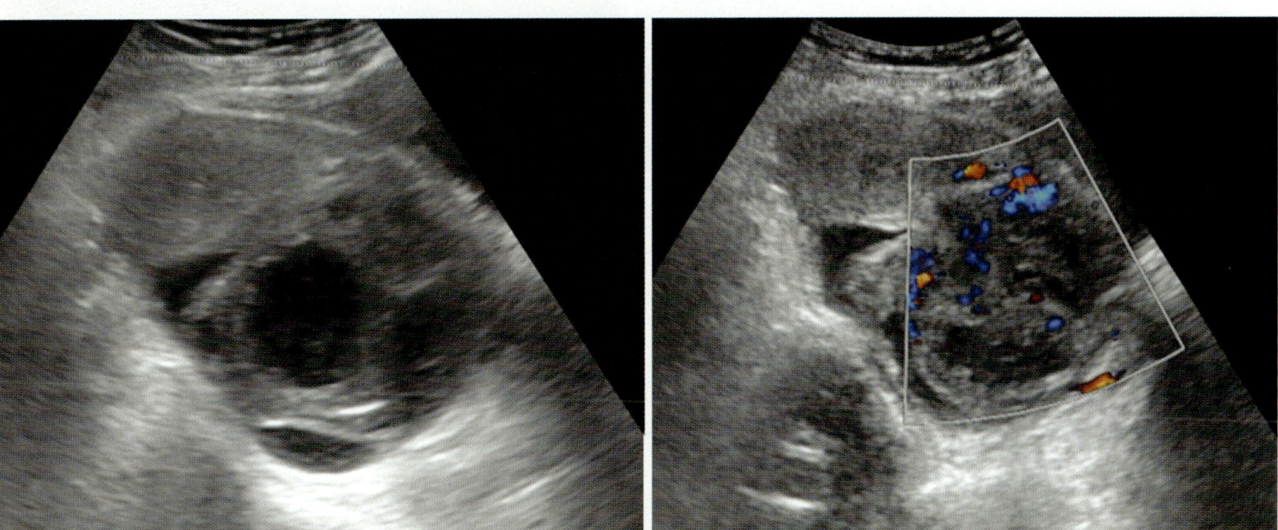

Figs. 43A and B

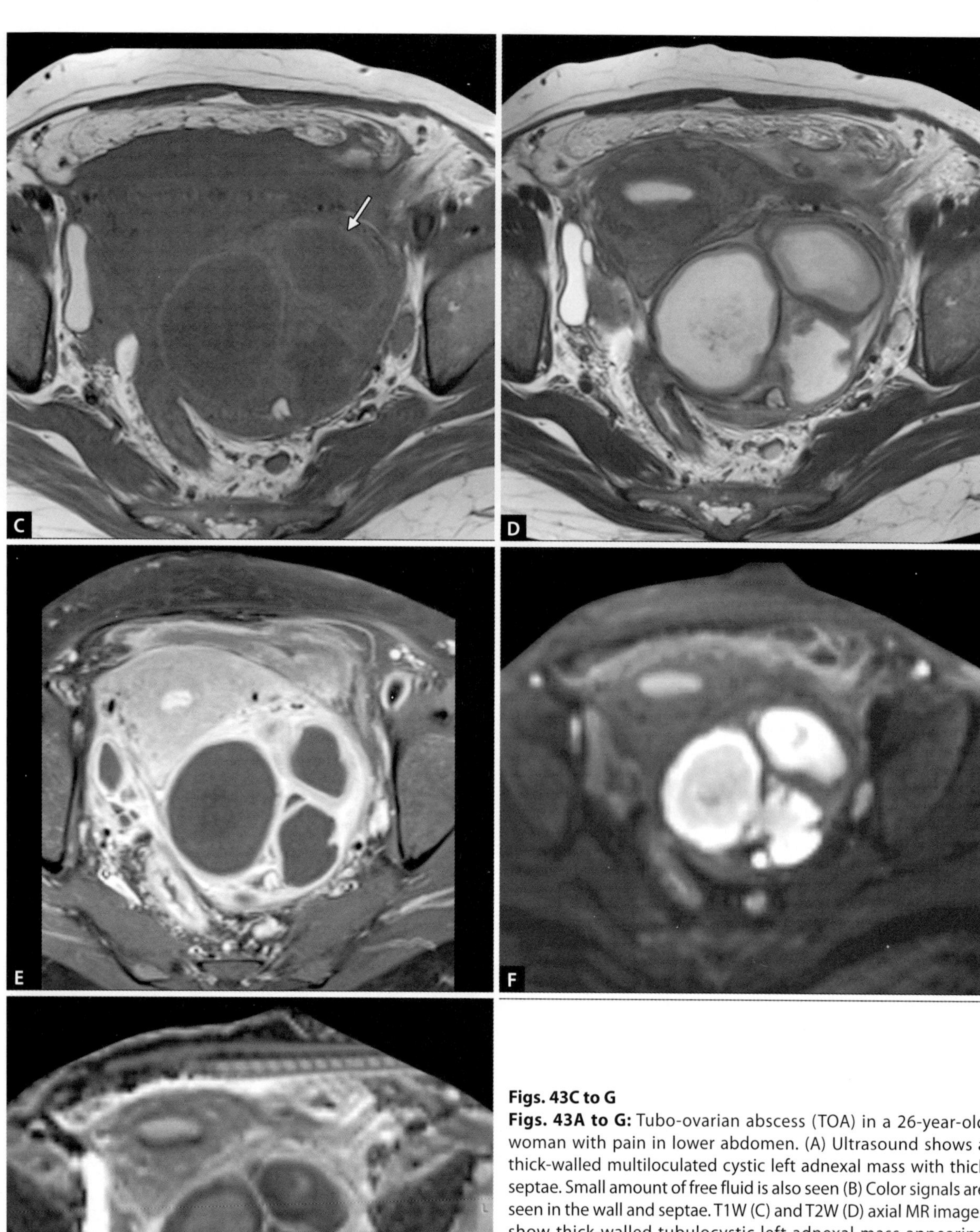

Figs. 43C to G

Figs. 43A to G: Tubo-ovarian abscess (TOA) in a 26-year-old woman with pain in lower abdomen. (A) Ultrasound shows a thick-walled multiloculated cystic left adnexal mass with thick septae. Small amount of free fluid is also seen (B) Color signals are seen in the wall and septae. T1W (C) and T2W (D) axial MR images show thick-walled tubulocystic left adnexal mass appearing iso- to hypointense on T1W and hyperintense on T2W images. A T1 hyperintense rim is seen along the inner walls of the cystic areas representing granulation tissue. (E) Intense enhancement is seen in the wall and septae and in the surrounding soft tissues. Culture of pus confirmed a tubercular TOA. (F) Axial DWI at b = 800 sec/mm^2 and corresponding apparent diffusion coefficient (ADC) map (G) shows evidence of restricted diffusion in the cystic spaces (bright on DWI, and dark on the ADC map) with a low ADC value of $<0.6 \times 10^{-3}$ mm^2/sec due to purulent material.

best seen on CT and is the most specific sign of an abscess, however, it is unusual in a TOA. On MRI, the abscess fluid has a variable signal depending on the viscosity and protein concentration. It is heterogeneous and usually low (equal to muscle) on T1WI, high on fat suppressed T1WI and T2WI. A rim of hyperintensity maybe seen along the inner margin of the wall on T1WI, which is due to a layer of granulation tissue with focal areas of hemorrhage **(Figs. 43C and D)**. On postcontrast CT and MRI, enhancement of the thickened irregular wall, septations and adjacent inflammation is a hallmark of PID **(Fig. 43E)**. Restricted diffusion with low ADC values is seen in the pus-filled abscess cavities **(Figs. 43F and G)**.

Specific Pelvic Inflammatory Disease

Tuberculosis is a very common cause of chronic pelvic inflammatory disease (PID) in our country. Infection generally spreads from an extragenital source. It can be hematogenous, via lymphatic vessels or from the peritoneal cavity. Tubercular PID often shows bilateral adnexal involvement with salpingitis, TOAs, endometritis, peritoneal spread in the form of free, and/or loculated ascites, peritoneal, mesenteric, and omental thickening. It can mimic peritoneal carcinomatosis from ovarian carcinoma **(Figs. 44 and 45)**. It is important to remember that CA-125 levels may also be raised in tubercular PID, although not as high as in malignant carcinomatosis.

Associated lymphadenopathy, sometimes necrotic, can be seen. Generally, tubercular adnexal masses are not tender on US probe pressure. Dense adhesions with uterus and adjacent organs can occur. Calcifications maybe seen in the adnexal lesions and/or in the lymph nodes, best visualized on CT. Florid enhancement of the adnexal masses and adjacent tissues on CT and MRI, is characteristic of tubercular infection.

Actinomycosis is an uncommon pelvic infection usually seen in the presence of an intrauterine device. The findings mimic tuberculosis. The adnexal mass in actinomycosis is predominantly a solid lesion with low SI on T2-weighted images. Cystic elements are less common. There is diffuse infiltration of the uterus, adnexa, and pelvic muscles with loss of fascial planes. The presence of an IUCD further corroborates the diagnosis. Identification of sulfur granules in the aspirate is diagnos is of actinomycotic infection.[61]

Xanthogranulomatous inflammation (XGI) can also rarely involve the female genital tract. It is an uncommon form of chronic inflammation in which there is destruction of the tissues of affected organs, which are replaced by lipid-containing macrophages and lymphocytes, plasma cells, multinucleated giant cells, and neutrophils. It is more commonly seen to affect the kidney and gallbladder. The proposed causes are infection, ineffective antibiotic therapy, endometriosis, abnormality in lipid metabolism or ineffective clearance of bacteria by phagocytes. The uterus is more commonly affected. Adnexal involvement is seen as a complex adnexal mass with multiple internal cystic lesions on US and MRI. The imaging findings are nonspecific, resembling a chronic PID or even a malignant lesion. It is almost impossible to make a diagnosis of XGI on imaging, however the pathological findings show the characteristic xanthogranulomas.[62]

Complications

A common sequela of PID is damage to the fallopian tubes, due to scarring and adhesions within the lumen and in the peritubal fat, which leads to obstruction of the tubes. Tubal damage leads to ectopic pregnancies, hydrosalpinx formation and infertility. About 40–50% of cases of infertility can be attributed to previous PID.[63] There can be formation of peritoneal adhesions which can lead to small or large bowel obstruction, or ureteric obstruction. Peritoneal inclusion cysts can also occur secondary to PID.

Fitz-Hugh-Curtis syndrome is a rare complication of PID that is seen in 1–30% of cases, associated with PID caused by *N. gonorrhoeae* and *C. trachomatis*.[62] It is seen as an inflammation of the peritoneal capsule of the liver and is believed to result from peritoneal spread of pelvic infection along the right paracolic gutter. On CT, an intense enhancement and thickening of the anterior liver capsule is seen with geographic areas of variable perfusion in the subcapsular and periportal locations. Loculated perihepatic fluid may be seen and classic "violin string" adhesions may be found between the liver capsule and the anterior abdominal wall. Associated gallbladder wall thickening can occur.

Differential Diagnosis

Pelvic endometriosis

Endometriomas can mimic ovarian abscesses, hematosalpinx can be difficult to differentiate from pyosalpinx. Associated adhesions can occur in both conditions. At MRI, the presence of T1 hyperintensity within the lesions or in the fallopian tube can help confirm the diagnosis of endometriosis and differentiate it from PID.

Hemorrhagic cysts are common mimics of PID. Clinical manifestations are frequently nonspecific and unhelpful in distinguishing between these entities. Characteristic

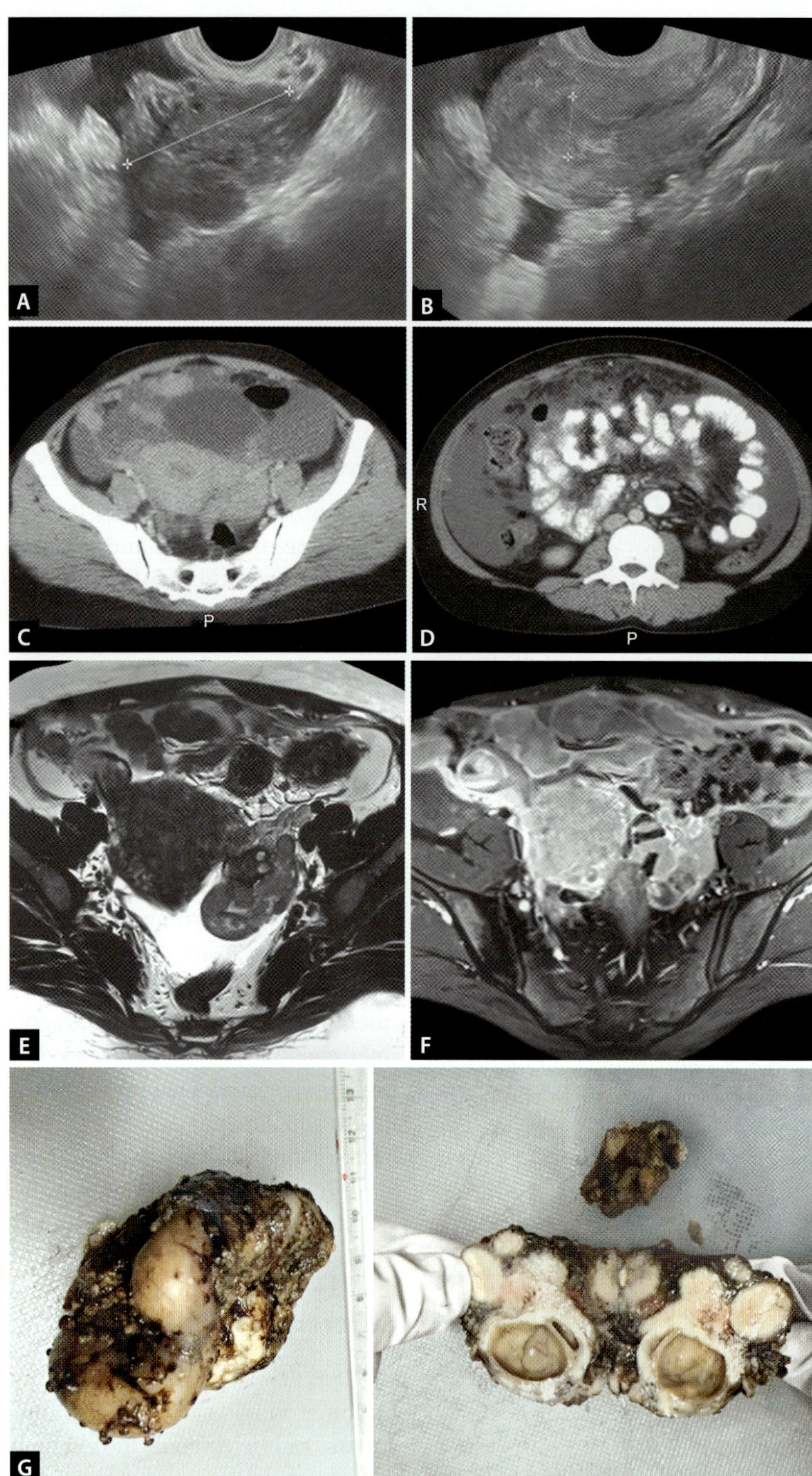

Figs. 44A to G: Tubercular pelvic inflammatory disease (PID). A 35-year-old woman with abdominal distension, loss of weight, and appetite. Transvaginal ultrasound (A and B), axial contrast-enhanced computed tomography (CECT) section pelvis (C) shows an irregular heterogeneous predominently solid mass in left adnexa, with associated ascites. Ill-defined endometrial thickening is seen in the uterus—endometritis. There is peritoneal thickening and omental stranding seen in axial CECT section of abdomen (D) T2W axial MR pelvis (E) shows a predominantly hypointense left adnexal mass with ascites; Contrast-enhanced MRI (F) shows marked enhancement of the mass, uterus, and adjacent tissues; (G) On surgery, the left adnexal mass seen to be a thickened tube wrapped around left ovary with multiple small caseous nodules studding outer surface of mass and peritoneum.

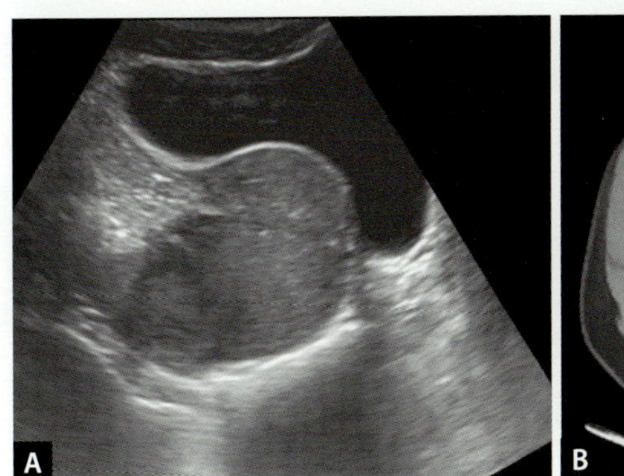

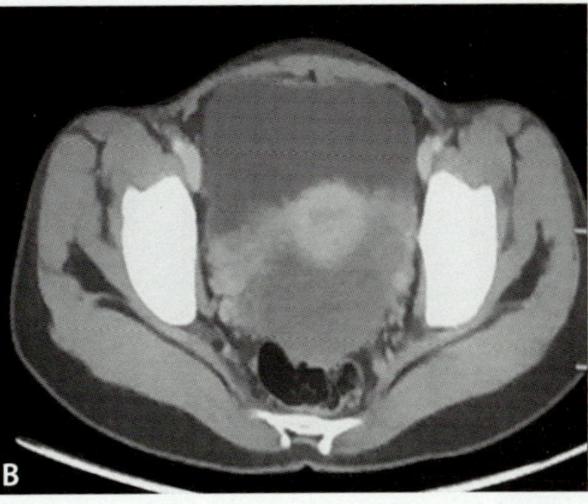

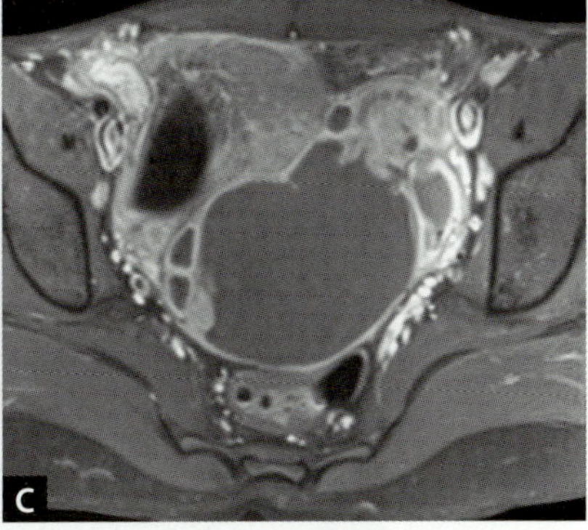

Figs. 45A to C: Tubercular tubo-ovarian abscess in a 16-year-old girl with low-grade fever and constitutional symptoms for 2 months. Transabdominal ultrasound (A); CECT axial scan (B); and CEMR scan (C) through the pelvis show a large abscess involving bilateral ovaries and tubes posterior to the uterus.

features of hemorrhagic cysts include the presence of a unilocular adnexal cyst with a ring of peripheral contrast enhancement and an internal high-attenuation component with or without a fluid-hematocrit level.

Ovarian neoplasms can mimic the complex cystic-solid masses of PID, especially in chronic cases, where peritoneal and mesenteric involvement may also be present.

Ovarian Torsion

Distinguishing features include an enlarged ovary with a diameter of more than 5 cm, a lack of enhancement on contrast administration, and uterine deviation toward the affected side.

Other adjacent inflammatory conditions such as acute appendicitis or diverticulitis can mimic PID. An inflamed pus-filled pelvic appendix maybe impossible to differentiate from a pyosalpinx. The presence of an appendicolith, cecal origin of the tubular structure, and the presence of cecal wall thickening are helpful distinguishing features of appendicitis.

Management

In the absence of complications, PID is generally treated conservatively with a short course of oral antibiotics. However, complicated PID frequently requires hospitalization of patients with intravenous administration of antibiotics, in addition to percutaneous or surgical drainage of pelvic abscesses, if present. Specific PIDs like tubercular or actinomycotic infection have to be treated as per protocol.

EXTRAOVARIAN DISEASE

TUBAL PATHOLOGY

Tubal dilatation/Hydrosalpinx

Tubal dilatation results from an accumulation of secretions when the tube is occluded at its distal end, fimbrial/ampullary end, or both ends, with dilatation of the proximal portion of the tube. Hydrosalpinx is used as a generic term for a dilated tube. It can contain serous fluid, blood, or pus may accumulate, depending on the cause of the dilatation. *Serous hydrosalpinx* occurs when the tube gets occluded by postinflammatory or postsurgical adhesions, or due to tubal ligation and contains serous fluid. A fallopian tube distended with blood is referred to as *hematosalpinx*, is seen commonly with endometriosis, in an ectopic tubal pregnancy, in obstructive developmental lesions in association with hematometra and rarely in association with a tubal malignancy. A tube filled with pus is referred to as *pyosalpinx* which is commonly associated with acute or chronic PID.

Clinical Features

Clinically, the patient may present with lower abdominal pain or with symptoms of the underlying cause of the tubal dilatation. In others, hydrosalpinx may be incidental finding in an asymptomatic woman.

Imaging Features

On imaging, the objective is to first recognize the tubal origin of a cystic mass in the adnexal region, and then to characterize its nature and if possible, the cause. Sonographically, dilated fallopian tubes are seen as tubular, fluid-filled structures that are folded upon themselves to form a C or S shape **(Figs. 40 and 46A)** or, at times, a multilocular mass, in the adnexal region, separate from the uterus and ovary. Incomplete septations, which result from segments of distended tube folding over/adhering to other tubal segments, are a characteristic appearance. Longitudinal folds present in a normal tube may become thickened in the presence of a hydrosalpinx, seen as small round nodules less than 3 mm in size—the characteristic *cogwheel* or *beads on a string* sign appearance when

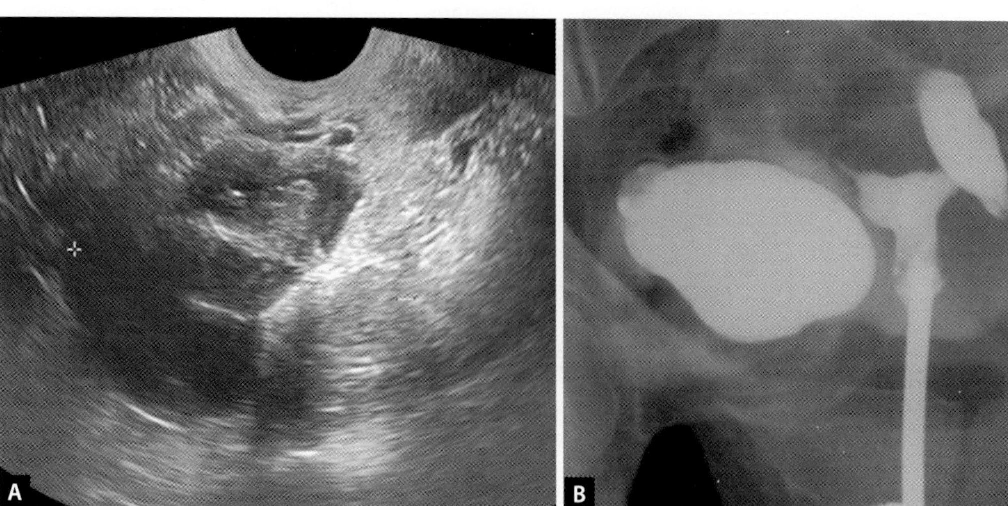

Figs. 46A and B: Hydrosalpinx. TVUS (A) showing fluid-filled, C-shaped tortuous dilated tube with incomplete septation; (B) HSG, in another case, showing both the fallopian tubes to be markedly dilated (right more than left), with no tubal spill.

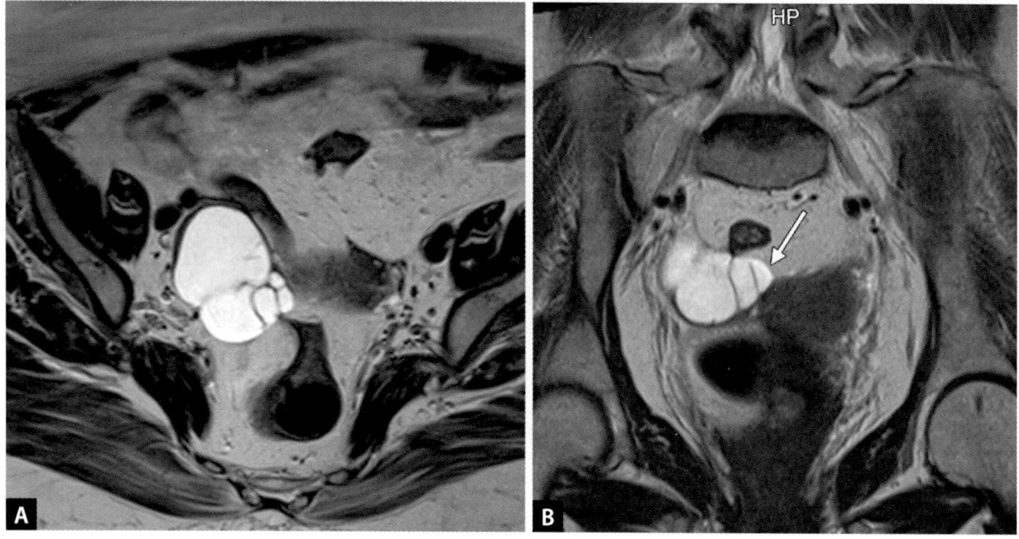

Figs. 47A and B: Hydrosalpinx. T2W axial (A) and coronal (B) MR images show a well-defined multiloculated cystic mass on the axial images which can be identified as a hydrosalpinx on the coronal scan, as the convoluted nature of tube with incomplete septae (arrow) can be well seen.

imaged in cross section (***see* Fig. 40**). The *waist* sign can be seen as indentations on the opposite sides of the wall and is pathognomonic of a hydrosalpinx.[64] A 3D US can depict the tubular nature of the dilated tube better than the 2D examination.

A hysterosalpingogram will show a dilated fallopian tube, filling with contrast and with absence of free spillage. It can be tubular or retort-shaped (**Fig. 46B**).

Multiplanar imaging can be helpful in confirming the tubular nature of an adnexal mass or demonstrating incomplete septations, thus confirming it to originate from the fallopian tube (**Figs. 47A and B**). In case of a complex cystic adnexal mass, it may not be possible to establish the tubular nature by US. MR can help to show the incomplete septations and to identify the separate normal ovary. MR can also assist in determining the etiology of the tubal dilatation. If hydrosalpinx is due to endometriosis, SI characteristics of the tubal fluid are similar to those in endometriomas, i.e. high T1 and low T2 signal intensities (**Figs. 48A and B**). In a patient with adhesions, SI of the dilated tube follows that of simple fluid—low on T1 and high on T2W images.

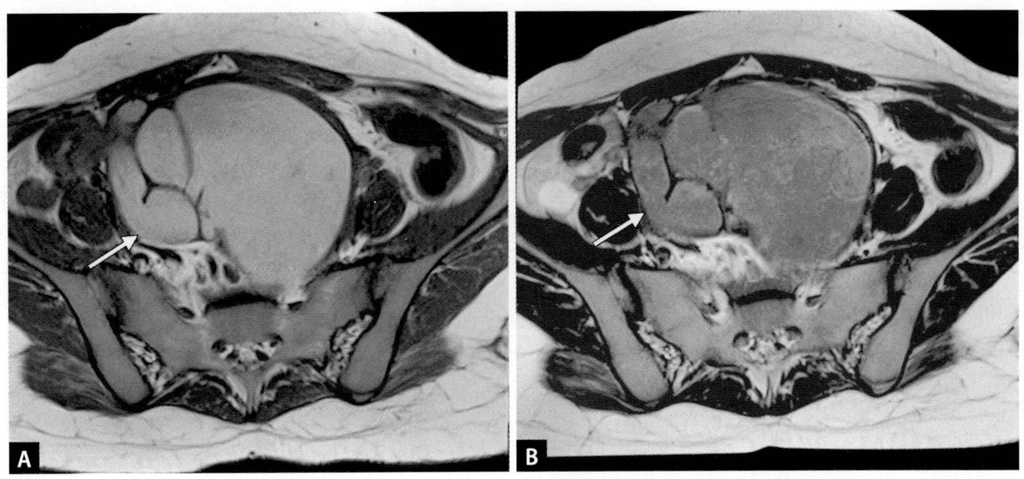

Figs. 48A and B: Hematosalpinx in a case of endometriosis. A dilated tortuous structure with incomplete septations appearing hyperintense on axial T1W MR image (A) and hypointense on T2W MR image (B) consistent with the dilated, blood filled left fallopian tube.

Complications and Differential Diagnosis

Dilated tubes can lead to infertility due to obstruction. They can also undergo torsion. If the tubular nature of the cystic adnexal mass is not recognized, they can be confused with benign cystic neoplasms, PICs, paravarian or functional ovarian cysts. Management will depend on the cause of the tubal dilatation.

Ectopic Pregnancy

A tubal ectopic pregnancy is another very important tubal pathology that presents as an adnexal mass lesion. A detailed discussion of this topic is beyond the scope of this chapter. A few salient features are mentioned here.

The most common site for ectopic pregnancy is the fallopian tubes, occurring in up to 97% of cases of which 75–80% are located in the ampullary region.[65] The ovary, cervix, abdominal cavity, etc. are other less common sites of ectopic pregnancy. The diagnosis is usually reached by a combination of clinical presentation and correlation of last menstrual period, β-hCG levels, and findings on sonography.

The imaging findings will depend on the stage at which examined, i.e. whether there is: (1) unruptured live ectopic, (2) early embryonic demise without rupture, or (3) ruptured ectopic with hemoperitoneum.

In an unruptured live ectopic, the most specific finding for ectopic pregnancy is seen, i.e. presence of a live extrauterine pregnancy showing a fetal pole with cardiac activity. However, it is positive in only 8–26% of ectopic pregnancies on TVS.[66] The next most specific sign is the presence of an extrauterine gestation sac containing a yolk sac, with or without an embryo. The "tubal ring" of ectopic pregnancy is another finding which has been found to be 40–68% sensitive for ectopic pregnancy.[67] The tubal ring represents an extrauterine gestation sac with trophoblastic tissue. The use of color Doppler shows a "ring of fire" pattern and a high-velocity, low-impedance flow which is compatible with placental perfusion. The most important differential diagnosis is from a corpus luteum cyst which is also very vascular and shows a similar appearance on color flow imaging. However, the most common, but less specific finding of an ectopic pregnancy is a complex adnexal mass separate from the ovary which is most often seen in a nonviable ectopic pregnancy. In the case of ruptured ectopic, a hemoperitoneum may be seen along with a complex adnexal mass.

On MRI, a heterogeneous adnexal mass separate from the ovary and/or a hematosalpinx, with or without hemoperitoneum can be seen.

Differential Diagnosis

The important considerations in the differential diagnosis are corpus luteum cyst, hydrosalpinx, endometrioma, or a ruptured hemorrhagic ovarian cyst.

Paraovarian and Paratubal Cysts

Paraovarian and paratubal cysts represent 10–20% of all adnexal masses and most commonly occur in the 3rd to 4th decade. Paraovarian cysts are remnants of the mesonephric (Wolffian) ducts and are seen close to the ovary, whereas paratubal cysts include hydatid cysts of Morgagni (fimbrial cysts), cysts arising from the paramesonephric (MÜllerian) ducts and mesosalpingeal cysts, and are situated a little away from the ovary.[3]

Imaging Features

Paraovarian cysts are unilocular cysts of variable size, with an average diameter of 8 cm at diagnosis, but may reach very large sizes even occupying the whole abdomen. Sonographically, these cysts are round to oval in shape, anechoic with good sound transmission and morphologically indistinguishable from simple functional cysts. A normal ovary seen separately from the cyst is a pointer to a paraovarian cyst **(Fig. 49)**. They may indent the ovary mimicking an intraovarian cyst, but US probe pressure may show separation from ovary. Fimbrial cysts or hydatid cysts of Morgagni can be seen as multiple, small, thin walled, anechoic cysts. Occasionally, their attachment to the fibrial end of tube may become evident in the presence of fluid in the pelvic cavity.

On CT, a round or oval cystic structure is seen close to the ovary, but separate from it. MRI shows the cyst as a well-defined homogeneous structure, with high SI on T2-wieghted images and low SI on T1-weighted images. MRI can clearly depict the independent relationship of the ovary to an adjacent paraovarian cyst **(Figs. 50A and B)**. Complicated cyst (torsion or hemorrhage) may demonstrate high SI on T1-weighted images and have thick walls.

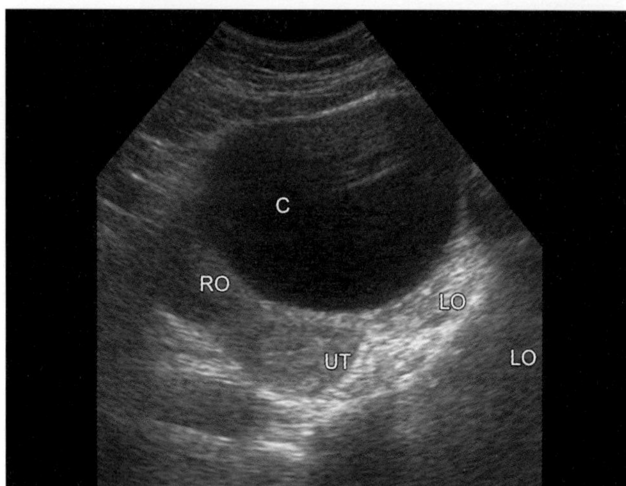

Fig. 49: Paraovarian cyst in a 22-year-old woman with right iliac fossa pain. Transabdominal US image shows a unilocular, thin-walled, cyst (C) adjacent to the right ovary (RO). Both ovaries are seen separately. (UT: uterus; LO: left ovary).

Differential Diagnosis and Complications

Simple paraovarian cysts need to be differentiated from follicular cyst, PIC, simple benign epithelial neoplasm, benign teratoma or a hydrosalpinx. Rarely, these cysts may be complicated by torsion, infection or hemorrhage, in which case they can show thick walls and turbid internal echoes. A complicated paraovarian cyst may resemble an endometrioma, a hemorrhagic cyst or a serous cystadenoma. Malignancy is rare in cysts less than 5 cm. The presence of soft-tissue component within the cyst, which shows vascularity on US, and/or enhancement on contrast-enhanced magnetic resonance imaging (CEMRI) is indicative of a neoplasm.[67]

Management

Simple, asymptomatic paratubal or paraovarian cysts are generally managed conservatively. Surgical removal

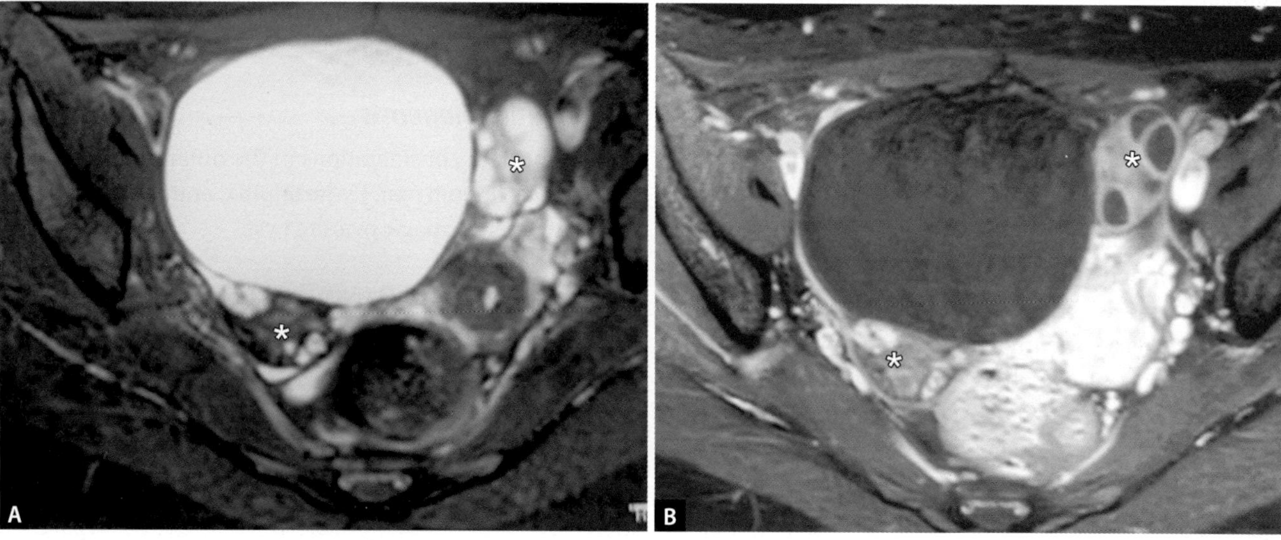

Figs. 50A and B: Paraovarian cyst. T2WFS (A) and T1FSCE (B) axial MR images show a large, simple cyst hyperintense on T2W and hypointense on T1W scans with no enhancing focus. Both the ovaries are seen separately (*).

is indicated if they are symptomatic (persistent pain or pressure symptoms), undergo torsion or appear neoplastic.

Peritoneal Inclusion Cyst

Peritoneal inclusion cysts are also known as cystic mesotheliomas, peritoneal pseudocysts or inflammatory cysts of the peritoneum. They were first described by Mennemeyer and Smith in 1979.[68] They are relatively occurring lesions which are frequently misdiagnosed.

Pathophysiology

The ovary is responsible for secretion of fluid into the peritoneum, contributing to the normally occurring peritoneal fluid. This fluid, in turn, is absorbed by the normal peritoneum. When the peritoneum is damaged, its absorption properties become slower, leading to a decrease in the clearance of the ovarian fluid, which collects in the peritoneal cavity in the form of fluid containing cysts. The development of a PIC, thus depends on the presence of peritoneal adhesions and an active ovary.[69,70]

A PIC maybe a unilocular or multilocular lesion containing clear or yellow-colored serous or gelatinous fluid or sometimes even a hemorrhagic pulp-like material. Histologically, the cyst is lined by one or several layers of mesothelial cells. Although these cells may undergo squamous metaplasia, a PIC does not have any malignant potential.[71]

Clinical Features

Peritoneal inclusion cysts are most commonly seen in premenopausal women with a history of previous abdominal or pelvic surgery, trauma, PID (especially tuberculosis), inflammatory bowel disease or endometriosis.[72] Patients present with chronic or intermittent lower abdominal or pelvic pain, abdominal distension, tenderness, mass, and pressure symptoms like dyspareunia, urinary hesitancy, or constipation. Cancer antigen 125 (CA 125) is usually normal. In 10% cases, these may be detected incidentally in asymptomatic patients.

Imaging Features

On US, they are seen as variable sized (few mm to large masses almost filling the abdominal cavity), multiseptated, cystic structures which are in close contact with the ovaries and uterus. They are frequently anechoic, but sometimes may show internal echoes due to debris or hemorrhage. The ovary may, at times, be completely surrounded by the PIC. Septations may be complete, incomplete, of varying thickness, and maybe nodular or polypoid. Unilocular and multifocal cysts may also be seen. A characteristic feature of these cysts is the irregular shape with projections around the normal structures, conforming to the peritoneal space, which is explained by the fact that these are not true cysts, but collections of fluid within peritoneal adhesions **(Figs. 51A and B)**.

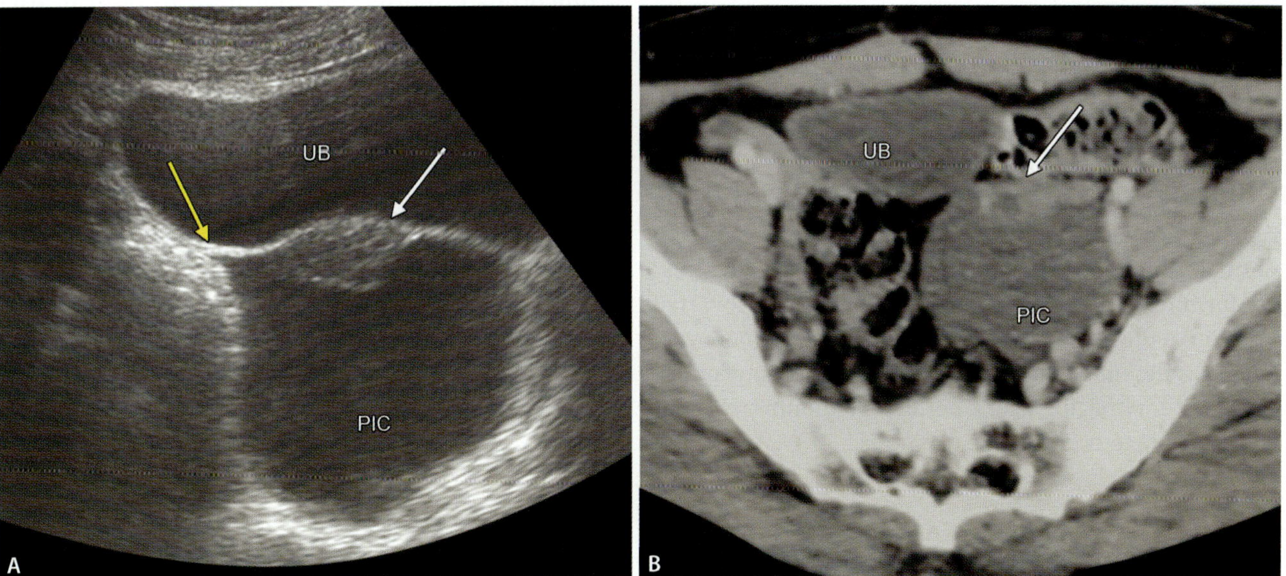

Figs. 51A and B: Peritoneal inclusion cyst in a 32-year-old woman with history of previous pelvic surgery. Transabdominal US (A) and axial CECT pelvis (B) show an anechoic, unilocular cystic lesion behind the bladder. The left ovary is seen to lie within the cyst along its anterior margin (white arrows). US scan shows the angular margins very well (yellow arrow). (UB: urinary bladder; PIC: peritoneal inclusion cyst).

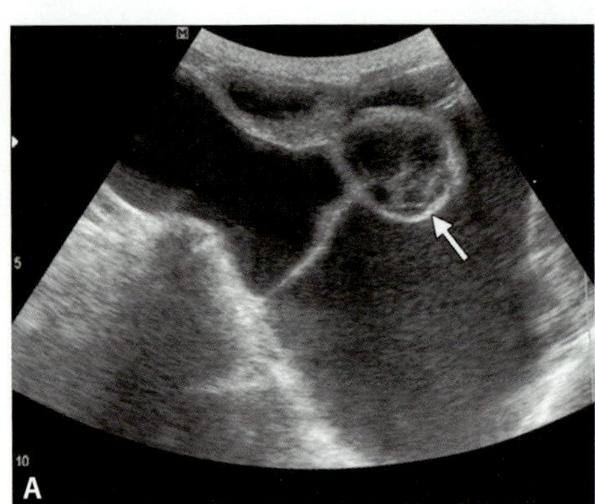

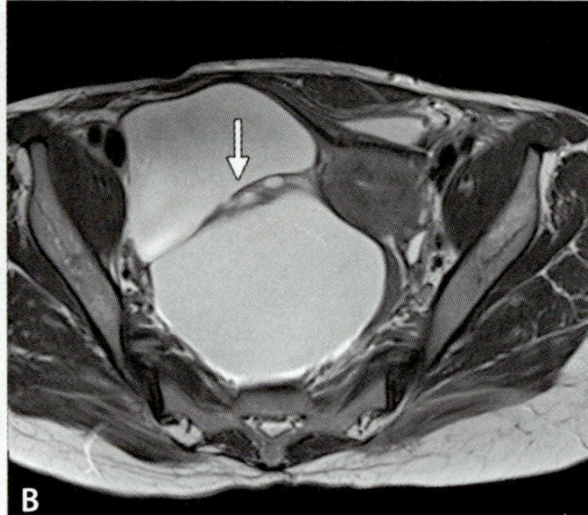

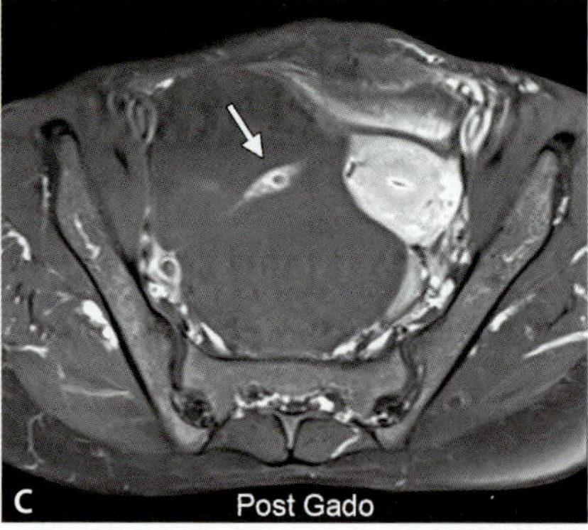

Figs. 52A to C: Peritoneal inclusion cyst in a 35-year-old woman with chronic pelvic pain. She had been treated 3 years back for abdominal tuberculosis. (A) Transabdominal sonogram shows a multiseptated cystic mass in the right adnexal region with thin walls, with the ovary suspended within it. The ovary shows a hemorrhagic corpus luteal cyst (arrow); (B) On T2W MRI done 6 weeks later, the large cystic mass is well seen to the right of the uterus with the ovary within (arrow). The hemorrhagic cyst in the ovary has resolved; (C) CEMR shows contrast uptake by the ovarian tissue within the cyst (arrow).

Computed tomography and MR are useful in defining the exact extent of the lesion and for identifying presence of multiple cysts. Large multiseptated cysts with fluid attenuation can be seen on CT, while MR shows homogeneous fluid SI that is hypointense on T1 and hyperintense on T2W images. If the protein content of the cyst is high or hemorrhage has occurred into the cyst, intermediate to hyperintense T1 signal can be seen. The fluid can be better seen to conform to the shape of the peritoneal cavity with these imaging techniques. On contrast administration, the septations are seen to enhance **(Figs. 52A to C)**.

Differential Diagnosis

Cystic ovarian neoplasms—benign and malignant, functional cysts of the ovary, paraovarian cysts, hydro- or pyosalpinx, lymphangioma, complex loculated ascites, early stages of pseudomyxoma peritonei can all be considered in the differential diagnosis of PICs.

The diagnosis of PICs should be suspected in the right clinical setting, and depends on the presence of normal ipsilateral ovary with surrounding loculated fluid conforming to the peritoneal space. The extra-ovarian location of the lesion and identification of a normal ovary enables a definitive diagnosis. Stable imaging appearance on follow-up imaging over a period of 6 months to 1 year can also help to establish the diagnosis.[73]

Management

Peritoneal inclusion cysts tend to grow slowly, and although they are not associated with any increased mortality, they are a cause of long-term morbidity. The treatment options are varied and will depend on the clinical symptoms, imaging findings, confidence of diagnosis, and the clinician's choice: (1) Conservative approach, with use of hormonal therapy to suppress ovulation, thus reducing formation of ovarian fluid; (2) Image-guided aspiration of cyst fluid with or without sclerotherapy, if symptomatic; and (3) Surgical resection, only in selected cases as the recurrence rate ranges between 30% and 50%.[73]

UTERINE LESIONS

A few benign uterine masses can also be present in the adnexal region, the most common being a subserosal or pedunculated fibroid, a broad ligament fibroid and an obstructed or nonobstructed rudimentary horn of a unicornuate uterus. Identification of both ovaries separately, connection of fibroid with the uterus, bridging vessel sign, and the morphological characteristics of the fibroid can all help in differentiating fibroids from an ovarian mass. Multiplanar imaging capability of MRI is an important adjunct in establishing the uterine origin of the mass.

IMAGING APPROACH TO AN ADNEXAL LESION

Adnexal lesions are commonly encountered in clinical practice. It is important to determine the nature of the lesion and especially to categorize the benign or malignant potential of an adnexal lesion, to be able it to manage it properly.

Sonography is the first line of investigation for detection, establishing the origin, and for characterizing the nature of the lesion. Transvaginal US is the preferred technique, however the transabdominal route has its own advantages. Wherever possible, it is better to evaluate the lesion with

Box 2: Morphological and color Doppler features on transvaginal sonography used by the International Ovarian Tumour Analysis group for qualitative classification of adnexal masses.[75]

Morphological characteristics

- Size of mass
- Cystic content—anechoic/low level echoes/ground-glass/ hemorrhagic/mixed
- Septations—complete or incomplete
- Internal walls—smooth or irregular
- Papillary projections >3 mm
- Solid component—present or absent
- Acoustic shadow—present or absent
- Ascites present or absent

Based on above features, mass classified qualitatively into six categories

1. Unilocular cyst—no complete septum, solid component or papillary projection
2. Multilocular cyst—≥ 1 complete septum, no solid component or papillary projection
3. Unilocular solid cyst—unilocular cyst with solid component or ≥ 1 papillary projection
4. Multilocular solid cyst—multilocular cyst with solid component or >1 papillary projection
5. Solid—>80% solid component
6. Not classifiable—due to poor visualization

Color Doppler sonography

Score 1—no blood flow
Score 2—minimal flow
Score 3—moderate flow
Score 4—very strong flow

both transabdominal and transvaginal routes. Over the years, various approaches have been used to categorize an adnexal mass lesion on US, including the subjective assessment or the pattern recognition approach, simple scoring systems, probability predictors based on logistic regression analysis, etc. Of these, the pattern recognition approach has been found to be the most superior, with a sensitivity of 88–100% and specificity of 62–96% for predicting malignancy.[74] However, this approach works best in experienced hands.

A consensus opinion paper was published by the International Ovarian Tumour Analysis (IOTA) group in which objective criteria were put forward to standardize the terminology, definitions, and measurements used for describing the various morphological features of adnexal masses on gray scale and Doppler USG **(Box 2)**.[75] Using these terms and definitions, the IOTA group also described *simple rules* for categorizing the lesions into three categories—benign , malignant and indeterminate lesions on US—which has become the most used method and has shown the best validation reports. They described five benign and five malignant descriptors as elaborated in

Box 3: Benign and malignant features as described by the International Ovarian Tumour Analysis group.[76]

Benign features	
B1	Unilocular Cyst
B2	Presence of solid components with largest diameter <7 mm
B3	Presence of acoustic shadows
B4	Smooth multilocular tumor with largest diameter <10 cm
B5	No blood flow—color score 0
Malignant features	
M1	Irregular solid tumor
M2	Presence of ascites
M3	At least four papillary projections
M4	Irregular multilocular—solid tumor with largest diameter >10 cm
M5	Very strong blood flow—color score 4

Box 3. In the presence of one or more benign features with no malignant feature, the mass was categorized as benign; if one or more malignant features was seen, with no benign feature, the mass was categorized as malignant; the mass was deemed indeterminate if one or more features of both benign and malignant were seen, or if no features of benign or malignant were seen.[76] Using these simple rules, about 77% of the masses could be categorized as benign or malignant with a specificity of 96% and sensitivity of 92%, while the rest were labeled as the indeterminate masses.[77]

Sonographically indeterminate masses are those masses that (1) appear complex and even after a thorough evaluation with gray scale and Doppler assessment, cannot be confidently placed into either the benign or malignant category or (2) one whose site of origin, from the ovary, uterus, or another pelvic structure cannot be established. It has been found that majority of the indeterminate masses are not malignant, but common benign adnexal conditions with a complex or unusual appearance, e.g. mature teratomas with no or little fat, hemorrhagic lesions with clot or debris mimicking a solid nodule or fibrous masses which appear solid on US and thus cause a concern for malignancy, etc.[78] Various methods have been adopted for further confirmation of the nature of the indeterminate masses including (a) a review US by an expert in the field of gynecological US, (b) MRI, (c) a diagnostic laparoscopy or (d) a "wait and watch" policy with follow-up sonography **(Flowchart 3)**. Amongst these options, MRI is the least invasive and offers the earliest solution with a high accuracy.

Flowchart 3: Algorithm for imaging evaluation of an adnexal mass.

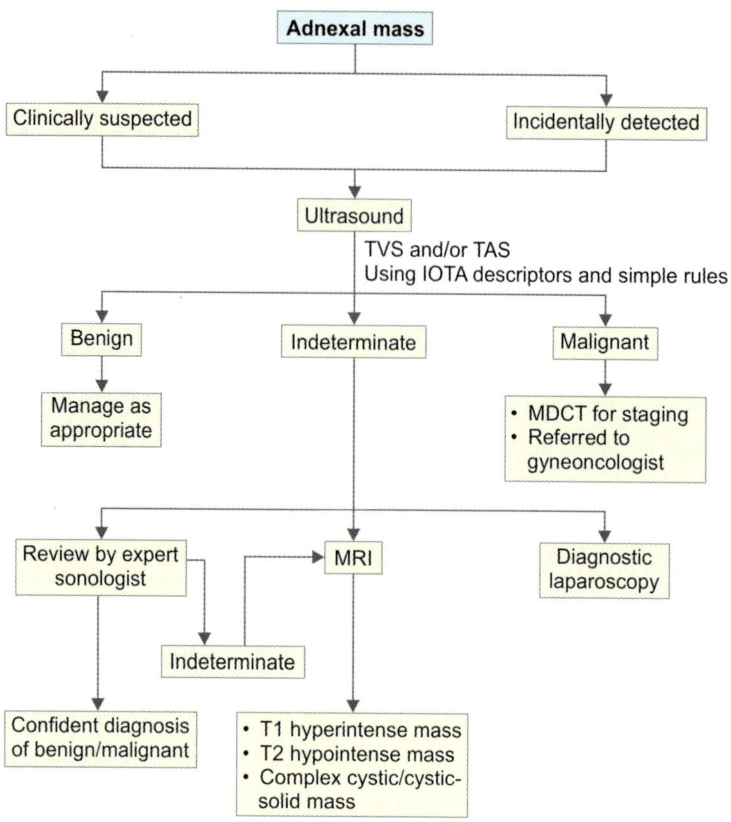

Magnetic resonance imaging has been found to be a useful complementary imaging modality for assessing the indeterminate lesions allowing a confident differentiation between benign and malignant etiology in majority of the cases. A number of scoring systems have been devised for systematic MR evaluation (MR ADNEX scoring system, EURAD-MR classification, etc.). The 2017 European Society of Urogenital Radiology (ESUR) recommendations for MRI incorporates the use of both conventional and functional MRI techniques.[79] As a general rule, malignant tumors show restricted diffusion on DWI, whereas benign tumors do not. However, some benign lesions can also show restricted diffusion: teratomas, endometriomas, hemorrhagic cysts, ovarian abscesses, ovarian infarction, and some benign sex cord-stromal tumors. On DCE-MRI, malignant solid components generally show a rapid rate and high level of enhancement, whereas a slow rate and low level of enhancement is seen in benign lesions.

The ESUR advocates that an initial basic series of MRI should be done in all patients, i.e. (1) A T2W

Flowchart 4A: MRI of sonographically indeterminate ovarian lesions—T1 "bright" mass. (ESUR recommendations, 2017).[79]

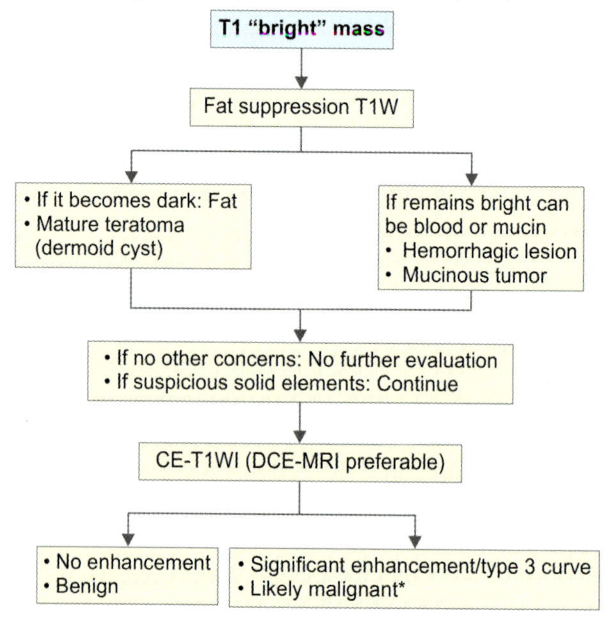

(*Mature teratoma can show enhancement at times)

Flowchart 4B: MRI of sonographically indeterminate ovarian lesions—T2WI "dark" or "intermediate" solid mass. (ESUR recommendations, 2017).[79]

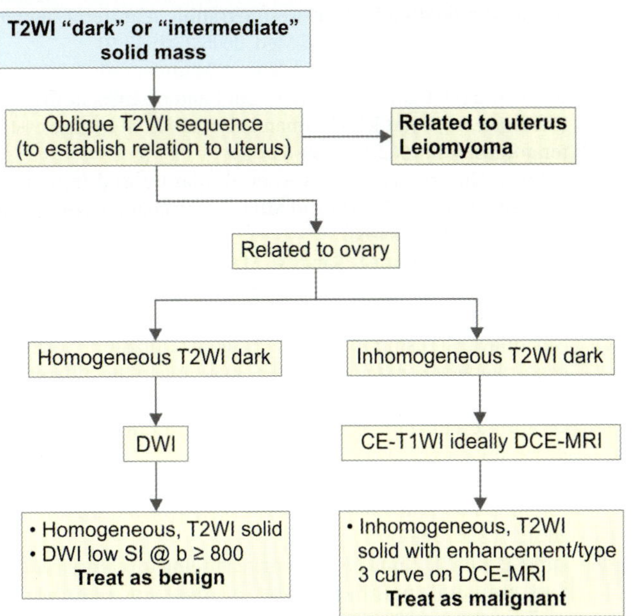

Flowchart 4C: MRI of sonographically indeterminate ovarian lesions—Complex cystic or cystic/solid mass. (ESUR recommendations, 2017).[79]

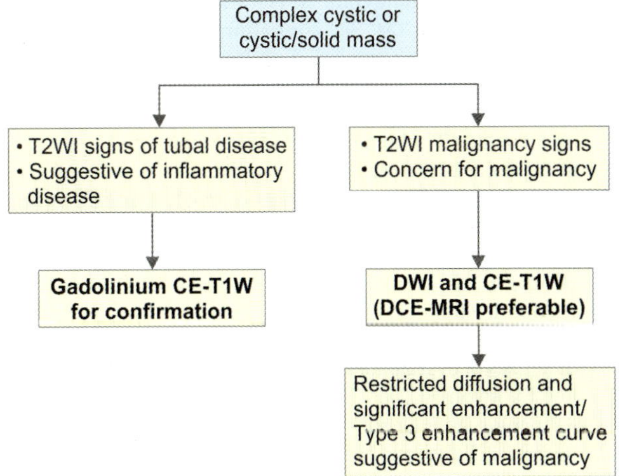

sagittal sequence to look at the uterus and the position of the adnexal mass, and (2) a pair of T1W and T2W sequences in an orthogonal plane for morphological evaluation of the mass. These sequences will establish the likely site and origin of the mass. At the same time, depending on the morphological characteristics on the T1- and T2W sequences, the masses can be divided into three broad categories: (1) T1W hyperintense mass, (2) the T2W low-SI mass, and (3) the complex-cystic or cystic-solid mass. Further sequences will be decided based on these categories. The subsequent algorithmic approach is given in the **Flowcharts 4A to C**, which will help in narrowing the differential diagnosis still further.

CONCLUSION

Although the large majority of adnexal lesions are benign, a significant number do turn out to be malignant. Being able to characterize the adnexal mass is important as it may lead to a more conservative management approach in benign masses, whilst ensuring an early and appropriate referral to a gynecological oncologist in the case of malignancy. Imaging plays a very significant role in establishing the origin of the lesion as well as in predicting whether it is benign or malignant. A thorough knowledge of the usual and unusual imaging appearances of the various conditions, correlation with the clinical details, laboratory parameters and use of a systematic step-by-step imaging algorithm will allow us to establish a short meaningful diagnosis or even a definitive diagnosis.

REFERENCES

1. Lee JH, Jeong YK, Park JK, et al. "Ovarian vascular pedicle" sign revealing organ of origin of a pelvic mass lesion on helical CT. Am J Roentgenol. 2003;181:131-7.
2. Modesitt SC, Pavlik EJ, Ueland FR, et al. Risk of malignancy in unilocular ovarian cystic tumors less than 10 centimeters in diameter. Obstet Gynecol. 2003;102:594-9.
3. Joshi M, Ganeshan K, Munshi HN. Ultrasound of adnexal masses. Semin Ultrasound CT MRI. 2008;29:72-97.
4. Siddall KA, Rubens DJ. Multi-detector CT of the female pelvis. RCNA. 2005;43:1097-118.
5. Jain KA. Sonographic spectrum of hemorrhagic ovarian cysts. J Ultrasound Med. 2003;21(8):879-86.
6. Potter AW, Chandrasekhar CA. US and CT evaluation of acute pelvic pain of gynecologic origin in nonpregnant premenopausal patients. Radiographics. 2008;28:1645-59.
7. Levine D, Brown DL, Andreotti RF, et al. Management of asymptomatic ovarian and other adnexal cysts imaged at US: Society of radiologists in Ultrasound Consensus. Radiology. 2010;256:943-54.
8. Chamié LP, Blasbalg R, Pereira RM, et al. Findings of pelvic endometriosis at transvaginal US, MR imaging, and laparoscopy. Radiographics. 2011;31(4):E77-100.
9. Patel MD, Feldstein VA, Chen DC, et al. Endometriomas: diagnostic performance of US. Radiology. 1999;210(3):739-45.
10. Dogan MM, Ugur M, Soysal SK, et al. Transvaginal sonographic diagnosis of ovarian endometrioma. Int J Gynaecol Obstet. 1996;52(2):145-9.
11. Alcázar JL, Laparte C, Jurado M, et al. The role of transvaginal ultrasonography combined with color velocity imaging and pulsed Doppler in the diagnosis of endometrioma. Fertil Steril. 1997;67(3):487-91.
12. Glastonbury CM. The shading sign. Radiology. 2002; 224(1):199-201.
13. Takahashi K, Okada S, Ozaki T, et al. Diagnosis of pelvic endometriosis by magnetic resonance imaging using "fat-saturation" technique. Fertil Steril. 1994;62(5):973-7.
14. Corwin MT, Gerscovich EO, Lamba R, et al. Differentiation of ovarian endometriomas from hemorrhagic cysts at MR imaging: utility of the T2 dark spot sign. Radiology. 2013;271(1):126-32.

15. Namimoto T, Awai K, Nakaura T, et al. Role of diffusion-weighted imaging in the diagnosis of gynecological diseases. Eur Radiol. 2009;19:745-60.
16. Thomassin-Naggara I, Daraï E, Cuenod CA, et al. Contribution of diffusion-weighted MR imaging for predicting benignity of complex adnexal masses. Eur Radiol. 2009;19:1544-52.
17. Turocy JM, Benacerraf BR. Transvaginal sonography in the diagnosis of deep infiltrating endometriosis: a review. J Clin Ultrasound. 2017;45(6):313-8.
18. Bennett GL, Slywotzky CM, Cantera M, et al. Unusual manifestations and complications of endometriosis—spectrum of imaging findings: pictorial review. Am J Roentgenol. 2010;194(6):WS34-46.
19. Kobayashi H. Ovarian cancer in endometriosis: epidemiology, natural history, and clinical diagnosis. Int J Clin Oncol. 2009;14(5):378-82.
20. Asch E, Levine D. Variations in appearance of endometriomas. J Ultrasound Med. 2007;26(8):993-1002.
21. Moghissi KS. Medical treatment of endometriosis. Clin Obstet Gynecol. 1999;42(3):620-32.
22. Valentini AL, Gui B, Miccò M, et al. Benign and suspicious ovarian masses-mr imaging criteria for characterization: pictorial review. J Oncol. 2012;2012:481806.
23. Hart WR. Mucinous tumors of the ovary: a review. Int J Gynecol Pathol. 2005;24(1):4-25.
24. Imaoka I, Wada A, Kaji Y, et al. Developing an MR imaging strategy for diagnosis of ovarian masses. Radiographics, 2006;26:1431-48.
25. Okada S, Ohaki Y, Inoue K, et al. Calcifications in mucinous and serous cystic ovarian tumors. J Nippon Med Sch. 2005;72(1):29-33.
26. Tanaka YO, Nishida M, Kurosaki Y, et al. Differential diagnosis of gynaecological "stained glass" tumours on MRI. Br J Radiol. 1999;72(856):414-20.
27. Cho SM, Byun JY, Rha SE, et al. CT and MRI findings of cystadenofibromas of the ovary. Eur Radiol. 2004;14:798-804.
28. Wasnik A, Elsayes K. Ovarian cystadenofibroma: A masquerader of malignancy. IJRI. 2010;20(4):297-9.
29. Dierickx I, Valentin L, Van Holsbeke C, et al. Imaging in gynecological disease: clinical and ultrasound features of Brenner tumors of the ovary. Ultrasound Obstet Gynecol. 2012;40:706-13.
30. Zhao Y, Mao X, Yao L, et al. Computed tomography imaging features of benign ovarian Brenner tumors. Oncology letters. 2018;16(1):1141-6.
31. Rha SE, Byun JY, Jung SE, et al. Atypical CT and MRI manifestations of mature ovarian cystic teratomas. AJR. 2004;183:743-50.
32. Togashi K, Nishimura K, Itoh K, et al. Ovarian cystic teratomas: MR imaging. Radiology. 1987;162:669-73.
33. Comerci JT Jr, Licciardi F, Bergh PA, et al. Mature cystic teratoma: clinicopathologic evaluation of 517 cases and review of the literature. Obstet Gynecol. 1994;84:22-8.
34. Ismail SR. An evaluation of the incidence of right-sided ovarian cystic teratoma visualized on sonograms. JDMS. 2005;21:336-42.
35. Quinn SF, Erickson S, Black WC. Cystic ovarian teratomas: The sonographic appearance of the dermoid plug. Radiology. 1985;155:477-8.
36. Beller MJ. The "tip of the iceberg" sign. Radiology. 1998;209(2): 395-6.
37. Vyas B, Dyer RB. The "dot-dash" sign. Abdom Imaging. 2015;40:2901-2.
38. Tongsong T, Wanapirak C, Khunamornpong S, et al. Numerous intracystic floating balls as a sonographic feature of benign cystic teratoma. J Ultrasound Med. 2006;25:1587-91.
39. Guinet C, Ghossain MA, Buy J-N, et al. Mature cystic teratomas of the ovary: CT and MR findings. Eur J Radiol. 1995;20:137-43 .
40. Friedman AC, Pyatt RS, Hartman DS, et al. CT of benign cystic teratomas. AJR. 1982;138:659-65.
41. Saba L, Guerriero S, Sulcis R, et al. Mature and immature ovarian teratomas: CT, US and MR imaging characteristics. Eur J Radiol. 2009;72:454-63.
42. Sahin H, Abdullazade S, Sanci M. Mature cystic teratoma of the ovary: a cutting edge overview on imaging features. Insights Imaging. 2017;8(2):227-41.
43. Nakamaya T, Yoshimitsu K, Irie H, et al. Diffusion-weighted echo-planar MR imaging and ADC mapping in the differential diagnosis of ovarian cystic masses: usefulness of detecting keratinoid substances in mature cystic teratomas. J Magn Reson Imaging. 2005;22:271-8.
44. Outwater EK, Siegelman ES, Hunt JL. Ovarian teratomas: tumor types and imaging characteristics. Radiographics. 2001;21(2):475-90.
45. Park SB, Kim JK, Kim K, et al. Imaging findings of complications and unusual manifestations of ovarian neoplasms. Radiographics. 2008;28:969-83.
46. Haroon S, Zia A, Idrees R, et al. Clinicopathological spectrum of ovarian sex cord-stromal tumors; 20 years' retrospective study in a developing country. J Ovarian Res. 2013;6(1):87.
47. Horta M, Cunha TM. Sex cord-stromal tumors of the ovary: a comprehensive review and update for radiologists. Diagn Interv Radiol. 2015;21(4):277-86.
48. Duigenan S, Oliva E, Lee SI. Ovarian torsion: diagnostic features on CT and MRI with pathologic correlation. Am J Roentgenol. 2012;198(2):W122-31.
49. Bider D, Mashiach S, Dulitzky M, et al. Clinical, surgical and pathologic findings of adnexal torsion in pregnant and nonpregnant women. Surg Gynecol Obstet. 1991;173(5): 363-6.
50. Hibbard LT. Adnexal torsion. Am J Obstet Gynecol. 1985;152:456-61.
51. Sibal M. Follicular ring sign: a simple sonographic sign for early diagnosis of ovarian torsion. JUM. 2012;31(11):1803-9.
52. Lee EJ, Kwon HC, Joo HJ, et al. Diagnosis of ovarian torsion with color Doppler sonography: depiction of twisted vascular pedicle. J Ultrasound Med. 1998;17(2):83-9.
53. Albayram F, Hamper UM. Ovarian and adnexal torsion: spectrum of sonographic findings with pathologic correlation. J Ultrasound Med. 2001;20:1083-9.
54. Nizar K, Deutsch M, Filmer S, et al. Doppler studies of the ovarian venous blood flow in the diagnosis of adnexal torsion. J Clin Ultrasound. 2009;37(8):436-9.
55. Shalev J, Goldenberg M, Oelsner G, et al. Treatment of twisted ischemic adnexa by simple detorsion. N Engl J Med. 1989;321(8):546.
56. Huang C, Hong M-K, Ding D-C. A review of ovary torsion. Ci Ji Yi Xue Za Zhi. 2017;29(3):143-7.
57. Umesaki N, Tanaka T, Miyama M, et al. Sonographic characteristics of massive ovarian edema. Ultrasound Obstet Gynecol. 2000;16(5):479-81.
58. Coakley FV, Anwar M, Poder L, et al. Magnetic resonance imaging of massive ovarian edema in pregnancy. J Comput Assist Tomogr. 2010;34(6):865-7.

59. Takeuchi M, Matsuzaki K, Sano N, et al. Ovarian fibromatosis: magnetic resonance imaging findings with pathologic correlation. J Comput Assist Tomogr. 2008;32(5):776-7.
60. Revzin MV, Mathur M, Dave HB, et al. Pelvic inflammatory disease: multimodality imaging approach with clinical-pathologic correlation. Radiographics. 2016;36(5): 1579-96.
61. Kim SH, Kim SH, Yang DM, et al. Unusual causes of tubo-ovarian abscess: CT and MR imaging findings. Radiographics. 2004; 24:1575-89.
62. Sam JW, Jacobs JE, Birnbaum BA. Spectrum of CT findings in acute pyogenic pelvic inflammatory disease. Radiographics. 2002;22(6):1327-34.
63. Lareau SM, Beigi RH. Pelvic inflammatory disease and tubo-ovarian abscess. Infect Dis Clin North Am. 2008;22(4):693-708.
64. Patel MD, Acord DL, Young SW. Likelihood ratio of sonographic findings in discriminating hydrosalpinx from other adnexal masses. Am J Roentgenol. 2006;186(4):1033-8.
65. Eyvazzadeh AD, Levine D. Imaging of Pelvic Pain in the First Trimester of Pregnancy. Radiol Clin North Am. 2006;44:863-77.
66. Nuberg DA, Mack LA, Jeffrey RB Jr, et al. Endovaginal sonographic evaluation of ectopic pregnancy: A prospective study. Am J Roentgenol. 1987;149:1181-6.
67. Kishimoto K, Ito K, Awaya H, et al. Paraovarian cyst: MR imaging features. Abdom Imaging. 2002;27(6):685-9.
68. Mennemeyer R, Smith M. Multicystic, peritoneal mesothelioma: a report with electron microscopy of a case mimicking intra-abdominal cystic hygroma (lymphangioma). Cancer. 1979;44:692-8.
69. Sohaey R, Gardner TL, Woodward PJ, et al. Sonographic diagnosis of peritoneal inclusion cysts. J Ultrasound Med. 1995;14:913-7.
70. Kim JS, Lee HJ, Woo SK, et al. Peritoneal inclusion cysts and their relationship to the ovaries: evaluation with sonography. Radiology. 1997;204:481-4.
71. Jain KA. Imaging of peritoneal inclusion cysts. Am J Roentgenol. 2000;174:1559-63.
72. Ross MJ, Welch WR, Scully RE. Multilocular peritoneal inclusion cysts (so-called cystic mesotheliomas). Cancer. 1989;64:1336-46.
73. Vallerie AM, Lerner JP, Wright JD, et al. Peritoneal inclusion cysts: a review. Obstet Gynecol Surv. 2009;64(5):321-34.
74. Brown DL, Dudiak KM, Laing FC. Adnexal masses: US characterization and reporting. Radiology. 2010;254(2):342-54.
75. Timmerman D, Valentin L, Bourne TH, et al. Terms, definitions and measurements to describe the sonographic features of adnexal tumors: a consensus opinion from the International Ovarian Tumor Analysis (IOTA) Group. Ultrasound Obstet Gynecol. 2000;16:500-5.
76. Timmerman D, Testa AC, Bourne, T et al. Simple ultrasound-based rules for the diagnosis of ovarian cancer. Ultrasound Obstet Gynecol. 2008;31:681-90.
77. Timmerman D, Ameye L, Fischerova D, et al. Simple ultrasound rules to distinguish between benign and malignant adnexal masses before surgery: prospective validation by IOTA group. BMJ. 2010;341:c6839.
78. Ameye L, Timmerman D, Valentin L, et al. Clinically oriented three-step strategy for assessment of adnexal pathology. Ultrasound Obstet Gynecol. 2012;40:582-91.
79. Forstner R, Thomassin-Naggara I, Cunha TM, et al. ESUR recommendations for MR imaging of the sonographically indeterminate adnexal mass: an update. Eur Radiol. 2017;27(6):2248-57.

15

Chapter

Malignant Ovarian and Tubal Disease

Smita Manchanda, Surabhi Vyas, Manisha Jana

INTRODUCTION

Cervical cancer, endometrial cancer, and ovarian cancer constitute the spectrum of gynecologic malignancies. Ovarian malignancy is the second most common gynecologic cancer and the fourth leading cause of cancer deaths in females in the United States.[1] It accounts for 3.6% of all cases with a mortality of 4.3%.[2] It is a leading cause of mortality predominantly because of the late diagnosis. Majority of the patients present in stage III or stage IV disease as the symptoms are often nonspecific.

ETIOPATHOGENESIS

For ovarian malignancy, the etiopathogenesis appears to be multifactorial. Risk factors include a first-degree relative with ovarian cancer, nulliparity, early menarche, and late menopause. Hereditary cases are seen in the premenopausal age group usually as the breast-ovarian cancer syndrome (mutations in the *BRCA1* and *BRCA2* tumor suppressor genes).[2] Pregnancy, lactation, and the use of oral contraceptives appear to be protective factors for ovarian malignancy.

CLASSIFICATION

WHO Histological Classification

The World Health Organization (WHO) histological classification for ovarian tumors is based on the most probable tissue of origin: surface epithelial (65%), germ cell (15%), sex cord-stromal (10%), metastases (5%), and miscellaneous. Further classification is done on the basis of cell type, cellular atypia, malignant potential, and invasion. Among these, the surface epithelial tumors comprise most of the malignant tumors (around 90%). The main entities in the 2014 WHO classification[3] are given in **Table 1**.

STAGING

The 2014 revised staging system by the international Federation of Gynaecology and Obstetrics (FIGO) provides prognostic as well as personalized management guidance in the ovarian malignancies and also recognizes the heterogeneity of ovarian malignancies, which may arise from the ovaries, fallopian tubes, or peritoneum.[4,5]

Although imaging modalities like computed tomography and chest radiography, and biochemical tests like CA-125 levels in the serum, may have prognostic implications, the staging is based on the findings of surgical exploration.

The 2014 FIGO staging is summarized below:

- *Stage I*: Tumor is confined to the ovaries; limited to one ovary capsule intact (*stage IA*); tumor involves both ovaries; rest as IA (*stage IB*); tumor involves one or both ovaries (*stage IC*), with either surgical/intraoperative spill (*stage IC1*), capsule ruptured before surgery, or tumor on ovarian or fallopian tube surface (*stage IC2*) or malignant cells in the ascites or peritoneal washings (*stage IC3*).
- *Stage II*: Tumor involves one or both ovaries with pelvic or peritoneal extension; involvement of the uterus and/or fallopian tubes (*stage IIA*); involvement of other pelvic intraperitoneal tissue (*stage IIB*).
- *Stage III*: Tumor involves one or both ovaries or fallopian tubes with extension to extrapelvic peritoneum and/or retroperitoneal (RP) lymph nodes metastasis:

Table 1: World Health Organization classification of ovarian neoplasms (2014).[3]

Histological categories	*Subcategories*		*Individual entities*
Epithelial tumors	Serous tumors	Benign	• Serous cystadenoma • Serous adenofibroma • Serous surface papilloma
		Borderline	• Serous borderline tumor/atypical proliferative serous tumor • Serous borderline tumor—micropapillary variant/noninvasive low-grade serous carcinoma
		Malignant	• Low-grade serous carcinoma • High-grade serous carcinoma
	Mucinous tumors	Benign	• Mucinous cystadenoma • Mucinous adenofibroma
		Borderline	Mucinous borderline tumor/atypical proliferative mucinous tumor
		Malignant	Mucinous carcinoma
	Endometrioid tumors	Benign	• Endometriosis cyst • Endometrioid cystadenoma • Endometrioid cystadenofibroma
		Borderline	Endometrioid borderline tumor/atypical proliferative endometrioid tumor
		Malignant	Endometrioid carcinoma
	Clear cell tumors	Benign	• Clear cell cystadenoma • Clear cell adenofibroma
		Borderline	Clear cell borderline tumor/atypical proliferative clear cell tumor
		Malignant	Clear cell carcinoma
	Brenner tumors	Benign	Brenner tumor
		Borderline	Borderline Brenner tumor/atypical proliferative Brenner tumor
		Malignant	Malignant Brenner tumor
	Seromucinous tumors	Benign	• Seromucinous cystadenoma • Seromucinous adenofibroma
		Borderline	Seromucinous borderline tumor/atypical proliferative seromucinous tumor
		Malignant	Seromucinous carcinoma
	Undifferentiated carcinoma		
Mixed epithelial and mesenchymal tumors			• Carcinosarcoma • Adenosarcoma
Sex cord—stromal tumors	Pure stromal tumors		• Fibromas • Fibrothecomas • Thecomas • Leydig cell tumors
	Pure sex cord tumors		• Adult granulosa cell tumor • Juvenile granulosa cell tumor • Sertoli cell tumors • Sex cord tumor with annular tubules
	Mixed sex cord—stromal tumors		Sertoli-Leydig cell tumors
Germ cell tumors			• Mature teratoma • Immature teratoma • Yolk sac tumor (endodermal sinus tumor) • Dysgerminoma • Nongestational choriocarcinoma • Embryonal carcinoma • Mixed germ cell tumors • Monodermal (e.g. struma ovarii, carcinoid)
Malignant not otherwise specified	Metastatic cancer from nonovarian primary		• Colonic, appendiceal • Gastric • Breast

- *Stage IIIA*: Positive RP lymph nodes only; if node size ≤10 mm in greatest dimension—*stage IIIA1* (i); if size > 10 mm in greatest dimension *stage IIIA1* (ii). *Stage IIIA2*: There is microscopic extrapelvic peritoneal involvement with or without RP lymph node involvement.
- *Stage IIIB*: Extrapelvic peritoneal metastasis ≤2 cm in greatest dimension, with or without RP lymph nodes metastasis.
- *Stage IIIC*: Macroscopic extrapelvic peritoneal metastases >2 cm in greatest dimension, with or without RP lymph node metastasis, including tumor extension to liver and splenic capsules only.
- *Stage IV:* Distant metastasis, excluding peritoneal metastases; with positive pleural effusion cytology (*stage IVA*), distant metastases to parenchyma of extra-abdominal organs or inguinal lymph nodes or lymph nodes outside of the abdominal cavity (*stage IVB*).

Few salient features of the 2014 FIGO staging include:

- The ovarian and peritoneal fallopian tube origin of ovarian carcinomas are dealt collectively.
- Stage IC is subdivided into three to specify the nature and timing of capsular rupture like preoperative or intraoperative rupture or positive peritoneal washings.
- In up to 30% patients with bilateral disease, either with one-sided dominant mass or multiple small masses may be due to metastasis.
- The Stage IIC is eliminated in the 2014 FIGO staging.
- The presence of metastatic nodes rather than the number of metastatic nodes has prognostic significance.[6]
- New subdivisions of stage IV, i.e. IVA and IVB, were introduced for positive pleural cytology and distant parenchymal metastasis, respectively.

ROLE OF IMAGING MODALITIES

The role of imaging in a suspected adnexal lesion is to detect, characterize, and stage the mass. Ultrasonography (USG), computed tomography (CT), magnetic resonance imaging (MRI), and positron emission tomography CT (PET-CT) are used in various combinations to evaluate adnexal masses.

Ultrasonography

Ultrasonography, being a low-cost, noninvasive, and widely available modality, is the initial investigation of choice in the evaluation of a suspected adnexal mass. Both transabdominal and endovaginal scanning in combination with Doppler are used for adnexal mass assessment.[7,8] The morphological features **(Figs. 1A to D)** suggestive of malignancy are thick walls and septations (>2–3 mm), irregular walls/septations, and presence of solid areas/papillary projections/mural nodules. Other signs such as presence of ascites, peritoneal nodules, and metastases also indicate malignant etiology. Reported sensitivity of USG in predicting malignancy is 85–97% and specificity varies from 56% to 95%.[7,9-12]

Color Doppler

Color Doppler in the qualitative mode has greater utility to demonstrate flow within a solid component or septum. Solid component with no detectable flow likely represents a blood clot. Presence of central and strong color flow is more suggestive of malignancy. However, it is important to remember that benign lesions also show internal color flow. Spectral Doppler parameters have been used variably in the past for the prediction of malignancy in an adnexal mass with varying sensitivity and specificity. A resistive index (RI) value of 0.4 was reported by Timor-Tritsch et al. to have a sensitivity of 93.8% and specificity of 98.7% and in 2007,[13] Laban et al.[14] reported the best RI cutoff value as <0.48 with a sensitivity of 90% and specificity of 89%. $P < 1.0$ has also had low reported sensitivity and specificity (52.8% and 77.6%, respectively).[15] Since there is a significant overlap in these values in benign and malignant masses, they are not much used in lesion characterization. In general, lower RI, lower pulsatility index (PI), and higher peak systolic velocity (PSV) suggest malignancy **(Figs. 2A and B)**.

IOTA Simple Rules

The International Ovarian Tumor Analysis (IOTA) Simple Rules (2008) consist of B-features (five features typical for benign tumors) and M-features (five features typical for malignant tumors) for preoperative classification of ovarian tumors.[16-18] These are summarized in **Table 2** and depicted in **Figures 3 and 4**. These are used to diagnose ovarian malignancy in women who have at least one persistent adnexal (ovarian, paraovarian, and tubal) tumor and are considered to require surgery.

ADNEX Model

There are various diagnostic models available for adnexal tumors [e.g. IOTA models, Risk of Malignancy Index (RMI), Risk of Ovarian Malignancy Algorithm (ROMA), Assessment of Different NEoplasias in the adneXa (ADNEX)]. However, when creating these models the patients selected for expectant management

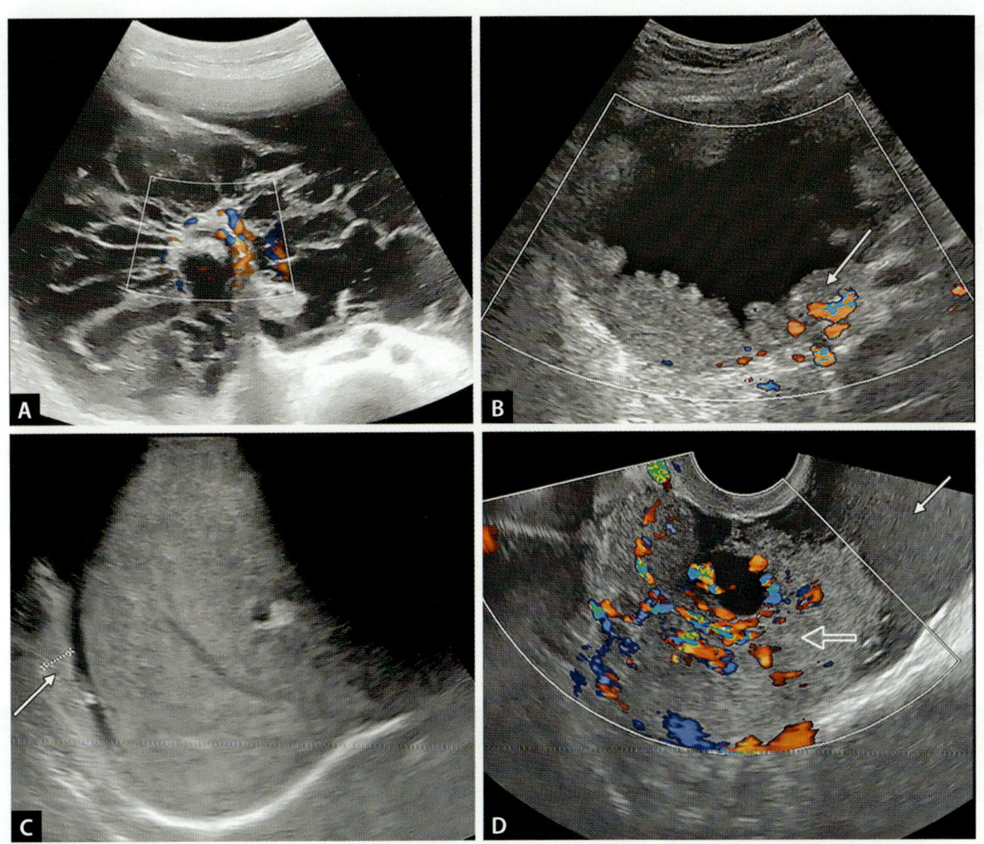

Figs. 1A to D: USG features of malignancy. (A) Thick septations with internal color flow. (B) Papillary projections and mural nodules (arrow). (C) Peritoneal deposits in subphrenic location (arrow). (D) Solid mass with cystic component and marked neovascularity (block arrow) with ascites (arrow).

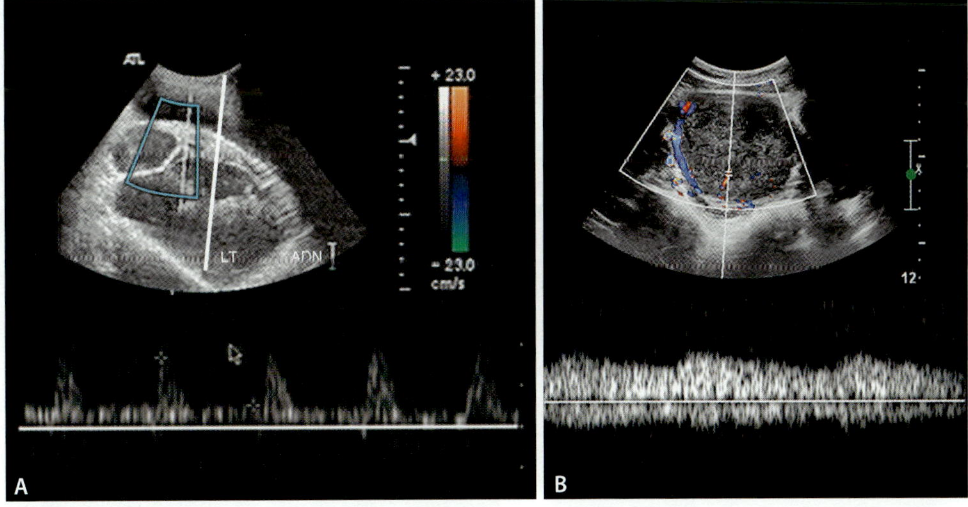

Figs. 2A and B: Doppler features of benign versus malignant lesion. (A) Multilocular cystic lesion with high resistance flow in septation in a case of serous cystadenoma. (B) Solid mass with low resistance internal flow in case of dysgerminoma.

were excluded. It is therefore important to remember that these cannot be applied to adnexal tumors being conservatively treated. ADNEX is a risk model, which uses nine predictors **(Table 3)** to diagnose ovarian malignancy in females with persistent adnexal tumor (ovarian/paraovarian/tubal), which is considered to need surgical management. ADNEX estimates the probability of adnexal tumor to be benign, borderline, stage I malignancy, stage II-IV malignancy, or secondary metastatic disease (i.e. metastasis of nonadnexal tumor to the ovary). This model

Table 2: International Ovarian Tumor Analysis (IOTA) simple rules.

Benign features (B)		*Malignant features (M)*	
B1	Unilocular	M1	Irregular solid tumor
B2	Presence of solid components with largest diameter <7 mm	M2	Presence of ascites
B3	Presence of acoustic shadows	M3	At least four papillary structures
B4	Smooth multilocular tumor with largest diameter <100 mm	M4	Irregular multilocular—solid tumor with largest diameter >100 mm
B5	No blood flow (color score 1)	M5	Very strong blood flow (color score 4)

Benign: Only B-features apply.
Malignant: Only M-features apply.
Inconclusive: No features apply, or both B- and M-features apply.

developed by clinicians and statisticians from the IOTA group is based on clinical and USG data from almost 6,000 women recruited at 24 centers in 10 countries (Italy, Belgium, Sweden, Czech Republic, Poland, France, UK, China, Spain, and Canada).[19]

Computed Tomography

The role of CT is primarily two-fold:

1. To stage the disease preoperatively
2. To assess resectability and identify patients suitable for primary cytoreductive surgery vis-a-vis patients who will require neoadjuvant chemotherapy prior to surgery.

In addition, the staging CT is used to plan image-guided biopsy for histological subtyping prior to primary chemotherapy.

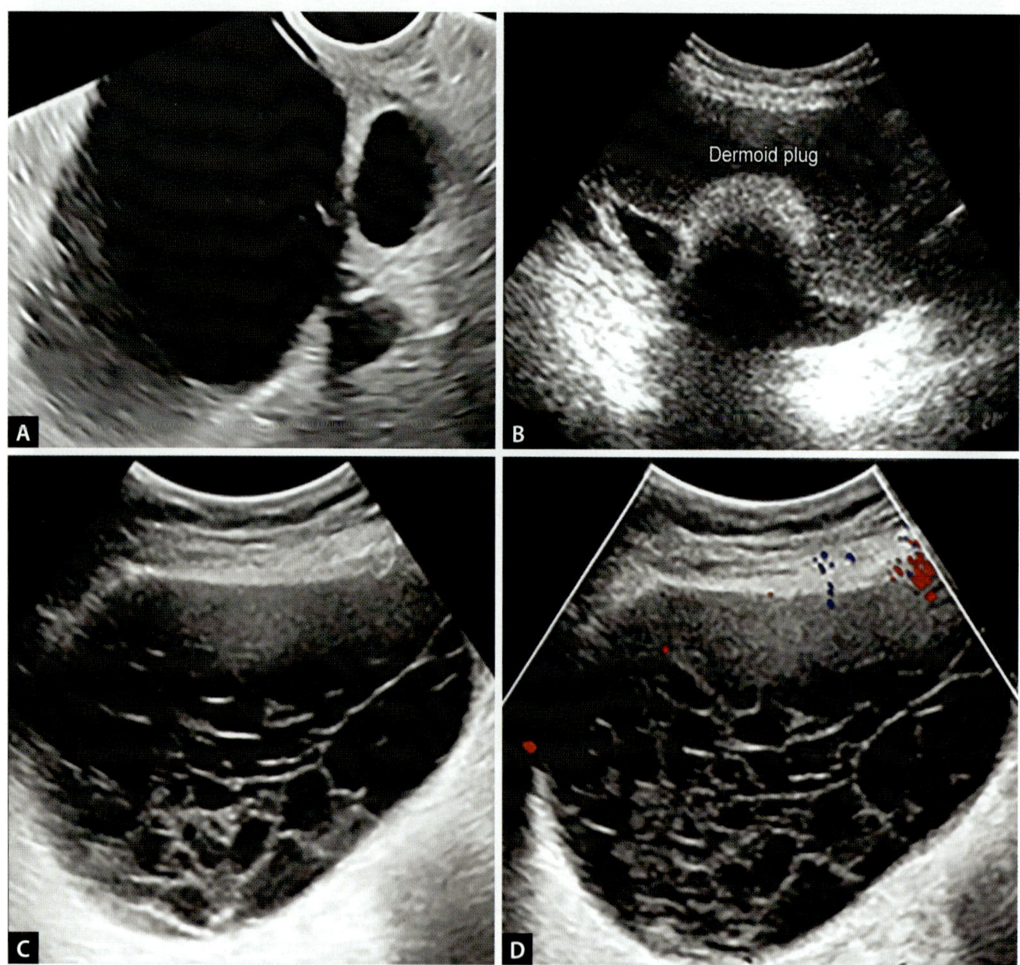

Figs. 3A to D: Benign features (IOTA simple rules, 2008). (A) Unilocular tumor: B1. (B) Presence of acoustic shadows: B3. (C) Smooth multilocular tumor with largest diameter <100 mm: B4. (D) No blood flow (color score 1): B5. (IOTA: International Ovarian Tumor Analysis).

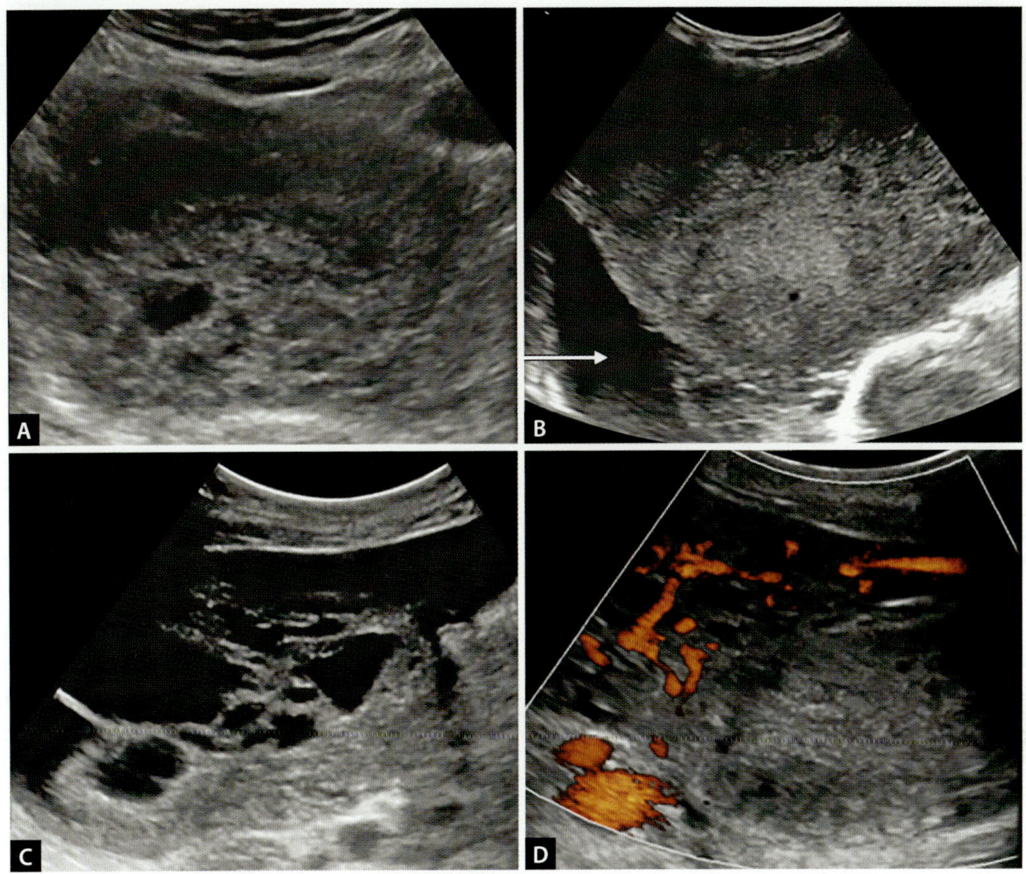

Figs. 4A to D: Malignant features (IOTA simple rules, 2008). (A) Irregular solid tumor: M1. (B) Presence of ascites (arrow): M2. (C) Irregular multilocular solid tumor: M4. (D) Very strong color flow: M5. (IOTA: International Ovarian Tumor Analysis).

Table 3: ADNEX risk model predictors.

Clinical variables	*USG variables*
• Age • Serum CA-125 level • Type of center (oncology referral center vs other)	• Maximal diameter of lesion • Proportion of solid tissue • >10 cyst locules • Number of papillary projections • Acoustic shadow • Ascites

CT Technique

Contrast-enhanced CT (CECT) abdomen is planned with oral and intravenous contrast administration. Positive oral contrast media is used to distinguish between luminal lesions and mesenteric/serosal deposits. Some institutions prefer oral water (negative contrast medium) as the small, calcified deposits may get obscured by positive oral contrast. Acquisition is in the venous phase 70 seconds after injection of contrast medium from the domes of diaphragm to the inguinal regions.[20] Axial thin reconstructions (1.5 mm) are then used to generate 3D coronal and sagittal multiplanar images.

CT chest: Many centers now routinely perform CT chest to detect pleural deposits, lung metastases, paracardiac, and mediastinal lymph nodes (these findings are detected in approximately 30% of the patients at presentation). In addition, the presence of moderate or large pleural effusions or enlarged paracardiac lymph nodes is a predictor of poor post-treatment outcome.[21]

Routes of Dissemination

Direct pelvic invasion and transcoelomic peritoneal disease extension are the most common ways of dissemination.[21] **Table 4** summarizes the various routes of dissemination in ovarian malignancy.

Limitation of CT in Assessing Disease Burden

The reported accuracies for detection of disease at all stages have been in the range of 70–90% with a good CT acquisition and reading.[22]

Only limited evaluation is possible with noncontrast CT, and inability to use intravenous contrast adversely affects CT staging accuracies.

It is difficult to detect small-volume extraovarian deposits (<5 mm) on mesentery, peritoneum, and bowel serosa, especially in the absence of ascites. This emphasizes the complementary role of laparoscopy in preoperative assessment of ovarian cancer.

Table 4: Routes of dissemination in ovarian malignancy.

Direct invasion in pelvis	Adnexa, uterus, pelvic side walls, bladder, and rectum
Transcoelomic spread	Peritoneal, subdiaphragmatic mesenteric and serosal surfaces
Lymphatic metastases	Pelvic, abdominal, retroperitoneal, para-aortic, paracardiac, and mediastinal lymph nodes
Hematogenous metastases (least common)	Liver, lung, bone, and brain

Box 1: Signs of peritoneal disease.

- Subtle thickening of peritoneum
- Fine reticular nodular pattern along peritoneal surface
- Abnormal enhancement of peritoneum
- Large nodular deposits
- Calcified deposits in serous cystadenocarcinomas
- Omental nodularity/omental caking

CECT Assessment

- *Pelvic disease*: In the pelvis, it is important to evaluate the size, location, and extent of primary disease including bladder, ureteric, and rectal invasion. Pelvic sidewall invasion is likely if the disease is less than 3 mm from the muscular sidewall and there is encasement or invasion of the iliac vessels.[21]
- *Peritoneal/omental disease*: It is important to identify peritoneal disease and document the extent of omental or peritoneal involvement. The signs of peritoneal disease are detailed in **Box 1** and depicted in **Figures 5A to D**.

Apart from the peritoneum or omentum, mesenteric disease and deposits along the *upper abdominal ligaments* **(Figs. 6A to D)** are important to document. Presence of small nodules or a misty stranded mesentery is seen in early disease whereas plaque-like thickening with retraction and distortion of the bowel loops is a feature of advanced disease. Disease in the lesser omentum, lesser sac, and perihepatic space along with the associated upper abdominal ligaments **(Table 5)** complicates surgical approach with associated increased morbidity. Nodular or plaque-like disease greater than 2 cm is considered unresectable disease.[21] Similar criteria apply

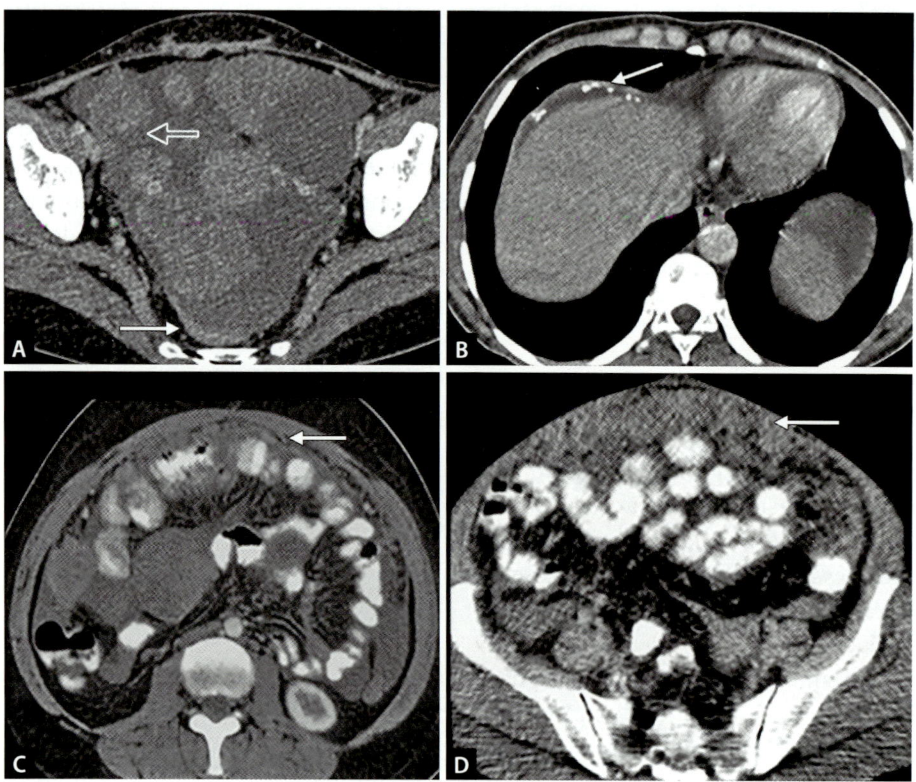

Figs. 5A to D: CT signs of peritoneal disease. (A) Thickening of peritoneum (arrow) and peritoneal deposits (block arrow). (B) Calcified deposits (arrow) in serous cystadenocarcinoma. (C) Omental nodularity (arrow). (D) Omental caking (arrow).

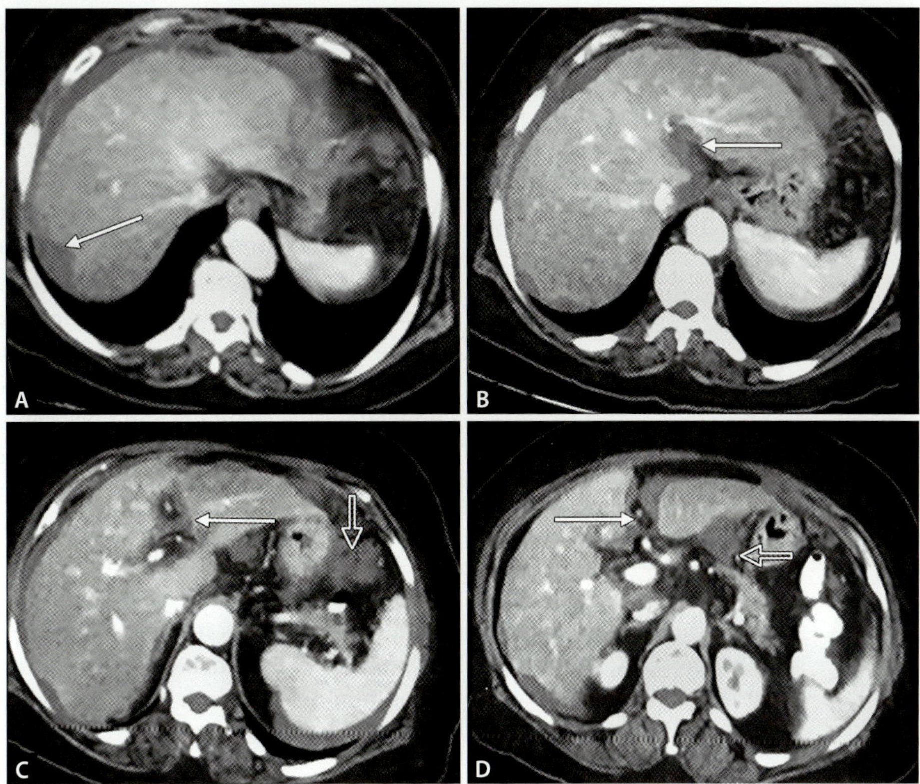

Figs. 6A to D: Peritoneal disease: Upper abdominal ligament involvement. (A) Large subphrenic deposit (arrow). (B) Horizontal hepatoduodenal ligament deposit (arrow). (C) Deposit along vertical gastrohepatic ligament (arrow) and lesser sac (block arrow). (D) Deposit along falciform ligament (arrow) and hepatoduodenal ligament (block arrow).

Table 5: Computed tomography (CT) landmarks for the upper abdominal ligaments.

Space	*Abdominal ligament associated*	*CT identification*
Lesser omentum	Horizontal hepatoduodenal ligament	• Between porta hepatis and first part of the duodenum • Contains common bile duct, portal vein, hepatic artery, lymph nodes
	Vertical gastrohepatic ligament	Identified by recognizing left gastric artery
Lesser sac	Splenorenal and splenogastric ligaments	Lies between stomach and pancreas
Perihepatic space	• Falciform ligament • Morrison's pouch • Gallbladder fossa	• Falciform ligament • Morrison's pouch: Hepatorenal space • Gallbladder fossa

for subdiaphragmatic disease extension and both the subphrenic spaces should be carefully looked for in axial and coronal planes.

- *Lymphadenopathy*: The criterion for malignant lymphadenopathy is nodal short axis diameter (SAD) of 1 cm. Pelvic, RP, and paracardiac nodal disease should be clearly documented. Diffuse RP suprarenal nodal disease and paracardiac nodes ≥1 cm may preclude surgery.
- *Visceral metastases*: Hematogenous parenchymal liver metastases are rare with invasive serosal surface implants being more common. Splenic surface implants and splenic hilar disease should also be clearly mentioned in CT report as they increase the likelihood of a splenectomy.
- *Bowel metastases*: Involvement of bowel is commonly seen in advanced disease. The mode of involvement can be:
  - Direct invasion from the pelvic carcinomas
  - Along mesenteric fascial planes
  - Intraperitoneal seeding of tumor
  - Through lymphatic channels
  - Embolic hematogenous spread.

Bowel involvement is seen as nodular or plaque-like lesions along serosal surfaces and with bowel wall invasion, obstruction is a common complication.

Criteria for Nonresectability

Optimal cytoreduction is not currently defined, though at most centers less than 1 cm of residual tumor present at completion of cytoreductive surgery is considered as a better predictor of long-term survival.[23]

Table 6 summarizes the sites considered potentially nonresectable disease (may be regarded resectable at some centers with specialty surgeons) and nonresectable disease (where resection is unlikely to achieve optimal cytoreduction).[21] **Figures 7A to D** illustrate an example of nonresectable high-grade serous papillary carcinoma. Extensive surgical resections increase the risk of surgical morbidity and mortality.

Table 6: Criteria for nonresectability.

Potentially nonresectable disease	*Nonresectable disease*
• Disease in the lesser omentum, lesser sac, and perihepatic space along with the associated upper abdominal ligaments • Gastric and duodenal serosa • Rectal and sigmoid diffuse serosal, wall and luminal invasion • Vascular side wall invasion • Ureteric invasion	• Pleural infiltration • Paracardiac nodes • Subdiaphragmatic plaque-like disease greater than 2 cm • Parenchymal liver metastases • Invasive surface implants • Diffuse large volume mesenteric disease • Root of small bowel mesentery • High retroperitoneal lymph nodes • Bony and muscular side wall invasion • Diffuse presacral disease

Magnetic Resonance Imaging

MRI has a superior contrast resolution and can accurately characterize adnexal masses with fat/hemorrhagic/fibrotic components.

Findings highly predictive of malignancy **(Figs. 8A to D)** are the demonstration of solid component, solid/cystic masses, or cystic lesions with the presence of papillary projections (vegetations) and thick septations. Secondary features of malignancy include peritoneal, mesenteric or omental involvement, pelvic side wall invasion, and lymphadenopathy.[24]

MRI features most predictive of malignancy are vegetations in a cystic lesion, tumor diameter greater than 6 cm, necrosis in a solid lesion, and the presence of ascites.[25,26] Presence of ascites anterior to the uterus or abdominal ascites is highly suggestive for malignant ascites.[24]

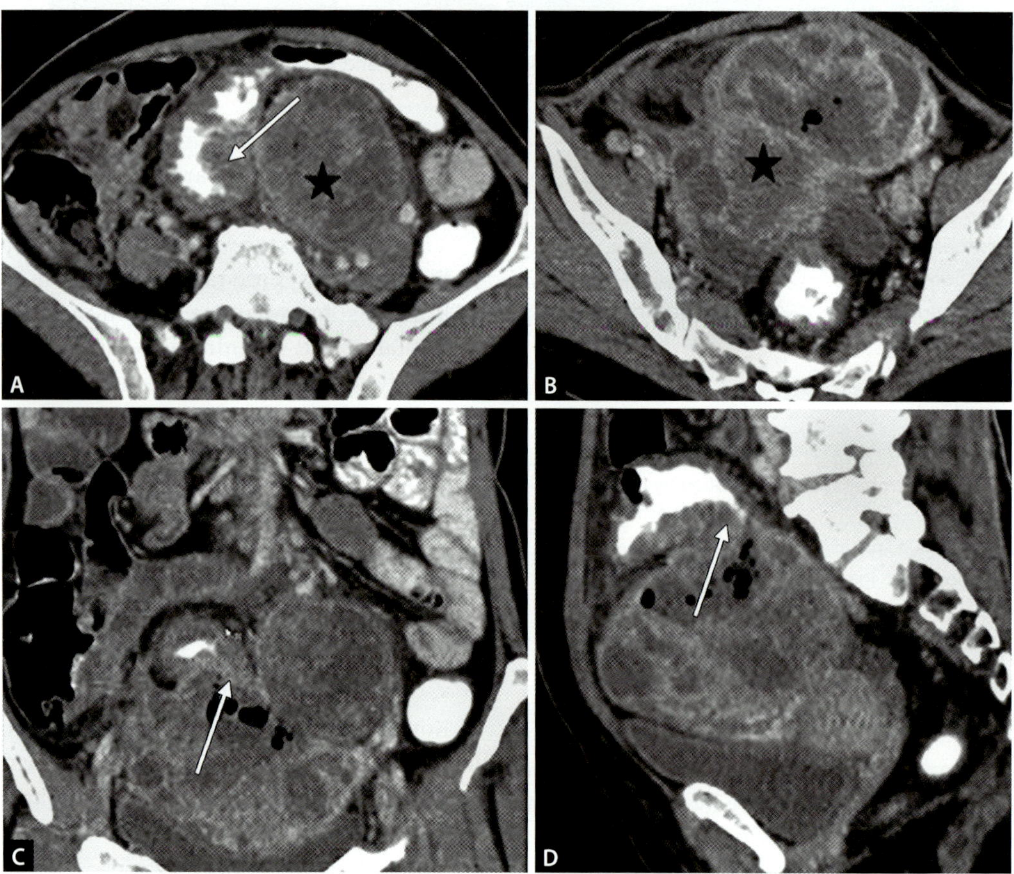

Figs. 7A to D: Nonresectable high-grade serous papillary carcinoma: bowel metastases. (A and B) Axial CT pelvis images reveal high-volume peritoneal disease (asterisk in A), adjacent sigmoid mural invasion (arrow in A). (C) Coronal and (D) sagittal multiplanar reconstructed images reveal infiltration of the sigmoid (arrows) by the mass, as evidenced by contiguous extension and presence of gas within the mass.

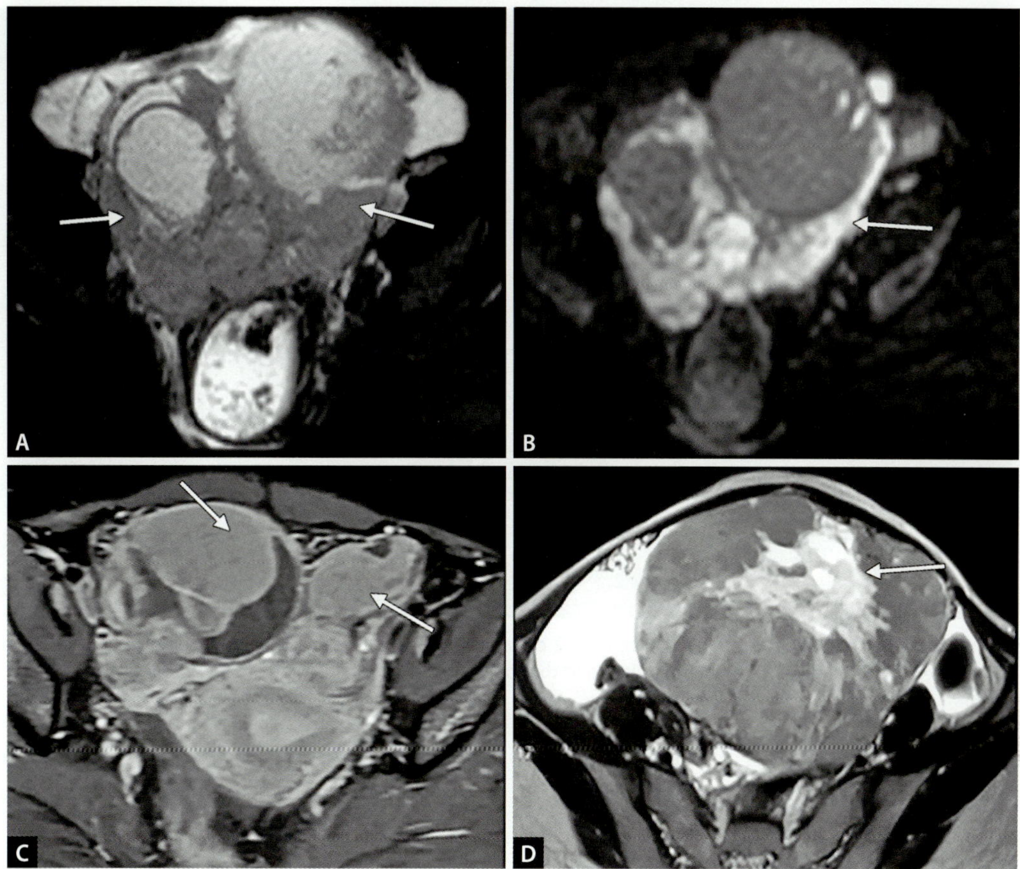

Figs. 8A to D: MRI features of malignant ovarian mass. (A) Bilateral complex solid cystic adnexal masses (arrows) and vegetations in a cystic lesion. (B) Diffusion restriction in the solid component (arrow). (C) Enhancing solid component (arrows) in bilateral complex solid cystic adnexal masses. (D) Large solid mass with internal necrosis (arrow) and the presence of ascites.

Imaging features for the staging of disease are similar on CT and MRI. MRI can also accurately delineate the extent of intra-abdominal and pelvic disease including involvement of peritoneum and mesentery, urinary tract, visceral and bowel metastases, lymph nodes, and ascites.

MRI Technique

For evaluation of female pelvis, patient preparation includes fasting for 4 hours, use of an antiperistaltic agent (Buscopan), and instructing the patient to void 15–30 minutes prior to imaging.[27]

The following sequences are suggested:

- Sagittal and axial non-fat-suppressed T2-weighted turbo spin-echo sequences.
- Coronal and axial non-fat-suppressed T2-weighted turbo spin-echo sequences.
- T1-weighted gradient-echo sequences with and without fat suppression in axial plane.
- *Diffusion-weighted imaging (DWI):* Axial plane by using a single-shot echo-planar imaging sequence; b values 0 and 1000 sec/mm^2.
- *MR perfusion:* Dynamic contrast-enhanced T1-weighted gradient-echo sequence is performed with a temporal resolution of 15 seconds; through the mass at the level of "solid tissue."[28] Solid tissue[29,30] comprises vegetation/solid portion/irregular thickened septa. This sequence is performed through the mass and adjacent myometrium after injection of Gadolinium chelate (0.2 mL/kg) at a rate of 2 mL/sec, followed by 20 mL of normal saline in the optimal plane. Images are obtained successively at 2.4-second intervals starting 10 seconds before the bolus injection, for a total duration of 320 seconds.
- Delayed postcontrast axial and sagittal T1-weighted gradient-echo images are obtained.

The perfusion images are used to generate the time-intensity curve of the solid tissue.[28] These curves are defined as follows:

- *Curve type 1*: A gradual increase in the signal intensity of the solid tissue, without a well-defined "shoulder".
- *Curve type 2*: A moderate initial increase in the signal intensity of solid tissue relative to that of myometrium

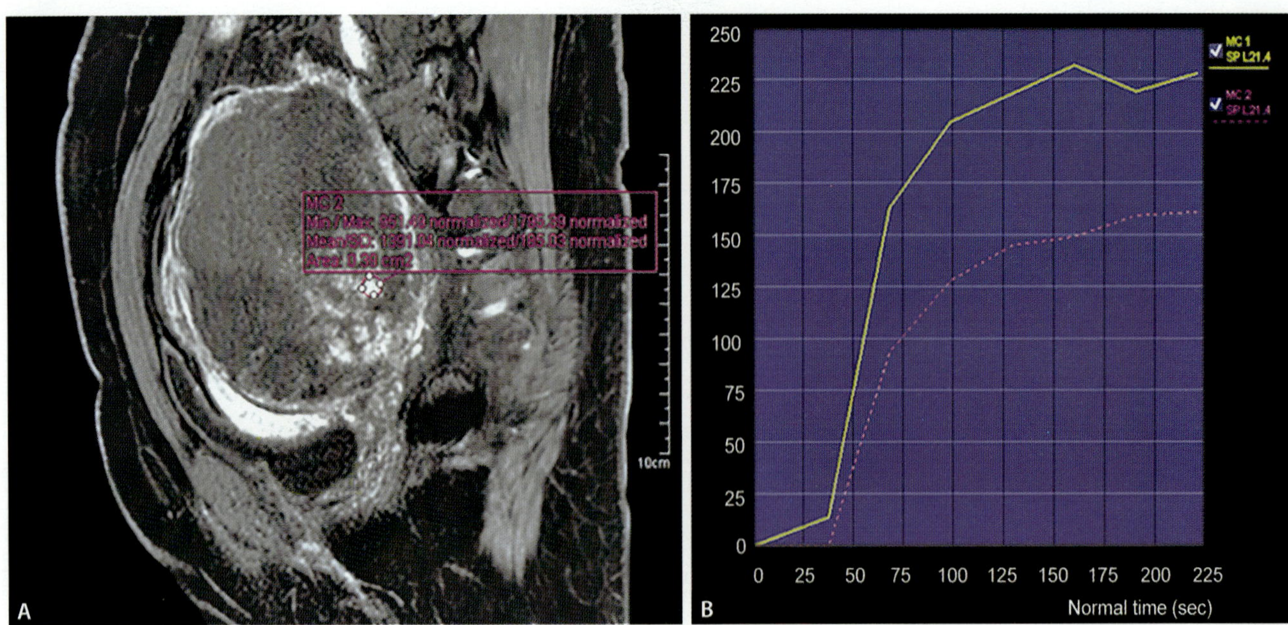

Figs. 9A and B: ADNEX MR score 4 (Indeterminate mass). Type 2 curve in left ovarian solid cystic complex mass. There is a moderate initial increase in the signal intensity of solid tissue (pink line) relative to that of myometrium (yellow line), followed by a plateau.

(enhancement of solid tissue has an initial slope less than the myometrium), followed by a plateau **(Figs. 9A and B)**.

- *Curve type 3*: An initial marked increase in the signal intensity of solid tissue steeper than that of myometrium (enhancement of solid tissue has an initial slope more than the myometrium), followed by a plateau.

MRI can be used as a problem-solving tool in sonographically indeterminate ovarian masses by providing better tissue characterization. For borderline/invasive tumors versus benign ovarian lesions the reported sensitivity of MRI is 92% and specificity is 85%.[31] Recently, the ADNEX MR scoring system **(Table 7)** was proposed which incorporates MR perfusion and DWI sequences into an algorithm for the assessment of adnexal masses.[28] Use of the ADNEX MR scoring algorithm has increased the sensitivity to 93.5% and specificity to 96.6% for the diagnosis of ovarian cancer.[28]

Key Points about MRI Signal of Ovarian Lesions[2]

- T1WI with and without fat suppression are crucial for identification of fat (teratoma) or hemorrhage.
- Endometriotic cysts are usually multifocal and bilateral with high SI on T1WI and characteristic shading and layering on T2WI. However, a complex and rapidly growing mass with contrast enhancement in preexisting endometriotic cyst suggests the possibility of endometrioid or clear cell tumor.
- Varying SI is suggestive of mucinous content and presence of solid, enhancing component in such a lesion raises the possibility of malignancy.
- A very-low SI on T2WI suggests a fibrotic component (thecoma/fibroma group, Brenner tumor or cystadenofibroma).
- Bilateral complex solid/solid cystic enhancing mass is suspicious for metastases; however, serous epithelial tumors can be also be bilateral.

PET-CT

Role in Diagnosis

Fluorodeoxyglucose (FDG) PET-CT is not routinely used in the diagnosis of ovarian cancer. USG and CT remain the primary investigation modalities. While studies have reported high specificity for detection of malignancy larger than 5 mm in size, FDG PET-CT has been shown to have lower sensitivity, especially in tumors less than 5 mm.[32,33] The pitfalls in the diagnosis of ovarian carcinoma by FDG PET-CT include:

- *Normal physiological ovarian uptake:* Typically observed in the early luteal phase. In order to avoid it, scan should ideally be performed in the early few days of the menstrual cycle. The characteristic appearance of a physiological uptake is summarized in **Box 2**.
- *Small tumors <5 mm:* PET-CT has less sensitivity in small tumors.

Table 7: ADNEX MRI scoring system.[27]

Score	*Type*	*Definition*
1	No ovarian mass	
2	Benign mass	• Unilocular cyst of any type, with no wall enhancement • Unilocular simple cyst without solid tissue; wall may enhance • Unilocular endometrioma without solid tissue; wall may enhance • Unilocular/multilocular fat-containing cystic lesion without solid tissue; wall may enhance • Cyst with solid tissue where the solid tissue is homogenously low SI on T2WI and low SI on high B-value images, with mild or moderate enhancement (type 1 or 2 curve)
3	Probably benign mass	• Unilocular hemorrhagic/ proteinaceous cyst with wall enhancement and without solid tissue • Multilocular cyst without solid tissue • Cyst with solid tissue which has intermediate SI on T2WI, is hyperintense on the high B-value DWI, and has a type 1 enhancement curve
4	Indeterminate mass	• Cyst with solid tissue which has intermediate SI on T2WI, is hyperintense on the high B-value DW image, and has a type 2 enhancement curve **(*see* Figs. 9A and B)**
5	Probably malignant mass	• Obvious peritoneal implants • Cyst with solid tissue which has intermediate T2 signal, is hyperintense on the high B-value DW image, and has a type 3 enhancement curve

Role in Staging

- PET-CT has high sensitivity in detecting peritoneal metastases **(Figs. 10A to D)** larger than 1 cm and lymph nodes larger than 7 mm.[34] When compared to CT alone, it increases the staging accuracy by almost 15–20%.[32]
- Another important role of PET-CT is differentiating patients who can undergo optimal debulking (FIGO stages I-IIIB) from patients who need neoadjuvant chemotherapy (stage IIIC-IV).[33]

Role in Post-treatment Follow-up

Various studies have quoted widely variable sensitivity and specificity of FDG PET-CT in recurrent ovarian cancer.[35-37] A recent study has shown that PET-CT has much higher sensitivity in detecting extrapelvic recurrence, compared to pelvic recurrence.[38])This is explained by the presence of high physiological activity in the urinary bladder and normal postoperative inflammatory changes in the pelvis. Some studies[39,40] have documented that PET-CT can change the management in a significant number of recurrent ovarian cancer; and can play an important role in determining who will benefit from optimal cytoreduction.

Box 2: Imaging appearance of physiological uptake in ovary.[34]

- Seen in premenopausal women (any ovarian uptake in postmenopausal women is abnormal)
- In early luteal phase
- Round or oval shape
- Smooth margin
- Located superior to the urinary bladder or close to the uterus
- SUV >3 is considered abnormal

(SUV: standardized uptake value)

KEY IMAGING FEATURES OF OVARIAN MALIGNANCIES

Epithelial tumors comprise 60% of all ovarian neoplasms and 85% of ovarian malignant neoplasms.[41] They are most commonly seen in the sixth and seventh decades of life.[41] The histological subtypes include serous, mucinous, endometrioid, clear cell, and Brenner tumors and the imaging findings of these are summarized in **Table 8**.[41,42]

These can be further classified as benign (60% of cases), borderline (5%) or malignant (35%) depending on their histologic characteristics.[41-43]

Germ cell tumors are the second most common group of ovarian neoplasms, and comprise 15–20% of all ovarian tumors and <5% of malignant ovarian neoplasms.[41] These maybe associated with elevated levels of serum α-feto-protein and human chorionic gonadotropin (βhCG). The key imaging findings of these are summarized in **Table 9**.[41-43]

Sex cord-stromal tumors are composed of cells of coelomic epithelium (sex cords) or mesenchymal cells (theca cells, granulosa cells, Leydig cells, Sertoli cells, and fibroblasts). Majority of these are benign like fibrothecoma and malignant lesions like granulosa cell tumor and Sertoli-Leydig cell tumor are also confined to the ovary at the time of diagnosis. The key imaging findings of these are summarized in **Table 10**.[2,41,42]

Collision Tumors

Collision tumor represents the simultaneous occurrence of two histologically distinct tumors with no histologic admixture at the interface. Teratoma and cystadenoma or

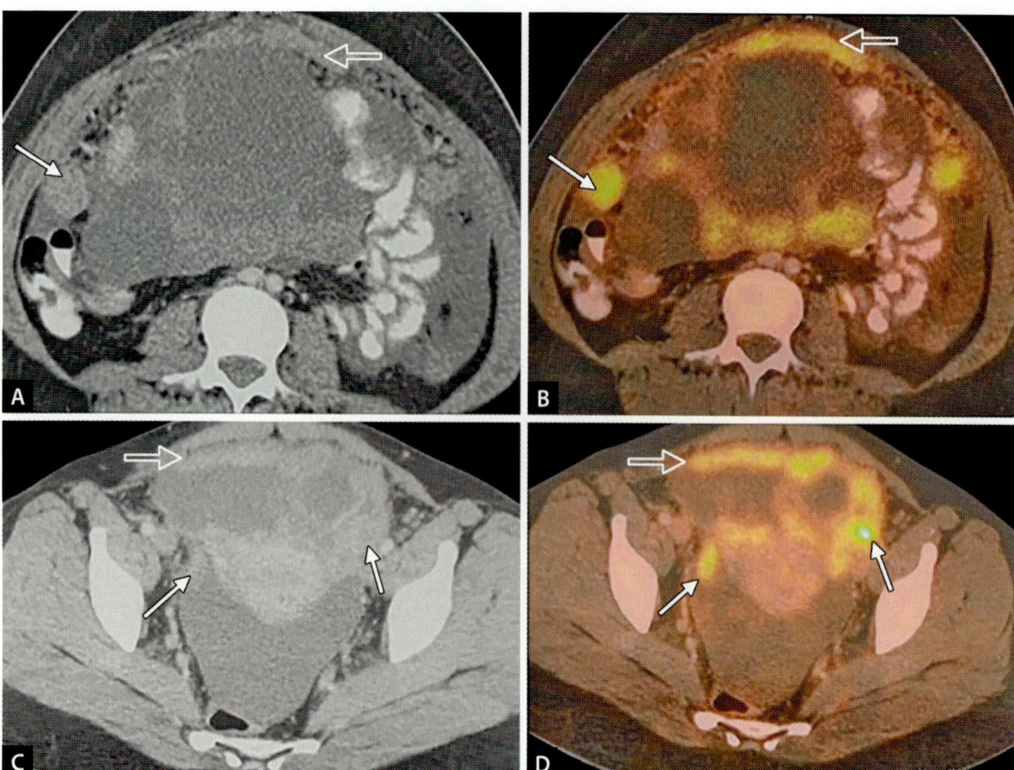

Figs. 10A to D: PET-CT in serous papillary cystadenocarcinoma. Axial CECT (A) and corresponding PET-CT image (B) reveal enhancing peritoneal deposits (arrow) and omental thickening (block arrow) with PET uptake. Axial CECT (C) and corresponding PET-CT image (D) show the bilateral solid adnexal masses (arrows) with diffuse peritoneal thickening (block arrow) with PET uptake. (CECT: contrast-enhanced computed tomography; PET: positron emission tomography).

Table 8: Key imaging features of epithelial tumors.

Histological type	*Clinical*	*Key imaging features*
Serous tumors **(Figs. 11 and 12)**	Often bilateral— 60% benign, 15% borderline, 25% malignant	• Small lesions • B-Unilocular cyst with thin regular wall, no internal septations, linear calcification (infrequent) • M-Solid component, papillary projections, peritoneal carcinomatosis
Mucinous tumors **(Figs. 13A to D)**	Often unilateral— 80% benign, 10–15% borderline, 5–10% malignant	• Large lesions • Multilocular cystic lesions with variable echoes/density/signal intensity (stained glass appearance), psammomatous calcification • M-Solid component • Pseudomyxoma peritonei
Endometrioid tumors	Almost always malignant— Bilateral: 30–50% cases	• Complex, solid cystic mass • Associated endometrial hyperplasia/carcinoma • Most common malignancy arising from endometriosis, followed by clear cell carcinoma
Clear cell tumors	Always malignant	• Second most common malignancy arising from endometriosis • Unilocular or large cyst with solid enhancing, protrusions
Brenner tumors	• Composed of transitional cells with dense stroma • Rarely malignant • Commonly incidental lesion on imaging	• Small lesions • Usually solid mass with mild enhancement • T2 hypointense stroma • Extensive amorphous calcification may be seen

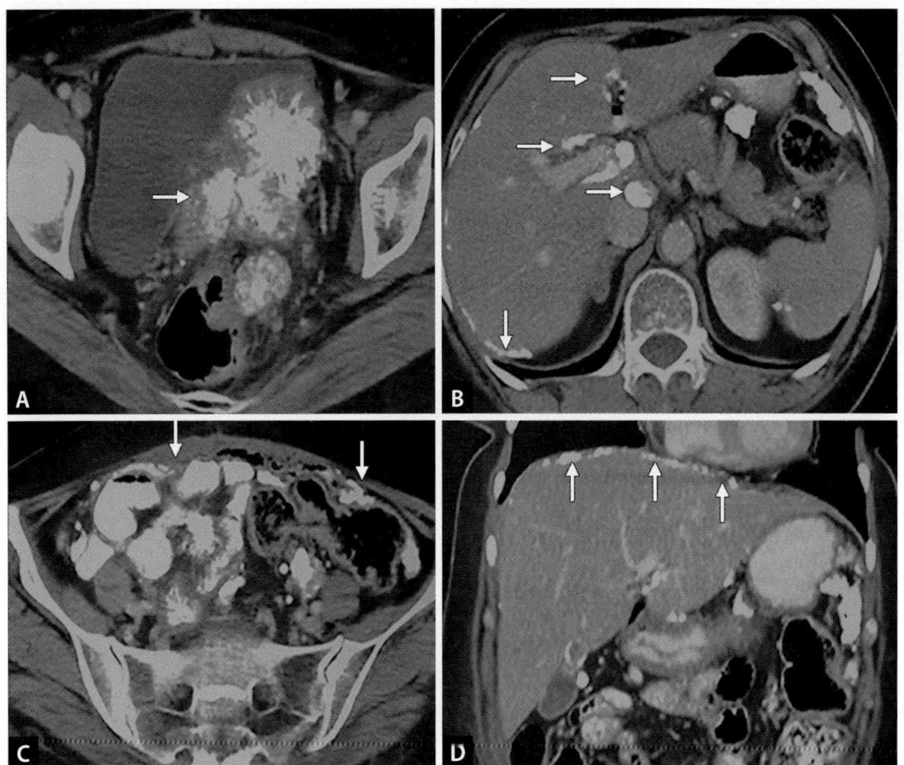

Figs. 11A to D: Serous cystadenocarcinoma ovary with calcified peritoneal deposits. Axial contrast-enhanced CT pelvis (A) shows left adnexal mass (arrow) with dense calcification. Calcified peritoneal deposits in upper abdomen (arrows in B) and pelvis (arrows in C). Coronal multiplanar reconstructed image (D) reveals calcified subphrenic deposits (arrows).

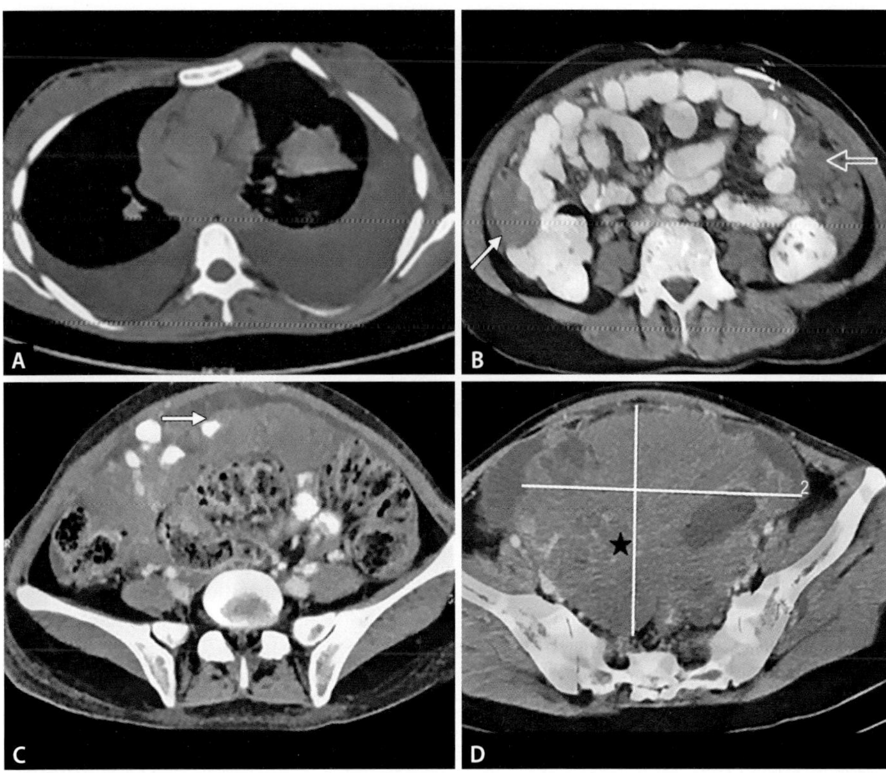

Figs. 12A to D: High-grade serous papillary carcinoma. (A) Axial CT chest reveals bilateral pleural effusion. (B to D) Axial contrast-enhanced CT abdomen and pelvis reveals multiple large solid peritoneal deposits (arrow in B), omental caking (block arrow in B), diffuse peritoneal thickening (arrow in C); and a large solid enhancing pelvic mass (asterisk in D).

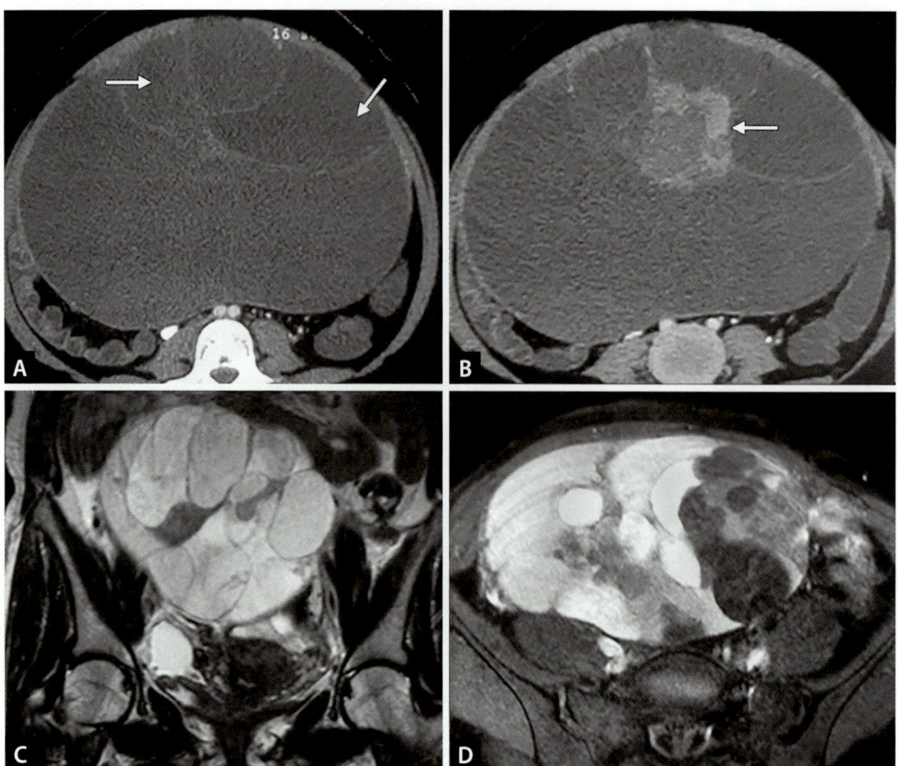

Figs. 13A to D: Mucinous cystadenocarcinoma ovary. (A) Axial contrast-enhanced CT shows multiloculated right adnexal cystic mass with different densities (arrows). (B) Solid-enhancing component within the lesion (arrow). (C) T2W coronal MRI shows loculi of variable signal intensities in the mass. (D) Axial T1W fat-suppressed MR image reveals multiple loculi to be hyperintense.

Table 9: Key imaging features of germ cell tumors.

Histological type	*Clinical*	*Key imaging features*
Mature teratoma	Most common benign ovarian tumor in <45-year-old females	• Varied spectrum (detailed in Chapter 14) • Cystic mass with fat, calcification • *Complications:* Torsion, rupture, or malignant degeneration
Immature teratoma	• First two decades of life • May have normal α-fetoprotein and βhCG levels	• Cystic solid mass with poorly defined capsule • Internal necrosis/hemorrhage • *Fat:* Small foci • *Calcification:* Small, irregular, scattered
Dysgerminoma **(Figs. 14A and B)**	• Young women • Elevated LDH • Elevated βhCG levels if syncytiotrophoblastic giant cells within the tumor	• Large, multilobulated sold mass • Fibrovascular septa characteristic
Yolk sac tumor **(Figs. 15A and B)**	• Second decade • Poor prognosis • Elevated serum α-fetoprotein • Elevated LDH may be seen	• Large solid cystic mass • "Bright dot sign" due to foci of enhancement (dilated vessels) in wall or solid component
Embryonal carcinoma	• Adolescent age group • May present as precocious puberty • Elevated βhCG and α-fetoprotein levels may be seen	• Predominantly solid mass • Nonspecific imaging features

cystadenocarcinoma are the most common occurrence as collision tumors.[44] These should be suspected on imaging if the imaging features are not typical for any particular entity.

Metastatic Ovarian Tumors

Metastases to the ovary are most commonly from colon and stomach followed by the breast, lung, and contralateral ovary.

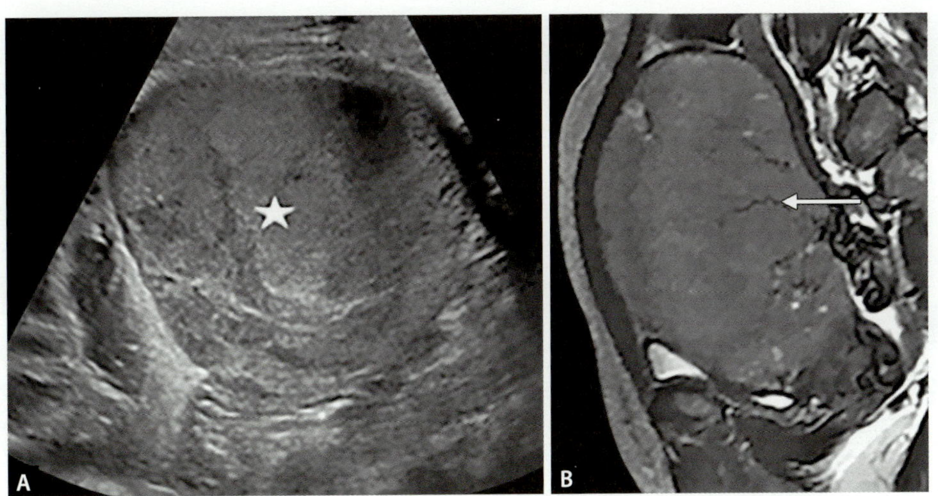

Figs. 14A and B: Ovarian dysgerminoma. (A) Solid echogenic mass on USG (asterisk). (B) Sagittal T2WI MRI reveals large, multilobulated solid T2 intermediate SI mass with characteristic fibrovascular septa (arrow).

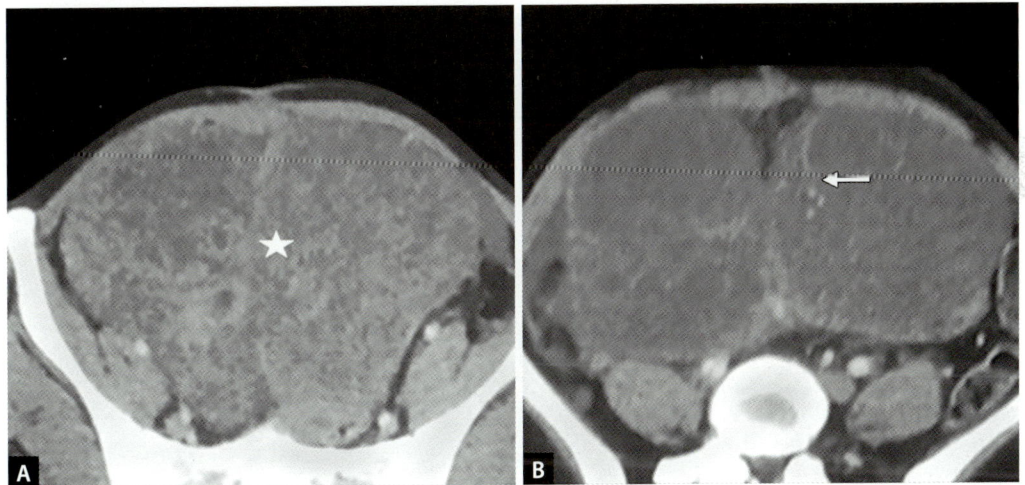

Figs. 15A and B: Yolk sac tumor. (A) Heterogeneously enhancing solid abdominopelvic mass (asterisk). (B) Foci of enhancing vessels: Bright dot sign (arrow).

Table 10: Key imaging features of sex cord–stromal tumors.

Histological type	*Clinical*	*Key imaging features*
Fibromas Fibrothecomas Thecomas	Associations: Meig syndrome	Solid masses CT: Homogenous, solid mass with delayed enhancement; dense calcifications may be seen MRI: Low SI on T1WI and markedly hypointense on T2WI
Granulosa cell tumors **(Figs. 16A and B)**	Most common estrogen producing tumor	Associated endometrial hyperplasia, polyps, or carcinoma Wide imaging spectrum: Solid masses, tumors with hemorrhage or fibrosis, multilocular cystic tumors or completely cystic tumors Compared to epithelial malignancies, these are usually confined to ovary with less peritoneal seeding and do not have intracystic papillary projections
Sertoli-Leydig cell tumors	<30 years age Most common virilizing tumor Low-grade malignancy	Well-defined, enhancing solid mass Intratumoral cysts maybe seen

Imaging findings: Nonspecific findings varying from predominantly solid masses to cystic and solid masses.

Krukenberg tumors ***(Figs. 17A and B)****:* Metastatic tumors to the ovary containing mucin-secreting "signet ring" cells and originating in the gastrointestinal tract commonly.[45,46] On imaging, these appear as bilateral solid masses with T1 hyperintensity due to mucin and T2 hypointensity (stromal reaction).

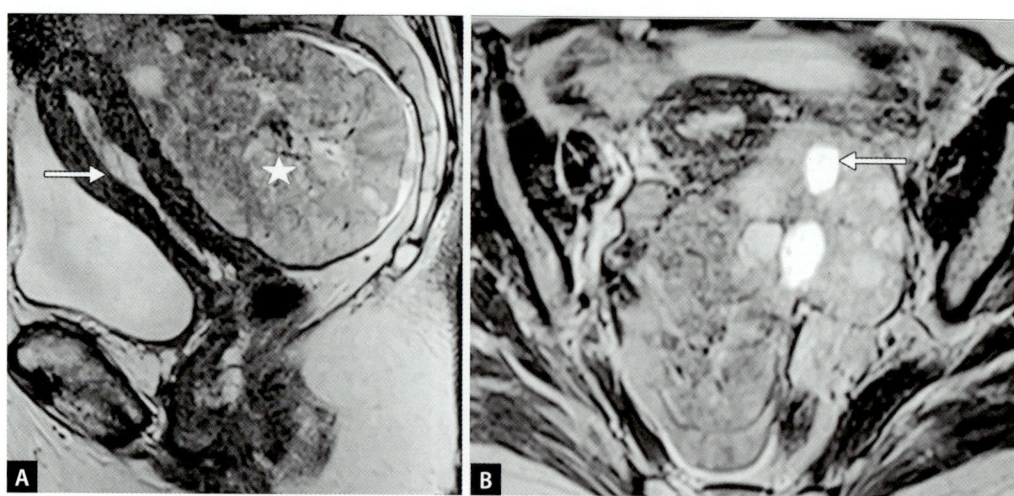

Figs. 16A and B: Granulosa cell tumor in 65/F. (A) Sagittal T2WI shows solid mass in pouch of Douglas (asterisk) with endometrial thickening (arrow). (B) Axial T2WI reveals lobulated, solid mass with cystic areas (arrow) in left adnexa and pouch of Douglas.

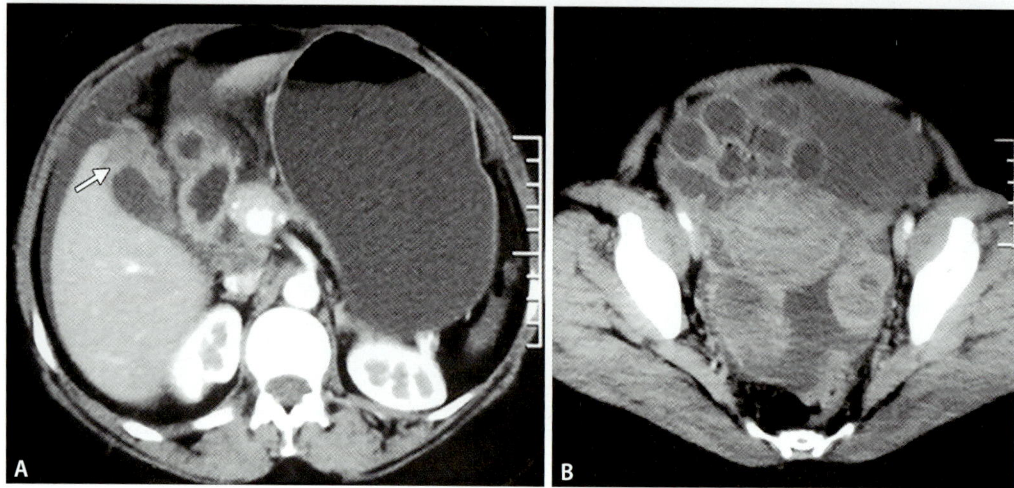

Figs. 17A and B: Krukenberg's tumor from carcinoma gallbladder. (A) Irregular mass-like GB wall thickening (arrow) and presence of ascites. (B) Bilateral solid ovarian masses with maintained ovarian shape.

Fallopian Tube Malignancies

These are uncommon neoplasms, seen mostly in the postmenopausal age group. Primary fallopian tube carcinomas arise from the ampulla with endoluminal growth leading to hydrosalpinx formation (because of obstruction). The classically described *Latzko's triad* of abdominopelvic mass, intermittent sudden and profuse watery serosanguineous vaginal discharge, and pelvic spasmodic pain relieved by discharge is seen in only 15% of the cases. Imaging features are indistinguishable from ovarian malignancies (typically solid cystic pelvic mass with peritoneal dissemination and lymph node metastases). Hydrosalpinx adjacent to the mass maybe seen in some cases.

Key point: It is important to note that in the new staging FIGO classification system the ovarian, fallopian, and primary peritoneal cancers are seen as one entity. This revision takes into account the concept of a common origin of high-grade serosal tumors from tubal cells.[3]

TUMOR MARKERS IN OVARIAN NEOPLASMS

Tumor markers include various proteins and other molecules which are produced, expressed, or metabolized by tumor tissue and are characterized in blood, serum, or urine. They are utilized in early diagnosis and screening of ovarian cancers and are also useful in follow-up, treatment response evaluation, and prediction of recurrence. *The important tumor markers are discussed briefly:*

- *CA-125 (Cancer antigen 125):* Currently, it the most widely used biomarker in diagnosis and follow-up of ovarian cancer. It is a glycoprotein expressed by epithelial cells and has a sensitivity and specificity of around 85% and 66%, respectively. Normal values range from 0 U/mL to 45 U/mL.[47]

- *BRCA 1/BRCA2*: Mutation in these tumor suppressor genes is associated with 20-60% risk of ovarian cancer, in addition to the breast malignancies.
- Alpha fetoprotein (AFP)—associated with germ cell tumors (endodermal sinus tumor, embryonal carcinoma).[48]
- Beta hCG—associated with choriocarcinoma and germ cell tumor (embryonal carcinoma).
- HE4—human epididymis protein 4, associated with ovarian carcinoma, more in endometrioid and serous cancers. Increased CA-125 and HE4 levels both increase the specificity for epithelial malignancies.
- Lactate dehydrogenase—associated with germ cell tumors (dysgerminoma).
- Inhibin A/B—granulosa cell tumors.
- Carcinoembryonic antigen (CEA)—mucinous epithelial tumors.

There are multiple other biomarkers, for which initial research has suggested potential benefits in disease detection and follow-up. These are however in an experimental stage and not part of standard evaluation. These include:

Haptoglobin, osteopontin, prostatin, macrophage colony stimulating factor and OVX1, vascular endothelial growth factor (VEGF), HER 2/neu, Ras homologue member 1 (ARHI), insulin-like growth factor binding protein 3 (IGFBP-3), metastasis-related gene synuclein gamma (SNCG), p53, mesothelin, IL-6, and IL-8.[49]

RECENT ADVANCES IN IMAGING BIOLOGY

The conventional concept of considering epithelial ovarian cancer as a single disease has been replaced by the new concept of considering them as a group of different disease entities. This concept is based on new insights into tumor biology, genetic mutations, and identification of specific precursor lesions for different groups.[50-52] Whereas high-grade serous carcinoma (HGSC) is an aggressive tumor, can develop within a short span of time, and has a poor prognosis, low-grade serous carcinoma (LGSC) is much less aggressive and develops from preexisting serous cystadenoma.[50]

High-grade Serous Carcinoma

High-grade serous carcinoma is the commonest of all epithelial ovarian cancers. It presents with an advanced stage, widespread peritoneal dissemination, and a poor prognosis. *BRCA1* and *BRCA2* mutations are found in about 10% patients. The patients with the mutations have better prognosis and can have new therapeutic options.[53] Studies have shown that HGSC with *BRCA* mutation has peritoneal metastases with a "pushing" pattern whereas the tumors lacking the mutation have a more infiltrative pattern of metastases.[54] A new concept in the pathogenesis of HGSC is that it originates from serous tubal intraepithelial carcinoma (STIC). According to this new concept, HGSC, tubal carcinoma, and primary peritoneal carcinoma have the same origin from STIC.[55] Typical imaging findings in HGSC include ascites and bulky peritoneal disease. With the advances in knowledge about tumor genetics, even more detailed subtyping of HGSC has been studied. One such notable study by Vargas et al.[56] attempted to establish association CT imaging patterns and ovarian cancer subtypes based on gene signatures (*Classification of ovarian cancer; CLOVAR*). Depending on different marker gene expression, various HGSCs were divided into four groups: differentiated, immunoreactive, mesenchymal, and proliferative. The study described that the mesenchymal subtype was more often associated with diffuse peritoneal spread and poor survival. The mesenchymal subtype was also found to be more commonly associated with resistance to platinum-based chemotherapy (e.g. cisplatin).

A detailed description of these is beyond the scope of this chapter.

Low-Grade Serous Carcinoma

Low-grade serous carcinoma constitutes of a small percentage of epithelial ovarian cancer and is much less aggressive in behavior compared to HGSC. It has better prognosis than HGSC and shows intermediate sensitivity to platinum-based chemotherapy.

Other Subtypes

Other subtypes of epithelial ovarian cancer include mucinous, endometrioid, and clear cell carcinoma. Mucinous cystadenoma is considered a precursor to mucinous cancer, and endometriosis a precursor to the other two variants. All of them have separate genetic mutations (similar to *BRCA1* and *BRCA2* in HGSC). An overview of the clinical, radiological, and pathological features is given in **Table 11**.

CONCLUSION

The role of imaging in ovarian malignancies is to detect, characterize, and stage the disease. It is important for the radiologist to be able to accurately characterize an adnexal

Table 11: Comparison of clinico-patho-radiological features of ovarian cancer subtypes.[50,57]

	HGSC	*LGSC*	*Mucinous*	*Endometrioid*	*Clear cell*
Biological behavior	Aggressive, poor prognosis	Less aggressive, intermediate prognosis	Good prognosis	Good prognosis	Intermediate prognosis
Disease spread	Extensive peritoneal spread in the abdomen	Peritoneal spread	Localized to ovary	Spread limited to pelvis	Spread limited to pelvis
Mutation	*TP53, BRCA1/2*	*BRAF, KRAS*	*KRAS*	*PTEN, CTNNB-1*	*KRAS, PTEN, PIK3CA*
Precursor lesion	STIC	Serous cystadenoma	Mucinous cystadenoma	Endometriosis	Endometriosis
Radiologic appearance	Solid/cystic or solid mass	Solid-cystic mass with papillary projection and psammoma bodies	• Large solid-cystic mass with smooth outline • Different attenuations within the tumor	• Solid-cystic with smooth outline • In pre-existing endometrioma, it is seen as a solid nodule in endometrioma wall	Large thick-walled cystic mass with mural nodules

(HGSC: high-grade serous carcinoma; LGSC: low-grade serous carcinoma; STIC: serous tubal intraepithelial carcinoma)

mass as benign or malignant. Preoperative staging by imaging is important for definitive patient management and surgical planning.

REFERENCES

1. Iyer VR, Lee SI. MRI, CT, and PET/CT for ovarian cancer detection and adnexal lesion characterization. Am J Roentgenol. 2010;194:311-21.
2. Foti PV, Attinà G, Spadola S, et al. MR imaging of ovarian masses: classification and differential diagnosis. Insights Imaging. 2016;7:21-41.
3. Kurman RJ, Carcangiu ML, Herrington CS, et al. WHO Classification of Tumors of Female Reproductive Organs. Lyon: IARC; 2014.
4. Prat J. FIGO Committee on Gynecologic Oncology. Staging classification for cancer of the ovary, fallopian tube, and peritoneum. Int J Gynaecol Obstet. 2014;124:1-5.
5. Mutch DG, Prat J. 2014 FIGO staging for ovarian, fallopian tube and peritoneal cancer. Gynecol Oncol. 2014;133:401-4.
6. Javadi S, Ganeshan DM, Qayyum A, et al. Ovarian cancer, the revised FIGO staging system, and the role of imaging. Am J Roentgenol. 2016;206:1351-60.
7. Leibman AJ, Kruse B, McSweeney MB. Transvaginal sonography: comparison with transabdominal sonography in the diagnosis of pelvic masses. Am J Roentgenol. 1988;151:89-92.
8. Hata K, Hata T, Manabe A, et al. A critical evaluation of transvaginal Doppler studies, transvaginal sonography, magnetic resonance imaging, and CA 125 in detecting ovarian cancer. Obstet Gynecol. 1992;80:922-6.
9. Reles A, Wein U, Lichtenegger W. Transvaginal color Doppler sonography and conventional sonography in the preoperative assessment of adnexal masses. J Clin Ultrasound. 1997;25:217-25.
10. Ferrazzi E, Zanetta G, Dordoni D, et al. Transvaginal ultrasonographic characterization of ovarian masses: comparison of five scoring systems in a multicenter study. Ultrasound Obstet Gynecol. 1997;10:192-7.
11. Kurjak A, Predanic M. New scoring system for prediction of ovarian malignancy based on transvaginal color Doppler sonography. J Ultrasound Med. 1992;11:631-8.
12. Franchi M, Beretta P, Ghezzi F, et al. Diagnosis of pelvic masses with transabdominal color Doppler, CA 125, and ultrasonography. Acta Obstet Gynecol Scand. 1995;74:734-9.
13. Timor-Tritsch IE, Lerner JP, Monteagudo A, et al. Transvaginal ultrasonographic characterization of ovarian masses by means of color flow-directed Doppler measurements and a morphologic scoring system. Am J Obstet Gynecol. 1993;168:909-13.
14. Laban M, Metawee H, Elyan A, et al. Three-dimensional ultrasound and three-dimensional power Doppler in the assessment of ovarian tumors. Int J Gynecol Obstet. 2007;99:201-5.
15. Ueland FR, DePriest PD, Pavlik EJ. Preoperative differentiation of malignant from benign ovarian tumors: the efficacy of morphology indexing and Doppler flow sonography. Gynecol Oncol. 2003;91:46-50.
16. Timmerman D, Testa AC, Bourne T, et al. Simple ultrasound-based rules for the diagnosis of ovarian cancer. Ultrasound Obstet Gynecol. 2008;31:681-90.
17. Alcázar JL, Pascual MÁ, Olartecoechea B, et al. IOTA simple rules for discriminating between benign and malignant adnexal masses: prospective external validation. Ultrasound Obstet Gynecol. 2013;42:467-71.
18. Timmerman D, Van Calster B, Testa A, et al. Predicting the risk of malignancy in adnexal masses based on the simple rules from the International Ovarian Tumor Analysis group. Am J Obstet Gynecol. 2016;214(4):424-37.
19. Van Calster B, Van Hoorde K, Valentin L, et al. Evaluating the risk of ovarian cancer before surgery using the ADNEX model to differentiate between benign, borderline, early and advanced stage invasive, and secondary metastatic tumors: prospective multicentre diagnostic study. BMJ. 2014;349:g5920.

20. Forstner R, Sala E, Kinkel K, et al. ESUR guidelines: ovarian cancer staging and follow-up. Eur Radiol. 2010;20:2773-80.
21. Sahdev A. CT in ovarian cancer staging: how to review and report with emphasis on abdominal and pelvic disease for surgical planning. Cancer Imaging. 2016;16:19-27.
22. Tempany CM, Zou KH, Silverman SG, et al. Staging of advanced ovarian cancer: comparison of imaging modalities–report from the Radiological Diagnostic Oncology Group. Radiology. 2000;215(3):761-7.
23. Chang SJ, Hodeib M, Chang J, et al. Survival impact of complete cytoreduction to no gross residual disease for advanced-stage ovarian cancer: a meta-analysis. Gynecol Oncol. 2013;130:493-8.
24. Sohaib SAA, Reznek RH. MR imaging in ovarian cancer. Cancer Imaging. 2007;7:S119-29.
25. Sohaib SA, Sahdev A, Van Trappen PO, et al. Characterization of adnexal mass lesions on MR imaging. Am J Roentgenol. 2003;180:1297-304.
26. Hricak H, Chen M, Coakley FV, et al. Complex adnexal masses: detection and characterization with MR imaging-multivariate analysis. Radiology. 2000;214:39-46.
27. Sadowski EA, Robbins JB, Rockall AG, et al. A systematic approach to adnexal masses discovered on ultrasound: the ADNEx MR scoring system. Abdom Radiol. 2018;43:679-96.
28. Thomassin-Naggara I, Aubert E, Rockall A, et al. Adnexal masses: development and preliminary validation of an MR imaging scoring system. Radiology. 2013;267:432-43.
29. Thomassin-Naggara I, Daraï E, Cuenod CA, et al. Dynamic contrast-enhanced magnetic resonance imaging: a useful tool for characterizing ovarian epithelial tumors. J Magn Reson Imaging. 2008;28(1):111-20.
30. Timmerman D, Valentin L, Bourne TH, et al. Terms, definitions, and measurements to describe the sonographic features of adnexal tumors: a consensus opinion from the International Ovarian Tumor Analysis (IOTA) Group. Ultrasound Obstet Gynecol. 2000;16(5):500-5.
31. Medeiros LR, Freitas LB, Rosa DD, et al. Accuracy of magnetic resonance imaging in ovarian tumor: a systematic quantitative review. Am J Obstet Gynecol. 2011;204:67.e61-10.
32. Castellucci P, Perrone AM, Picchio M. Diagnostic accuracy of 18F-FDG PET/CT in characterizing ovarian lesions and staging ovarian cancer: correlation with transvaginal ultrasonography, computed tomography, and histology. Nucl Med Commun. 2007;28:589-95.
33. Kitajima K, Murakami K, Yamasaki E. Diagnostic accuracy of integrated FDG-PET/contrast-enhanced CT in staging ovarian cancer: comparison with enhanced CT. Eur J Nucl Med Mol Imaging. 2008;35:1912-20.
34. Prakash P, Cronin CG, Blake MA. Role of PET/CT in ovarian cancer. Am J Roentgenol. 2010;194:W464-70.
35. Sironi S, Messa C, Mangili G, et al. Integrated FDG PET/CT in patients with persistent ovarian cancer: correlation with histological findings. Radiology. 2004;233:433-40.
36. Chung HH, Kang WJ, Kim JW, et al. Role of [18F] FDG PET/CT in the assessment of suspected recurrent ovarian cancer: correlation with clinical or histological findings. Eur J Nucl Med Mol Imaging. 2007;34:480-6.
37. Sebastian S, Lee SI, Horowitz NS, et al. PET-CT vs CT alone in ovarian cancer recurrence. Abdom Imaging. 2008;33:112-8.
38. Iagaru AH, Mittra ES, McDougall IR, et al. 18F-FDG PET/CT evaluation of patients with ovarian carcinoma. Nucl Med Commun. 2008;29:1046-51.
39. Mangili G, Picchio M, Sironi S. Integrated PET/CT as a first-line restaging modality in patients with suspected recurrence of ovarian cancer. Eur J Nucl Med Mol Imaging. 2007;34:658-66.
40. Simcock B, Neesham D, Quinn M. The impact of PET/CT in the management of recurrent ovarian cancer. Gynecol Oncol. 2006;103:271-6.
41. Jung SE, Lee JM, Rha SE, et al. CT and MR imaging of ovarian tumors with emphasis on differential diagnosis. Radiographics. 2002;22:1305-25.
42. Jeong YY, Outwater EK, Kang HK. Imaging evaluation of ovarian masses. Radiographics. 2000;20:1445-70.
43. Heo SH, Kim JW, Shin SS, et al. Review of ovarian tumors in children and adolescents: radiologic-pathologic correlation. Radiographics. 2014;34:2039-55.
44. Kim SH, Kim YJ, Park BK, et al. Collision tumors of the ovary associated with teratoma: clues to the correct preoperative diagnosis. J Comput Assist Tomogr. 1999;23:929-33.
45. Brown DL, Zou KH, Tempany CM, et al. Primary versus secondary ovarian malignancy: imaging findings of adnexal masses in the Radiology Diagnostic Oncology Group Study. Radiology. 2001;219:213-8.
46. Ha HK, Baek SY, Kim SH, et al. Krukenberg's tumor of the ovary: MR imaging features. Am J Roentgenol. 1995;164:1435-9.
47. Bast RC Jr, Badgwell D, Lu Z, et al. New tumor markers: CA125 and beyond. Int J Gynecol Cancer. 2005;15(Suppl 3):274-81.
48. Taskinen S, Fagerholm R, Lohi J, et al. Pediatric ovarian neoplastic tumors: incidence, age at presentation, tumor markers and outcome. Acta Obstet Gynecol Scand. 2015;94(4):425-9.
49. Rein BJD, Gupta S, Dada R, et al. Potential markers for detection and monitoring of ovarian cancer. J Oncol. 2011;2011:475983.
50. Forstner R, Meissnitzer M, Cunha TM. Update on imaging of ovarian cancer. Curr Radiol Rep. 2016;4:31.
51. Lawrenson K, Gyther SA. Ovarian cancer: a clinical challenge that needs some basic answers. PLoS Med. 2009;6(2e):1000025.
52. Kurman RJ, Shih IeM. Molecular pathogenesis and extraovarian origin of epithelial ovarian cancer–shifting the paradigm. Hum Pathol. 2011;42:918-31.
53. Bolton KL, Chenevix-Trench G, Goh C, et al. Association between BRCA1 and BRCA2 mutations and survival in women with invasive epithelial ovarian cancer. JAMA. 2012;307:382-90.
54. Reyes MC, Arnold AG, Kauff ND, et al. Invasion patterns of metastatic high-grade serous carcinoma of ovary or fallopian tube associated with BRCA deficiency. Mod Pathol. 2014;27(10):1405-11.
55. Nik NN, Vang R, Shih IM, et al. Origin and pathogenesis of pelvic (ovarian, tubal, and primary peritoneal) serous carcinoma. Annu Rev Pathol. 2014;9:27-45.
56. Vargas HA, Micco M, Hong SI, et al. Association between morphologic CT imaging traits and prognostically relevant signatures in women with high-grade serous ovarian cancer. A hypothesis-generating study. Radiology. 2015;274:742-51.
57. Lalwani N, Prassad SR, Vikram R, et al. Histologic, molecular, and cytogenetic features of ovarian cancers: implication for diagnosis and treatment. Radiographics. 2011;31:625-46.

Chapter 16

Benign Diseases of the Uterus and Vagina

Rashmi Dixit, Anju Garg, Alpana Manchanda

INTRODUCTION

A wide variety of benign lesions involve the uterus. These may be congenital or acquired. The clinical presentation is often nonspecific, hence imaging has an important role in establishing an accurate diagnosis. Ultrasound (US), especially transvaginal sonography (TVS) is the investigation of choice for initial evaluation. MRI is an excellent problem-solving tool and helps guide management decisions. The role of computed tomography (CT) is limited in the evaluation of benign disease of the female pelvis due to its poor soft tissue differentiation.

CONGENITAL ANOMALIES

The uterus arises from paired embryologic structures—the Müllerian ducts that undergo fusion and resorption, between 6 weeks and 11 weeks in utero, to give rise to the uterus, fallopian tubes, cervix, and upper two-thirds of the vagina. Disruption at any stage, i.e. ductal development, ductal fusion, or septal resorption can result in anomalies of these structures referred to as Müllerian duct anomalies (MDAs). Since the ovaries arise from the primitive yolk sac while the distal one-third of the vagina arises from the sinovaginal bud, anomalies of the external genitalia or ovary are not associated with MDAs. The reported prevalence varies widely from 1% to 5% in the general population to 13%–25% in women with recurrent pregnancy loss.[1-3]

Ultrasound, especially three-dimensional US (3D US) and MR imaging play an important role in the diagnosis and evaluation of suspected MDA. Hysterosalpingography (HSG), usually a part of the initial workup infertility, may suggest a MDA, but it cannot reliably differentiate subtypes. 3D US is recommended as the initial investigation for the diagnosis of female genital anomalies in "symptomatic" patients of the reproductive age suspected to have an anomaly of a female genital tract and for any suspicious findings on routine US.[4] It is preferable to do the US during the second half of the menstrual cycle, since the endometrium is thick and echogenic during this period, making visualization of the MDAs easier.[5] MR is generally the most preferred imaging modality especially for complex anomalies and is recommended as the first-line diagnostic procedure for symptomatic adolescents.[4] MR imaging decreases the number of invasive procedures, costs, and guides management decisions.[5] Concomitant renal anomalies like agenesis, horseshoe kidney, renal dysplasia, ectopic kidney, and duplicated collecting systems have been reported in 29% of patients. Associated skeletal anomalies may also be present.[1,3,6]

Classification

There is no universally accepted MDA classification system; each having its limitations. The system proposed by the American Society for Reproductive Medicine (ASRM)[7] has been the most widely accepted until recently. *The ASRM classification* ***(Fig. 1)*** *of congenital anomalies*:

- *Class I—agenesis or hypoplasia*: Failure of development of the Müllerian ducts in the early stages (around 5 weeks' of gestation) results in varying degrees of agenesis or hypoplasia of uterus, cervix, and the proximal two-thirds of the vagina. In *agenesis*, there is no uterus or small amount of rudimentary tissue without any differentiation. This anomaly is part of the *Mayer-Rokitansky-Küster-Hauser (MRKH) syndrome.*

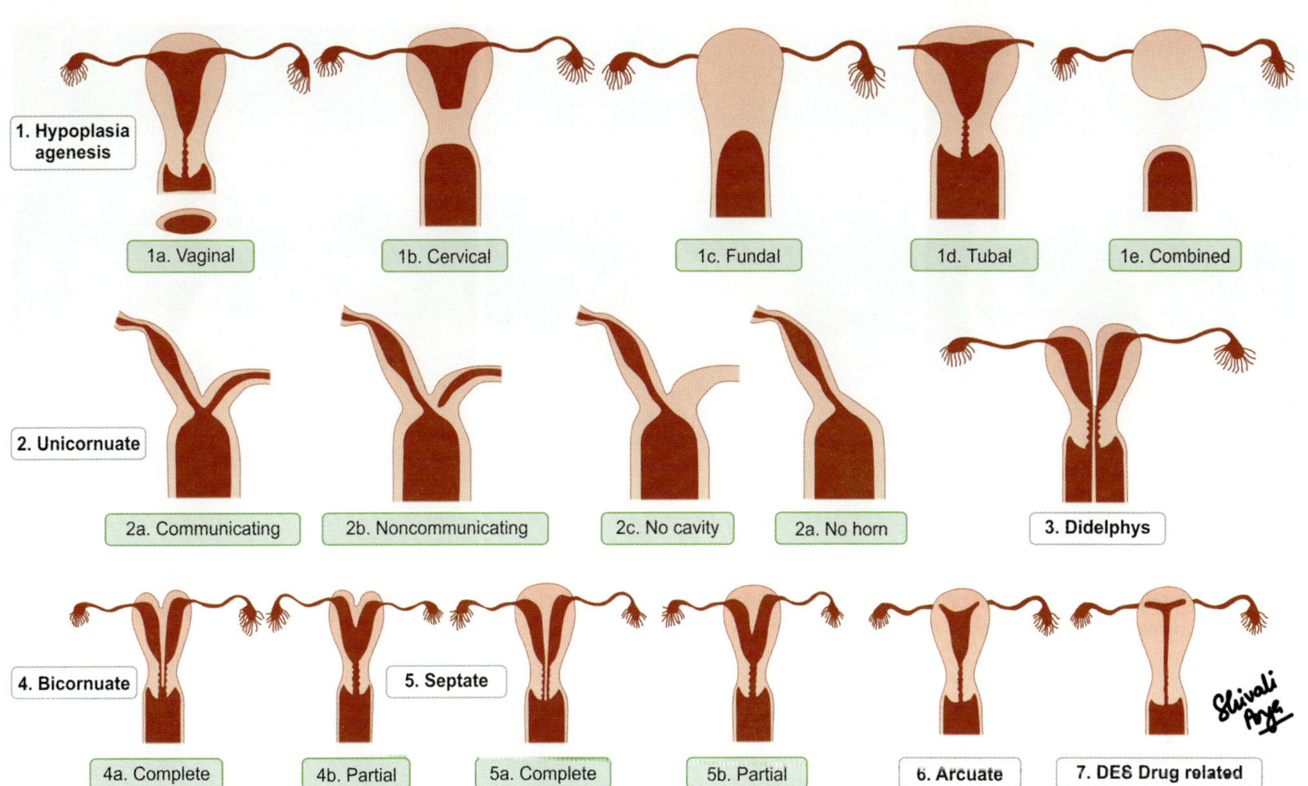

Fig. 1: The ASRM classification of female genital tract congenital anomalies (ASRM: American Society for Reproductive Medicine; DES: diethylstilbestrol).

It is the most severe type of MDA, i.e. complete agenesis of the proximal vagina, cervix, and uterus. The patients mostly manifest at puberty as primary amenorrhea with normal secondary sexual characteristics, since ovarian function is preserved. Isolated involvement of reproductive organs is classified as MRKH syndrome type 1 while if patients also have extragenital, e.g. renal, skeletal, vertebral, otologic, or cardiac anomalies, it is classified as MRKH syndrome type 2. A small but fully differentiated organ is visualized in uterine *hypoplasia*.[5,8]

Ultrasound reveals normal-appearing ovaries and absence of a normal uterus. However, definitive diagnosis of uterine agenesis or hypoplasia is challenging since the uterine position may be variable. MR is excellent for investigating primary amenorrhea, helping to differentiate uterine hypoplasia or agenesis from other causes. On sagittal T2W images, the expected location of the cervix and uterus can be extrapolated from the position of the urethra, lower vagina, and bladder, making them very useful for the diagnosis of uterine agenesis or hypoplasia. There is no identifiable uterus in complete uterine agenesis **(Figs. 2A to C)**. A hypoplastic uterus is visualized as a soft-tissue mass with signal pattern of normal myometrium, i.e. slightly hyperintense on T2-weighted images and it may be possible to identify zonal anatomy after puberty, due to the influence of female hormones. In younger females, the myometrium is T2-hypointense with poorly defined zonal anatomy.[6] In general, the endometrial cavity is small and intercornual diameter is less than 2 cm.[9] Vaginal agnesis is well seen on the axial images with no normal vaginal zonal anatomy identified between the rectum and the urethra. The length of the atretic vaginal segment may affect surgical approach in cases of isolated vaginal agenesis, and is best determined in the sagittal plane.[6]

- *Class II—unicornuate uterus*: Normal development of one Müllerian duct and near complete or complete arrest in development of the other duct results in unicornuate uterus. This can occur in four subtypes: (1) unicornuate uterus with no contralateral rudimentary horn, (2) contralateral rudimentary horn with no endometrial cavity (nonfunctioning), (3) contralateral rudimentary horn with an endometrial cavity communicating with the normal side, and (4) contralateral rudimentary horn with a noncommunicating endometrial cavity.

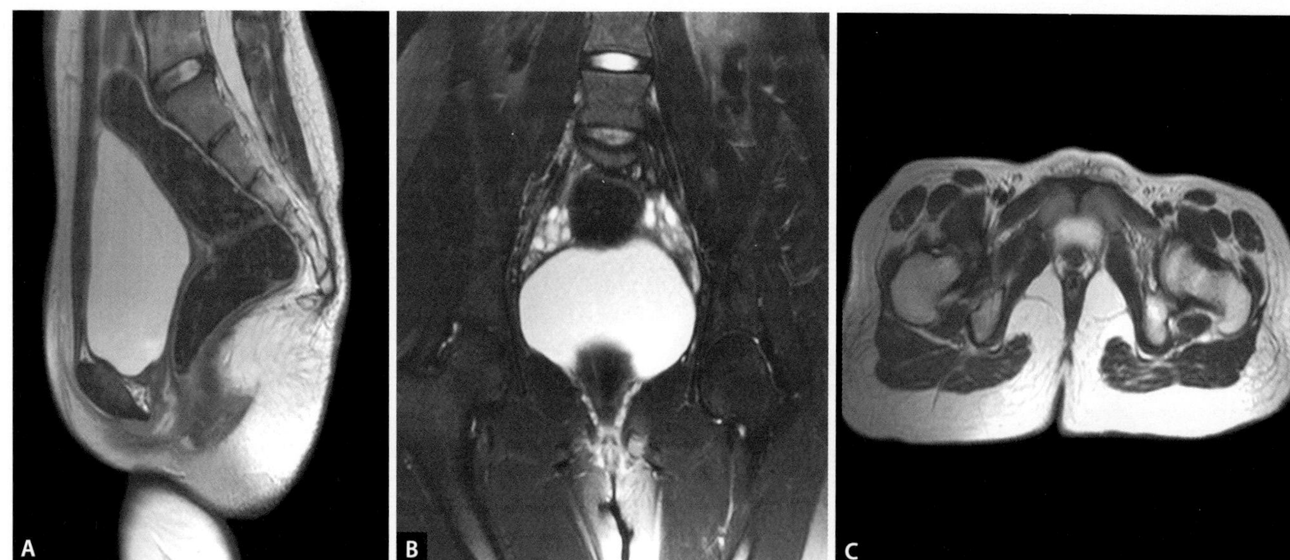

Figs. 2A to C: Müllerian agenesis T2W sagittal and coronal MR images. (A and B) No uterine tissue is visualized posterior to the bladder. Both ovaries are normal; (C) T2W axial image shows lower one-third of vagina between the bladder and rectum.

Renal anomalies on the same side as the rudimentary horn may be seen in nearly 40% of patients with unicornuate uteri, renal agenesis accounting for most of these (67% of cases).

The first two subtypes have minimal risk and do not require surgical management. Endometrium in a rudimentary horn is important to report. When present in a noncommunicating rudimentary horn, it can present with pelvic pain either due to an obstructed, distended horn or due to endometriosis consequent to retrograde flow of menstrual flow.[10,11] In addition, when endometrium is present in a rudimentary horn, both when it does or does not communicate with the uterine cavity, there is an increased risk of complications like ectopic pregnancy, miscarriage, preterm labor, and uterine rupture.[12]

A fusiform, banana-shaped off midline uterine cavity is seen with a single fallopian tube on HSG. However, presence of a noncommunicating rudimentary horn cannot be excluded. A small, oblong, off-midline structure is seen on US, and the rudimentary horn may be difficult to identify. On MR, the unicornuate uterus shows normal zonal anatomy and the rudimentary horn is best delineates. When there is no endometrium in the rudimentary horn, it shows diffuse low signal intensity with no zonal anatomy, while preserved zonal anatomy is evident when endometrial tissue is present **(Fig. 3)**. A functioning rudimentary horn may become distended with blood after menarche when noncommunicating.[5,13]

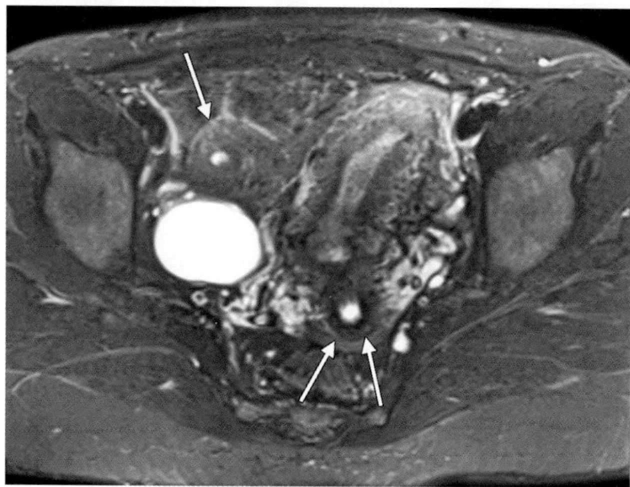

Fig. 3: Unicornuate uterus with noncommunicating functional horn: Axial T2 fat saturated MR image showing a banana-shaped uterine cavity on the left and a rudimentary horn with non-communicating cavity on the right side (single arrow). The unicornuate uterus is seen to be continuous with the cervix posteriorly (arrows). A cyst is also seen in the right ovary. Vagina was normal—European Society of Human Reproduction and Embryology (ESHRE) class U4aC0V0.

- *Class III—uterus didelphys*: Complete failure of Müllerian duct fusion results in uterus didelphys producing duplication of the uterus, cervix, and proximal vagina. Vaginal duplication has been reported in 75% of patients.[14] A transverse vaginal septum on one side may be present in addition, resulting in ipsilateral obstruction.

Two separate, elongated endometrial cavities with contrast opacification of both fallopian tubes is seen on HSG. However, if only one cervix is cannulated or if one side is obstructed due to a transverse septum, nonopacification of the ipsilateral uterine horn occurs, resulting in a fallacious impression of unicornuate uterus.[15,16] On ultrasonography and MR, two widely divergent uterine horns with separate, noncommunicating endometrial cavities and two cervices are seen. Duplication of the vagina (hemivaginal septum) may not be seen on US; in such cases, differentiation between uterus didelphys and a bicornuate bicollis uterus may be difficult. Duplication of the proximal vagina is better visualized on MR, which may be aided by introduction of a viscous liquid, like US gel, into the vagina prior to imaging. If a septum obstructing one side is present, that horn will be distended with blood products producing hematometrocolpos. It is often associated with ipsilateral renal agenesis. This is referred to as **Herlyn-Werner-Wunderlich syndrome, also known as obstructed hemivagina and ipsilateral renal anomaly (OHVIRA) (Fig. 4)**.

- *Class IV—bicornuate uterus*: This is due to partial nonfusion of the Müllerian ducts accounting for nearly 10% of MDAs. The horns of the bicornuate uteri are not as fully developed and are smaller than those in the didelphys uteri.[8] The endometrial cavity is duplicated with or without cervical duplication, referred to as bicornuate bicollis and bicornuate unicollis uteri, respectively.

  Hysterosalpingography shows opacification of two symmetric fusiform uterine cavities and fallopian tubes with an intercornual angle of more than 105°. However, differentiation of the unicollis variety from a septate uterus is impossible at HSG due to overlapping features.[15,16] On MR/3D US, bicornuate uterus is characterized by the presence of a fundal cleft (>1 cm in depth) in the external contour, similar to uterus didelphys, best identified on oblique coronal images **(Figs. 5A to C)**. *This has been reported to be 100% sensitive and specific in differentiation of didelphys and bicornuate uteri, which are fusion anomalies, from septate and arcuate (reabsorption anomalies)*.[1,17] Normal zonal anatomy on MR is seen in both uterine horns. In a bicornuate bicollis uterus, the duplicated cervix gives an "owl eyes" appearance on axial section. An associated longitudinal vaginal septum may be present in one-fourth of cases, making a bicornuate bicollis uterus indistinguishable from a uterus didelphys.
- *Class V—septate uterus*: Septate uterus constitutes nearly 55% of cases, making it the most common MDA.[15,16,18-21] The septum occurs due to complete or partial failure of reabsorption of the uterovaginal septum. It arises from the midpart of the uterine fundus and is variable in length and composition. A complete septum extends to the external cervical os and may even extend into the vagina in approximately 25% of cases.[9,22,23] It may be fibrous, myometrial, or consists of varying proportions of fibrous tissue and myometrium. Septate uterus has a strong association with repeated midtrimester miscarriage. It may at times be challenging to differentiate between a septate and bicornuate uterus. Correct diagnosis is important because the former requires surgical correction to improve reproductive outcomes. The most important difference is the appearance of the uterine fundus; a septate uterus has a normal convex external fundal contour. The external fundal contour cannot be seen on HSG hence reliable differentiation of septate from bicornuate uterus is not possible. Conventionally, an angle below 75° between the uterine horns is said to be seen in septate rather than bicornuate uterus but this is not reliable.[9,22-25]

  On US, a septum arising from fundus, dividing the endometrial cavity, is seen. The fibrous component tends to be less echogenic compared to myometrium.

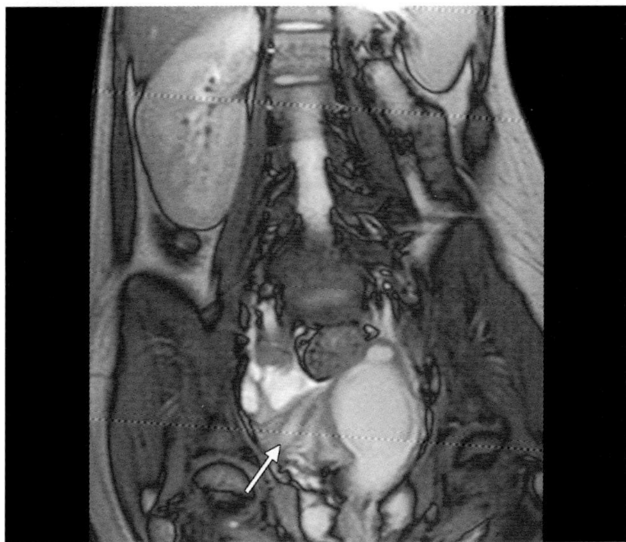

Fig. 4: OHVIRA syndrome. Coronal T2W MR image showing left hematometra and hematocolpos due to an obstructing hemivaginal septum. Note the normal right uterine cavity and cervix (arrow) and absent left kidney—ESHRE class U3bC2V2.

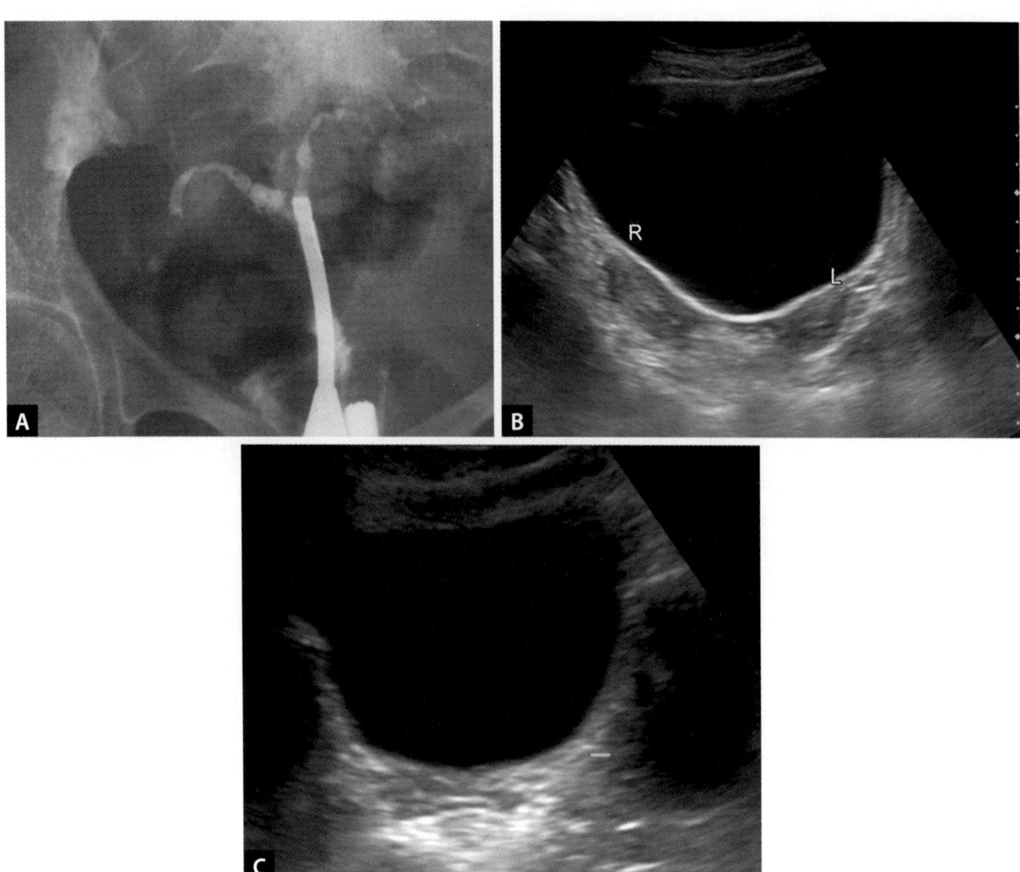

Figs. 5A to C: Bicornuate uterus. (A) Hysterosalpingography showing two widely divergent uterine cavities; (B) Midline transverse ultrasound image showing two widely separated uterine horns; (C) Transverse section at a lower level shows the normal vagina.

The external uterine contour is well-evaluated with 3D imaging, as it allows coronal views of the uterus.[22,26] The fundus either has a normal convex external contour **(Figs. 6A to D)** or a fundal cleft <1 cm deep.[27] Some authors have reported that if a line is drawn between the uterine ostia and the apex of the external fundal contour is >5 mm above this line, it suggests a septate uterus. On the other hand, if it is below or <5 mm above the interostial line, it suggests a bicornuate or didelphys uterus.[5,19]

On MR, the external fundal contour is well seen on oblique coronal images planned along the uterine plane. MR can also help to differentiate myometrium (which has a higher T2 signal and is usually seen closer to the fundus in a complete septum) from fibrous tissue (which has a low signal intensity). This is important as a hysteroscopic septoplasty is offered for a fibrous septum, but a transabdominal surgical approach is needed for a muscular septum **(Figs. 7A and B)**. Rarely, a complete septate uterus may also be associated with cervical duplication.[28] Careful evaluation of the outer uterine contour should be done to avoid a wrong diagnosis of a bicornuate bicollis uterus.

- *Class VI—arcuate uterus*: Arcuate uterus is characterized by only a mild indentation of the endometrium at the uterine fundus and occurs due to near complete reabsorption of the uterovaginal septum.[27] Ludwin et al. have suggested that if the distance between the interostial line and endometrial-myometrial junction at uterine fundus is >15 mm on 3D-US, it suggests a septate configuration; on the other hand, in case of arcuate uterus, this is more than 10 mm but less than 15 mm.[29] As per the modification of ASRM criteria in 2016, a septate uterus has an internal indentation of greater than 15 mm and an indentation angle less than 90° while in a normal/arcuate uterus, both the indentation depth should be less than 10 mm and angle more than 90°. Values in between these are considered to lie in the gray zone.

Hysterosalpingography reveals a single uterine cavity with a broad saddle-shaped indentation at the uterine fundus.[5,22] On US and MR imaging, the external fundal

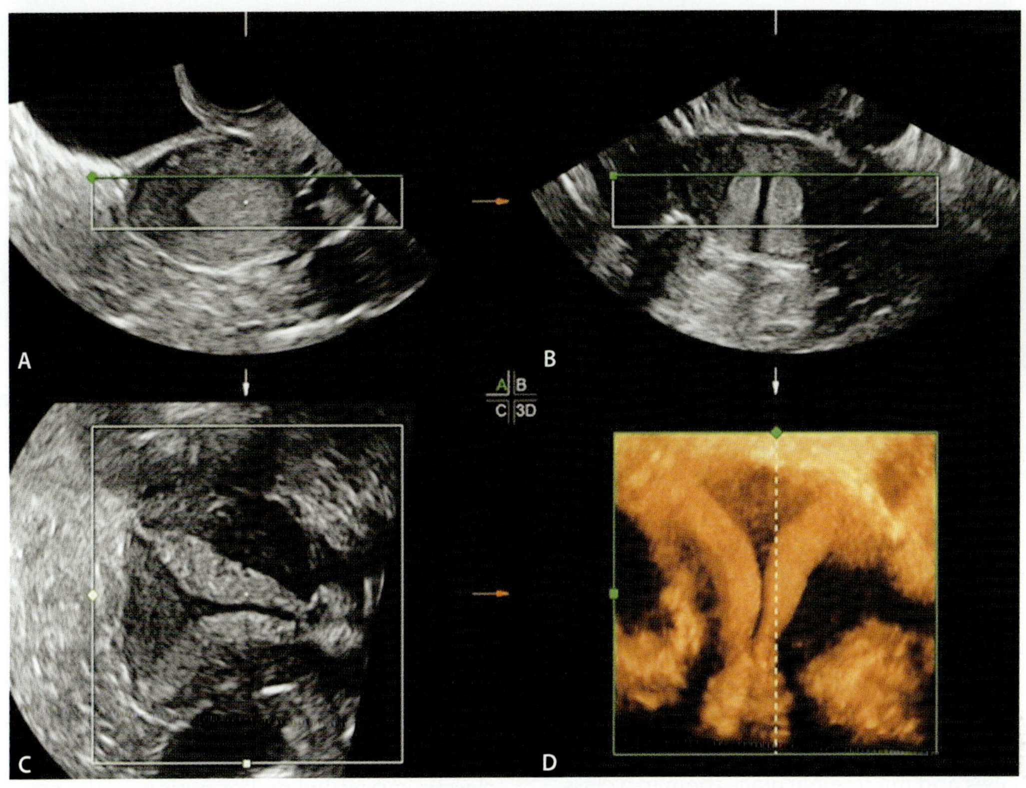

Figs. 6A to D: (A and B) Septate uterus on 3D USG. Normal external fundal contour is well-appreciated on the coronal images (C and D) with a hypoechoic septum arising from the fundus, dividing the endometrial cavity into two up to the level of external os—ESHRE class U2bC1V0.

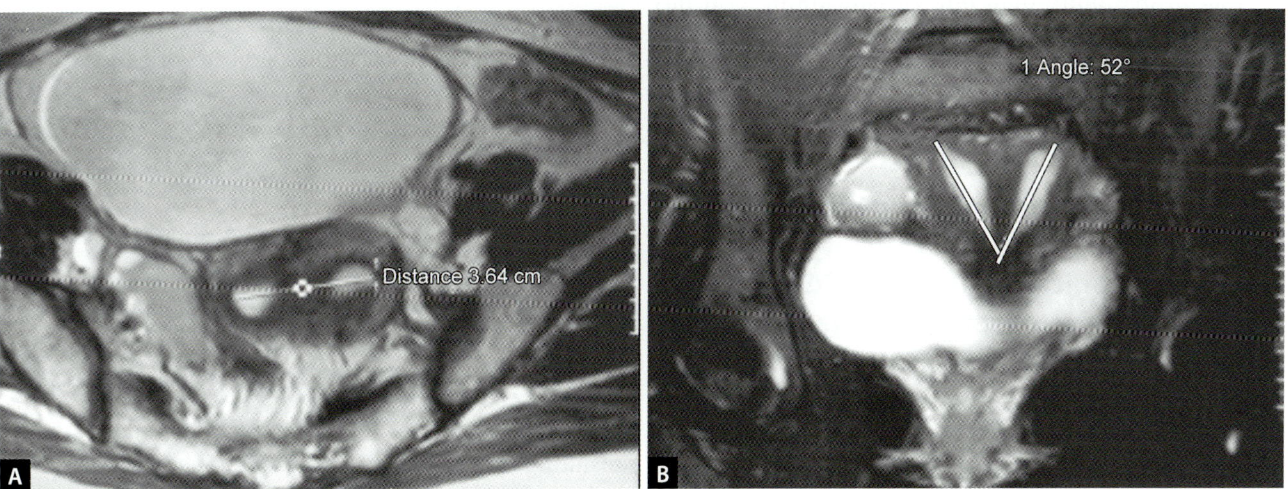

Figs. 7A and B: Septate uterus. (A) Axial and (B) coronal T2W MR images depict a uterus with a normal external fundal outline, well seen on the coronal image. The septum shows signal similar to the myometrium, dividing the endometrial cavity till the internal os suggesting a muscular septum.

contour is normally convex with a broad-based, smooth prominence of inner myometrium, at the fundus, indenting the endometrial cavity. On MR, the signal is consistent with myometrium without low signal intensity on T2-weighted images to suggest any fibrous tissue.

- *Class VII—diethylstilbestrol (DES)-related uterus*: DES is a synthetic nonsteroidal estrogen that was used to prevent miscarriage between 1940s and 1971s. DES produces a T-shaped hypoplastic uterus or, which is now mainly of historical interest since its usage was stopped in 1975 as it was linked to vaginal clear cell

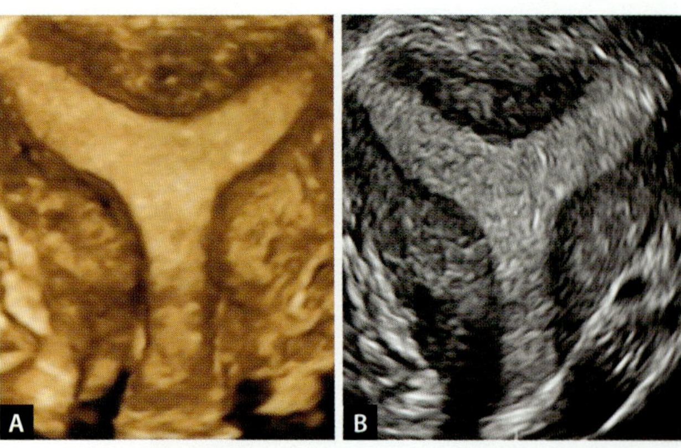

Figs. 8A and B: T-shaped uterus. 3D USG coronal reconstructions showing a T-shaped uterine cavity with a normal corpus-to-cervix ratio in a patient with no history of DES exposure (ESHRE: U1a).

carcinoma and uterine, cervical, and vaginal congenital malformations. Very rarely, the same spectrum of anomalies is noted among women without history of DES exposure **(Figs. 8A and B)**.[30,31]

It is important to classify MDAs accurately, as surgical planning differs. In case of uncertainty or presence of multiple subtypes, it is advisable to describe the anomalies and not forcibly place them in a class.[5] The major limitation of the ASRM classification is its lack of categorization of vaginal and other anomalies that bridge more than one classification.[28,32] It has also been criticized for absence of clear definitions and objective diagnostic criteria, lack of clarity on which diagnostic methods should be used introducing subjectivity in diagnosis and differential diagnosis.

European Society of Human Reproduction and Embryology/European Society for Gynaecological Endoscopy (ESGE) Classification System of Congenital Anomalies

The European Society of Human Reproduction and Embryology (ESHRE) and the *European Society for Gynaecological Endoscopy (ESGE)*, under a common Working Group—CONgenital UTerine Anomalies (CONUTA), have developed a new ESHRE/ESGE classification system of female genital anomalies in 2013 subsequently modified in 2015 in an attempt to overcome the limitations of the ASRM classification.[4,8] This was done mainly based on 3D US.

In the ESHRE/ESGE classification, systematic classification of anomalies into six main classes, is done primarily on anatomic basis. Deviation of uterine anatomy arising from the same embryological origin is the basis for division of the main classes. Anatomical variations of the main classes with different degrees of uterine deformity which are clinically significant are the basis of the main subclasses. The less severe variants are placed in the beginning, and the more severe ones at the end. Cervical and vaginal anomalies are classified in independent supplementary subclasses **(Fig. 9)**.

Definitions: Uterine Main Classes and Subclasses—Smaller than ESHRE/ESGE

Class U0—or normal uterus.

A normal uterus is one with a straight or curved interostial line, with a midline internal fundal indentation not exceeding 50% of the uterine wall thickness. Uterine wall thickness is the distance between interostial line and external uterine profile on the midcoronal plane of the uterus; if a coronal plane is not feasible, the average anterior and posterior uterine wall thickness in the longitudinal plane can be used.[8] Since uterine wall thickness may vary from patient to patient, percentage measurement is used rather than absolute numbers in millimeters. The inclusion of normal uterus is useful to independently classify congenital malformations of the cervix and vagina.

Class U1 or dysmorphic uterus: It includes all cases with an abnormal shape of uterine cavity, except for septa and normal uterine outline. Usually, dysmorphic uteri are smaller in size. *Class I* has three subcategories:

1. *Class U1a or T-shaped uterus* has narrow uterine cavity due to thickened lateral walls with a two-thirds uterine corpus and one-third cervix ratio **(*see* Figs. 8A and B)**.
2. *Class U1b or uterus infantilis* also has a narrow uterine cavity, no lateral wall thickening, and an inversion of uterine body and cervix ratio (1/3:2/3).
3. *Class U1c or others* includes all minor deformities of the uterine cavity including those with an inner midline fundal indentation of <50% uterine wall thickness.

Class U2 or septate uterus: It includes all anomalies resulting from complete or partial nonabsorption of the midline septum and normal fusion. The uterus has a normal external outline. There is an internal indentation in the midline fundal region exceeding 50% of the uterine wall thickness which is referred to as a septum. *Class U2* is divided into two subclasses:

1. *Class U2a or partial septate uterus* has a septum ending above the level of the internal cervical os dividing the uterine cavity partially.
2. *Class U2b or complete septate uterus* has a septum which completely divides the endometrial cavity up

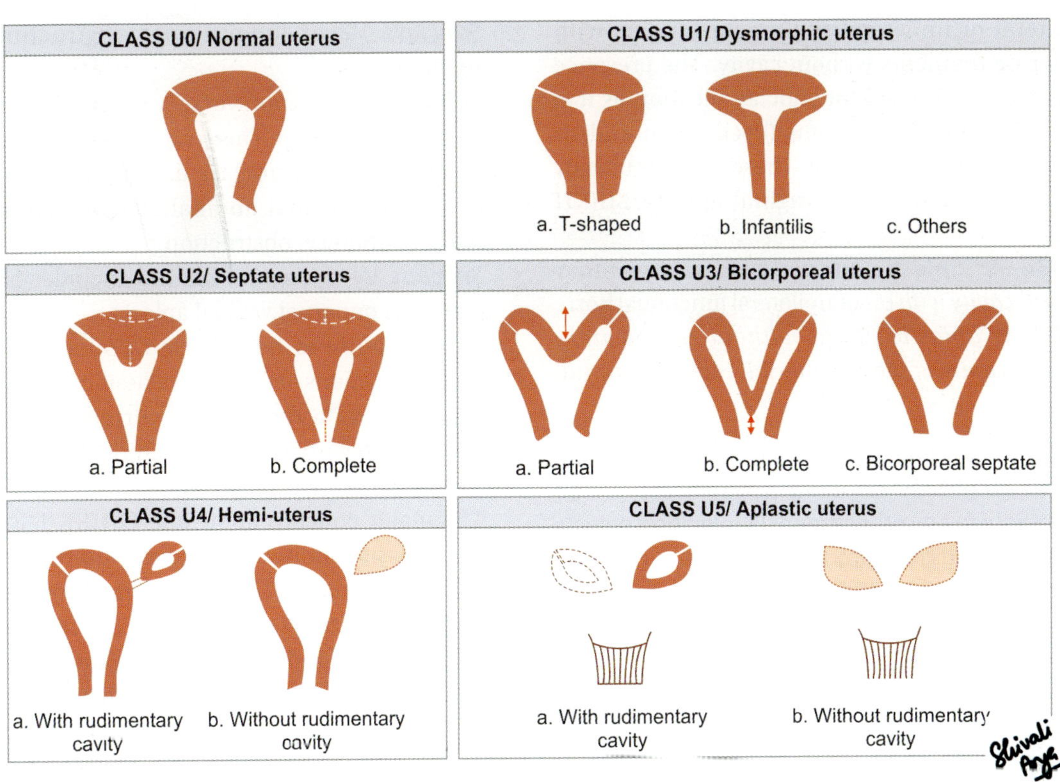

Fig. 9: Schematic representation of the ESHRE/ESGE classification of congenital uterine anomalies (ESGE: European Society for Gynaecological Endoscopy; ESHRE: European Society of Human Reproduction and Embryology).

to the level of the internal cervical os. These patients (Class U2b) may or may not have cervical (e.g. bicervical septate uterus) and/or vaginal anomalies **(*see* Figs. 6 and 7)**.

Class U3 or bicorporeal uterus includes all fusion defects; it is characterized by the presence of an external indentation at the fundal midline >50% of the uterine wall thickness.

1. *Class U3a or partial bicorporeal uterus*: The external fundal indentation only partly divides the uterine corpus above the level of the cervix.
2. *Class U3b or complete bicorporeal uterus*: The external fundal indentation reaches up to the level of the cervix, completely dividing the uterine corpus. This subgroup may have coexistent cervical (e.g. double cervix or didelphys uterus of the ASRM) or vaginal anomalies (e.g. vaginal septum—obstructing or nonobstructing) **(*see* Fig. 4)**.
3. *Class U3c or bicorporeal septate uterus* has an absorption defect in addition to the fusion anomaly. In this case, the width of the midline fundal indentation exceeds the uterine wall thickness by 150%. Treatment by hysteroscopic resection of the septate component is possible to some extent.

Class U4 or hemi-uterus includes all cases of unilateral uterine development; the contralateral part is absent or incompletely formed. It is a formation defect; included in a different class from aplastic uterus (also formation defect) because of the presence of a fully developed functional uterine hemi-cavity. Class U4 is divided into two subclasses depending on the presence or absence of a functional uterine cavity:

1. *Class U4a or hemi-uterus with a rudimentary (functional) cavity*: There is a functional contralateral horn which may be communicating or noncommunicating. These are clubbed together (unlike ASRM) since the presence of an endometrial cavity in the contralateral horn is the sole predictor of complications, like hematocavity or ectopic pregnancy in the rudimentary horn. Treatment is always advisable even in a communicating horn **(*see* Fig. 3)**.
2. *Class U4b or hemi-uterus with no rudimentary (functional) cavity* has either a nonfunctional contralateral uterine horn or no contralateral horn.

Class U5 or aplastic uterus includes all cases of uterine aplasia. There is absence of any fully or unilaterally developed uterine cavity. In some patients, however, there may be bilateral or unilateral rudimentary horns with cavity, or uterine remnants without cavity. The presence of a horn with cavity is used for subclassification as it is associated with clinical symptoms (cyclic pain and/or hematocavity) requiring treatment. These patients usually have concomitant defects (e.g. vaginal aplasia/MRKH syndrome).

1. *Class U5a or aplastic uterus with rudimentary (functional) cavity with* bi- or unilateral functional horn.
2. *Class U5b or aplastic uterus without rudimentary (functional) cavity* is seen as uterine remnants or full uterine aplasia.

Class U6 or unclassified cases are infrequent, subtle anomalies, or combined anomalies which cannot be allocated correctly to any other group. Duplication defects or ectopic Müllerian tissue anomalies, if present, could be put in this class.

Coexistent Cervical Anomalies

- *Subclass C0* or normal cervix.
- *Subclass C1 or septate cervix* includes cervical absorption defects. The cervix shows a normal externally rounded contour with presence of a septum.
- *Subclass C2 or double cervix* includes cases of cervical fusion anomalies. Two distinct externally rounded cervices (fully divided or partially fused) are seen. It may occur with a complete bicorporeal uterus as a Class U3b/C2 (uterus didelphys).
- *Subclass C3 or unilateral cervical aplasia* includes patients with unilateral cervix formation. The contralateral part is either incompletely formed or absent. This is obvious in Class U4 patients, and not necessary to mention in the final report (Class U4 is adequate instead of Class U4/C3). However, this gives a chance to classify other rarely seen anomalies like complete bicorporeal uterus with unilateral cervical aplasia as Class U3b/C3, a severe obstructing anomaly.
- *C4 or cervical aplasia* includes patients with complete cervical aplasia and severe cervical formation defects. There is either no cervical tissue or severely defective cervical tissue like cervical cord, obstruction, or fragmentation. This subclass may be combined with a normal or abnormal uterine corpus and helps in classification of all obstructing anomalies caused by cervical defects.

Coexistent Vaginal Anomalies

- *Subclass V0 or* normal vagina
- *Subclass V1* or longitudinal nonobstructing vaginal septum
- *Subclass V2 or* longitudinal obstructing vaginal septum
- *Subclass V3* or transverse vaginal septum and/or imperforate hymen. These vaginal anomalies classified together in this subclass as they generally present as isolated vaginal anomalies with similar clinical manifestation i.e. obstruction
- *Subclass V4 or vaginal aplasia* includes all cases of complete or partial vaginal aplasia.

Various authors have raised concerns about the clinical implications of the ESGE classifications, as specific diagnostic criteria that clearly correlate to pregnancy have not yet been validated in clinical practice by any prospective or retrospectives studies.[33]

The major concern about the ESHRE/ESGE criteria is the reclassification of the arcuate uterus into normal (U0) or septate uterus (U2), which modifies the number of diagnosed uterine septa. There is concern that it leads to overdiagnosis and perhaps overtreatment of septate uteri. Authors have reported that no significant difference was found in the past reproductive outcomes in women diagnosed with normal or partial septate uteri by these criteria. It has been suggested that clinicians should be cautious in offering surgical correction to women diagnosed to have partial septate uteri as per the new ESHRE/ESGE classification.[33]

UTERINE LEIOMYOMAS

Epidemiology

Leiomyomas, or fibroids, represent the most common benign tumors of the uterus. The incidence reported in literature varies between 25% to 50% of women of reproductive age. However, in autopsy studies, uterine leiomyomas have been found in up to 77% of women.[17,34,35]

Pathogenesis

Genetic factors, steroid hormones (i.e. estrogen and progesterone), and growth factors play a role in the development and growth of leiomyomas. They occur in women of reproductive age. They do not occur before puberty and fibroid-related symptoms reduce or resolve after menopause as a result of decreasing levels of female hormones. Early menarche and obesity are risk factors possibly due to increased estrogen exposure.[36]

Pathological Features

Leiomyomas are benign smooth muscle tumors. They usually form in the uterine corpus/fundus, less often in the cervix (<8%) and rarely in the broad ligament. Two-thirds of cases have multiple fibroids, size varying from microscopic to large tumors filling the abdomen. Leiomyomas that are no longer continuous with the uterus and develop an atypical blood supply are often referred to as parasitic leiomyomas. It is thought that a pedunculated subserosal leiomyoma becomes vascularized by the adjacent peritoneum, loses its attachment to the uterus and its vascular supply to become a parasitic leiomyoma. They are well-defined round lesions compressing the surrounding myometrium to form a pseudocapsule, which allows surgical enucleation of the tumors. Macroscopically, the cut surface has a whitish, whorled appearance, but the color (red, brown, or yellow) and texture may be different if degeneration is present. On microscopy, they are composed of intertwined smooth muscle cells, organized in fascicles, forming whorl-like patterns, embedded in a stroma of collagen fibers. The smooth muscle cells have eosinophilic cytoplasm and a centrally located cigar-shaped nucleus. Mitosis and atypia are not found in fibroids.[37-39]

As leiomyomas enlarge, they may outgrow their vascular supply. This results in different types of degeneration: hyaline, myxoid, cystic, red (hemorrhagic), or fatty degeneration and calcification, depending on the degree and rapidity of the onset of vascular insufficiency.[40,41]

Rare manifestations include diffuse leiomyomatosis of the uterus, benign metastatic leiomyomatosis, peritoneal disseminated leiomyomatosis, and intravenous leiomyomatosis, the last three being varieties that extend beyond the uterus.[42,43] These are benign leiomyomas.

Clinical Features

Most women with leiomyomas (up to 80%) are asymptomatic and require no treatment.[3] About 20–50% of women with leiomyomas present with symptoms such as menorrhagia, dysmenorrhea, urinary frequency, pelvic and back pain, dyspareunia, constipation, or obstipation depending on the size and location.[34,36]

Classification

According to their location, leiomyomas are classified as submucosal, intramural, or subserosal. This classification has clinical significance since the clinical presentation and treatment vary. *Submucosal leiomyomas* lie below the mucosal lining and protrude into the endometrial cavity. Though the least common, they are usually associated with dysmenorrhea, menorrhagia, or infertility. *Intramural leiomyomas*, the most common type, are located completely within the wall of the uterus. They are usually asymptomatic, but may occasionally produce symptoms similar to submucosal lesions. *Subserosal leiomyomas* are situated beneath the serosa, distort the outer uterine contour. They may be pedunculated, being attached to the uterus by a stalk. Subserosal leiomyomas are also mostly asymptomatic; however, pedunculated subserosal leiomyomas may undergo torsion, resulting in infarction and pain.[44,45] The FIGO classifications is often used to describe the relationship of fibroids to both the serosal and mucosal uterine surfaces and is summarized in **Figure 10**.

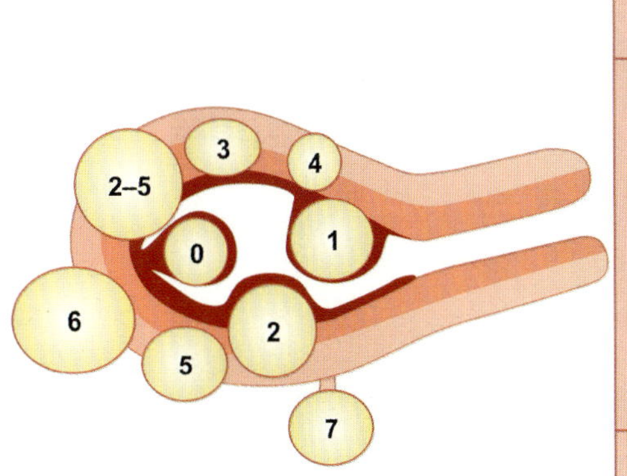

SM—Submucosal	0	Pedunculated intracavitary
	1	<50% intramural
	2	≥50% intramural
O—Other	3	Contacts endometrium; 100% intramural No distortion
	4	Intramural
	5	Subserosal ≥50% intramural
	6	Subserosal <50% intramural
	7	Subserosal pedunculated
	8	Other (specify, e.g. cervical, parasitic)
Hybrid leiomyomas	2–5	Submucosal and subserosal, each with less than half the diameter in the endometrial and pertioneal cavities, respectively

Fig. 10: The International Federation of Gynecology and Obstetrics (FIGO) classification of fibroids.

Imaging

Imaging of leiomyomas allows classification by location in the uterus and pretreatment planning. US is the first-line imaging and a combination of transabdominal sonography (TAS) and TVS may be required depending on size and uterine position.

Leiomyomas are round or oval well-circumscribed hypoechoic (or isoechoic) solid lesions **(Figs. 11A and B)** with associated areas of posterior shadowing at the interface of the leiomyoma with the normal myometrium or due to calcifications. Cystic areas, echo-poor foci, and heterogeneity suggest degeneration, while a hyperechoic appearance may be seen in lipoleiomyomas. Doppler US depicts tumor vascularity and typically demonstrates a marginal vascular network **(Figs. 12A and B)**.[36] Hysterosonography with the instillation of fluid/saline into the endometrial cavity can improve the accuracy of TVS in detecting and differentiating submucosal fibroids from endometrial polyps. It is also more accurate in demonstrating degree of myometrial component. 3D US is also an excellent technique to demonstrate the relationship between the fibroid and the endometrial cavity.[46-49]

CT is not a recommended imaging modality for the evaluation of leiomyomas, but they may be incidentally seen, as variably enhancing masses **(Fig. 13)**, sometimes with popcorn or rim calcifications (4%) **(Fig. 14)**.[36,46]

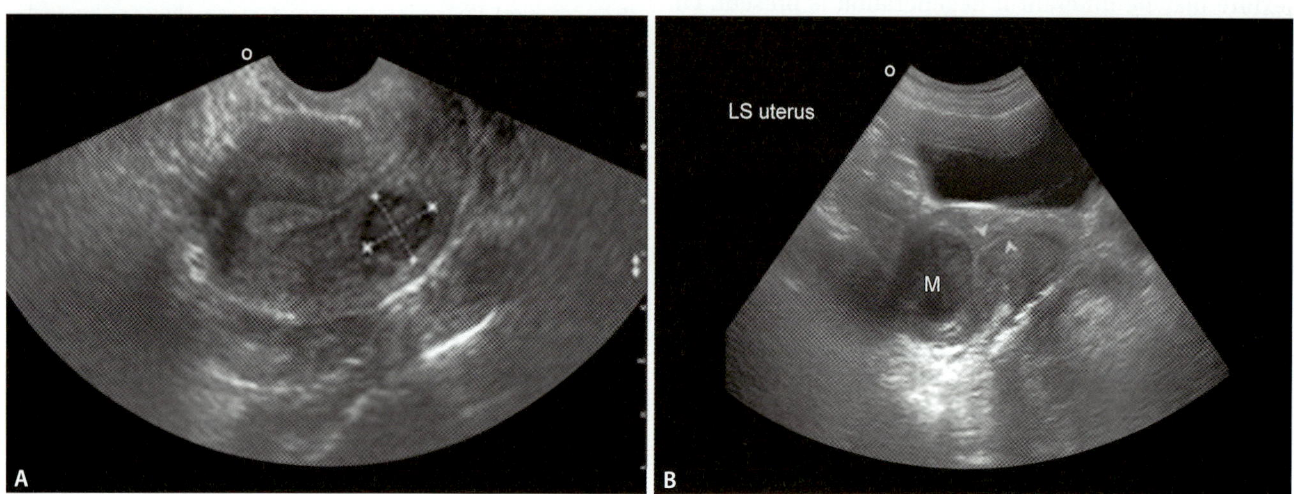

Figs. 11A and B: Uterine fibroids. (A) TVS shows well-defined, round, and hypoechoic mass in posterior myometrium—intramural fibroid; (B) TAS in another patient reveals homogeneous, hypoechoic well-marginated round to oval mass lesion in the uterus consistent with fibroid (TAS: transabdominal sonography; TVS: transvaginal sonography).

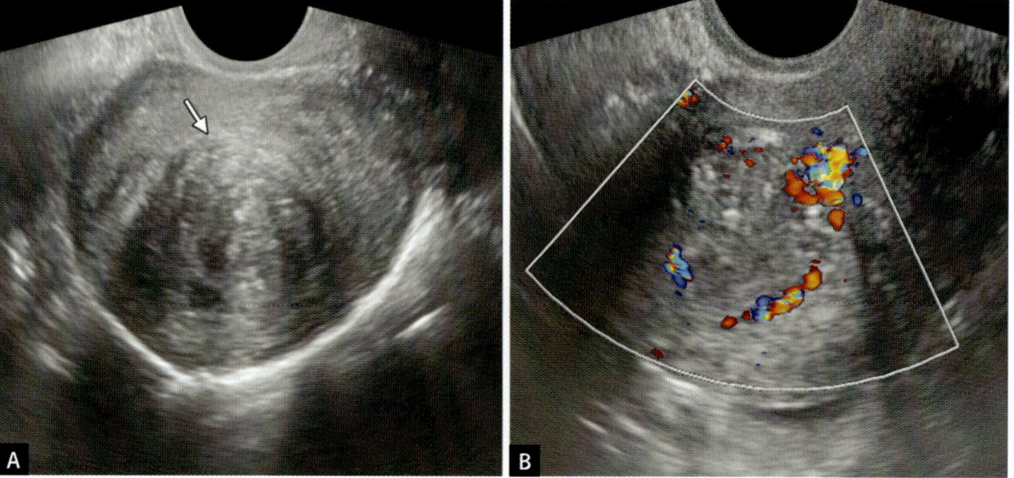

Figs. 12A and B: Fibroid uterus. (A) Transverse section of the uterus on transvaginal sonography shows a well-defined iso- to heteroechoic lesion displacing the endometrial echo anteriorly due to mass effect (arrow). Multiple coarse posterior acoustic shadows are well seen; (B) Color Doppler reveals peripheral vascularity.

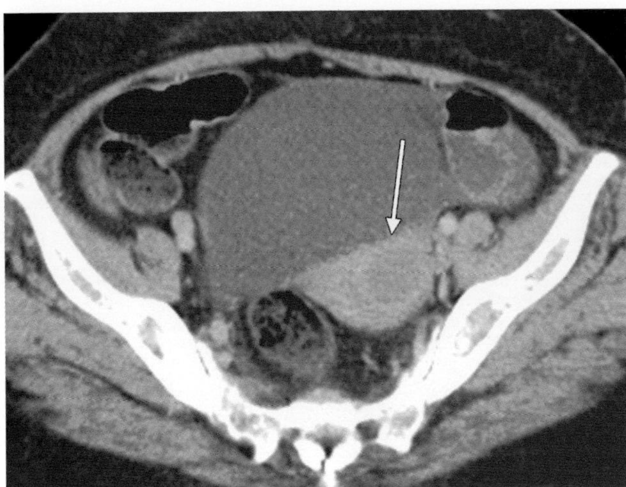

Fig. 13: Fibroid uterus. Axial contrast-enhanced CT scan shows a well-defined hypodense fibroid, enhancing less than the adjacent myometrium (arrow).

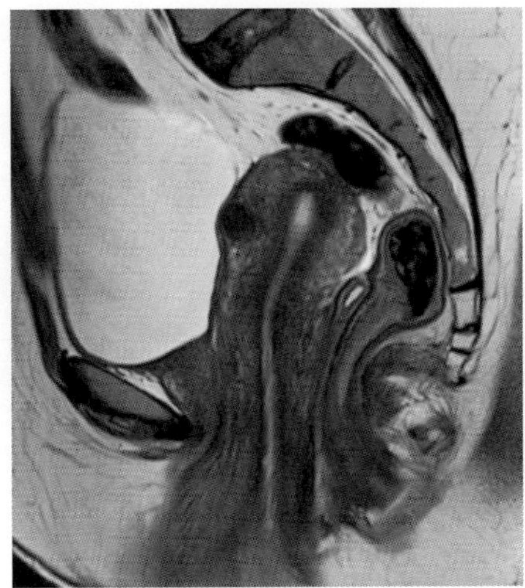

Fig. 15: T2W sagittal MR image showing a small hypointense fibroid in the anterior wall, and subserosal location. Note the subtle deformity of the uterine outline, despite the small size.

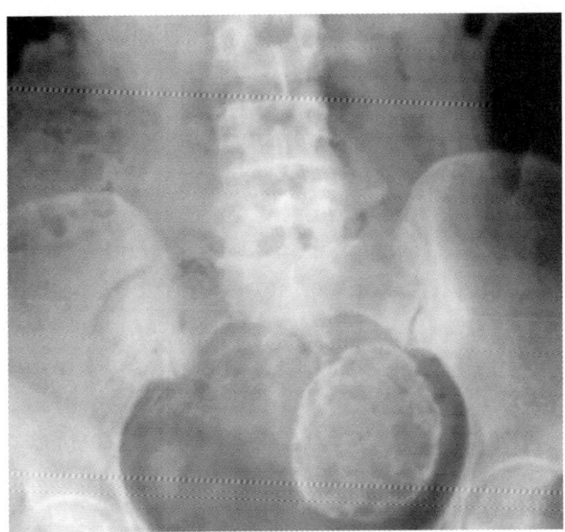

Fig. 14: Plain radiograph of pelvis shows a large fibroid with rim calcification.

MRI is the most accurate and preferred tool for pretreatment planning of leiomyomas, showing the exact number, size, location, and character of leiomyomas, a process also known as (*fibroid mapping*). The excellent soft-tissue contrast enables accurate localization of lesions as submucosal, intramural, or subserosal and fibroids as small as 5 mm in diameter can be demonstrated. Nondegenerated leiomyomas are seen as well-circumscribed round or oval masses. They are isointense on T1, homogeneously low signal on T2W compared to the outer myometrium. A T2-hyperintense rim, indicating a pseudocapsule of edema, due to some degree of venous or lymphatic obstruction may be seen in some cases. On contrast-enhanced scans, fibroids usually show lesser degree of enhancement relative to the myometrium, although, occasionally they may be of the same or of higher attenuation. Routine use of gadolinium is, however, not required. Areas of calcification are poorly detected on MR but can appear as signal voids. Diffuse leiomyomatosis is characterized by the presence of many small ill-defined leiomyomas that may be confluent.[36,46-48,50]

Leiomyomas do not infiltrate surrounding structures, but show expansile growth and already have a mass effect when they are still small therefore, distorting the shape of the uterus **(Fig. 15)**. In patients with large exophytic, subserosal leiomyomas, or a markedly enlarged uterus due to multiple fibroids, it may sometimes be difficult to differentiate fibroids from extrauterine or ovarian lesions. The presence of a beak, or claw-like extension of myometrium surrounding the lesion (*claw sign*) and multiple flow voids on noncontrast images or enhancing tubular channels on contrast-enhanced T1W images, at the interface between lesion and normal uterine tissue, indicate uterine fibroids with a high degree of confidence **(Figs. 16A and B)**.[36-39] These flow voids represent the arteries arising from the uterine artery and feeding the fibroid and have been referred to as the *bridging vascular sign* (originally described on Doppler). **Table 1** summarizes the MR findings of leiomyomas.

Fibroids that have undergone degeneration show great variation in their MRI appearance.[36,44,45,49,51,52] *Hyaline degeneration* is the most common type of degeneration seen in about 60% of all leiomyomas. It is characterized by the collection of high-protein eosinophilic material, in the extracellular space, between strands of muscle cells.

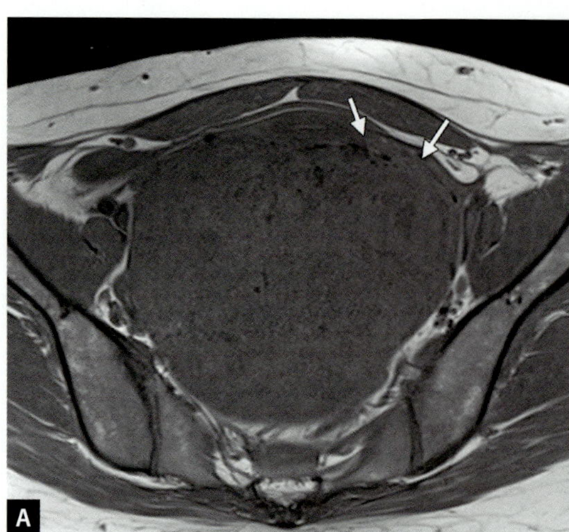

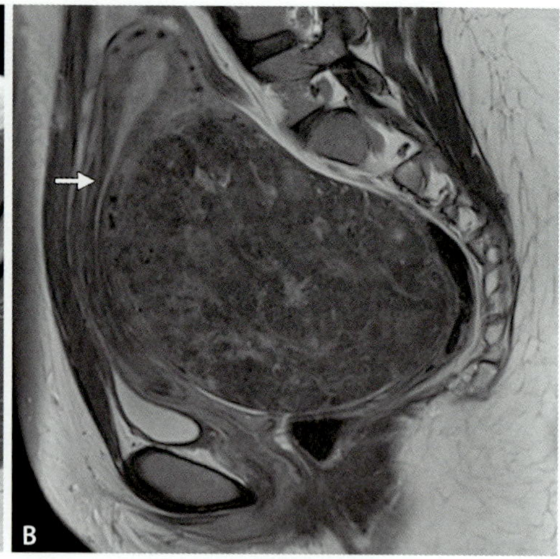

Figs. 16A and B: Subserosal fibroid uterus. (A) T1W axial and (B) sagittal T2W MR images depict a large posterior wall subserosal fibroid with less than 50% intramyometrial component appearing isointense on T1, hypointense on T2, stretching the myometrium and displacing the endometrial cavity anteriorly (arrow in B). Note the flow voids at the interface between the lesion and the uterus on T1W (arrows in A).

Table 1: MRI features of leiomyoma.

Location	Corpus, less often cervical or within uterine ligaments Subserosal, intramural, submucous
Morphology	• Spherical, sharply marginated, pseudocapsule may be present, mass effect even if small, deforming the uterine outline, and/or cavity may be singular but often numerous • Size 0.5 cm to >20 cm • Claw-like extension of myometrium surrounding the lesion
Appearance on T1	• Isointense to the myometrium • Hyperintense areas related to hemorrhage
Appearance on T2	• Variable, in general hypointense relative to myometrium • Homogeneously, high SI often seen in cellular leiomyomas • High SI rim represents dilated lymphatics in large leiomyoma
Appearance on gadolinium-enhanced T1	• hypo-, iso-, and hyperintense relative to myometrium.
Additional findings	• Flow voids in the periphery representing perifibroid plexus vessels • A vascular stalk may be seen in pedunculated leiomyomas (bridging vessel sign)

Hyaline degeneration produces low signal on T2W images, making it difficult to distinguish from nondegenerated fibroids, however, decreased enhancement, especially on triphasic dynamic scans has been reported with hyaline degeneration.

Other types of degeneration that can be differentiated are *cystic, myxoid, and hemorrhagic (red) degeneration. Cystic degeneration* results in internal areas of T2 hyperintensity and T1 hypointensity with no enhancement **(Figs. 17A and B)**. *Myxoid degeneration* is seen as areas of very high signal intensity on T2-weighted images, intermediate to low signal on T1-weighted images. These can be difficult to differentiate from fibroids that have undergone cystic degeneration; however, they appear as more complex cystic masses. They tend to show intense enhancement of the stroma. Minimal enhancement of the high signal areas, indicating that these are not necrotic or cystic areas, can be seen.

Hemorrhagic or carneous or red degeneration usually occurs during pregnancy or in women on oral contraceptives. It is thought to occur due to obstructed draining veins with sudden infarction and secondary intralesional hemorrhage. MRI is extremely useful to confirm the diagnosis of acute hemorrhagic degeneration of a leiomyoma, especially in conjunction with the clinical presentation of acute pain, subfebrile temperature, and leukocytosis. This is seen as a variably heterogeneous signal depending on the age of blood products. Commonly described patterns include, high signal on T1 and moderate to high signal on T2-weighted scans; there can also be a hyperintense rim on T1 and a markedly hypointense rim on T2-weighted scans. Hemorrhagic fibroids show no enhancement after contrast.

Lipoleiomyoma or fatty degeneration is rare. It is thought to be due to fatty metamorphosis of the smooth muscle cells of a leiomyoma **(Fig. 18)**. At USG, they are

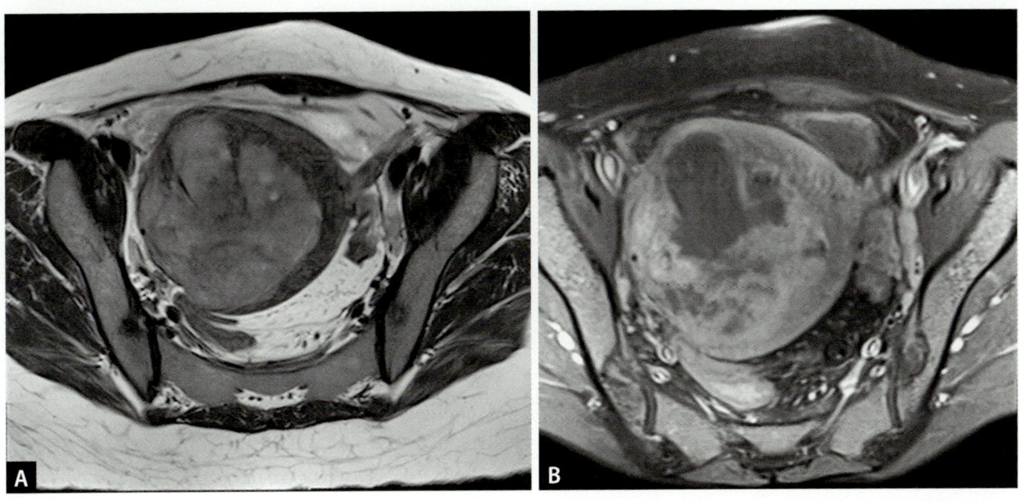

Figs. 17A and B: Fibroid with areas of cystic degeneration which appear hyperintense on T2 (A) and do not enhance on the postcontrast image (B).

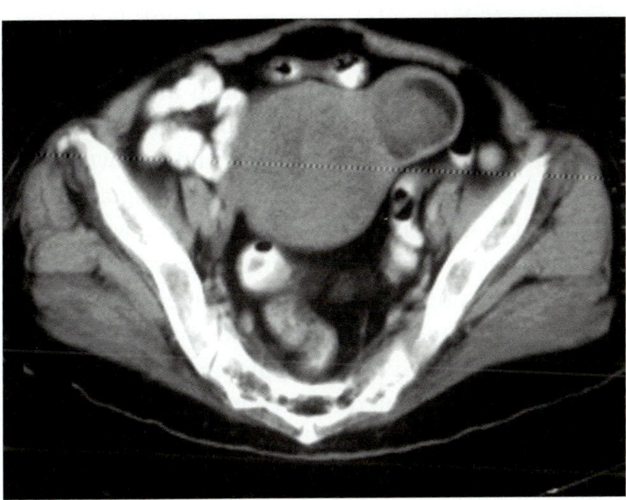

Fig. 18: CT scan of pelvis showing a lobulated uterine mass with fatty degeneration—lipoleiomyoma.

typically echogenic masses, unlike the usually hypoechoic appearance. If pedunculated, they can be mistaken for ovarian dermoids. On MR, they display a signal similar to subcutaneous fat on all pulse sequences due to the presence of variable amounts of fat cells. Fat suppression is useful to determine the fatty nature of these leiomyomas.

The MRI features of degenerating uterine leiomyomas are summarized in **Table 2**.

Table 2: MRI features of degenerated (but ordinary) leiomyomas.

Types of degeneration	*T1-weighted imaging*	*T2-weighted imaging*	*IV contrast-enhanced imaging*
Cystic	Hypointense relative to myometrium	Internal areas of high T2 signal intensity	With corresponding areas of nonenhancement
Hemorrhagic	Areas of high T1 signal intensity	Variable T2 signal intensity	Variable
Fatty	Moderate T1 signal intensity, which suppresses on fat-saturated sequence	Moderate	Variable
Hyaline	Isointense	Hypointense	Decreased enhancement (compared with ordinary leiomyomas)
Myxoid	iso to Hypointense	Markedly high T2 signal intensity Complex appearance	Some enhancement seen

Leiomyoma Variants

Besides the ordinary leiomyomas discussed above, there are several leiomyoma variants, such as mitotically active, cellular, and atypical leiomyomas, as well as smooth muscle tumors of uncertain malignant potential (STUMP) which lie between the ordinary benign leiomyomas and the malignant leiomyosarcomas **(Box 1)**. In contrast to ordinary leiomyomas, imaging features of leiomyoma variants are neither well-studied nor understood due to their rarity.

Cellular leiomyomas, a subgroup of leiomyomas, on microscopy show compact smooth muscle cells with little intervening collagen. According to one study, they are more likely to be single and larger than ordinary fibroids; there

Box 1: Uterine leiomyomas and their variants.

- *Ordinary leiomyomas—benign*:
  - Nondegenerated
  - *With degeneration*:
    - Hyaline
    - Myxoid
    - Cystic
    - Hemorrhagic (carneous)
    - Fatty (lipoleiomyoma).
- *Leiomyoma variants—in between*:
  - Cellular
  - Atypical
  - Mitotically active
  - Smooth muscle tumors of uncertain malignant potential (STUMP)
- *Leiomyosarcoma—malignant*

is also a greater probability that the patient is symptomatic and that the indication for imaging is "enlarging lesion". Cellular leiomyomas have a homogeneously high signal intensity on T2-weighted scans, are isointense to surrounding myometrium on T1, and tend to enhance homogeneously. Studies report that cellular leiomyomas can significantly decrease in size following gonadotropin-releasing hormone (GnRH) therapy compared with degenerated leiomyomas.

Atypical leiomyomas, mitotically active leiomyomas, as well as STUMPs are very rare; hence, their imaging appearances are not well-described.[45]

Differential Diagnosis

Differential diagnostic considerations include adenomyosis, solid adnexal masses, endometrial polyp, and the rare leiomyosarcoma.

Adenomyosis may mimic intramural leiomyomas. Adenomyosis tends to be poorly marginated, with multiple cystic spaces (anechoic on US, T2 hyperfoci on MR), is mostly in contact with the junctional zone, and does not produce as much mass effect.

Submucosal leiomyomas may have to be distinguished from endometrial polyps. On color Doppler, a feeding vessel is more often seen in endometrial polyp, while fibroids tend to show circumferential vascularity. On MR, submucosal leiomyomas are differentiated from endometrial polyps by their more spherical shape, their connection to the myometrium, and lower signal intensity on T2-weighted images.

Solid adnexal or ovarian masses must be considered in the differential diagnosis of subserosal leiomyomas. The claw sign and/or presence of bridging vessels is useful to establish the diagnosis of leiomyoma.

Uterine contractions can appear as transient T2 hypointense lesions which may simulate leiomyomas or focal adenomyosis at MR.

Leiomyosarcomas of the uterus are rare, most are thought to arise de novo unrelated to benign leiomyomas. Due to overlapping of imaging features, differentiation of benign degenerating cellular leiomyomas and leiomyosarcomas is challenging.[52-57] The distinction, however, may be important as recently leiomyoma morcellation has been reported to have a negative impact on the survival of patients who were found to have malignant instead of benign uterine masses following the procedure (morcellation is a technique to reduce the size of the uterus or myomas by creating smaller pieces, so that they can be removed through small incisions or laparoscopically). Leiomyosarcomas occur in an older age group (6th decade) as compared with leiomyoma (4th decade/premenopausal). Traditionally, rapid enlargement of leiomyomas has been interpreted as a sign of malignancy, but the results of some large studies have not supported this. Although rapid growth is not considered, an indicator of malignancy in premenopausal women, it is suspicious in postmenopausal women. On US, the detection of hypervascularity in a large solitary uterine mass can raise the suspicion of leiomyosarcoma. According to a study, a cutoff value of 41.0 cm/s [peak systolic velocity (PSV)] on Doppler markedly increased the detection rate of uterine sarcomas.[52,53] However, there are no US findings that reliably differentiate ordinary leiomyomas from leiomyoma variants and leiomyosarcomas. Lakhman et al. recently reported four discriminative features on MR: (1) nodular borders, (2) intralesional hemorrhage, (3) T2W dark areas, and (4) central unenhanced areas. They reported that combination of more than three MR features provided a specificity of >95% **(Table 3)**.[57]

Treatment

Asymptomatic fibroids may be left alone with a wait and watch policy. Treatment of uterine fibroids is indicated when they are symptomatic. Treatment depends on symptomatology, age, and patients' desire for gestation and has to be tailored on a case-to-case basis. Treatment can be medical, surgical, or interventional. *Medical therapy* is usually done to relieve abnormal menstrual bleeding, and bulk symptoms. This may include nonsteroidal anti-inflammatory drugs (NSAIDs), oral contraceptives (OCs), tranexamic acid and GnRH analogs, and the recently introduced selective progesterone receptor modulators

Table 3: Differentiation between leiomyoma and leiomyosarcoma.

	Leiomyoma	*Leiomyosarcoma*
Age	Premenopausal	Peri-/postmenopausal
Borders	Well-delineated	Often nodular*
DWI	Variable	Restricted diffusion, low ADC
Invasiveness	No	Adjacent tissues
Number	Commonly multiple	Solitary
Size	Variable	Large (>10 cm)
T2WI	Mostly low, high in degeneration, and whorled pattern	Inhomogeneous with areas of hemorrhage*, intralesional vessels; T2 dark areas*
Vascularity	Variable; often parallels myometrium	Hypervascularization, peripheral early enhancement, and central necrosis*

*Discriminative features on MR.
(ADC: apparent diffusion coefficient; DWI: diffusion-weighted imaging)

(sPRMs) like ulipristal acetate (UPA). Levonorgestrel-releasing intrauterine device (IUD) and endometrial ablation are other techniques to reduce the severity of menstrual bleeding.

Surgical techniques include hysterectomy, hysteroscopic, or laparoscopic myomectomy.

Hysterectomy is the definitive cure, especially in patients with a symptomatic multiple fibroids not wanting to preserve fertility. *Myomectomy* is a uterus-sparing operative technique, where myomas are resected or enucleated using a laparoscopic, hysteroscopic access or via open laparotomy. Here, imaging plays an important role in accurate localization prior to myomectomy. Submucosal leiomyomas (FIGO 0, 1, and 2) with minimal intramural component can be removed by hysteroscopic resection. Hysteroscopic resection is usually considered difficult or unsuitable if the submucosal leiomyoma is larger than 5 cm in size, if there are more than three fibroids, or if the uterine cavity is very large (length of uterine probe >12 cm). A large intramural component with thin residual myometrium increases the risk of perforation during hysteroscopic resection.[58] Laparoscopic removal can be done for subserosal visible leiomyomas, but intramural tumors are not easily accessible to laparoscopic removal. Incision of the uterine cavity may be necessary for the removal of transmural fibroids which is associated with the risk of synechia. Laparotomy is primarily used in patients with one or more large fibroids.

Interventional techniques that are available include uterine artery embolization (UAE) or uterine fibroid embolization (UFE) and MRI-guided focused US. MRI can be used to both predict and assess the response of fibroids to UAE-MR prior to UAE helps in identification of tumors in which embolization is associated with a higher risk, such as subserosal pedunculated fibroids with a narrow stalk (<2 mm stalk width) or those which are likely to show poor response to embolization, e.g. those with a parasitic blood supply, cervical leiomyomas, and those with high signal on T1W images (hemorrhagic necrosis). On the other hand, high signal on T2W images and gadolinium enhancement indicating vascularity have been shown to be a predictor of good response.[36,51]

ADENOMYOSIS OF THE UTERUS

Epidemiology

According to the classical teaching, adenomyosis or endometriosis genitalis interna is mainly seen in multiparous, premenopausal women generally more than 30 years of age. Currently, however, adenomyosis is not uncommonly diagnosed between 20 years and 30 years of age, and even during adolescence with availability of hysteroscopic or laparoscopic biopsy. Hysterectomy specimens demonstrate adenomyosis in 19–63% of cases. A prevalence of 34% has been reported in nulliparous females between 18 years and 30 years, who presented for contraception advice.[59-61]

Pathogenesis

Adenomyosis is a common non-neoplastic benign uterine condition resulting from the displacement of basal endometrial glands and stroma into the underlying myometrium. While the exact reason for the displacement is unclear, estrogen-mediated and mechanical effects have been implicated. High estrogen levels in pregnancy and breakdown of the basal endometrial layer as well as inner myometrium (due to postpartum endometritis) have been postulated as possible reasons in multiparous women. Early menarche, short menstrual cycles, and high body mass index—other features associated with high estrogen levels, are also associated with an increased risk of adenomyosis. Increased incidence of adenomyosis is seen in postmenopausal women on tamoxifen, a nonsteroidal antiestrogen agent.[59-63]

Histopathology

Adenomyosis may produce focal or diffuse involvement of the uterus. It occurs more often in the posterior wall and the fundus and does not involve the uterine cervix. The cut surface has a whorled texture produced by irregular trabeculations of the thickened myometrium. Cyst-like lesions and hemorrhagic foci within the myometrium are commonly seen. On histologic examination, dispersed endometrial glandular tissue is seen in the myometrium. The pathologic diagnosis is dependent on visualization of endometrial glands and stroma in more than one low-power field, 2.5 mm from the endometrial basalis layer.[64,65]

Clinical Presentation

The clinical presentation is nonspecific and includes dysmenorrhea, menorrhagia, and pelvic pain, hence its incidence is underestimated. The uterus may be enlarged in adenomyosis but does not show distortion in its shape unlike with leiomyomas. Adenomyosis, however, often occurs along with fibroids and endometriosis.

Imaging

Ultrasound (TAS or TVS) is generally used as the initial imaging modality in suspected adenomyosis. The reported sensitivity and specificity of TAS vary between 32.5–63% and 95–97%, respectively. TVS has a higher sensitivity and specificity for diagnosing adenomyosis in the range of 53–89% and 67–98%, respectively.[60,66] Saline infusion sonohysterography (SIS) may be useful in selected cases.

Some authors have categorized the US findings into three groups, paralleling the histology of adenomyosis: (1) ectopic endometrial glands and stroma, (2) muscular hyperplasia/hypertrophy, and (3) increased vascularity.

1. *Ectopic endometrial glands* are seen as echogenic nodules or striations which radiate from the endometrium into the myometrium. Myometrial cysts, lakes, and fluid-filled striations are seen when these glands contain fluid. Myometrial cysts are generally anechoic, 1–5 mm in size, but may be variable in size or have echogenic contents representing blood. Myometrial cysts are reported to be most sensitive and specific US feature of adenomyosis. Reducing the field of view and using magnification improve the depiction of these cysts. At times, an entire striation may be fluid filled referred to as *lollipop diverticulum*. Cystic changes in the outer myometrium on gray-scale may actually be small arcuate veins and rather than myometrial cysts of adenomyosis which can be differentiated with color Doppler imaging.[64]
2. The ectopic endometrial glands are hormonally sensitive and produce a "local reaction" within the adjacent myometrium, producing *smooth muscle hyperplasia and hypertrophy*. This results in asymmetric uterine wall thickening in focal disease. A globular uterine enlargement, up to 12 cm in uterine length, is commonly associated with the diffuse variety. Thickening of the junctional zone >12 mm (seen as a hypoechoic halo surrounding the endometrium) may be seen but is less apparent than on MR. Coronal views on 3D US may allow better measurement of the junctional zone. Blurring of the normally distinct endometrial/myometrial border can be seen. There is alteration of myometrial echotexture, becoming heterogeneous and coarse, with thin vertical posterior acoustic shadows, producing a *venetian blind appearance* **(Figs. 19A and B)**. This combination of heterogeneity, thin shadows, small hyperechoic nodules, and striations gives an appearance similar to end-stage liver disease and described as *cirrhosis of the uterus* by some authors.[64]
3. *Myometrial vascularity* is generally increased due to muscular hyperplasia and hypertrophy in adenomyosis. Color Doppler demonstrates an increased number of intramural vessels, which are randomly scattered, penetrate the involved myometrium and may be tortuous. This is different from the pattern typically seen in leiomyomas, which tend to displace vessels and demonstrate peripheral vascularity rather than a penetrating pattern **(Fig. 19C)**.

MRI is an accurate technique for diagnosing adenomyosis with a high sensitivity (78–88%) and specificity (67–93%).[63-69] It may be more useful than TVS in delineating the location and extent of disease, especially in an enlarged uterus. MR is also very useful in distinguishing adenomyosis from a leiomyoma in patients with enlarged uterus and in monitoring response to hormonal therapy. Many of the features of adenomyosis, seen on US, are depicted more clearly on MR, which is superior in showing changes in zonal anatomy **(Figs. 20A and B and Table 4)**.

Adenomyosis is visualized as either diffuse or focal thickening of the junctional zone forming an ill-defined area of low signal intensity, which represents smooth muscle hyperplasia. A junctional zone thickness of >12 mm has been reported to be highly accurate for diagnosing adenomyosis. Adenomyosis can be excluded if the junctional zone thickness is 8 mm or less. Bright foci on T2-weighted images within the lesion are seen in >50% of cases, which represent islands of ectopic endometrial tissue and cystic dilatation of glands. When menstrual

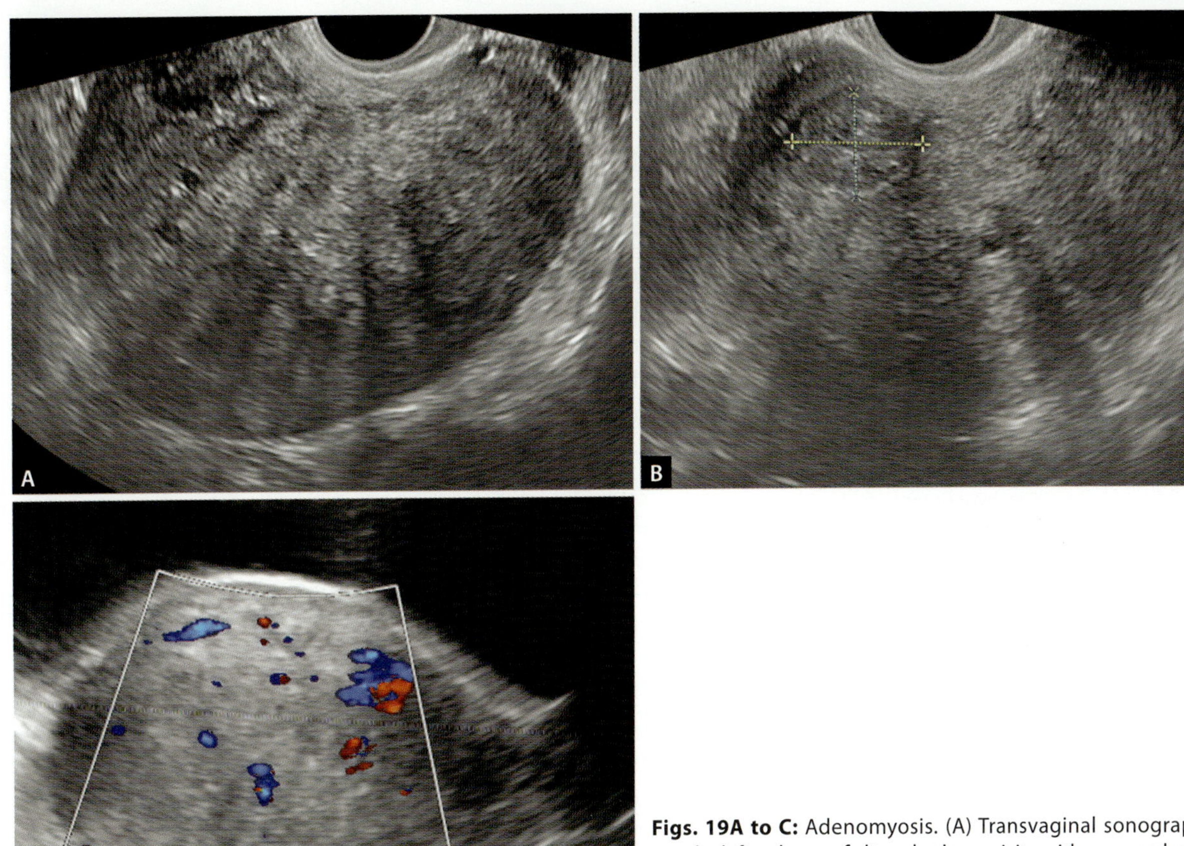

Figs. 19A to C: Adenomyosis. (A) Transvaginal sonography shows a poorly defined area of altered echogenicity with a coarse heterogeneous echotexture, multiple thin Venetian blind acoustic shadows, small anechoic cystic areas, and indistinct endometrial-myometrial junction; (B) Note an associated fundal fibroid marked by calipers; (C) Penetrating pattern of intralesional vascularity is noted on the transabdominal scan.

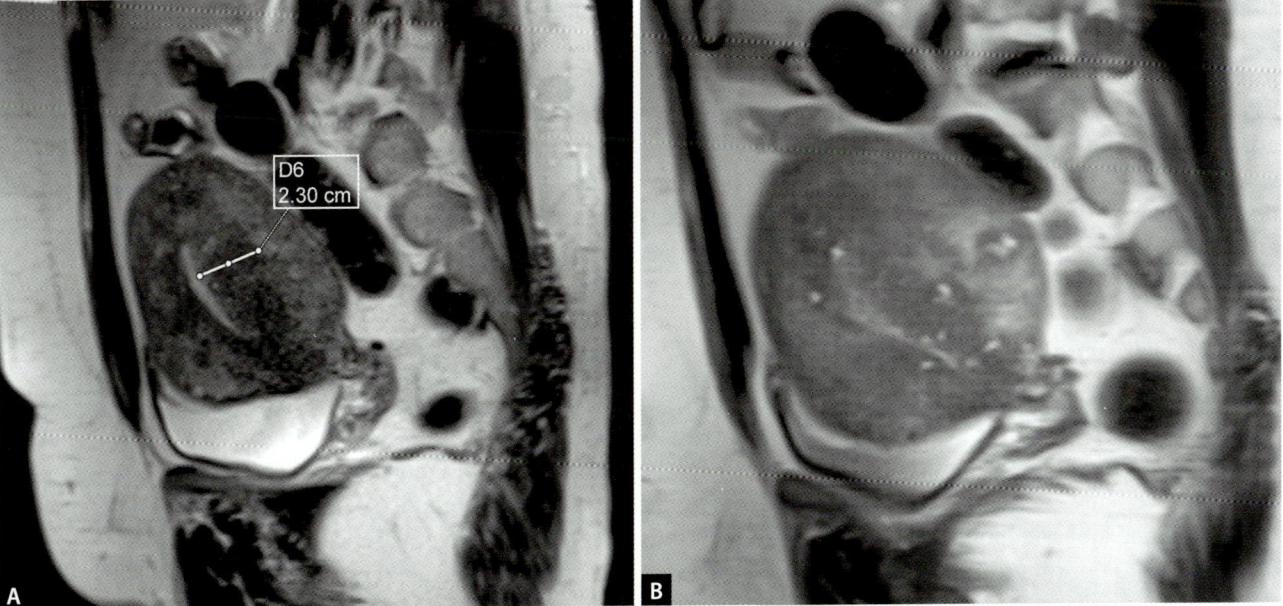

Figs. 20A and B: Adenomyosis. Sagittal T2W MR images of the same patient as in Figure 19 show globular enlargement of the uterus. The junctional zone is markedly widened with heterogeneous myometrium showing multiple variable-sized cystic areas.

Table 4: MRI criteria for adenomyosis.

Location	• Focal or diffuse widening of junctional zone >12 mm • More often found in the posterior uterine wall • Not seen in the cervix
Morphology	• Ill-defined margins blending with the surrounding myometrium • Poor definition of endomyometrial junction • *Focal:* May be globular, elliptical but usually not round or spherical • Significant mass effect missing, even if large lesion present • Mild distortion of endometrium, but marked enlargement of the uterus in diffuse adenomyosis
Appearance on T1	• Mostly isointense to the myometrium • May show hyperintense foci corresponding to small areas of hemorrhage
Appearance on T2	• Low SI uterine lesion with or without punctuate high signal intensity (SI) foci • High SI linear striations extending from the endometrium that may lead to a pseudowidening of the endometrium • Rarely large cystic spaces within a lesion (cystic adenomyosis)
Appearance on gadolinium-enhanced T1	Can appear hypo-, iso-, and hyperintense relative to myometrium
Additional findings	• No pseudocapsule • Adenomyosis is seen in combination with finding of endometriosis

bleed occurs in these ectopic endometrial glands, these foci appear bright on T1-weighted images and are highly suggestive of endometriosis. In addition, striations of high signal on T2W images extending from the endometrium into the myometrium, producing pseudowidening of the endometrium, may be seen. The appearance of adenomyosis and the amount of bright foci may fluctuate with or without treatment. Contrast-enhanced imaging does not increase the accuracy in diagnosing adenomyosis although perfusion abnormalities have been reported **(Figs. 21A to C)**.[66-70]

Atypical/Unusual Patterns of Adenomyosis

Adenomyoma is a localized, circumscribed form of adenomyosis. The lesion is generally seen as a polypoid mass protruding into the endometrial cavity, or as a myometrial or subserosal mass without any connection to the junctional zone. Adenomyoma may be misdiagnosed as a leiomyoma or other tumors. An *adenomyotic cyst* is another extremely rare variation of adenomyosis which is thought to be caused by extensive hemorrhage into the ectopic endometrium. This produces a well-defined cystic myometrial lesion with different stages of blood degradation products.

Differential Diagnosis

Pseudolesions: During menstruation (especially day 1 and 2), the uterus may demonstrate marked thickening of the junctional zone (>12 mm). Thus, MR imaging should be avoided during the menstrual phase. *Myometrial contraction* is another pseudolesion. This produces focal bulging of the myometrium into the uterine cavity. The contracted area shows ill-defined or well-marginated areas of low signal intensity on T2-weighted images[71] as blood is squeezed out, reducing the water content (due to the reduced blood volume). Sequential studies demonstrate their transient nature distinguishing them from true myometrial disease although, this is not always possible on a single study.

Leiomyoma is the most common lesion which resembles focal adenomyosis. Focal adenomyosis produces an oval or elliptical lesion which leads to thickening of the uterine wall, but differs from leiomyoma in that there is little mass effect or distortion of the uterine cavity or outline. Unlike leiomyomas, adenomyosis shows poorly defined margins and blends with surrounding myometrium. It also lacks the pseudocapsule and dilated vessels or signal voids at the periphery that may be seen with leiomyomas. The differences have been summarized in **Table 5**.

Adenomatoid tumor, which is a relatively rare benign mesothelial tumor, resembles a leiomyoma or adenomyoma. *Metastasis* to the uterine corpus and *myometrial invasion by endometrial cancer* may also produce appearances identical to adenomyosis. *Endometrial stromal sarcoma (ESS)* which involves both endometrium and myometrium with infiltrative margins and cystic changes and *adenocarcinoma arising in adenomyosis* are other rare differential diagnostic considerations.

OTHER BENIGN MESENCHYMAL TUMORS

Fatty or mixed mesenchymal tumors such as fibromyolipoma, and lipoma of the uterus are rare benign tumors.[72] They may arise from metaplasia of connective tissue or smooth muscle cells.

On US, lipoma is seen as a rounded lesion showing increased echogenicity with a hypoechoic rim.[73] On CT, the encapsulated fat density of uterine lipoma may mimics an ovarian dermoid (benign cystic teratoma).[74] Accurate diagnosis is important because teratomas are generally

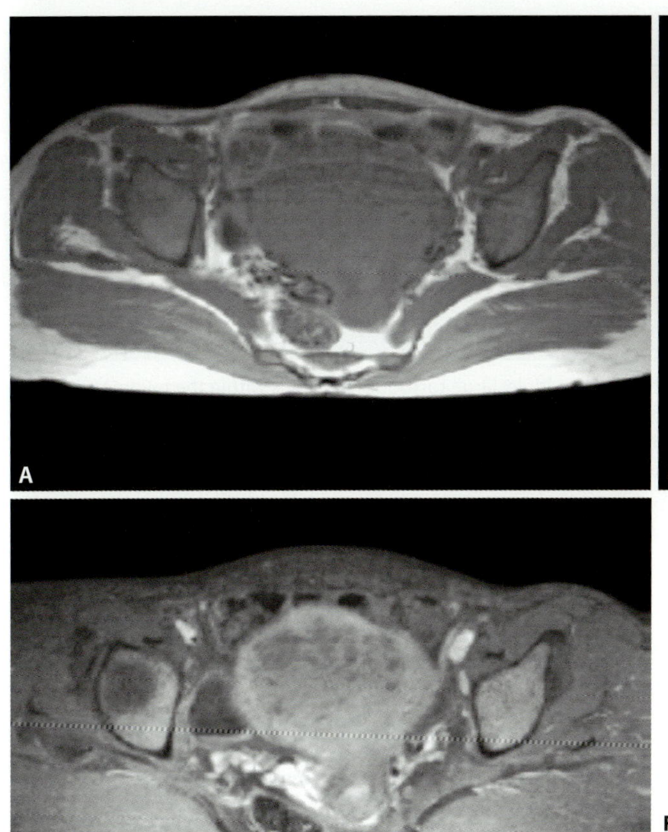

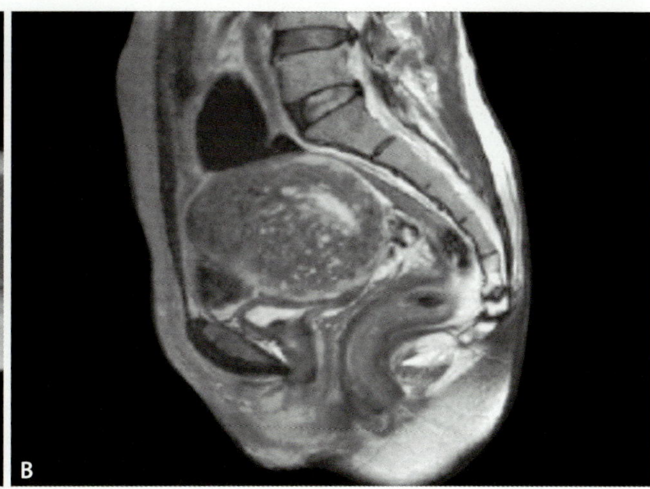

Figs. 21A to C: Adenomyosis. Axial and sagittal T1, T2, and postcontrast images reveal bulky uterus with thickening and heterogeneity of junctional zone, poorly defined endomyometrial junction, and multiple small T2 hyperintense foci with heterogeneous contrast enhancement in the anterior myometrium.

Table 5: Comparison of findings of focal adenomyosis and leiomyomas.

Categories	*Adenomyosis*	*Leiomyomas*
Borders	Indistinct	Distinct, usually round
Location	Generally contiguous with endometrium	Submucosal, intramural, or subserosal
Shadowing on US	Thin, parallel, vertical, and Venetian blind shadows	Edge shadowing; dense shadows from calcification
Mass effect	Absent	Present
Calcification	None	Common; rim and chunky
Cysts	Tiny cysts and cystic striations	Usually solid; may have macrocystic degeneration
Vascularity	Increased flow, penetrating vessels	Qualitatively variable, typically circumferential
Junctional zone	Thickened, with indistinct borders	Normal thickness

managed by surgical excision, whereas lipomatous uterine tumors require no therapy unless symptomatic.

UTERINE ARTERIOVENOUS MALFORMATION

Uterine arteriovenous malformations (AVMs) may be congenital, traumatic, malignant, or idiopathic. Congenital AVMs are thought to occur due to undifferentiated vascular structures from the arrest of embryonic development. Acquired AVMs are usually secondary to trauma caused by procedures such as curettage or uterine surgery or secondary to neoplasms.[75]

On grayscale imaging, appearance of AVMs is nonspecific and includes subtle, myometrial inhomogeneity, tubular spaces within the myometrium, or prominent parametrial vessels. Doppler findings reveal a low resistance flow with high PSVs. Spectral analysis of venous flow also shows high flow velocities and systolic velocity peaks similar to arterial pattern, suggesting an arteriovenous shunting.[76]

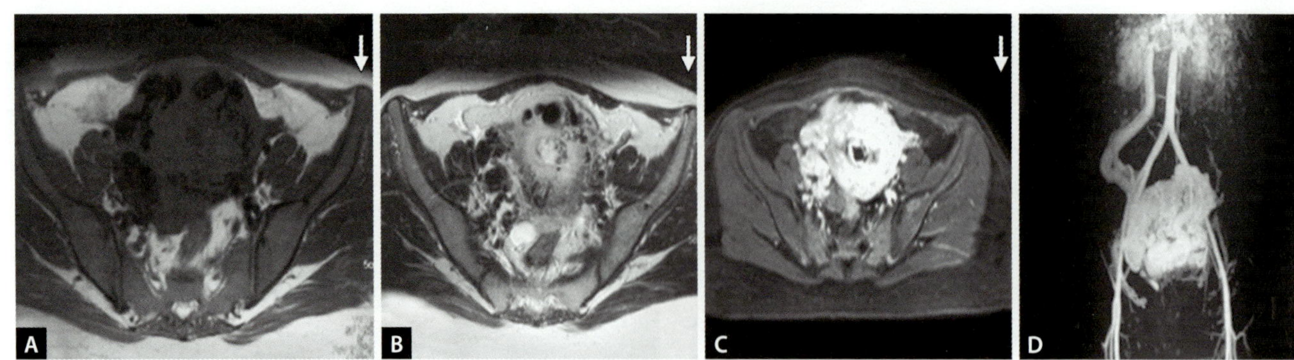

Figs. 22A to D: (A) T1W and (B) T2W axial MR images reveal a bulky uterus with multiple, large tortuous flow voids within the myometrium and bilateral parametrial regions; (C) Intense enhancement of the myometrium and the vascular channels is seen on postgadolinium images; (D) Magnetic resonance angiography reveals prominent arterial feeder channels arising from the internal iliac arteries. Enlarged, tortuous venous channels are seen draining into the iliac and right ovarian veins—uterine arteriovenous malformation.

Both computed tomography angiography (CTA) and magnetic resonance angiography (MRA) can be used to accurately assess the size, extent of AVMs and the degree of adjacent organ involved. On MRI, AVMs appear as focal uterine masses or as disruption of the junctional zones with serpiginous flow-related signal voids within the myometrium, showing intense enhancement on postgadolinium imaging with early draining veins **(Figs. 22A to D)**. Treatment of uterine AVM consists of either surgery or transcatheter embolization. The extent of involvement of adjacent pelvic viscera is important in deciding between the two treatment options.[77]

UTERINE INVERSION

Uterine inversion is most often attributed to excessive traction on the cord during delivery or a fundal location of the placenta. Nonpuerperal causes of uterine inversion include a benign or malignant uterine mass, but it is extremely rare.[78]

On longitudinal US scans, the uterine fundus is poorly seen due to the folding of the uterus on itself sometimes referred to as the "*fallen fundus*" sign. The central uterine echoes appear to have a "Y" configuration with the limbs of the "Y" formed by the inverted endometrial lining extending both anteriorly and posteriorly and the base by the noninverted endometrial lining. The miduterus gives a "*bull's eye*" appearance on transverse scans consisting of a hyperechoic ring representing the inverted endometrial lining surrounding the geographic center of the uterus. With complete inversion into the vagina, a mirror reflection of the uterus projecting into the vagina and a central pseudostripe may be seen, as the interface between the two opposing serosal surfaces may mimic an endometrial stripe. On MRI, V- or U-shaped uterine cavity and an inverted uterine fundus on sagittal images, and a *bull's eye* configuration on axial images have been reported. At times, the uterine anatomy may be completely distorted.

ENDOMETRIAL PATHOLOGY

Endometrial Polyps[79-81]

Endometrial polyps usually occur in perimenopausal/postmenopausal women, and are multiple in 20% of cases. Women on tamoxifen therapy for breast cancer treatment have an increased relative risk for developing endometrial polyps. Most patients are asymptomatic; however, they may cause menorrhagia, intermenstrual bleeding, or postmenopausal bleeding.

Endometrial polyps represent localized hyperplastic overgrowth of endometrial glands and stroma, covered by endometrium. They may be sessile or pedunculated and are usually attached to the uterine fundus or cornua. They are variable in size and may be small or so large as to protrude into the endocervical canal. Histologically, they are of three types: (1) hyperplastic (resembling glands of endometrial hyperplasia), (2) atrophic (cystically dilated atrophic glands), and (3) functional (undergo cyclical endometrial changes). Malignancy is seen in 0.5% of endometrial polyps.

On US, endometrial polyps are visualized as nonspecific, echogenic endometrial thickening or as a focal, echogenic endometrial mass. It may be broad based and sessile or pedunculated. The point of attachment should not disrupt the endometrial lining[30] anechoic regions within the polyps may be seen and correspond histologically to dilated glands.[17] *An interrupted mucosa sign* has been described where the highly echogenic linear interface of opposing endometrial surfaces is focally interrupted by an endometrial polyp. This is best

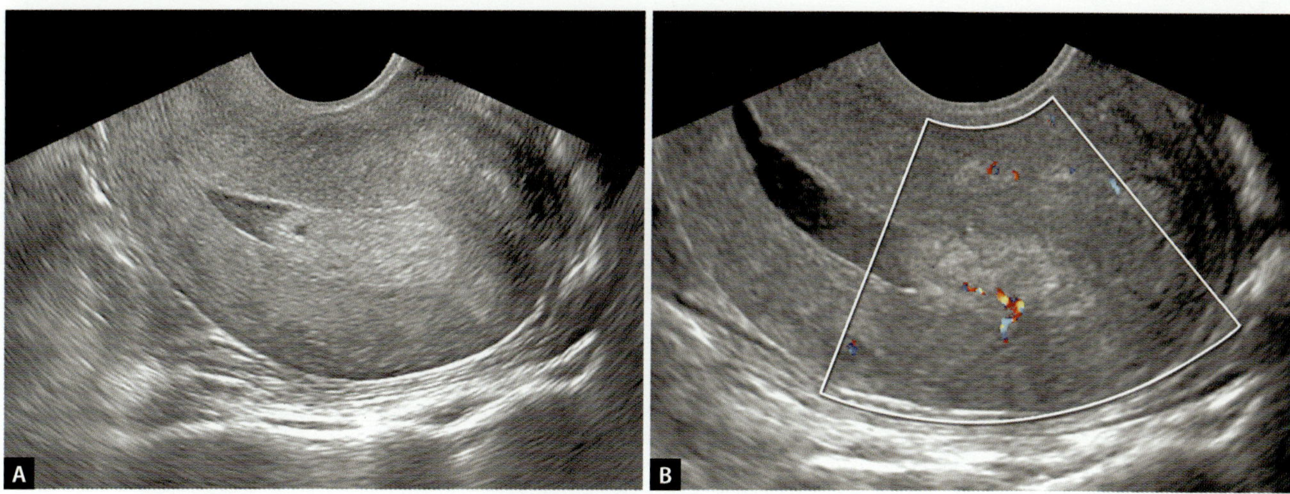

Figs. 23A and B: Endometrial polyp. (A) Saline infusion sonohysterography (SIS) demonstrates a well-defined echogenic mass in the endometrial cavity near the fundus; (B) A characteristic single feeding vessel is well seen on color Doppler.

appreciated on transvaginal transverse or longitudinal images in the first half of the menstrual cycle. Color Doppler imaging demonstrates a single feeding vessel, which is reported to be fairly specific for endometrial polyps and better seen with SIS. On SIS, endometrial polyps are seen as smooth, well margined, echogenic masses protruding into the endometrial canal surrounded by fluid **(Figs. 23A and B)**.

Most commonly, endometrial polyps show a slightly hypointense signal compared to endometrium on T2-weighted MR images, but may also be isointense to endometrium, appearing as focal or diffuse thickening of the endometrium. They may show intratumoral cystic areas or have a low T2-signal intensity fibrous core or stalk, features which have been reported more often in benign lesions than malignant ones. On T1-weighted images, endometrial polyps are isointense to endometrium. On postcontrast images, moderate to strong enhancement, generally less than normal endometrium, but more than normal myometrium is seen **(Figs. 24A to D)**. On dynamic examination, early persistent enhancement or a gradually increasing enhancement has been reported. These MRI features may be useful to differentiate endometrial polyps from other endometrial lesions but overlap may be seen with hyperplasia and malignancy.

A submucosal fibroid/fibroid polyp may mimic an endometrial polyp but may be differentiated by a broader base and more irregular contour of the former on SIS. A normal layer of endometrium is seen overlying a submucosal fibroid while the polyp can be seen arising from the endometrium. A single feeding vessel as opposed to a circumferential vascular supply in fibroids is also a useful distinguishing feature. Endometrial hyperplasia may also be impossible to distinguish from a polyp, especially when the former is focal and the latter is large.

Endometrial Hyperplasia

Excessive proliferation of the endometrial glands is termed as endometrial hyperplasia. The endometrial gland-to-stroma ratio is increased when compared with normal proliferative endometrium[82] and the glands can be cystically dilated. It may be focal or diffuse. Unopposed estrogen stimulation is the underlying cause in most cases of endometrial hyperplasia. Endometrial hyperplasia commonly presents as postmenopausal bleeding.

Two types have been described: with or without cellular atypia. Patients with cellular atypia may have foci of endometrial carcinoma in 25% of cases or develop it in future, while only approximately 2% patients without cellular atypia may develop malignancy.

On US, endometrial hyperplasia usually appears as a diffusely thickened, echogenic endometrium occasionally with small cysts representing dilated cystic glands at histology.[83] Focal, asymmetric thickening may also be seen in endometrial hyperplasia **(Fig. 25)**. The US and SIS features of endometrial hyperplasia are nonspecific and endometrial hyperplasia cannot be differentiated from endometrial carcinoma based on imaging alone.

On MRI, endometrial hyperplasia usually appears as diffuse thickening of the endometrium appearing iso- to hypointense on T2 sequences compared to normal endometrium, but the signal tends to be brighter than that in carcinoma. Small foci of increased T2 signal, attributable to cystically dilated glands, may be seen.

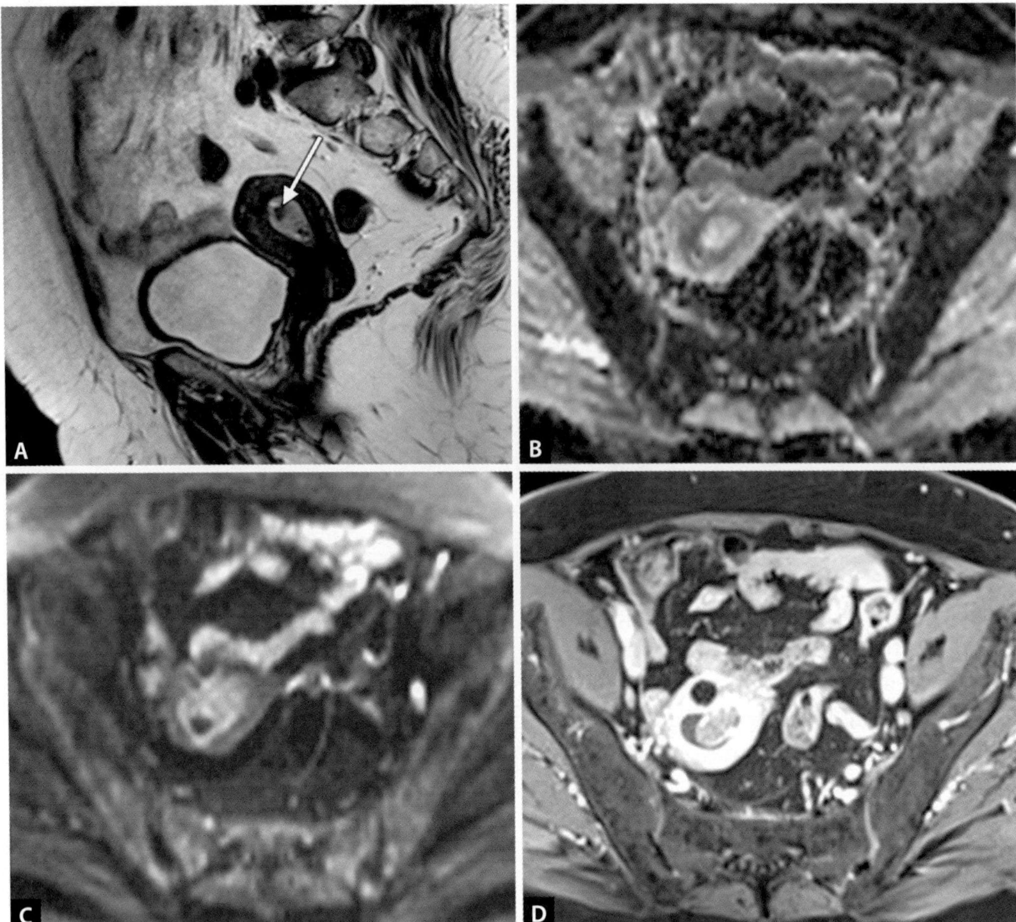

Figs. 24A to D: Endometrial polyp. (A) Sagittal T2W MR image reveals a focal lesion in the endometrial cavity, marginally lower in signal than expected for the normal endometrium. A few markedly hypointense areas (arrow) are also seen, representing fibrous core; (B and C) No diffusion restriction is seen on the DWI and ADC images with the lesion remaining bright on ADC; (D) Postcontrast image reveals mild enhancement of the polyp attached to the left lateral wall, well-delineated by the surrounding nonenhancing fluid. Note an incidental fibroid in the anterior myometrium (ADC: apparent diffusion coefficient; DWI: diffusion-weighted imaging).

Hyperplastic endometrium enhances less than the adjacent normal myometrium. On diffusion-weighted imaging (DWI), higher apparent diffusion coefficient (ADC) values have been reported in benign lesions as opposed to malignancy but stage 1A endometrial cancer cannot be reliably distinguished from endometrial hyperplasia based on imaging alone.

Infection

Endometritis is the most common cause of fever in the postpartum period, occurring in 2–3% of vaginal deliveries and in up to 85% of cesarean sections. The uterus and endometrium may appear normal on US, or may show a thickened, heterogeneous endometrium, intracavitary fluid, and/or intrauterine air as dirty shadowing.[84]

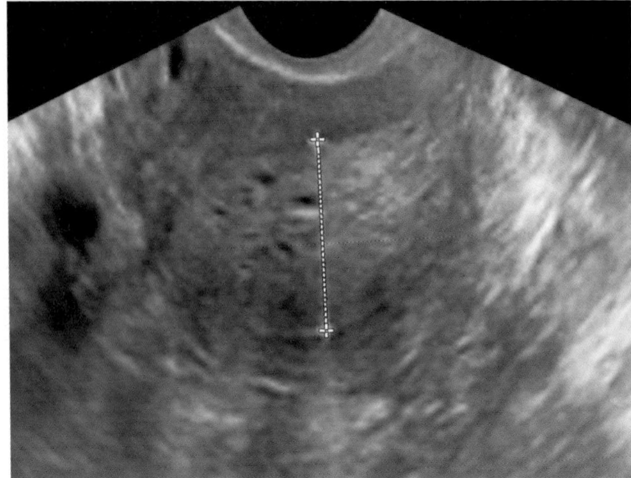

Fig. 25: Endometrial hyperplasia. Transvaginal sonography reveals diffusely thickened echogenic endometrium with small cysts within.

Tuberculosis is also an important cause of endometritis in India, usually secondary to primary infection elsewhere. Tuberculosis of the genital tract may often be associated with tubo-ovarian abscesses. It has been discussed elsewhere in this text.

BENIGN VAGINAL LESIONS

Benign lesions of the vagina are very rare. Tumors occurring in other locations in the genital tract may also occur in the vagina. They usually produce no symptoms until large in size which include feeling of pressure, dyspareunia, vaginal or urethral obstruction, or vaginal bleeding. Vaginal neoplasms may be cystic or solid.

Vaginal cysts include Gartner's cysts, usually found in the anterolateral wall of upper vagina and Bartholin's cysts which occur below the pubic symphysis in the vaginal introitus posterolaterally. They are well-defined cystic lesions following fluid signal on MR unless the contents are proteinaceous.

Vaginal leiomyomas or fibromyomas are rare usually situated in the anterior vaginal wall and very few cases have been reported in the world literature.[1]

Fibroepithelial polyps of the vagina are uncommon and usually asymptomatic. They are usually small and may be multiple. During pregnancy, they may become enlarged and edematous with a bizarre in appearance. In infants and young girls, sarcoma botryoides is a differential consideration.

CONCLUSION

Benign diseases of the uterus and vagina encompass a wide variety of conditions. Uterine lesions are very common and often produce overlapping symptoms. Some of there may be extremely distressing for the patients, besides the associated morbidity. Imaging, thus, has an invaluable role in establishing an accurate diagnosis and ensuring appropriate management.

ACKNOWLEDGMENT

The authors would like to gratefully acknowledge the contribution of Dr Shivali Arya in drawing the illustrations for Figures 1 and 9.

REFERENCES

1. Chan YY, Jayaprakasan K, Zamora J, et al. The prevalence of congenital uterine anomalies in unselected and high-risk populations: a systematic review. Hum Reprod Update. 2011;17:761-71.
2. Grimbizis GF, Camus M, Tarlatzis BC, et al. Clinical implications of uterine malformations and hysteroscopic treatment results. Hum Reprod Update. 2001;7:161-74.
3. Acién P. Incidence of Müllerian defects in fertile and infertile women. Hum Reprod. 1997;12:1372-6.
4. Grimbizis GF, Gordts S, Di Spiezio Sardo A, et al. The ESHRE-ESGE consensus on the classification of female genital tract congenital anomalies. Gynecol Surg. 2013;10:199-212.
5. Behr SC, Courtier JL, Qayyam A. Imaging of Müllerian duct anomalies. Radiographics. 2012;32:E233-50.
6. Miller RJ, Breech LL. Surgical correction of vaginal anomalies. Clin Obstet Gynecol. 2008;51:223-36.
7. The American Fertility Society classifications of adnexal adhesions, distal tubal occlusion, tubal occlusion secondary to tubal ligation, tubal pregnancies, Müllerian anomalies and intrauterine adhesions. Fertil Steril. 1988;49:944-55.
8. Grimbizis GF, Gordts S, Di Spiezio Sardo A, et al. The ESHRE/ESGE consensus on the classification of female genital tract congenital malformations. Hum Reprod. 2013;28:2032-44.
9. Carrington BM, Hricak H, Nuruddin RN, et al. Müllerian duct anomalies: MR imaging evaluation. Radiology. 1990;176:715-20.
10. Uğur M, Turan C, Mungan T, et al. Endometriosis in association with Müllerian anomalies. Gynecol Obstet Invest. 1995;40:261-4.
11. Olive DL, Henderson DY. Endometriosis and Müllerian anomalies. Obstet Gynecol. 1987;69:412-5.
12. Jayasinghe Y, Rane A, Stalewski H, et al. The presentation and early diagnosis of the rudimentary uterine horn. Obstet Gynecol. 2005;105:1456-67.
13. Chandler TM, Machan LS, Cooperberg PL, et al. Mullerian duct anomalies: from diagnosis to intervention. Br J Radiol. 2009;82:1034-42.
14. Sarto GE, Simpson JL. Abnormalities of the Müllerian and Wolffian duct systems. Birth Defects Orig Artic Ser. 1978;14:37-54.
15. Ott DJ, Fayez J, Zagoria R, et al. Congenital anomalies. In: Ott DJ, Fayez JA, Zagorian RJ (Eds). Hysterosalpingography: A Text and Atlas, 2nd edition. Philadelphia: Lippincott Williams & Wilkins; 1998. pp. 59-69.
16. Zanetti E, Ferrari LR, Rossi G. Classification and radiographic features of uterine malformations: hysterosalpingographic study. Br J Radiol. 1978;51:161-70.
17. Buttram VC, Reiter RC. Uterine leiomyomata: etiology, symptomatology, and management. Fertil Steril. 1981;36:433-45.
18. Fedele L, Dorta M, Brioschi D, et al. Magnetic resonance evaluation of double uteri. Obstet Gynecol. 1989;74:844-7.
19. Homer HA, Li TC, Cooke ID. The septate uterus: a review of management and reproductive outcome. Fertil Steril. 2000;73:1-14.
20. Raga F, Bauset C, Remohi J, et al. Reproductive impact of congenital Müllerian anomalies. Hum Reprod. 1997;12:2277-81.
21. Fedele L, Bianchi S. Hysteroscopic metroplasty for septate uterus. Obstet Gynecol Clin North Am. 1995;22:473-89.
22. Pellerito JS, McCarthy SM, Doyle MB, et al. Diagnosis of uterine anomalies: relative accuracy of MR imaging, endovaginal sonography, and hysterosalpingography. Radiology. 1992;183:795-800.
23. Propst AM, Hill JA. Anatomic factors associated with recurrent pregnancy loss. Semin Reprod Med. 2000;18:341-50.

24. Zreik TG, Troiano RN, Ghoussoub RA, et al. Myometrial tissue in uterine septa. J Am Assoc Gynecol Laparosc. 1998;5:155-60.
25. Reuter KL, Daly DC, Cohen SM. Septate versus bicornuate uteri: errors in imaging diagnosis. Radiology. 1989;172:749-52.
26. Fischetti SG, Politi G, Lomeo E, et al. Magnetic resonance in the evaluation of Müllerian duct anomalies. Radiol Med. 1995;89:105-11.
27. Brucker SY, Rall K, Campo R, et al. Treatment of congenital malformations. Semin Reprod Med. 2011;29:101-12.
28. Troiano RN, McCarthy SM. Müllerian duct anomalies: imaging and clinical issues. Radiology. 2004;233:19-34.
29. Ludwin A, Ludwin I, Kudla M. Differentiating between septate and bicornuate uterus: bi-dimensional and 3-dimensional power Doppler findings. J Minim Invasive Gynecol. 2014;21:1123-6.
30. Herbst AL, Ulfelder H, Poskanzer DC. Adenocarcinoma of the vagina: association of maternal stilbestrol therapy with tumor appearance in young women. N Engl J Med. 1971;284:878-81.
31. Rennell CL. T-shaped uterus in diethylstilbestrol (DES) exposure. Am J Roentgenol. 1979;132:979-80.
32. Olpin JD, Heilbrun M. Imaging of Müllerian duct anomalies. Clin Obstet Gynecol. 2009;52:40-56.
33. Knez J, Saridogan E, van Den Bosch T, et al. ESHRE/ESGE female genital tract anomalies classification system—the potential impact of discarding arcuate uterus on clinical practice. Hum Reprod. 2018;33:600-6.
34. Uterine leiomyomata. Number 192—May 1994. ACOG technical bulletin. Int J Gynaecol Obstet. 1994;46:73-82.
35. Cramer SF, Patel A. The frequency of uterine leiomyomas. Am J Clin Pathol. 1990;94:435-8.
36. Sue W, Scott-Barrett S. Radiological appearances of uterine fibroids. Indian J Radiol Imaging. 2009;19:222-31.
37. Kebapci M, Aslan O, Kaya T, et al. Pedunculated uterine leiomyoma associated with pseudo-Meigs' syndrome and elevated CA-125 level: CT features. Eur Radiol. 2002;12:S127-9.
38. Lurie S, Gorbacz S, Caspi B, et al. Parasitic leiomyoma: a case report. Clin Exp Obstet Gynecol. 1991;18:7-8.
39. Yeh HC, Kaplan M, Deligdisch L. Parasitic and pedunculated leiomyomas: ultrasonographic features. J Ultrasound Med. 1999;18:789-94.
40. Novak ER, Woodruff JD. Myoma and other benign tumors of the uterus. In: Novak ER, Woodruff JD (Eds). Novak's Gynecologic and Obstetric Pathology. Philadelphia: Saunders; 1979. pp. 260-79.
41. Okizuka H, Sugimura K, Takemori M, et al. MR detection of degenerating uterine leiomyomas. J Comput Assist Tomogr. 1993;17:760-6.
42. Hayasaka K, Tanaka Y, Fujii M, et al. Intravenous leiomyomatosis. J Comput Assist Tomogr. 2000;24:83-5.
43. Robboy SJ, Bentley RC, Butnor K, et al. Pathology and pathophysiology of uterine smooth-muscle tumors. Environ Health Perspect. 2000;108:779-84.
44. Gompel C, Silverberg SG. The corpus uteri. In: Gompel C, Silverberg SG (Eds). Pathology in Gynecology and Obstetrics. Philadelphia: Lippincott; 1994. pp. 163-283.
45. Arleo EK, Schwartz PE, Hui P, et al. Review of Leiomyoma Variants. Am J Roentgenol. 2015;205:912-21.
46. Gross BH, Silver TM, Jaffe MH. Sonographic features of uterine leiomyomas: analysis of 41 proven cases. J Ultrasound Med. 1983;2:401-6.
47. Dodd GD, Budzik RF. Lipomatous uterine tumors: diagnosis by ultrasound, CT, and MR. J Comput Assist Tomogr. 1990;14:629-32.
48. Vlahos N, Economopoulos K, Skarpidi E, et al. Bizarre leiomyoma of the posterior vaginal fornix. Int J Gynaecol Obstet. 2008;102:296-7.
49. Mittl RL, Yeh IT, Kressel HY. High-signal-intensity rim surrounding uterine leiomyomas on MR images: pathologic correlation. Radiology. 1991;180:81-3.
50. Casillas J, Joseph RC, Guerra JJ. CT appearance of uterine leiomyomas. Radiographics. 1990;10:999-1007.
51. Murase E, Siegelman ES, Outwater EK, et al. Uterine leiomyomas: histopathologic features, MR imaging findings, differential diagnosis, and treatment. Radiographics. 1999;19:1179-97.
52. Exacoustos C, Romanini ME, Amadio A, et al. Can gray-scale and color Doppler sonography differentiate between uterine leiomyosarcoma and leiomyoma? J Clin Ultrasound. 2007;35:449-57.
53. Hata K, Hata T, Maruyama R, et al. Uterine sarcoma: can it be differentiated from uterine leiomyoma with Doppler ultrasonography? A preliminary report. Ultrasound Obstet Gynecol. 1997;9:101-4.
54. Kubik-Huch RA, Weston M, Nougaret S, et al. European Society of Urogenital Radiology (ESUR) Guidelines: MR Imaging of Leiomyomas. Eur Radiol. 2018;28:3125-37.
55. Sudderuddin S, Helbren E, Telesca M, et al. MRI appearances of benign uterine disease. Clin Radiol. 2014;69:1095-104.
56. Kinkel K, Vincent B, Balleyguier C, et al. Value of MR imaging in the diagnosis of benign uterine conditions. J Radiol. 2000;81:773-9.
57. Lakhman Y, Veeraraghavan H, Chaim J, et al. Differentiation of uterine leiomyosarcoma from atypical leiomyoma: diagnostic accuracy of qualitative MR imaging features and feasibility of texture analysis. Eur Radiol. 2017;27:2903-15.
58. Wamsteker K, Emanuel MH, de Kruif JH. Transcervical hysteroscopic resection of submucous fibroids for abnormal uterine bleeding: results regarding the degree of intramural extension. Obstet Gynecol. 1993;82:736-40.
59. Parazzini F, Vercellini P, Panazza S, et al. Risk factors for adenomyosis. Hum Reprod. 1997;12:1275-9.
60. Cunningham RK, Horrow MM, Smith RJ, et al. Adenomyosis: A Sonographic Diagnosis. Radiographics. 2018;38:1576-89.
61. Struble J, Reid S, Bedaiwy MA. Adenomyosis: a clinical review of a challenging gynecologic condition. J Minim Invasive Gynecol. 2016;23:164-85.
62. Siegler AM, Camilien L. Adenomyosis. J Reprod Med. 1994;39:841-53.
63. Tamai K, Togashi K, Ito T, et al. MR Imaging findings of adenomyosis: correlation with histopathologic features and diagnostic pitfalls. Radiographics. 2005;25:21-40.
64. Sakhel K, Abuhamad A. Sonography of adenomyosis. J Ultrasound Med. 2012;31:805-8.
65. Katz VL. Benign gynecologic lesions. In: Katz VL, Lobo RA, Lentz G, Gershenson D (Eds). Comprehensive Gynecology, 5th edition. Philadelphia: Elsevier; 2007. pp. 419-71.
66. Bazot M, Cortez A, Darai E, et al. Ultrasonography compared with magnetic resonance imaging for the diagnosis of adenomyosis: correlation with histopathology. Hum Reprod. 2001;16:2427-33.

67. Reinhold C, McCarthy S, Bret PM, et al. Diffuse adenomyosis: comparison of endovaginal US and MR imaging with histopathologic correlation. Radiology. 1996;199:151-8.
68. Togashi K, Ozasa H, Konishi I, et al. Enlarged uterus: differentiation between adenomyosis and leiomyoma with MR imaging. Radiology. 1989;171:531-4.
69. Outwater EK, Siegelman ES, van Deerlin V. Adenomyosis: current concepts and imaging considerations. Am J Roentgenol. 1998;170:437-41.
70. Reinhold C, Tafazoli F, Mehio A, et al. Uterine adenomyosis: endovaginal US and MR imaging features with histopathologic correlation. Radiographics. 1999;19:S147-60.
71. Togashi K, Kawakami S, Kimura I, et al. Uterine contractions: possible diagnostic pitfall at MR imaging. J Magn Reson Imaging. 1993;3:889-93.
72. Soyer P, Harry G, Cazier A. Uterine fibromyolipoma: uncommon imaging features. Eur J Radiol. 1991;13:67-8.
73. Houser LM, Carrasco CH, Shelhan LR. Lipomatous tumour of the uterus: radiographic and ultrasonic appearance. Br J Radiol. 1979;52:992-3.
74. Lehrman BJ, Nisenbaum HL, Glasser SA. Uterine myolipoma. Magnetic resonance imaging, computed tomographic, and ultrasound appearance. J Ultrasound Med. 1990;9:665-8.
75. Dixit R, Prakash A, Chowdhury V, et al. Pelvic arteriovenous malformation. radiological quiz: GU imaging. Indian J Radiol Imaging. 2000;10:177-9.
76. Huang MW, Muradali D, Thurston WA, et al. Uterine arteriovenous malformations: gray-scale and Doppler US features with MR imaging correlation. Radiology. 1998;206:115-23.
77. Joshi M, Ganeshan K, Munshi HN. Ultrasound of adnexal masses. Semin Ultrasound CT MRI. 2008;29:72-97.
78. Rana KA, Patel PS. Complete uterine inversion: an unusual yet crucial sonographic diagnosis. J Ultrasound Med. 2009;28:1719-22.
79. Sadro CT. Imaging the endometrium: a pictorial essay. Can Assoc Radiol J. 2016;67:254-62.
80. Kamaya A, Yu PC, Lloyd CR, et al. Sonographic evaluation for endometrial polyps: the interrupted mucosa sign. J Ultrasound Med. 2016;35:2381-7.
81. Hase S, Mitsumori A, Inai R, et al. Endometrial polyps: MR imaging features. Acta Med Okayama. 2012;66:475-85.
82. Salem S, Wilson SR. Gynaecologic ultrasound. In: Rumack CM, Wilson SR, Charbonean JW (Eds). Diagnostic Ultrasound, 3rd edition. Elsevier: Mosby; 2005. pp. 527-87.
83. Nalaboff KM, Pellerito JS, Ben-Levi E. Imaging the endometrium: disease and normal variants. Radiographics. 2001;21:1409-24.
84. DePalma R, Leveno, K, Cunningham F, et al. Identification and management of women at high risk for pelvic infection following cesarean delivery. Obstet Gynecol. 1980;55: 185S-92.

Chapter 17

Malignant Diseases of the Uterus and Vagina

Alpana Manchanda, Anju Garg, Gaurav Shanker Pradhan

INTRODUCTION

Gynecologic cancers consist of tumors which develop in the uterus, ovaries, cervix, vagina, vulva and rarely the fallopian tubes. The two most common uterine malignancies are endometrial cancer (arising from the glandular epithelium of the uterus) and cervical cancer. Though they both arise in the uterus, endometrial and cervical cancer differ from each other in their epidemiology, etiology and clinical features.[1,2] Uterine sarcomas are uncommon and heterogeneous tumors of the uterus arising from the mesenchymal or stromal tissue. Lymphoma, metastasis to uterus and vaginal cancers are much rarer gynecologic malignancies. Imaging has an important role in the staging, treatment planning and post-treatment evaluation of these malignancies.

ENDOMETRIAL CANCER

Epidemiology

Endometrial cancer is the most common gynecologic malignancy in developed countries. In India, its incidence is 4.3/100,000 women,[3] which is rising because of increased prevalence of obesity. A number of risk factors are associated with endometrial cancer such as nulliparity, early menarche, late menopause, exposure to unopposed estrogen therapy, obesity and polycystic ovarian disease.

The effect of long-lasting unopposed estrogen leads to endometrial hyperplasia which increases the chance of developing atypical hyperplasia, and ultimately endometrial cancer.[4] Most endometrial cancers occur sporadically, with some having a hereditary basis such as Lynch syndrome being caused by germline mutations.

Pathogenesis and Histology

The traditional histological classification of endometrial cancer based on clinical and hormonal features was proposed by Bokhman in 1983, according to which endometrial cancers are of two types: (1) Type I and (2) Type II endometrial cancers.

Type I endometrial cancer or endometrioid adenocarcinoma is the most common type, accounting for 80–85% of all endometrial cancers.[5] They are called endometrioid as they resemble the proliferative phase of endometrium. Type I tumors are estrogen-dependent, include grade 1 and 2 endometrioid adenocarcinomas, are of low malignant potential and have a good prognosis. Based on their degree of differentiation endometrioid endometrial cancer can vary from poorly-differentiated to well-differentiated cancers. In contrast, *Type II endometrial cancers or nonendometrioid adenocarcinomas* are nonestrogen-dependent, occur in older females and include clear cell carcinoma, serous papillary carcinoma, and carcinosarcoma and arise in the setting of endometrial atrophy. They are poorly differentiated, present at a higher stage, are more aggressive, have a poorer prognosis and spread-like ovarian cancer.

Table 1 outlines the differences between the two types of endometrial cancers.[5,6]

All type II and grade 3 endometrioid tumors are high-grade tumors and tend to have a poor prognosis.

The histological classification of endometrial cancer by World Health Organization (WHO) is based on tumor morphology and tumor grade. **Box 1** depicts the histological classification of endometrial cancer.[7]

Table 1: Differences between type I and type II endometrial cancer.

Type I (endometrioid) endometrial cancer	*Type II (nonendometrioid) endometrial cancer*
• Comprises of 85% of all endometrial cancers	• Comprises of 15% of all endometrial cancers
• Premenopausal/perimenopausal age group	• Older patients (postmenopausal)
• Low-grade malignancy with endometrioid morphology (grades 1 and 2)	• High-grade malignancy with endometrioid grade 3, nonendometrioid subtypes, e.g. (Serous; Clear cell; Undifferentiated carcinoma)
• Good prognosis as diagnosed early	• Poor prognosis, account for 40% of endometrial cancer deaths
• Hormone receptor positive cancers	• Hormone receptor negative cancers
• More common in obese women, related to long-term estrogen therapy	• More common in nonobese women
• Originate from endometrial hyperplasia	• Associated with an atrophic endometrium
• Present as localized disease (low stage)	• Biologically aggressive with higher risk of metastasis
• Surgery is curative in early endometrial cancers	• Surgery with adjuvant chemoradiation
• Associated with *PTEN* or *KRAS* gene mutation	• Associated with P53 mutation
• 5-year survival is ~ 80%	• 5-year survival is ~ 40%

Sources: 1. Faria SC, Devine CE, Rao B, et al. Imaging and staging of endometrial cancer. Semin Ultrasound CT MRI. 2019;40:287-94.
2. Nougaret S, Lakhman Y, Vargas HA, et al. From staging to prognostication: achievements and challenges of MR imaging in the assessment of endometrial cancer. Magn Reson Imaging Clin N Am. 2017;25:611-33.

Box 1: Histological classification of endometrial cancer.

- Endometrioid (~80% of all endometrial cancers)
- Serous (~10%)
- Clear cell (<6%)
- Mixed cell adenocarcinoma

Rare types:

- Mucinous adenocarcinoma
- Neuroendocrine tumor (small cell, large cell or carcinoid)
- Dedifferentiated carcinoma
- Undifferentiated carcinoma

Source: Yen TT, Wang TL, Fader AN, et al. Molecular classification and emerging targeted therapy in endometrial cancer. Int J Gynecol Pathol. 2019.

Molecular Classification

The histological classification is useful in determining the appropriate surgical and adjuvant treatment. The dual classification of endometrial cancer (into type I and II) has been found to have its own limitations as all well-differentiated endometrial cancers do not have a good outcome and some poorly differentiated endometrial cancers have a good outcome. Often an overlap between histologic subtypes and grading has been seen, thereby causing a dilemma in clinical decision making. To overcome this drawback, the Cancer Genome Atlas (TCGA) in 2013 proposed a new molecular classification which by understanding the molecular alteration involved in endometrial cancer, may be useful in allowing early detection of endometrial cancer or precursor lesions and help in guiding targeted therapies.[7]

Clinical Presentation

Patients most commonly present in the 6th and 7th decades of life with history of postmenopausal bleeding. As a result, majority of endometrial cancers are diagnosed at an early stage (80% stage I) with 5-year survival > 95%.[6]

Diagnosis

The diagnosis of endometrial cancer is histopathological, by endometrial tissue sampling or aspiration. With adequate tissue sampling, detection rate of endometrial cancer is up to 99%.[4] Prognosis is affected by age of the patient, stage of disease, histological tumor grade, cell type and lymph node status. Deep myometrial and cervical invasion carry an adverse prognosis.

Imaging

Ultrasound

Transvaginal sonography (TVS) is usually the first and most common investigation performed as more than 95% women present with postmenopausal bleeding. However, only around 10% of women with postmenopausal bleeding develop endometrial cancer.[8]

Sonographic evaluation is quick, easily available and does not involve any ionizing radiation. TVS provides noninvasive, high-resolution imaging of the endometrium. The normal endometrium in postmenopausal women should be thin, homogeneous and echogenic. A cut-off value of 5 mm is considered as upper limit of normal in postmenopausal women presenting with abnormal uterine bleeding with a sensitivity and specificity of 96% and 61% respectively in diagnosing endometrial cancer **(Fig. 1)**. However, in postmenopausal women who are asymptomatic, an endometrial thickness of up to 8 mm is considered normal and biopsy should be considered only, if the endometrium is more than 11 mm thick.[8]

The margins of endometrial cancer may be well delineated on ultrasound, if it is a focal mass or thickening. The endometrial thickness should be measured in the anteroposterior dimension in the sagittal plane and a thickened endometrium must be considered as cancer until it is proven otherwise. Sonographic appearance of a uniformly thickened endometrium is the most common appearance seen **(Fig. 2)**. When the thickening is well defined, uniform and echogenic, it may be indistinguishable from endometrial hyperplasia or polyp. The diagnosis of endometrial cancer is more likely if the thickened endometrium is irregular or has poorly defined margins with a heterogeneous echotexture **(Fig. 3)**.[8] Due to overlapping features on TVS which may favor a benign or malignant etiology, an endometrial biopsy is required for a definitive diagnosis.

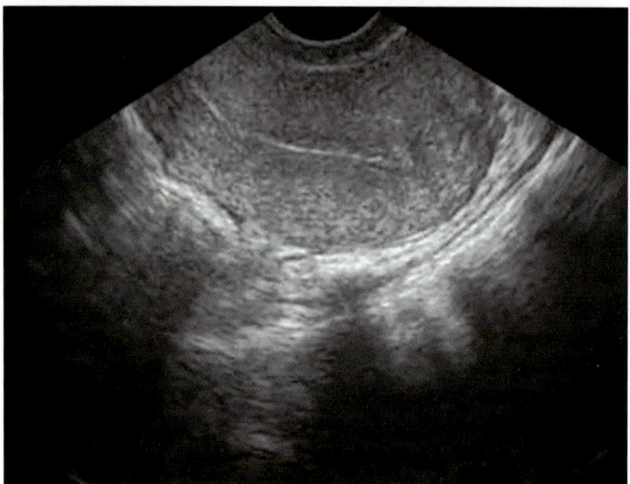

Fig. 1: Longitudinal transvaginal sonography image shows a uniformly thin (1.5 mm) well-defined endometrial echo. This appearance of the endometrium excludes malignancy in a postmenopausal woman with vaginal bleeding.

Ultrasound is limited in the evaluation of depth of myometrial invasion. Myometrial invasion can be suggested on TVS when there is asymmetric extension of the tumor into the myometrium, the endometrial-myometrial junction appears irregular or the subendometrial halo (inner myometrial layer) is disrupted.

On Doppler ultrasound, a normal or benign endometrium is characterized by high resistance flow, while an endometrial cancer by low resistance flow. Studies have shown that Doppler evaluation of uterine, subendometrial or intra-endometrial arteries are not reliable in the differentiation of benign and malignant endometrial processes and measurement of endometrial thickness is a better method of discrimination.

The limitations of TVS are that it is (1) operator-dependent; (2) the endometrium may not be visualized in around 10% cases; (3) it may be difficult to evaluate cervical or extrauterine extension due to its limited field of view; and (4) it may overestimate myometrial invasion in case of concomitant pathology such as adenomyosis or leiomyoma.[1]

Saline infusion sonography (SIS) or sonohysterography has been found to increase the accuracy of TVS.

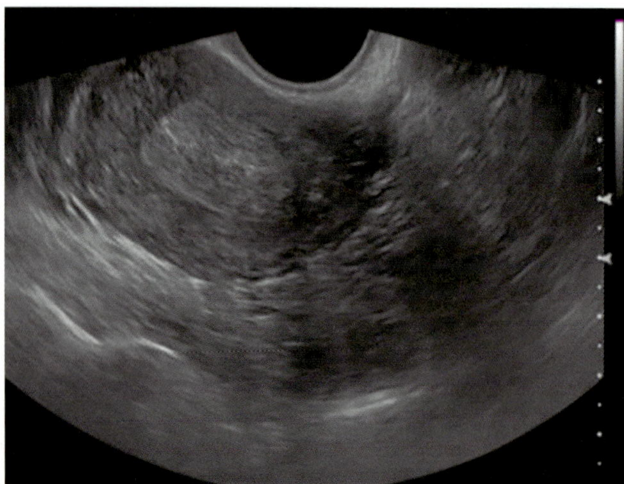

Fig. 2: Axial grayscale transvaginal sonography image reveals nonspecific diffusely thickened hyperechoic endometrium measuring 26 mm.

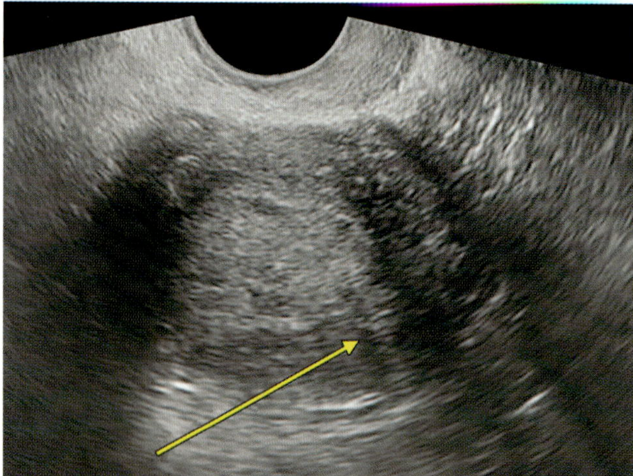

Fig. 3: Transvaginal sonography in a patient presenting with postmenopausal bleeding reveals diffuse thickening (30 mm) of the endometrium appearing heterogeneously hyperechoic with ill-defined endomyometrial junction posteriorly (arrow).

Endometrial cancer can appear as an intracavitary polyp or an asymmetric thickening of the endometrial lining on SIS. The depth of myometrial invasion has been found to be predicted with a greater accuracy on SIS than by TVS alone.[1]

A thin endometrium on TVS virtually excludes endometrial cancer, i.e. the negative predictive value of a thin endometrium is very high.[9]

Flowchart 1 depicts the various endometrial appearances on transvaginal sonography in postmenopausal women presenting with abnormal uterine bleeding and their workup.[10]

Such a TVS-based approach not only helps in excluding endometrial cancer, but also allows for better clinical management.

Computed Tomography

Due to its poor soft tissue differentiation, CT is not used in the local staging of endometrial cancer. On contrast-enhanced CT, endometrial cancer may be seen as a dilated endometrial cavity with a hypodense mass, which may be indistinguishable from an endometrial polyp or submucosal fibroid **(Fig. 4)**. CT has shown to have low sensitivity and specificity in evaluating myometrial invasion and cervical extension as compared to magnetic resonance imaging (MRI).[11]

Computed tomography is mainly indicated when the endometrial cancer is in a more advanced stage for assessing extrauterine spread, lymphadenopathy and extrapelvic metastasis. Lymph nodes, lungs and ovaries are the most common sites of metastasis of endometrial cancer.[5]

A recent study has shown dual energy CT to be a promising tool for assessing myometrial invasion with 50 KeV images being superior to 70 KeV images.[12]

Magnetic Resonance Imaging

Magnetic resonance imaging is the most accurate noninvasive imaging modality for preoperative assessment of endometrial cancer due to its excellent soft tissue contrast resolution. Although MR imaging is not a part of the standard International Federation of Gynecology and Obstetrics (FIGO) staging of endometrial cancer, MR imaging has been recommended by the National Cancer Institute of France, the European Society of Radiology guidelines and the Royal College of Radiologists.[13,14]

Technique: MRI is performed using a phased array body coil with high-resolution T2-weighted imaging being the mainstay of imaging. Nonfat suppressed images should be acquired because of the inherent contrast between the signal intensity of the uterus and surrounding fat.[15]

Flowchart 1: Endometrial assessment on TVS with history of postmenopausal bleeding.

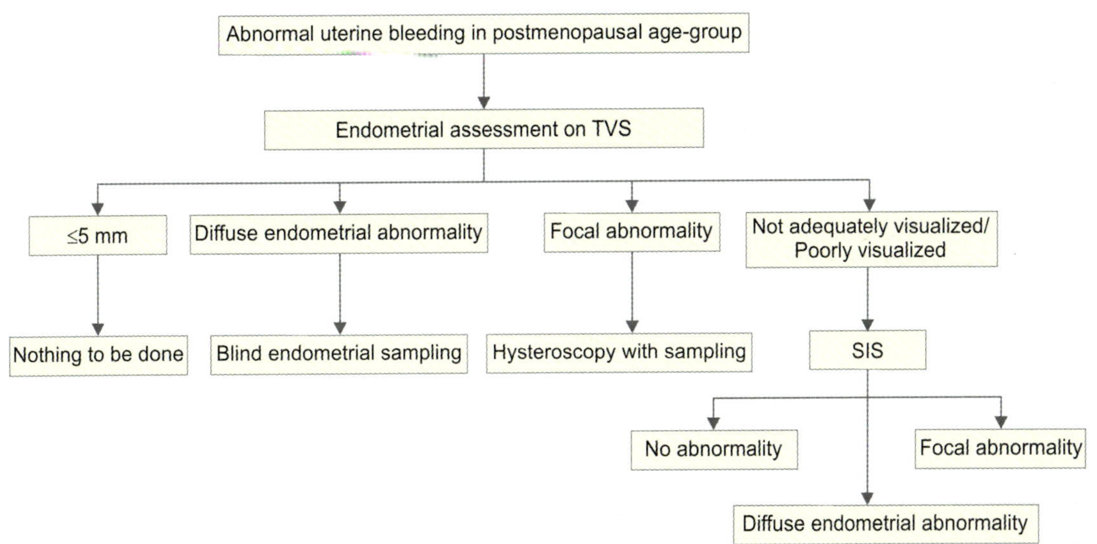

(SIS: saline infusion sonography)

Source: Rezvani M, Winter TC. Abnormal uterine bleeding: the role of ultrasound. In: Norton ME (Ed). Callen's Ultrasonography in Obstetrics and Gynecology, 6th edition. Philadelphia: Elsevier; 2017. pp. 835-45.

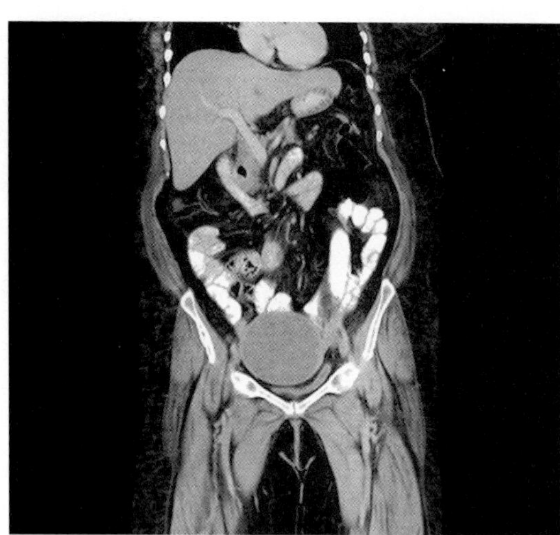

Fig. 4: Coronal contrast-enhanced CT in a 70-year-old woman with biopsy proven endometrial cancer reveals a large soft tissue mass expanding the endometrial cavity: **Type II endometrial cancer**.

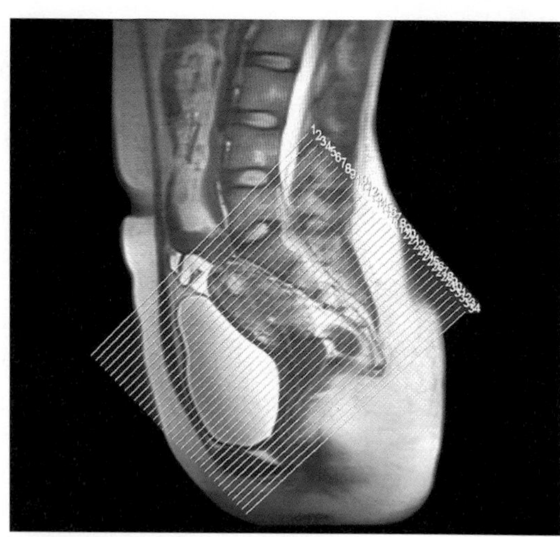

Fig. 5: Sagittal localizer image with reference lines depicting proper planning for image acquisition according to the uterine axis. The images should be acquired in a plane perpendicular to the endometrial lining.

The MRI sequences of the pelvis should be planned according to the uterine axis with the plane perpendicular to the endometrial lining to allow evaluation of depth of myometrial and cervical invasion **(Fig. 5)**. Multiparametric MR imaging is the preferred technique of MR imaging in endometrial cancer. A combination of three sequences, i.e. sagittal and axial oblique T2 weighted, diffusion-weighted imaging (DWI), and dynamic contrast-enhanced MR imaging (DCE-MRI) provides the most comprehensive evaluation by accurately delineating the extent of local disease and lymph node involvement if any. Staging of endometrial cancer by MR Imaging is found to be accurate in the range of 85–93%. By combining disease extent at MR imaging with the histologic subtype and grade obtained at endometrial biopsy, assessment of risk stratification and prognosis can be done precisely.[14]

Endometrial cancer appears hypo- to isointense mass on T1-weighted images, with intermediate signal intensity lower than the normal endometrium on T2-weighted images. On DCE-MRI, endometrial cancer enhances less than the myometrium. It shows restricted diffusion, showing high signal intensity on DWI, and low signal intensity on apparent diffusion coefficient (ADC) maps **(Figs. 6A to E)**. Both DCE-MRI and DWI increase the accuracy of T2-weighted imaging in assessment of depth of myometrial imaging. DW imaging has a role in endometrial cancer by showing the primary tumor better, depicting drop metastasis in cervix and vagina, extrauterine spread to the peritoneum and lymph nodes especially when intravenous gadolinium contrast is contraindicated and it can detect tumor when histopathology findings are inconclusive or endometrial biopsy is not possible.[16]

Diffusion-weighted imaging should always be evaluated together with the corresponding ADC maps and conventional T2-weighted images to avoid any pitfall. The ADC values of malignant lesions are found to be less than benign lesions and normal tissue. In a study by Rechichi et al., using two b values of 0 and 1,000 an ADC value of 1.05×10^3 mm^2/sec as cut-off was obtained which could differentiate endometrial cancer from normal endometrium. However a connection between ADC value and tumor grade could not be established.[17]

Bonatti et al. in 2018 documented the evidence of deep myometrial invasion and a tumor to uterus volume ratio ≥ 0.13 correlated with high-grade endometrial cancer, while ADC values were not found to be helpful in predicting the histological grade of endometrial cancer.[18]

Several features have been found to be associated with a poor prognosis in endometrial cancer, such as deep myometrial invasion (i.e. >50% depth of myometrial involvement or stage I B), cervical stromal involvement, and lymph nodal involvement.[5]

The depth of myometrial invasion is the most significant indicator for survival. The relation between depth of myometrial invasion and nodal involvement is given in **Table 2**.

Sagittal T2-weighted images depict the uterine anatomy well and are the best for optimal depiction of depth of myometrial invasion with a greater accuracy

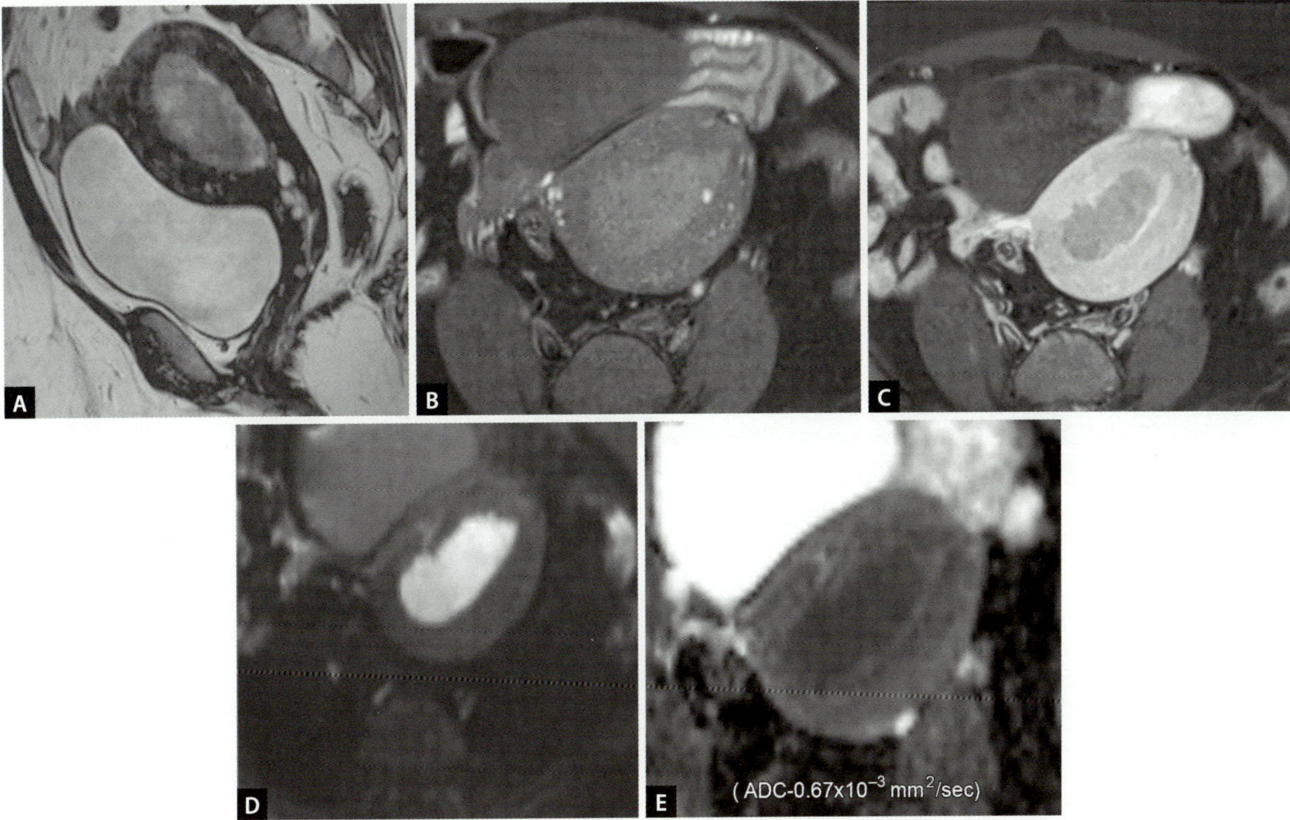

Figs. 6A to E: Multiparametric MR images of pelvis reveal (A) diffuse endometrial thickening of 28 mm showing intermediate hyperintense signal on T2W sagittal image (B) isointense on axial T1W image. Delayed post-contrast (3 minutes) axial T1 fat suppressed image depicts (C) endometrial lesion to be hypoenhancing to the myometrium and DWI and ADC map at the same level shows the mass to be hyperintense on DWI (D) with (E) loss of signal on corresponding ADC map with ADC value of 0.67×10^{-3} mm^2/sec. Both DWI and CEMR images depict the irregular endomyometrial junction very well: **Stage IA endometrial cancer** (ADC: apparent diffusion coefficient; CEMR: contrast-enhanced magnetic resonance; DWI: diffusion-weighted imaging).

Table 2: Relation of depth of myometrial invasion with lymph node involvement and 5-year survival in endometrial cancer patients.[5]

Depth of myometrial invasion	*Lymph node involvement*	*5-year survival*
<50%	3–9%	95%
>50%	20–40%	68%

in premenopausal than postmenopausal age group.[14] This is because of poor definition of junctional zone in postmenopausal women which may also be seen in those who have any other pathology such as adenomyosis or leiomyoma. DCE-MRI should be a part of standard imaging protocol for endometrial cancer as it improves the delineation of tumor margins and enables accurate assessment of invasion as endometrial cancer enhances less than the normal myometrium. The maximum contrast between the tumor and myometrium has been described between 90 seconds and 150 seconds after intravenous contrast administration **(Figs. 7A to E)**.[19] DCE-MRI and T2-weighted imaging together have an accuracy of 98% for assessing myometrial invasion, hence are the two-key MR imaging sequences required for adequate staging of endometrial cancer.[5,13]

The presence of a smooth, uninterrupted band of early subendometrial enhancement (at 35–40 sec) on DCE-MRI helps to exclude superficial myometrial invasion. This is an important finding when fertility sparing management is being considered. Delayed DCE-MRI images (3–4 minutes after contrast administration) should be acquired to rule out cervical stromal invasion.

The presence of an intact enhancing cervical mucosa excludes cervical invasion. It is important to diagnose cervical stromal invasion as it is associated with a high risk

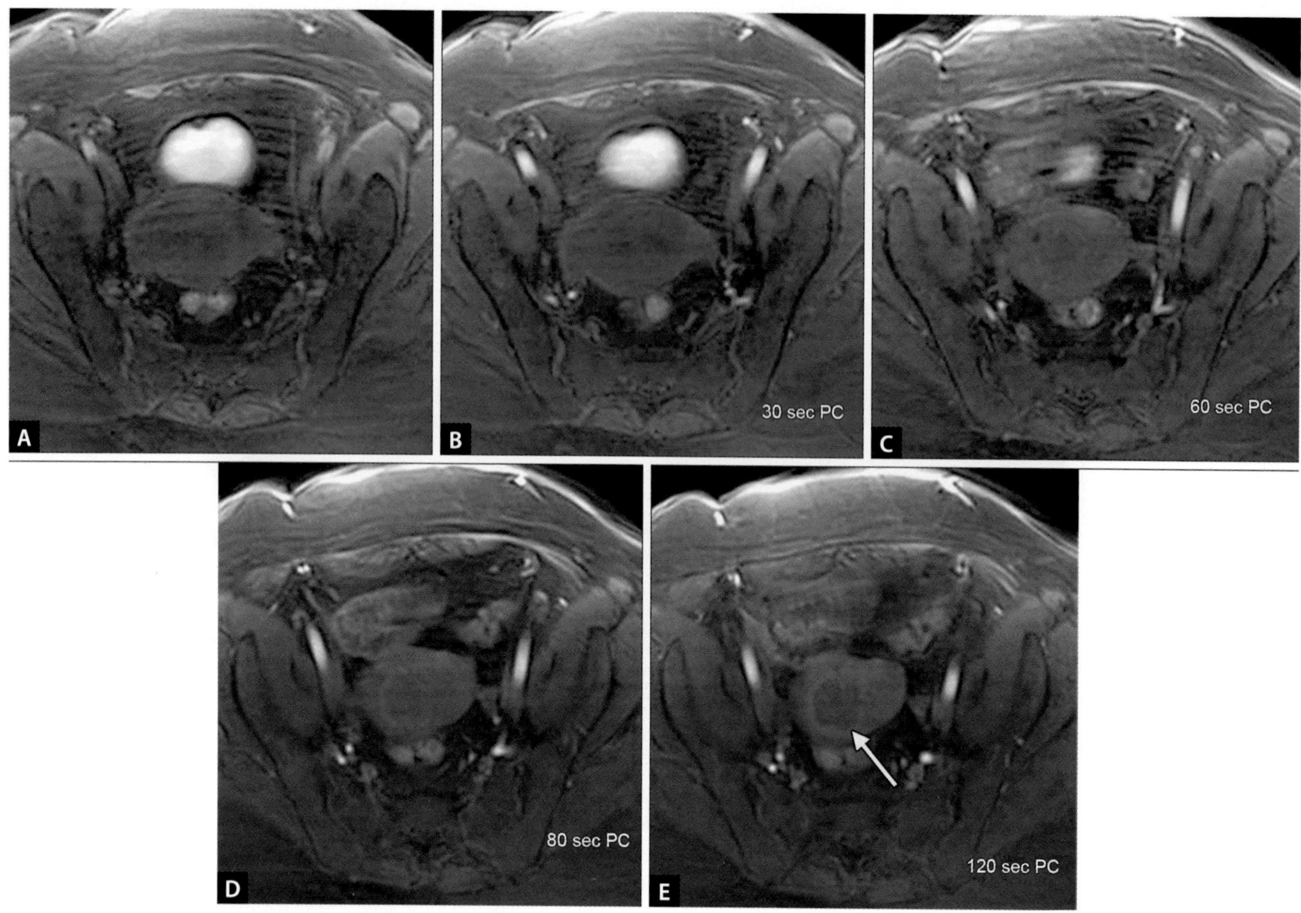

Figs. 7A to E: (A) Noncontrast and dynamic contrast enhanced MRI; (B to E) Axial T1-weighted fat suppressed images through the uterus reveal an endometrial mass with maximum enhancement between the mass and myometrium at 120 seconds (E) after intravenous contrast administration, appearing hypoenhancing (arrow) compared to the myometrium.

for lymphovascular space invasion (LVSI) which thereby infers a poorer prognosis. A widened internal os with tumor protruding into the endocervical canal does not represent stromal invasion.

Staging

Staging of endometrial cancer is surgicopathological as the primary treatment is surgical. Also, clinical staging often underestimates the disease extent.[16] Staging is based on the FIGO staging system which was first established in 1958, then updated in1988. It was revised in 2009 as a result of better understanding of the clinicopathological characteristics and prognostic factors. **Table 3** gives the revised FIGO staging of endometrial cancer.[3,6]

The standard surgical procedure for staging of endometrial cancer consists of findings from exploratory laparotomy, i.e. total abdominal hysterectomy with bilateral salpingo-oophorectomy, peritoneal lavage and pelvic and para-aortic lymphadenectomy. In patients who are at increased risk of mortality or severe morbidity, the surgical staging is not performed. Para-aortic lymphadenectomy is usually performed in patients with high-grade histologic tumor or where there is deep myometrial invasion.[3]

The five-year survival of endometrial cancer varies with the stage at which it is diagnosed. Patients in whom the tumor is confined to the uterus, the reported five-year survival rate is ≥95%.This decreases once the tumor has spread outside the uterus with five-year survival rates of 69% and 17% with regional and distant metastasis, respectively.[5] **Figures 8A to D** give the diagrammatic representation of various stages of endometrial cancer.

MRI Features of Endometrial Cancer as per FIGO Staging

Stage I: Stage I endometrial cancers are confined to the uterus. Stage IA tumors appear as a focal or diffuse

Table 3: Revised FIGO staging of endometrial cancer (2009).

FIGO	*Stage*	*Description*
I	IA IB	Tumor confined to uterus, ≤50% myometrial invasion ≥50% myometrial invasion
II		Cervical stromal invasion
IIIA IIIB IIIC	 IIIC1 IIIC2	Tumor invades serosa of uterus and/or adnexa Vaginal or parametrial involvement Metastasis to pelvic and/or para-aortic lymph nodes Pelvic node involvement Para-aortic lymph node involvement
IV	IVA IVB	Tumor invasion of bowel and/or bladder mucosa Distant metastasis (including abdominal metastasis and/or inguinal lymph nodes)

Source: 1. Nougaret S, Lakhman Y, Vargas HA, et al. From staging to prognostication: achievements and challenges of MR imaging in the assessment of endometrial cancer. Magn Reson Imaging Clin N Am. 2017;25:611-33.
2. Faria SC, Sagebiel T, Balachandran A, et al. Imaging in endometrial carcinoma. Indian J Radiol Imaging. 2015;25(2):137-47.

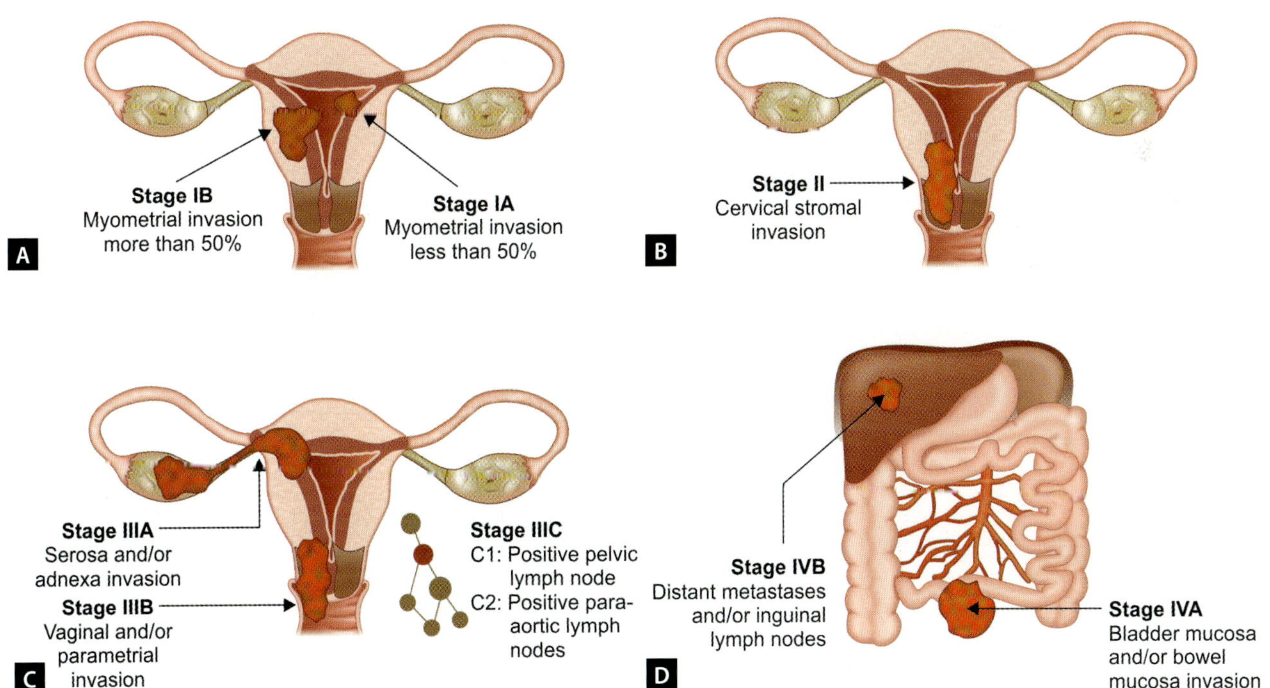

Figs. 8A to D: Diagrammatic representation depicting the FIGO staging of endometrial cancer.

intermediate signal intensity lesion within the high-signal endometrial lining or involve less than 50% of the myometrium. Superficial myometrial invasion is seen as disruption or irregularity of the low signal intensity junctional zone on T2-weighted images and loss of smooth subendometrial enhancement on DCE-MR imaging. Stage IB tumors are seen as low signal intensity tumor which invade greater than 50% of the myometrial thickness but do not extend beyond the outer myometrial margin **(Figs. 9A to G)**.

It is important to differentiate stage IA from stage IB disease because stage IB is associated with high risk of LVSI which has a direct bearing with the risk of lymph node metastasis and relapse.

Accurate evaluation of depth of myometrial invasion is possible on axial oblique images on MR imaging. An objective method of assessment has been described. First a line is drawn parallel to the presumed inner edge of the myometrium. Then two perpendicular lines are drawn, one measuring the thickness of the entire myometrium

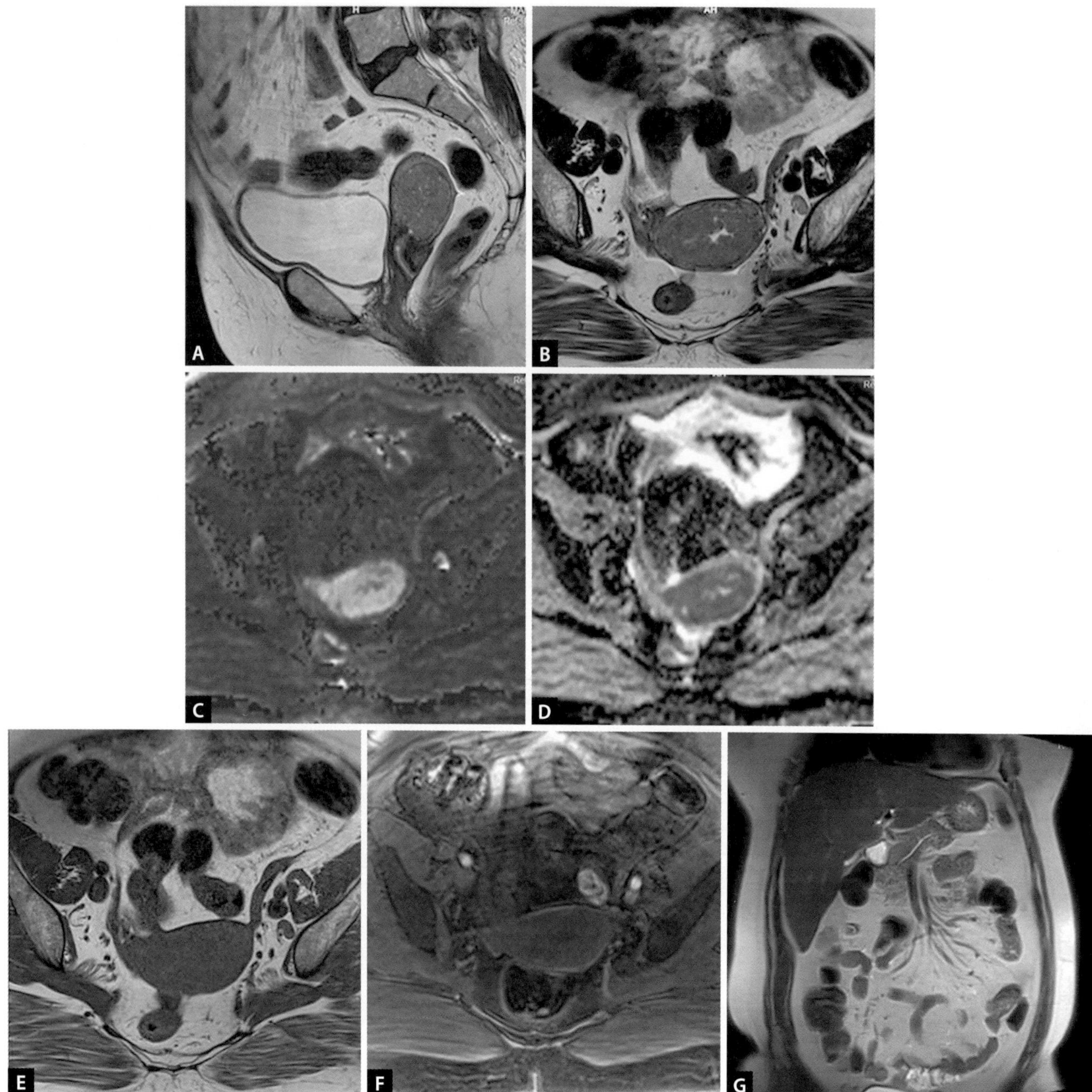

Figs. 9A to G: Stage IB endometrial cancer: (A and B) sagittal and axial T2-weighted images show a homogeneous mass of intermediate signal intensity expanding the endometrial cavity with thinned out myometrium. (C and D) the mass shows diffusion restriction on diffusion-weighted imaging. The mass is isointense on T1W image (E) and hypoenhancing on CE-MRI (F). (G) T2 coronal HASTE sequence reveals normal liver with no evidence of any enlarged nodes or deposits (HASTE: half-fourier acquisition single-shot turbo spin-echo).

and the other line measuring the maximum tumor extent within the myometrium. The ratio of the two lines described above represents the depth of myometrial invasion **(Fig. 10)**.

Stage II: Stage II endometrial cancer is characterized by the tumor invading the cervical stroma. Stromal invasion is best depicted on delayed DCE–MR images by the low signal intensity of the cervical stroma being replaced by the intermediate signal intensity tumor **(Figs. 11A to F)**.

Stage III: Stage IIIA tumors invade the serosa and/or adnexa and appear as disruption of the hypointense serosa, irregular uterine contour with or without enhancing adnexal masses. In stage IIIB disease, the tumor extends into the upper vagina with disruption of the hypointense vaginal wall signal. Stage IIIC tumors are characterized by lymph node metastasis with involvement of pelvic nodes (IIIC1) and/or para-aortic nodes (IIIC2). This reflects the different prognosis associated with lymph node metastasis.

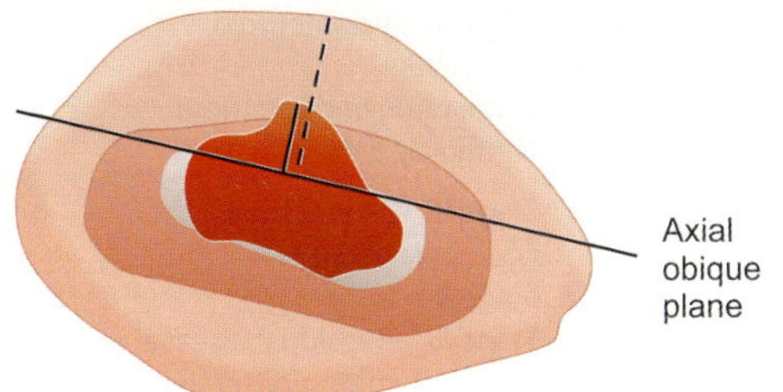

Fig. 10: Schematic diagram to show depth of myometrial invasion in axial oblique plane of uterus. A line is drawn parallel to the inner edge of the myometrium. Two perpendicular lines are drawn, one measuring the thickness of the entire myometrium and the other line measuring the maximum tumor extent within the myometrium. The ratio of the two lines described above represents the depth of myometrial invasion.

Risk factors for nodal metastasis consist of type 2 tumors, grade 3 tumors, lymphovascular spread invasion, and deep myometrial invasion. Lymph nodal distribution is influenced by the tumor location. The upper part of uterus drains to the common iliac and para-aortic lymph nodes while the middle and lower parts of the uterus drains to the parametrial and the paracervical and obturator nodes. Inguinal nodes are not in the regional lymphatic drainage pathway for endometrial cancer, and if present, represent stage IV disease. There is rarely direct drainage to para-aortic lymph nodes.[3]

The sensitivity of CT/MRI for lymph node metastasis is low because of size cut-off. Recent studies have described an increased sensitivity of CEMRI (82–93%) compared to size (29%) using ultra small paramagnetic iron oxide (USPIO) particles which is a lymph node specific MR contrast.[6]

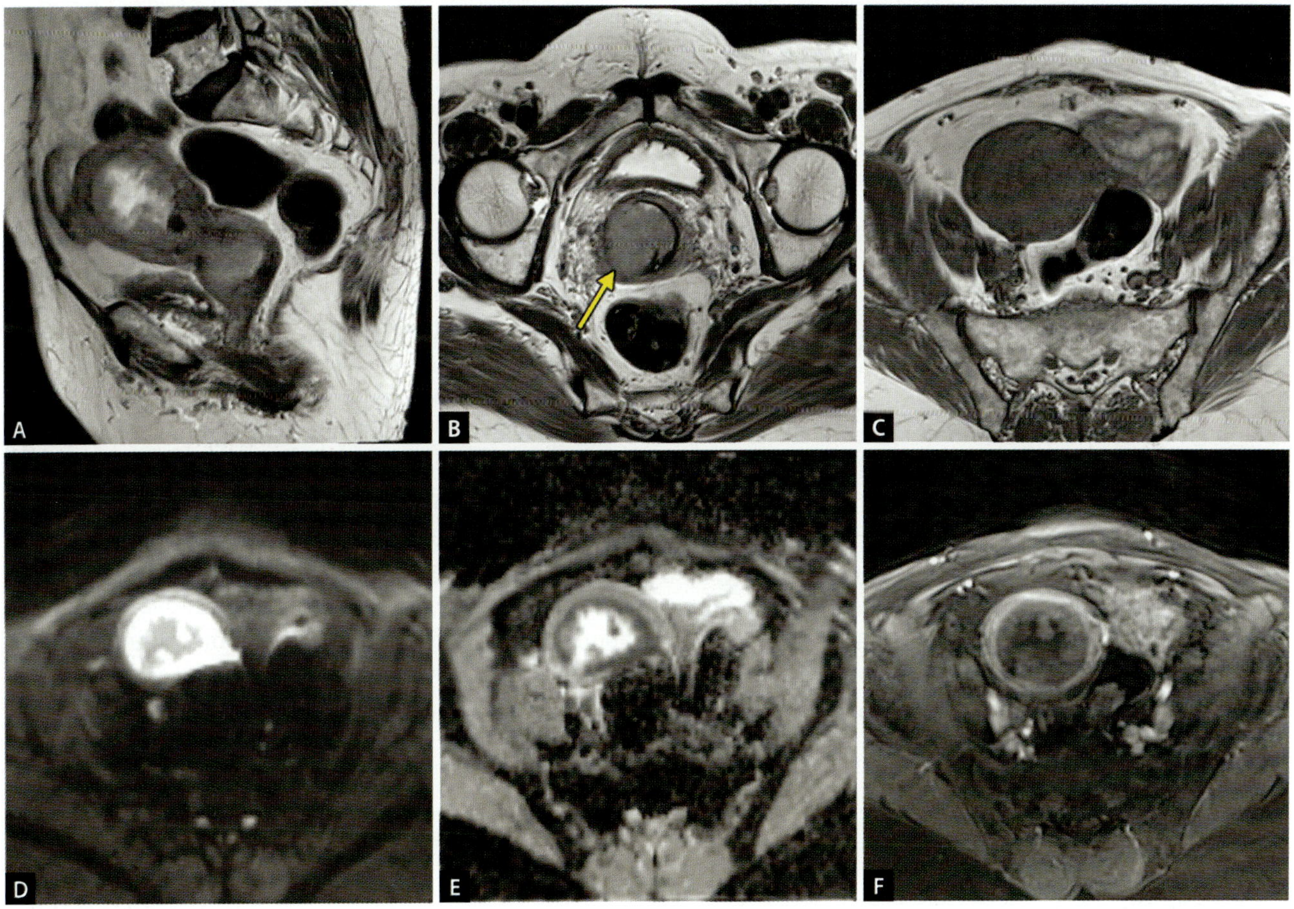

Figs. 11A to F: MRI pelvis in a 60-year-old woman with postmenopausal bleeding reveals a heterogeneously hyperintense mass with central necrosis expanding the endometrial cavity (A) with cervical stromal invasion (arrow in B) on T2-weighted sagittal and axial images. (C) The mass appears isointense on axial T1W image. Diffusion-weighted imaging and apparent diffusion coefficient map at the same level show diffusion restriction in the mass (D and E) and appears hypoenhancing as compared to the myometrium on contrast-enhanced-MRI (F): **Stage II endometrial cancer.**

Magnetic resonance imaging features which are suspicious for lymph involvement are node with a short axis diameter ≥10 mm or ≥8 mm but round configuration, multiple nodes, nodes with an irregular contour, necrosis, and an abnormal signal intensity similar to the primary tumor.

Diffusion-weighted imaging can be utilized for preoperative lymph node mapping as lymph nodes can be easily detected on DWI. However as per literature, none of the studies have been able to differentiate benign from malignant lymph nodes due to an overlap in ADC values.[6]

Stage IV: In stage IVA disease, the tumor invades bladder or bowel mucosa which is seen as tumor extending directly into the hyperintense vesical or rectal mucosa. Bullous edema (i.e. thickening of the high signal intensity mucosal layer) does not indicate mucosal invasion. Stage IVB disease is characterized by intra-abdominal metastasis and para-aortic lymph nodes above renal vessels and/or inguinal lymph nodes. Malignant ascites and peritoneal deposits are more common in type II endometrial tumors and high-grade type I tumors. Serous papillary and clear cell adenocarcinoma (both type II endometrial cancers) are characterized by omental-like and serosal deposits, a pattern of metastatic spread which is similar to that of ovarian cancer.[6]

FDG–PET

FDG–PET or PET/CT has not shown to be of value in the initial staging of patients of endometrial cancer. However, it may have a role in staging of more aggressive endometrial tumors (higher grade histology, type II endometrial cancer) such as serous papillary carcinoma, clear cell carcinoma for identifying extranodal metastatic disease in the thorax or abdomen.[20] PET-MR has been found to be comparable to PET-CT for detecting local lymph nodes and distant metastasis (i.e. N and M staging). For evaluating local tumor extent, PET-MR is superior while for evaluation of lung parenchyma PET-CT scores over PET-MR.[21]

Management of Endometrial Cancer

Stage I Endometrial Cancer

Endometrial cancer is primarily treated by surgery. The standard surgical procedure is total hysterectomy (TH) with bilateral salpingo-oophorectomy (BSO) along with cytology of peritoneal washings.

The addition of systemic lymphadenectomy to the surgical procedure in all patients is regarded as controversial as it leads to increased anesthesia and operative time with risk of development of lymphocele (7–10%) and lymphedema of the lower extremity (23%). From the various clinical trials and studies, it has been shown that only high-risk patients are likely to benefit from such an aggressive surgery. The National Comprehensive Cancer Network (NCCN) guidelines recommend sentinel lymph node mapping for the surgical staging of endometrial cancer which is confined to the uterus with no metastasis seen on imaging or no evidence of extrauterine disease at surgical exploration.[6]

Table 4: Risk stratification in endometrial cancer.

Risk category	*Type of endometrial cancer*
Low risk	Stage IA, endometrioid, G1 and G2, LVSI (–)
Intermediate risk	Stage IB, endometrioid G1 and G2, LVSI (–)
High intermediate risk	1. Stage IA, endometrioid G3, ± LVSI 2. Stage I A/B, endometrioid G1 and G2, LVSI (+)
High risk	1. Stage IB, endometrioid G3, ± LVSI 2. Stage II 3. Stage III, no residual disease 4. Non-endometrioid (serous, clear cell, undifferentiated carcinoma)

G: Grade of differentiation at histology
Stage: As per the revised 2009 FIGO staging of endometrial cancer
LVSI: Lymphovascular space invasion
Source: Nougaret S, Lakhman Y, Vargas HA, et al. From staging to prognostication: achievements and challenges of MR imaging in the assessment of endometrial cancer. Magn Reson Imaging Clin N Am. 2017;25:611-33.

Stage I endometrial cancers are stratified into four risk categories—low risk, intermediate risk, high intermediate risk, and high risk based on histology (grade and type) and depth of myometrial invasion as described in **Table 4.**[6]

As per the European Society for Medical Oncology (ESMO) Practice Guidelines, systemic/para-aortic lymphadenectomy is recommended for the intermediate- and high-risk categories. Hence, preoperative information about depth of myometrial invasion on MR imaging and histologic grade by endometrial sampling are essential to tailor the surgical approach in these patients.

Stage II Endometrial Cancer

The treatment of stage II endometrial cancer is hysterectomy, bilateral salpingo-oophorectomy, and lymphadenectomy.

Stage III and IV Endometrial Cancer

For stage III and IV cancers, extensive debulking is advocated with external radiotherapy with or without tumor directed brachytherapy.

The management of serous papillary and clear cell endometrial cancer is on the same lines as ovarian cancer with omentectomy and peritoneal biopsies in addition to TH, BSO, and lymphadenectomy.[1]

Recurrent Endometrial Cancer

Endometrial cancer is known to recur in two-thirds of patients within 2 years of surgery. The most common sites of recurrent endometrial cancer are lymph nodes, vaginal vault, peritoneum, and lungs. Patients with isolated vaginal recurrence are considered to have a better prognosis than pelvic or abdominal metastasis.[20]

Pelvic and para-aortic lymph nodes are the most common lymph nodes to be involved. Peritoneal involvement reported in 28% may be in the form of large masses, nodules or serosal implants.[20]

Patients with risk factors such as advanced age, higher grade of tumor at primary surgery, multiple sites of disease, and rapid presentation of relapse are known to have a less favorable outcome in recurrent disease. Compared to other gynecologic malignancies, endometrial cancer has the highest frequency of lung secondaries in up to 20–25%.[22]

Role of MRI in Fertility Preservation in Endometrial Cancer Patients

Around 5% of women who are diagnosed with endometrial cancer are below 40 years of age. If they wish to preserve their fertility, then MR imaging is found to be very useful by confirming that the disease is confined to the endometrium. **Box 2** shows the eligibility criteria for fertility preservation.[23]

In 2017, the European Society of Urogenital Radiology (ESUR) updated the 2009 ESUR endometrial cancer guidelines to recommend an MR imaging protocol for endometrial cancer. As per the recommendations, MR imaging should be tailored according to the tumor histology and grade, patients' desire for fertility preservation and the availability of a radiologist to monitor the MR investigation. The ESUR recommendations for MR imaging of endometrial cancer are given in the **Table 5**.[23]

UTERINE SARCOMA

Uterine sarcomas are rare, aggressive, and heterogeneous group of uterine tumors that arise from the mesenchymal or stromal elements.

They account for around 8% of uterine malignancies and have been seen to have a higher incidence than the earlier reported incidence of 2–3%, due to the longevity of the population and advancements in diagnostic techniques.[24]

Uterine sarcomas are the most malignant group of uterine tumors and differ from endometrial cancer with

Box 2: Eligibility criteria for fertility preservation in patients with endometrial cancer.

All criteria to be met
Histopathology: • Histologic diagnosis with dilatation and curettage • Grade I (well differentiated) endometrioid adenocarcinoma Or • Premalignant conditions such as atypical hyperplasia or endometrial intraepithelial neoplasia
MRI: Tumor confined to the endometrium (absence of myometrial invasion, cervical stromal invasion, ovarian metastases or synchronous primary ovarian cancer, and absence of lymphadenopathy)
Clinical: Patient compliance for close follow-up during and after conservative treatment

Table 5: ESUR recommendations for MR imaging of endometrial cancer.

Type and grade of endometrial cancer (EC)/patient population	*Role of MRI*	*MRI protocol recommendation*
1. Grade 3 EC and nonendometrioid EC (carcinosarcoma, serous carcinoma, clear cell carcinoma)	To detect extrauterine disease	• DWI of whole abdomen and pelvis to be performed • DCE–MRI—not required CEMR is recommended
2. Grade 1 or 2 endometrioid EC	To evaluate myometrial invasion and cervical stromal invasion	MRI protocol depends on MR acquisition • *Unsupervised MR imaging:* DWI + CEMRI are recommended • *Supervised MR imaging:* DCE–MRI as an adjunct to DWI in challenging cases
3. Patients' of childbearing age with grade I endometrioid EC, who wish to preserve their fertility	To rule out myometrial invasion	• DCE–MRI should be added to T2WI and DWI • An intact subendometrial enhancement rules out myometrial invasion

respect to their clinical behavior and spread. They are associated with a poorer prognosis even when detected early.

They comprise of malignancies which may arise from myometrial smooth muscle such as leiomyosarcoma, those arising from the endometrial stroma are endometrial stromal sarcoma (ESS) and undifferentiated endometrial sarcoma (UES) or arise from both (adenosarcoma). Carcinosarcoma (previously known as malignant mixed müllerian tumor) was earlier categorized as uterine sarcoma but is now regarded as a variant of endometrial carcinoma. This change led the FIGO to develop independent staging criteria for uterine sarcomas in 2010 which has separate staging system for leiomyosarcoma **(Table 6)** and another for endometrial stromal sarcoma and adenosarcoma **(Table 7)**. Carcinosarcomas are included in the same FIGO staging system as endometrial cancer.[25]

Clinical Presentation

The clinical presentation of uterine sarcomas is nonspecific. Patients may present with a rapidly growing pelvic mass with abdominal or pelvic pain, along with vaginal bleeding.

The various subgroups of uterine sarcoma cannot be distinguished clinically, from each other or from other uterine tumors. As uterine sarcomas arise from uterine muscle or mesenchymal tissue, they are not amenable to endometrial sampling and are difficult to diagnose preoperatively. Hence, cross-sectional imaging studies have a major role in the assessment of these tumors and in their staging.

Mixed Epithelial and Mesenchymal Tumors

Carcinosarcoma

Carcinosarcomas, also known previously as malignant mixed müllerian tumor (MMMT), constitute around 50% of all uterine sarcomas. They were originally classified as part of uterine sarcomas, but are now believed to be high grade endometrial cancers with sarcomatous/stromal differentiation due to their biological behavior being similar to high-grade endometrial cancer. Advanced age, obesity, pelvic radiation, and long-term tamoxifen use are some of the risk factors for developing uterine carcinosarcoma.[25]

Patients of carcinosarcoma are mostly postmenopausal, presenting with vaginal bleeding and bulky polypoidal mass in the endometrial cavity that prolapse through the cervical os. Elevated CA125 levels may predict myometrial invasion or extrauterine spread and also aid in monitoring for tumor recurrence.[26]

Carcinosarcomas are aggressive tumors with nearly 60% of patients presenting with metastatic disease. As compared to other sarcomas that spread hematogenously, they show lymphatic dissemination. Lungs, peritoneum, pelvic, and para-aortic lymph nodes are the most common sites of metastases **(Fig. 12)**.[27]

Table 6: FIGO staging of uterine leiomyosarcoma.

Stage		*Definition*
I		Tumor confined to uterus
	IA	<5 cm
	IB	>5 cm
II		Tumor extends beyond the uterus, within the pelvis
	IIA	Adnexal involvement
	IIB	Involvement of other pelvic tissues
III		Invasion of abdominal tissues (not just protruding into the abdomen)
	IIIA	One site
	IIIB	More than one site
	IIIC	Metastasis to pelvic and/or para-aortic lymph nodes
IV	IVA	Tumor invades bladder and/or rectum
	IVB	Distant metastasis

Source: Sala E, Rockall AG, Freeman SJ, et al. The added role of MR imaging in treatment stratification of patients with gynecologic malignancies: what the radiologist needs to know. Radiology. 2013;266(3):717-40.

Table 7: FIGO staging of uterine endometrial stromal sarcoma and adenosarcoma.

Stage		*Definition*
I		*Tumor limited to uterus:*
	IA	Tumor limited to endometrium/endocervix with no myometrial invasion
	IB	<50% myometrial invasion
	IC	>50% myometrial invasion
II		*Tumor extends beyond the uterus, within the pelvis:*
	IIA	Adnexal involvement
	IIB	Involvement of other pelvic tissues
III		*Tumor invades abdominal tissues (not just protruding into the abdomen):*
	IIIA	One site
	IIIB	More than one site
	IIIC	Metastasis to pelvic and/or para-aortic lymph nodes
IV	IVA	Tumor invades bladder and/or rectum
	IVB	Distant metastasis

Source: Sala E, Rockall AG, Freeman SJ, et al. The added role of MR imaging in treatment stratification of patients with gynecologic malignancies: what the radiologist needs to know? Radiology. 2013;266(3):717-40.

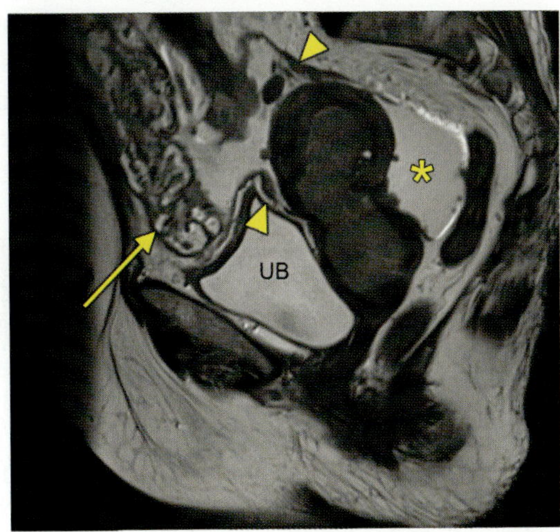

Fig. 12: T2W sagittal MRI image of pelvis shows soft tissue mass in the endometrial cavity extending into the endocervical canal. There is stranding and thickening of mesentery and omental caking (arrow). Nodular thickening also seen along peritoneal reflection (arrowheads) along with gross ascites(*): **Serous papillary endometrial cancer on HPE**.

On imaging, carcinosarcomas most commonly present as endometrial masses that expand the endometrial cavity and are difficult to differentiate from endometrial cancer. Certain imaging features which may help in differentiating that two are:[4]

- Carcinosarcomas are larger masses that distend endometrial cavity **(Figs. 13A to E)**. An anteroposterior tumor ratio >0.63 has been described to differentiate carcinosarcoma from endometrial cancer.[27]
- Carcinosarcomas are more heterogeneous tumors with areas of intratumoral hemorrhage and necrosis that have intermediate to high signal on T2-weighted images.
- They show significant contrast enhancement compared to endometrial cancer which are hypovascular.
- Carcinosarcomas have a poorer prognosis as they more often show deep myometrial invasion, cervical stromal invasion, and metastatic nodal disease at presentation.

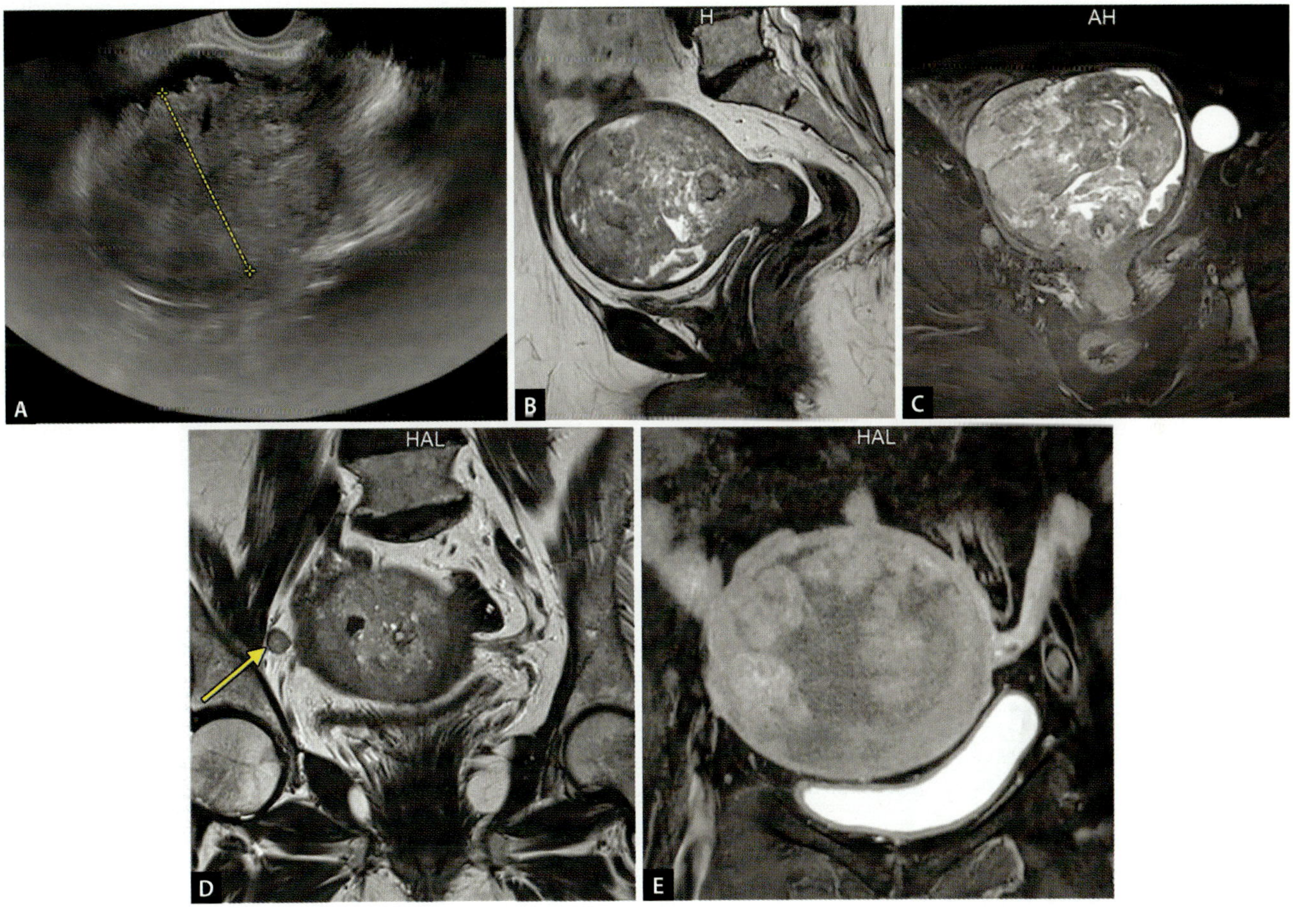

Figs. 13A to E: Transvaginal sonography of the uterus (A) reveals a large heterogeneous mass expanding the endometrial cavity. On T2 weighted sagittal (B) and coronal (C and D) images, the heterogeneous mass with few areas of necrosis are well visualized. A rounded lesion is seen adjacent to the uterus suggestive of nodal metastasis (arrow in D). On post-contrast MR image (E), the mass shows heterogeneous enhancement with loss of planes with the myometrium in the right lateral aspect: **Carcinosarcoma on histopathology**.

Imaging feature which aids in differentiation from leiomyosarcoma is a lower incidence of hemorrhage and necrosis in carcinosarcoma.[26]

Five-year survival of carcinosarcoma is <5%. Surgery is the mainstay of treatment consisting of total hysterectomy with bilateral salpingo-oophorectomy and lymphadenectomy. Radiotherapy has shown to decrease local recurrence and chemotherapy is advocated for recurrent or metastatic disease.

Smooth Muscle Tumors

Leiomyosarcoma

Leiomyosarcoma comprises around 40% of uterine sarcoma and occur in women more than 40 years of age. Most arise de novo from uterine musculature or connective tissue of uterine blood vessels but very rarely can occur due to sarcomatous transformation of leiomyoma. They may mimic leiomyomas clinically, with a history of abnormal vaginal bleeding, pelvic mass and/or pelvic pain. Pathologically, leiomyosarcomas are large, irregular masses with hemorrhage, necrosis, extrauterine extension, and nuclear atypia.

Ultrasound may show a large heterogeneous mass with irregular margins, mixed hypo- and hyperechoic areas with distortion of endometrial cavity. Both leiomyosarcomas and degenerated/cellular leiomyoma can present as nonspecific heterogeneous solitary masses with high vascularity.[28]

On MRI, leiomyomas usually present as well-defined lesions with low-signal intensity on T1- and T2-weighted images, while sarcomas are ill-defined with irregular margins and show intermediate-to-high signal intensity on T2-weighted images. Leiomyosarcomas show presence of extensive necrosis (>50%) with hemorrhage also being common. They show heterogeneous contrast enhancement **(Figs. 14A to G)**. Features suggestive of malignancy are a large mass with rapid growth, irregular margins, and necrosis.[24]

It is important to distinguish leiomyosarcoma from leiomyoma because of difference in treatment. Leiomyomas are treated more conservatively by myomectomy, uterine artery embolization or high-intensity focused ultrasound (HIFU) while sarcomas require surgical treatment.

Diffusion-weighted imaging and ADC maps have been used for differentiating the two, with a mean ADC value

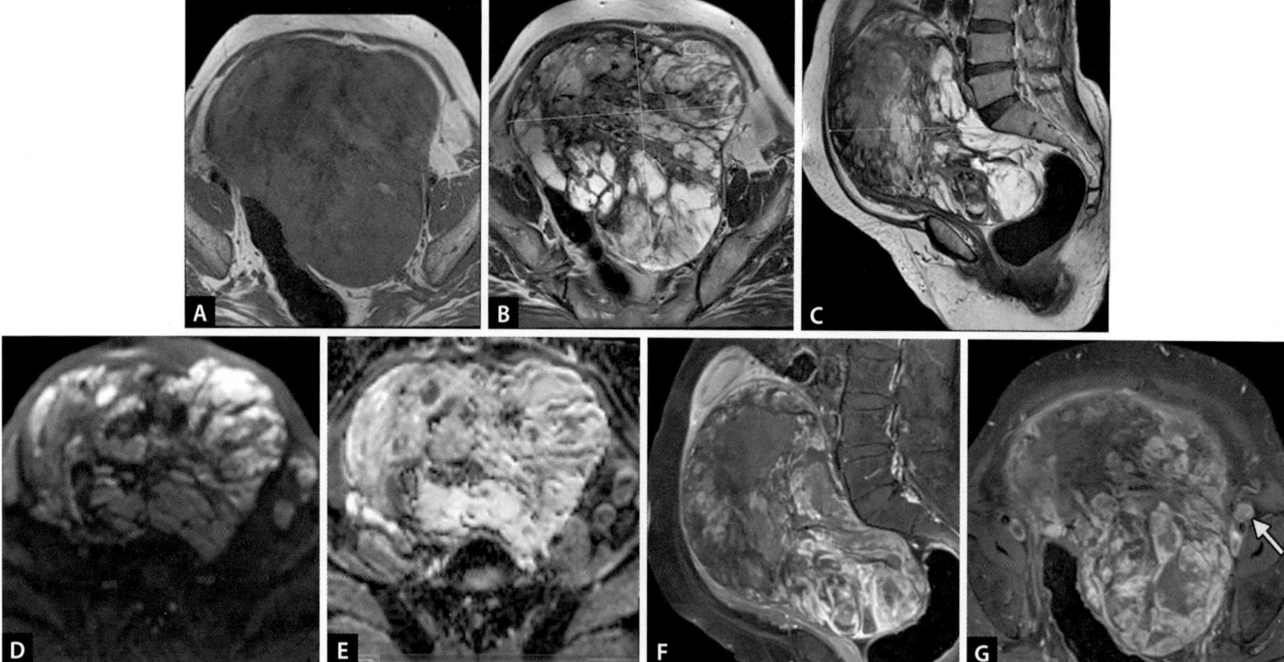

Figs. 14A to G: MRI of the lower abdomen and pelvis reveals (A) a large well-defined smoothly margined predominantly solid abdominopelvic mass which measures 14 × 12 × 14 cm arising from posterior myometrium. It appears hypointense on T1WI (A) and heterogeneous on T2WI (B and C) with a well-defined T2 hypointense capsule. Few foci of restricted diffusion are seen with the mass (D and E) with heterogeneous enhancement on postcontrast scans (F and G). Uterus is stretched along the anterosuperior aspect of the mass with mild fluid in endometrial cavity. The mass is compressing the cervix, vagina, and urinary bladder anteriorly and abutting the lumbar vertebrae posteriorly and rectum posteroinferiorly. An internal iliac lymph node is enlarged (arrow in G): **Uterine leiomyosarcoma**.

of uterine sarcoma being significantly lower than that of leiomyoma (0.83×10^{-3} mm^2/sec vs 1.37×10^{-3} mm^2/sec).[28]

In patients with suspicion of uterine sarcoma on MRI, a PET-CT has been found to be effective. A SUV max >7.5 has shown to exclude leiomyoma with 100% specificity.[29] However, an overlap may occur.

Stromal Tumors

They are classified as endometrial stromal nodule (noninvasive which is benign), endometrial stromal sarcoma (low-grade), and undifferentiated endometrial stromal sarcoma (high-grade).

Endometrial Stromal Sarcoma

They account for 10–15% of all uterine myometrial tumors and affect patients in the 40–55 years age group. Their cells resemble the stromal elements of proliferative endometrium and are characterized by low cellular atypia and a low mitotic rate.[26]

Patients may be asymptomatic or present with abnormal uterine bleeding. There has been reported association of endometrial stromal sarcoma (ESS) with polycystic ovaries, estrogen use, and tamoxifen therapy.

On imaging, ESS appears as a polypoidal endometrial mass which typically shows myometrial involvement, which may be well-defined or diffuse. On MRI, they appear as low signal on T1-weighted images and have heterogeneously increased T2 signal.

These tumors have a tendency for lymphatic and vascular invasion and show mild heterogeneous contrast enhancement. When myometrial invasion is present, worm-like bands of low T2 signal intensity may be seen in the high signal tumor representing preserved normal myometrium. This "bag of worms" appearance is more common in higher grade tumors and is best seen on DWI.[30]

As compared to endometrial cancer, ESS appears larger, with greater enhancement, irregular margins, and marginal nodularity with nodular extension into myometrium. They may rarely present as a myometrial mass and mimic a leiomyoma with cystic degeneration or invasive adenomyosis.

These tumors have a favorable prognosis with metastasis and recurrence occurring late. Five-year survival is around 50–65%. Nodal metastasis is uncommon and does not affect survival. Treatment is by hysterectomy with bilateral salpingo-oophorectomy. Adjuvant hormonal therapy in patients with advanced disease and chemotherapy has also been used.

Undifferentiated Endometrial Sarcoma

They are aggressive tumors, earlier called high-grade ESS. Undifferentiated endometrial sarcomas (UES) occur in an older age group as compared to ESS and are characterized by myometrial invasion, severe nuclear polymorphism, and high mitotic activity.

On imaging, UES appear as a large polypoidal mass in an expanded endometrial cavity. They infiltrate the myometrium in a more destructive manner and are associated with areas of necrosis and hemorrhage resulting in heterogeneous signal intensity on both T1- and T2-weighted images. Due to marked lymphatic and vascular invasion, UES show extensive invasion into the myometrium with marginal irregularity and nodularity, much more frequently than seen in ESS.[30]

Adenosarcoma

Adenosarcomas are rare mixed tumors consisting of a benign epithelial component and a malignant sarcomatous stromal component. They are slow growing with a low malignant potential. Most patients present early (stage 1) with a five-year survival of approximately 80%.

At imaging, adenosarcoma are seen as predominantly endometrial based well-circumscribed, multiseptated, cystic masses with multiple well-defined cystic spaces or clefts, hemorrhage, necrosis, and heterogeneous solid component. The intervening septae give a lattice-like appearance on MRI.[30] This appearance on imaging may resemble that seen in gestational trophoblastic disease.

There is heterogeneous enhancement with septae and solid component showing enhancement similar to myometrium.

Adenosarcoma with sarcomatous overgrowth (ASSO) is said to occur when the sarcomatous component constitutes more than 25% of the tumor. On imaging, there is myometrial invasion with areas of hemorrhage and necrosis. Adenosarcomas with sarcomatous overgrowth have a poorer prognosis than adenosarcoma without sarcomatous overgrowth.[30]

CERVICAL CANCER

Cervical cancer is the second most common cancer in women in India after breast cancer and the fourth most common cancer in women in the world as per the latest data from Global Cancer Statistics 2018. Around 85% of the cases occur in developing countries such as Central and South America, parts of Africa and South

Central Asia.[31] There has been a significant decrease in its incidence in developed countries due to effective screening programs which detect preinvasive disease on cervical smear.

Clinical Presentation

Cervical cancer affects women of reproductive age group, mainly in the 3rd and 4th decades. Noninvasive cancer may not produce any symptoms and may be detected by the Pap smear. Invasive cervical cancer patients typically present with a history of intermenstrual, postcoital bleeding, metrorrhagia, and/or foul swelling vaginal discharge.[32]

Etiopathogenesis

The main etiologic factor for developing cervical cancer is infection of the lower genital tract by the human papillomavirus (HPV) which is sexually transmitted. HPV 16 and 18 account for 70% of cervical cancer worldwide with HPV 16 associated with squamous cell carcinoma. HPV vaccination of adolescents has been approved to prevent persistent infection with HPV, and is recommended by major health organizations around the world with the goal of reducing the incidence of HPV related cervical cancer.[32,33] Other risk factors include low socioeconomic background, early sexual activity, multiple partners, multiparity, immunosuppression, cigarette smoking, and use of oral contraceptive pills.[1]

Histopathology

Squamous cell carcinoma (SCC) accounts for around 85% of cervical cancer and arises from the ectocervix at the squamocolumnar junction. The remaining 15% cervical cancer is of nonsquamous type which arises from the endocervix and includes adenocarcinoma, adenosquamous carcinoma, adenocystic carcinoma, small cell carcinoma, and lymphoma.

Adenoma malignum is a very rare type of cervical adenocarcinoma which has a very poor prognosis though histologically it is well differentiated.[33]

Squamous cell carcinoma of cervix spreads most commonly by direct extension to lower uterine segment and vagina. With advanced disease, the tumor invades paracervical space along the uterosacral and broad ligaments to invade adjacent organs. Lymphatic dissemination to the draining lymph nodes is the next common pattern of spread. Hematogenous spread is rare which can occur to lung, liver, and bone.

Detection and Diagnosis

Early cervical cancer is diagnosed clinically based on results of Pap smear and colposcopic-guided biopsies. Imaging alone is not adequate for the diagnosis of cervical cancer as it cannot differentiate between invasive cancer or its precursor, i.e. intraepithelial neoplasia. Hence, biopsy of suspicious lesions on colposcopy is the gold standard for diagnosis.[34]

Staging

Traditionally, the staging of cervical cancer has been clinical according to the FIGO staging system (2009) and was mainly based on tumor diameter and local extent of tumor. Unlike ovarian and endometrial cancers, it was not based on surgicopathological findings. This was because cervical cancer is more prevalent in developing countries with only clinical methods available for staging and evaluation and limited access to advanced technology. However, clinical staging was found to have several limitations. It was found to be inaccurate in evaluating important prognostic parameters such as precise evaluation of tumor size, depth of stromal invasion, and parametrial or pelvic sidewall invasion. Lymph node assessment which is an important prognostic parameter, was also not a part of FIGO (2009) staging and distant metastasis could not be assessed clinically.

Accurate tumor staging is very important not only for prognosis, but also for guiding appropriate management. Treatment of cervical cancer depends on the stage of disease, therefore, accurate staging is of prime importance.

In order to evaluate the local tumor extent and assess distant spread of disease accurately, the 2009 FIGO staging recommended the use of diagnostic imaging (CT/MRI) where available. The staging of cervical cancer has continued to be clinical but clinicians all over the world started relying more on cross sectional imaging modalities (CT/MRI) to guide treatment planning.

In 2018, the FIGO Gynecologic Oncology Committee revised the 2009 FIGO staging of cervical cancer with incorporation of imaging and pathological findings where available to assign the stage so as to maintain uniformity worldwide. The revised FIGO staging of cancer cervix is given in **Box 3**.[35]

The amendments to the staging of cancer of the cervix uteri were made by the FIGO committee for gynecologic oncology in 2018 and the general recommendations are as follows.

Box 3: FIGO staging of cancer of the cervix uteri (2018).

Stage I:
The carcinoma is limited to the cervix (extension to the uterine body should be ignored)
- *IA:* Invasive carcinoma which can be diagnosed only by microscopy, with maximum depth of invasion <5 mm[a]
  - *IA1:* Measured stromal invasion <3 mm in depth
  - *IA2:* Measured stromal invasion ≥3 mm and <5 mm in depth
- *IB:* Invasive carcinoma with measured deepest invasion ≥5 mm (greater than stage IA), lesion limited to the cervix uteri[b]
  - *IB1:* Invasive carcinoma ≥5 mm depth of stromal invasion and <2 cm in greatest dimension
  - *IB2:* Invasive carcinoma ≥2 cm and <4 cm in greatest dimension
  - *IB3:* Invasive carcinoma ≥4 cm in greatest dimension

Stage II:
The carcinoma invades beyond the uterus, but has not extended onto the lower third of the vagina or to the pelvic wall
- *IIA:* Involvement limited to the upper two-thirds of the vagina without parametrial involvement
  - *IIA1:* Invasive carcinoma <4 cm in greatest dimension
  - *IIA2:* Invasive carcinoma ≥4 cm in greatest dimension
- *IIB:* Parametrial involvement but not up to the pelvic wall

Stage III:
The carcinoma involves the lower third of the vagina and/or extends to the pelvic wall and/or causes hydronephrosis or nonfunctioning kidney and/or involves pelvic and/or para-aortic lymph nodes[c]
- *IIIA:* Carcinoma involves the lower third of the vagina, with no extension to the pelvic wall
- *IIIB:* Extension to the pelvic wall and/or hydronephrosis or nonfunctioning kidney (unless known to be due to another cause)
- *IIIC:* Involvement of pelvic and/or para-aortic lymph nodes, irrespective of tumor size and extent (with r and p notations)[c]
  - *IIIC1:* Pelvic lymph node metastasis only
  - *IIIC2:* Para-aortic lymph node metastasis

Stage IV:
The carcinoma has extended beyond the true pelvis or has involved (biopsy proven) the mucosa of the bladder or rectum
- *IVA:* Spread of the growth to adjacent organs
- *IVB:* Spread to distant organs

[a]Imaging and pathology can be used, when available, to supplement clinical findings with respect to tumor size and extent, in all stages.
[b]The involvement of vascular/lymphatic spaces does not change the staging. The lateral extent of the lesion is no longer considered.
[c]Adding notation of r (imaging) and p (pathology) to indicate the findings that are used to allocate the case to stage IIIC. For example, if imaging indicates pelvic lymph node metastasis, the stage allocation would be stage IIIC1r and, if confirmed by pathological findings, it would be Stage IIIc1p. The type of imaging modality or pathology technique used should always be documented. When in doubt, the lower staging should be assigned.

Source: Bhatla N, Berek JS, Fredes MC, et al. Revised FIGO staging for carcinoma of the cervix uteri. Int J Gynecol Obstet. 2019;143(Suppl 3):43 991.

- It allows the use of any imaging modality (Ultrasound, CT, MRI, PET, PET-CT, PET-MRI, etc.) and pathological findings for the measurement of size of the lesion in all stages and its extent.
- Lymph nodal involvement, previously not a part of FIGO staging has been incorporated into the 2018 staging of cervical cancer. The presence of pelvic or para-aortic lymph nodes on imaging or pathological finding upstages it to stage IIIC, regardless of other findings. A notation of "*r*" or "*p*" is to be given depending on whether the staging was assigned on the basis of imaging or pathology.
- There are no recommendations for routine investigations. They are to be decided on the basis of clinical findings and standard of care.

Imaging

Imaging is not useful for establishing diagnosis, but for staging.

Ultrasound

Ultrasound is not routinely used in assessing the primary tumor or local extent of disease. Advanced cervical cancer can be visualized on transabdominal sonography and appears as an enlarged, irregular hypoechoic mass with resultant hydrometra or hematometra if tumor obstructs the cervical canal.[36] Small masses may be visualized only on TVS **(Figs. 15A to D)**. Ultrasound can show hydronephrosis secondary to the involvement of vesicoureteric junction by the growth. However, its main limitation is that it is unable

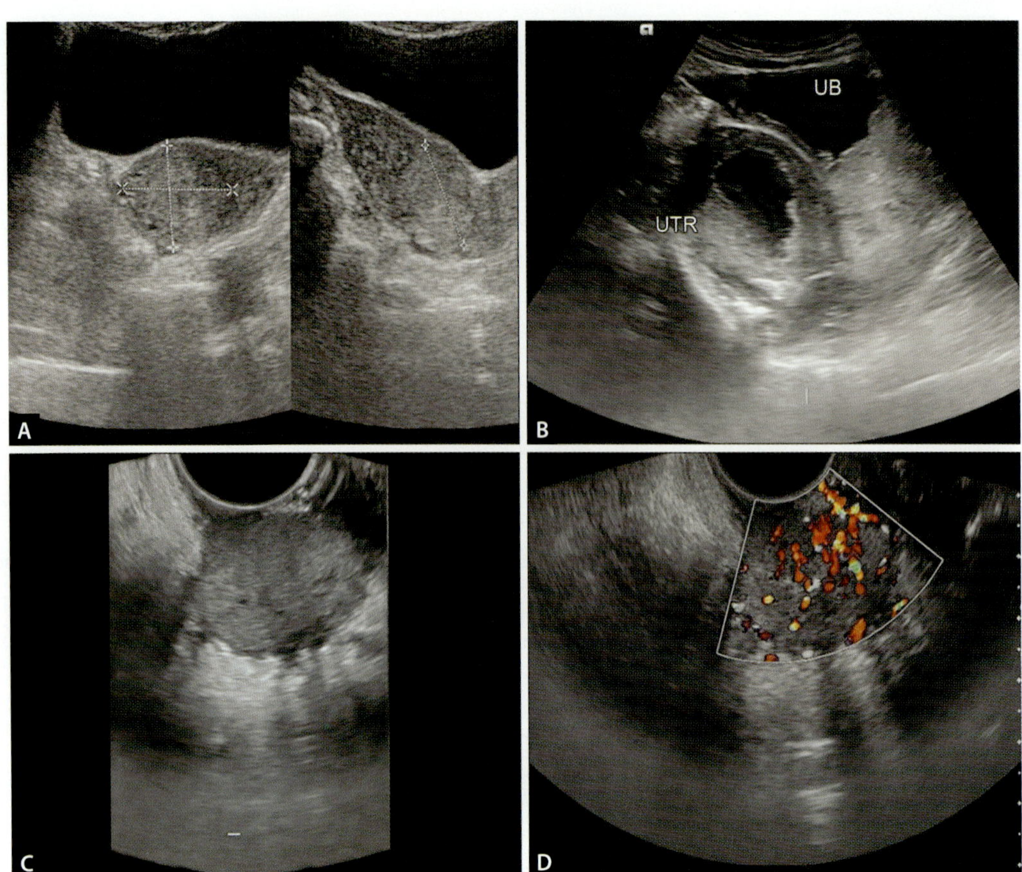

Figs. 15A to D: Transabdominal sonography of the pelvis reveals (A) a solid mass of 3.8 × 4.3 × 4 cm in the cervix extending into the lower uterine segment; (B) Sagittal view of the uterus depicting pyometra secondary to a cervical mass obstructing the internal os. TVS in another patient shows (C) the cervix to be replaced by a large, irregular hypoechoic mass which is (D) highly vascular on color doppler flow imaging.

to detect the invasion of pelvic side walls and metastatic lymph nodes.

Recent studies have reported TVS and TRUS (transrectal ultrasound) as a potentially useful tool for tumor detection and parametrial invasion, comparable to MRI.[37] TRUS has shown to detect bladder invasion based on the intact mobility of bladder over cervix with accuracy greater than that of CT or MRI.[1]

Magnetic Resonance Imaging

MRI is the preferred imaging modality for staging cervical cancer as it can distinguish between early disease that can be surgically treated, from advanced disease that is treated with chemoradiotherapy. MRI accurately depicts the location (exophytic or endocervical) of tumor, the tumor size, depth of stromal invasion, parametrial and pelvic sidewall invasion, bladder or rectal involvement and lymph node metastasis, which are important prognostic parameters that determine whether treatment would be palliative or curative. The role of MR imaging in cervical cancer is well established and given in **Box 4**.

Box 4: Role of MR imaging in cervical cancer.

- Localization and staging the tumor
- Assess feasibility of fertility sparing surgery (trachelectomy)
- Treatment planning
- Identify complications of disease and treatment
- Monitor treatment response
- Detect recurrence

MRI technique: The tumor extent is best assessed on T2-weighted imaging. The sagittal plane depicts the tumor extension into the body of uterus and vagina very well. The axial-oblique T2-weighted FSE (fast spin echo) sequence obtained perpendicular to the long axis of the cervix is valuable in assessing parametrial invasion.[16] DCE-MRI is not routinely recommended as part of protocol for cervical cancer. However, in the guidelines given by the ESUR, contrast administration is indicated for the detection of small tumors, when findings are equivocal on T2-weighted imaging and to differentiate tumor recurrence from post-radiotherapy fibrosis. DWI is useful as it improves tumor detection and characterization and aids in visualization of small peritoneal implants. ADC values are known to precede reduction of tumor size following treatment with neoadjuvant chemotherapy.

MRI Correlation with Revised FIGO (2018) Staging

Localization and staging of tumor: The tumor appears isointense to the normal cervix on T1-weighted images and intermediate-to-high signal intensity mass on T2-weighted images that replaces the low signal intensity cervical stroma. The tumor growth pattern may be exophytic, infiltrative or endocervical. In younger women, the tumor usually arises from the squamocolumnar junction and is exophytic, while in older women, it mostly originates from the endocervical canal and is endophytic. For an accurate size determination, the tumor should be measured in two orthogonal views in all three dimensions. Tumor size is often underestimated at clinical imaging compared with MRI, especially of endocervical lesions. The reported accuracy of MRI for determining tumor size is 93%, within 5 mm of the surgical size.[34]

Tumor size determines the type of treatment, with fertility sparing surgery (trachelectomy) possible in tumors <2 cm size, while in patients with tumors >4 cm, chemoradiation in the treatment even in the absence of parametrial spread.

- *Stage I:* Stage I cervical cancers are confined to the cervix and any extension to the body of the uterus is disregarded as it does not change the tumor stage.
  Stage IA tumors are microinvasive with <5 mm stromal invasion which are diagnosed only by microscopy and not by any imaging modality. MRI is not indicated for their evaluation as these tumors do not show any signal alteration.
  Stage IB tumors are defined as clinically visible tumors which are limited to the cervix. This stage has been revised and subdivided into IB1–IB3 on the basis of tumor size.
  - IB1 is ≥5 mm of invasive and <2 cm in greatest dimension
  - IB2 is ≥2.0 cm and <4.0 cm in greatest dimension
  - IB3 is ≥4.0 cm in greatest dimension.

  The above subdivisions of stage IB have been introduced based on oncologic data from fertility sparing surgery such as conization in stage IA and radical trachelectomy in stage IB.
  Assessment of feasibility of fertility sparing surgery (trachelectomy): MRI helps in assessing the cervical length and distance from the internal os in patients planned for fertility sparing surgery. For undergoing trachelectomy (cervix is removed and uterine body is left intact), the tumor should be <2 cm size, length of cervix should be >2 cm and the distance from the internal os should be >1 cm. Involvement of internal os by the tumor is a contraindication to the treatment.[33]
  The recurrence rates of patients with primary tumors <2.0 cm have been found to be significantly lower than those with tumors between 2.0 cm and 4.0 cm.[35]
- *Stage II:* Stage II tumors extend beyond the cervix into the upper vagina or parametrium but do not extend to the pelvic side walls or lower one-third of vagina. They are further subdivided into stage IIA and IIB according to whether parametrium is spared (IIA) or there is infiltration of tumor into the parametrium (IIB).
  Stage IIA tumors show involvement of upper two-thirds of vagina which on T2-weighted images is seen as a high signal intensity lesion disrupting the low signal intensity vaginal wall **(Figs. 16A and B)**. The maximum tumor diameter has a bearing on the prognosis of patients with stage IIA tumors. Hence, they are subdivided by size into IIAI (<4 cm in greatest dimension) and IIA2 (>4 cm in greatest dimension), both having different treatment strategies.[16,36]
  Stage IIB tumors are not further subdivided by size as presence of parametrial invasion itself is indicative of a poor prognosis as it precludes surgical treatment. On MRI, parametrial invasion is seen as the breech of low signal intensity stromal ring on T2-weighted imaging **(Figs. 17A to D)**. An intact stromal ring of >3 mm on MRI known as "hypointense rim sign" has a negative predictive value of >96% for parametrial invasion. Other reliable signs on MRI which suggest parametrial invasion are irregular or spiculated interface between tumor and parametrium, soft tissue extension into parametrium and uterine ligaments, encasement of parauterine vessels, and distortion of cervix with displacement to the side of parametrial invasion.[1]
  Overestimation in assessment of parametrial invasion on MRI can occur due to post-biopsy stranding or hemorrhage, peripheral stromal edema in large tumors, and endometriosis or bulky intravaginal tumors. In such cases, DWI and ADC maps may help to determine the true extent of tumor.
- *Stage III:* Stage III disease occurs when there is direct extension of the tumor to the lower third of vagina (IIIA) **(Figs. 18A to E)** and /or pelvic side walls (IIIB) **(Figs. 19A to D)** which is very well-depicted on MRI. Pelvic side wall invasion is diagnosed when the tumor is within 3 mm of the obturator internus,

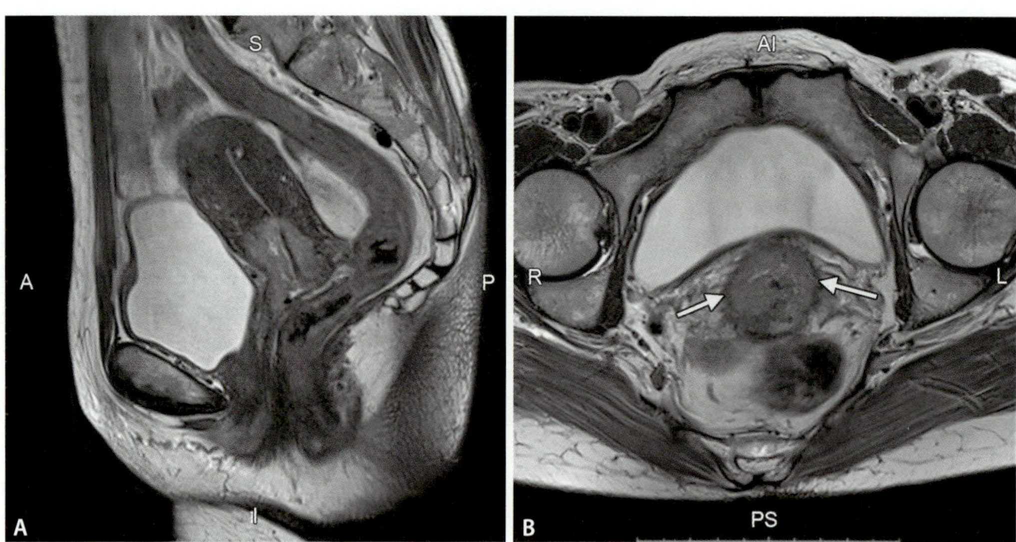

Figs. 16A and B: (A) Sagittal and (B) axial T2W images reveal a well-defined hyperintense mass in the cervix extending into the upper vagina and lower uterine segment. On T2W axial image, the hypointense stromal ring is intact (arrows) indicating that parametrium is spared: **Stage IIA carcinoma cervix**.

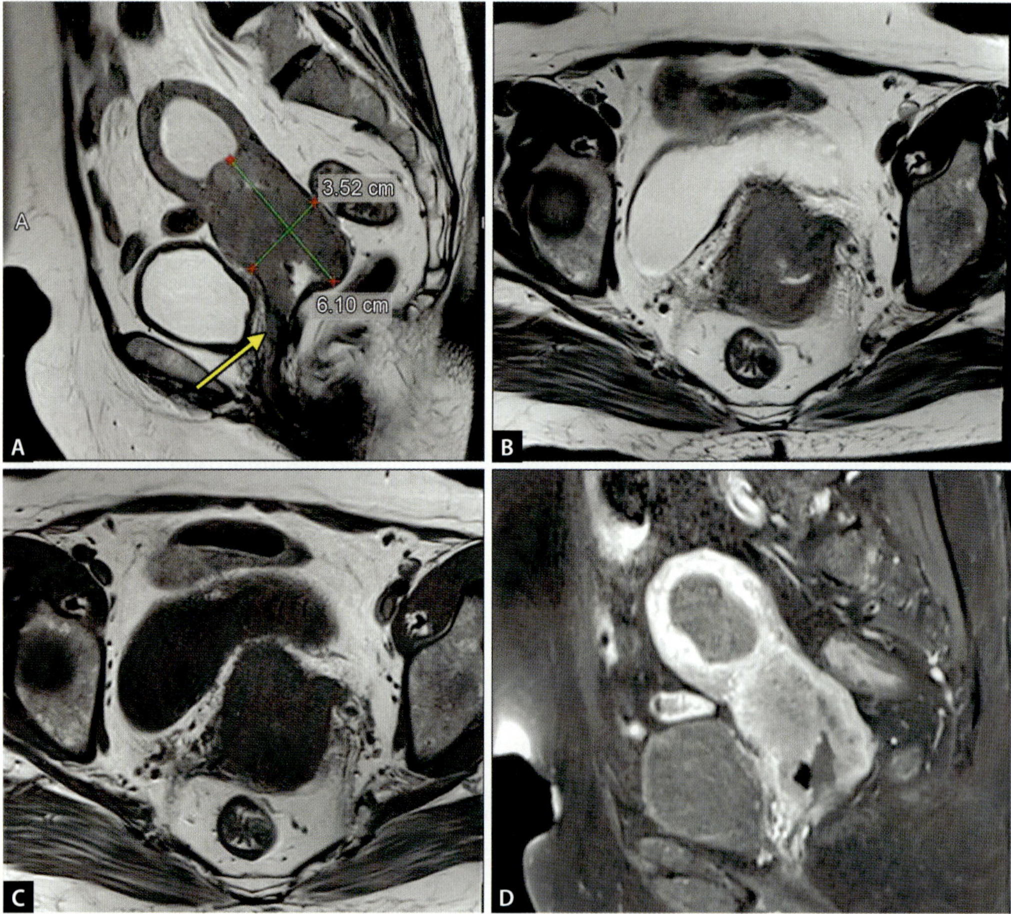

Figs. 17A to D: Stage IIB carcinoma cervix: (A) Sagittal and (B) axial T2W images of the pelvis reveal an infiltrating hyperintense lesion measuring 6.1 cm × 3.5 cm in the cervix extending to the upper vagina (arrow) and bilateral parametrium. The lesion appears (C) hypointense on axial T1W image and shows (D) heterogeneous enhancement and enhancing less than myometrium on postcontrast scan.

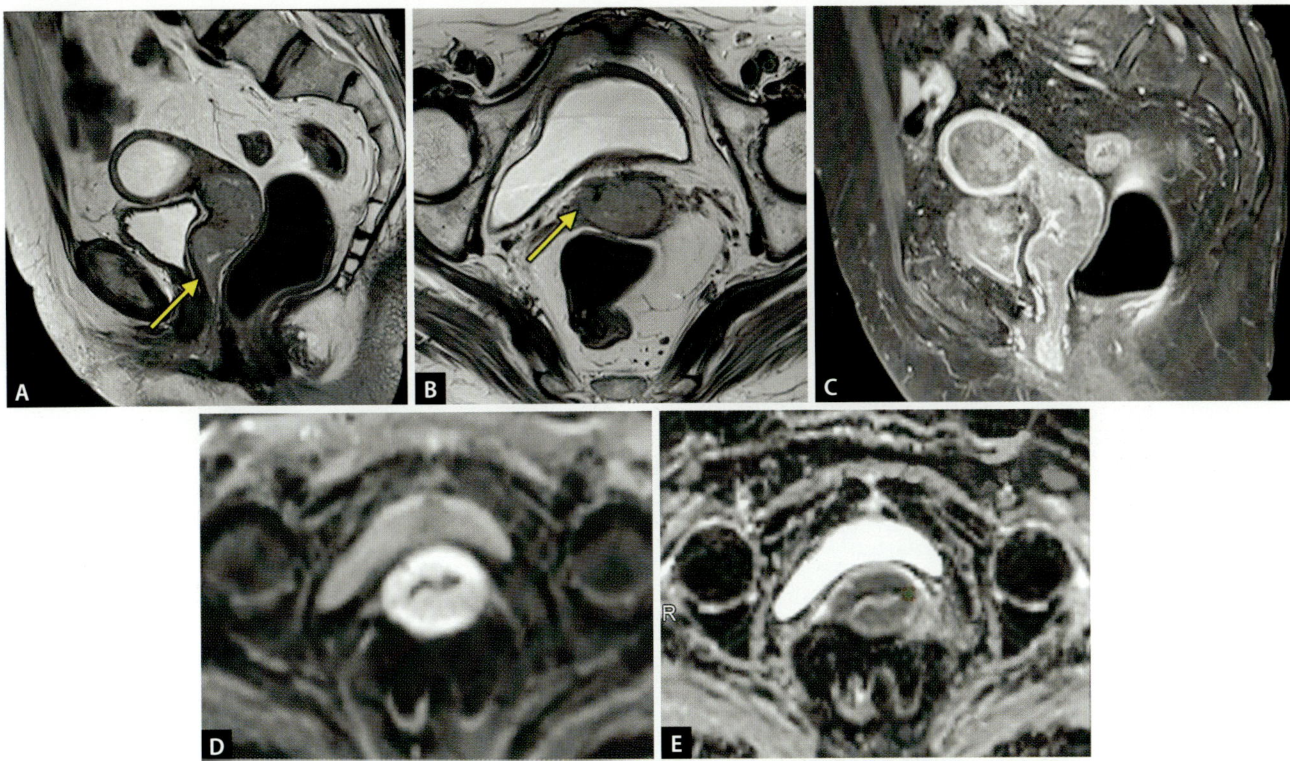

Figs. 18A to E: Multiparametric MR imaging in a 67-year-old presenting with foul smelling discharge and bleeding per vagina reveals (A) a well-defined hyperintense mass lesion involving the cervix and extending up to lower third of vagina (arrow in A) and parametrium (arrow in B) with associated pyometra (A). Postcontrast sagittal image (C) shows heterogeneous contrast enhancement. On diffusion-weighted image (D) and ADC map (E), the lesion shows diffusion restriction with mean ADC value 0.74×10^{-3} mm^2/sec: **Stage IIIA carcinoma cervix** (ADC: apparent diffusion coefficient).

levator ani or piriformis muscle or it encases the iliac vessels. The presence of hydroureteronephrosis due to ureteric encasement by the growth also indicates stage IIIB disease. Hence, MRI should always include a T2-weighted coronal sequence of the upper abdomen for assessment of hydronephrosis.

Stage IIIC disease which consists of lymph nodal involvement is a new subdivision which has been included in the latest revision of FIGO staging of cervical cancer. This is because nodal metastasis is one of the most important prognostic factors in cervical cancer. The five-year survival rates have found to decrease from 85–90% to 30–60% if nodal metastasis is found at surgery.[32] Also, presence of metastatic pelvic nodes at surgery necessitates adjuvant chemoradiation.[33]

The initial lymphatic drainage from the tumor is to the parametrial nodes. From here the lymphatic drainage proceeds to the external iliac group (laterally), internal iliac nodes (inferiorly), and along sacral nodes (posteriorly). Stage IIIC1 disease represents pelvic lymph node metastasis **(Figs. 20A to F)**. From the pelvis, there is an orderly spread to the common iliac and para-aortic nodes. Stage IIIC2 disease is indicative of para-aortic lymph node metastasis. The lymphatic spread in cervical cancer has a more orderly progression as described above, in contrast to endometrial cancer which can show a more complex lymphatic drainage with involvement of para-aortic lymph nodes without any pelvic nodal enlargement.

Metastatic lymph node involvement on MRI is mainly based on size criteria with a short-axis diameter of 10 mm or more being indicative of abnormal nodes. However, this has some limitation as larger lymph nodes may represent reactive hyperplastic nodes and small nodes may harbor microscopic foci of disease. Other imaging features of abnormal nodes suggestive of metastasis are a round shape, irregular margins, and internal heterogeneity. Malignant nodes may show signal intensity similar to the primary tumor. Central nodal necrosis on CT or MRI has been found to have 100% positive predictive value (PPV) for metastasis in cervical cancer **(Figs. 21A and B)**.[33]

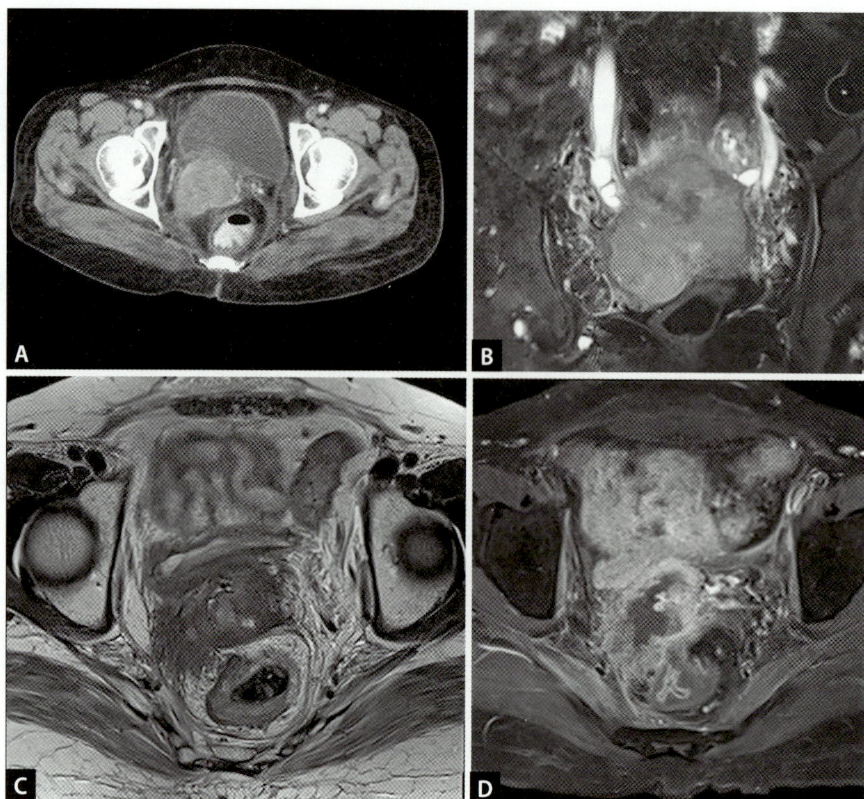

Figs. 19A to D: (A) Contrast-enhanced CT pelvis reveals hyperdense cervical mass extending into the right parametrium and lateral pelvic wall; (B) MRI pelvis shows bilateral hydronephrosis secondary to involvement of bilateral distal ureters; (C and D) Post-chemotherapy axial T2W image (C) depicts iso- to hypointense mass in cervix extending to right parametrium reaching till lateral pelvic wall; (D) On postcontrast axial image, the lesion shows heterogeneous enhancement with large necrotic area within.

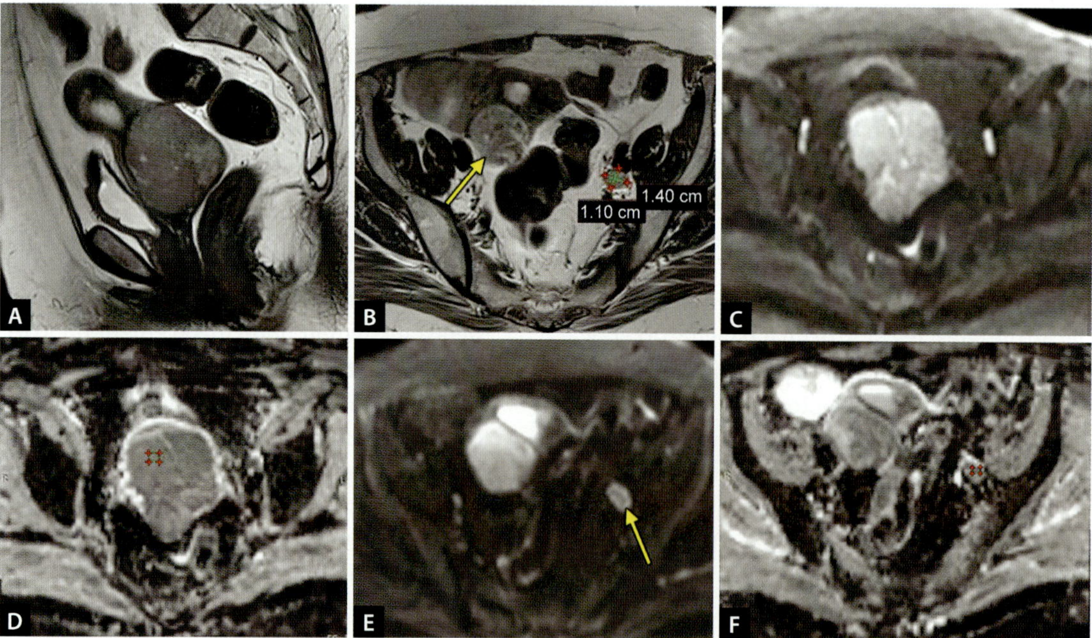

Figs. 20A to F: Carcinoma cervix Stage IIIC: (A) Sagittal T2W image reveals a well-defined hyperintense mass in cervix with (B) T2 axial image depicting an enlarged left external iliac lymph node measuring 1.4 cm × 1.1 cm. Note made of uterine fibroid (arrow). Cervical mass shows diffusion restriction on DWI and ADC map (C and D) with mean value 0.98 × 10^{-3} mm^2/sec; (E and F) Axial DWI and ADC map shows restricted diffusion in the left external iliac lymph node (arrow in E) with mean ADC value of 0.99 × 10^{-3} mm^2/s (ADC: apparent diffusion coefficient; DWI: diffusion-weighted imaging).

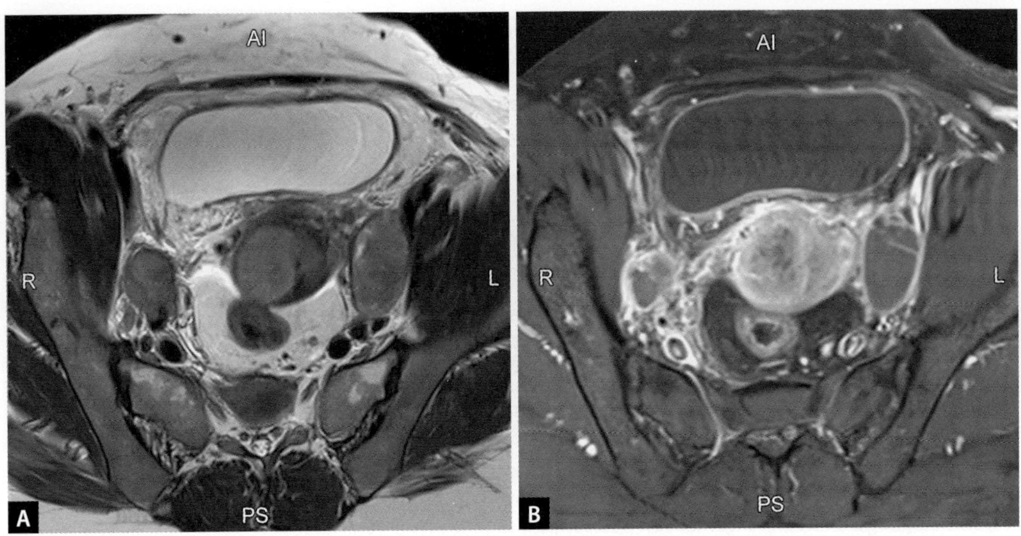

Figs. 21A and B: Squamous cell carcinoma cervix with bilateral internal iliac nodes: (A) Axial T2W and (B) T1FS axial images reveal an intermediate signal intensity cervical mass on T2W imaging with loss of stromal ring on right side. Bilateral low signal intensity internal iliac nodes are seen which show peripheral rim enhancement.

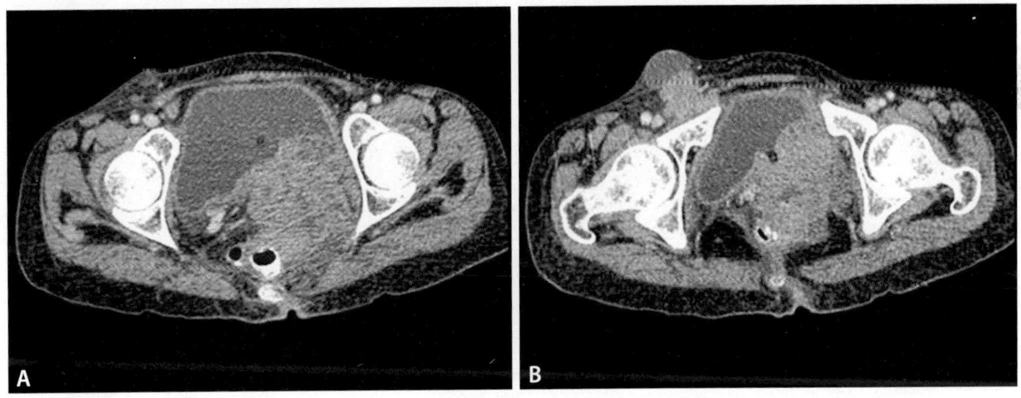

Figs. 22A and B: (A) CT pelvis shows a large irregular enhancing cervical mass infiltrating into urinary bladder with loss of planes with rectum and (B) There is enlargement of right inguinal node suggestive of metastasis: **Stage IVB cervical cancer.**

- *Stage IV:* In stage IVA disease, there is tumor invasion into the urinary bladder or rectal mucosa. MRI findings which suggest bladder invasion are disruption of the normal low signal intensity of posterior wall of bladder, nodular or irregular bladder wall or mass protruding into the lumen of the bladder, best seen on T2-weighted imaging **(Figs. 22A and B)**.[38] Bladder invasion is more common than infiltration of the rectal wall due to the relative "bare area" of bladder posteriorly below the level of peritoneal reflection **(Figs. 23A to C)**.[2]

  Rectal invasion is usually via the uterosacral ligaments. Direct invasion of the cervical tumor into the rectum is uncommon as the pouch of Douglas separates the posterior fornix from the rectum.[25]

  The presence of a fat plane between the cervical tumor and bladder and/or rectum on MRI excludes local invasion into the urinary bladder or rectum with a NPV of 100%.[16,25] Hence, the use of invasive cystoscopic or endoscopic procedures for staging can be eliminated.

  Stage IVB disease signifies distant metastasis. It is seen only in a small percentage of patients and involves spread to lungs, liver, bones, and adrenals by hematogenous route.[33] In patients of early cervical cancer, plain chest radiographs are sufficient for evaluation of any lung involvement, while chest CT should be performed in those with advanced stage of disease to rule out any lung secondaries. The metastasis of squamous cell type of cervical cancer may present as cavitating lung nodules. Bony metastasis in cervical cancer patients is rare with a reported incidence of around 1% **(Figs. 24A to E)**.[34]

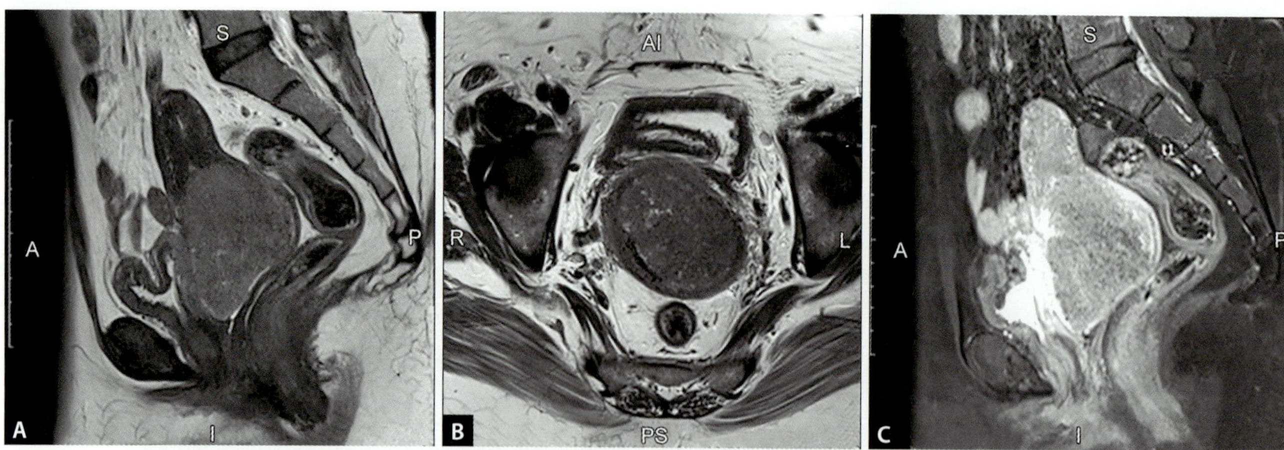

Figs. 23A to C: Carcinoma cervix with infiltration into urinary bladder, Stage IVA: Sagittal (A) and axial (B) T2-weighted images reveal a large well-defined hyperintense mass in the cervix extending into the vagina with parametrial involvement (B) and invasion into posterior wall of urinary bladder (A) with heterogeneous enhancement on postcontrast sagittal image (C).

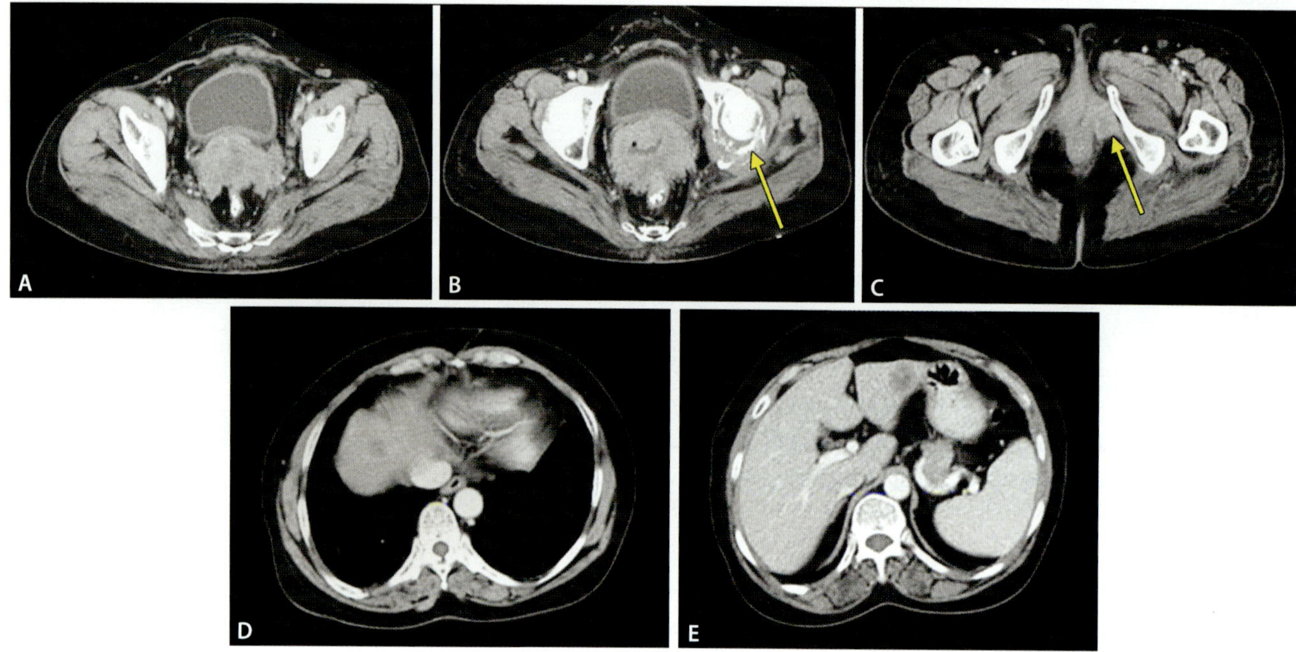

Figs. 24A to E: Contrast-enhanced CT of the abdomen and pelvis in a patient with advanced squamous cell carcinoma of the cervix reveals (A and B) a heterogeneous mass lesion in the cervix infiltrating into bilateral parametrium, with primary tumor showing loss of planes with rectum. A lytic lesion is noted in the left acetabulum (arrow in B). An enhancing soft tissue lesion in the perineum on the left side (arrow in C) suggestive of deposit. Sections through the upper abdomen (D and E) show hypodense lesions in the liver in segment VIII and (D) segment III (E): **Carcinoma cervix with hepatic and bony metastasis**.

Treatment

Treatment of cervical cancer depends on the stage of the disease and is stage-specific. Other factors which have an impact on treatment are age of the patient, patient's desire to have children, and overall health and accessibility to resources. Therapeutic options are available for different stages of cervical cancer as depicted in **Table 8.**[15,39]

Complications of Disease and Treatment

- *Tumor invasion* into pelvic side wall results in involvement of distal ureter and resultant hydronephrosis. Fistulous tract may form due to invasion of advanced tumor into urinary bladder or rectum. The most common fistulas in patients with cervical cancer are vesicovaginal or enterovaginal

Table 8: Management of cervical cancer patients.

Tumour Stage	*Management*
Early cancer FIGO IA1 without LVSI FIGO IA1 with LVSI	Conisation with negative margins Total extrafascial hysterectomy if family is complete Modified radical hysterectomy with pelvic lymphadenectomy. Fertility preserving procedures: • Conization with negative margins with pelvic lymphadenectomy • Radical trachelectomy with pelvic lymphadenectomy
FIGO IA2	Radical hysterectomy with pelvic lymphadenectomy, adjuvant chemoradiotherapy if required. Fertility preserving procedures: • Conization with negative margins with pelvic lymphadenectomy • Radical trachelectomy with pelvic lymphadenectomy
Invasive cancer FIGO IB1, IB2, IIA1	For tumor ≤2 cm: Radical trachelectomy with pelvic lymphadenectomy For tumor 2-4 cm: • Radical hysterectomy with pelvic lymphadenectomy, adjuvant chemoradiotherapy if required • Chemoradiation
Locally advanced cancer FIGO IB3, IIA2, IIB, III, IVA	Primary concurrent chemoradiation: CCRT (CTH + external beam RTH + brachytherapy). Chemotherapy – cisplatin or carboplatin based
FIGO IVB	Incurable – palliative treatment CTH + bevacizumab to improve survival
Recurrent cancer (Central and isolated)	Pelvic exenteration – may be curative
Non central recurrent/metastatic disease	Pelvic exenteration – not curable

(CCRT: concurrent chemoradiation therapy)
Source: Otero-Garcia MM, Mesa-Alvarez A, Nikolic O, et al. Role of MRI in staging and follow-up of endometrial and cervical cancer: pitfalls and mimickers. Insights Imaging. 2019;10:19.

fistulae. MRI precisely delineates the course, extent, and complex nature of fistulae.

- *Radiation fibrosis* is a known complication of radiotherapy to the tumor and can be distinguished from recurrent disease on MR studies by typical low signal of post-radiation fibrotic tissue on T2-weighted sequences. However, this distinction can be challenging, especially within the first 6 months of radiation treatment as high signal intensity due to coexistent inflammation and edema may mimic tumor recurrence. In such instances, functional imaging like DWI, DCE-MRI, and PET/CT can aid in the diagnosis. Tumor recurrence shows restricted diffusion on DWI and early enhancement (45–90 sec) on DCE-MRI, while fibrosis either does not enhance significantly or enhances in the late phase. On DWI, both tumor recurrence and inflammatory changes may appear hypointense at a high "b" value, but only recurrent tumors will have a lower signal intensity on the ADC map.[15]

Treatment Follow-up

Evaluation of Response

In patients with locally advanced cervical cancer who are treated with chemoradiation, MRI is routinely performed during and after completion of treatment to assess tumor response. A decrease in tumor size can be seen as early as 2 months following treatment and predicts a good prognosis. DW-MRI and DCE-MRI also complement the morphological assessment based on tumor size on conventional MRI **(Figs. 25A to C)**.[25]

MR criteria for complete response consists of resolution of cervical mass, a normal low signal intensity of cervical stroma (homogeneously hypointense), and postcontrast scans showing a uniform delayed enhancement of the cervix. All follow-up MRI should be compared with pretreatment images.[33]

Recurrent Cervical Cancer

Recurrent disease is said to occur when the local tumor regrows or distant metastasis develops at least 6 months after the regression of primary tumor. Residual disease is that which is evident within 6 months of the primary treatment.[2]

Cervical cancer recurrence can be either pelvic or nodal. The prevalence varies with stage of disease, histologic type, adequacy of therapy, and host response. Around 70% of cervical cancers are known to recur within 2 years of treatment, while 89–98% recur within 5 years of treatment. Local recurrence involves the cervix or vaginal vault after radical hysterectomy. This is well-depicted on MRI as a lobulated soft tissue mass of moderate-to-high signal intensity on T2-weighted sequences showing

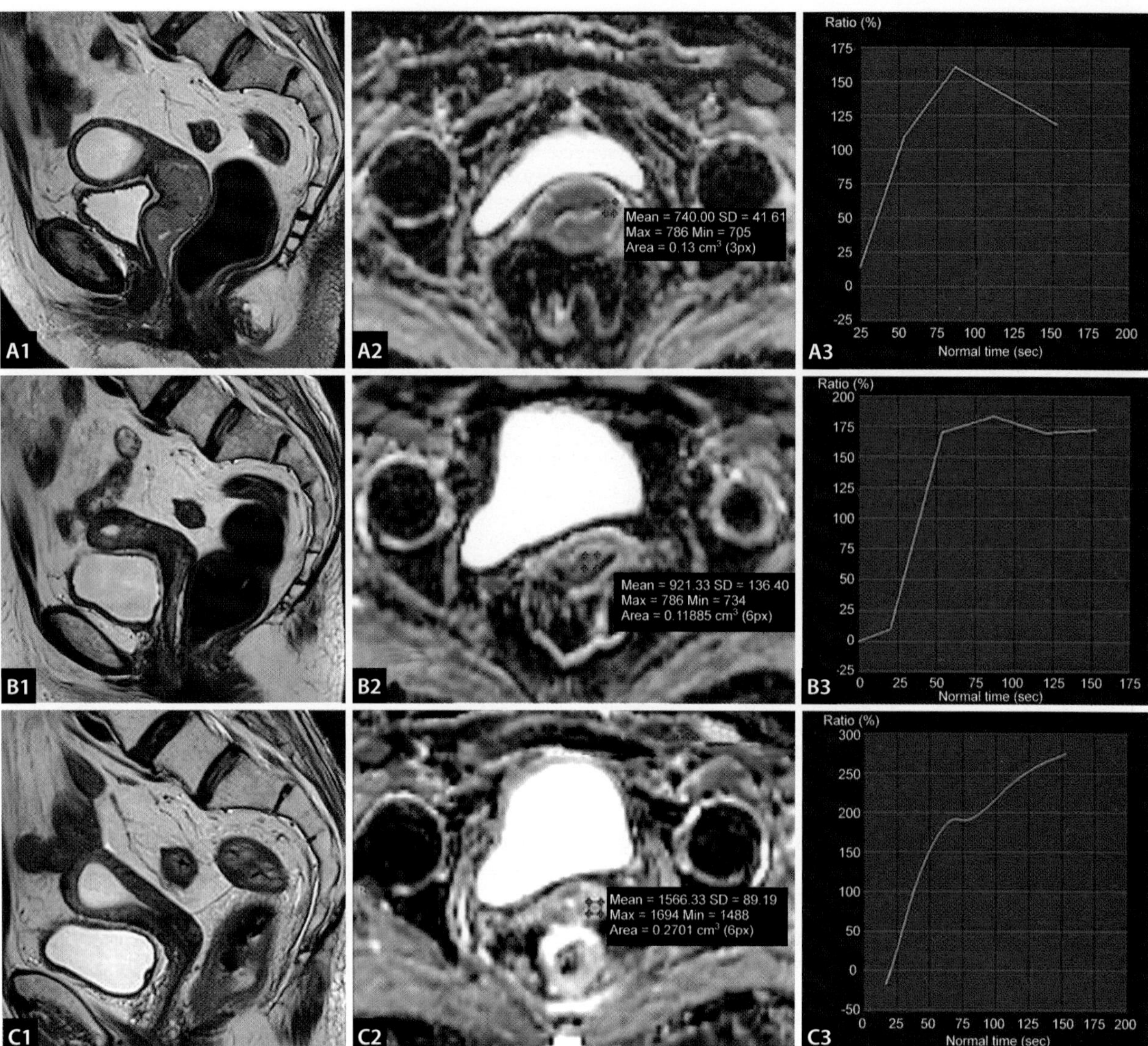

Figs. 25A to C: Multiparametric MRI showing post chemoradiation response: *Baseline MRI (A1 to A3):* T2 sagittal image (A1) of pelvis reveals well-defined hyperintense mass involving cervix extending up to lower one-third of vagina with associated pyometra. The mass shows restricted diffusion (A2) with washout pattern of enhancement (A3).

Post-chemotherapy MRI (B1 to B3): T2 sagittal image (B1) shows reduction in size of the cervical lesion. The lesion shows diffusion restriction on DWI (B2) with increase in mean ADC value to 0.92×10^{-3} mm^2/sec from baseline MRI. Time-intensity curve (TIC) (B3) shows plateau pattern of enhancement.

Post-chemoradiation therapy MRI (C1 to C3): On T2 sagittal image (C1) the cervix appears hypointense with no mass lesion seen and pyometra noted. Diffusion restriction is not seen in the cervical region on DW image (C2) with ADC value of 1.56×10^{-3} mm^2/sec. TIC (C3) depicts progressive enhancement of cervical stroma.

heterogeneous contrast enhancement, often similar to the primary mass **(Figs. 26A to F)**.

When nodal recurrence is seen in cervical cancer, the prognosis is seen to worsen when nodal involvement progresses from paracervical nodes to para-aortic nodes.

In the setting of recurrent disease, PET-CT is valuable for the evaluation of lymphadenopathy and distant metastasis.

Main factors predicting recurrence of cervical cancer are:

- Size >3 cm
- Adenocarcinoma on histology
- LVS1
- Deep stromal invasion.

Computed Tomography

On CT, cervical cancer appears as an enlarged cervix, with areas of low attenuation due to tumor necrosis.

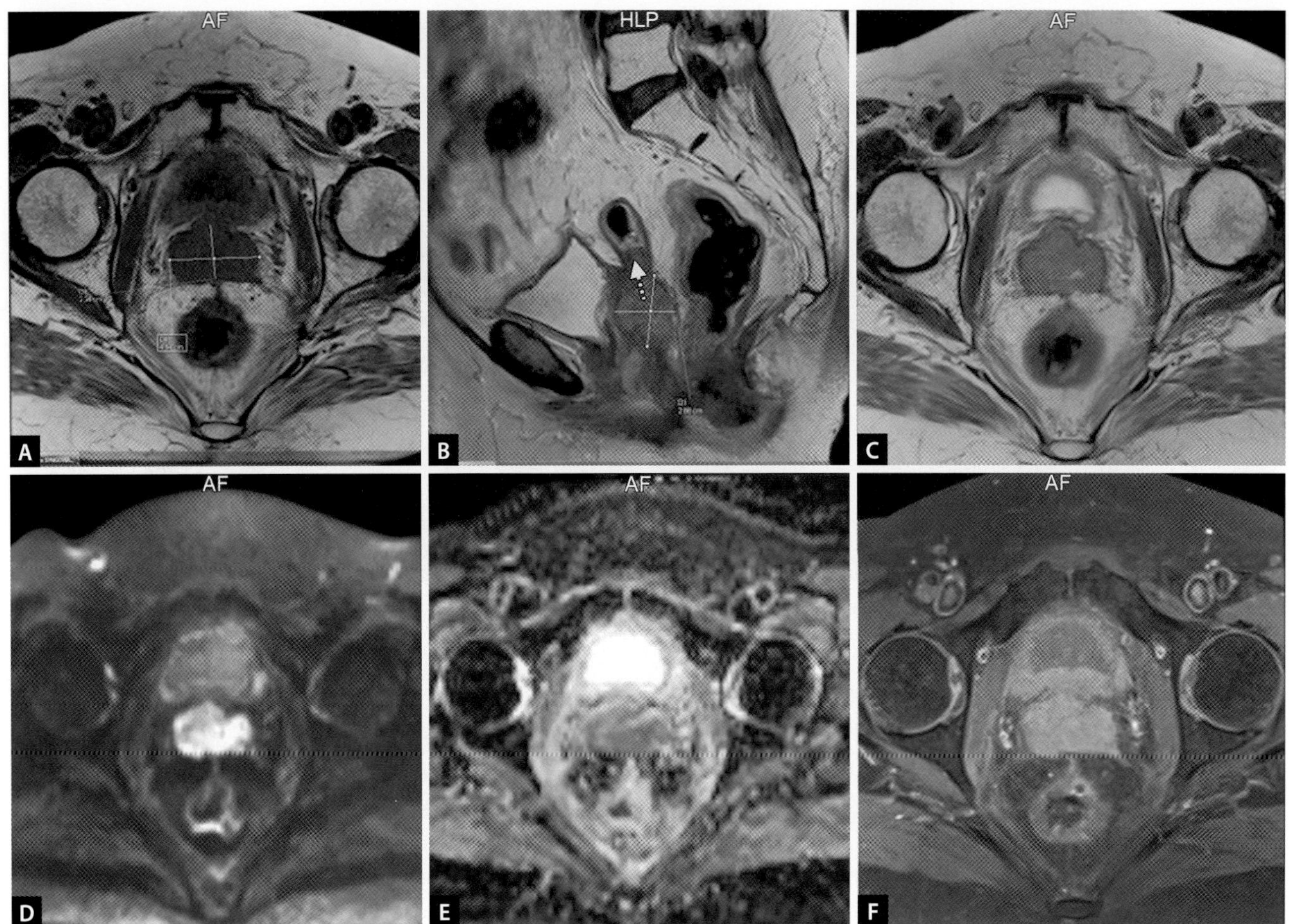

Figs. 26A to F: Vault recurrence in a postoperative patient of carcinoma cervix: (A to C) T1- and T2-weighted axial and sagittal images reveal a homogeneous lobulated mass isointense to muscle on T1WI and mildly hyperintense on T2WI images involving the vaginal vault abutting the urinary bladder anteriorly with loss of fat planes with sigmoid colon superiorly (arrow in B) showing restricted diffusion (D and E) homogeneous contrast enhancement (F).

It may not be easy to distinguish tumor from normal cervix and parametrium and parametrial invasion can be overestimated on CT because of poor soft tissue resolution. Hence, CT is not indicated in assessing local spread. CT is useful in diagnosing hydroureteronephrosis which is indicative of stage III disease or higher **(Figs. 27A and B)**. Presently, staging with CT is advocated where there is clinical evidence of advanced cervical cancer with a reported accuracy of 92% in depicting advanced disease.[26]

Hybrid Imaging (FDG–PET/CT and PET/MRI)

Fluorodeoxyglucose (FDG) PET/CT is a noninvasive tool which has a valuable role in staging, treatment planning, and assessing treatment response in cervical cancer patients. It is not indicated in early stage disease, i.e. FIGO stage IB1 or less.

PET/CT is recommended as a staging investigation in FIGO stage IIB or above disease as it helps in detecting both locoregional disease and distant metastasis in a single examination due to its wider anatomic coverage. Studies have shown FDG uptake on PET/CT to correlate with prognosis. Larger size, higher stage tumors, with parametrial invasion and nodal metastasis are seen to have higher maximum standardized uptake value (SUV). Dual phase imaging performed at 40 minutes and 3 hours after injection of tracer has enabled an increase in the sensitivity in detection of para-aortic lymph nodes from 81.6% to 100% in cervical cancer patients.

PET/MRI has evolved in recent years due to the inherent shortcoming of ionizing radiation and poor soft tissue contrast of PET/CT, especially in head and neck and gynecologic imaging. It is comparable to PET/CT in the evaluation of nodal involvement and distant metastasis and superior to PET/CT in assessment of local extent of tumor.[21]

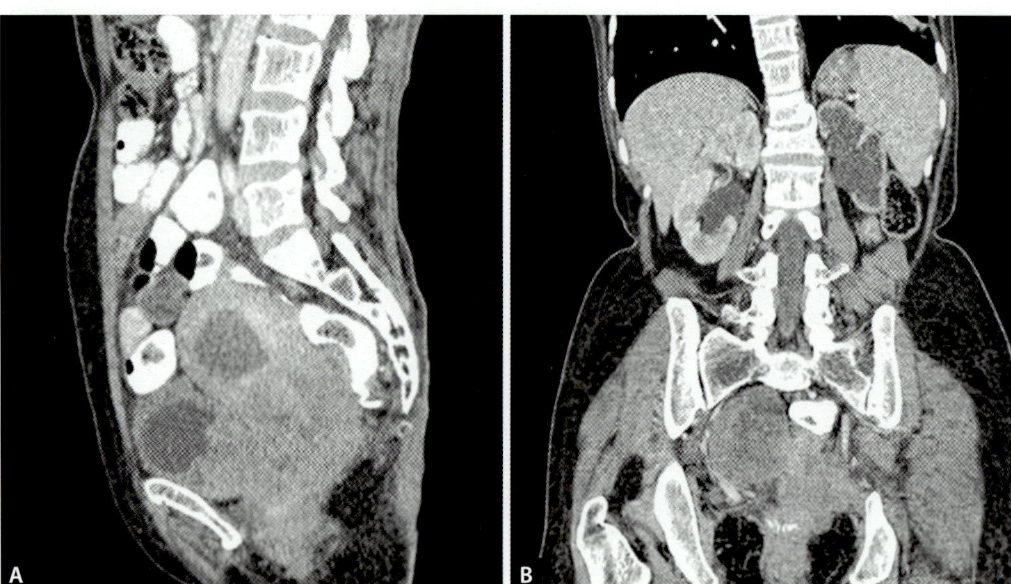

Figs. 27A and B: Sagittal (A) and coronal (B) CT reformations in advanced stage of cervical cancer reveal a large cervical mass infiltrating into the urinary bladder anteriorly (A) with resultant bilateral hydroureteronephrosis.

ENDOMETRIAL VERSUS CERVICAL ORIGIN OF UTERINE CANCER WHEN BIOPSY FINDINGS ARE INCONCLUSIVE OR INDETERMINATE

Endometrial and cervical cancer can be differentiated on the basis of their clinical presentation, location, and histology of biopsy specimen. An accurate distinction between both the malignancies must be made as both of them are treated differently. About 80–90% of endometrial cancer are adenocarcinoma on histology and a similar percentage (80–90%) of cervical cancer are squamous cell cancer on histology. Around 10% of cervical cancers that arise from the endocervix are adenocarcinoma. About 10–60% of endometrial cancers can extend into the cervix and can be misdiagnosed as cervical cancer.[40] There may be difficulty in differentiating an endocervical from an endometrial origin, especially when the histopathology suggests an adenocarcinoma.

Immunohistochemical staining may be helpful in case of unclear/indeterminate findings on conventional histology. Endometrial adenocarcinoma stains positive for ER (estrogen receptor), vimentin, PR (progesterone receptor), and are negative for carcinoembryonic antigen (CEA) or p16. Endocervical adenocarcinoma stains positive for p16 and CEA.[41]

Imaging features which help in differentiating such atypical endometrial cancer from cervical cancer are based on the epicenter of the lesions and different enhancement patterns of endometrial and cervical cancers. MR imaging, with use of T2-weighted and DCE MRI, can help in differentiating primary cervical cancer from primary endometrial cancer on the basis of the epicenter of the tumor and enhancement pattern.

The bulk or epicenter of the tumor in endometrial adenocarcinoma lies in the endometrial cavity, while that of the endocervical adenocarcinoma lies in the cervix. Contrast enhancement pattern of both differ significantly. Endometrial cancers are usually hypovascular and do not enhance in the early phase. While cervical cancers are hypervascular tumors and usually show early phase contrast enhancement compared to surrounding cervical stroma **(Figs. 28A to C)**.

VAGINAL CANCER

Primary vaginal cancer is very rare and accounts for around 2% of all gynecologic malignancies. Histologically, invasive vaginal cancer is mainly of squamous cell type (<95%), followed by adenocarcinoma (<5%) and melanoma (<1%). It more often affects women of 70 years of age or older. The risk factors for developing squamous cell cancer of the vagina are same as that seen in cervical cancer with infection with high-risk human papilloma virus (HR-HPV) being a major risk factor.

WHO defines squamous cell cancer of the vagina as a vaginal cancer without a previous cervical or vulvar cancer in the past 10 years before the present diagnosis. Otherwise

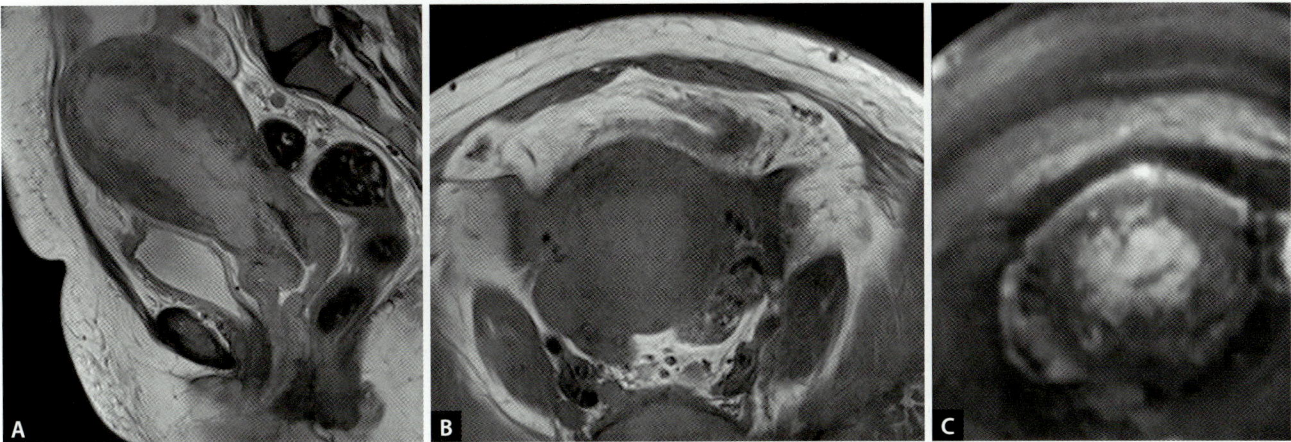

Figs. 28A to C: Sagittal T2W (A) and axial non-FS T1W images (B) reveal extensive intermediate signal intensity mass extending from endometrial cavity to cervix with dynamic postcontrast image revealing (C) hypervascular mass enhancing earlier than the cervical stroma: **Cervical adenocarcinoma** (FS: fat saturated).

the vaginal cancer is considered to be a recurrence of the previously treated cancer.

Staging of vaginal cancer by the FIGO staging system **(Table 9)**.[42]

Staging is determined by the findings at surgery along with histopathological findings of surgical specimen. The regional lymph nodes for the cancer in the upper two-thirds of vagina are the pelvic group of nodes, i.e. obturator, internal iliac, external iliac, while cancer of lower one-third of vagina drains into the inguinofemoral lymph nodes.

The diagnostic workup of a suspicious vaginal lesion should consist of clinical, cytological, and colposcopic examination. Pelvic MRI is the imaging modality of choice for local staging of vaginal cancer of FIGO stage II and beyond. In patients with advanced vaginal cancer or if there is a suspicion of metastasis, a contrast-enhanced CT of the chest and abdomen should be carried out for complete staging.

On MRI, vaginal cancer appears as a mass which appears isointense to muscle on T1-weighted images and intermediate signal intensity on T2-weighted images, distinct from the low signal intensity of the vaginal wall, and shows enhancement on contrast administration.

Surgery is used to treat FIGO stage I tumor. Radiotherapy is the standard treatment for tumors of FIGO stage II to IV for both local and advanced squamous cell and adenocarcinoma of vagina. The five-year survival rate correlates with the tumor stage and histological subtype.

Secondary vaginal cancer accounts for more than 80% of all vaginal cancers and occur most commonly due to direct spread from carcinoma of the cervix, endometrium, ovaries, and rectum.[42]

Table 9: FIGO staging of vaginal cancer.

FIGO	*Tumor spread*
I	Tumor is limited to the vagina and does not involve nearby lymph nodes or distant sites
II	Tumor has infiltrated paravaginal tissue (paracolpium), but has not reached the pelvic wall
III	Tumor extends to pelvic wall
IV	Tumor extends beyond the pelvic wall or involves mucosa of bladder or rectum
IVA	Tumor invades bladder and/or rectal mucosa
IVB	Tumor spread to distant organs

CONCLUSION

Imaging is an essential tool in the workup of uterine malignancies. MRI, especially multiparametric MRI is the mainstay of imaging as it has an invaluable role in accurate tumor localization, evaluation of tumor extent (staging), appropriate treatment planning, and follow-up of disease. Both CT and PET/CT have important roles in advanced cancers by detecting nodal and distant metastatic disease.

It is important for the radiologists to familiarize themselves with the revised staging classification of uterine malignancies, understand the treatment options, and be aware of the diagnostic performance, advantages, and limitations of imaging modalities.

ACKNOWLEDGMENTS

We wish to thank Dr Malavika Gulati and Dr Raghavendra HK for their help; and Mohit and Dr Shivali Arya for the illustrations.

REFERENCES

1. Tirumani SH, Shanbhogue AK, Prasad SR. Current concepts in the diagnosis and management of endometrial and cervical carcinomas. Radiol Clin North Am. 2013;51:1087-110.
2. Patel S, Liyanage SH, Sahdev A, et al. Imaging of endometrial and cervical cancer. Insights Imaging. 2010;1:309-28.
3. Faria SC, Sagebiel T, Balachandran A, et al. Imaging in endometrial carcinoma. Indian J Radiol Imaging. 2015;25(2):137-47.
4. Sohaib SA, Verma H, Attygalle AD, et al. Imaging of uterine malignancies. Semin Ultrasound CT MRI. 2010;31:377-87.
5. Faria SC, Devine CE, Rao B, et al. Imaging and staging of endometrial cancer. Semin Ultrasound CT MRI. 2019;40:287-94.
6. Nougaret S, Lakhman Y, Vargas HA, et al. From staging to prognostication: achievements and challenges of MR imaging in the assessment of endometrial cancer. Magn Reson Imaging Clin N Am. 2017;25:611-33.
7. Yen TT, Wang TL, Fader AN, et al. Molecular classification and emerging targeted therapy in endometrial cancer. Int J Gynecol Pathol. 2019.
8. Salem S. Gynaecology. In: Rumack CM, Wilson SR, Charboneau JW, Levine D (Eds). Diagnostic Ultrasound, 4th edition. Philadelphia: Elsevier/Mosby; 2011. p. 4.
9. Goldstein SR. Sonography in postmenopausal bleeding. J Ultrasound Med. 2012;31:333-6.
10. Rezvani M, Winter TC. Abnormal uterine bleeding: the role of ultrasound. In: Norton ME (Ed). Callen's Ultrasonography in Obstetrics and Gynecology, 6th edition. Philadelphia: Elsevier; 2017. pp. 835-45.
11. Hardesty LA, Sumkin JH, Hakim C, et al. The ability of helical CT to preoperatively stage endometrial carcinoma. Am J Roentgenol. 2001;176:603-6.
12. Rizzo S, Femia M, Radice D, et al. Evaluation of deep myometrial invasion in endometrial cancer patients: is dual energy CT an option? La Radiologica Medica. 2018;123(1):13-9.
13. Beddy P, O'Neill AC, Yamamoto AK, et al. FIGO staging system for endometrial cancer: added benefits of MR imaging. Radiographics. 2012;32:241-54.
14. Rauch M, Kaur H, Choi H, et al. Optimization of MR imaging for pretreatment evaluation of patients with endometrial and cervical cancer. Radiographics. 2014;34(4):1082-2014.
15. Otero-Garcia MM, Mesa-Alvarez A, Nikolic O, et al. Role of MRI in staging and follow-up of endometrial and cervical cancer: pitfalls and mimickers. Insights Imaging. 2019;10:19.
16. Freeman SJ, Aly AM, Kataoka MY, et al. The revised FIGO staging system for uterine malignancies: implications for MR imaging. Radiographics. 2012;32:1805-27.
17. Rechichi G, Galimberti S, Signorelli M, et al. Endometrial cancer: correlation of apparent diffusion coefficient with tumor grade, depth of myometrial invasion, and presence of lymph node metastases. Am J Roentgenol. 2011;197(1): 256-62.
18. Bonatti M, Pedrinolla B, Cybulski AJ, et al. Prediction of histological grade of endometrial cancer by means of MRI. Eur J Radiol. 2018;103:44-50.
19. Bonatti M, Stuefer J, Oberhofer N, et al. MRI for local staging of endometrial carcinoma: is endovenous contrast medium administration still needed? Eur J Radiol. 2015;84(2):208-14.
20. Kurra V, Krajewski KM, Jagannathan J, et al. Typical and atypical metastatic sites of recurrent endometrial carcinoma. Cancer Imaging. 2013;13(1):113-22.
21. Singurkar A, Poon R, Mester U. Comparison of 18F-FDG-PET/CT and 18F-FDG-PET/MR imaging in oncology: a systematic review. Ann Nucl Med. 2017;31(5):366-78.
22. Shoiab SA, Houghton SL, Meroni R, et al. Recurrent endometrial cancer: patterns of recurrent disease and assessment of prognosis. Clin Radiol. 2007;62:28-34.
23. Nougaret S, Horta M, Sala E, et al. Endometrial cancer MRI staging: updated guidelines of the European Society of Urogenital Radiology. Eur Radiol. 2019;29(2):792-805.
24. Santos P, Cunha TM. Uterine sarcomas: clinical presentation and MRI features. Diagn Interv Radiol. 2015;21:4-9.
25. Sala E, Rockall AG, Freeman SJ, et al. The added role of MR imaging in treatment stratification of patients with gynecologic malignancies: what the radiologist needs to know. Radiology. 2013;266:717-40.
26. Shah SH, Jagannathan JP, Krajewski K, et al. Uterine sarcomas: then and now. Am J Roentgenol. 2012;199:213-23.
27. Sagebiel TL, Bhosale PR, Patnana M, et al. Uterine carcinosarcomas. Semin Ultrasound CT MRI. 2019;40(4): 295-301.
28. Valdes-Devesa V, Jimenez MD, Sanz-Rosa D, et al. Preoperative diagnosis of atypical pelvic leiomyoma and sarcoma: the potential role of diffusion-weighted imaging. J Obstet Gynaecol. 2019;39(1):98-104.
29. Kusunoki S, Terao Y, Ujihira T, et al. Efficacy of PET/CT to exclude leiomyoma in patients with lesions suspicious of uterine sarcoma on MRI. Taiwan J Obstet Gynecol. 2017;56:508-13.
30. Tirumani SH, Ojili V, Shanbhogue AK, et al. Current concepts in the imaging of uterine sarcoma. Abdom Imaging. 2013;38(2):397-411.
31. Bray F, Ferlay J, Soerjomataram I, et al. Global cancer statistics 2018: GLOBOCAN estimates of cancer incidence and mortality for 36 cancers in 185 countries. CA Cancer J Clin. 2018;68:394-424.
32. Bhosale P, Devine C, Gardner CS, et al. Role of magnetic resonance imaging in the evaluation of gynecologic disorders. In: Norton ME (Ed). Callen's Ultrasonography in Obstetrics and Gynecology. Philadelphia: Elsevier; 2017. pp. 1045-75.
33. Devine C, Viswanathan C, Faria S, et al. Imaging and staging of cervical cancer. Semin Ultrasound CT MRI. 2019;40(4):280-6.
34. Bourgioti C, Chatoupis K, Moulopoulos LA. Current imaging strategies for the evaluation of uterine cervical cancer. World J Radiol. 2016;8(4):342-54.
35. Bhatla N, Berek JS, Fredes MC, et al. Revised FIGO staging for carcinoma of the cervix uteri. Int J Gynecol Obstet. 2019;143(Suppl 3):43-991.
36. Sala E, Freeman S, Ascher SM, et al. Gynecological cancer. In: Adam A, Dixon A, Gillard J, Schaefer-Prokop C, Grainger R (Eds). Grainger and Allison's Diagnostic Radiology, 6th edition. London: Churchill Livingstone; 2015. pp. 957-71.
37. Moloney F, Ryan D, Twomey M, et al. Comparison of MRI and high-resolution transvaginal sonography for the local staging of cervical cancer. J Clin Ultrasound. 2016;44(2):78-84.

38. Nicolet V, Carignan L, Bordon F, et al. MR imaging of cervical carcinoma: a practical staging approach. Radiographics. 2000;20(6):1539-49.
39. Tewari KS, Agarwal A, Pathak A, et al. Meeting report, "First Indian national conference on cervical cancer management - expert recommendations and identification of barriers to implementation". Gynecol Oncol Res Pract. 2018;5:5.
40. He H, Bhosale P, Wei W, et al. MRI is highly specific in determining primary cervical versus endometrial cancer when biopsy results are inconclusive. Clin Radiol. 2013;68:1107-13.
41. Bourgioti C, Chatoupis K, Panourgias E, et al. Endometrial vs. cervical cancer: development and pilot testing of a magnetic resonance imaging (MRI) scoring system for predicting tumor origin of uterine carcinomas of indeterminate histology. Abdom Imaging. 2015;40(7):2529-40.
42. Schnürch H, Ackermann S, Alt-Radtke CD, et al. Diagnosis, therapy and follow-up of vaginal cancer and its precursors. Guideline of the DGGG and the DKG (S2k-Level, AWMF Registry No. 032/042, October 2018). Geburtshilfe Frauenheilkd. 2019;79(10):1060-78.

Chapter 18

Female Infertility

Radhika Batra, Rashmi Dixit, Swati Gupta

INTRODUCTION

Infertility is defined as inability to achieve pregnancy after 12 months of regular unprotected intercourse.[1] Couples are evaluated together and in around 80% of the cases the etiology is identified. A male factor is ascribed in 40% of the cases and the rest 40% cases are ascribed to the female factor. Approximately 25% couples have more than one etiology.[2]

Workup for infertility in women less than 35 years of age is indicated after 1 year of regular unprotected sexual intercourse and if the woman is more than 35 years of age, it is indicated after 6 months of unprotected intercourse.[1] The work-up may commence earlier in women with irregular menstrual cycles, endometriosis, pelvic inflammatory disease (PID), reproductive tract malformations, and prior history of multiple miscarriages. Evaluation of female infertility has greatly progressed in the last few decades with imaging playing an important role. The various causes of female infertility are listed in **Table 1**.

Table 1: Causes of female infertility.

Cervical factors	• Abnormal cervical mucus • Cervical stenosis • Cervicitis
Uterine factors	• Leiomyomas • Developmental anomalies • Adhesions • Infections • Tumors
Peritoneal factors	Adhesions due to infection, endometriosis or surgery
Tubal factors	• Tubal occlusion • Peritubal adhesions • Salpingitis isthmica nodosa
Ovarian factors	• Polycystic ovary syndrome • Hypothalamic amenorrhea • Luteinized unruptured follicle • Ovarian tumors or infections
Endocrine factors	• Panhypopituitarism • Hypothyroidism • Adrenal insufficiency
Others	• Idiopathic • Drugs • Radiation

RISK FACTORS FOR INFERTILITY

These include age, women's fertility rapidly drops after the age of 37 years and this is due to lower number and quality of eggs. Other factors include tobacco and alcohol use, being overweight or underweight and lack of or very strenuous exercise.

INITIAL APPROACH

It is essential to evaluate both the partners for possible causes of infertility. A thorough diagnostic evaluation should be performed to detect the underlying cause. The infertility specialist uses this information to assess the etiology and subsequently offer a treatment plan.

History

The detailed history includes the duration of infertility alongwith any results of any previous evaluation and therapy, and duration and characteristics of menstrual cycle. It is important to note any medical, surgical or gynecological history. Other aspects include previous obstetrical history, family history, and personal and lifestyle history.

Physical Examination

Patient's body mass index (BMI) should be calculated. The body habitus and secondary sexual characters are assessed. Abnormalities of thyroid gland, galactorrhea or signs of androgen excess suggest the presence of an endocrinopathy. Pelvic examination may reveal tenderness or mass in pouch of Douglas, palpable tender nodules in the cul-de-sac and uterosacral ligaments, uterine enlargement, and irregularity in leiomyoma or uterine anomaly.

Imaging Modalities

Imaging modalities used in evaluation of female infertility include the following:

- Hysterosalpingography (HSG)
- Sonography including transvaginal sonography (TVS) and sonohysterosalpingography.
- Magnetic resonance imaging (MRI).

Hysterosalpingography

Hysterosalpingography is performed during the first 6–10 days of menstrual cycle and is best performed during the second to fifth day interval just after the cessation of menstruation. This minimizes the risk of infection and avoids interference from intrauterine blood clot. It also prevents the possibility of HSG being done in a conception cycle that has not been recognized. HSG does not require any specific preparation, although pretreatment with a nonsteroidal anti-inflammatory drug (NSAID) (approximately 30 minutes before) is helpful to limit discomfort associated with the procedure. HSG is best avoided altogether for at least several weeks following any episode of acute PID to minimize risk of infectious complications. Administration of intravenous buscopan (after ruling out contraindications to buscopan such as myasthenia gravis, mechanical stenosis in gastrointestinal tract, megacolon, and prior known hypersensitivity to drug) prior to HSG is effective in relieving tubal spasm and reduces the incidence of false positive tubal occlusion due to tubal spasm.

The basic technique for performing HSG is quite standard. The study should be performed using image intensification fluoroscopy with a limited number of radiographs. The average HSG requires only 20–30 seconds of fluoroscopic time with minimal radiation exposure and has very low risk. Usually, only 3–4 basic films are required—a scout, one film during early filling, third film to document the uterine contours with the uterus fully distended and assess tubal patency, and a fourth film to detect-free intraperitoneal spill not seen earlier or any areas of contrast loculation **(Figs. 1 and 2)**. Additional films may be required when the uterus obscures the tubes or the uterine cavity appears abnormal.[3]

Contrast can be introduced using a common metal "acorn" cannula or via a balloon catheter. In general, the latter technique is preferred as it requires less fluoroscopic time and smaller volumes of contrast, produces less pain, and is easier to perform. Slow injection of contrast (typically 3–10 mL) helps to minimize the discomfort associated with HSG.[4] Water-soluble contrast media are generally used. Oil-based contrast media have also been used in the past but these are generally too viscous to reveal internal tubal architecture and disperse poorly in pelvis, so adnexal adhesions cannot be detected. They are also associated with significant risk of granulomatous reaction, venous intravasation, and embolism and are generally not used.

Complications following HSG are relatively rare but may include light spotting, infection, and pain. The light spotting usually lasts less than 24 hours after the procedure. Rarely systemic reactions to contrast media and uterine or fallopian tube perforation have been reported.[3]

Hysterosalpingography is the standard of care to look for tubal occlusion in all patients, unless laparoscopy is planned. Diagnostic laparoscopy and chromotubation are performed in women with suspicion of endometriosis

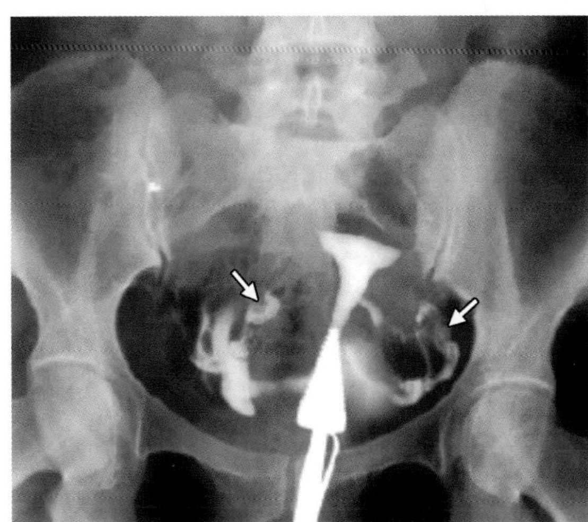

Fig. 1: Normal hysterosalpingography showing an inverted triangle-shaped smooth uterine outline. Both fallopian tubes are well outlined by contrast. Note the presence of longitudinal rugal folds in the ampullary portion (arrows). Free intraperitoneal spill is seen on both sides outlining the bowel loops.

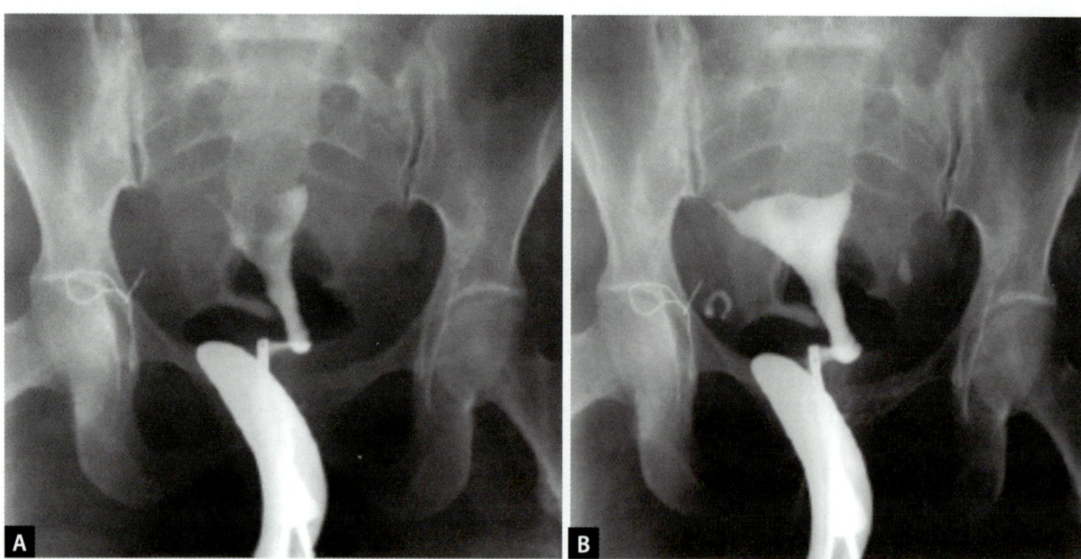

Figs. 2A and B: Uterine filling defect due to a fundal fibroid is much better appreciated on the early filling film (A) as compared with (B) where the uterine cavity is fully distended with contrast and the filling defect is much less apparent.

or pelvic adhesions as HSG is not useful for detecting peritubal adhesions or endometriosis.

Transvaginal Sonography

Ultrasonography (USG) allows morphological characterization of the uterus and ovaries. TVS can be performed for assessing uterine contour, endometrial and myometrial abnormalities, and ovaries. While evaluating patients for infertility by TVS, especially for follicular monitoring or oocyte retrieval, normal condoms with spermicidal gels should be avoided.[5] Even ultrasound gels may have a detrimental effect on sperm and embryo and should not be used during oocyte retrieval or embryo transfers (ETs).[6]

Saline Infusion Sonohysterography

Saline infusion sonohysterography (SIS) is a technique that enables improved depiction of the endometrial lining and intrauterine cavity. Saline is instilled within the endometrial cavity under sonographic guidance and improves detection of intrauterine cavity defects. It is a sensitive technique to detect uterine synechiae, endometrial polyps and can also be used to evaluate for tubal patency. This technique allows differentiation between intrauterine, endometrial, and submucosal abnormalities without the use of contrast agents or ionizing radiation. It can be done to look for tubal patency by visualizing the passage of fluid or contrast through the tubes or presence of fluid in the cul-de-sac.[7]

Hysterosalpingo Contrast Sonography (HyCoSy)

This procedure utilizes hyperechoic contrast agents for visualization of contrast flow through the fallopian tubes. Echovist 200 has been used as a contrast agent for this technique. One of its limitations includes rapid degeneration. However, Echovist is not Food and Drug Administration approved. Another alternative used as distending media is a mixture of saline and air. "Scintillations" are rendered possible by the positive pressure flow of echogenic contrast from the uterine cavity and into the pelvis through patent fallopian tubes. Tubal patency is then distinguished by visual intratubal flow of echogenic contrast using ultrasound scanning for at least 5–10 seconds duration or flow extending from the distal end of a tube and over the adjacent ovary.[7]

Magnetic Resonance Imaging

Magnetic resonance imaging is usually performed for indeterminate cases and it provides detailed assessment of pelvic soft tissues. MRI also plays an important role in presurgical planning.

THE NORMAL MENSTRUAL CYCLE

A basic understanding of the normal menstrual cycle is important before trying to image female infertility. There are three major stages, namely the follicular/proliferative phase, the ovulation phase, and the luteal phase.

The menstrual cycle is under the control of the hypothalamic-pituitary-ovarian axis. It consists of an average 28-day cycle. Day 1 of this average 28-day cycle is the start of menstruation. In the follicular phase, the follicle-stimulating hormone (FSH) level begins to increase. This in turn stimulates the growth of the ovarian follicles. One of the follicles becomes the dominant or Graafian follicle. The developing follicles secrete estradiol, leading to endometrial proliferation. The peak of estradiol occurs 12 hours before the luteinizing hormone (LH) ovulatory surge. The estradiol peak results in an increase in the levels of LH/FSH that leads to ovulation on or around the 14th day of the cycle.

The luteal phase, also known as the secretory phase, starts after ovulation. During this phase, the ruptured Graafian follicle becomes the corpus luteum (CL). Progesterone is produced by the CL. The endometrium is primed by progesterone for the fertilized egg. The CL degenerates if conception does not occur, resulting in a decrease in estradiol/progesterone levels and shedding of the endometrial lining (menstruation).[8]

CERVICAL FACTOR

The cervical factor infertility pertains to the properties of cervical mucus and sperm transport. Imaging cannot evaluate the hospitality of the cervix to the sperm and the patient can be assessed with a postcoital test. The timing and the methodology of performing the postcoital test is a controversial topic. Most of the recommendations state doing the postcoital test as close to ovulation as possible and after at least 8 hours of intercourse.[8,9] There is limited role of imaging in this assessment. Imaging might help in monitoring of follicle development, thereby helping in optimization of the timing of the test.[1] Its utility and predictive value has seriously been questioned over the years, but it is still considered to be a useful diagnostic test by some.[10,11]

Cervical Stenosis

Cervical stenosis is clinically defined as cervical narrowing that inhibits the insertion of a 2.5 mm wide dilator.[12] Causes of cervical stenosis may be congenital or consequent to infection or trauma. Cervical stenosis leads to obstruction of menstrual flow causing amenorrhea, dysmenorrhea, and potential infertility as the sperm is unable to enter the upper genital tract. Cervical stenosis also hinders the various techniques used in the treatment of infertility including intrauterine insemination and ET.

During HSG, cervical stenosis may be seen as narrowing of the endocervical canal (normal diameter is 0.5–3 mm) or there may be complete obliteration of the cervical os with inability to insert the HSG catheter. Cervical stenosis can cause hematometra, which can be seen as a fluid-filled endometrial cavity on USG. Fluid-fluid levels may be seen within, secondary to sedimentation of red blood cells. Additional imaging with MRI may also be performed if required. Gradual dilatation of the cervix, performed with ultrasound guidance, is an effective treatment for the problem.[13] Conditions such as cervical polyps, fibroids, and neoplasms also cause narrowing of the cervical lumen.

UTERINE FACTOR

Uterine and endometrial abnormalities account for less than 10% of cases of infertility.[8,9,14] Although a relatively uncommon cause of infertility, they should be considered as they can adversely affect the outcome of pregnancies achieved by treatment of other common factors.

The abnormalities can be anatomic or physiological. The anatomic factors include uterine adhesions, leiomyomas or fibroids, and congenital uterine malformations. The physiological factors include lack of normal endometrial response to hormonal stimulation.

There are four basic methods for the assessment of the uterine cavity: HSG, standard TVS, TVS with saline contrast (sonohysterography), MRI, and hysteroscopy. The choice of the investigation needs to be assessed according to the individual patient. HSG is the traditional method and still the best initial method because it also evaluates tubal patency. However, in women with no risk for tubal disease and whose tubal status is already known (say from previous laparoscopic surgery for some other cause), TVS offers a better tolerated and simpler alternative that can also reveal suspected ovarian pathology (cyst/endometrioma) with no radiation exposure. When uterine cavity detail is critical or when congenital anomalies are suspected, sonohysterography or MRI may be used. Hysteroscopy is the most definitive method but may be safely reserved for treatment of abnormalities identified by other less invasive methods.[4]

Endometrial Adhesions or Synechiae

The adhesions or synechiae may cause infertility by two mechanisms. Firstly, they may obstruct the cervical os or fallopian tube. Secondly, the environment provided for implantation of the embryo may be suboptimal. Synechiae usually form as sequelae of infection including tuberculosis or previous history of dilatation and curettage. The association of synechiae with hypomenorrhea or amenorrhea and infertility is known as Asherman's syndrome.

The imaging modality of choice in the evaluation of synechiae is HSG. On HSG, they appear as multiple irregular filling defects in the uterine cavity.[8] They are usually linear and irregular, extending from one uterine wall to the opposite side. They allow the contrast agent to flow around them in one dimension only. Thus, these can be easily differentiated from polyps, myomas or other masses that usually allow contrast agent to flow around them in two dimensions.[15] Adhesions at the margins of the cavity may cause distortion of the uterine outline or obscure cornua **(Fig. 3)**.[4] Adhesions are tough to visualize on TVS, but when visualized, they are seen as echogenic bridges in the endometrial cavity or as irregularities of the endometrium that are surrounded by cystic spaces.[8,14] In contrast, synechiae are easier to identify on sonohysterography, appearing as linear echogenic bridges in the fluid-filled endometrial cavity.

Leiomyoma

Leiomyoma (fibroid or myoma) is the most common neoplasm of the uterus found in up to 20–40% of women in the reproductive age group, they can be single or multiple.[16] Leiomyomas may be found in submucosal, intramural, and subserosal locations. Leiomyomas should only be considered as a primary reason of infertility after ruling out other possible causes. Pregnancy and implantation rates are significantly lower in women with submucosal myomas but not in patients with subserosal or intramural myomas that do not encroach or clearly distort the endometrial cavity, especially when modest in size (5–7 cm) **(Fig. 4)**. Suggested mechanisms by which myomas can adversely affect fertility include cornual occlusion by

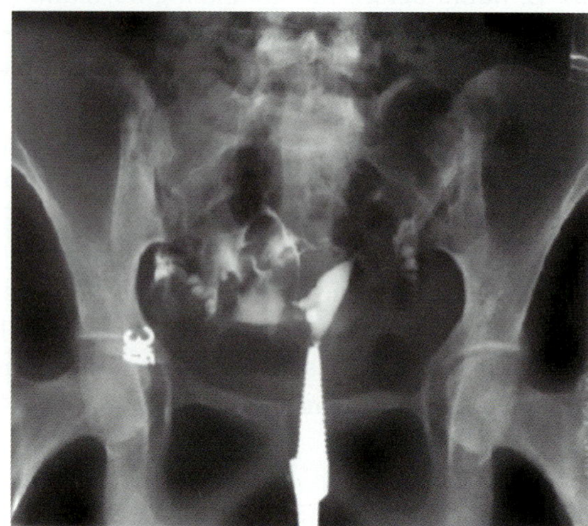

Fig. 3: Hysterosalpingography in a patient with secondary infertility following prior dilatation and curettage shows a distorted uterine cavity with irregular filling defects in the region of right cornu suggestive of intrauterine adhesions.

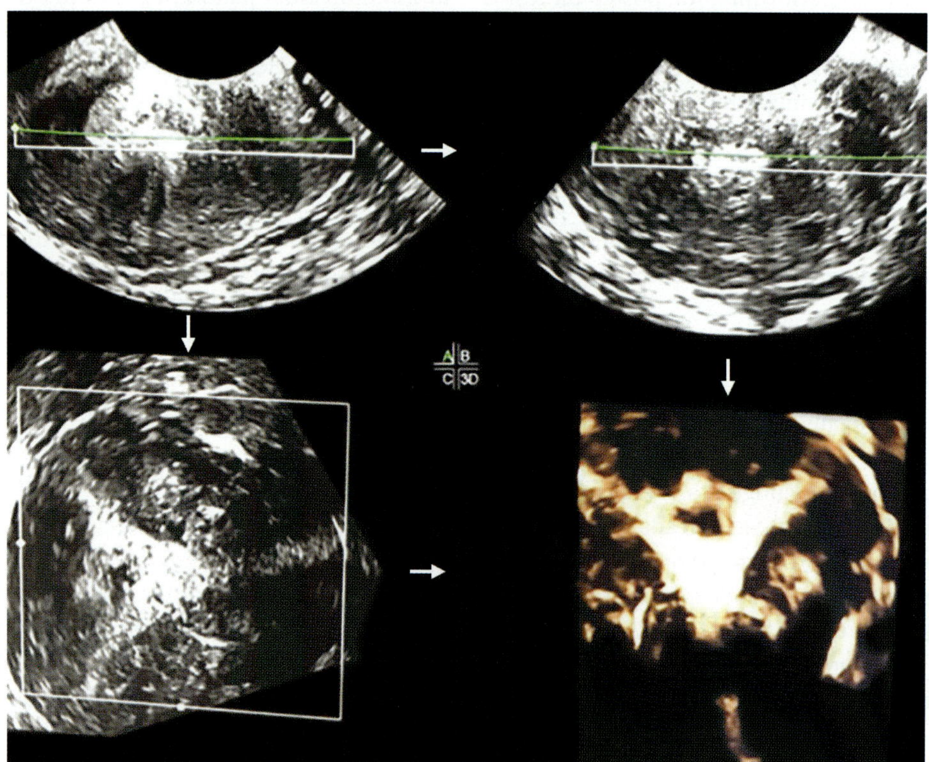

Fig. 4: Three-dimensional coronal view on ultrasound with three-dimensional reconstruction demonstrates a submucosal fibroid projecting into the mid aspect of the uterine cavity.

myomas that involve or compress the interstitial segment of the tube, dysfunctional uterine contractility interfering with ovum or sperm transport or embryo implantation and poor regional blood flow resulting in focal endometrial attenuation or ulceration.[4]

On HSG, leiomyomas are usually seen as filling defects in the endometrial cavity with enlargement of cavity when sufficiently large **(Fig. 5)**. It is essential to distinguish leiomyomas from other filling defects that include polyps, blood clots, and air bubbles. On USG, leiomyomas show a variable imaging appearance. They are usually hypoechoic, but can also be isoechoic or hyperechoic **(Fig. 6)**. Calcification causing posterior shadowing may also be seen. Limitations of USG in evaluating leiomyomas include inability to detect small lesions and difficulty in exact localization due to unfavorable uterine position, and poor uterine visualization due to patient body habitus. MRI has the highest sensitivity for picking up leiomyomas.[8,17] They show low to intermediate signal intensity on T1-weighted (T1W) images and low signal intensity on T2-weighted (T2W) images; however, the signal characteristics may be variable if degeneration is present **(Figs. 7A and B)**. MRI helps in distinguishing leiomyomas from adenomyosis; aids in better preoperative localization for surgical planning and better prediction of treatment outcome.

Treatment for fibroids includes myomectomy, uterine fibroid embolization, image-guided ablation, and medical management. When fertility is a concern,

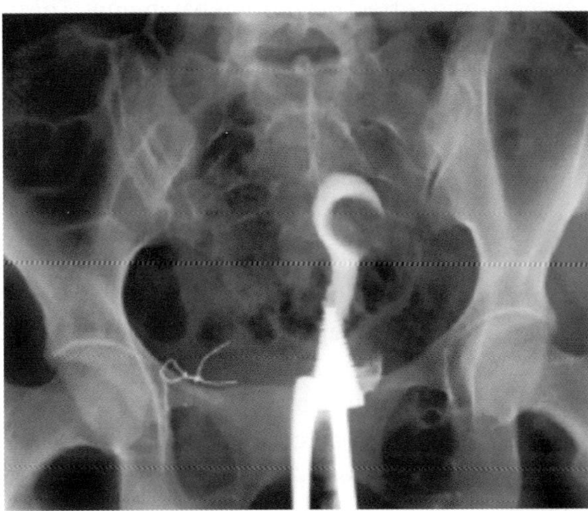

Fig. 5: A globular uterine cavity with a well-defined rounded filling defect consistent with a fibroid.

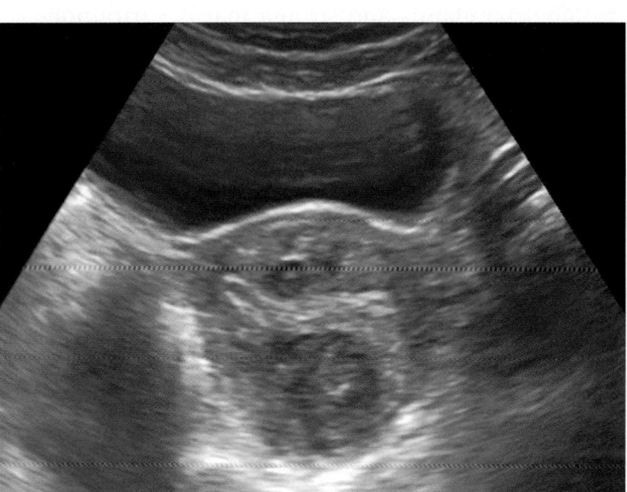

Fig. 6: Transverse ultrasound image shows few hypoechoic myomas in anterior and posterior myometrium causing mild distortion of the endometrium.

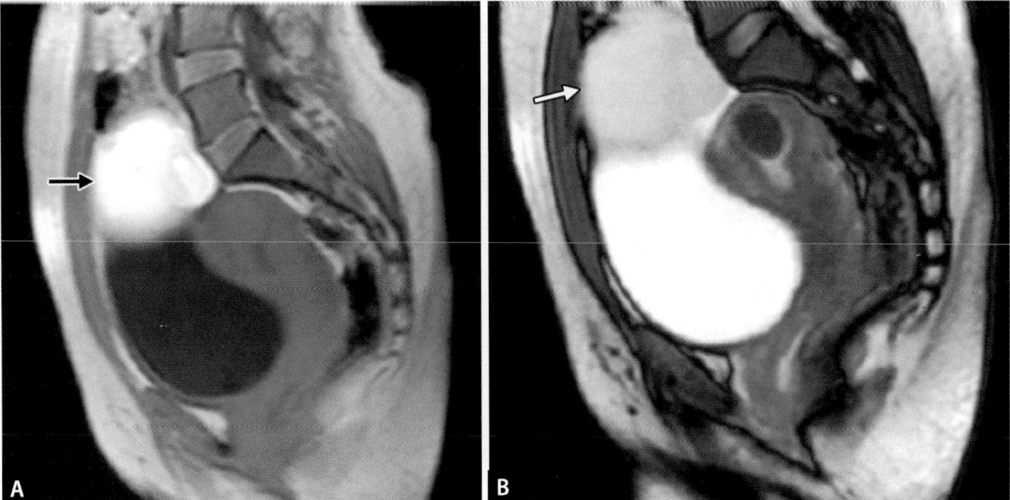

Figs. 7A and B: T1 (A) and T2 (B) weighted sagittal MR images reveal a small submucousal fundal fibroid appearing isointense on T1 and hypointense on T2W images causing distortion of the endometrial cavity. Note the presence of hemorrhagic cyst in one of the ovaries lying superior to the bladder and the uterus appearing hyperintense on both T1W and T2W images (arrows).

treatment includes myomectomy or image-guided ablation. Submucosal fibroids may be removed by a hysteroscope rather than laparotomy. When submucous myomas are single and small, the benefits of hysteroscopic myomectomy generally outweigh the few associated risks. When these are multiple and large, hysteroscopic myomectomy requires much greater technical expertise and poses greater risks including severe postoperative uterine adhesions.[8,18] Uterine fibroid embolization is not done in patients where fertility is to be preserved due to the risk of damage to the uterus and ovaries.[19]

Endometrial Polyps

Endometrial polyps are focal overgrowth of the endometrial glands and stroma that is surrounded by normal endometrium.[16] Endometrial polyps, even when very small, can interfere with ET and implantation. On HSG, polyps are best seen during early filling, however, differentiation from other causes, e.g. submucosal leiomyomas is limited. Endometrial lesions that are not seen on pelvic ultrasound can be picked up with SIS, the latter also helps to differentiate between endometrial polyps and submucosal leiomyomas. It also helps in an accurate assessment of the number and location of endocavitary lesions and provides guidance for their management. Endometrial polyps are seen as echogenic intracavitary masses, which may contain cystic foci. A central vascular stalk may be seen with color Doppler ultrasound. On MRI, they appear isointense to endometrium on T1W images, on T2W images, they appear hypointense with surrounding hyperintense fluid and endometrium **(Figs. 8A and B)**. Homogeneous or heterogeneous contrast enhancement may be seen on postgadolinium scans.

Müllerian Duct Abnormalities

Congenital malformations of the female genital tract are defined as deviations from the normal anatomy due to maldevelopment of the Müllerian or paramesonephric ducts with a prevalence of 4–7%.[20] Approximately 25% of females with Müllerian duct abnormalities have problems with reproduction,[21] although they have long been associated with pregnancy loss and complications, the ability to conceive is generally not affected.

As the treatment of Müllerian duct anomalies is dependent on the type of abnormality and because certain treatment options like in vitro fertilization (IVF) and super ovulation are associated with multifetal gestation which present even greater risk to women with uterine malformations, a correct diagnosis is paramount. The most accurate imaging modality for evaluation of Müllerian duct anomalies is MRI **(Fig. 9)**. Three-dimensional (3D) ultrasound is comparable in accuracy to MRI in evaluation of congenital malformations.[22,23] HSG mainly evaluates the internal morphology of the endometrial cavity and is less accurate for diagnosis.

An accurate classification system is very useful for the management and treatment of these disorders. The American Society of Reproductive Medicine (ASRM) system classified the Müllerian duct abnormalities into seven classes including class I—uterine hypoplasia or agenesis; class II—unicornuate uterus; class III—uterus didelphys; class IV—bicornuate uterus; class V—septate uterus; class VI—arcuate uterus; class VII—diethylstilbestrol (DES)-related anomalies.[21] This classification was used previously.

The European Society of Human Reproduction and Embryology (ESHRE) and the European Society for

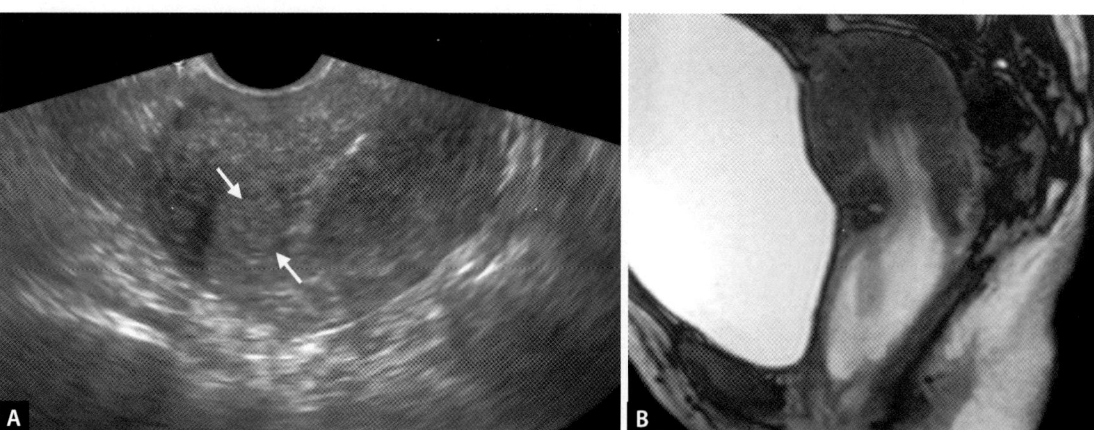

Figs. 8A and B: (A) TVS reveals a relatively well-defined hypoechoic mass within the upper endometrial cavity (arrows) due to an endometrial polyp which was resected hysteroscopically; (B) Sagittal T2W MR image (in another patient) reveals a large hyperintense endometrial polyp coming out through the cervix and bulging into the vagina.

Gynecological Endoscopy (ESGE) have established a common working group called CONUTA (CONgenital UTerine Anomalies) and have formulated a new updated classification system. These criteria were proposed to eliminate the subjective diagnosis of the original ASRM classification and to allow differentiation between septate uterus and other similar conditions independent of absolute morphometric criteria.[20] This classification has been discussed in detail elsewhere in the textbook.

Among the Müllerian duct anomalies, the highest rate of pregnancy loss is associated with septate uterus **(Figs. 10A and B)**. According to the ESHRE/ESGE 2016, there is a high proportion of overdiagnosis of septate uterus leading to avoidable surgeries and hence risk to women and burden on healthcare systems. The ESHRE/ESGE has recommended an indentation to wall thickness (I:WT) ratio >50% for diagnosis of septate uterus. According to a study conducted by Ludwin et al, the values for defining septate uterus include indentation depth >10 mm, indentation angle <140° and I : WT ratio >110%.[24]

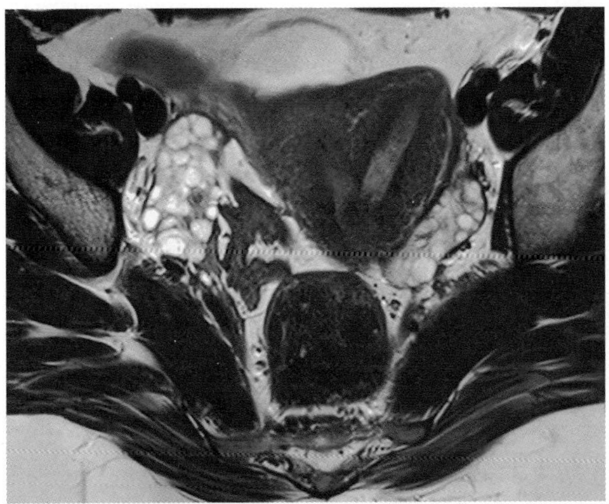

Fig. 9: Axial T2W MR image shows two uterine cavities separated by a hypointense septum—septate uterus. Bilateral polycystic ovaries are seen.

Adenomyosis

Adenomyosis is a benign condition in which the endometrial glands and stroma invade the myometrium. It may be diffuse in which the uterus becomes enlarged and globular in shape or focal where there is a well-circumscribed nodule known as adenomyoma. Initial imaging is performed using ultrasound, which shows the uterus to be enlarged and globular in shape with indistinct junctional zone. Increased echogenicity of the myometrium may be seen due to endometrial extension with multiple small hypoechoic myometrial cysts. Other findings include indistinct interface between the endometrium and myometrium, subendometrial echogenic nodules or linear striations, asymmetric myometrial thickening, and indistinct lesion borders **(Fig. 11)**. On HSG, adenomyosis is seen as multiple small diverticula extending into the myometrium **(Fig. 12)**. MRI reveals enlargement of uterus with thickening of the junctional zone (>12 mm), which shows poorly defined margins and low signal intensity on T2W images and small T2 bright foci secondary to dilated endometrial glands or foci of hemorrhage within the myometrium **(Figs. 13A and B)**. A junctional zone thickness of <8 mm rules out the

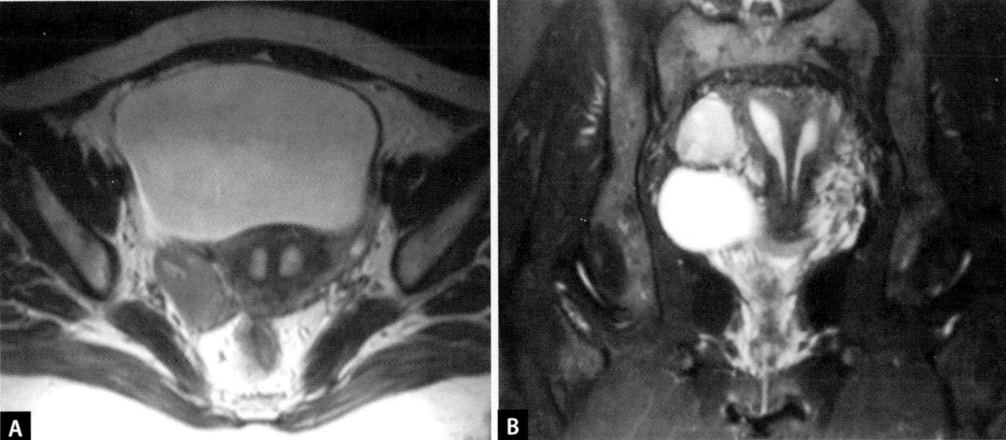

Figs. 10A and B: T2W axial and coronal MR images in a patient with complete uterine septum. Two uterine cavities are seen which are separated by a septum showing signal isointense to myometrium in its upper part and an inferior fibrous component which is T2 hypointense extending into the cervix, the external fundal contour is only mildly indented—septate uterus. Note the cyst in the right ovary.

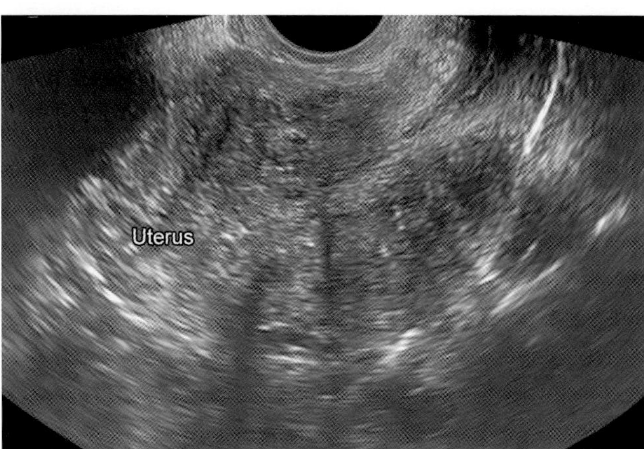

Fig. 11: Transvaginal ultrasound image shows an enlarged globular uterus with poorly defined endomyometrial interface in a case of adenomyosis.

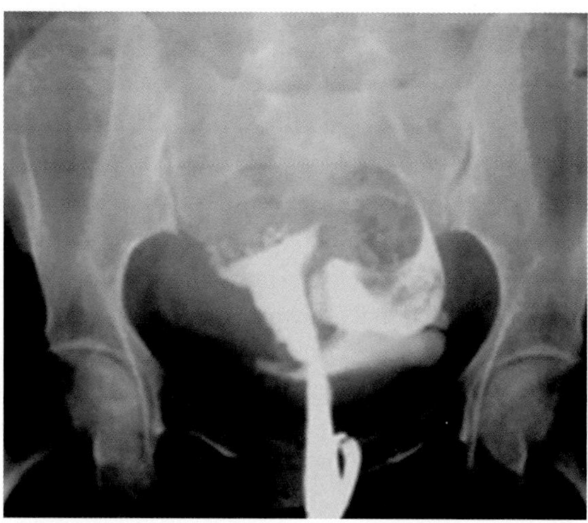

Fig. 12: HSG in a known case of adenomyosis shows multiple small irregular diverticulae in the region of fundus filling with contrast. Right-sided tube is not visualized—cornual block. Left tube is normal.

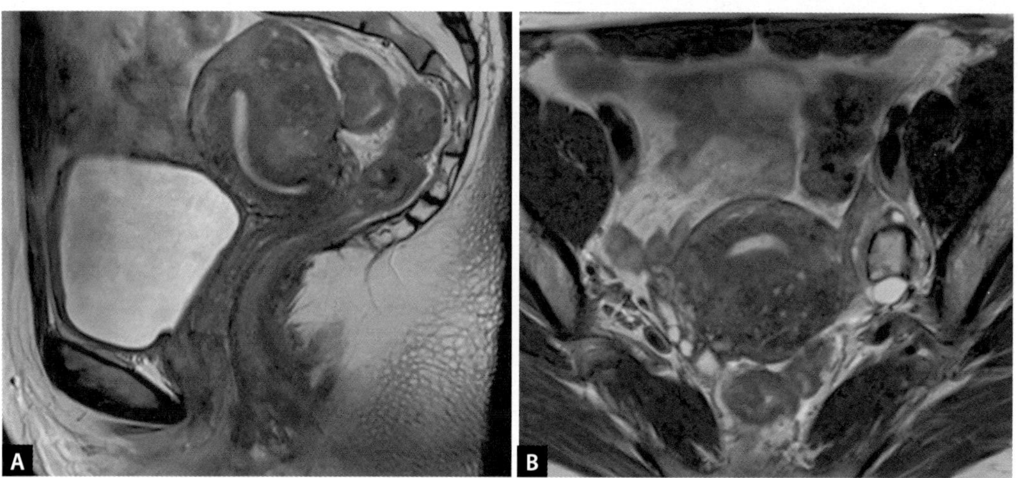

Figs. 13A and B: Sagittal (A) and axial (B) T2W MR images reveal ill-defined myometrial masses with indistinct margins, myometrial cysts, and widening of junctional zone—adenomyosis.

diagnosis and thickness between 8 mm and 12 mm and requires additional investigations.[21] A strong association between adenomyosis and pelvic endometriosis has been found in women <36 years of age with adenomyosis being reported in approximately 90% of these patients.[25] Adenomyosis is said to be the cause of infertility in these patients. Fertility is affected by impaired uterine contractility and focal adenomyomas in submucosal location.

The only functional uterine abnormality that is of particular interest in the evaluation of infertility is chronic endometritis.

Nontubercular Chronic Endometritis

Chronic endometritis results from loss of the coexistence between microorganisms and the host immune system in the endometrium. Majority of these patients have no or mild symptoms. However, association of chronic endometritis with conditions related to infertility like implantation failure and recurrent miscarriages is of concern.[26] Chronic endometritis is diagnosed by endometrial biopsy, which shows the presence of plasma cells in endometrial stroma, but in florid cases, TVS may reveal thin echogenic endometrium that does not thicken as follicular phase advances.

Sonography has also been used to study the usual developmental response of the endometrium to try and predict implantation. During menstruation, the endometrium is seen as a thin echogenic interface, which thickens during the proliferative phase of the menstrual cycle and is relatively hypo-to isoechoic yielding a prominent trilaminar pattern. During the secretory phase, the endometrium does not thicken further but becomes more echogenic.

In a study conducted by Khan et al no pregnancy was reported with an endometrial thickness of <7 mm. They also found that average pulsatility index (PI) of the uterine artery was higher in nonconception than in conception cycles. PI value of >2.8 was associated with no conception.[27] Tekay et al reported no pregnancy when the PI was more than 3.[28]

Calcific Endometritis

Calcific endometritis is an uncommon cause of infertility. It can occur postabortion, after chronic endometritis (due to genital tuberculosis, nonspecific chronic endometritis, and pyometra). An echogenic line may be seen along the endometrial cavity with posterior shadowing. Doppler studies show increased blood flow in the myometrium and endometrium with peak systolic velocity >60 cm/sec and resistive index (RI) <0.5 in subendometrial and myometrial vessels. MRI reveals a thin hypointense line along the endometrial cavity on T2W images.[29]

TUBAL FACTOR

The fallopian tubes connect the peritoneal cavity to the external environment through the uterus, cervix, and vagina. The normal length of the fallopian tube varies from 7 cm to 16 cm, with an average length of 12 cm. Ciliated mucosal epithelial layer surrounded by three smooth muscle layers lines the tube and the tube is divided into four segments: (1) the intramural or interstitial part, which lies in the wall of the fundus, it is 1–2 cm in length; (2) the isthmic part, which is around 2–3 cm in length; (3) the ampullary portion, which is 5–8 cm in length; and (4) the infundibulum, it is the distal end of the tube which is trumpet-shaped and terminates in the fimbria.[15] Fallopian tubes help in transport of sperms from the uterine end toward the ampulla and transport of the ova in the other direction, that is from the fimbriated end to the ampulla. They also provide support to the early embryo and enable conduction of the early embryo from the ampulla to the uterus for implantation.

Fallopian tube pathology accounts for infertility in up to 40% of women and is among the most common causes of infertility. Infection or endometriosis commonly result in tubal obstruction. Salpingitis isthmica nodosa (SIN) is also a cause of tubal infertility that has commonly been described in the Western literature.[8,15]

Evaluating patency of the fallopian tube is an important part of the workup for infertility. The techniques available to evaluate the fallopian tubes include HSG, sonohysterosalpingography and laparoscopy. HSG remains the most common initial imaging technique used to evaluate the fallopian tubes. It provides exquisite depiction of the fallopian tubes and enables delineation of tubal patency, tubal occlusion, tubal irregularity, and peritubal disease. Compared with laparoscopy (which is the gold standard test for assessing tubal patency), HSG has only moderate sensitivity but relatively high specificity. The clinical implications are that when obstruction is seen on HSG, there is still a relatively high probability (approximately 60%) that the tube is in fact open, but when HSG reveals patency, there is little chance that the tube is actually blocked (approximately 5%). In these cases, contrast in a dilated tube or vaginal fornix may be mistaken for peritoneal spill.[4] Sonohysterosalpingography and 3D ultrasound and Doppler techniques have been used to evaluate the tubes. However, the techniques provide no information regarding tubal anatomy and whether one or both tubes are patent. Although 3D ultrasound and Doppler techniques have improved visualization of fluid movement through fallopian tubes, it is unlikely that they will replace traditional HSG.

On HSG, the interstitial segment of the fallopian tube may be delicate and thread-shaped or it may be funnel-shaped, taking the configuration of a small triangle or diamond. The isthmic segment is usually thread-shaped. The diameter of both these segments is around 1 mm. Proximal tubal obstruction is obstruction seen in the first 3–4 cm of the tube.[8,15] Obstruction of the proximal end of the fallopian tube is seen in 20% of cases on HSG. The cause of proximal tubal obstruction is frequently unclear, however, all reported series implicate infection and subsequent inflammation as leading causes. Histopathology of the resected proximal tubal segments reveals plugs of amorphous debris, chronic inflammation, obliterative fibrosis, and SIN. All these lesions account for majority of anatomic occlusions at the uterotubal junction. Other causes include granulomatous or "giant cell" salpingitis secondary to tuberculosis, foreign bodies, certain parasitic infestations, intraluminal endometriosis, and congenital atresia of fallopian tubes. Around 10% of tubes resected for proximal occlusion reveal intraluminal endometriosis and may exist without relation to visible lesions anywhere else in the pelvis. Müllerian anomalies of the fallopian tube are not seen frequently, but cornual occlusion is seen with variants of unicornuate uterus, where atresia of tubal segments, including the proximal isthmus, can occur.

Proximal tubal obstruction on HSG can also be seen with "tubal spasm". The cornual portion of the fallopian tube is encased by smooth muscle of the uterus. If the muscle goes into spasm during HSG, one or both tubes may not be opacified beyond the interstitial portion. A spasmolytic agent, such as glucagon or scopolamine, if administered can occasionally result in uterine muscle relaxation and consequent tube opacification. According to some authors, however, tubal spasm is the cause of proximal tubal obstruction much less often than originally proposed. They postulate that temporary nonvisualization of the tube may be due to some easily dislodged entity such as amorphous debris in the lumen of the tube.[30,31] In some cases, it may be helpful to place the patient in prone position and wait for 5 minutes before slowly reinjecting contrast. If proximal tubal obstruction persists in spite of these maneuvers, tubal catheterization with selective salpingography can be performed.

Proximal tubal obstruction can be diagnosed and treated with fluoroscopically guided selective salpingography.[15,32-34] Selective salpingography is a technique which is minimally invasive, and it involves placing the tip of the catheter in the tubal ostia and injecting contrast directly into the tube. The obstruction can usually be overcome by the injection alone. In case the obstruction is not relieved, a guidewire can be directed into the tube fluoroscopically through the catheter. Tubal recanalization may be achieved either through forceful injection of contrast or by clearing the obstruction with a guidewire. A technical success rate of 75% has been reported and in 10–22% of these patients, pregnancy is achieved without further management.[35] Traditionally, this procedure was performed for patients with bilateral proximal tubal occlusions but there is a lower threshold for considering fallopian tube recanalization in patients with unilateral occlusion. It is essential to exclude distal tubal disease especially noncommunicating hydrosalpinx. Complications include tubal perforation, infection, and tubal pregnancy. Ultrasonographic guidance has also been used for this procedure in a few cases.

Salpingitis isthmica nodosa is a tubal pathology commonly described in Western literature. An association between SIN and PID exists, however, it is unclear whether SIN is caused by pelvic inflammation or it is congenital and predisposes to inflammation. It mostly affects the isthmic portion and occasionally the interstitial and ampullary segments. On HSG, it is seen as characteristic multiple small diverticula present in the proximal two-thirds of the tube. It leads to infertility and is also associated with increased risk of ectopic pregnancy. Tuberculous salpingitis can have similar imaging appearance but may be associated with calcified lymph nodes or calcifications of the tube itself. SIN associated with tubal obstruction may be treated by tubal catheterization and recanalization under fluoroscopic guidance.[8,15]

The longest part of the fallopian tube is the ampullary segment. It measures 1–2 mm at its proximal end and widens to approximately 15 mm, where it joins the fimbriated infundibular portion. Subtle ampullary rugal folds can be seen with salpingography, and sometimes the fimbriae may be outlined by contrast material. Damage to the epithelium secondary to infection causes abnormal rugal folds and these usually coexist with a dilated and at times a distally obstructed tube. Abnormal rugal folds may be found in a patent tube, and they imply decreased chances for conception. The presence of abnormal rugal folds needs optimal tubal imaging, because the normal rugal folds are subtle. Rugal folds may be best seen before the dilated tube is fully distended with contrast, i.e. during early filling.[8]

Dilation of the ampullary portion of the tube is seen with obstruction in the fimbrial portion of the fallopian tube, which sometimes can be massive, with absence of free peritoneal spill of contrast agent in spite of adequate filling of the tubes and rolling the patient **(Fig. 14)**. It may

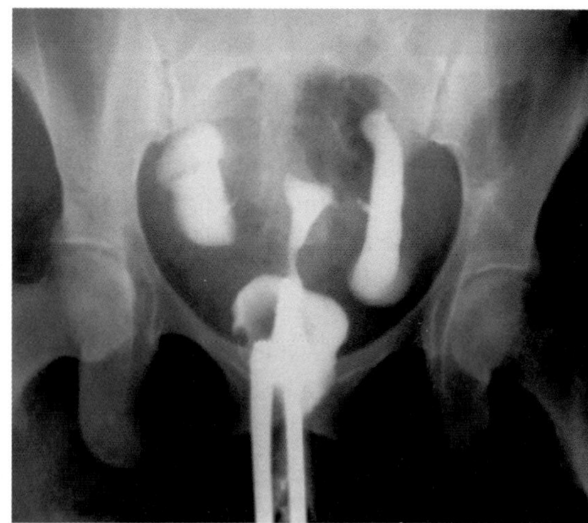

Fig. 14: HSG in a patient with bilateral fimbrial block shows markedly dilated ampullary segments (hydrosalpinx) with absence of free intraperitoneal spill.

be difficult to distinguish a dilated tube from loculated spill of contrast agent sometimes. If hydrosalpinx is seen on HSG, postprocedural antibiotic prophylaxis should be prescribed to prevent infection secondary to stasis of contrast material in the obstructed tube.

The degree of tubal dilatation does not predict results of surgery. The epithelium may be intact in a dilated tube which is soft and pliable, and thus amenable to surgery. An obstructed tube, which is mildly dilated, may not be amenable to reconstruction as the wall can be thickened and indurated. Improved chances of successful tubal reconstruction are associated with visualization of normal ampullary rugal folds. Dilatation of the ampullary part of the tube in the absence of complete occlusion suggests perifimbrial phimosis or adhesions around the fimbria that hinder egress of fluid.

Fimbrial phimosis can be mild or severe, but mostly the presence of at least a pinpoint opening in the distal tube is associated with a more favorable prognosis after surgery than complete occlusion. It also increases the risk of post HSG peritonitis.

Although ultrasound is unable to visualize normal fallopian tubes, blockage of the fallopian tube with fluid accumulation (hydrosalpinx) is easily seen on ultrasound **(Figs. 15A and B)**. The distended tube coiled around the ovary with folds producing septa which do not completely cross the lumen. A hydrosalpinx may occasionally be visible on ultrasound, distended with fluid only at midcycle, under the estrogenic influence of a preovulatory follicle.[36]

A woman with severely damaged fallopian tubes but a normal uterine cavity is a good candidate for IVF and ET. However, presence of hydrosalpinx in a woman being treated by IVF is associated with poor embryo uptake which may be improved after treatment of hydrosalpinx. Even a unilateral hydrosalpinx is capable of disrupting natural fertility and preventing the success of IVF.[36-38] The mechanism is as follows: Estradiol produced by the preovulatory and ovulating follicle stimulates both ampullary transudation of fluid and isthmic secretion of dense mucus which along with an estrogen mediated increase in isthmic myosalpingeal tone functionally occludes the tube's communication with the cavity of the uterus. Thus, the hydrosalpinx gathers fluid. With ovulation, increasing progesterone secretion from the luteinizing follicle relaxes the isthmus, allowing passage of accumulated hydrosalpinx fluid down the endometrial cavity just at the time that a normal tube allows passage of preembryo to the uterus. This cascade from a single tube is likely to displace any preembryos that might have reached through the contralateral patent one or through IVF and transcervical transfer. Conceptions rates following salpingostomy are less than 25% if the hydrosalpinx has a thick wall or a diameter greater than 15 mm.[5,39]

PERITONEAL FACTOR

The peritoneal factor responsible for infertility is due to pelvic adhesions resulting from previous infection, endometriosis or surgery.[8,9,15] Adhesions can cause problems in oocyte pick up and transfer due to alteration of the normal anatomy, restriction of fimbrial motility and obstruction of fallopian tubes. Imaging techniques are limited in their ability to diagnose pelvic adhesions. The gold standard for visualization of pelvic adhesions and endometriosis is laparoscopy.[8]

With HSG, the presence of peritubal adhesions and endometriosis is under diagnosed with reported sensitivities ranging from 34% to 75%. Peritubal adhesions can be suggested if loculated spill of contrast is seen in the peritoneal cavity, or it is seen to track along the outside of the tube producing "a halo effect" or double contour appearance to tubal wall.[40] Peritubal adhesions can also be

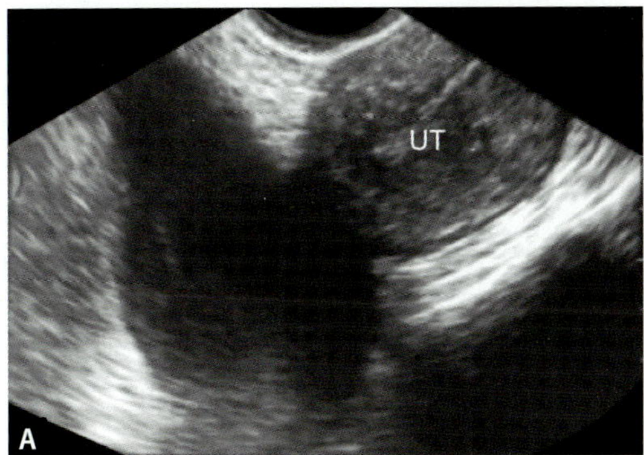

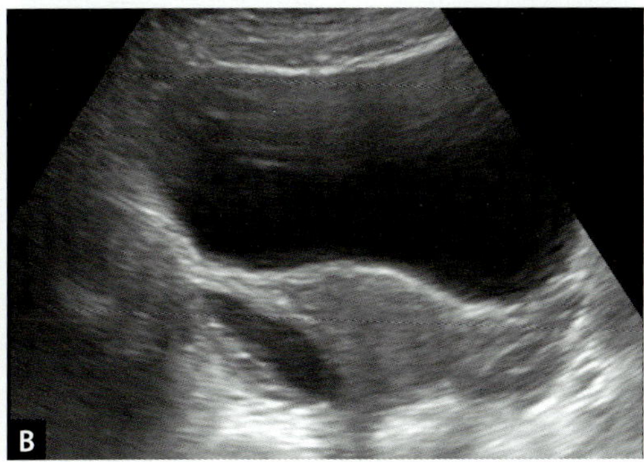

Figs. 15A and B: USG showing a cystic hypoechoic retort-shaped dilated tube with incomplete septations—Hydrosalpinx (A); In another case, an oblong cystic structure is seen in the right adnexa adjacent to the right ovary consistent with hydrosalpinx (B).

diagnosed if a persistently convoluted, kinked, stretched or vertically oriented fallopian tube is seen **(Fig. 16)**. Delayed films or film obtained after rolling the patient may be useful to confirm loculated spill in doubtful cases. Normally, the contrast should flow freely to outline the bowel loops.[8,15,41] A tug and release maneuver has also been described to confirm the presence of adhesions. If traction is applied on the HSG system both a fixed laterodeviated uterus (due to adhesions) as well as a normal nonmedian uterus initially follow the traction direction, however, during the releasing phase the fixed laterodeviated uterus tends to keep the original deviated position while the nonmedian uterus keeps the pelvis midline.[40]

Ultrasound, especially TVS may also detect pelvic adhesions and loculated fluid collections in the adnexae. Adhesions may be suggested by *en masse* movement of the tethered organs when pressure is applied simultaneously by the operator's hand transabdominally and by the probe transvaginally.

Endometriosis

Endometriosis is found in 25–50% of infertile women and 30–50% of women with endometriosis are infertile.[42] Endometriosis results from ectopic foci of secretory endometrium situated outside the uterus. It can impair fertility through formation of adhesions and hormonally medicated mechanisms. Endometriosis may occur as diffuse peritoneal implants or focal endometriomas (chocolate cysts). TVS is the preferred technique to identify ovarian endometriomas which are seen as complex adnexal or cul-de-sac masses. Diffuse low level internal echoes may be seen **(Fig. 17)**. However, TVS has limited ability to identify generalized disease producing subtle changes such as obliteration of margins between pelvic organs and a generalized increase in echogenicity.[41,43]

On MRI, endometriomas may be seen as adnexal cysts with high signal on both T1W and T2W images or high signal on T1 and low signal on T2W images (T2 shading) with indistinct margins due to adhesions **(Figs. 18A to C)**. Evaluation of adhesions is difficult and these may be seen as low signal intensity stranding that obscures organ interfaces, posterior displacement of uterus, kissing ovaries, angulated bowel loops, an elevated posterior vaginal fornix, loculated fluid collections, and hydro/hematosalpinx **(Fig. 19)**. Hormonal therapy is occasionally used to treat endometriosis and shading on T2W images is the most important negative predictor for volume reduction with medical treatment, such therapy should be discontinued should low T2 signal be seen in a case on hormonal treatment. It is important to remember that small implants and adhesions that may cause infertility are not well visualized by any imaging technique. Laparoscopy remains the gold standard for diagnosis and staging of endometriosis and is also the mainstay for diagnosis.[10,15]

Genital Tuberculosis

About 18% of female infertility in India is attributed to genital tuberculosis.[44] Tuberculosis commonly results in

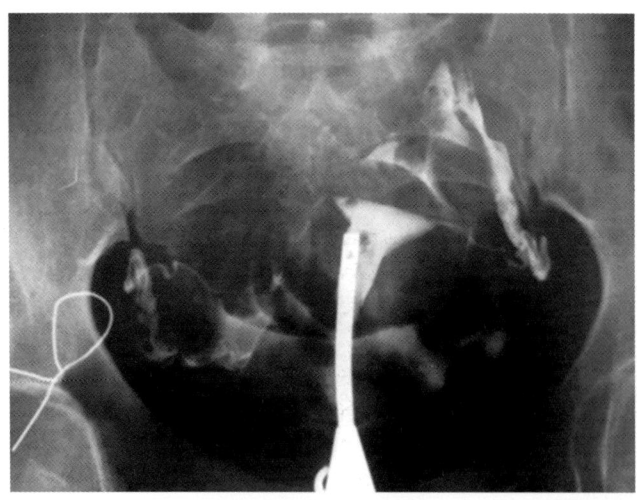

Fig. 16: HSG film reveals an irregular filling defect in the uterine body just adjacent to the cannula due to adhesions. An air bubble is seen in the right cornu. The ampullary portion of the left fallopian tube is vertically stretched with evidence of both peritubal and free spill due to peritubal adhesions.

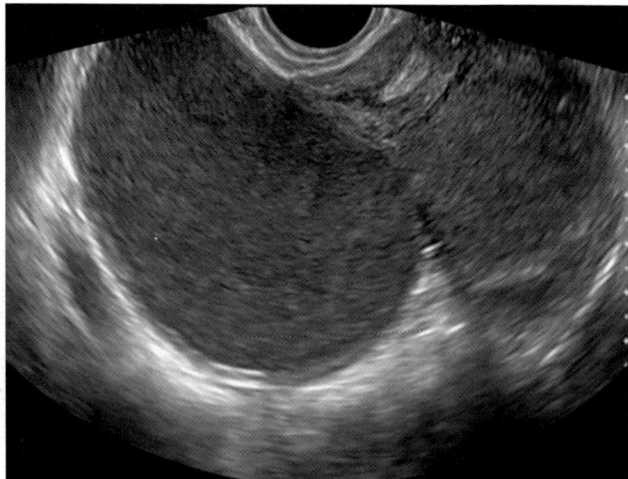

Fig. 17: Transvaginal ultrasound image shows bilateral adnexal lesions with homogeneous diffuse low level internal echoes consistent with bilateral endometriomas. The uterus is displaced anterolaterally.

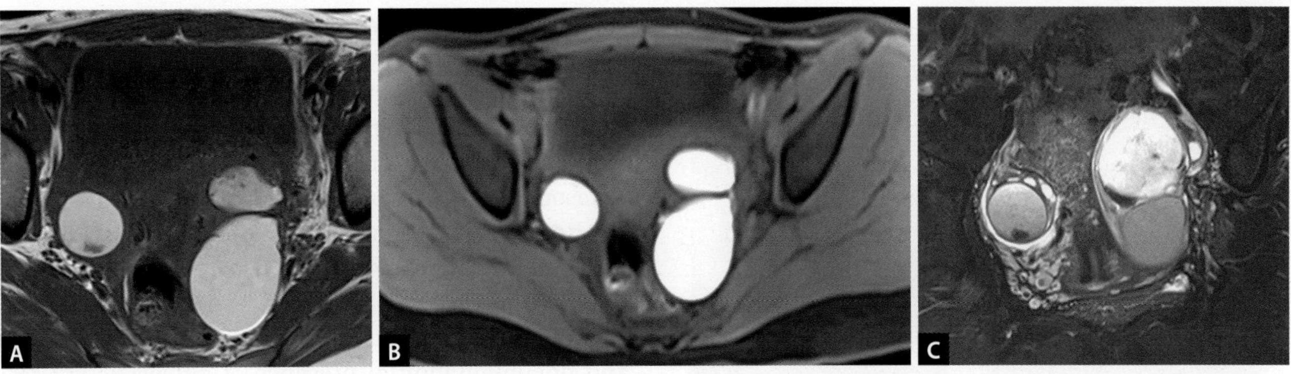

Figs. 18A to C: Bilateral adnexal lesions are seen appearing hyperintense on axial T1W (A) and axial T1W fat saturated (B) images. The lesions show T2 shading on T2W coronal images as well as T2 dark spots (C)—bilateral endometriomas.

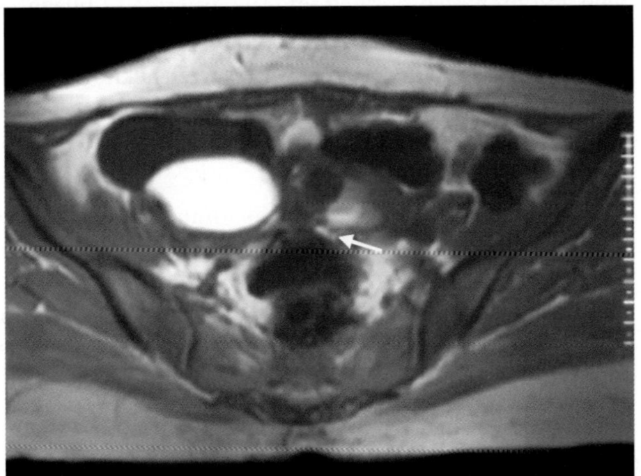

Fig. 19: T1W MR image reveals bilateral adnexal cysts with high signal due to hemorrhage and angulation of the anterior rectal surface due to adhesions (arrow).

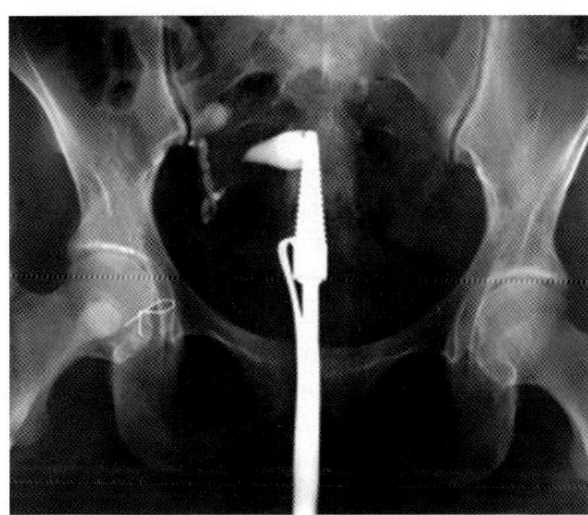

Fig. 20: A HSG showing a mildly dilated beaded right fallopian tube with evidence of loculated spill. Left tube is not visualized due to cornual block—sequelae of tuberculosis.

changes in the endometrium, the fallopian tubes, and pelvic peritoneum.

Scarring in uterine tuberculosis is well demonstrated by HSG. This can take few specialized forms namely: T-shaped uterus, asymmetric uterus, and pseudounicornuate uterus.[45] A significant number of patients with uterine tuberculosis show a T-shaped uterus and it is virtually diagnostic of this condition in the appropriate setting. A T-shaped uterus has usually been labelled as a DES uterus in the Western literature. The DES and the tuberculous uterus reveal irregular margins. However, tubal changes are not seen in DES uteri, but are mostly seen in T-shaped uteri due to tuberculosis. The normal uterine cavity shows a triangular configuration with straight or concave lateral walls. In tuberculous endometritis due to scarring along the long as well as the short axis of the uterus; this triangular shape is converted into a T shape.[45] DES was discontinued in the 1970s, so these cases are not seen now.

Scarring is also recognizable by the asymmetric uterine contour it produces. An asymmetric, small-sized uterine cavity is usually due to tuberculosis. Sometimes, the scarring may be more unilateral leading to obliteration of that part of the uterine cavity leading to a unicornuate uterus-like appearance—"the pseudounicornuate uterus". Comparison with previous films, laparoscopy, and awareness about this type of scarring would be essential in differentiating tuberculosis from a true unicornuate uterus. A good pointer towards endometrial tuberculosis is myometrial extravasation and/or venous intravasation. This finding in association with any other endometrial or tubal change **(Figs. 20 and 21)** is very suggestive of a tuberculous etiology of endometritis.[45]

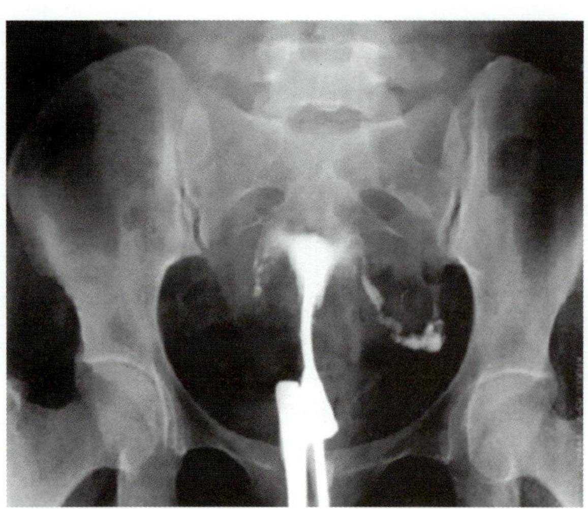

Fig. 21: HSG demonstrating a beaded left fallopian tube with no free spill. Only the proximal (isthmic and interstitial portion) of the right fallopian tube is visualized. Note the presence of myometrial extravasation suggestive of tubercular involvement.

OVARIAN FACTOR

Ovarian dysfunction accounts for up to 40% of infertility in women.[46] Adequate reproductive function requires normal ovarian follicular development, ovulation, and formation of functional CL. It is essential to evaluate these ovulatory factors while investigating infertility. TVS is an excellent imaging modality to evaluate the ovaries, which is used to detect both ovarian pathology and monitor ovulation. Functional ovarian cysts or other benign ovarian cysts and tumors like dermoid cysts or fibromata may occasionally interfere with ovarian function particularly when large. Endometriomas have already been discussed.

Gonadal Dysgenesis

Gonadal dysgenesis is a congenital condition characterized by abnormal gonadal organization and function. There is replacement of the gonadal tissue by fibrous stroma, no germ cells are present. The most common form of this condition is secondary to Turner syndrome. Diagnosis can be made on clinical, biochemical, and karyotype identification, imaging when performed demonstrates small oval to linear fibrous tissue within the broad ligament with absence of normal appearing ovaries, best seen on MRI, although detection is limited with the gonads found only in approximately 40–65% of cases.[16]

Polycystic Ovary Syndrome

Polycystic ovary syndrome (PCOS) is the most common cause of ovarian infertility. It is the most common endocrinopathy affecting women in the reproductive age group with prevalence between 8% and 13%.[47] PCOS is a complex disorder with reproductive, metabolic, and psychological features and is also known as Stein-Leventhal syndrome. Previously used criteria for PCOS on ultrasound include round, enlarged ovaries, with multiple small cysts, absence of cysts measuring more than 1.5 cm in diameter, smooth contours, and hyperechoic appearance of ovarian stroma.

The aim of imaging in PCOS is proper identification and documentation of presence of polycystic ovaries. In 2003, a joint ESHRE/ASRM meeting in Rotterdam created a definition for polycystic ovaries which was reaffirmed by the Androgen Excess and PCOS society in 2009 and then incorporated into the American College of Obstetricians and Gynecologists guidelines. Two criteria for identification of polycystic ovaries were acknowledged and these include 12 or more follicles measuring 2–9 mm in diameter in one or both ovaries and ovarian volume >10 cc.[48]

Reasons for revision of this diagnostic criteria include inadequate initial evidence, advances in ultrasound technology with greater resolution, lack of standard reporting, ill-defined cut-offs between normal ovaries and polycystic ovarian morphology, impact of approach (e.g. TVS), body habitus, and age. Natural changes in antral follicle count (AFC) occur during prepubertal and menopausal transitions and up to 70% adolescents have polycystic ovary morphology on original criteria **(Figs. 22A and B)**. Diagnosis of PCOS mandates not only polycystic ovarian morphology but presence of associated features of hyperandrogenism and/or ovulatory dysfunction. Recommendations from the international evidence-based guidelines for the assessment and management of PCOS were given in 2018. According to these, endovaginal ultrasound transducers with a frequency bandwidth that includes 8 MHz should be used and threshold for polycystic ovarian morphology should be on either ovary, a follicle number (follicle size measuring 2–9 mm) per ovary of more than or equal to 20 and/or volume more than or equal to 10 mL, ensuring no corpus lutea, cysts or dominant follicles are present **(Figs. 23 and 24)**. USG should not be used for the diagnosis of PCOS in <8 years after menarche as the incidence of multifollicular ovaries is high in this life stage. Threshold for polycystic ovary morphology should be revised regularly with advancing USG technology and age specific cut-off values for polycystic ovarian morphology should be defined.

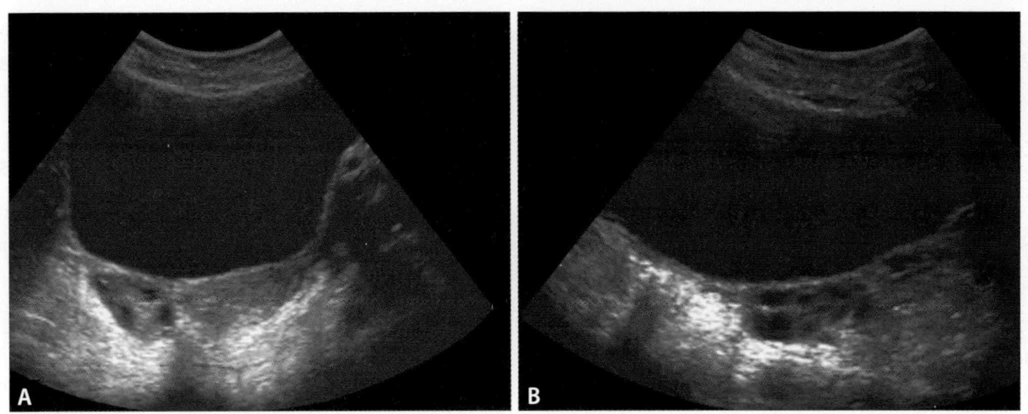

Figs. 22A and B: Multifollicular ovarian morphology seen in a prepubertal female.

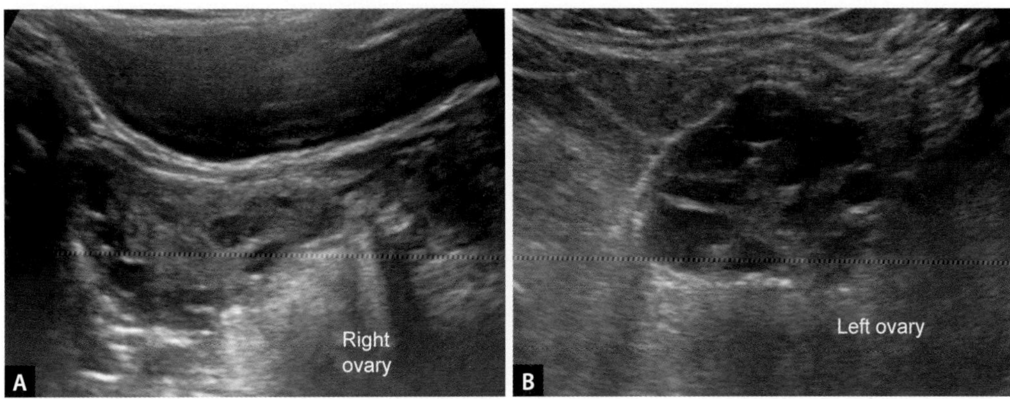

Figs. 23A and B: Ultrasound images reveal bilateral enlarged ovaries with multiple small follicles within. Note the peripherally arranged small follicles in the right ovary.

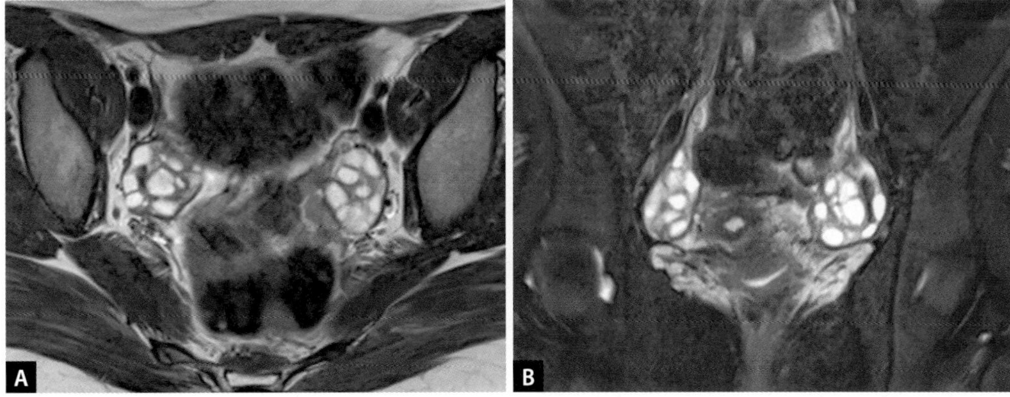

Figs. 24A and B: T2W (axial) and T2W fat saturated (coronal) images show bilateral enlarged ovaries showing multiple small follicles within.

In patients with irregular menstrual cycles and hyperandrogenism, USG is not essential for PCOS diagnosis, however, it identifies the complete PCOS phenotype. In transabdominal sonogram reporting is best focused on ovarian volume with threshold of more than or equal to 10 mL, given the difficulty of reliably assessing follicle number with this approach.

The following factors are important to consider while reporting: last menstrual period, transducer bandwidth frequency, approach/route assessed, total follicle

number per ovary measuring 2–9 mm, three dimensions and volume of each ovary, endometrial thickness and appearance, and other ovarian and uterine pathology. The presence of a thickened echogenic endometrium (due to estrogen excess) is also seen with PCOS.[47]

Ovulatory Function Tests

Ovulation can be monitored using basal body temperature recordings, endometrial biopsy (for documenting secretory changes in the endometrium), measurement of a serum progesterone (generally done 1 week before the expected onset of next menses), urinary LH determination using ovulation predictor kits to identify midcycle LH surge which occurs 1–2 days before ovulation and follicular monitoring using USG. The latter follows the development of the follicle till its disappearance and is the most accurate method for documentation of ovulation.

Development and Evolution of Ovarian Follicles

Ultrasonography is an excellent modality for monitoring the follicles during spontaneous and induced cycles. TVS is used for monitoring the follicles during ovarian induction using clomiphene citrate or human menopausal gonadotropin (hMG). This is done from the 7th day of the menstrual cycle and preferably on a daily basis, which can help in adjustment of the patient's medication. A follicle is considered mature when it measures 15–18 mm in mean diameter. Presence of fine echoes within the mature follicle is an indication of ovulation and is associated with serum estradiol value of 400 pg/mL or urine estrogen levels of 80–150 µg/day. Other features that help predict ovulation include sudden collapse of the preovulatory follicle, a loss of clearly defined follicular margins and increase in cul-de-sac fluid volume.

Follicular Monitoring: Spontaneous Cycles

Starting with menarche, during spontaneous cycles there is usually development of one or sometimes two dominant follicles. Sonography can show the developing follicles starting at the time measure 3–5 mm. In the spontaneous cycle, by unknown mechanisms, one or at the most two follicles develop to approximately 10 mm. At this time (about 7 days before LH surge), a dominant follicle takes over and there is a very little further growth of other follicles. Occasionally, two dominant follicles develop. During the 5 days prior to ovulation the dominant follicle grows at the rate of 2–3 mm/day. As a follicle reaches maturity, its inner dimensions range from 17 mm to 25 mm. However, within the same person the size of the mature follicle is relatively constant cycle to cycle.[5,49]

Follicular Monitoring: Induced Cycles

Ovulation induction is indicated in patients in whom infertility can be ascribed to an ovulation abnormality or anovulation. Ovulation induction or super ovulation therapy is also used in women with normal ovulation before assisted conception techniques such as IVF-ET or gamete intrafallopian transfer to increase the number of oocytes aspirated. This increases the number of fertilized conceptions that may be transferred thereby increasing the chances of pregnancy.[5,10]

Before starting treatment, a baseline scanning of the pelvis should be done. If one or more cysts, larger than approximately 2 cm in diameter are found, especially if accompanied by serum estradiol concentration of more than 100 pg/mL, it may interfere with treatment and induction may be postponed to the next cycle or cysts treated by aspiration.

The most commonly used medications for ovulation induction include clomiphene citrate, aromatase inhibitors (e.g. letrozole), and gonadotropins [FSH, LH, hMG, hCG]. Patients undergoing this treatment are usually examined every other day starting at day 10. Patients undergoing IVF-ET are examined by sonography starting earlier and usually daily in an attempt to carefully monitor their follicular development.

Clomiphene citrate is an estrogen antagonist, its action is to indirectly promote secretion of FSH and LH. In some patients ovulation occurs due to elevated serum levels of FSH and LH, without further therapy. In other patients, hCG may be required to induce ovulation. Follicular development with clomiphene citrate can be quite different from that seen in natural cycles. Each follicle seems to develop at an individual rate and at times may be accelerated or slowed down. Hence, the larger follicles on a given date may not be the same one that is the largest 2 days later and it may not even be the same one that is most mature. Furthermore, correlation of estradiol levels (E2) and follicle size is poor and maximum preovulatory diameter can range from 19 mm to 24 mm. In clomiphene stimulated cycles, the growth rate in the last few days preceding ovulation is higher.

In contrast to clomiphene citrate, treatment with hMG does not require an intact hypothalamic-pituitary axis. This contains both FSH and LH and induces follicle development. hCG is then administered to induce ovulation of mature follicles. The follicle growth can be evaluated by serial measurement of serum or urinary estradiol levels; however, multiple, small, and immature follicles may produce as much estradiol as a large mature follicle. Therefore, TVS is used to predict the optimal timing for giving an ovulation inducing dose of hCG.[8,50-52] Sonographic assessment of follicle size is critical because hCG is best administered once follicles reach 15–18 mm.[8]

Prediction of Ovulation

Follicular rupture occurs at a wide range of diameters between 2 cm and 2.7 cm. In the unstimulated ovary, follicles are approximately spherical. They may, however, be flattened in one plane by either pressure of the transducer or bladder so a mean of the maximum diameter in three planes is a better estimate of follicular size than measurements only in two planes.[5] In superovulation cycles, pressure from abutting follicles distorts the follicle so exact measurements are often difficult. Serial follicular measurement is best done by the same observer using the TVS route. In a recent study, assessment of follicular volume using 3D ultrasound was found to correlate better with oocyte retrieval than two-dimensional (2D) ultrasound alone. The authors found that a follicular size of >22 mm or a volume >5 mL was correlated with poor oocyte retrieval probably due to postmature follicle.[53]

Ovulation can also be predicted by noting collapse of a follicle that was previously seen, development of internal echoes within the follicle, crenation of follicular walls, visualization of cumulus, perifollicular halo, and visualization of fluid in the cul-de-sac (if not previously seen). However, fluid may commonly be seen in the pouch of Douglas in the periovulatory period and only a small percentage of women have a detectable increase with ovulation. Contrary to popular belief, ovulation need not alternate between two ovaries. Unfortunately, the variable appearance of ovulation makes the use these of ultrasound signs problematic in the management of infertility.[5]

Ultrasound Doppler studies reveal an increase in blood flow to the ovary carrying the dominant follicle[54-57] (and later, the CL)—an increase that precedes other indicators of follicular dominance. With maturation of the follicle, increased flow is directed to the follicle itself within the dominant ovary. Intrafollicular neovascularization occurs over the hours preceding ovulation and becomes massive after follicular collapse as blood vessels invade the luteinizing follicular (or granulosa) cells and the CL forms and impedance in intraovarian arterioles drops while velocities reach up to 40 cm/sec. These changes do not occur in nonovulatory cycles. A study was undertaken to investigate, if corpus luteal function could be improved by increasing CL blood flow in women with luteal phase defect (LPD) and high CL-RI ($\geq$0.51).[58] They concluded that vitamin E or L-arginine treatment improved luteal function by decreasing CL blood flow impedance.

Ovarian Reserve

Ovarian reserve describes the reproductive potential as a function of the number and quality of oocytes. Diminished ovarian reserve refers to women of reproductive age group having regular menses whose response to ovarian stimulation or fecundity is reduced as compared to those women of comparable age.

Various tests utilized to assess ovarian reserve include cycle-day 3 serum FSH and estradiol measurements (high values of >10–20 IU/L have been found to be associated with poor ovarian stimulation and failure to conceive) and the clomiphene citrate challenge test (CCCT), which involves serum FSH evaluation before and after treatment with clomiphene citrate (100 mg daily, days 5–9 of cycle) on day 3 and day 10. Elevated FSH concentration after this test suggests diminished ovarian reserve.[59] Other and more frequently done tests include AFC and serum anti-Müllerian hormone (AMH) levels.

Serum AMH Level

Serum AMH is produced by the granulosa cells of the antral follicles and is a marker for ovarian reserve. Its levels remain stable throughout the menstrual cycle and therefore it can be evaluated on any day of the cycle. Low AMH levels (<1 ng/mL) have been associated with poor responses to ovarian stimulation, poor embryo quality, and poor pregnancy outcomes in IVF.[59]

Antral Follicle Count

Antral follicle count (AFC) is a good surrogate marker for evaluating ovarian reserve. AFC is used for work up of infertility and assisted reproduction techniques, prediction of risk of menopause and to raise doubt of ovulatory dysfunction secondary to hyperandrogenism anovulation.

Four different types of follicles are found in the ovary at distinct stages of development—primordial, primary, secondary, and tertiary (or antral). The first three stages are too small to be visualized on USG. The antral follicles are identified by USG when they reach 2 mm in diameter, coinciding with higher sensitivity to FSH. Antral follicles measuring between 2 mm and 10 mm are "recruitable" while antral follicles >10 mm are "dominant follicles". AFC includes follicles that have a mean diameter varying from 2 mm to 10 mm.[60]

The follicles should preferably be counted in the early follicular phase of the menstrual cycle, however, it may be performed at any time of the menstrual cycle. It is important to consider that counting follicles in the early follicular phase is simpler as this decreases the chance of presence of an ovarian cyst or CL, which may mask some of the follicles. AFC <5–7 is associated with small number of oocytes retrieved and reduced pregnancy rate, whereas AFC more than or equal to 20 is associated with risk of ovarian hyperstimulation syndrome (OHSS).[60]

Indications for counting ovarian follicles include the following:

- Woman >35 years of age attempting pregnancy for >6 months
- Risk for diminished ovarian reserve—history of cancer treatment with gonadotoxic drugs or history of irradiation
- Surgery for endometriosis.

Antral follicle count can be performed with both 2D and 3D-USG.

Real-time Two-dimensional Ultrasonography

Transvaginal sonography is performed and after centering the ovary on screen, all the follicular structures measuring between 2 mm and 10 mm in diameter are identified and counted. Only one measurement is needed for round follicles and the mean of two diameters is calculated for oval follicles. Imaging quality can be improved by using tissue harmonic imaging. Real-time 2D USG requires the presence of the patient during the entire span of examination as follicular dimensions are obtained one at a time. However, real-time imaging helps in distinguishing between a follicle and parovarian cysts/hydrosalpinx and with Doppler a vascular structure can be differentiated from a follicle. In cine loop 2D USG, a single continuous sweep of each ovary is performed and the loops are saved and images can be analyzed. This shortens the duration of examination. The loops can be replayed and assessed in case of any doubt.[60]

Three-dimensional Manual Mode

Using the 3D manual mode, AFC can be performed while visualizing three perpendicular planes simultaneously. Automatic acquisition of the ovaries occurs and the volumes are stored and studied using the three orthogonal planes simultaneously. Cross-linking of follicles in different planes provides better reliability compared with 2D methods. Volume contrast imaging (VCI) is a 3D US tool that helps to improve contrast enhancement and speckle suppression, enabling better definition between tissues and/or organs and improves the contrast between fluid and surrounding structures. Inversion mode enables visualization of 3D arrangement of follicles and all of them can be seen at the same time. However, this is time consuming and requires specifically trained observers.

Sono Automated Volume Calculations (SonoAVC)

SonoAVC is a semi-automated technique that permits counting and measuring of diameters and volumes of anechoic structures within a particular region of interest of an acquired 3D dataset. Manual postprocessing may be required to include unidentified follicles and to exclude extraovarian structures or tissue that have been inaccurately identified as follicles. This requires particular ultrasound systems and specifically trained sonologists **(Figs. 25A and B)**.[60] **Table 2** lists the interpretation of AFC.

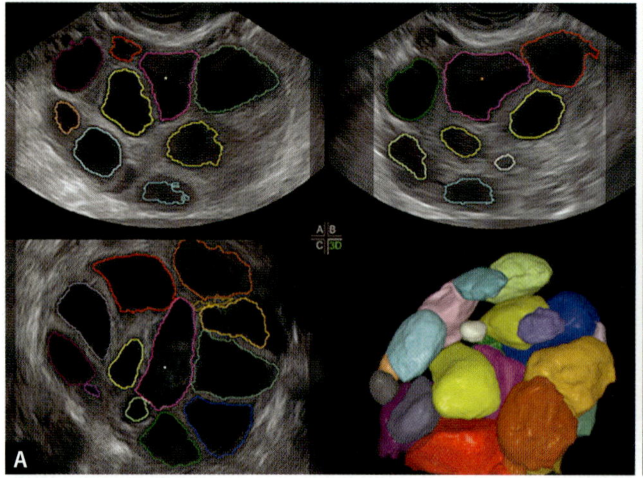

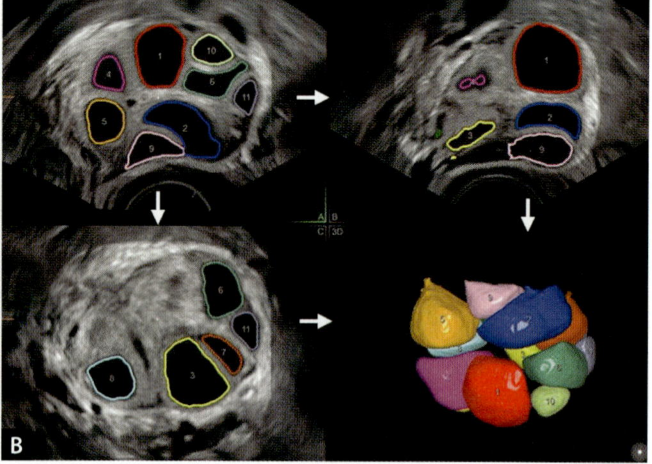

Figs. 25A and B: Sono AVC mode shows individual identification and automated volume calculation of the follicles, each depicted in a different color.

Table 2: Interpretation of AFC.

Nomenclature	*Total AFC*	*Interpretation for ovarian stimulation*
Very low functional reserve or very small number of recruitable follicles	0–4	Very high risk of poor response to ovarian stimulation and reduced chance of pregnancy
Low functional reserve or small number of recruitable follicles	5–8	High risk of poor response to ovarian stimulation
Normal functional reserve or normal number of recruitable follicles	9–19	Expected normal response to ovarian stimulation
High functional reserve or large number of recruitable follicles	>20	High risk of excessive ovarian response and OHSS
(AFC: antral follicle count; OHSS: ovarian hyperstimulation syndrome)		

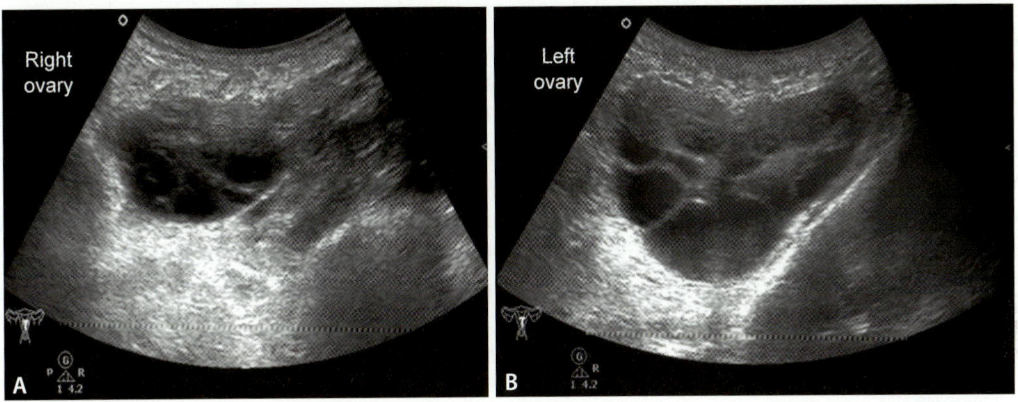

Figs. 26A and B: Transvaginal scans of both ovaries in a patient on ovulation induction reveals enlarged ovaries with a myriad of cysts varying in size consistent with ovarian hyperstimulation syndrome.

Luteinized Unruptured Follicle

The CL formed after ovulation may have a variety of ultrasound appearances. It may be imperceptible from the surrounding ovarian stroma, it may show a small cystic component with echoes or may be large (>40 mm) and be hemorrhagic.[5]

Failure to detect follicular collapse but with infilling of the follicle suggests luteinization without ovulation. The luteinized unruptured follicle (LUF) syndrome occurs more commonly in infertile patients than in fertile patients and may be a cause of unexplained infertility. However, ultrasound diagnosis has a 15% false positive rate. Great care should be taken in diagnosing this condition because ovulation may be associated with an increase in size of follicles and these cystic corpora lutea may indicate a conception cycle.

Ovarian Hyperstimulation Syndrome

Ovarian hyperstimulation syndrome is a potentially life-threatening complication of ovulation induction or ovarian stimulation. It occurs during the luteal phase of menstrual cycle or in early pregnancy and mostly follows administration of endogenous or exogenous LH or hCG. It occurs after hCG administration to patient with a large number of immature follicles and high serum estradiol levels and is more likely to occur in those with a polycystic ovarian morphology.

Ovarian hyperstimulation syndrome results when hyperstimulation of the ovaries is associated with an aberration of the fluid balance. It is characterized by third-space fluid accumulation and electrolyte abnormalities. The severity of the syndrome is variable, but it is usually more severe if pregnancy follows ovulation. The clinical features that cause concern are: nausea, vomiting, ascites, and pleural and pericardial effusion. These worsen hemoconcentration causing hyperviscosity and hypercoagulability which predispose to thrombosis, embolism, and renal failure.

On imaging, symmetric enlargement of bilateral ovaries is seen which contain multiple cystic areas of varying sizes which represent enlarged follicles or corpus luteal cysts in the presence of ascites. The "spoke wheel" appearance has been described with peripherally located follicles surrounding a central core of ovarian stroma. The cysts are usually anechoic but may contain hemorrhage **(Figs. 26A and B)**. On MRI, the cysts are hypointense on TIW images and hyperintense on T2W images. The enlarged ovaries can be differentiated from ovarian neoplasms by absence of any abnormal enhancing soft tissue in or around the cystic ovarian mass and the normal central ovarian stroma should be recognizable. Other imaging features related to complications associated with OHSS include pleural effusion, ascites, and thromboembolism. Gradual decrease in the size and number of cysts, resolution of the ascites, and pleural effusions may be seen on follow up scans.[61]

Ovarian hyperstimulation syndrome is classified according to the modified Golan classification scheme as shown in **Table 3**.

Mild and moderate OHSS is seen with clomiphene induction whereas the severe form is rarely seen in this situation.

A similar appearance of bilateral enlarged ovaries with multiple cysts resulting in a "spoke wheel" appearance can be seen with *theca lutein cysts*. They develop in response to raised levels of beta-hCG that occur with complete molar pregnancy. They may also be seen with singleton or multiple pregnancy or fetal hydrops.[62]

TREATING INFERTILITY

Increasingly assisted conception with IVF or one of its related therapeutic modalities is being used to treat infertility. These acronyms are summarized[36] in **Table 4**.

Follicle Aspiration

In the first successful IVF, oocytes were collected during laparoscopy which is an expensive procedure associated with complications such as periovarian adhesions, hemorrhage, infection, etc.

Ultrasound directed follicle aspiration (UDFA) has reduced costs considerably and can be done as an outpatient technique. Various approaches have been used in the past for follicular aspiration including direct transabdominal, transabdominal through full bladder, transvaginal, transvesical, and per-urethral approach.[5] Oocyte collection using TVS, first described by Wikland in 1985 has become the technique of choice, however, the actual method used can be tailored according to each patient depending on where the ovaries are situated.

Table 3: Modified Golan classification scheme for ovarian hyperstimulation syndrome.

Category	*Ovarian size (cm)*	*Grade*	*Signs and symptoms*
Mild	<6	I II	Abdominal distension Abdominal distension, nausea, vomiting, and diarrhea
Moderate	6–12	III	Abdominal distension, nausea, vomiting, diarrhea, ascites at USG, and weight gain
Severe	>12	IV V	Ascites/hydrothorax Ascites/hydrothorax, hypovolemia, hemoconcentration, coagulation disorder, and oliguria, shock

Table 4: Acronyms used in assisted conception.

IVF	Recovered eggs are fertilized with prepared sperm in the laboratory and transferred back to the genital tract after usually several days' culture.
IUI	Washed and concentrated sperms are placed inside the uterus around the time of ovulation to facilitate fertilization.
GIFT	Recovered eggs are almost immediately transferred, with prepared sperm, into the fallopian tubes, so that fertilization and early development occur in the normal situation; generally, a higher pregnancy rate than after IVF, provided the tube used is normal and normal sperm function can be assumed.
ZIFT	IVF in which 1 day fertilized eggs, or zygotes, are transferred to the fallopian tube.
Uterine ET	Conventional procedure with IVF: 2-day pre-embryos are transferred through the cervix to the endometrial cavity.
FET, FrET	Transfer of IVF pre-embryos previously cryostored.
TEST	2-day IVF pre-embryos are transferred to the tube instead of the uterus.
ICSI	Laboratory refinement for IVF in cases of severely depressed sperm function, in which a single sperm is selected and microinjected into each egg.
MESA	A means of obtaining sperm for ICSI in men with obstructive azoospermia.
TESE	A means of obtaining sperm cells from testicular tubules for ICSI in some men with nonobstructive azoospermia.

IVF: *in vitro* fertilization; IUI: intrauterine insemination ; GIFT: gamete intrafallopian transfer; ZIFT: zygote intrafallopian transfer; ET: embryo transfer; FET, FrET: frozen embryo transfer; TEST: tubal embryo-stage transfer; ICSI: intracytoplasmic sperm injection; MESA: microepididymal sperm aspiration; TESE: testicular sperm extraction

With all these aspiration techniques, a long (30 cm) 18-gauge needle is used that is scored at the tip, which results in its enhanced sonographic visualization. The procedure for follicle aspiration is performed under local anesthesia and with supplemental intravenous or intramuscular medication.

A needle guide is secured with the transvaginal transducer for aspiration through the transvaginal approach. This permits the needle to transverse in the beam path of the transducer. The cursor is seen on the scanning screen, which indicates the path of the needle. A condom containing sterile gel is placed over the transducer and a sterile needle guide is attached to it, the operator then manipulates the transducer to delineate the ovary optimally. The desired follicle is focused into the "line of sight" and the needle is introduced through the transvaginal route. After the initial aspiration, the follicle may be filled with buffered medium and flushed so that there are maximum chances of retrieving a mature oocyte. The technique has been associated with low complication rates that include vaginal hemorrhage and pelvic infection. When a transvesical or transurethral approach is used postoperative clot retention or occasionally urine extravasation may occur.

Transabdominal ultrasound-guided follicular aspiration is considered a safe option in women with ovaries that are not accessible by TVS. This approach is used in women with history of laparoscopic or pelvic laparotomy surgery, transposed ovaries, PCOS, fibroids, and Müllerian agenesis. Increased use of this approach due to increasing BMI in some populations has also been reported. No significant difference between pregnancy rates and associated complications was seen between transabdominal ultrasound and transvaginal ultrasound procedures.

Ultrasound has also been used to guide ET to the uterine cavity, to assist accurate placement of the embryos in the uterine cavity rather than cervical canal.

CONCLUSION

The causes of female infertility include abnormalities involving the uterus, cervix, tubes, peritoneum, and ovaries. Imaging plays a valuable role in evaluation of infertility and a multimodality approach is essential to establish the cause of infertility and guide further management and treatment. HSG is usually the initial investigation to be performed to assess for tubal patency, which may be followed by pelvic ultrasound, pelvic MRI or both as required. Imaging is also vital for guidance in various reproductive techniques such as oocyte collection and gamete transfer IVF programs.

REFERENCES

1. Pfeifer S, Goldberg J, Lobo R, et al. Definitions of infertility and recurrent pregnancy loss: a committee opinion. Practice Committee of American Society for Reproductive Medicine. Fertil Steril. 2013;99(1):63.
2. Jeelani R, Puscheck EE. Imaging and the Infertility Evaluation. Clin Obstet Gynecol. 2017;60(1):93-107.
3. Simpson WL, Beitia LG, Mester J. Hysterosalpingography: A reemerging study. Radiographics. 2006;26:419-31.
4. Speroff L, Fritz MA. Female Infertility. In: Speroff L, Fritz MA (Eds). Clinical gynecologic endocrinology and infertility, 7th edition. Philadelphia: Lippincott Williams and Wilkins; 2005. pp. 1013-67.
5. Steer CV, Parsons JH. Infertility. In: Dewbury K, Meire H, Cosgrove D, Farrant P (Eds). Ultrasound in Obstetrics and Gynaecology, 2nd Edition. London: Churchill Livingstone; 2001. pp. 99-122.
6. Hill LM. Transvaginal Sonography in an assisted conception program. In: Anderson JC (Ed). Gyneologic Imaging. London: Churchill Livingstone; 1999. pp. 585-99.
7. Saunders RD, Shwayder JM, Nakajima ST. Current methods of tubal patency assessment. Fertil Steril. 2011;95(7):2171-9.
8. Collins JI, Woodward PJ. Radiological evaluation of infertility. Semin Ultrasound CT MR. 1995;16(4):304-16.
9. Jaffe SB, Jewlewicz R. The basic infertility investigation. Fertil Steril. 1991;56:599-613.
10. ASRM Practice Committee. Optimal evaluation of the infertile female. Fertil Steril. 2006;86(4):264-7.
11. Glatstein IZ, Harlow BL, Hornstein MD. Practice patterns among reproductive endocrinologists: further aspects of the infertility evaluation. Fertile Steril. 1998;70:263-9.
12. Baldauf JJ, Dreyfus M, Wertz JP, et al. Consequences and treatment of cervical stenoses after laser conization or loop electrosurgical excision. J Gynecol Obstet Biol Reprod. 1997;26:64-70.
13. Christianson MS, Barker MA, Lindheim SR. Overcoming the challenging cervix: techniques to access the uterine cavity. J Low Genit Tract Dis. 2008;12:24-31.
14. Krysiewicz S. Infertility in Women: Diagnostic evaluation with hysterosalpingography and other imaging techniques. Am J Roentgenol. 1992;159:253-61.
15. Thurmond AS. Imaging of female infertility. Radiol Clin N Am. 2003;41:757-67.
16. Kaproth-Joslin K, Dogra V. Imaging of female infertility: a pictorial guide to the hysterosalpingography, ultrasonography and magnetic resonance imaging findings of the congenital and acquired causes of female infertility. Radiol Clin North Am. 2013;51(6):967-81.
17. Dudiak CM, Turner DA, Patel SK, et al. Uterine leiomyomas in the infertile patient: Preoperative localization with MR imaging versus US and hysterosalpingography. Radiol. 1988;167:627-30.
18. Woodward PJ. Wagner BJ, Farley TE. MR imaging in the evaluation of female infertility. Radiographics. 1993;13:293-310.
19. Vickramarajah S, Stewart V, Ree K, et al. Subfertility: What the Radiologist Needs to Know? Radiographics. 2017;37:1587-602.
20. Grimbizis GF, Gordts S, Sardo ADS, et al. The ESHRE/ESGE consensus on the classification of female genital tract congenital anomalies. Hum Reprod. 2013;28(8):2032-44.

21. Steinkeler JA, Woodfield CA, Lazarus E, et al. Female infertility: a Systematic approach to Radiologic Imaging and Diagnosis. Radiographics. 2009;29:1353-70.
22. Olphin JD, Heilbrum M. Imaging of Müllerian duct anomalies Clin Obstet Gynaecol. 2007;52(1):40-56.
23. Deutch TD, Abuhamad AZ. The role of 3D-USG and MR imaging in the diagnosis of MDA: a review of literature. J Ultrasound Med. 2008;27(3):413-23.
24. Ludwin A, Martins WP, Nastri CO, et al. Congenital Uterine Malformations by Experts (CUME): better criteria for distinguishing between normal/arcuate and septate uterus? Ultrasound Obstet Gynecol. 2018;51(1):101-9.
25. Kunz G, Beil D, Huppert P, et al. Adenomyosis in endometriosis: prevalence and impact on fertility. Evidence from magnetic resonance imaging. Hum Reprod. 2005;20:2309-16.
26. Park HJ, Kim YS, Yoon TK, et al. Chronic endometritis and infertility. Clin Exp Reprod Med. 2016;43(4):185-92.
27. Khan MS, Shaikh A, Ratnani R. Ultrasonography and Doppler Study to Predict Uterine Receptivity in Infertile Patients Undergoing Embryo Transfer. J Obstet Gynaecol India. 2016;66(1):377-82.
28. Tekay A, Martikainen H, Jouppilas P. The clinical value of transvaginal colour Doppler ultrasound in assisted reproductive technology procedures. Hum Reprod. 1996;11(8):1589-91.
29. Dev G, Ilyas M, Khurana A. Calcific endometritis as a cause of infertility: Ultrasonography as the main diagnostic modality. Egypt J Radiol Nucl Med. 2016;47(3):1133-6.
30. Thurmond AS, Novy MJ, Rosch J. Terburaline in diagnosis of interstitial fallopian tube obstruction. Invest Radiol. 1988;23:209-10.
31. Sulak PJ, Letterie, GS, Coddington CC, et al. Histology of proximal tubal occlusion. Fertil Steril. 1987;48:437-40.
32. Thurmond AS. Selective salpingography and fallopian tube recanalization. Am J Roentgenol. 1991;156:33-8.
33. Rösch J. Thurmond AS, Vchida BT, et al. Selective transcervical fallopian tube catherterization: Technique update. Radiol. 1988;168:1-5.
34. Thurmond AS, Rösch J. Nonsurgical fallopian tube recanalization for treatment of infertility. Radiol. 1990;174:371-4.
35. National Institute for Health and Care Excellence. (2004). Fallopian tube recanalisation by guidewire: guidance and guidelines. [online] Available from: https://www.nice.org.uk/guidance/ipg71. [Last accessed November, 2019].
36. Jansen RPS, Ramsay PA. Imaging in gynecologic infertility. In: Anderson JC (Ed). Gynecologic Imaging. London: Churchill Livingstone; 1999. pp. 567-80.
37. Strandell A, Waldenstrom U, Nilsson L, et al. Hydrosalpinx reduces *in vitro* fertilization/embryo transfer pregnancy rates. Hum Reprod. 1994;9:861-3.
38. Andersen AN, Yue Z, Meng FJ, et al. Low implantation rate after in-vitro fertilization in patients with hydrosalpinges diagnosed by ultrasonography. Hum Reprod. 1994;9:1935-8.
39. Donnez J, Casanas-Roux E. Prognostic factors of fimbrial microsurgery. Fertil Steril. 1986;46:200-4.
40. Valentini AL, Muzuil L, Marana R. Improvement of hysterosalpingographic accuracy in the diagnosis of peritubal adhesions. AJR. 2000;175:1173-6.
41. Krysiewicz S. Infertility in women: Diagnostic evaluation with hysterosalpingography and other imaging techniques. AJR. 1992;158:253-61.
42. Schenken RS. Endometriosis. In: Scott JR, Di Saia PJ, Hammona CB, Spellacy WN (Eds). Danforth's Obstetrics and Gynaecology, 8th edition. Philadelphia, PA: Lippincott Williams and Wilkins; 1999. pp. 669-75.
43. Imaka I, Wada A, Matsuo M, et al. MR imaging of disorders associated with female infertility: use in diagnosis, treatment and management. Radiographics. 2003;23:1401-21.
44. Das P, Ahuja A, Gupta SD. Incidence, etiopathogenesis and pathological aspects of genitourinary tuberculosis in India: a journey revisited. Indian J Urol. 2008;24:356-61.
45. Merchant SA. Tuberculosis of the genitourinary system. Ind J Radiol Imag. 1993;3:253-74.
46. Quaas A, Dokras A. Diagnosis and Treatment of unexplained infertility. Rev Obstet Gynecol. 2008;1(2): 69-76.
47. Teede HJ, Misso ML, Costello MF, et al. Recommendations from the international evidence-based guideline for the assessment and management of polycystic ovary syndrome. International PCOS Network. Hum Reprod. 2018;33(9):1602-18.
48. Lee TT, Rausch ME. Polycystic Ovarian Syndrome: Role of Imaging in Diagnosis. Radiographics. 2012;32:1643-57.
49. Fleischer AC, Daniell JF, Rodein J, et al. Sonographic monitoring of ovarian follicular development. J Clin Ultrasound. 1981;9:275-80.
50. Fleischer AC, Herbert CM, Hill GA, et al. Transvaginal sonography of the endometrium during induced cycles. J Ultrasound Med. 1991;10:93-5.
51. Haning RV, Zwiebel WJ. Ultrasound assistance in clinical management of infertility. Semin Ultrasound CT MR. 1983;4:226-34.
52. Hann LE, Crivello M, McArdle C, et al. In vitro fertilization: Sonographic perspective. Radiol. 1987;163:665-8.
53. Shmorgun D, Hughes E, Mohida P, et al. Prospective cohort study of three versus two dimensional ultrasound for prediction of oocyte maturity. Fertil Steril. 2010;93(4):1333-7 .
54. Campbell S, Bourne TH, Waterstone J, et al. Transvaginal colour blood flow imaging of the periovulatory follicle. Fertil Steril. 1993;60:433-8.
55. Taylor KJ, Wells PN, Conway DI, et al. Ultrasound Doppler flow studies of the ovarian and uterine arteries. Br J Obstet Gynaecol. 1985;92:240-6.
56. Deutinger J, Reinthaller A, Bernaschek G. Transvaginal pulsed Doppler measurement of blood flow velocity in the ovarian arteries during cycle stimulation and after follicle puncture. Fertil Steril. 1989;51:466-70.
57. Collins W, Jurkovic D, Bourne T, et al. Ovarian morphology, endocrine function and intrafollicular blood flow during the peri-ovulatory period. Hum Reprod. 1991;6:319-24.
58. Takasaki A, Tamura H, Taniguchi K, et al. Luteal blood flow and luteal function. J Ovarian Res. 2009;2:1.
59. Practice Committee of the American Society for Reproductive Medicine. Diagnostic evaluation of the infertile female: a committee opinion. Fertil Steril. 2015;103(6):e44-50.
60. Coelho Neto MA, Ludwin A, Borrell A, et al. Counting ovarian antral follicles by ultrasound: a practical guide. Ultrasound Obstet Gynecol. 2018;51(1):10-20.
61. Baron KT, Babagbemi KT, Arleo EK, et al. Emergent complications of assisted reproduction: expecting the unexpected. RadioGraphics. 2013;33:229-44.
62. Brown DL, Dudiak KM, Laing FC. Adnexal masses: US characterization and reporting. Radiol. 2010;254:342-54.

SECTION 4

Male Genital Tract

Chapter 19

Imaging Techniques and Radiological Anatomy of the Male Genital Tract

Anmol Bhatia, Paramjeet Singh, Sameer Vyas

MALE GENITAL TRACT

The male genital tract consists of the prostate, testes with epididymis, vas deferentia, seminal vesicles, and penis. The present chapter aims to discuss the various imaging techniques and the normal radiological anatomy of the organs constituting the male genital tract.

PROSTATE GLAND

Prostate gland is a pyramidal-shaped fibromuscular gland which surrounds the urethra from the bladder base up to the urogenital diaphragm. It has a thin capsule and is surrounded by fibrous sheath of pelvic fascia. Posterior to the prostate, paired seminal vesicles are present. The ejaculatory ducts penetrate the superior part along the posterior surface of the prostate gland and then open into the prostatic urethra along the lateral margin of the prostatic utricle. The prostate gland can be divided into two major zones—the peripheral and the central zones. The central gland comprises periurethral glandular tissue, and transitional and central zones.

IMAGING MODALITIES

Ultrasound

The prostate is routinely imaged using transabdominal and transrectal approaches. Transabdominally, a 3–5 MHz transducer is used with the full bladder acting as an acoustic window. The suprapubic approach allows for gross evaluation of the prostate size but does not provide images of sufficient quality to visualize the zonal anatomy **(Fig. 1)**.

Transrectal ultrasonography (TRUS) is the preferred sonological technique as it demonstrates the zonal anatomy, as well as helps in visualization of seminal vesicles and ejaculatory ducts. The most commonly used transducers (frequency ranging from 5 MHz to 8 MHz) fire from the end. The advantages of end-viewing probe designs include patient convenience, ease of use, and biopsy capability at the time of the diagnostic examination.

The patient is examined with empty bladder in the left lateral decubitus position with the knees flexed up to the abdomen. The probe is lubricated and covered by a rubber balloon or condom, and is then inserted gently into the rectum. In the sagittal plane, the gland is systematically evaluated from right to midline to left;

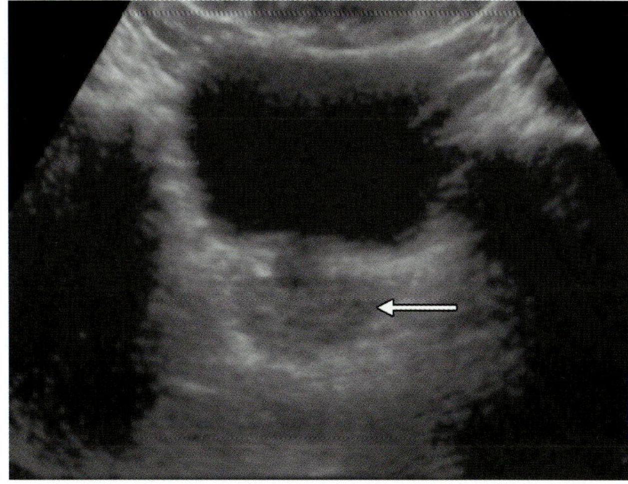

Fig. 1: Transabdominal axial scan showing a normal prostate gland (arrow) without any zonal demarcation behind the urinary bladder.

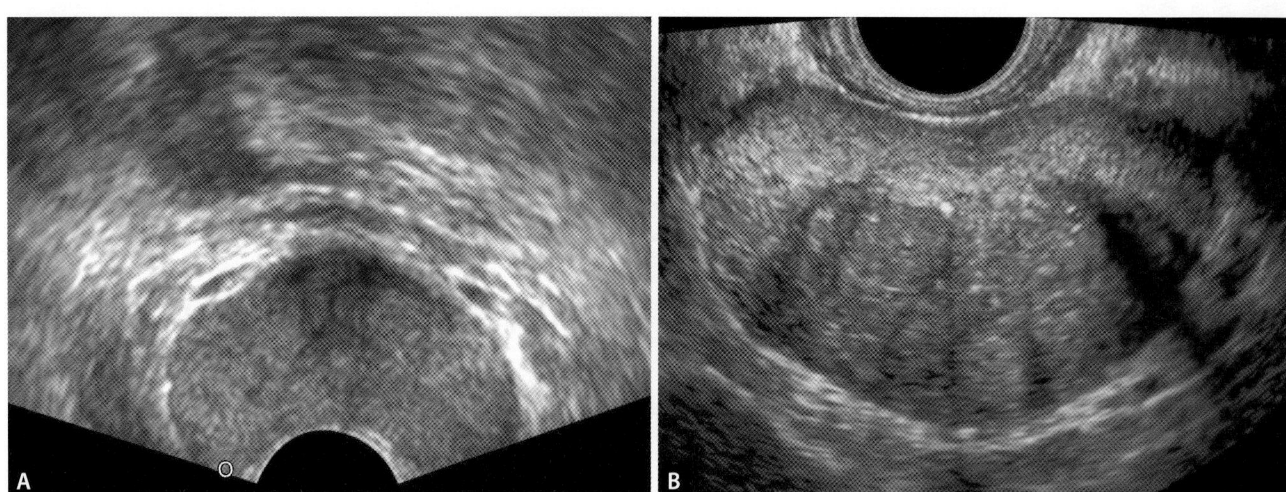

Figs. 2A and B: Transrectal axial images of normal prostate at midgland level in a young (A) and a middle age male (B). Demarcation of the central and peripheral zone is seen in middle age male.

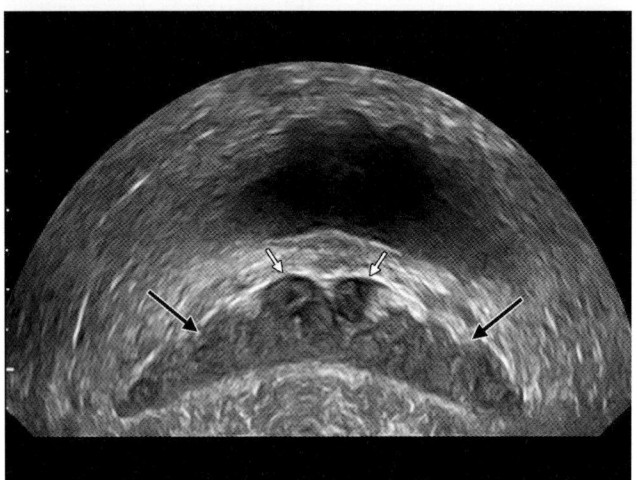

Fig. 3: Transrectal axial image showing paired seminal vesicles (black arrows) and vas (white arrows).

while in the axial plane, cranial to caudal viewing is done from a plane starting cranially just superior to the prostate and extending caudally to the apex of the prostate. The central and peripheral zones form the bulk of prostate gland and appear uniformly hyperechoic with only subtle differentiation in their echogenicity. The hypoechoic periurethral area corresponds to the transitional zone **(Figs. 2A and B)**. The posterior urethra and its surrounding smooth muscle and glandular area appear relatively hypoechoic and can be quite prominent measuring up to 2 cm in diameter. Near the apex of the gland most of the tissue is the peripheral zone.

The seminal vesicles are paired, symmetric hypoechoic structures and seen cephalic to the base of prostate **(Fig. 3)**. They normally measure up to 1 cm in thickness, but sometimes may be of larger size in normal men.[1]

Prostatic volume can be calculated on transabdominal ultrasound and TRUS by using the Dodd's formula (0.523 × length × width × height).

Computed Tomography

Computed tomography is not a preferred modality to evaluate the prostate gland. A normal prostate appears as homogeneous hyperdense on CT. It is not possible to differentiate normal prostate from hyperplastic gland or detect the tumor which is limited to the prostate gland.

Magnetic Resonance Imaging

Magnetic resonance imaging (MRI) has a unique ability for delineating the zonal anatomy of the prostate gland.[2] The zonal anatomy is of clinical importance, as most carcinoma arises in the peripheral zone, while the benign hyperplasia affects the transition zone.[3] The relationship of the zones of the gland normally changes with age. The central gland predominantly consists of central zone in young population, whereas in older population with benign hyperplasia of prostate, most of the central gland is transitional zone. The prostate is described based on the division of the gland into thirds in the craniocaudal direction (base, midgland, and apex), and then into left and right side. Since surgery is potentially curable in a tumor confined to the gland, it is important to diagnose the extracapsular tumor spread, seminal vesicle, and other adjacent visceral involvement and pelvic lymphadenopathy. The primary role of MRI is not for tumor detection, but for staging diagnosed cancer. In addition, it helps in cancer localization, in treatment planning, and post-treatment follow-up.[3]

MR spectroscopic examination is helpful for showing normal and altered tissue metabolism. Functional MR techniques on 3T-MRI such as diffusion-weighted images (DWI) and dynamic contrast-enhanced MRI have evolved as promising new techniques in the assessment of prostate cancer. Multimodality MRI which includes T2-weighted images (T2WI), functional imaging, and spectroscopic imaging may be able to accurately characterize and stage the carcinoma.[4]

Technique and Recommended Sequences

Magnetic resonance imaging provides one-stop examination for detailed evaluation of prostate gland, periprostatic and pelvic anatomy. The results of prostate imaging using body coil are not very satisfactory. Use of an endorectal coil along with a pelvic phased-array coil markedly improves the quality of images. A balloon-mounted endorectal coil placed in the rectum provides the best contrast and spatial resolution for prostate imaging, and the pelvic phased array coil provide good pelvic coverage and simultaneously assess pelvic side walls and lymphadenopathy.

Axial spin-echo T1-weighted images (T1WI) are taken of the entire pelvis, i.e. from the level of aortic bifurcation to the pubic symphysis for the detection of nodal disease.[5] High spatial resolution [thin sections with a small field of view (FOV)] T2W fast spin-echo (FSE) sections in the axial, coronal, and sagittal planes including prostate and seminal vesicles are useful for the detection of tumor, its localization, and staging. Axial T2WI is important in differentiating peripheral and central zones, whereas coronal and sagittal images are useful to assess the base and apex of the gland, pelvic muscles, rectum, and seminal vesicles.

Prostate imaging should not be performed for at least 4–8 weeks (preferably 6 weeks) of biopsy, as hemorrhage can lead to a false positive and negative interpretation of cancer. Routine use of gadolinium and fat suppression is not recommended. However, contrast may be used in evaluation of prostatic infections and abscesses. Enhancement of prostate cancer during the first pass of contrast during dynamic scanning has indicated its potential for the detection of cancer, especially the more aggressive ones. For dynamic contrast-enhanced MRI, the data may be evaluated in a semiquantitative (contrast arrival, time to peak, peak enhancement, and wash-in-washout gradient) or quantitative approach using pharmacokinetic modeling method. MR spectroscopy is performed by chemical shift imaging with point resolved spectroscopy voxel excitation and band selective inversion with gradient rephrasing for water and lipid suppression.[5] Diffusion imaging with value from 0 to 800 have been applied to obtain data and create apparent diffusion coefficient maps which show restriction in high cellularity of tumors.

Normal Appearance of Prostate on MRI

The appearance of prostate varies depending on the coil type and the technique used. On T1WI the zonal anatomy cannot be appreciated well and the gland is of uniform low signal intensity but postbiopsy hemorrhage is better seen in these images. T1WI also show cysts and abscesses well. The zonal anatomy is well-demonstrated on T2WI, where the peripheral zone is seen as a relatively bright area compared to the central gland[2] **(Figs. 4A and B)**. It is surrounded by a thin uninterrupted hypointense line comprising true prostatic capsule. The anterior fibromuscular stroma is dark on all pulse sequences **(Fig. 5)**. The central and transitional zones show intermediate signal due to sparse glandular elements. These cannot be differentiated from each other but in older men the transitional zone stands out due to hypertrophy. The verumontanum may be seen on T2WI, where it has high signal intensity. The anterior fibromuscular stroma is dark on all pulse sequences. The periprostatic fat is hyperintense on both T1WI and T2WI and allows easy assessment of periprostatic spread of growth. The pelvic bone marrow shows high signal. The neurovascular bundles are seen at 5 and 7 o'clock position on axial images and are outlined by periprostatic fat, pelvic fascia, and muscles.[2] The seminal vesicles and vas can be well seen on in both the axial and coronal planes **(Figs. 6A and B)**. Seminal vesicle fluid appears bright on T2WI due to water content, while the walls are hypointense. Loss of signal in these structures indicate invasion by malignancy. The prostate volume can be assessed on MR images by using the Dodd's formula.

Prostate spectroscopic examination shows relative concentrations of citrate, creatinine, choline, and polyamines inside the contiguous voxels. Normal prostate tissue shows high levels of citrate **(Fig. 7)**.[5] High field strength imaging may improve the quality of the spectra.

SCROTUM AND PENIS

The scrotum consists of skin, muscle and fascial layers, and the tunica vaginalis. The tunica vaginalis is a two-layered serous membrane which develops from the processus vaginalis during the development. The outer

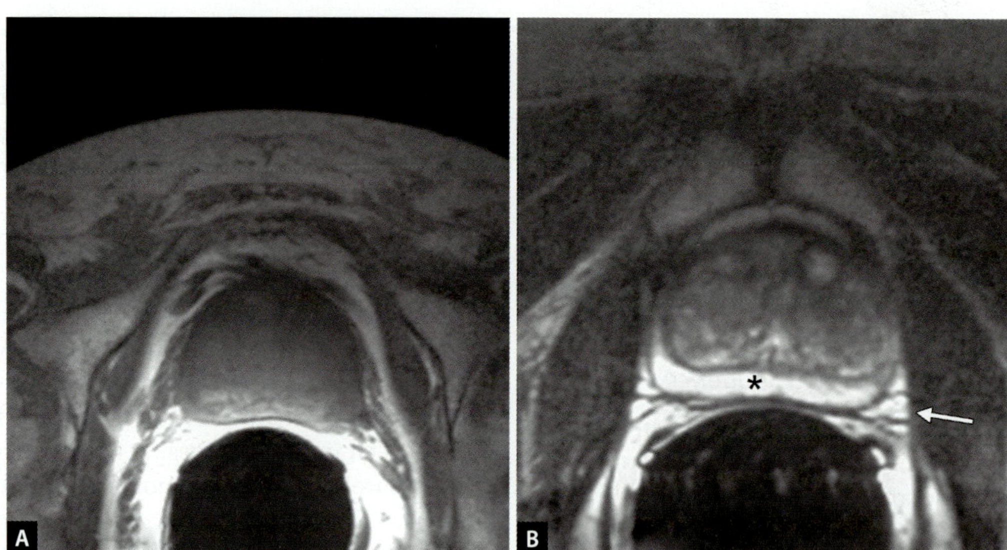

Figs. 4A and B: T1 (A) and T2 (B) weighted axial sections of prostate using endorectal coil. The zonal anatomy of prostate is not made out on T1 but the gland contour is well-outlined against bright periprostatic fat. The neurovascular bundle (arrow) is seen at 5 and 7 o'clock positions. T2WI (B) shows zonal anatomy, i.e. hyperintense peripheral gland (*) and heterogeneous central zone due to hyperplastic changes. The bright nodule represents glandular hyperplasia and dark areas being stromal hyperplasia. The surgical and anatomical capsules are seen as hypointense structures. The near field signal amplification is seen in proximity of the coil.

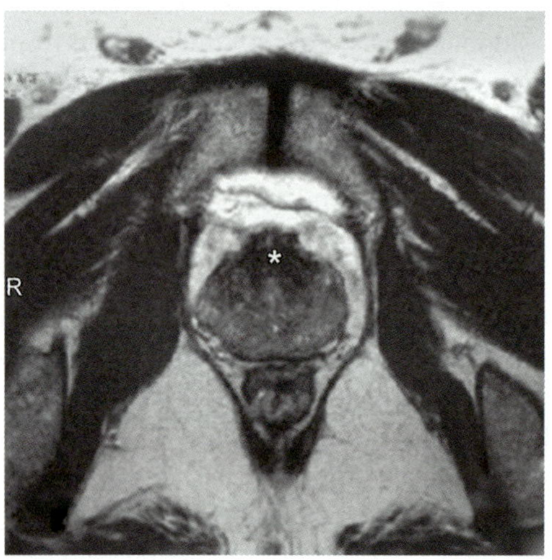

Fig. 5: T2-weighted axial section in a young adult. The gland does not show central and peripheral zone distinction or any hyperplastic central gland changes. The fibromuscular stroma anteriorly appears hypointense (*).

parietal layer forms the inner lining of the scrotum, while the inner visceral layer encloses the testis and epididymis.[6]

The penis contains paired corpora cavernosa dorsally and a midline corpus spongiosum ventrally. Tunica albuginea which is a fascial sheath surrounds both the corpus spongiosum and the corpora cavernosa. The corpora cavernosa contains venous sinusoids which are filled with blood during erection. The deep cavernosal arteries run centrally through the length of each corpus cavernosum with dorsal arteries lying superficially. The dorsal vein of the penis lies between the two dorsal arteries. The corpus spongiosum encases the penile urethra and forms the glans penis distally.[6]

IMAGING MODALITIES

Ultrasound

A high-frequency (7.5–15 MHz) linear probe is used for scanning the scrotum and penis.

Normal Appearance

The layers of the normal scrotal wall cannot be identified separately on ultrasound and are seen as a single 5–7 mm thick hyperechoic stripe. The testis is seen as an ovoid structure with homogeneous granular echotexture having medium level echoes surrounded by an echogenic capsule **(Fig. 8)**. The mediastinum testis (which is a longitudinal condensation of fibrous tissue on one side of the testis) is seen as a thin echogenic band on the same side as the epididymis with fine hypoechoic strands of septa radiating from it into the testicular parenchyma **(Fig. 9)**. The appearance of mediastinum testis depends on the amount of fibrous and fatty tissue.[7] The head of the epididymis is relatively isoechoic or slightly hyperechoic to the adjacent testis, while the main body is hypoechoic and lies along the posterolateral aspect of testis.

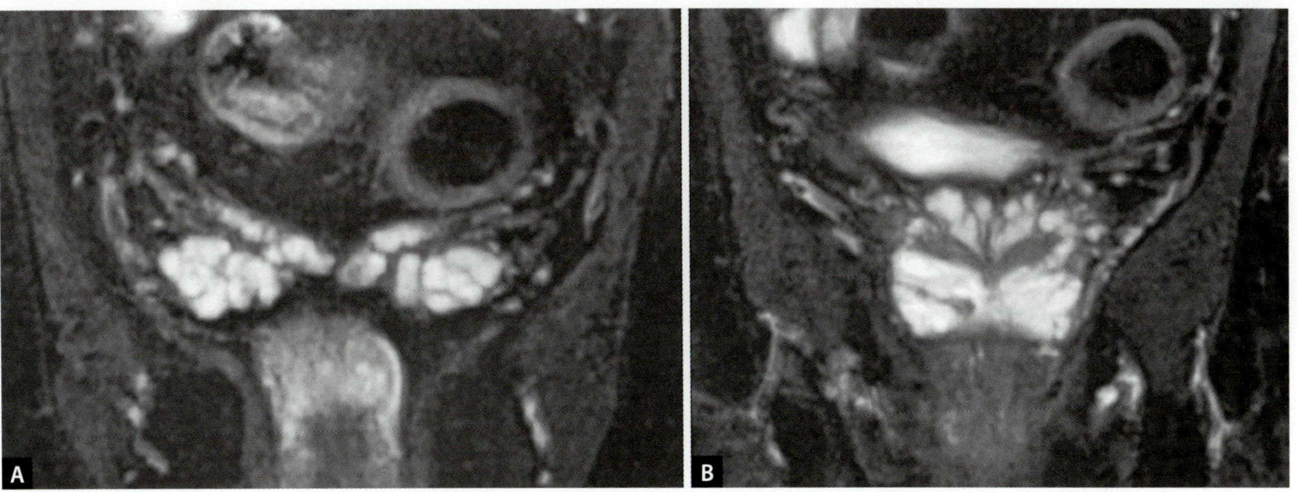

Figs. 6A and B: Coronal T2 images showing junction of the vas deferens and the seminal vesicle (A) both appearing normally bright due to fluid. More anteriorly (B) the ejaculatory ducts are seen approaching the verumontanum, where they open into the urethra.

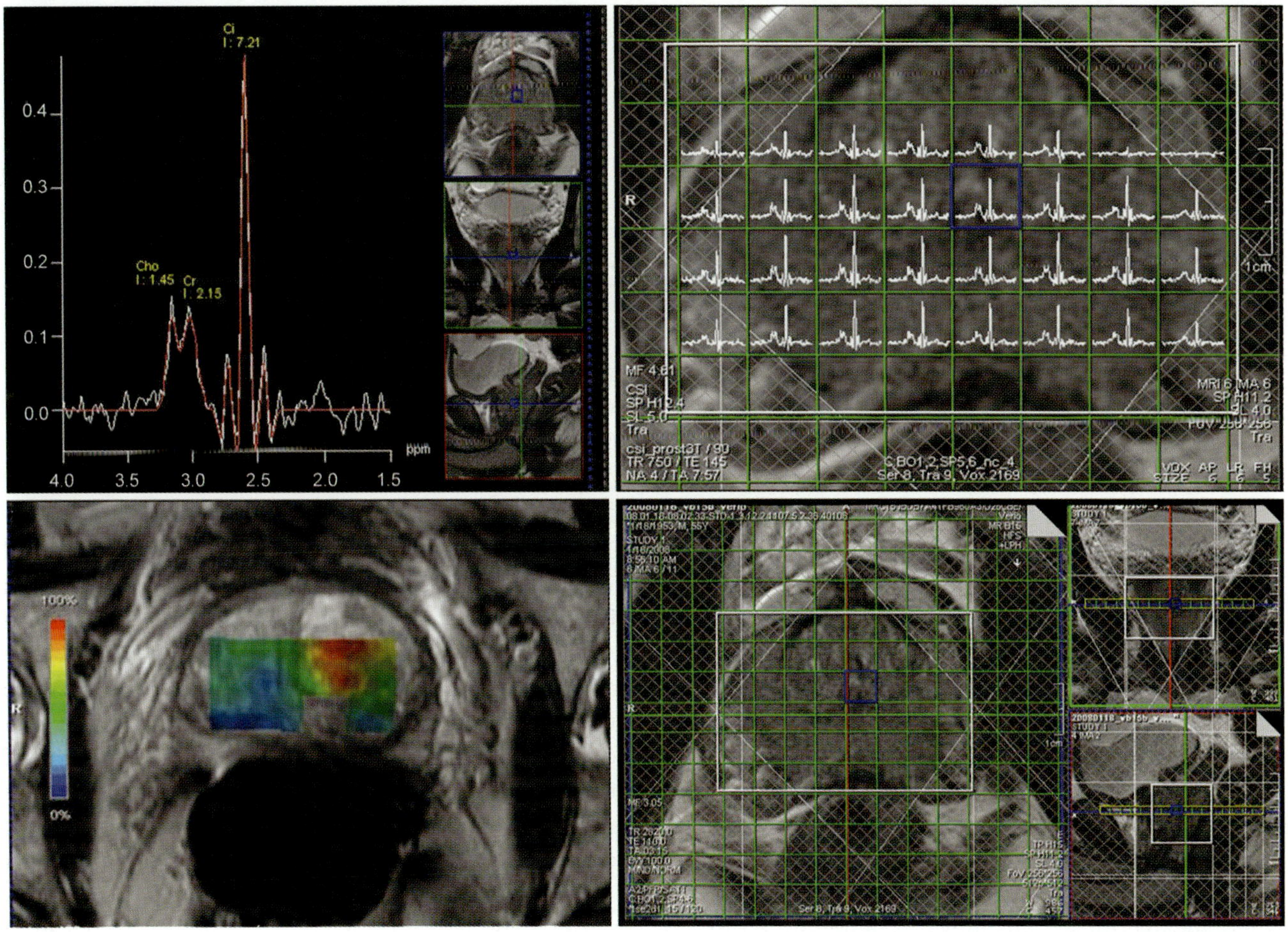

Fig. 7: Proton magnetic resonance spectroscopic imaging (3DCSI-voxel size 8 × 8 × 8, spin echo TE 145, TR 750, total acquisition time 7.57 minutes). Spectra from normal prostate tissue shows dominant citrate peak at 2.6 ppm and choline/creatinine complex at 3–3.2 ppm. Metabolite map (lower left) and spectral map (upper right) are seen over laid on the T2 axial image. Volume selection (lower right) with presaturation slabs is to suppress periprostatic fat.

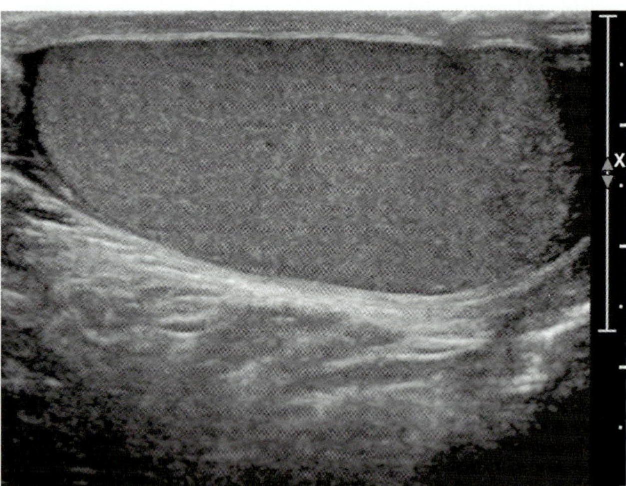

Fig. 8: Ultrasound image showing a normal testis.

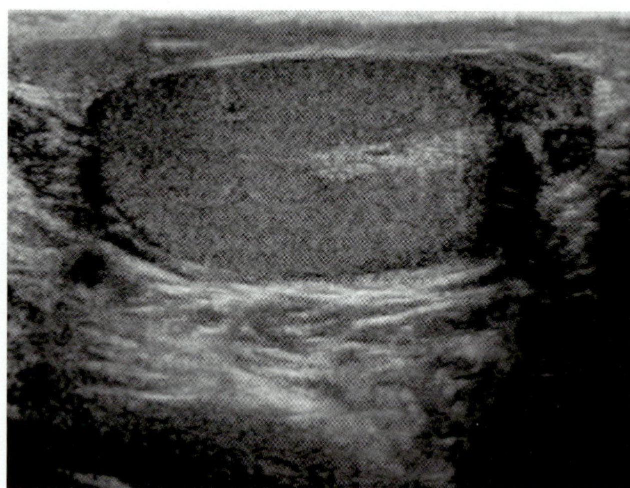

Fig. 9: Ultrasound image showing echogenic stripe of mediastinum testis.

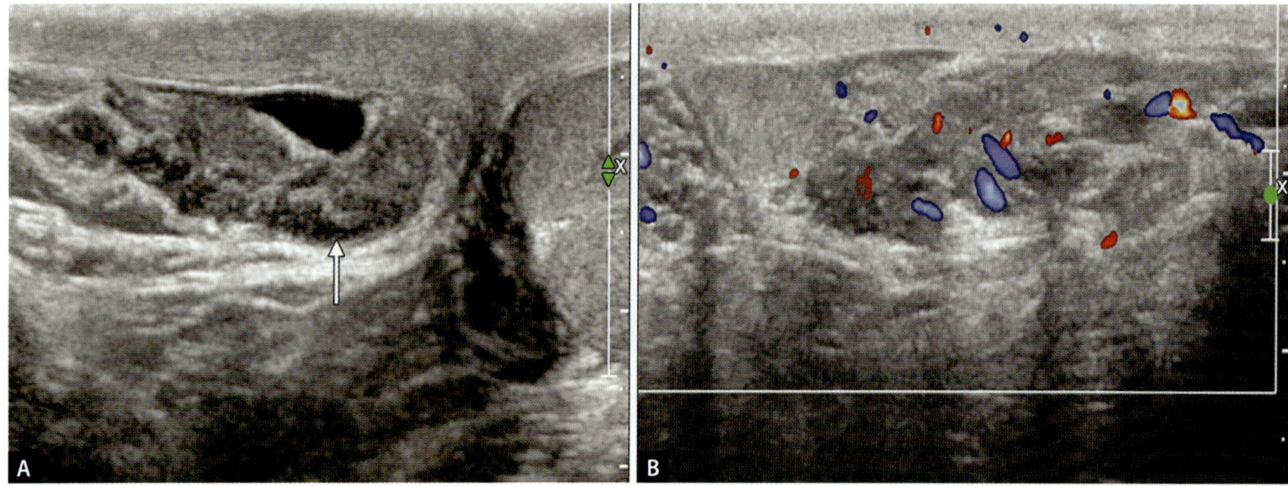

Figs. 10A and B: Ultrasound images showing a hypoechoic spermatic cord (arrow in A) with vascularity within on color Doppler (B).

The appendix testis is a remnant of the paramesonephric duct, and may be seen as a small ovoid structure seen along the superior pole of the testis, or in the groove between the testis and the head of the epididymis.[8]

The vas is difficult to identify and is seen as a fine hypoechoic tubular structure with a hyperechoic lumen running along the epididymis. The spermatic cord contains the vas deferens; the deferential, cremasteric and testicular arteries; pampiniform venous plexus; the lymphatics; and the nerves of the testis **(Figs. 10A and B)**. The normal spermatic cord is difficult to distinguish from the adjacent soft tissues of the inguinal canal sonologically, but its position can be identified by the pulsations of the testicular artery within it.

Examination of penis is performed in transverse and longitudinal planes. Scanning should be done from the glans to the base of the penis. A transperineal approach may be used for assessing the base of the penis.

The corpora cavernosa are seen as two circular structures adjacent to each other, of medium echogenicity with the deep arteries lying medially within them on the transverse section.[9] The corpus spongiosum is difficult to visualize optimally from the ventral aspect as it is usually compressed. It is more hypoechoic with the urethra seen as an anechoic central area within it. The tunica albuginea is seen as a hyperechoic capsule encasing all the three corporal structures **(Fig. 11)**.

Doppler Evaluation

On color Doppler, the normal testis shows little flow in the testicular tissue, but larger centripetal and centrifugal vessels are seen in the lobular septa and around the

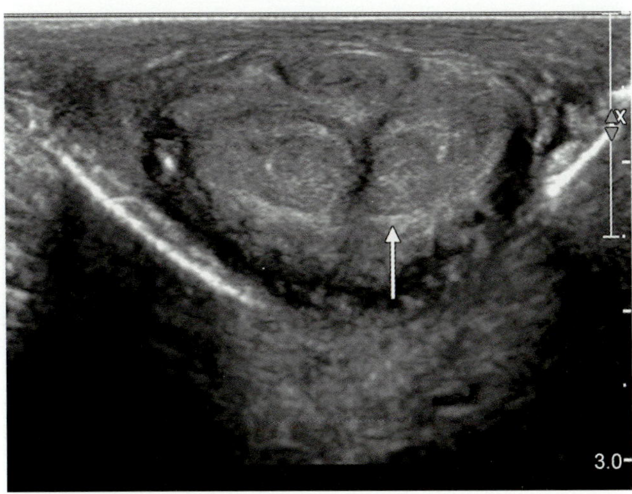

Fig. 11: Transverse ultrasound image of the penis showing corpora spongiosum and paired corpora cavernosa encased by echogenic tunica albuginea (arrow).

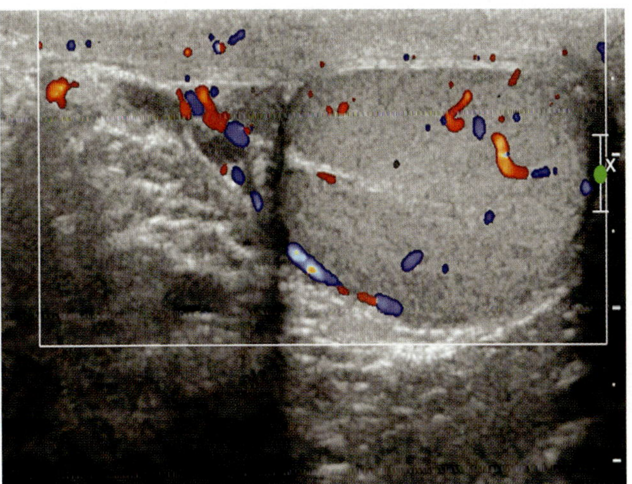

Fig. 12: Ultrasound image showing normal vascularity pattern of testis on color Doppler.

capsule **(Fig. 12)**. The velocity waveforms of the normal capsular and intratesticular arteries show high levels of antegrade diastolic flow, reflecting the low vascular resistance of the testis. The peak systolic flow velocities in intratesticular arteries, including capsular arteries, range from 4 cm/sec to 23.4 cm/sec (mean 10.8), end-diastolic velocities from 1.6 cm/sec to 9.2 cm/sec (mean 3.8) and resistive index (RI) from 0.46 to 0.78 (mean 0.64).[10] Supratesticular arterial waveforms vary in their appearance. Two main types of waveform exist: (1) A low resistance waveform (testicular artery and its branches) and (2) a high-resistance waveform with a sharp, narrow systolic peak and little or no diastolic flow which is believed to reflect the high vascular resistance of the extratesticular tissues (supplied by the branches of cremasteric and deferential arteries).[10]

The Doppler evaluation of the penis will be dealt in detail in the chapter on male infertility and sexual dysfunction.

Magnetic Resonance Imaging

Patients should be positioned supine, with a support placed between thighs in the upper part which will elevate the scrotum. The penis should be dorsiflexed against the anterior pelvic wall and secured using a bandage or a dressing in order to avoid its motion during the scan. A multiple phased array surface coil is used and kept covering the lower abdominopelvic wall as well as scrotum. To scan the penis and/or scrotum, a small FOV (up to 16 cm) and thin slices (4 mm) nonfat-suppressed FSE T2 should be used having a high resolution (matrix of at least 256 ×192 or higher).[9] The scan should be performed in all the three planes (sagittal, axial, and coronal). A full-FOV T2WI through the pelvis should be added in patients with known/suspected malignancy or infection. Use of dual-echo (in- and opposed-phase) spoiled Gradient Echo (GRE) T1W (11) sequence will help to identify the lesions that contain lipid, and also will improve the depiction of blood products because of the T2* effects of these substances. In cases of a suspicion of mass or a palpable abnormality, at least one FS sequence should also be included to identify macroscopic fat. Fat-suppressed FSE or short-tau inversion recovery T2WI helps in identification of fluid collections or soft-tissue edema. A three-dimensional (3D)-FS spoiled GRE T1WI should be done in the axial plane before as well as after the administration of intravenous contrast. Postcontrast 3D spoiled GRE imaging should also be done in coronal and/or sagittal planes for staging of cancer or delineating the extent of an infectious process. Axial DWI may be added in patients with suspected infection or a tumor.[9]

A normal adult testis is homogeneously hyperintense ovoid structure on T2WI **(Fig. 13)** and hypo- to isointense on T1WI. Tunica albuginea is seen as T1/T2 hypointense rim. The epididymis is hypointense on T2WI and isointense on T1WI compared to the testis. The testis and epididymis show enhancement following the intravenous contrast administration.[9]

The corpora spongiosum and the corpora cavernosa show bright signal on T2WI and intermediate signal on T1WI. The urethral musculature is hypointense relative to the encasing corpus spongiosum. The tunica albuginea shows hypointense signal on T1WI and T2WI. Following

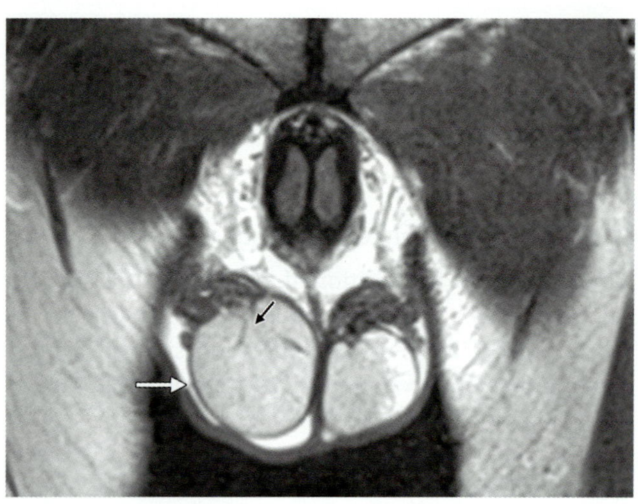

Fig. 13: T2 coronal magnetic resonance image of the scrotum showing testes as high signal intensity structures within the scrotum. Note the hypointense rim of tunica albuginea (white arrow) around the testes and the mediastinum testis (black arrow) within it.
Courtesy: Dr Anupam Lal and Dr Manphool Singhal, PGIMER, Chandigarh.

contrast administration, the corpora cavernosa shows a gradual enhancement with a centrifugal pattern, while early enhancement is seen in the corpora spongiosum.[9]

REFERENCES

1. Rickards D, Hare C. The lower urinary tract. In: Meire HB, Cosgrove D, Dewbury KC, Farrant P (Eds). Abdominal and General Ultrasound. Edinburgh: Churchill Livingstone; 2001. pp. 585-611.
2. Somford DM, Futterer JJ, Hambrock T, et al. Diffusion and perfusion MR imaging of the prostate. Magn Reson Imaging Clin N Am. 2008;16:685-96.
3. Akin O, Hricak H. Imaging of prostate cancer. Radiol Clin North Am. 2007;45:207-22.
4. Bonekamp D, Jacobs MA, El-Khouli R, et al. Advancements in MR imaging of the prostate: from diagnosis to interventions. Radiographics. 2011;31:677-703.
5. Rajesh A, Coakley FV. MR imaging and MR spectroscopic imaging of prostate cancer. Magn Reson Imaging Clin N Am. 2004;12:557-80.
6. Avery LL, Scheinfeld MH. Imaging of penile and scrotal emergencies. Radiographics. 2013;33:721-40.
7. Rifkin MD, Foy PM, Goldberg BS. Scrotal ultrasound: acoustic characteristics of the normal testis and epididymis defined with higher resolution superficial scanners. Med Ultrasound. 1984;8:91-7.
8. Johnson KA, Dewbury KC. Ultrasound imaging of the appendix testes and appendix epididymis. Clin Radiol. 1996;51:335-7.
9. Parker RA 3rd, Menias CO, Quazi R, et al. MR imaging of the penis and scrotum. Radiographics. 2015;35:1033-50.
10. Middleton WD, Thorne DA, Melson GL. Colour Doppler ultrasound of the normal testis. Am J Roentgenol. 1989;152: 293-7.

Chapter 20

Disorders of the Prostate Gland

Ujjwal Gorsi, Paramjeet Singh, Anupam Lal

INTRODUCTION

The prostate gland is a common cause of urinary symptoms in elderly men. Two most important diseases of aging men affecting the prostate gland are benign prostatic hyperplasia (BPH) and malignancy. In addition, few congenital and inflammatory pathologies also affect the gland. Imaging techniques and radiological anatomy of the prostate have been discussed in detail in Chapter 19.

BENIGN PROSTATIC HYPERPLASIA

Prostate gland enlargement is common in older men. This is the most common type of prostatic pathology. About 50–75% of men over 50 years will be affected by BPH which increases to 80% for men over 70 years of age.[1]

Pathology: In BPH, transitional zone (TZ) and periurethral region of the prostate show increased glandular epithelial cells as well as increased stromal volume. Androgens (testosterone and dihydrotestosterone) and estrogens play a major role in the proliferation of glandular epithelial elements. BPH starts in the transition zone in form of nodules which progressively enlarge in number and size, subsequently compressing the adjacent central and peripheral zones (PZs).

Clinical features: Men usually seek medical consultation when lower urinary tract symptoms (LUTS) are caused by enlarging prostate. LUTS can be irrititative or obstructive. Urgency, frequency of urination, and nocturia are common irrititative symptoms whereas hesitancy, weak urinary stream, incomplete voiding, and straining during micturition are examples of obstructive symptoms. Although LUTS are more likely to be caused by prostate glands which are large, the gland size does not always correlate with symptoms of prostatism. Some men with severe LUTS will have only mild to moderately enlarged glands (≤50 cm)[3] whereas in others, very large glands may not be associated with significant symptoms. Left untreated, significant problems may be caused by BPH. Urinary retention, recurrent stones, recurrent infection, obstructive uropathy, and renal failure may occur in chronic long-standing nontreated BPH.

Imaging: In routine clinical practice, evaluation of men with prostatitis does not require imaging. Indications for imaging are: (1) symptoms which suggest complications of BPH, (2) if malignancy is suspected clinically or on digital rectal examination (DRE), and (3) symptomatic patients with history of previous urologic surgery.[3] Imaging usually shows enlargement and nodules of the prostate. Secondary findings of BPH are also demonstrated. In young men, whether by transrectal ultrasonography (TRUS), computed tomography (CT), or magnetic resonance imaging (MRI), the prostate gland measures about 3 cm in diameter on axial images.[2]

Primary Findings in Benign Prostatic Hyperplasia

Computed Tomography

Computed tomography can demonstrate enlarged prostate and reveal its relation with other pelvic organs. However, zonal anatomy of the prostate is not well delineated. Thus, it has limited value in patients of BPH. Changes of BPH are often detected incidentally in patients undergoing CT for unrelated indication.

Ultrasonography

Transrectal ultrasonography can show internal prostatic anatomy in detail and prostate volume can be measured accurately. However, the sonographic appearance of BPH is varied and depends on the histopathologic changes and proportion of glandular and stromal elements. Central gland can be diffused enlarged or distinct nodules may be present. The typical sonographic feature of BPH is enlargement of the inner gland, which appears relatively hypoechoic to the PZ. The border between central and peripheral gland which is indistinct in young men, becomes more distinct due to presence of BPH. Nodules can be fibroblastic, muscular, fibromuscular, hyperadenomatous, and fibroadenomatous.[4] Depending on the combination, the nodules may appear either isoechoic, hyperechoic or hypoechoic. Nodules may be surrounded by a hypoechoic rim **(Fig. 1)** and can sometimes distort the capsule but without disrupting it. Cystic dilation of the glands of the TZ may be seen due to blockage of prostatic ducts by stromal hyperplasia.[5]

Because the growth of the gland is primarily anterior, the volume or weight cannot be estimated well by digital palpation. Prostatic ultrasound provides an accurate and reproducible method to determine the prostatic volume and the effect of the hyperplasia on the anterior urethra that correlates with the symptoms of prostatism.

Magnetic Resonance Imaging

Magnetic resonance imaging will depict enlargement of TZ clearly. The TZ will typically become heterogeneous and contain numerous nodules. The signal characteristics of BPH nodules on T2-weighted images (T2WI) are quite variable depending on the proportion of glandular and stromal elements. Glandular nodules will be hyperintense on T2WI due to accumulated secretions. They may show early enhancement and rapid washout, similar to both stromal nodules and tumors. However, because of their higher extracellular content, they typically do not show diffusion restriction.[6] Stromal nodules have lower signal on T2WI and can be very difficult to distinguish from TZ carcinoma. Like TZ carcinomas, stromal nodules may show diffusion restriction and early enhancement on dynamic postcontrast images. Due to overlapping imaging characteristics on T2WI, diffusion-weighted imaging (DWI), and postcontrast images, margins of the nodule are the key distinguishing features. BPH nodules have smooth well-defined margins with convex shapes **(Fig. 2)** whereas malignant lesions are ill-marginated and have typical erased charcoal appearance.

Secondary Findings in Benign Prostatic Hyperplasia

As the prostate enlarges, its mass effect on the bladder as well as morphologic changes of outlet obstruction may emerge. Findings include indentation of the bladder base, thickening of bladder wall and formation of trabeculations **(Fig. 3)**. The bladder starts to dilate when detrusor hypertrophy cannot compensate for bladder outlet obstruction. Long-standing outlet obstruction will lead to formation of bladder calculi and diverticula.[2]

Ultrasound with combination of transabdominal and transrectal scan can demonstrate most of the secondary

Fig. 1: *Benign prostatic hyperplasia:* Grayscale transrectal ultrasound scan shows enlarged heterogeneous central gland with variable echogenicity nodules. Hypoechoic rim (arrow) is noted around one of the nodule.

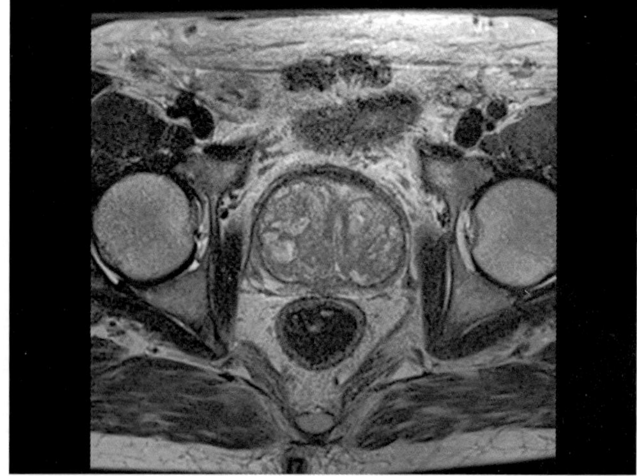

Fig. 2: Benign prostatic hyperplasia: T2-weighted axial image shows multiple nodules with varying internal signal. Well-circumscribed convex margin is noted around all nodules.

findings of BPH. It allows measurement of prostate size, bladder wall thickening, and postvoid residual bladder volume. Bladder wall trabeculations, diverticula, and calculi are easily demonstrated. Backpressure changes in form of bilateral hydroureteronephrosis may be seen in long-standing obstruction.

The median lobe of the prostate is particularly prone to enlargement in BPH, and may prolapse into the bladder neck causing obstruction during voiding **(Figs. 4A to C)**. Enlargement of median lobe of the gland predicts risk of urinary retention better than overall prostate volume.

Alpha-blockers and 5α-reductase inhibitors are usually prescribed as first line of treatment in BPH. However, persistent symptoms may require surgical intervention most commonly, transurethral resection of the prostate.

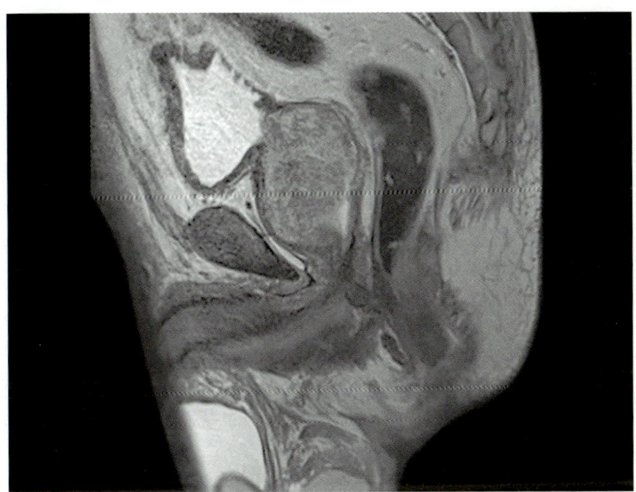

Fig. 3: Benign prostatic hyperplasia: T2-weighted sagittal image showing enlarged prostate bulging into bladder neck. Morphological changes of bladder outlet obstruction are apparent in form of bladder wall thickening and trabeculations.

Open surgery is rarely performed but may be considered in situations in which the gland is very large.

PROSTATE CANCER

Introduction

Cancer of the prostate is now the second most commonly occurring malignancy affecting men and also the fifth most common cause of cancer-related deaths in men worldwide. In 2018, an estimated 1.3 million new cases were there and 359,000 deaths related to the disease. In more than 50% of the countries of the world (105 out of 185), prostate cancer (PCa) is the most common malignancy among men with highest rates of incidence seen in the Americas, Sub-Saharan Africa, Australia/New Zealand, and Northern and Western Europe.[7]

Around 10–15% of younger men who develop PCa have a positive family history. However, the etiology still remains unclear. The only established risk factors for PCa are a positive family history, ethnicity, and increasing age.[8]

Clinical Features

Many-a-time, clinical manifestations of PCa are absent when a diagnosis is made. The spectrum of clinical behavior of PCa ranges from a screen-detected asymptomatic, microscopic, well-differentiated tumor that might never become clinically significant to the rarer screen-detected or clinically symptomatic high-grade aggressive cancer that causes metastases, morbidity, and death. When symptomatic, patients usually present with nonspecific complaints such as those of LUTS, hematuria, hematospermia, pelvic pain, malaise or weight loss. In patients who have metastases at presentation, the only symptom may be bone pain as bone is the predominant

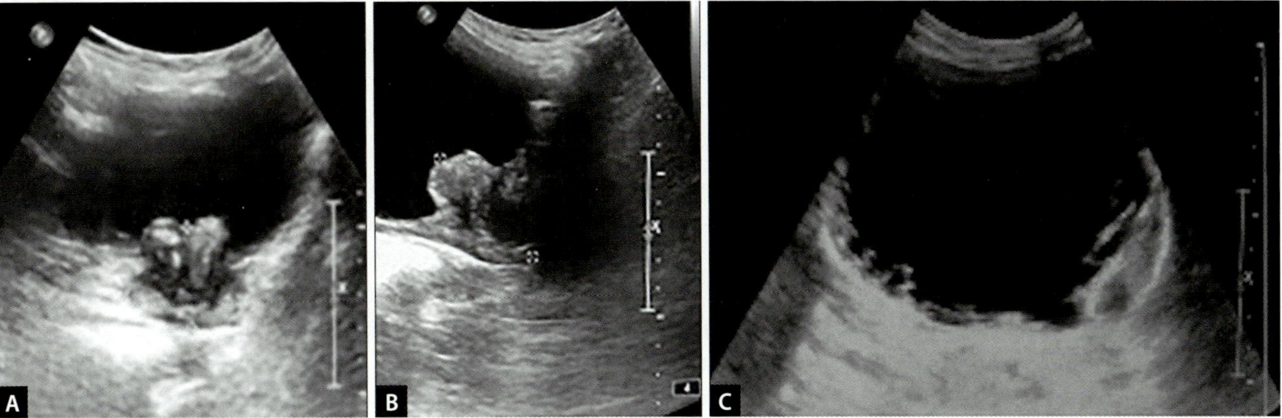

Figs. 4A to C: Median lobe enlargement: Transabdominal ultrasound axial (A) and sagittal (B) images show median lobe of prostate projecting into bladder base; (C) Axial image of urinary bladder shows thickening and trabeculations of bladder wall.

site of disseminated PCa, and pain is the most common manifestation of bone metastases.

Pathology

Adenocarcinoma is the most common histologic type, encountered in approximately 95% of patients. Other prostate tumors are rare but include squamous cell carcinomas, endometrioid carcinomas arising from the prostatic utricle, carcinosarcomas, melanomas, and mesenchymal neoplasms such as rhabdomyosarcoma, leiomyosarcoma, or fibrosarcoma. Around 70% of the prostatic cancer originates in the PZ, 10–20% in the TZ, and 5–10% in the central zone. Multicentricity of the tumor is quite common. Approximately, 30–46% men above 50 years of age may harbor a cancer focus but less than 20% of those develop clinical disease which is largely related to variability in aggressiveness.

Screening

Digital rectal examination (DRE) and serum prostate-specific antigen (PSA) levels have been used in conjunction for screening men for PCa for last many decades. Neither DRE nor PSA is highly sensitive, but their combined use improves screening performance. If both DRE and PSA are positive, 60% of those patients will have PCa; if both DRE and PSA are normal, only 2% of those patients will have the disease. PSA density (obtained by dividing the PSA by the prostate size), PSA velocity (rate of increase of the PSA level), and ratio of free PSA to total PSA are found to be more useful in predicting the risk of harboring PCa as compared to single reading of serum PSA.

Studies have also found that a novel biomarker which is measured in the urine sediment attained after prostatic massage—the Prostate Cancer Antigen 3 (PCA3) may also be useful tool for screening of PCa.[9]

At present, there is no evidence of using any imaging modality in PCa screening. Broadly speaking, ultrasound, CT, MRI, scintigraphy, and positron emission tomography (PET) are insufficiently accurate and/or too expensive to be used for screening.

Diagnosis

Individuals with any abnormal findings on DRE and/or a raised (>4 ng/mL) or increasing PSA level are taken up for a standard 12-core biopsy guided by TRUS. Because accurate prognosis depends upon histologic information, tissue diagnosis is obtained prior to treatment even when disease is obviously locally advanced or metastatic clinically.

The current gold-standard investigation for the diagnosis of PCa is a 12-core TRUS-guided biopsy.[10] In a typical transrectal biopsy, passes are taken at 3 levels—the base, mid gland and apex. At each of these levels, 4 cores are to be taken—2 from the right and 2 from the left with 1 core taken medially (in parasagittal location) and the other laterally on each side. The National Comprehensive Cancer Network (NCCN) has recently suggested the concept of an "extended-pattern 12-core biopsy" which would include, apart from the standard sites, the lesion-directed palpable nodules or suspicious images as well.

The Gleason scoring system, which is based on the architectural growth patterns of adenocarcinoma of prostate was first described in 1966. Five histological patterns were described.[11] It was however observed that many adenocarcinomas of the prostate demonstrated ≥2 patterns. Because of this, the Gleason score was formulated and it was shown that this score demonstrated better correlation with the behavior of the cancer. The final Gleason score is arrived at by adding up the scores of the primary and secondary patterns. For example, if the primary pattern has a Gleason score of 3 and the secondary pattern has a Gleason score of 4, the final Gleason score will be 3 + 4 = 7. The World Health Organization has recently incorporated a new "Grade Group" system for classifying prostate cancers. According to this new system, groups have been made as follows:[12-14]

- Grade group I—Gleason scores ≤ 6
- Grade group II—Gleason score 3 + 4 = 7
- Grade group III—Gleason score 4 + 3 = 7
- Grade group IV—Gleason score 4 + 4 = 8
- Grade group V—Gleason score 9–10.

ROLE OF VARIOUS IMAGING MODALITIES IN DIAGNOSIS OF PROSTATE CANCER

Transrectal Ultrasound

Transrectal ultrasonography alone is insufficient in diagnosing prostatic malignancy because of various reasons. Prostatic cancer can have variable appearance on gray scale mimicking benign tissue, substantial percentage of cancers are isoechoic and PCa can be multifocal.[15]

Against the background of normal PZ glandular tissue, small prostatic cancer usually appears hypoechoic because of closely packed cells in the tumor nodule. Larger tumors may appear isoechoic or hyperechoic. This appearance may be caused by a desmoplastic response of adjacent normal tissue or due to infiltration of the neoplasm into a background of BPH.[16]

The sensitivity and specificity of gray scale imaging alone is limited and has not improved the accuracy of PCa detection with an overall positive predictive value for cancer remaining <50%. TRUS is predominantly used to establish position and borders of the prostate during biopsy, rather than for lesion detection, characterization or targeting. Color Doppler, ultrasound-contrast agents, and elastography have improved diagnostic performance of TRUS for detecting and characterizing prostatic lesions.

Contrast-enhanced ultrasound (CEUS) involves the administration of an ultrasound-contrast agent (UCA) by the intravenous route which allows us to visualize the changes in vascularity (especially angiogenesis) within the prostate, some of which are characteristic for significant PCa. Shear wave elastography (SWE) is based on the measurements of the speed of shear waves through the tissue of interest. With these measurements, we can then map tissue stiffness properties (as Young's modulus). Young's modulus is significantly greater in PCa as compared to that in benign prostatic tissue as malignant tissue has more stiffness as compared to rest of gland **(Figs. 5A to C)**.

Magnetic Resonance Imaging

Indications of Magnetic Resonance Imaging

Most common situation in which MRI is requested for diagnostic work-up of suspected prostate malignancy is when repeated TRUS-guided biopsy results are negative or equivocal but occult high-risk tumor is suspected. MRI has an important role in lesion localization and risk stratification. Suspicious areas can be biopsied under direct MRI guidance or with fusion biopsy in which real-time coregistration of magnetic resonance (MR) images with TRUS guidance for biopsy is performed.

Multiparametric Magnetic Resonance Imaging

The introduction of multiparametric MRI (mp-MRI) has increased the ability of MRI in detecting and characterizing prostatic malignancies. It has also lead to improvement in lesion localization and targeted biopsy. mp-MRI combines high-resolution T2WI with ≥2 functional MRI sequences. The two sequences which we use most commonly are DWI and dynamic contrast-enhanced (DCE) perfusion

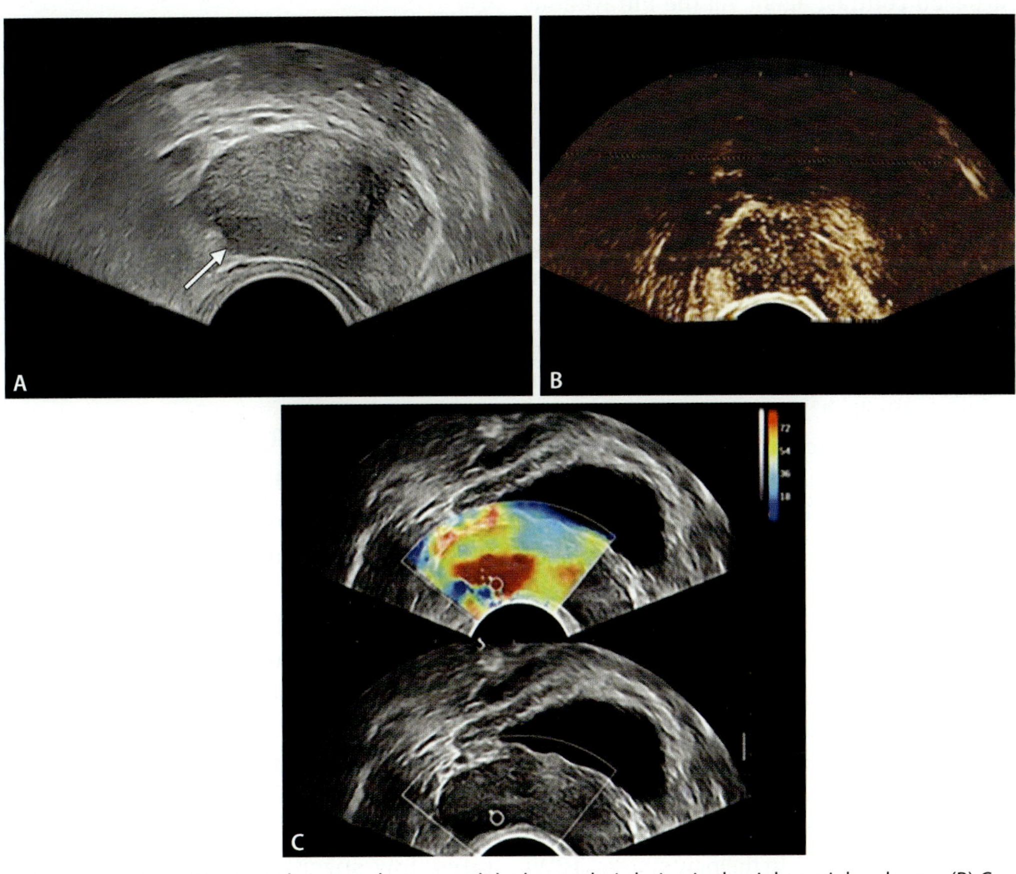

Figs. 5A to C: Carcinoma prostate: (A) Grayscale image shows a nodular hypoechoic lesion in the right peripheral zone; (B) Contrast-enhanced ultrasound image showing asynchronous early wash-in of contrast; (C) Shear-wave elastography image showing increased stiffness of the malignant lesion.

imaging. Prostate imaging using a 3T magnet provides the benefit of attaining a higher signal to noise ratio, and it is not an absolute requirement to use an endorectal coil (ERC) in cancer detection protocols, but should preferably be used when working with a 1.5T magnet.

With T2WI, The PZ is seen as a T2 hyperintense area due to its high water content. Because of this, a cancerous lesion in the PZ can easily be picked up as it would appear as a low signal intensity area. This, however, is a nonspecific feature as low T2 signal may also be seen in nonmalignant conditions such as fibrosis, prostatitis, postirradiation, and also in patients with postbiopsy hemorrhage.

On DWI, a cancerous lesion can be identified by the hallmark findings of low apparent diffusion coefficient (ADC) with an associated iso-to-high signal value on DWI images (keeping b-value ≥1,400 sec/mm^2). Unlike T2WI, functional imaging (especially DWI) is very helpful in differentiating a malignant lesion from nonmalignant abnormalities (like the ones stated above) and therefore, increase the overall performance of mp-MRI in diagnosing PCa.

In DCE MRI, T1-weighted sequences are acquired before, during, and after the rapid administration of a bolus of gadolinium-based contrast agent via the intravenous (IV) route to assess tumor angiogenesis. PCa, on this sequence, may show early postcontrast enhancement (which usually has a high amplitude) followed by rapid washout. A limitation associated with this sequence is that it cannot be definitively used in isolation for diagnosing PCa because of similar enhancement patterns noted in benign conditions such as prostatitis and BPH. It however plays an important role in detecting residual/recurrent tumor following therapy.[17]

Magnetic resonance spectroscopy measures citrate, creatine, and choline to provide specific information regarding prostate metabolism. PCa is characterized by an elevated choline level and/or decreased citrate level at MR spectroscopy. Unlike the previous version, findings from MR spectroscopic imaging are not incorporated into Prostate Imaging-Reporting and Data System (PI-RADS) version 2.

Prostate Imaging-Reporting and Data System

For standardizing the assessment and reporting of the mp-MRI prostate findings, the European Society of Urogenital Radiology (ESUR) published a set of guidelines, termed the Prostate Imaging-Reporting and Data System (PI-RADS).[18] In 2015, a revised version (PI-RADS version 2) was introduced which brought about a few important alterations to the original system. In the new system, T2WI and DWI-ADC combination are scored by using a 5-point scale.[19]

Table 1: PI-RADS v2.1 assessment categories.

PI-RADS 1	Very low (clinically significant cancer is highly unlikely to be present)
PI-RADS 2	Low (clinically significant cancer is unlikely to be present)
PI-RADS 3	Intermediate (the presence of clinically significant cancer is equivocal)
PI-RADS 4	High (clinically significant cancer is likely to be present)
PI-RADS 5	Very high (clinically significant cancer is highly likely to be present)

(PI-RADS: Prostate Imaging-Reporting and Data System)

Newest version (Version 2.1) updated in 2019 recommends several minor adjustments which aim to simplify assessment and reduce inter-observership variability, without modifying the overall principles and scope of the original system.[20]

In PI-RADS™ v2.1, clinically significant cancer is defined on pathology/histology as the cancer with Gleason score ≥7 (including 3 + 4 with prominent but not predominant Gleason 4 component), and/or volume >0.5 cc, and/or extraprostatic extension.

PI-RADS™ v2.1 assessment uses a 5-point scale which is based on the probability that a combination of mp-MRI findings derived from T2WI, DWI, and DCE correlates with the presence of a clinically significant cancer. These assessment categories are given in **Table 1**.

Biopsy should not be considered for PI-RADS 1 or 2 lesions **(Figs. 6A and B)** but should be considered for PI-RADS 4 or 5 lesions **(Figs. 7 and 8)**. For findings with PI-RADS assessment Category 3, biopsy may or may not be considered depending on clinical scenario.

Prostate Imaging-Reporting and Data System Assessment

Guidance for assignment of overall PI-RADS-v2.1 score in PZ and TZ lesions are summarized in **Tables 2 and 3**. As it is obvious in given tables, DW1 is the dominant sequence for PZ lesions whereas T2WI is the dominant sequence for TZ lesions. Detailed PI-RADS assessment for T2WI and DWI, and DCE sequences is given in **Tables 4 to 7**.

Despite various studies validating the fairly high diagnostic performance of mp-MRI in PCa, it is still not recommended as a first-line investigation in the work-up of the disease, because of its high cost, high false-positive rates, low specificity, moderate inter-reader reproducibility, and contraindications such as claustrophobia and *in situ* metallic implants.[21]

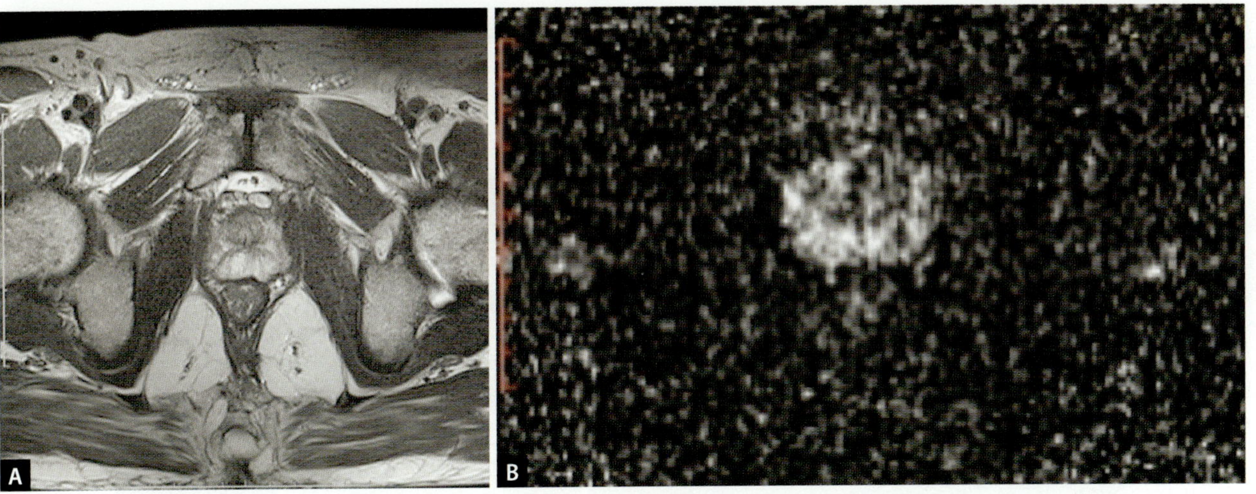

Figs. 6A and B: PI-RADS 2 lesion: (A) T2-weighted axial image showing multiple linear hypointensities with indistinct margin in peripheral zone; (B) On apparent diffusion coefficient map, these areas of abnormal signal appear dark.

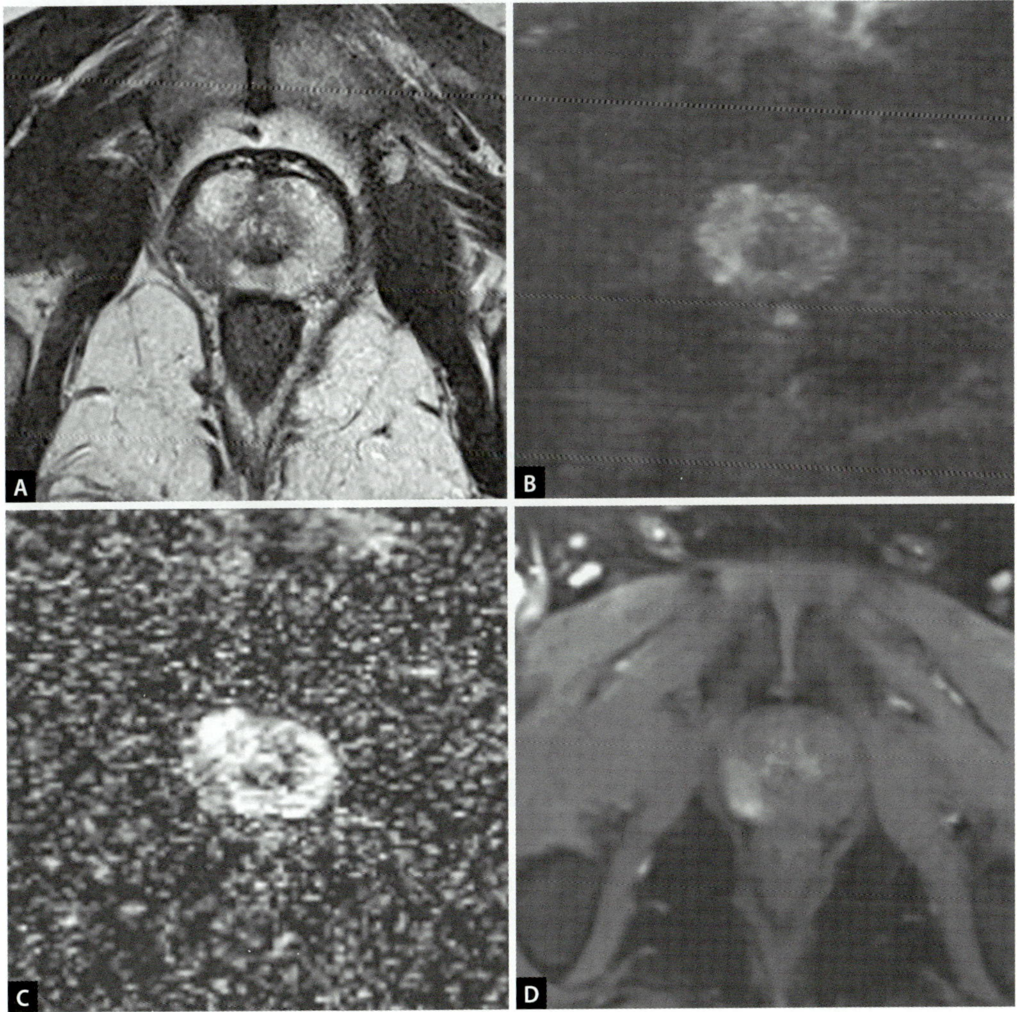

Figs. 7A to D: PI-RADS 5 lesion: (A) T2-weighted axial image shows a nodular hypointense lesion in the peripheral zone of the prostate on the right side; (B) On diffusion-weighted imaging, lesion shows hyperintensity and (C) on apparent diffusion coefficient map, it appears hypointense; (D) Postcontrast T1-weighted image shows early enhancement of the lesion. On biopsy, lesion turned out to be Gleason 8 adenocarcinoma.

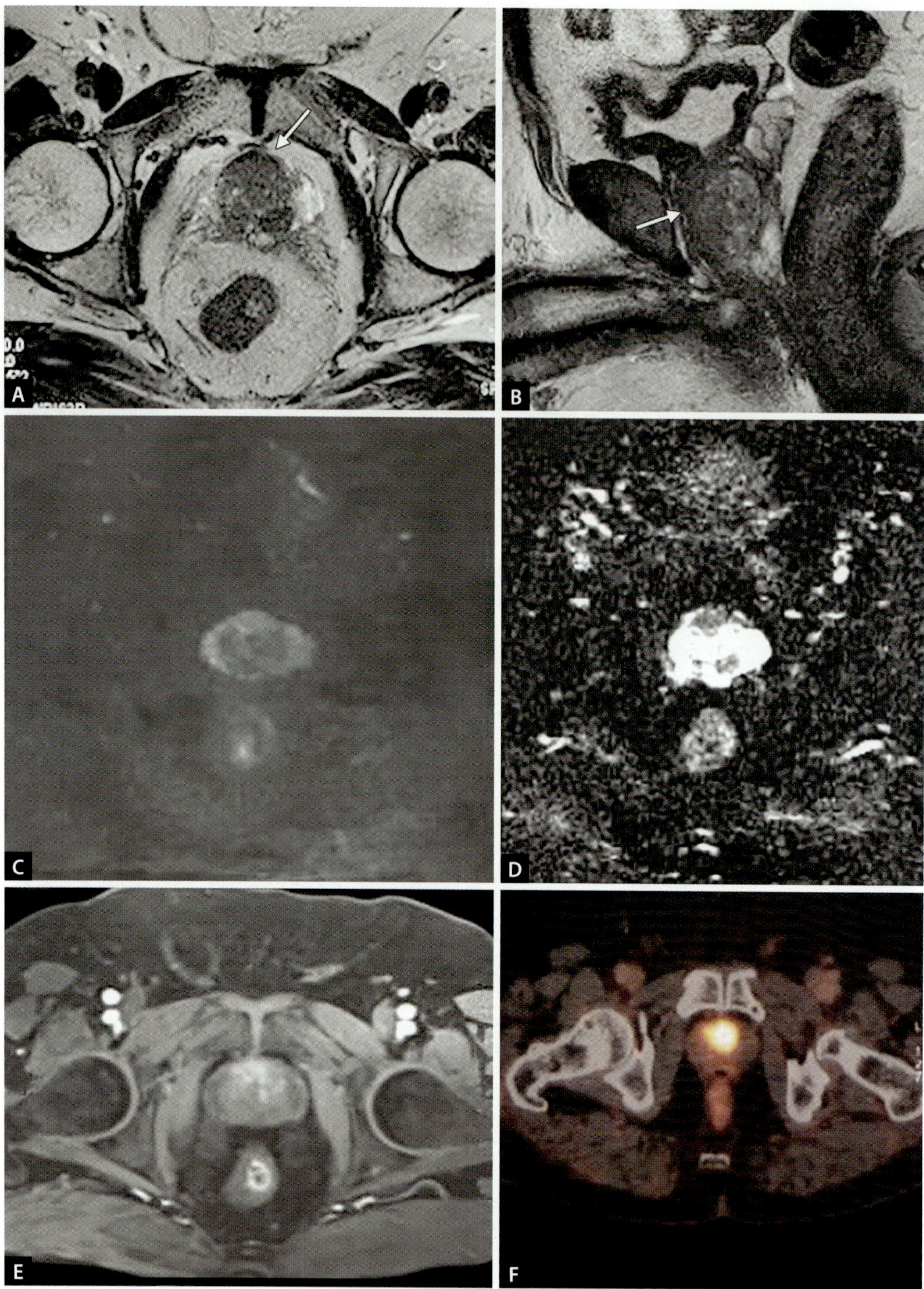

Figs. 8A to F: Biopsy proven transition zone Gleason 9 adenocarcinoma: T2-weighted axial (A) and sagittal (B) images demonstrating focal lenticular hypointense signal (arrows) in the anterior transitional zone of the mid-gland showing erased charcoal appearance. On diffusion-weighted imaging (C) lesion appears hyperintense and on apparent diffusion coefficient (D) it shows hypointense signal. On post-contrast T1-weighted image (E) it shows early enhancement. Prostate specific membrane antigen PET (F) done for staging shows intense uptake in the lesion. No distant metastasis, however, was seen.

Tumor Spread and Staging

Spread of prostatic carcinoma occurs by: (1) Direct extension; (2) lymphatic spread; and (3) hematogeneous spread.

Local spread is usually to the seminal vesicles, the urethra, the urinary bladder, and rectum. Later levator muscles and pelvic wall may get involved. Lymphatic spread involves initially the obturator, the external iliac,

Table 2: PI-RADS score—peripheral zone.

DWI	*T2W*	*DCE*	*PI-RADS*
1	Any*	Any	1
2	Any	Any	2
3	Any	–	3
		+	4
4	Any	Any	4
5	Any	Any	5

* indicates 1–5.
(DWI: diffusion-weighted imaging; T2W: T2-weighted; DCE: dynamic contrast-enhanced; PI-RADS: prostate imaging-reporting and data system)

Table 3: PI-RADS score—transition zone.

T2W	*DWI*	*DCE*	*PI-RADS*
1	Any*	Any	1
2	≤3	Any	2
	≥4	Any	3
3	≤4	Any	3
	5	Any	4
4	Any	Any	4
5	Any	Any	5

*indicates 1–5.

Table 4: PI-RADS assessment for T2W in peripheral zone.

Score	*Peripheral zone*
1	Uniform hyperintense signal intensity (normal)
2	Linear or wedge-shaped hypointensity or diffused mild hypointensity, usually indistinct margin
3	Heterogeneous signal intensity or noncircumscribed, rounded, moderate hypointensity Includes others that do not qualify as 2, 4, or 5
4.	Circumscribed, homogeneous moderate hypointense focus/mass confined to prostate and <1.5 cm in greatest dimension
5	Same as 4 but ≥1.5 cm in greatest dimension or definite extraprostatic extension/invasive behavior

(T2W: T2-weighted; PI-RADS: prostate imaging-reporting and data system)

Table 5: PI-RADS assessment for T2W in transition zone (TZ).

Score	*Transition zone*
1	Normal appearing TZ (rare) or a round, completely encapsulated nodule ("typical nodule")
2	A mostly encapsulated nodule OR a homogeneous circumscribed nodule without encapsulation ("atypical nodule") OR a homogeneous mildly hypointense area between nodules
3	Heterogeneous signal intensity with obscured margins includes others that do not qualify as 2, 4, or 5
4	Lenticular or noncircumscribed, homogeneous, moderately hypointense, and <1.5 cm in greatest dimension
5	Same as 4, but ≥1.5 cm in greatest dimension or definite extraprostatic extension/invasive behavior

Table 6: PI-RADS assessment of DWI.

Score	*Peripheral zone or transition zone*
1	No abnormality (i.e. normal) on ADC and high b-value DWI
2	Linear or wedge-shaped hypointense on ADC and/or linear or wedge-shaped hyperintense on high b-value DWI
3	Focal (discrete and different from the background) hypointense on ADC and/or focal hyperintense on high b-value DWI; may be markedly hypointense on ADC or markedly hyperintense on high b-value DWI, but not both
4	Focal markedly hypointense on ADC and markedly hyperintense on high b-value DWI; <1.5 cm in greatest dimension
5	Same as 4 but ≥1.5 cm in greatest dimension or definite extraprostatic extension/invasive behavior

(PI-RADS: prostate imaging-reporting and data system; DWI: diffusion-weighted imaging; ADC: apparent diffusion coefficient)

Table 7: PI-RADS Assessment for DCE.

Score	*Peripheral zone or transition zone*
(–)	No early or contemporaneous enhancement; or diffuse multifocal enhancement NOT corresponding to a focal finding on T2WI and/or DWI or focal enhancement corresponding to a lesion demonstrating features of BPH on T2WI (including features of extruded BPH in the PZ)
(+)	Focal and earlier than or contemporaneously with enhancement of adjacent normal prostatic tissues, and corresponds to suspicious finding on T2W and/or DWI

(PI-RADS: prostate imaging-reporting and data system; DCE: dynamic contrast-enhanced; T2WI: T2-weighted image; DWI: diffusion-weighted imaging; BPH: benign prostatic hyperplasia; PZ: peripheral zone)

and the internal iliac nodes. The common iliac, and para-aortic nodes may be involved in advanced disease. Hematogenous spread is to the axial skeleton or viscera. Sites of skeletal metastases are the lumbar spine, proximal femur, bony pelvis, thoracic spine, ribs, sternum, skull, and proximal humerus in order of decreasing frequency. More than 90% of prostatic metastatic lesions to bone are blastic. Spread to organs other than lymph nodes and bones is rare unless there is wide dissemination of the disease.[2]

Table 8: Prostate adenocarcinoma—TNM staging classification.

TX	Primary tumor cannot be assessed
T0	No evidence of primary tumor
T1	Clinically inapparent tumor not palpable or visible by imaging
T1a	Tumor incidental histologic finding in ≤5% of tissue resected (at time of TURP)
T1b	Tumor incidental histologic finding in >5% of tissue resected (at time of TURP)
T1c	Tumor identified by needle biopsy (because of elevated PSA level)
T2	Tumor confined within prostate (*Note:* Tumors found in one or both lobes by needle biopsy but not palpable on DRE or reliably visible by imaging are classified as T1c)
T2a	Tumor involves one-half of one lobe or less
T2b	Tumor involves more than one-half of one lobe but not both lobes
T2c	Tumor involves both lobes
T3	Tumor extends through the prostatic capsule (*Note:* Invasion into the prostatic apex, or into—but not beyond—the prostatic capsule is classified as T2)
T3a	Extracapsular extension (unilateral or bilateral)
T3b	Tumor invading seminal vesicle(s)
T4	Tumor fixed or invades adjacent structures other than seminal vesicles (e.g. bladder, levator muscles, and/or pelvic wall)

(TNM: tumor, node, and metastasis; TURP: transurethral resection of the prostate; PSA: prostate specific antigen; DRE: digital rectal examination)

The clinical staging of PCa is based on the tumor, node, and metastasis (TNM) system given by the American Joint Committee on Cancer (AJCC). The pathological staging is performed after prostatectomy and it depends on various factors such as the status of surgical margins, extracapsular disease, tumor burden, and also on whether or not the seminal vesicles and/or pelvic lymph nodes are involved. The clinical T-staging is as follows **(Table 8)**.[22]

The 5-year survival rate among patients with localized PCa and in those with just regional spread is almost 100% while those diagnosed at a stage with distant metastasis have a relative 5-year survival of just 29.3%.

After PCa is initially diagnosed, imaging plays a definite role in staging. CT, like ultrasound, is relatively inaccurate in local staging, because it cannot detect early-stage cancers. CT may depict local invasion and lymphadenopathy.[23] Use of CT is recommended for staging in patients who have Gleason score greater than 7, PSA greater than 20 ng/mL, and cancer stage T3 or higher.[23]

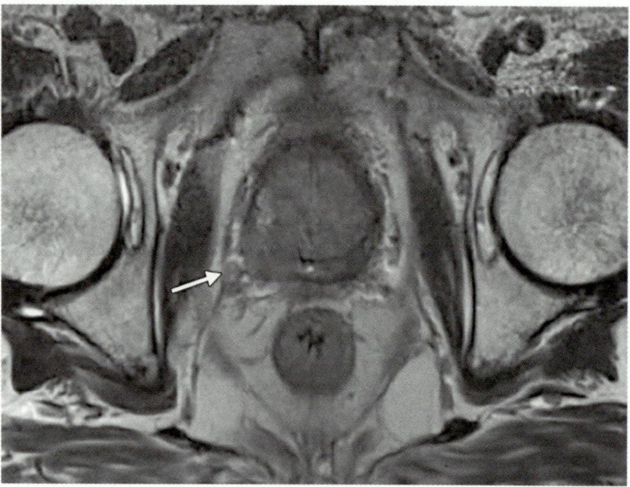

Fig. 9: Extracapsular spread: T2-weighted axial image showing focal disruption of capsule in right peripheral zone cancer with encasement of ipsilateral neurovascular bundle (arrow).

Magnetic resonance imaging is by far the most accurate method for local anatomic staging of PCa. T2WI in addition to DWI and DCE are the commonly used sequences. Prostate MRI aids in the staging evaluation by verifying organ-confined status, evaluating the status of the pelvic lymph nodes, and establishing the location and local extent of the tumor in patients being considered for radiation therapy.

The ability to distinguish between organ-confined tumors (≤T2c) and those that extend beyond the prostate (≥T3a) is an important component of treatment decision-making. It is often used to define the relationship of the tumor to the neurovascular bundle and to determine the need or risk of sacrificing the nerves either unilaterally or bilaterally. The neurovascular bundle is present postero-lateral to the prostate gland (at the 5 and 7 positions) on either side. It is hypointense on T1- and T2-weighted imaging and is surrounded by high-signal periprostatic fat.[23] Nerve-sparing surgery may be attempted in an effort to preserve potency if the neurovascular bundle is not involved.[24]

Few features predict extracapsular extension of PCa. These features are an irregular, spiculated, or angulated prostate margin **(Fig. 9)**, broad tumor contact with capsule, capsular retraction, tumor bulge into the periprostatic fat, asymmetry of the neurovascular bundle, and obliterated rectoprostatic angle.[23] Features of seminal vesicle involvement in a prostatic malignancy include focal hypointensity of the seminal vesicle which may be enlarged, hypointensity in ejaculatory ducts which may show increased size, obliteration of the angle between the prostate and the seminal vesicle and direct tumor extension from the prostate into seminal vesicle **(Fig. 10)**.[23] Accuracy of MRI in detecting seminal vesicle involvement

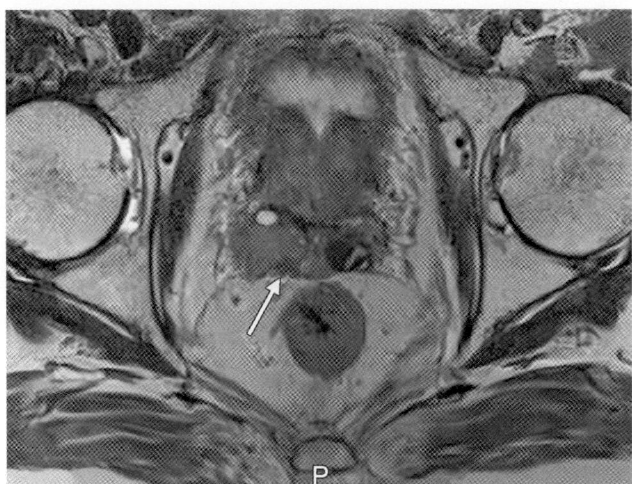

Fig. 10: Seminal vesicle involvement: T2-weighted axial image showing enlarged seminal vesicles with presence of low-signal intensity mass (arrow).

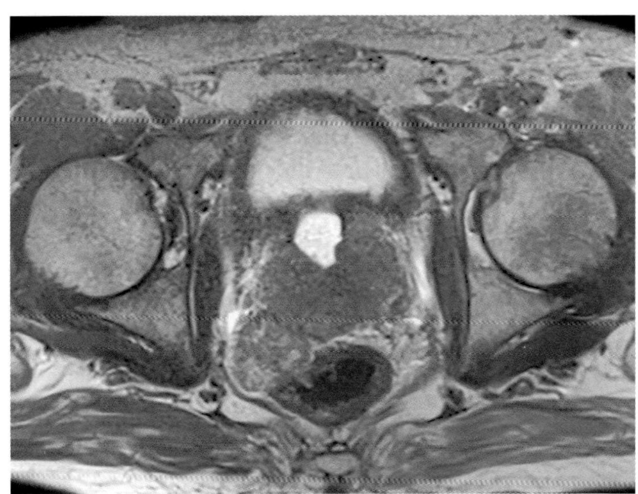

Fig. 11: Extracapsular spread: T2-weighted axial image showing lesion in right posterior peripheral zone with obvious extracapsular extension and complete encasement of right neurovascular bundle. Infiltration of anterior wall of rectum is also seen.

in prostatic malignancy is reported as >90%. In later stages, other pelvic organs may also get infiltrated **(Fig. 11)**.

Lymph nodes are hyperintense on both T2WI and DWI and can readily be detected and measured by MRI. Nodal staging currently relies on assessment of lymph node size and shape. The relatively new technique of MR lymphangiography demonstrates potential to detect metastases in lymph nodes which are not enlarged using lymphotropic ultrasmall superparamagnetic iron oxide (USPIO) nanoparticles.[25]

Nuclear Medicine

Radionuclide bone scans have very good sensitivity but low specificity for metastatic prostate tumor. Bone scan **(Fig. 12)** and MRI spine **(Figs. 13A and B)** will reveal osteoblastic metastasis. The American College of Radiology recommends bone scintigraphy when the PSA level is greater than 10 ng/mL and the Gleason score is greater than 6.[26]

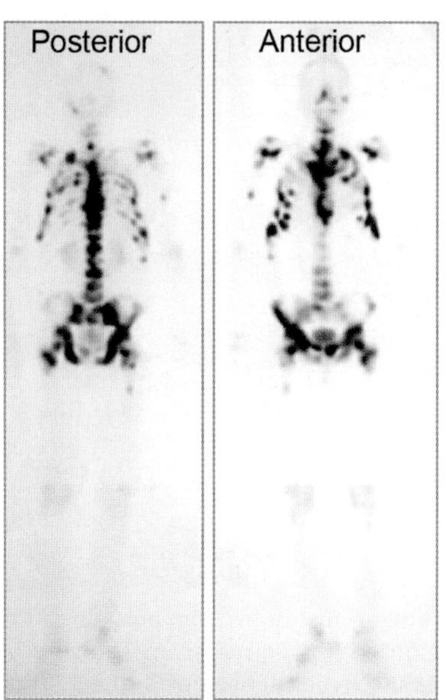

Fig. 12: Bony metastasis in carcinoma prostate: Nuclear scan anterior and posterior views showing multiple osteoblastic metastatic deposits involving axial skeleton from cancer prostate.

Role of 18-fluorodeoxyglucose (FDG)-PET in PCa is limited due to poor resolution and noise from the proximity to the bladder. Prostate specific membrane antigen (PSMA)-PET has shown promise in evaluation of lymph node metastasis and biochemical recurrence.

Active Surveillance and Surveillance after Treatment

Very low-risk and low-risk tumors may not need treatment at all, but may be managed by active surveillance. Active surveillance may also be the preferred approach in patients with higher risk tumors but relatively short life expectancies. Active surveillance consists of periodic DRE and PSA, intermittent repeat biopsies, and MRI if suspicious findings emerge through other means of surveillance.

Localized tumors are managed with surgery (usually radical prostatectomy) or radiotherapy (brachytherapy or external beam irradiation). Tumors that are metastatic usually require antiandrogen drugs, surgery, and/or chemotherapy.[2]

After treatment for localized PCa, surveillance for recurrence is primarily performed by serial PSA

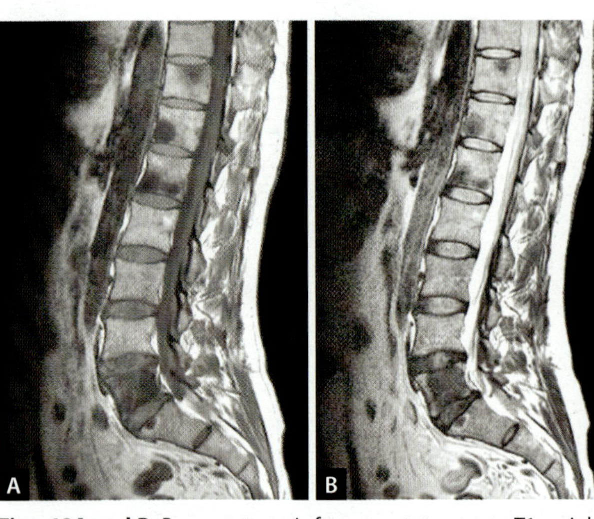

Figs. 13A and B: Bony metastasis from prostate cancer: T1-weighted (A) and T2-weighted (B) sagittal scans showing blastic marrow deposits appearing hypointense on T1 and T2 images involving dorsolumbar spine.

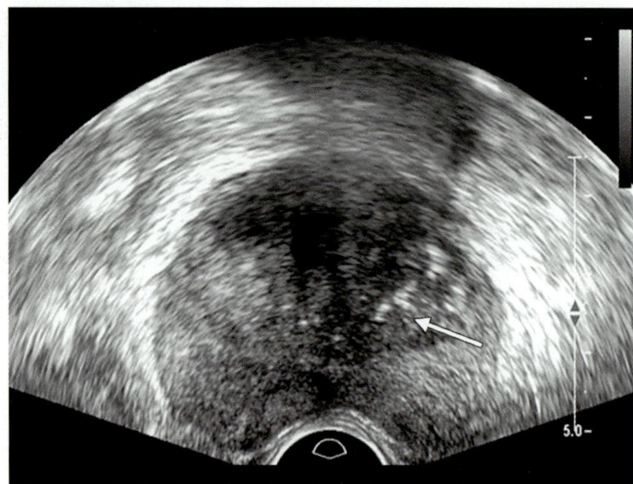

Fig. 14: Prostatic calcifications: Transrectal ultrasound scan showing areas of calcification (arrow) in transition zone.

determinations. If a continued rise in PSA is encountered, selection of treatment depends to a great degree upon whether the tumor has reappeared in the site of original treatment or has produced distant metastases. CT or MRI can demonstrate local recurrence, usually evident as an enhancing soft tissue mass in the surgical bed.

Prostatic Calcifications

The PZ of the prostate gland is the seat of the corpora amylacea, where calcifications with no known etiology and without pathologic effects tend to occur. Calcification is also noted in some BPH nodules in the TZ. Prostatic calcifications have little clinical significance and are not useful in differentiating between benign and malignant diseases **(Fig. 14)**.

PROSTATITIS AND PROSTATIC ABSCESS

Acute prostatitis occurs commonly due to ascending infection from the urethra. Sometimes, it may be involved by descent of organisms from the upper urinary tract or bladder. Distant focus of infection may sometimes lead to prostatitis via hematogenous or lymphogenous route. The common pathogens are those which cause urinary tract infection like *Escherichia coli*, *Klebsiella pneumoniae*, *Proteus*, *Pseudomonas*, etc.

In contrast to PCa, acute prostatitis is associated with significant symptoms. Patients may present with urinary frequency, urgency, dysuria, fever, perineal pain, and urethral discharge. DRE will reveal an extremely swollen and tender prostate.[2] In acute prostatitis, generally the glands are hypoechoic. Color Doppler shows a very vascular focus in areas of prostatitis, mimicking carcinoma.

Chronic prostatitis is caused in much the same way and by the same bacterial pathogens as acute prostatitis, however, it may be associated with certain other pathogens such as mycobacteria, chlamydia or *Mycoplasma*. A high index of suspicion for malignancy is necessary, because both PCa and prostatitis tend to occur in the PZ. Sonographic findings of chronic prostatitis include variable echogenicity focal masses, calcifications of ejaculatory duct, and irregularity and thickening of capsule. In addition, dilatation of periprostatic veins and distended seminal vesicles may be seen. Chronic granulomatous prostatitis can mimic sonographic features of prostatic carcinoma. TRUS does not reliably distinguish chronic prostatitis from cancer.

On MRI, certain morphologic features are helpful in differentiating prostatitis from malignancy. When focal, it is characteristically band-like, triangular or geographic in morphology compared with the typical nodular or mass like configuration of cancer **(Figs. 15A to D)**. When diffuse, the entire PZ may be "grayed out" or lower in signal than the very high signal expected in the PZ on T2WI. Prostatitis may be hyperintense on DWI but usually lacks the marked low-signal intensity which is seen in PCa on ADC maps. Prostatitis usually shows hyperenhancement on arterial phase DCE.[2]

On ultrasound, development of an anechoic lesion with or without internal echoes suggests the development of an abscess, which on color Doppler shows a highly vascular wall. The abscess cavity may also contain air due to gas-producing organisms. In doubtful cases,

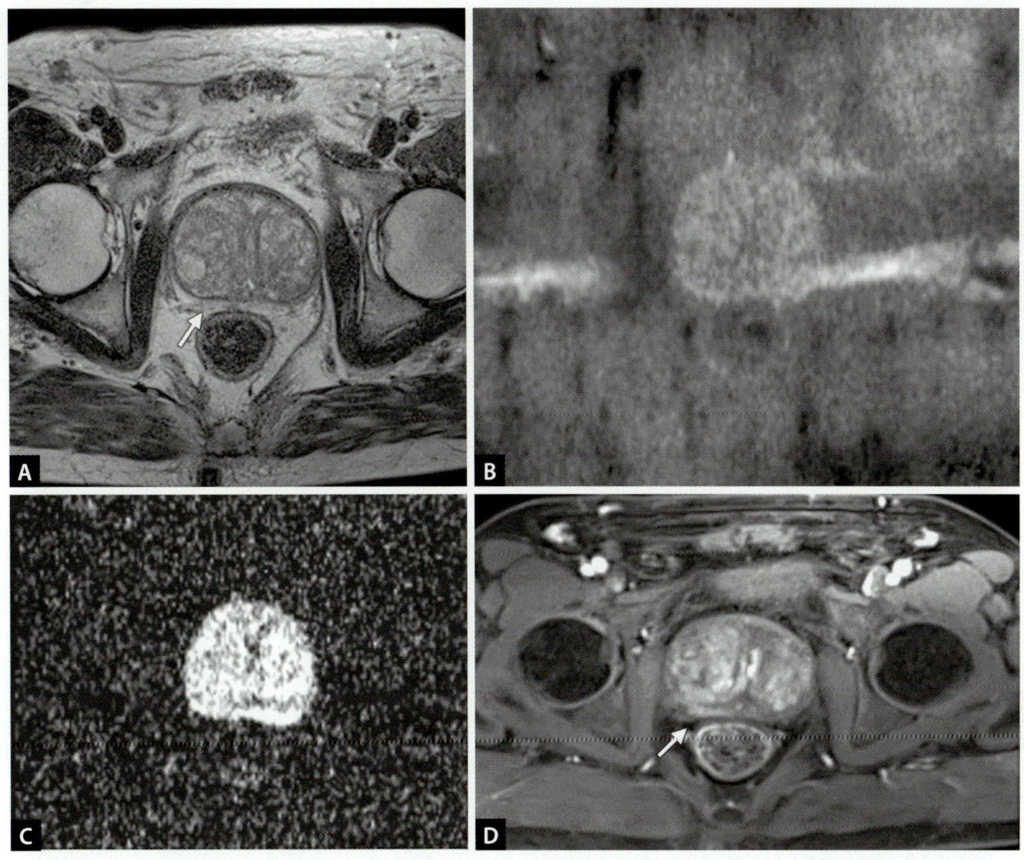

Figs. 15A to D: Focal prostatitis: (A) T2-weighted image shows noncircumscribed hypointense area (arrow) in right posterior peripheral zone; (B) Diffusion-weighted imaging shows mild hyperintense signal whereas on apparent diffusion coefficient; (C) corresponding area is hypointense; (D) Postcontrast T1-weighted image illustrates focal early enhancement (arrow) equal to that of the TZ. Lesion was reported as PIRADS 3 and final diagnosis of prostatitis was confirmed on biopsy.

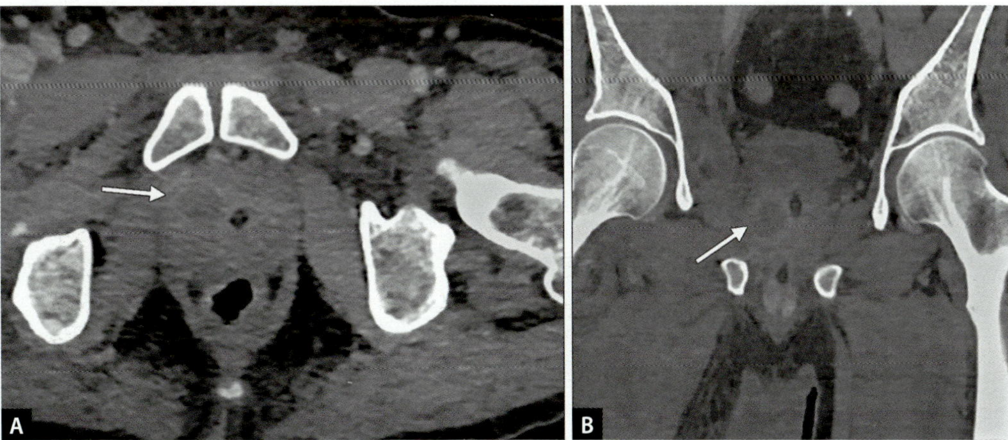

Figs. 16A and B: Prostatic abscess: Contrast-enhanced CT axial (A) and coronal (B) images showing hypodense collection with irregular enhancing walls (arrows).

contrast-enhanced CT and MRI can show the abscess cavity with enhancement of its wall **(Figs. 16 and 17)**. TRUS guidance can be used to diagnose as well as drain these prostatic abscesses **(Figs. 18A and B)**.

PROSTATIC CYSTS

Midline prostatic cysts can be Müllerian duct cysts or utricle cysts. Müllerian duct cysts do not contain sperms and can cause infertility due to compression of the

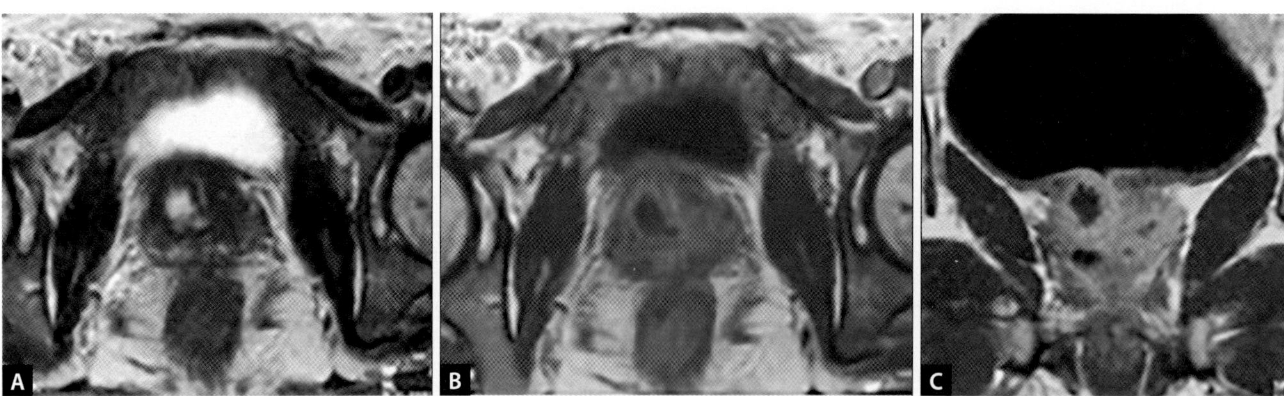

Figs. 17A to C: Prostatic abscess: T2 axial (A), T1 postcontrast axial (B) and coronal (C) sections show a bacterial intraprostatic abscess appearing hyperintense on T2 and showing enhancing peripheral margins in the right half of the gland.

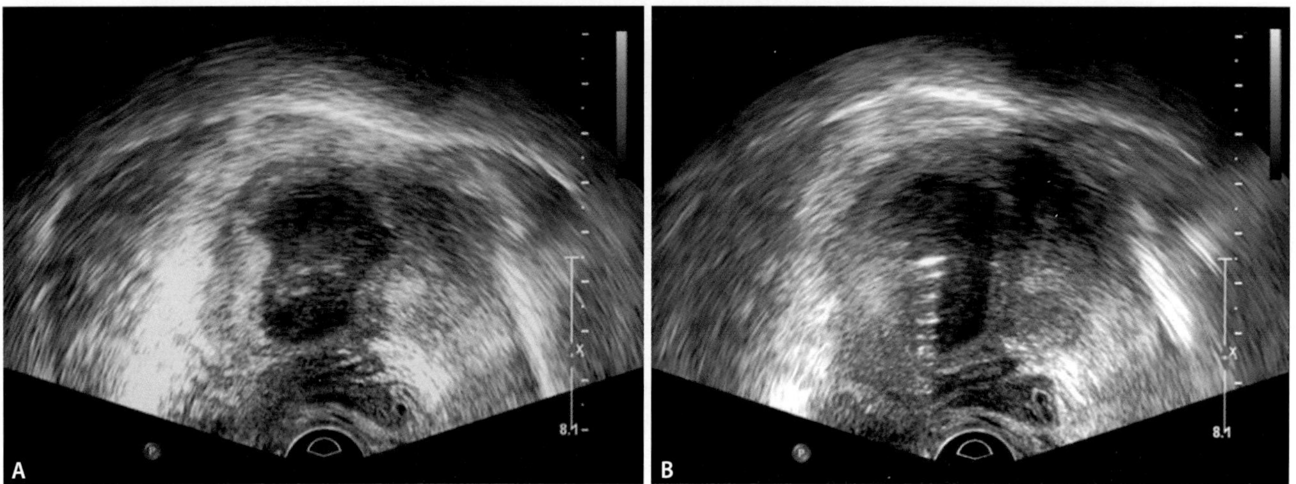

Figs. 18A and B: Prostatic abscess: (A) Transrectal ultrasound image showing abscess with thick irregular walls in right half of prostate; (B) Aspiration needle is seen with in the abscess.

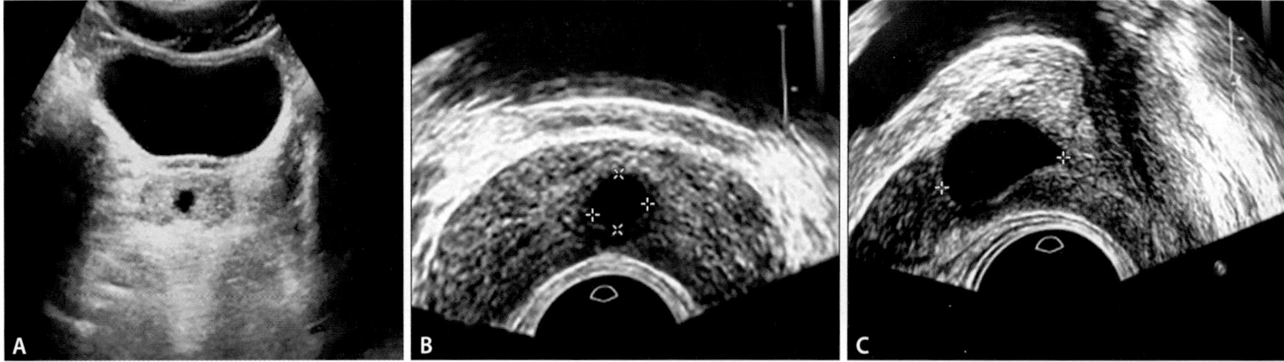

Figs. 19A to C: Utricle cyst: Transabdominal ultrasound (A), transrectal ultrasound axial (B), and sagittal (C) images showing small midline utricular cyst in prostate.

ejaculatory ducts. Utricle cysts contain sperms but unlike former do not extend beyond prostate **(Figs. 19 and 20)**. The paramidline cysts are Wolffian cysts, seminal vesicle cysts or ejaculatory duct cysts which contain sperms. Associated Wolffian duct anomalies, i.e. renal anomalies may be seen in these patients. Peripheral cysts are

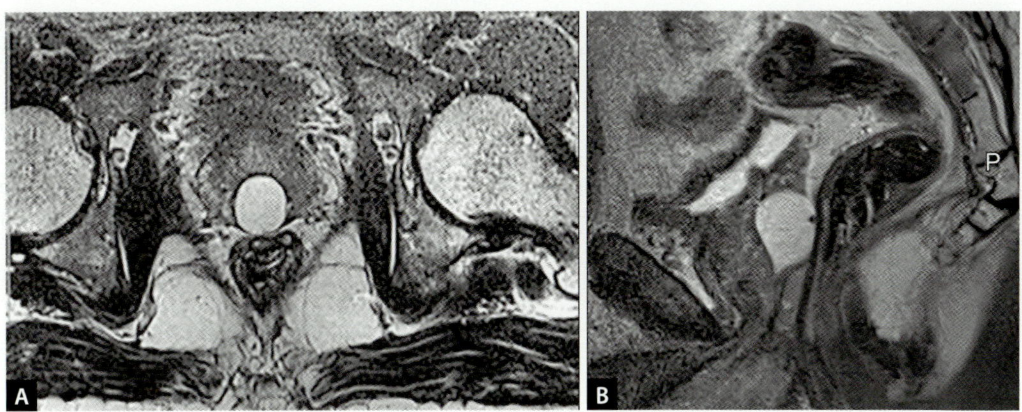

Figs. 20A and B: Utricle cyst: T2-weighted axial (A) and sagittal (B) images showing midline intraprostatic cyst which does not extend beyond the prostatic base.

acquired retention cysts and may be associated with BPH. Cowper's gland cysts are also acquired cysts associated with urogenital diaphragm. Cystic lesions appear smooth walled, hypoechoic on USG and hyperintense on T2WI unless complicated by infection or hemorrhage.[27]

ACKNOWLEDGEMENT

Sincere thanks to Dr Prabhjyot Singh Chowhan, Department of Radiodiagnosis.

REFERENCES

1. O'Brien WM. Benign prostatic hypertrophy. Am Fam Physician. 1991;44:162-71.
2. Dunnick NR, Newhouse JH, Cohan RH, et al. Prostate and seminal vesicles. In: Dunnick NR, Newhouse JH, Cohan RH, Maturen KE (Eds). Genitourinary Radiology. Philadelphia: Wolters Kluwer; 2018. pp. 321-38.
3. Grajo JR, Cronin C. Benign prostatic hyperplasia. In Sahani DV, Sameer AE (Eds). Abdominal Imaging. Philadelphia, Elsevier; 2017. pp. 896-904.
4. Shinohara K, Scardino PT, Carter SS, et al. Pathologic basis of the sonographic appearance of the normal and malignant prostate. Urol Clin North Am. 1989;16:675-91.
5. Kawashima A, Glockner J, King B. CT urography and MR urography. Radiol Clin North Am. 2003;41:945-61.
6. Pokharel SS, Patel NU, Garg K, et al. Multi-parametric MRI findings of transitional zone prostate cancers: correlation with 3-dimensional transperineal mapping biopsy. Abdom Imaging. 2015;40:143-50.
7. Bray F, Ferlay J, Soerjomataram I, et al. Global cancer statistics 2018: GLOBOCAN estimates of incidence and mortality worldwide for 36 cancers in 185 countries. CA Cancer J Clin. 2018;68:394-424.
8. Gann PH. Risk factors for prostate cancer. Rev Urol. 2002;4:S3-10.
9. Heidenreich A, Bellmunt J, Bolla M, et al. EAU guidelines on prostate cancer. Part 1: screening, diagnosis, and treatment of clinically localised disease. Eur Urol. 2011;59:61-71.
10. Guo G, Xu Y, Zhang X. TRUS-guided transperineal prostate 12+X core biopsy with template for the diagnosis of prostate cancer. Oncol Lett. 2017;13:4863-7.
11. Gleason DF. Histologic grading of prostate cancer: A perspective. Hum Pathol. 1992;23:237-79.
12. Kryvenko ON, Epstein JI. Changes in prostate cancer grading: Including a new patient-centric grading system. The Prostate. 2016;76:427-33.
13. Epstein JI, Egevad L, Amin MB, et al. The 2014 International Society of Urological Pathology (ISUP) Consensus Conference on Gleason Grading of Prostatic Carcinoma: Definition of Grading Patterns and Proposal for a New Grading System. Am J Surg Pathol. 2016;40:244-52.
14. Pierorazio PM, Walsh PC, Partin AW, et al. Prognostic Gleason grade grouping: data based on the modified Gleason scoring system. BJU Int. 2013;111:753-60.
15. Clements R. The role of transrectal ultrasound in diagnosing prostate cancer. Curr Urol Rep. 2002;3:194-200.
16. Yu KK, Hricak H. Imaging prostate cancer. Radiol Clin North Am. 2003;38:59-85.
17. Kitajima K, Murphy RC, Nathan MA, et al. Detection of recurrent prostate cancer after radical prostatectomy: comparison of 11C-choline PET/CT with pelvic multiparametric MR imaging with endorectal coil. J Nucl Med Off Publ Soc Nucl Med. 2014;55:223-32.
18. Barentsz JO, Richenberg J, Clements R, et al. ESUR prostate MR guidelines 2012. Eur Radiol. 2012;22:746-57.
19. Weinreb JC, Barentsz JO, Choyke PL, et al. PI-RADS prostate imaging—reporting and data system: 2015, version 2. Eur Urol. 2016;69(1):16e40.
20. Turkbey B, Rosenkrantz AB, Haider MA, et al. Prostate imaging reporting and data system version 2.1: 2019 update of prostate imaging reporting and data system version 2. Eur Urol. 2019; 76(3):340-51.
21. Mertan FV, Greer MD, Shih JH, et al. Prospective Evaluation of the Prostate Imaging Reporting and Data System Version 2 for Prostate Cancer Detection. J Urol. 2016;196:690-6.
22. Buyyounouski MK, Choyke PL, McKenney JK, et al. Prostate cancer—major changes in the American Joint Committee on Cancer eighth edition cancer staging manual. CA Cancer J Clin. 2017; 67(3):245-53.

23 Grajo JR, Lee LK, Cronin C. Benign and malignant focal prostate lesions. In: Sahani DV, Sameer AE (Eds). Abdominal Imaging. Philadelphia: Elsevier; 2017. pp. 905-22.
24. Somford DM, Hamoen EH, Fütterer JJ, et al. The predictive value of endorectal 3 Tesla multi parametric magnetic resonance imaging for extra prostatic extension in patients with low, intermediate and high risk prostate cancer. J Urol. 2013;190:1728.
25. Harisinghani MG, Barentsz J, Hahn PF, et al: Noninvasive detection of clinically occult lymph-node metastases in prostate cancer. N Engl J Med. 2003;348:2491-9.
26. Amis ES Jr, Bigongiari LR, Bluth EI, et al. Pre-treatment staging of clinically localized prostate cancer. Radiology. 2000;215 Suppl:703-8.
27. Parsons RB, Fisher AM, Bar-Chama N, Mitty HA. MR imaging in male infertility. RadioGraphics. 1997;17:627-37.

Chapter 21

Scrotal Diseases

Anupam Lal, Manphool Singhal, Sreedhara BC

ANATOMY

The scrotum is a cutaneous pouch which contains the testes and parts of the spermatic cords. It is formed by the fusion of two scrotal sacs separated by an inner septum that corresponds to a midline ridge or raphe on the surface, and extends anteriorly along the under surface of the penis, and posterior along the middle line of the perineum to the anus. The following structures form the wall of scrotum, from superficial to the deep layers: skin, fascia (superficial), muscle (dartos), external spermatic fascia, cremasteric fascia, and internal spermatic fascia. The testes are suspended in the scrotal sac by the spermatic cord and are anchored to scrotal wall caudally by gubernaculum testis. Gubernaculum testis is cord-like structure located caudal to the testis and guides the testicular descent. The left testis lies lower than the right, corresponding with bigger length of the left-sided spermatic cord.

Each testis is in oval form, lying obliquely in the scrotal sac; the upper pole is directed anterior and a little lateral; the lower pole is directed posterior and medial; the anterior border is convex, oriented forward and downward, and the posterior border is relatively straight oriented backward and upward, to which the spermatic cord is attached. The lateral surfaces, anterior border and extremities (both) of the testes are convex, smooth, free, and invested by the tunica vaginalis (visceral layer). There is only partial investment of tunica vaginalis along the posterior border, to which the cord is attached. Epididymis body is seen lying upon the posterior border (lateral edge). Visceral and parietal layers of tunica vaginalis surround the testis and epididymis. Between these two layers there lies vaginal cavity containing minimal amount of fluid, derived from the "saccus vaginalis" of the peritoneum. Saccus vaginalis in the fetus precedes the testis descent into the scrotum from abdomen. The testicular capsule is formed by tunica albuginea. Tunica albuginea is covered by the tunica vaginalis, except at the attachment points of the epididymis and spermatic vessels entry into the gland along its posterior border. It is attached to the tunica vasculosa, and is reflected into the interior of the gland along its posterior border, leading to formation of incomplete vertical septum, defined as mediastinum testis. From the mediastinum testis, numerous fibrous septa are seen to extend into the testis, dividing it into multiple lobules containing one to three seminiferous tubules each, supporting the Sertoli cells, spermatocytes, and "Leydig" cells within the interstitium.

All tubules drain into larger ducts called tubuli recti. These tubuli recti converge to form the rete testis, an anastomosing network of draining tubules, and enter into mediastinum testis, which carries the sperms from testis to the epididymis. The mediastinum testis consists of invagination of tunica albuginea and the rete testis. It also contains branches of testicular arteries, centripetal veins and lymphatics of the testis and hence is the anatomical hilum of the testis.

Testicular size varies with age and sexual development stage. It measures approximately 1.5 cm × 1 cm (length × width) at birth. Before 12 years of age, the average volume of testis is about 1-2 cm^3. Clinically, a male individual is considered to have reached puberty once the testis achieves a volume of 4 cm^3. The

postpubertal testis of average dimensions varies from 4 cm to 5 cm in length, 2.5 cm in transverse diameter, 3 cm in the AP dimension, and 10.5–14 g in weight.

The epididymis consists of a head (globus major), body and tail (globus minor). The head lies cranial to the testis and it consists of 8–12 efferent ducts converging into a single larger duct called as vas deferens in the body and tail, which continues in the spermatic cord.

There are four testicular appendages (remnants of embryonic ducts), which have been described: (1) appendix testis, (2) appendix epididymis, (3) paradidymis and (4) vas aberrans.[1] The appendix testis and appendix epididymis can be visualized on ultrasonography (USG). The testicular appendage (hydatid of Morgagni) is a remnant of Müllerian duct, a minute oval, sessile body visualized on the upper pole of testis, and the appendix epididymis (pedunculated hydatid) is seen on the head of the epididymis. The spermatic cord is composed of arteries (the internal and external spermatics; and the artery to the ductus deferens), veins, nerves, lymphatics, and the excretory duct of the testis.

The arteries supplying the testicular coverings are: the superficial and deep external pudendal arteries, cremasteric branch from the inferior epigastric artery and superficial perineal branch of internal pudendal. The veins follow the corresponding arteries. The nerves are lumboinguinal and ilioinguinal branches from the lumbar plexus, pudendal branch of the posterior femoral cutaneous nerve and superficial perineal branches of the internal pudendal nerve.

IMAGING MODALITIES

Ultrasonography with a high-frequency (7.5-14 MHz) transducer is the imaging modality of choice to examine scrotum. Sonography combined with color Doppler and power Doppler has evolved into an all-encompassing scrotal imaging technique as both structural and perfusion abnormalities can be detected. Magnetic resonance imaging (MRI) and nuclear scan are other important complementary modalities. Computed tomography (CT) scan and MRI have important role in staging of testicular cancer and for the localization of testis in patients with cryptorchidism.

Technique of Sonography

Scrotal ultrasound (US) is performed in the supine position, with a cloth between the thighs supporting the scrotum. A high-frequency (7–14 MHz) linear array transducer is optimal for visualization of scrotal structures, and a stand-off pad is useful for superficial lesions. The testes are examined in both longitudinal and transverse axes, and dimension and echogenicity are compared with the opposite side. In acute scrotum evaluation, normal side should be scanned first in order to set the grayscale and color Doppler gain settings, which helps in comparison with the affected side. While assessing small palpable nodules, placing the finger beneath the nodule with the transducer placed directly over the nodule, or placing the finger on the nodule and the transducer opposite should be considered for optimal imaging. Scrotal skin thickness (normal 2–8 mm, depends on the cremasteric muscle contraction) should be evaluated. Additional techniques like upright positioning or Valsalva maneuver can be used for venous evaluation.

Prepubertal testes are of low to medium echogenicity, whereas pubertal and postpubertal testes are of medium homogeneous echogenicity, indicating tubular maturation and development of germ cell elements.[2] The mediastinum testis is visualized as an echogenic band (variable length and thickness) extending in a caudocranial direction **(Fig. 1)**. The small amount of fluid in the space between leaves of the tunica vaginalis is seen as thin echo-free rim adjacent to the head. This minimal amount of fluid should not be misinterpreted as hydrocele. Longitudinal view is best to evaluate epididymis, where the epididymal head (5–12 mm in length) is seen as a pyramidal structure lying above the superior pole of the testis and is usually isoechoic to the testis.[3] The body (2–4 mm in diameter) is usually indistinguishable from the surrounding peritesticular tissue, and the tail

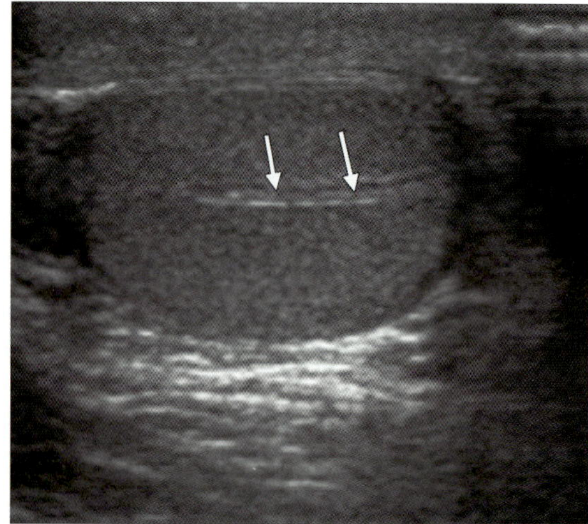

Fig. 1: US image of the test is in its long axis showing echogenic line of mediastinum testes (arrows).

(2-5 mm) is seen as a curved structure at the inferior pole of the testis, where it becomes the ductus deferens.

The spectral waveform of the intratesticular arteries characteristically has a low-resistance pattern,[4] with a mean resistive index (RI) of 0.62 (range, 0.48-0.75);[2] however, for a testis with volume less than 4 cm^3, this may not be true,[3] as in prepubertal boys, where diastolic arterial flow may not be detectable.[5]

Contrast-enhanced US (CEUS) role in depicting minimal vascular flow, vascular morphology along with "washout" characteristics of a lesion is well established and is increasingly being used in scrotal US evaluation with focus on a particular lesion characterization. A rapid enhancement and washout of a lesion usually depicts an aggressive or malignant lesion. In case of benign vascular pattern, recommendation of monitoring with follow-up can be provided confidently.

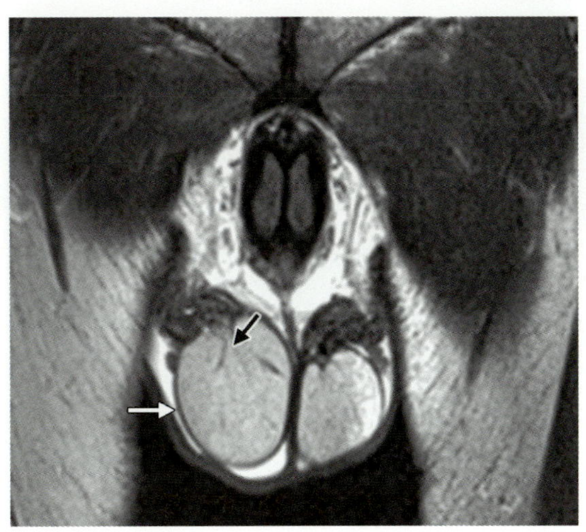

Fig. 2: T2 coronal MR image of the scrotum showing testes as high-signal intensity structures within the scrotum. Note the hypointense rim of tunica albuginea (white arrow) around the testes and the mediastinum testis (black arrow) within it.

Magnetic Resonance Imaging of Scrotum

Magnetic resonance imaging (MRI) of the scrotum is extremely valuable as a problem-solving modality. The MRI examination is performed in supine position with scrotum supported by towel. Symmetric placement of testis is important for optimal coronal scans. The scrotum is then covered by small cloth or gauze and the surface coil is placed over it in a flat position. T1-weighted (T1W) and T2-weighted (T2W) spin-echo images are obtained in coronal and axial planes. Contrast-enhancement or fat suppression sequences are also obtained when further tissue characterization is required. Optimum coverage is provided by thin (4-5 mm) slices with 1-2 mm interslice gaps and 8-20 cm field of view. The scan area must be extended to lower pole of kidneys when looking for undescended testis and up to the diaphragm when MRI is performed for staging of testicular cancer.

On MRI, the testis is seen as an oval, sharply defined structure with homogeneous intermediate signal intensity on T1W images and high-signal intensity on T2W images **(Fig. 2)**. The tunica albuginea is seen as a thin hypointense rim around the testis.

The mediastinum testis is also hypointense and it is seen as a dark stripe invaginating into the testis. The signal intensity of the epididymis is similar to testis on T1W images and much lower on T2W images. The pampiniform plexus is seen as a tortuous tubular structure extending from upper pole of testis up to the inguinal canal. Vas deferens can sometimes be seen as a low-intensity tubular structure that can be traced from epididymis to inguinal canal.

CONGENITAL ANOMALIES OF THE TESTIS

Cryptorchidism

Cryptorchidism is a condition where either one or both testes fails to descend to the base of the scrotum from abdomen, affects 4-5% of full-term and 9-30% of premature males at birth. In cryptorchidism, testis can be found in any position along the line of descent (abdominal, inguinal, prescrotal, or gliding); however, in about 80%, the nonpalpable undescended testis is located in inguinal canal and intra-abdominal in 20%.[6] Normal complete descent is necessary for full maturation of the testis. Complications of undescended testis include infertility, malignant degeneration, torsion and inguinal hernia. Orchiopexy performed later, even after puberty, is advocated for better surveillance of the testis. If orchiopexy is not feasible, orchidectomy is considered in patients after puberty. Recent epidemiologic studies indicate a 2.5 to 8 times greater risk of developing malignancy in cryptorchid testis.[7] Most common malignancy in the cryptorchid testis is seminoma. Orchiopexy does not reduce the risk of malignant degeneration of the once cryptorchid testis; however, it allows easier surveillance. In cases of seminoma of cryptorchid testis prompting unilateral orchiectomy, the remaining normal testis remains at a higher risk of developing cancer.

Ultrasound examination is indicated for the localization of undescended testis and also for the follow-up after orchiopexy. The undescended testis is often smaller and iso- or hypoechoic in echogenicity. Identification

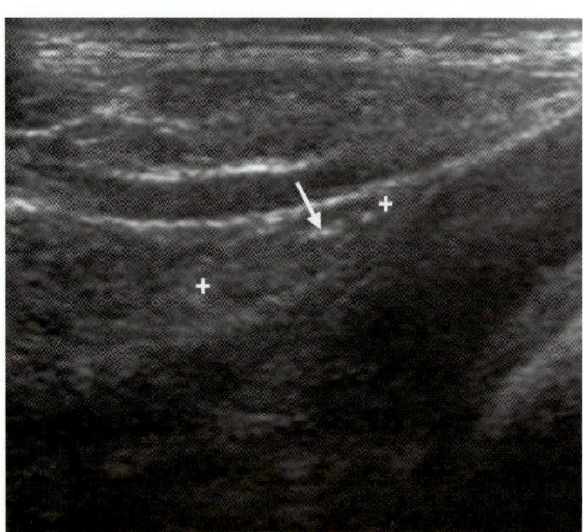

Fig. 3: US image of left undescended testis in a 24-year male: The testis is atrophic and located distal to external inguinal ring anterior to the pubic tubercle. Mediastinum testes are identified within the testis (arrow).

of mediastinum testis helps in differentiating this with other similar appearing structures like lymph nodes. The undescended testis is most commonly located distal to external inguinal ring anterior to the pubic tubercle. Even small rudimentary testis can be identified, if it is located here and hence, US is the primary imaging modality used for the localization of undescended testis **(Fig. 3)**. If testis is not located in the inguinal canal or base of the scrotum, then suprapubic, femoral and perineal regions should also be scanned. Intra-abdominal testis is difficult to locate on sonography.

Magnetic resonance imaging is an excellent modality for demonstration of penoscrotal or intracanalicular testis, but is not very satisfactory for demonstration of high intra-abdominal testis. Bladder should be emptied before the scanning. Fast T1W and T2W axial and coronal images are obtained from scrotum to the level above seminal vesicles. The examination is extended up to lower pole of the kidneys if testis is not located in the pelvis. The undescended testis can be easily identified with its characteristic signal intensity pattern. It tends to be oval in inguinal canal and round in intra-abdominal position. Sometimes the gubernaculum testis may be misdiagnosed as the undescended testis. While testis typically is hypointense on T1W and hyperintense on T2W images, the gubernaculum testis is hypointense on both T1W and T2W images. Hypertrophied inguinal lymph nodes may also have the signal characteristics similar to the testis; however, typical location of the nodes (adjacent to vessels or below the inguinal ligament) and demonstration of mediastinum in undescended testis help to differentiate testis from the lymph nodes. CT, like MRI, also allows precise identification of the undescended testis.

Miscellaneous Congenital Anomalies

Retractile or migratory testis is seen in 5- to 6-year-old boys and is due to a hyperactive reflex of cremaster muscle. The testis slides back and forth between scrotum and external inguinal ring. By puberty these usually take normal intrascrotal position and no treatment is required. The ectopic testis, i.e. location outside the descent path, is rare and is believed to be due to misdirected attachment to the scrotum. The usual sites of testicular ectopia are superficial inguinal pouch (lateral to external inguinal ring), femoral canal, suprapubic area, perineum, and contralateral scrotal pouch.[8] Unilateral absence of testis (monorchia) is usually left sided.[9] Unlike cryptorchidism, the testis in the patients with monorchia is not at increased risk of malignancy. Polyorchidism or testicular duplication is very rare.[8]

ACUTE SCROTUM

Acute scrotum is a clinical condition characterized by sudden onset of pain, swelling and redness of the scrotum that may occur alone or in any combination. It is important to differentiate surgical conditions like testicular torsion or rupture from those that can be managed conservatively (epididymo-orchitis) as early as possible. Clinical examination alone may not be helpful or it may be difficult to perform in patients with acute tender scrotum. Acute inflammation and testicular torsion are most important causes of acute scrotal pain. Other causes include torsion of appendix of testis or epididymis, trauma, tumor, incarcerated inguinal hernia and thrombophlebitis of the pampiniform plexus.

Epididymitis and Orchitis

Epididymitis is the most common cause of acute scrotum in postpubertal adults. Acute epididymitis is almost always caused by descending lower urinary tract infection. In children and older men, *Escherichia coli*, *Pseudomonas* and *Proteus* are the usual causative organisms. In young men, sexually transmitted organisms such as *Chlamydia and gonococci* are responsible. Rare causes of epididymitis and orchitis include tuberculosis, sarcoidosis,[10] brucellosis,[11] mumps and *Cryptococcus*. Chemical epididymitis can be seen due to drugs like amiodarone.[12] Direct extension of the inflammation in testis, resulting in epididymo-orchitis occurs in about 20% of patients with epididymitis.[13] Isolated orchitis is rare except when caused by viral infections such as mumps and acquired immunodeficiency syndrome (AIDS).[14] Complications of acute epididymitis include abscess, chronic pain, infarction, gangrene, atrophy, pyocele and infertility.

Patients present with insidious pain and scrotal swelling. Fever, dysuria and urethral discharge may also be present. Clinically, scrotal pain associated with epididymitis is usually relieved when the testes are elevated over the symphysis pubis (the Prehn's sign).[15] US findings of acute epididymitis include enlarged hypoechoic or hyperechoic (presumably secondary to hemorrhage) epididymis[2] **(Fig. 4)**. Indirect signs of inflammation, such as reactive hydrocele, pyocele and scrotal wall thickening can be seen. Diffuse testicular involvement is confirmed by inhomogeneous testicular echotexture and enlargement. Orchitis is characterized by heterogeneous echogenicity due to testicular edema contained within a rigid tunica albuginea.[16] It may be seen as focal or diffuse involvement, with the former manifesting as multiple hypoechoic lesions within the parenchyma **(Fig. 5)**. Lymphoma and leukemia of the testis have a similar appearance and are often bilateral (but not always), whereas infections (excluding mumps) are usually unilateral.

The sensitivity of color Doppler US (CDUS) imaging in detecting scrotal inflammation is almost 100%.[17] In acute epididymitis, there is a high-flow, low resistance pattern due to increase in the number of vessels with hyperemia.[18] In healthy volunteer, the RI in the testis is rarely less than 0.5; however, in more than 50% of epididymo-orchitis patients, the RI is less than 0.5.[19] Use of a peak systolic velocity (PSV) threshold of 15 cm/s results in a diagnostic accuracy of 93% for epididymitis and 90% for orchitis.[20] Reversal of flow during diastole is suggestive of venous infarction in acute epididymo-orchitis.[21] Follow-up sonography is necessary in patients who do not respond to therapy. However, it is not required in patients with uncomplicated epididymitis.

Contrast-enhanced US can be a problem-solving tool in acute inflammation for assessment of secondary complications like abscess formation, hemorrhage, spermatic cord thrombosis, or venous infarction. In testicular abscesses or venous infarction, CEUS demonstrates nonenhancement of a central avascular component, with enhancement of peripheral rim and septa.[22] It also shows absence of flow in the thrombosed spermatic vessels.

In acute epididymitis, enlarged epididymis with high-signal intensity on T2W images is seen on MRI. Areas of hemorrhages and hypervascularity (in the form of engorged vessels with signal void) can also be demonstrated. The inflamed epididymis shows marked enhancement on postcontrast images. Associated orchitis, if present, is seen as homogeneous or heterogeneous hypointense areas in testis on T2W images.

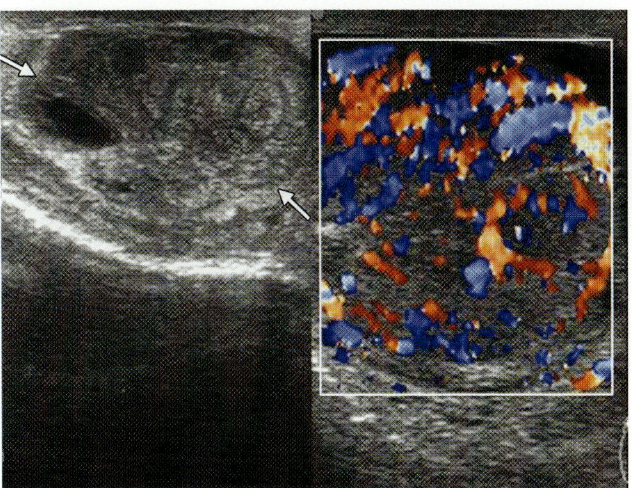

Fig. 4: US and color Doppler image of acute epididymitis showing enlarged heterogeneous epididymal head (arrows) with increased vascularity.

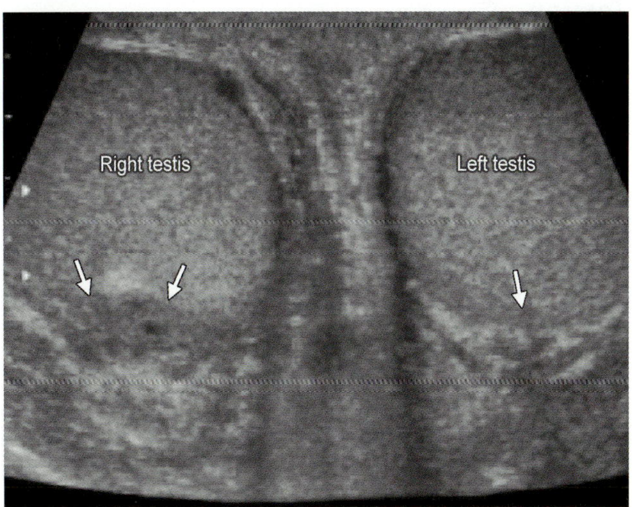

Fig. 5: Bilateral epididymo-orchitis: US image showing enlarged heterogeneous epididymis posterior to both testes and hypoechoic areas within the testes (arrows).

The sonographic findings in chronic epididymitis are nonspecific and diagnosis is usually made on the basis of clinical findings. It is characterized by persistent pain in the scrotal region and on grayscale US, an enlarged epididymis with increased echogenicity can be seen.[23] Sometimes calcifications within the epididymis can be seen. Tuberculosis, leprosy, sarcoidosis, brucellosis and syphilis can cause granulomatous epididymo-orchitis **(Fig. 6)**.

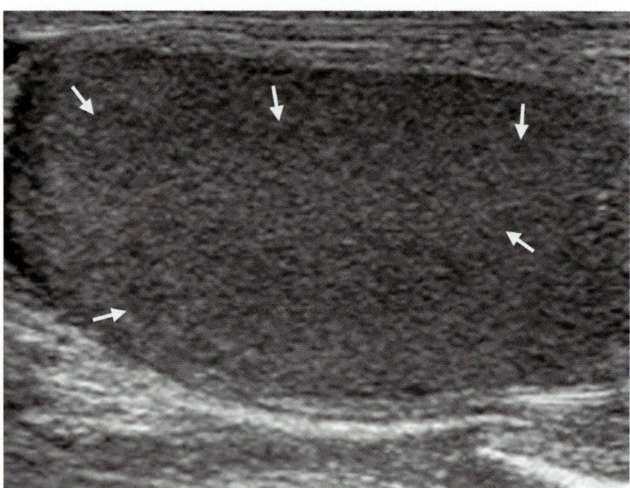

Fig. 6: Granulomatous orchitis in a case of syphilis: US image showing multiple ill-defined hypoechoic lesions (arrows) within the testis.

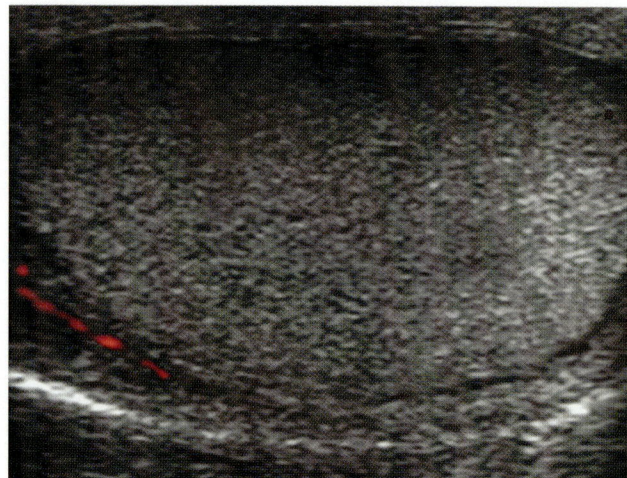

Fig. 7: Power Doppler US image showing heterogeneous appearing testis with reduced intratesticular flow in a case of torsion of testis.

Torsion

Testicular torsion occurs due to rotation of testis along the longitudinal axis of spermatic cord. Initially, venous drainage is stopped resulting in edema and hemorrhages. Subsequently arterial flow is also impaired resulting in ischemia and hemorrhagic necrosis of the gonad. It is a surgical emergency, as delay in diagnosis and intervention leads to irreversible damage to the testis. The extent of testicular ischemia depends on the degree of torsion, which ranges from 180° to 720° or greater, and the degree of torsion and duration of ischemia determines testicular salvage rate. Nearly 100% salvage rate exists when the surgery is done in first 6 hours after the onset of symptoms; which reduces to 70% within 6–12 hours, and 20% at 12–24 hours.[24]

There are two types of testicular torsion: (1) Extravaginal; and (2) Intravaginal. Extravaginal torsion is rare and occurs almost exclusively in neonates. It occurs when testis and gubernaculum are not fixed and are free to rotate in the scrotum. The entire vaginal sac including testis rotates at the level of external inguinal ring. It often presents as a mass in the groin in newborns. Intravaginal torsion occurs within the vaginal sac. It results from anomalous suspension of testis by a long stalk of spermatic cord and most commonly occurs in boys around the puberty. There is ten-fold increased incidence of torsion in undescended testis after orchiopexy.[25]

Approximately two-thirds of the cases of torsion are seen in adolescents between 12 years and 18 years of age. Acute torsion patients present with scrotal pain of sudden onset, followed by nausea, vomiting and low-grade fever. On physical examination, swollen, edematous, tender, and inflamed hemiscrotum can be seen. US is considered the first step in evaluation, and its findings vary with the degree and duration of rotation of the cord. Grayscale images are nonspecific and often appear normal, if the torsion has just occurred. In first 4–6 hours, most commonly encountered findings are testicular swelling and decreased echogenicity **(Fig. 7)**. After 24 hours of onset, the testis shows diffusely heterogeneous echotexture due to congestion, hemorrhage, and infarction (late or missed torsion). An enlarged hypoechoic epididymal head may also be seen as the deferential artery supplying the epididymis is often involved in the torsion.[26] In the setting of complete torsion, normal echogenicity of testis on US is a strong predictor of viability. Other indicators include reactive hydrocele and scrotal wall thickening.

Torsion may be transient, incomplete or complete. Partial or transient torsion pose a diagnostic challenge, and the ability of CDUS to enable accurate diagnosis of incomplete torsion remains undetermined. The presence of color or power Doppler signal in a patient with the clinical manifestation of torsion does not exclude torsion.[27]

For accurate diagnosis the US scanner should be optimized for detection of slow flow and be adjusted for the lowest possible threshold setting and lowest repetition frequency. On color Doppler, detection of testicular torsion and ischemia in painful scrotum by using the only criteria of absence of identifiable intratesticular flow is 86% sensitive, 100% specific and 97% accurate.[17] Scintigraphy and color Doppler are comparable with regard to diagnosis of torsion in adolescent and adult populations.[17] Scintigraphy is a reasonable alternative for evaluation of

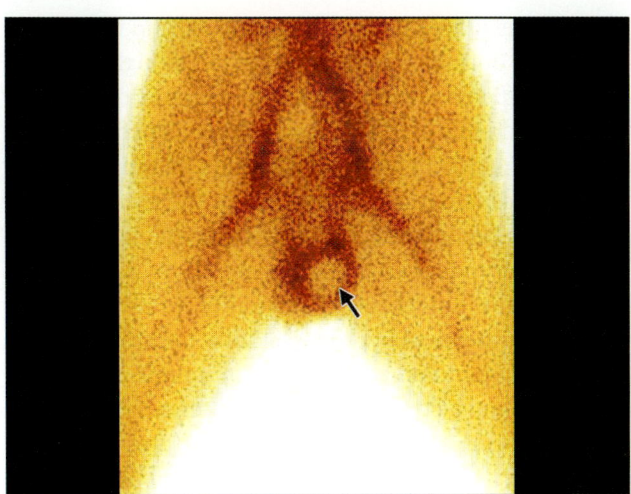

Fig. 8: Tc-99m pertechnetate scan showing photopenic area (arrow) in scrotum due to torsion of left testis.

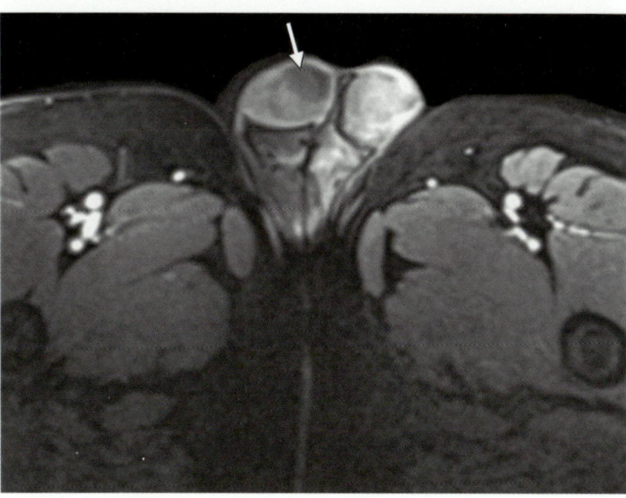

Fig. 9: Intermittent torsion: Contrast-enhanced magnetic resonance (CEMR) axial image showing hypoenhancing area within the right testis (arrow).

acute scrotal pain and should be used when diagnosis of torsion remains in question and CDUS sensitivity for low-velocity, low-volume testicular blood flow is inadequate **(Fig. 8)**.

Torsion of the testicular and epididymal appendages also present with acute scrotal pain with no other physical symptoms usually. On physical examination, a small firm nodule, palpable along the superior aspect of the testis exhibiting bluish discoloration through the overlying skin can be seen; defined as "blue dot" sign.[28] The appendix of testis is the most commonly twisted testicular appendices, seen in nearly 90% of cases and most often occur in boys of 7–14 years of age. Torsion of the appendages of the testes on US usually reveals a hyperechoic mass with a central hypoechoic area adjacent to the epididymis or testis. Skin thickening and reactive hydrocele are common in these cases. On color Doppler, increased peripheral flow may be seen around the twisted testicular appendage.[17] Management is conservative aimed at pain reduction. The pain usually subsides within 2–3 days, with atrophy of the appendix, which may calcify. The role of US examination in testicular appendage torsion is to exclude acute epididymo-orchitis and testicular torsion.

Magnetic resonance imaging in testicular torsion can show twisted cord as multiple low intensity curvilinear structures radiating in a "whirlpool" pattern. The torsion knot may be seen as an area of signal void. In patients with intermittent torsion, the testis is enlarged and hyperintense on both T1W and T2W images owing to subacute hemorrhages **(Fig. 9)**. Phosphorus magnetic resonance spectroscopy has been reported to be helpful in evaluation of acute torsion. It demonstrates decreased levels of β-ATP and phosphomonoester and increased levels of inorganic phosphorus.[13]

Scrotal Trauma

Scrotal trauma usually results from either direct injury or from straddle injuries. History is very helpful in the diagnosis; however, marked scrotal swelling, pain and open injuries limit adequate clinical examination. Patients with penetrating and open scrotal injuries undergo immediate surgery and are not candidates for US.

In cases of blunt trauma, sonography is used to confirm or exclude testicular rupture, differentiate a hematoma from hematocele and for follow-up of patients undergoing conservative management. Testicular rupture is a surgical emergency and such patients are taken up for immediate surgery whereas patients with small hematomas or hematocele are managed conservatively. Hence scrotal sonography has a decisive influence on clinical management.[29]

On sonography, intratesticular hematoma is seen as sharply defined hypoechoic space-occupying lesion (SOL). Irregularities of testicular contour and hypo- or hyperechoic heterogeneous areas suggest testicular rupture. These parenchymal areas correspond to hemorrhages and infarction. Visualization of solid and cystic intrascrotal mass and absence of testis like structure is a characteristic feature of testicular fragmentation. Sometimes a distinct fracture line may also be identified. Hematocele usually accompanies testicular rupture but its absence does not exclude the possibility of rupture.[14] Scrotal hematoma between the layers of scrotal wall is seen as nonspecific soft tissue thickening. If the urethra is injured, extravasation of urine between the layers of scrotal wall produces "onion peel" thickening of scrotal wall.

Acute hematocele or accumulation of blood in vaginal sac contains numerous small internal echoes. In chronic hematocele, thick septae and wall thickening are demonstrated.

There is good correlation of CEUS findings with extent of injury, which can clear demonstrate the fracture lines, interruption of tunica albuginea, and scrotal hematoma. It also quantifies viable parenchyma more reliably compared to conventional sonography or CDUS.[30] CEUS allows a more confident assessment of two clinically important features: (1) the presence of testicular rupture, and (2) the extent of viable testicular tissue which may influence the surgical decision.

Magnetic resonance imaging may be required in patients with scrotal injury when satisfactory sonographic examination is not possible. It is also indicated, if testicular rupture cannot be confidently excluded on the sonography. The diagnosis of testicular rupture is facilitated by unequivocal depiction of tunica albuginea on MRI.

The integrity of tunica albuginea is best assessed on T2W or contrast-enhanced T1W images. Intratesticular injuries demonstrate decreased contrast enhancement. MRI is also valuable in demonstration of hematomas.

Testicular Tumors

Testicular cancer is the most common solid malignancy affecting the young men between the age group of 18 years and 35 years, accounting for 1% of all cancers in men. Incidence of the testicular neoplasms is increasing from last decade and European men possess greater risk as compared to the other ethnicity. The germ cell tumors account for more than 90% of the testicular tumors. Risk factors for testicular cancer include cryptorchidism, testicular atrophy (e.g. mumps), testicular microlithiasis, Klinefelter's syndrome, Down syndrome, family history and maternal use of diethylstilbestrol.[31] The etiology of testicular cancer is not known till date; however; characteristic genetic alteration affecting the isochromosome of the short arm of the chromosome 12 (i(12p)) is implicated in the sporadic cases.

Localized testicular cancer presents as a painless nodule or a bump/swelling in the testicle or as a vague lower abdominal discomfort. Advanced disease or disseminated disease may present with lymphatic or hematogenous spread.

However, developments in diagnostic and therapeutic modalities during past decade have led to high cure rate, even for patients who present with metastatic disease.[16]

The main role of USG in the testicular cancer diagnosis is to distinguish between the lesions of intratesticular and extratesticular origin, as most of the extratesticular masses are benign and, intratesticular masses are more likely to be malignant.[32] Grayscale US is nearly 100% sensitive for detection of testicular tumors.[33] Many benign intratesticular processes like orchitis, abscess, hematoma, granuloma and infarction mimic malignancy and hence must considered in the differential diagnosis. Color Doppler examination demonstrates increased vascularity in the majority of malignant lesions and helps to better define testicular involvement. A suspicion of testicular cancer mandates radiological workup to ascertain the extent or spread of the disease with the help of chest and abdominopelvic cross-sectional imaging modalities. The lymph nodal metastasis into the pelvis, chest and supraclavicular nodal stations is considered as distant metastasis.

The radical inguinal orchiectomy is performed rather than a biopsy of the testis mass for histopathological evaluation as well as to achieve local tumor control. The testicular cancer stage, risk stratification and histopathological nature of tumor guide in selection of initial modality of the treatment. Definitive cure can be achieved by inguinal orchiectomy procedure alone in the patients with stage I seminoma. The adjuvant chemotherapy or radiation therapy is required in the advanced stages of the disease. With modern chemoradiation therapeutics development, it is not difficult to achieve complete cure rate even in presence of metastatic testicular cancer. Radiologists play a pivotal role in the initial detection, staging and active surveillance of the patients with testicular neoplasm.

Classification of the Testicular Tumors

Testicular cancers are broadly divided into the three categories as germ cell tumors, sex cord stromal tumors, and miscellaneous tumors **(Table 1)**. In young male, germ cell tumors account for 95% and sex cord stromal tumors for 5%, and miscellaneous tumors, including the most common entities like lymphoma or metastasis are encountered in the older age group. Among the germ cell tumors, seminoma constitutes ~50% of the prevalence and rest half is constituted by the nonseminomatous germ cell tumors which are enlisted in **Table 1** with percentage of each entity. Differentiation of seminomatous versus nonseminomatous germ cell tumor is important as treatment and prognosis is different.

Approach to Testicular Cancers

A suspected case of testicular cancer evaluation begins with complete history elicitation and systemic physical examination. The value of imaging and laboratory tests is invaluable in evaluation of testicular cancer. The USG (grayscale as well as Doppler mode), CT of chest, MRI or CT of abdomen and pelvis, MRI of brain and nuclear scans are utilized in workup of the subjects with testicular cancer based on the extent of the disease. Laboratory tests including the serum alpha-fetoprotein (AFP), serum beta-human chorionic gonadotropin (β-hCG), lactate dehydrogenase (LDH) and other chemistry profile are utilized in evaluation of patients.

Germ Cell Tumors

Germ cell tumors account for 90–95% of testicular cancer. Germ cell tumors are divided into two groups: (1) seminomatous and (2) nonseminomatous germ cell tumor (NSGCT). The later includes embryonal cell carcinoma, teratoma, choriocarcinoma, endodermal sinus tumor or mixed components of these tumors. The distinction of these tumors is primarily from the histological analysis, and immunohistochemical methods to be reserved for difficult cases. This distinction determines treatment and prognosis.

Table 1: Classification and prevalence (germ cell tumors) of the testicular tumors.

Testicular tumor	*Subtypes of testicular tumors*
Germ cell tumors	• Seminoma (50%) • Mixed germ cell tumor (33%) • Embryonal carcinoma (10%) • Teratoma (4%) • Yolk sac tumor (1%) • Choriocarcinoma (0.3%)
Sex cord stromal tumors	• Leydig cell tumor • Sertoli cell tumor • Granulosa cell tumor • Thecoma
Miscellaneous	• Metastasis (8–15%) • Lymphoma • Leukemia • Sarcoma • Leiomyoma • Vascular tumor • Fibroma • Neurofibroma

Serum tumor markers are important in diagnosis, staging and follow-up. These include LDH, AFP and hCG. LDH may increase in any type of tumor and it correlates well with the extent of the disease. The seminoma does not show elevated tumor marker AFP, if the elevated AFP in the patient with the histological analysis suggestive of seminoma warrants for consideration and treatment as for that of the nonseminomatous tumor.[34] Elevated hCG is encountered in subjects with choriocarcinoma, most of the NSGCT and a few subjects of seminomas.[31]

Seminomas

The most common tumor among the germ cell tumors is seminoma, approximately contributing to the 50% of the prevalence. Usually, it manifests in the young- and middle-aged adults in their 2nd to 3rd decade and almost never reported in the infants.[35] Best prognosis of seminomatous tumor is by virtue of its sensitivity to chemotherapeutic agents and radiation therapy.[7] The seminoma is subclassified into typical seminoma (~85%), anaplastic (~5–10%) and spermatocytic (~4–6%) histological variants. The spermatocytic variant of seminoma is seen in elderly (~60–70 years) males with excellent prognosis. On scrotal sonographic examination, seminoma of testis is visualized as a homogeneous, hypoechoic, nodule or mass, which matches the uniform appearance of gross pathological specimen **(Fig. 10)**. Infrequently, cystic changes (~10%) or calcification foci are also demonstrated in the seminoma.[36] Intralesional color uptake by the internal vascularity increases the diagnostic probability of malignant nature of the lesion of interest in appropriate clinical scenario. More advancements in the sonography modality has

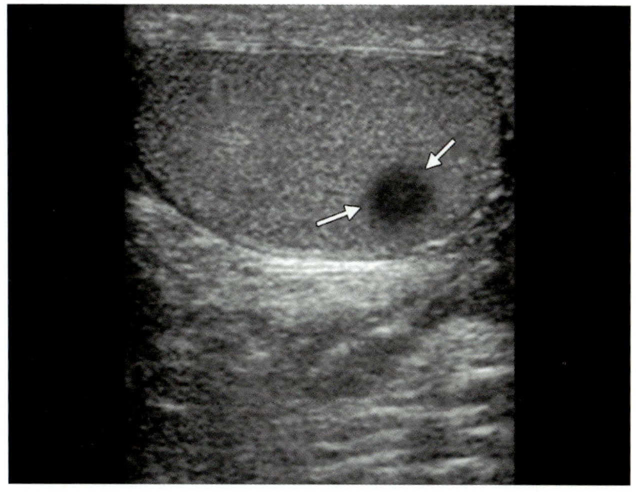

Fig. 10: US image showing a nonpalpable seminoma (arrows) of testis.

resulted in the advent of contrast-enhanced sonographic technique, which showed rapid uptake and washout characteristic of the seminoma lesion relative to the background parenchyma, along with the distortion of linear course of the intratesticular vascular channels.[37] Testicular mass may replace the whole of the testis in half of the cases, but still seminoma remains limited by the tunica albuginea, and rarely extends into the paratesticular substance/structures. Lymphatic and hematogenous dissemination of the seminoma is known phenomenon in testis oncology, which may be evident in the form of retroperitoneal or mediastinal lymph nodal enlargement and SOLs in the lung, liver and brain respectively, accounting for 25% of the population with seminoma.

Nonseminomatous Germ Cell Tumors

The NSGCTs constitute for the rest half of the prevalence of the germ cell tumors, the mixed germ cell tumor accounts for the most common (~30–60%) single variant tumor among the other NSGCTs. The embryonal carcinoma (10%), teratoma (4%), yolk sac tumor (1%), and choriocarcinoma (0.3%) are the other components of the NSGCTs. On histology, different proportions of the mixtures of tissue components or pure composition of lesions are seen, which reflect the similar characteristics on sonography resulting heterogeneous (71%) and irregular (45%) tumor lesions in testis. These lesions also demonstrate cystic (~61%) and calcification (~35%) changes more frequently as compared to the seminoma.[36] Most of the NSGCTs population presents with advanced disease.[32]

Embryonal Carcinoma

The pure component of the embryonal cells is rarely (~2%) seen in embryonal carcinoma, rather embryonal cellular component is most frequently (~85%) expressed in the mixed germ cell tumors, accounting for the ~10% of NSGCTs. Usually, this tumor is seen in middle-aged adults in their 3rd decade and rarely seen in the prepubertal males. On sonographic evaluation, irregular, heterogeneous lesions with calcific and cystic changes are seen with testicular distortion, breach of tunica albuginea and paratesticular extension frequently.[7]

Teratoma

Teratoma constitutes for the ~3–4% of the NSGCTs, and shows the cellular components derived from all the three-germ cell layers.[32] Teratomatous tumors can be present in any group, and it is the second most common testicular tumor in prepubertal boys. The mature teratoma in children is considered as benign, where as a teratoma in adults is treated as malignant. On sonologic evaluation, teratoma may be visualized as a heterogeneous lesion **(Fig. 11)**, with echogenic contents (fat, bone and cartilage) or hypoechoic components (soft tissue or fibrotic component). As compared to other tumors in the NSGCTs, the teratoma shows frequent cystic changes.

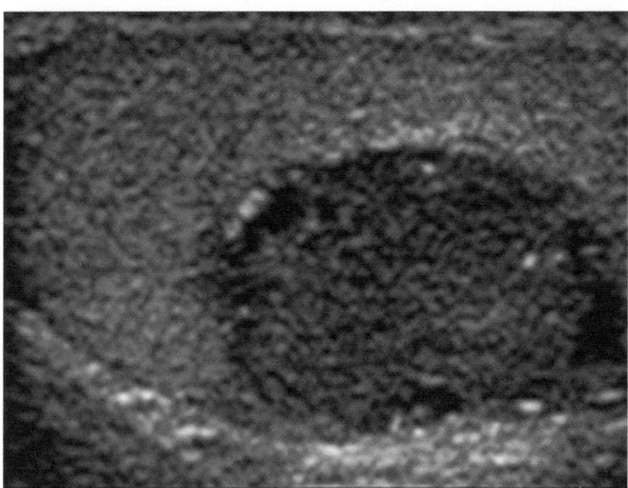

Fig. 11: US image showing teratoma of testis. Note small cystic areas and foci of calcification within the lesion.

Yolk Sac Tumor

Yolk sac tumors constitute ~1% of the NSGCTs, and this tumor is alternatively known an endodermal sinus tumor or infantile embryonal carcinoma. Usually, the children less than 5 year of age are most frequently involved by this tumor. Tumor marker AFP is elevated and its measurements adds in diagnosis (modest raise) as well as in prognostication of subjects with yolk sac tumor.[35] In adults, yolk sac component is encountered in the mixed germ cell tumors with associated poor prognosis. On sonographic evaluation, heterogeneous tumors with echogenic areas are seen scattered at places secondary to the hemorrhagic components.

Choriocarcinoma

The choriocarcinoma, syncytial cells containing tumor, is seen rarely, in ~0.5% subjects of NSGCTs. The choriocarcinoma is an aggressive malignant tumor, which shows microvascular invasion with early metastasis into the distant sites including the lungs and brain. Extensive tumoral hemorrhage is common in the choriocarcinoma, and exhibits poor prognosis. On US examination, mixed solid cystic mass is seen in the testis.[38] Cross-sectional imaging is warranted in the evaluation of the chest, abdominal and central nervous system metastases. The characteristic tumor marker β-hCG is used for establishing diagnosis as well as monitoring of the affected patients.

Burned-out Germ Cell Tumor

This is a biological magical phenomenon, where a rapidly growing tumor (usually the teratocarcinoma or choriocarcinoma) gets depleted of nutritional supply due to inadequate neoangiogenesis resulting the regression or vanishing of the primary tumor. The histopathological examination of such a testicular structure reveals scar or fibrotic component corresponding to the mixed echogenic or ill-defined hypoechoic lesion noted on USG.[39]

Non-germ Cell Testicular Tumors

The sex cord stromal tumors (including Leydig cell tumors, Sertoli cell tumor, granulosa cell tumors and thecoma) and miscellaneous tumors (such as lymphoma, metastasis, leukemia, and other mesenchymal tumors) are the non-germ cell tumors of testis accounting for the 5% of the testicular cancer.[40] The sex cord stromal tumors usually benign, and affect the prepubertal boys with mixed component of the tumor cells, and sometimes these tumors may biologically active with resultant secretion of endocrine substances resulting precocious puberty, scrotal enlargement and gynecomastia.

Gonadoblastoma is a rare tumor which is encountered in subjects with gonadal dysgenesis and associated intersex problems.

Sonographically, stromal tumors are seen as small, smoothly demarcated, homogeneous hypoechoic intratesticular masses[31] **(Fig. 12)**. Any lesion with rapid or aggressive growth patterns and intratumoral vascularity should suggest malignant behavior which reflects in histopathology analysis as cell atypia and high mitotic figures. Relatively newer sonological technique involving administration of US contrast agents showed persistent enhancement of the stromal tumors as opposed to the rapid enhancement and washout characteristic described in seminoma.[41]

Lymphomas constitute 5% of testicular tumors and are almost exclusively diffuse non-Hodgkin's lymphoma B-cell tumors **(Fig. 13)**. In men older than 60 years, lymphoma is the most common testicular tumor, accounting for nearly 50% of cases.[42] Sonographically, these tumors resemble seminomas but synchronous involvement of the contralateral testis and involvement of the spermatic cord and epididymis suggest lymphoma more than it does seminoma. Leukemic infiltration to the testis has been found at autopsy in 40–65% of patients with acute leukemia and in 20–35% of patients with chronic leukemia.[43] In boys with acute lymphoblastic leukemia, testicular involvement is reported in 5–10% of patients, with the majority found during clinical remission. Bilateral testicular involvement is seen in about 50% of the patients. Sonographically, lymphoma/leukemia deposits are seen as focal or diffuse hypoechoic areas. The testis is usually enlarged.

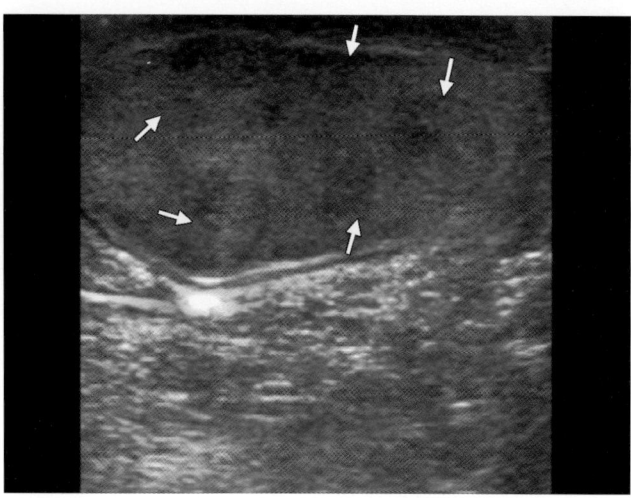

Fig. 12: US image showing multicentric rhabdomyosarcoma of testis (arrows).

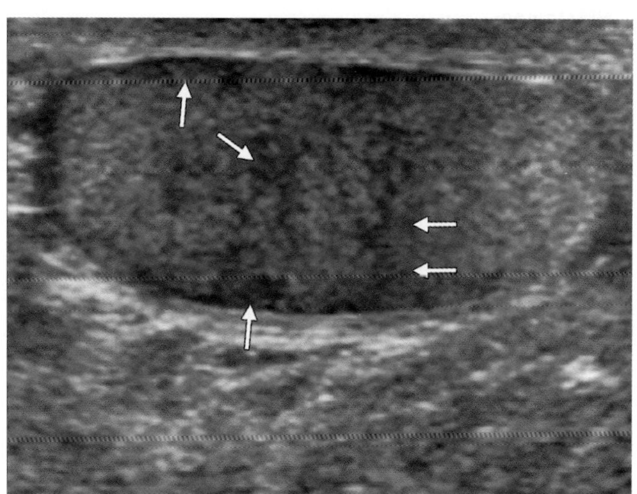

Fig. 13: US image showing sheet-like hypoechoic areas within the testis (arrows) due to lymphoma (NHL).

Intrascrotal metastases from tumors of other organs are rare and are usually found in older patients. Most frequent primaries are from lung, kidney, prostate and melanoma.[14] Sonographic appearances are nonspecific.

Staging of Testicular Cancer

T (Tumor) N (Node) M (Metastasis) staging by the American Joint Committee on Cancer (AJCC) is followed for testicular cancer **(Box 1)**. Extent of primary tumor (pT) is classified after radical orchiectomy, and nodal staging can be done clinically (N) or by pathological (pN) analysis.[44]

Serum Tumor Markers

Serum tumor markers(s) are also used in staging of testicular cancer. Blood tests are done before and after surgery, and for patients receiving chemotherapy, tumor markers on 1st of therapy are used for risk group determination **(Table 2)**.

CANCER GROUP STAGING

Considering all the above parameters [T (tumor), N (nodes), M (metastasis) and S (serum levels of tumor markers)], final staging of the tumor is done, which helps in treatment planning and prognostication of tumors **(Table 3)**.

Risk Group Classification

Another application of the TNM system is, it is used in risk stratification of advanced disease, taking into consideration of tumor markers and classifies the cancer as low, medium, and poor outlook. This helps in determining treatment plan and the likelihood of cure **(Table 4)**.

Box 1: TNM staging for testicular cancer.

TNM staging

Primary tumor

- pTx: Primary tumor cannot be assessed (if radical orchiectomy has not been performed, Tx is used)
- pT0: No evidence of primary tumor (e.g. histologic scar in testis)
- pTis: Intratubular germ cell neoplasia (carcinoma *in situ*)
- pT1: Tumor limited to the testis and epididymis without vascular/lymphatic invasion, or tumor invasion into the tunica albuginea but not the tunica vaginalis
- pT2: Tumor limited to the testis and epididymis with vascular/lymphatic invasion, or tumor extending through the tunica albuginea with involvement of the tunica vaginalis
- pT3: Tumor invades the spermatic cord with or without vascular/lymphatic invasion
- pT4: Tumor invades the scrotum with or without vascular/lymphatic invasion

Nodal staging

- NX or pNX: Regional lymph nodes cannot be assessed
- N0 or pN0: No regional lymph node metastasis
- N1 or pN1: Metastases with a lymph node mass 2 cm or less in greatest dimension; or multiple lymph nodes, none more than 2 cm in greatest dimension
- N2 or pN2: Metastases with a lymph node mass more than 2 cm but not more than 5 cm in greatest dimension; or multiple lymph nodes, any one mass greater than 2 cm but not more than 5 cm in greatest dimension
- N3 or pN3: Metastases with a lymph node mass more than 5 cm in greatest dimension

Metastasis

- MX: Distant metastasis cannot be assessed
- M0: No distant metastasis
- M1: Distant metastasis
- M1a: Nonregional nodal or pulmonary metastasis
- M1b: Distant metastasis other than to nonregional lymph nodes and lungs

(pT: primary tumor; N: clinical nodal staging; pN: pathological nodal staging)

Table 2: Blood levels of tumor markers for staging of testicular cancer.

	LDH (U/L)	*hCG (mIU/mL)*	*AFP (ng/mL)*
Sx	Marker studies not available or not performed		
S0	Normal	Normal	Normal
S1	<1.5 × Normal	<5,000	<1,000
S2	1.5–10 × Normal	5,000–50,000	1,000–10,000
S3	>10 × Normal	>50,000	>10,000

[LDH: lactate dehydrogenase (measured in units per liter); hCG: human chorionic gonadotropin (measured in milli-international units per milliliter); AFP: alpha-fetoprotein (measured in nanograms per milliliter)]

Table 3: Stage grouping.

Stage	*T*	*N*	*M*	*S*
Stage 0	Tis (*in situ*)	N0	M0	S0
Stage I	T1–T4	N0	M0	Sx
Stage IA	T1	N0	M0	S0
Stage IB	T2–T4	N0	M0	S0
Stage IS	Any T	N0	M0	S1–S3
Stage II	Any T	N1–N3	M0	Sx
Stage IIA	Any T	N1	M0	S0–S1
Stage IIB	Any T	N2	M0	S0–S1
Stage IIC	Any T	N3	M0	S0–S1
Stage III	Any T	Any N	M1	Sx
Stage IIIA	Any T Any T	Any N Any N	M1a M1a	S0–S1 S1
Stage IIIB	Any T Any T	N1–N3 Any N	M0 M1a	S2 S2
Stage IIIC	Any T Any T Any T	N1–N3 Any N Any N	M0 M1a M1b	S3 S3 Any S

Table 4: Risk group classification.

Risk status	*Nonseminoma*	*Seminoma*
Good outlook	No nonpulmonary metastasis: • AFP < 1000 ng/mL • hCG < 5000 IU/mL • LDH < 1.5 ULN (upper limit of normal)	• No non-pulmonary metastasis • Any tumor marker
Intermediate outlook	Nonpulmonary metastasis: • AFP: 1000–10000 ng/mL • hCG: 5000–50000 IU/mL • LDH: 1.5–10 ULN	• Nonpulmonary metastasis • Any tumor marker
Poor outlook	No nonpulmonary metastasis: • AFP > 10000 • hCG > 50000 • LDH > 10 ULN	• None (seminoma is never classified as poor outlook)

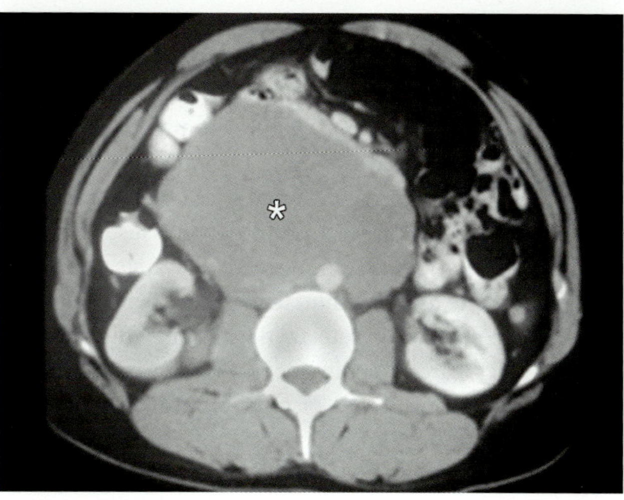

Fig. 14: Axial CECT image at the level of renal hilum showing a large metastatic homogeneous lymph nodal mass (star) in a case of seminomas testis.

Imaging in Evaluation of Testicular Cancer

Magnetic Resonance Imaging

Magnetic resonance imaging is used as a problem-solving modality. MRI of scrotum is more sensitive than sonography for detection of testicular tumors; however, the findings are variable and nonspecific. Most testicular tumors are isointense to testis on T1W images and hypointense on T2W images. On dynamic gadolinium-enhanced MRI, the tumor enhancement is often earlier and greater than the normal testicular parenchyma. Similar to their sonographic appearances, seminomas tend to be homogeneous, whereas NSGCTs are heterogeneous on MRI. Lymphoma and leukemia are characterized by testicular enlargement with diffuse, homogeneous decrease in signal intensity on T2W images. MRI is also useful in staging workup of testicular tumors when CT is inconclusive or contraindicated. It is also useful for follow-up after the treatment. In future, molecular imaging in fusion with MRI, with the help of iron oxide nanoparticles containing contrast media can aid in early and definitive, distant lymph nodal metastatic spread.

Computed Tomography

Computed tomography (CT) is the most commonly used modality in evaluation of tumor spread, staging and follow-up. CT is useful for detection of enlarged retroperitoneal or mediastinal lymph nodes as well as extranodal metastases in lungs and liver. In testicular carcinoma, lymph nodes of less than 1 cm in short-axis diameter (SAD) located in the regional nodal drainage site (e.g. renal hilum on the left or aortocaval region on right side) should be considered suspicious **(Fig. 14)**. Cut-off nodal diameter of 7 mm has been suggested as more useful for testicular cancer.[31] The enlarged lymph nodes may demonstrate necrotic center or heterogeneous contrast enhancement, particularly in NSGCTs. After completion of the treatment, some lymph nodes may not decrease in size and instead, develop more necrosis and fibrotic strands. Majority of such lymph nodal masses do not contain viable tumor; however, it cannot be ruled out on the basis of CT alone.

Positron Emission Tomography

Nuclear scans employing fludeoxyglucose-positron emission tomography (FDG-PET) in the setting of testicular malignancy is most useful in three scenarios which are described here:

1. To differentiate active disease from post-treatment changes or mature teratoma in residual component of the disease in postchemotherapy surveillance.
2. Initial staging and recurrent disease assessment in postorchiectomy period with elevation of tumor markers.
3. To predict tumor response to therapy.

The role of PET scan is invaluable in evaluation of post-treatment testicular cancer subjects for detection of residual or recurrent disease at usual or unusual sites.[45]

However, validation of the nuclear studies in routine patient care is limited due to the lack of sufficient trials and knowledge.

BENIGN INTRATESTICULAR LESIONS

Cysts

Testicular cysts are incidentally detected on sonography. These need to be differentiated from cystic tumors.

Symptomatic or palpable testicular cysts or those with suspicious solid component need further evaluation and/or exploration. Others can be followed up. Two types of simple benign cysts can be identified: (1) cysts of tunica albuginea and (2) simple testicular cysts. Tunica albuginea cysts are typically small (less than 5 mm) and are usually palpated as firm nodular masses. These are located at the periphery. Simple testicular cysts are usually located near the mediastinum testis and are not palpable.

Tubular ectasia of rete testis may be mistaken for tumors. These are typically located at the mediastinum testis and consist of areas of multiple tiny cystic spaces with no flow on color Doppler flow imaging (CDFI) **(Fig. 15)**. It is usually associated with epididymal obstruction. Epidermoid and dermoid cysts of the testis are rare and these are also seen as palpable simple cysts with characteristic echogenic margins. They do not have malignant potential.

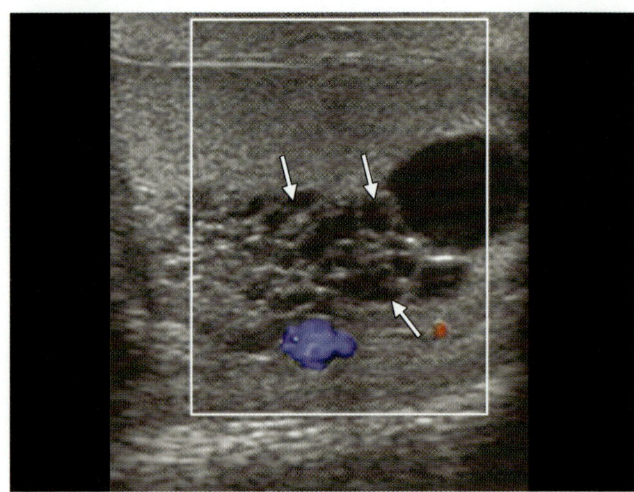

Fig. 15: US image showing tubular ectasia of rete testis (arrows). Note the absence of flow of color Doppler.

Adrenal Rests

Aberrant adrenal tissue rests may be found in testis in about 8% of patients with congenital adrenal hyperplasia. Pathogenesis may be related to the common embryonic origin of adrenals and gonads. On sonography, they are seen as multifocal and often bilateral hypoechoic lesions.

Calcifications

The consideration of testicular microlithiasis as a premalignant entity is a controversial topic, where multiple prospective studies failed to demonstrate the development of cancer in the surveillance of the subjects with testicular microlithiasis and at the same time ~18–75% patients with testicular malignancy are associated with the testicular microlithiasis.[45] Testicular microlithiasis is a condition where tiny calcification of the seminiferous tubules is seen, on sonographic examination these tiny calcifications fail to demonstrate posterior acoustic shadowing or rarely show in a few cases **(Fig. 16)**. Typically, testicular microlithiasis is seen as more than 5 calcific foci in single probe filed, whereas presence of less than 5 calcific foci per probe field is limited testicular microlithiasis. The self-examination or physical examination of the scrotum by the physician or regular sonological surveillance may be beneficial for those subjects with testicular microlithiasis.[46]

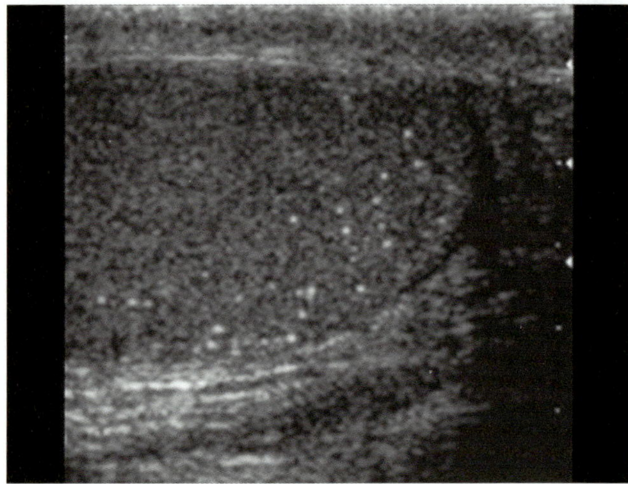

Fig. 16: US image showing multiple punctate hyperechoic nonshadowing foci of testicular microlithiasis.

Scrotoliths are the loose bodies in scrotum at extratesticular substance due to the torsion of the appendix testis and epididymis.[16] Detection of scrotoliths is easier, if fluid component is seen in the surrounding area **(Fig. 17)**. The macrocalcific changes in the testis may signify the suspicion of large cell calcifying Sertoli cell tumor, burned-out tumor or post-trauma alteration.

EXTRATESTICULAR PATHOLOGIES

Fluid Collections

Hydrocele is an abnormal accumulation of serous fluid in vaginal cavity. The congenital type is seen in infants and it is due to persistent communication between scrotal sac and the peritoneum. Acquired hydrocele is idiopathic or secondary to inflammation, torsion, trauma or tumor. Sonographically, a clear fluid is seen surrounding the testis. However, fine mobile echogenic concretions or a few thin septations can be seen in any long-standing

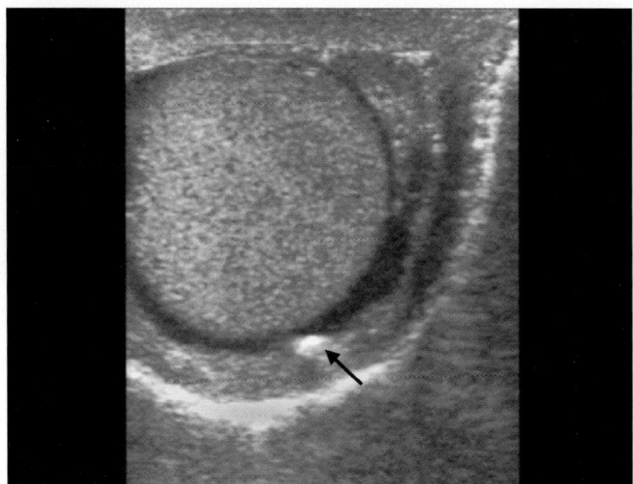

Fig. 17: US image showing a scrotal pearl (arrow).

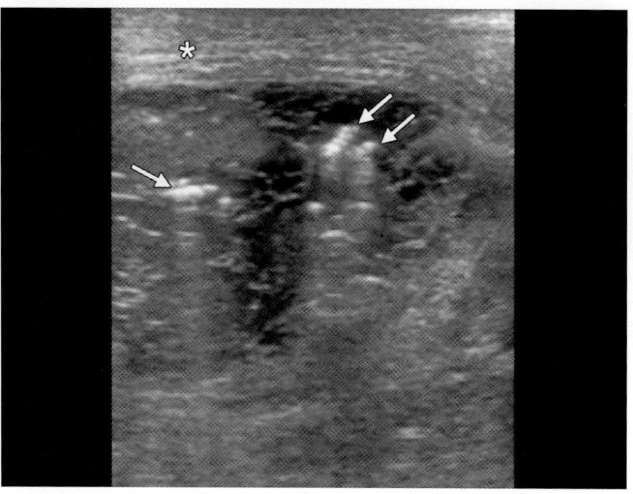

Fig. 18: Pyocele of scrotum: US image showing echogenic fluid collection within the scrotum and air foci (arrows) trapped within thin septations. Note the thickened skin of scrotum (star).

hydrocele and it does not necessarily suggest complicated collection. Rarely, the concretion may be fairly large when it gives a "bull's eye" appearance with central calcification surrounded by the hypoechoic layer.

Hematocele and pyocele result from hemorrhage and abscess formation respectively. Both contain multiple septations and echogenic debris. Thickening of scrotal skin and calcifications may be seen in both of these conditions[13] **(Fig. 18)**.

Inguinoscrotal hernia is usually diagnosed on the basis of clinical examination. Hernia may contain small bowel, large bowel and/or omentum.

On sonological evaluation, the inguinoscrotal hernia is appreciated as a breach in the inguinal canal fibers with abnormal protrusion of the peristaltic (bowel) or aperistaltic (omentum and other soft tissue) echogenic contents with their blood supply. The testes and appendages are localized separately from these protruded organs. Indirect inguinal hernia is more frequently associated with the bowel strangulation as compared to the direct inguinal hernia. Sonological evidence of the aperistaltic bowel loops in the hernial sac with associated dilatation and scrotum suggests bowel strangulation, which warrants immediate surgical management.[2]

Epididymal Cysts

Epididymal cysts and spermatoceles are the most common scrotal lesions and these may be encountered in up to 70% of all patients subjected to scrotal sonography.[12] Spermatoceles contain debris and sperms in addition to serous fluid and occur secondary to the obstruction of spermatic pathway. These are usually located in the head. Epididymal cysts are less common than spermatoceles

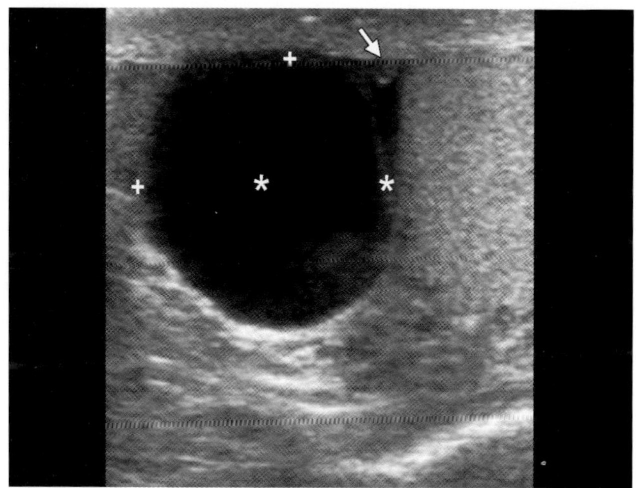

Fig. 19: US image showing an epididymal cyst. Appendix of testis (arrow) is seen between the cyst and the testis.

and do not contain sperms. These are usually smaller in size and are located anywhere in the epididymis. Spermatoceles and epididymal cysts are identical on sonography and are seen as anechoic, well-circumscribed cysts with no or few internal echoes **(Fig. 19)**. Sperm granulomas may be found in patients with epididymal obstruction or after vasectomy.[12] On sonography, these are seen as hypoechoic epididymal lesions, sometimes with focal calcification.

Postorchidectomy Scrotum

After orchidectomy, small amount of clear fluid is usually seen in the empty hemiscrotal sac, which resolves gradually. The scrotal wall appears thickened because of contraction. Hematomas are common in early post-operative period. Fresh hematomas are echogenic. These become hypoechoic or cystic as these resolve after 5–6 weeks. Tumor recurrence may be suspected if the mass develops several months after the orchidectomy.

On sonography, the recurrence is seen as a poorly defined hypoechoic lesion. Color Doppler, MRI or sonography guided biopsies are useful to differentiate recurrent tumor from hematoma.[46]

Testicular prosthesis is usually made up of silicone. On sonography, it is seen as a sharply defined, anechoic structure, frequently with excessive reverberations.[47]

Extratesticular Tumors

Extratesticular scrotal tumors are mostly benign and usually involve the epididymis. The most common is adenomatoid tumor constituting 30% of these tumors. It arises in epididymis or spermatic cord. On sonography, it is generally seen as solitary, well-defined, round to oval, small mass with variable echogenicity.[14] It may occasionally invade adjacent testicular parenchyma. Other benign paratesticular tumors include hemangioma, lipoma, neurofibroma and leiomyoma. Malignant paratesticular tumors include liposarcoma, fibrosarcoma and lymphoma in adults and rhabdomyosarcoma in children. The sonographic appearances of these tumors are nonspecific.[13]

Varicocele

Varicocele is an abnormal dilatation and tortuosity of the veins of the pampiniform plexus. It is described in detail in next chapter.

REFERENCES

1. Trainer TD. Testis and the excretory duct system. In: Sternberg S (Ed). Histology for Pathologists. New York, NY: Raven; 1992. pp. 744-6.
2. Siegel MJ. The acute scrotum. Radiol Clin North Am. 1997;35:959-76.
3. Bree RL, Hoang DT. Scrotal ultrasound. Radiol Clin North Am. 1996;34:1183-205.
4. Middleton WD, Thorne DA, Melson GL. Color Doppler ultrasound of the normal testis. Am J Roentgenol. 1989; 152:293-7.
5. Paltiel HJ, Rupich RC, Babcock DS. Maturational changes in arterial impedance of the normal testis in boys: Doppler sonographic study. Am J Roentgenol. 1994;163:1189-93.
6. Friedland GW, Chang P. The role of imaging in the management of the impalpable undescended testis. Am J Roentgenol. 1988;151:1107-11.
7. Heiken JP. Tumors of the testis and testicular adnexa. In: Pollack HM, McClennan BL (Eds). Clinical Urography. Philadelphia, PA: Saunders; 2000. pp. 1716-41.
8. Hricak H. Congenital anomalies of the testis. In: Hricak H, Hamn B, Kim B (Eds). Imaging of Scrotum. New York: Raven; 1995. pp. 37-48.
9. Levitt SB, Konyan SJ, Engel RM. The impalpable testis: a rational approach to management. J Urol. 1978;120:515-20.
10. Toyoshima M, Chida K, Masuda M. Testicular sarcoidosis. Nihon Kokyuki Gakkai Zasshi. 2000;38:63-6.
11. Bayram MM, Kervancioglu R. Scrotal gray-scale and color Doppler sonographic findings in genitourinary brucellosis. J Clin Ultrasound. 1997;25:443-7.
12. Cook JL, Dewbury K. The changes seen on high-resolution ultrasound in orchitis. Clin Radiol. 2000;55:13-8.
13. Gorman B, Carroll BA. The scrotum. In: Rummak CM, Wilson SR, Charhoneau JW (Eds). Diagnostic Ultrasound. St. Louis: Mosby; 2005. pp. 849-88.
14. Oyen RH. Scrotal ultrasound. Eur Radiol. 2002;12:19-34.
15. Noske HD, Kraus SW, Altinkilic BM, et al. Historical milestones regarding torsion of the scrotal organs. J Urol. 1998;159:13-6.
16. Dewbury KC. Scrotal ultrasonography: an update. BJU Int. 2000;86:143-52.
17. Burks DD, Markey BJ, Burkhard TK, et al. Suspected testicular torsion and ischemia: evaluation with color Doppler sonography. Radiology. 1990;175:815-21.
18. Horstman WG. Scrotal imaging. Urol Clin North Am. 1997;24: 653-71.
19. Jee WH, Choe BY, Byun JY, et al. Resistive index of the intrascrotal artery in scrotal inflammatory disease. Acta Radiol. 1997;38:1026-30.
20. Brown JM, Hammers LW, Barton JW, et al. Quantitative Doppler assessment of acute scrotal inflammation. Radiology. 1995;197:427-31.
21. Sanders LM, Haber S, Dembner A, et al. Significance of reversal of diastolic flow in the acute scrotum. J Ultrasound Med. 1994;13:137-9.
22. Lock G, Schmidt C, Helmich F, et al. Early experience with contrast-enhanced ultrasound in the diagnosis of testicular masses: a feasibility study. Urology. 2011;77(5):1049-53.
23. Rifkin MD. Inflammation of the lower genitourinary tract: the prostate, seminal vesicles, and scrotum. In: Pollack HM, McClennan BL (Eds). Clinical Urography, 2nd edition. Philadelphia, PA: Saunders; 2000. pp. 1058-87.
24. Patriquin HB, Yazbeck S, Trinh B, et al. Testicular torsion in infants and children: diagnosis with Doppler sonography. Radiology. 1993;188:781-5.
25. Williamson RC. Torsion of the testis and allied conditions. Br J Surg. 1976;63:465-76.
26. Berman JM, Beidle TR, Kunberger LE, et al. Sonographic evaluation of acute intrascrotal pathology. Am J Roentgenol. 1996;166:857-61.
27. Dogra VS, Sessions A, Mevorach A, et al. Reversal of diastolic plateau in partial testicular torsion. J Clin Ultrasound. 2001; 29:105-8.
28. Skoglund RW, McRoberts JW, Ragde H. Torsion of testicular appendages: presentation of 43 new cases and a collective review. J Urol. 1970;104:598-600.
29. Kratzik C, Hainz A, Kuber W. Has ultrasound influenced the therapy concept of blunt scrotal trauma? J Urol. 1989;142: 1243-6.
30. Moschouris H, Stamatiou K, Lampropoulou E, et al. Imaging of the acute scrotum: is there a place for contrast-enhanced ultrasonography? Int Braz J Urol. 2009;35(6):692-705.

31. Hari A, Grossfeld G, Hricak A. Tumors of the scrotum. In: Bragg DG, Rubin P, Hricak H (Eds). Oncologic Imaging. Philadelphia: WB Saunders; 2002. pp. 603-28.
32. Geraghty MJ, Lee FT Jr, Bernsten SA, et al. Sonography of testicular tumors and tumor-like conditions: a radiologic-pathologic correlation. Crit Rev Diagn Imaging. 1998;39:1-63.
33. Rifkin MD, Kurtz AB, Pasto ME, et al. Diagnostic capabilities of high-resolution scrotal ultrasonography: prospective evaluation. J Ultrasound Med. 1985;4:13-9.
34. Guthrie JA, Fowler RC. Ultrasound diagnosis of testicular tumours presenting as epididymal disease. Clin Radiol. 1992;46:397-400.
35. Cotran RS, Kumar P, Collins T. The male genital tract. In: Cotran RS, Kumar V, Collins T, Robbins SL (Eds). Robbins Pathologic Basis of Disease, 6th edition. Philadelphia, PA: Saunders; 1999. pp. 1011-34.
36. Schwerk WB, Schwerk WN, Rodeck G. Testicular tumors: prospective analysis of real-time US patterns and abdominal staging. Radiology. 1987;164:369-74.
37. Huang DY, Sidhu PS. Focal testicular lesions: colour Doppler ultrasound, contrast-enhanced ultrasound and tissue elastography as adjuvants to the diagnosis. Br J Radiol. 2012;85 Spec No. 1:S41-53.
38. Comiter CV, Renshaw AA, Benson CB, et al. Burned-out primary testicular cancer: sonographic and pathological characteristics. J Urol. 1996;156:85-8.
39. Hamm B. Differential diagnosis of scrotal masses by ultrasound. Eur Radiol. 1997;7:668-79.
40. Kim I, Young RH, Scully RE. Leydig cell tumors of the testis: a clinicopathological analysis of 40 cases and review of the literature. Am J Surg Pathol. 1985;9:177-92.
41. Jaffer O, Sidhu P. Contrast-enhanced ultrasonography of the testes. Ultrasound Clinics. 2013;8(4):509-23.
42. Nonomura N, Aozasa K, Ueda T, et al. Malignant lymphoma of the testis: histological and immunohistological study of 28 cases. J Urol. 1989;141:1368-71.
43. Richie JP. Neoplasms of the testis. In: Walch PC, Retik AB, Vaughan ED, Wein AJ (Eds). Campbell's Urology, 7th edition. Philadelphia, PA: Saunders; 1998. pp. 2411-52.
44. Amin MB, Greene FL, Edge SB, et al. The Eighth Edition AJCC Cancer Staging Manual: Continuing to build a bridge from a population-based to a more "personalized" approach to cancer staging. CA Cancer J Clin. 2017;67(2):93-9.
45. Basu S, Rubello D. PET imaging in the management of tumors of testis and ovary: current thinking and future directions. Minerva Endocrinol. 2008;33:229-56.
46. Ganem JP, Workman KR, Shaban SF. Testicular microlithiasis is associated with testicular pathology. Urology. 1999;53:209-13.
47. Eftekhari F, Smith JK. Sonography of scrotum after orchiectomy: normal and abnormal findings. Am J Roentgenol. 1993; 160;543-7.

Chapter 22

Male Infertility and Erectile Dysfunction

Deep Narayan Srivastava, Chandan J Das

MALE INFERTILITY

Infertility is defined as a failure to achieve pregnancy during 1 year of frequent, unprotected intercourse.[1] A multicenter study by the World Health Organization (WHO) found that in 20% of infertility cases, the male partner was the predominant cause whereas in 27% of cases abnormalities were found in both partners.[2] Hence, defects in male partner may be responsible for infertility in up to 50% of the infertile couples.[1] These defects account for a reduction in the quantity and quality of the semen. The evaluation of infertile male begins with a careful history and physical examination of the patient. This is followed by semen analysis in which ejaculate volume and its pH, sperms count, their motility, and morphology are studied. Average sperm count in normal fertile man is 70–80 million sperms per mL and it contains more than 60% motile sperms. Sperm count of less than 20 million per mL is termed as oligospermia, however, significant decrease in pregnancy rates occurs only at sperm concentration of less than 5 million per mL. Oligospermia is present in 80% and azoospermia is present in another 15–20% of the infertile men.[1,2]

Etiology

Male infertility results from many diverse conditions. Congenital anomalies include cryptorchidism, Klinefelter's syndrome, agenesis of vas deferens and/or seminal vesicles, and congenital ejaculatory duct cyst. Endocrinal abnormalities such as prolactinoma, Kallmann syndrome, Prader-Willi syndrome, and congenital adrenal hyperplasia are uncommon causes of the male infertility and these are diagnosed primarily on the basis of clinical examination and laboratory findings. Luteinizing hormone secreted by the pituitary gland regulates the *testosterone* secretion by Leydig cells of the testis. Low testosterone affects spermatogenesis, growth of the prostate, and seminal vesicle secretion.[2]

Acquired testicular abnormalities such as trauma, tumor, infection, and paratesticular abnormalities such as varicocele and epididymitis are responsible for infertility in significant number of patients. Tuberculosis and gonorrhea cause inflammation and obstruction of the ductal transport system. Other diseases such as mumps and syphilis may affect seminiferous tubules in the testicular parenchyma.[3]

IMAGING APPROACH IN MALE INFERTILITY

Male infertility is usually caused by azoospermia, which can be either due to obstructive cause [obstructive azoospermia—normal-sized testes, epididymal fullness, normal follicle-stimulating hormone (FSH)] or due to nonobstructive cause (nonobstructive azoospermia—small or soft testes, raised FSH).

Normal volume (more than 1 mL), fructose-positive ejaculate with azoospermia or oligospermia is usually caused by lesions of the testis or of paratesticular structures **(Box 1)** such as varicocele and epididymal diseases.[4] These lesions can be satisfactorily evaluated with scrotal ultrasonography, supplemented with color Doppler flow imaging. Although clinical examination is an integral part of diagnostic workup in these patients, up to 67% of scrotal pathologies detected on sonography are responsible for infertility which are not apparent clinically.[5]

Low-volume ejaculate (less than 1 mL) is caused by stenosis, obstruction, or congenital anomalies of distal sperm transport system, which include vas deferens,

Box 1: Testicular and paratesticular causes of nonobstructive azoospermia.[3]

- Cryptochidism
- Atrophy
- Torsion/Infarction
- Inflammation
- Mumps/TB
- Microlithiasis
- Hydrocele
- Varicocele
- Neoplasm
- Trauma

(TB: tuberculosis)

seminal vesicles, ejaculatory duct, and prostate. Abnormalities in these structures result in decreased semen volume and blockage of flow of sperms into the ejaculate leading to azoospermia or oligospermia. These abnormalities include agenesis of vas deferens or seminal vesicles or both, inflammatory strictures and obstruction of seminal vesicles and vas deferens, ejaculatory duct cysts, and obstruction.[6] Transrectal ultrasonography (TRUS) is the primary imaging modality of choice for distal ductal system.[1,7] It is now widely used to diagnose congenital and other obstructive lesions that produce low-volume ejaculate and azoospermia. Magnetic resonance imaging (MRI) is indicated only if TRUS findings are inconclusive.[8]

Varicocele

Varicocele is the most common surgically correctable cause of male infertility. There is abnormal dilatation of veins of the pampiniform plexus, which is due to venous reflux in these veins. The incidence of varicocele is 15% in general population and 35–40% in men presenting with infertility.[9,10] Primary varicocele is seen in young men and is due to incompetent testicular vein. It is mostly left-sided or bilateral. Left testicular vein is maximally predisposed to develop varicocele. Various factors responsible include right-angled entry of left testicular vein into left renal vein, the intermittent compression of left renal vein between aorta and the superior mesenteric artery (nutcracker syndrome), and pressure of the left colon.[11] Secondary varicocele results from left renal vein invasion by renal cancer, compression of testicular veins by adjacent masses such as tumor, lymph nodes, or hydronephrosis.[12] Cross-communications exist between veins of the pampiniform plexus and cremasteric veins as well as external spermatic veins and veins of vas deferens. In patients, subjected to high ligation, these communications may lead to recurrence.

Although most men with varicocele are not infertile, varicocele is present in up to 40% of infertile men. Repair of varicocele improves quality of semen in majority of patients.[13] Proposed mechanisms by which varicocele causes testicular dysfunction include hormonal imbalance, hypoxia secondary to venous stasis, reflux of adrenal and renal metabolites, and elevated testicular temperature.[13] During adolescence, when the testis is growing rapidly, it may be very susceptible to harmful effects of varicocele.

The simplest and most widely used method for diagnosis of varicocele is physical examination; however, subclinical varicocele cannot be diagnosed with physical examination alone. Ultrasonography with color duplex flow imaging is the preferred imaging modality for evaluation of varicocele. The patient is examined in supine and erect position during quite breathing, deep breathing, and Valsalva maneuver before interpreting the examination as normal.[9] Vessels are scanned on each side from the scrotal neck to the lower pole of testis. As the flow in pampiniform plexus is very slow, Doppler parameters must be adjusted to detect very slow flow during color Doppler examination. On grey scale ultrasonography, visualization of three or more dilated veins with at least one of them having a diameter of 3 mm or more is suggestive of varicocele.[13] These tortuous venous channels are easily compressible as opposed to other cystic abnormalities in this region. On color Doppler study, continuous retrograde flow toward testis during Valsalva maneuver, is taken as a positive sign for varicocele **(Figs. 1A to D)**.[13,14] A brief reflux in veins of pampiniform plexus followed by cessation of flow is physiological. A further scoring system described by Chiou et al. incorporating maximal venous diameter, the sum of six venous diameters, and change of flow velocity after a Valsalva maneuver allows greater sensitivity of 93% by using a total score >4 compared to merely measuring the venous diameter **(Table 1)**.[15] Some varicoceles can be demonstrated in erect position of the patient only and hence scanning in erect position is mandatory before the study is interpreted as normal.[13] Intratesticular varicocele is rare and always associated with paratesticular varicocele. It is usually located in subcapsular location or in the mediastinum testis which measures 2 mm or more.[16]

Size of the varicocele does not correlate with degree of impairment of spermatogenesis. Thus a small varicocele detected only on radiological assessment may have a

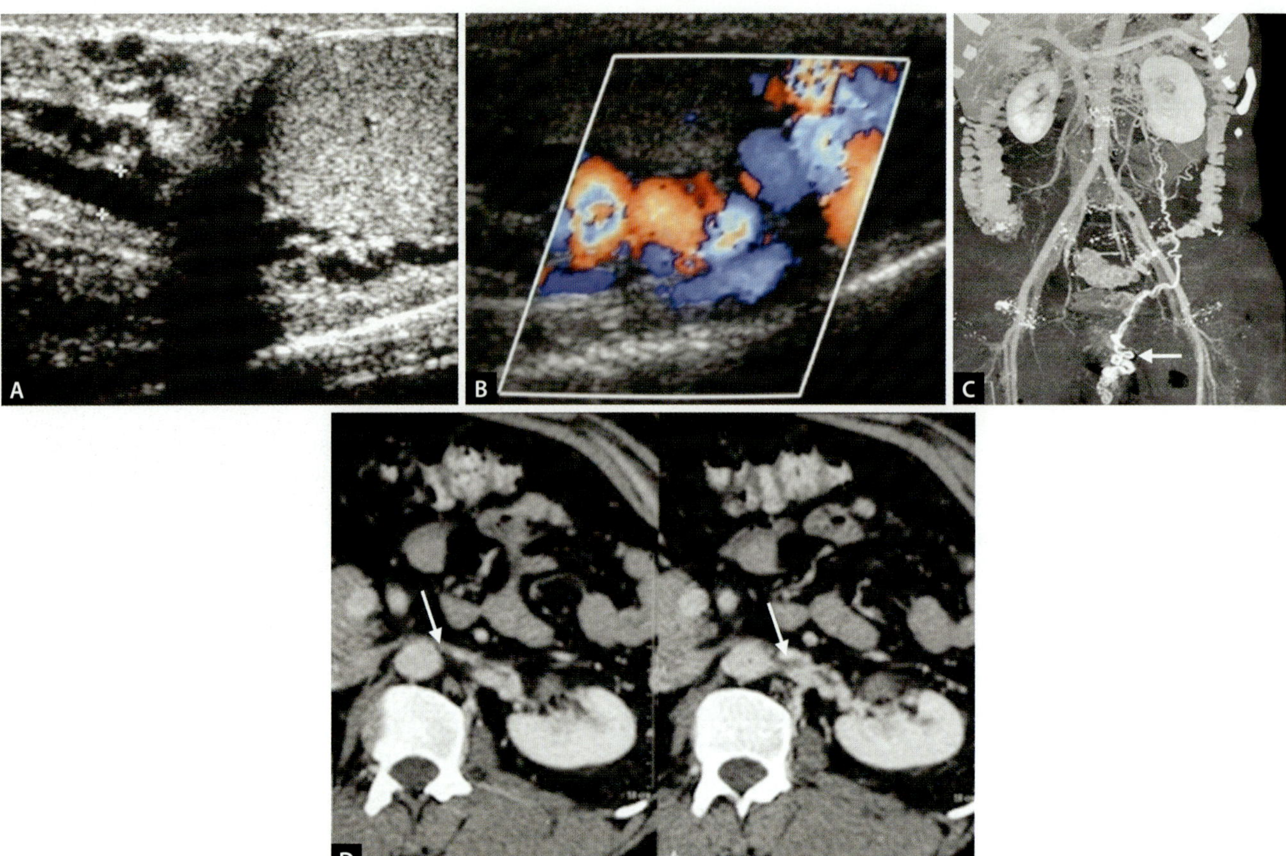

Figs. 1A to D: Varicocele: (A) Multiple dilated vascular channels measuring more than 3 mm on gray-scale USG at the lower pole of testes; (B) marked detectable flow is seen on this color Doppler scan which is exaggerated during Valsalva maneuver; (C) CECT coronal MIP images showing multiple dilated vessels in left scrotum (arrow) which is communicating through the left gonadal vein draining into left renal vein; (D) axial CECT showing thrombosed left renal vein (arrows) as cause of the left varicocele. (CECT: contrast-enhanced computed tomography; MIP: maximum intensity projection; USG: ultrasonography).

Table 1: Scoring system of Chiou et al. for color Doppler ultrasound diagnosis of varicocele.[15]

Parameter	*Score*
Maximum vein diameter:	
• <2.5 mm	0
• 2.5–2.9 mm	1
• 3.0–3.9 mm	2
• ≥4 mm	3
Plexus/sum of diameter of veins:	
• No plexus identified	0
• Plexus (+) with sum diameter <3 mm	1
• Plexus (+) with sum diameter 3–5.9 mm	2
• Plexus (+) with sum diameter ≥6 mm	3
Change in flow velocity of Valsalva maneuver:	
• <2 cm S^{-1} or duration <1 s	0
• 2–4.9 cm S^{-1}	1
• 5–9.9 cm S^{-1}	2
• ≥10 cm S^{-1}	3
Total score	*0–9*

profound effect on spermatogenesis.[17] The treatment of subclinical varicocele in infertility is still controversial, however, it has been demonstrated that sperm motility improvement after varicocele surgery is comparable in patients with both clinical and subclinical varicocele.[18]

Venography is rarely performed for diagnostic purpose but may be used when embolization is used as a procedure for treating varicocele.[13] When compared with venography, color Doppler ultrasonography had a sensitivity of 93% and specificity of 80% in a group of infertile patients with normal physical examinations.[19] In addition to the diagnosis, spermatic venography has therapeutic application for embolization of varicocele. In this technique, an angiographic catheter is placed into the testicular vein via transfemoral venous route. About 5–10 mL of contrast is injected during Valsalva maneuver and radiographs of abdomen and pelvis are taken. The venography can be followed by embolization performed using coils **(Figs. 2A and B)** or sclerosants such as sodium tetradecyl sulfate foam.[13] Correct identification of all venous collaterals with their selective embolization

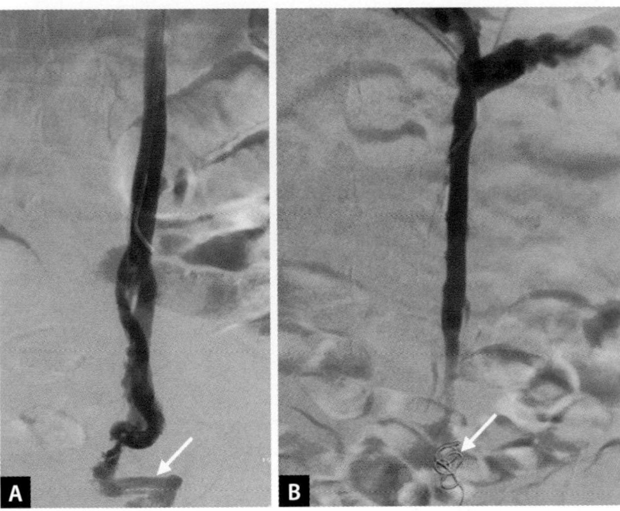

Figs. 2A and B: (A) Venography of left gonadal vein shows the varicocele (arrow). (B) Coil embolization (arrow) of the varicocele was performed in the same setting.

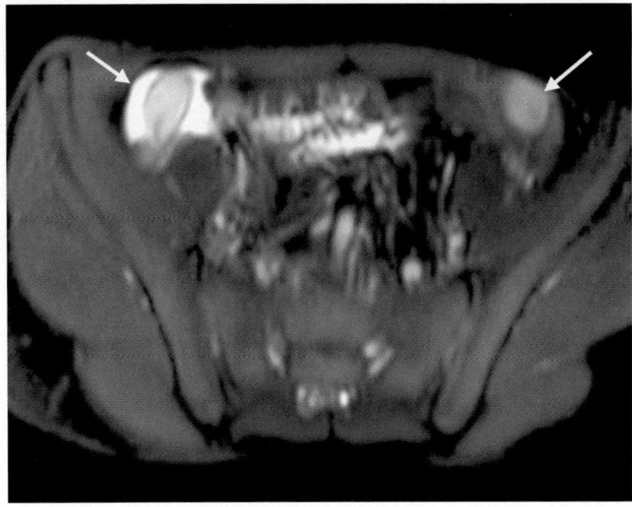

Fig. 3: T2W MRI image showing hyperintense structures (arrows) in both iliac fossa regions suggesting undescended testes. (MRI: magnetic resonance imaging).

is necessary. High technical success rate with significant improvement in semen quality can be achieved with this technique.[20] This technique is especially suitable for postsurgical recurrent varicocele.[21]

Testis

Sonographic examination of the testis is important in the evaluation of infertile male, specifically for measurement of testicular size for atrophy or for tumor identification. Normal adult testis is homogenous with low to medium echogenicity and measures 3–5 cm in length, 2–3 cm in width, and 2–3 cm in anteroposterior thickness. Testicular volume in cc can be calculated using the formula of length × width × thickness × 0.53. The normal volume of adult testis is 15–20 cc and testis is symmetrical on both sides.[21]

Cryptorchidism occurs in approximately 0.8% of all 1-year-old boys and if left untreated can represent a congenital cause of male infertility.[22] Progressive germ cell damage occurs in the cryptorchid testis secondary to the increased temperature at its extrascrotal location. Significant germ cell damage occurs by 2 years of age and untreated postpubertal undescended testis may be completely devoid of germ cells. It also has a deleterious effect on contralateral normal descended testis. Pregnancy rates in men who have undergone prepubertal treatment of unilateral cryptorchidism ranges between 65% and 80%.[22] In addition to infertility, undescended testis is highly susceptible for malignant transformation.

Most of the undescended testes are located at or close to the inguinal canal and ultrasonography is very sensitive to identify their location. Ultrasonography is less accurate in detection of undescended testis when it is located in the retroperitoneum. MRI scans of abdomen and pelvis **(Fig. 3)** from the level of inguinal rings to lower poles of the kidney are required for testicular localization in such situations. MRI is more accurate because of its high soft tissue contrast and multiplanner capabilities. The characteristic high-signal intensity of testis on T2-weighted sequences aid in easy recognition of undescended testis. MRI scores over ultrasonography (USG) in localization of atrophic undescended testis.

Testicular tumors are most common in the same age group in which fertility disorders of male are most prevalent. Testicular tumors may be identified in-patients presenting with oligospermia or azoospermia.[23] Seminomas are the most common testicular tumors and are usually homogeneously hypoechoic on sonography **(Fig. 4)**. Nonseminomatous tumors are complex and heterogeneous in echotexture. Testicular tumors are described in details in the chapter on imaging of scrotum.

Testicular torsion occurs most frequently during adolescence and therefore has the potential impact on fertility of affected young males. Acute testicular torsion is an emergency and torsed testis must be salvaged at the earliest. There are good chances of salvage when patients are operated within 7 hours. If it is delayed for more than 24 hours, virtually all testicular function is lost.

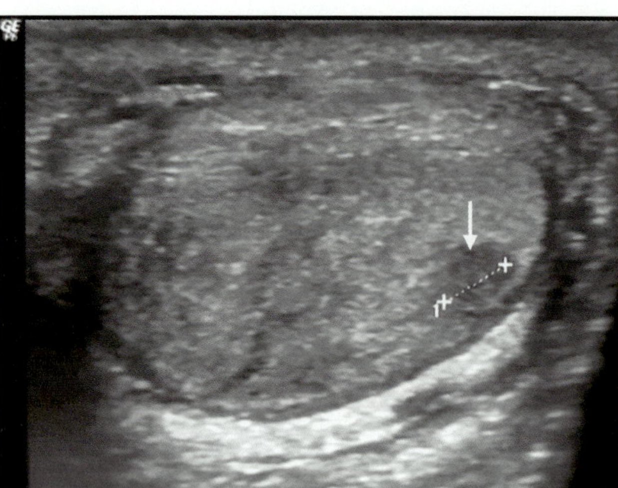

Fig. 4: USG showing a focal hypoechoic lesion in testis (arrow) and with elevated alpha-fetoprotein (AFP) level it is highly suspicious for seminoma. (USG: ultrasonography).

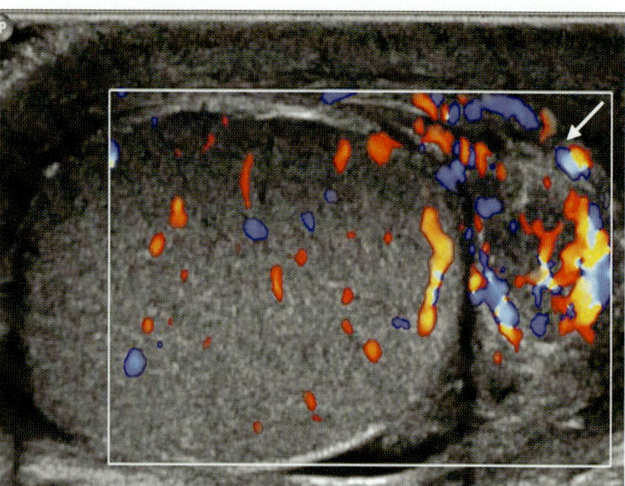

Fig. 5: USG showing enlarged epididymal head (arrow) with marked increase in vascularity in a case of acute epididymitis. Note is made of increased vascularity in adjacent testis. (USG: ultrasonography).

On sonography, the affected testis is hypoechoic and may be enlarged. Color Doppler shows decreased vascularity, which is best appreciated when compared with contralateral normal testis.

Testicular trauma has less impact on male fertility than the other testicular factors such as torsion or cryptorchidism.[22] Spermatogenic dysfunction may develop in testicular trauma patients, secondary to direct cell injury and the formation of antisperm antibodies from disruption of blood-testis barrier in them. Ultrasonography with color Doppler is most suitable investigation to determine the extent of testicular trauma; however, satisfactory ultrasonography examination may not be possible in acutely traumatized and painful scrotum. In such situations, MRI is more accurate to detect disruption of the testicular capsule; however, most of these patients will need surgical exploration.

Higher incidence of testicular microlithiasis is found on scrotal ultrasonography in infertile men; however, its relationship with infertility is not known.[10]

Epididymis

The epididymis is located along the posterolateral aspect of testis and runs parallel and posterior to the mediastinum testis. The head of the epididymis is pyramidal in shape and it is larger than rest of the epididymis. The head measures 5–12 mm in thickness.

Infertile man may have infection or inflammation of the epididymis. The normal epididymis has the echogenicity similar to the testis. In acute epididymitis, epididymis is enlarged and hypoechoic with increased vascularity on color Doppler **(Fig. 5)**. Adjacent increase in vascularity may be seen in testis also. Chronic inflammation results in an enlarged and heterogeneously hyperechoic epididymis, sometimes with foci of calcification.[12] Scarring in chronically inflamed epididymis may result in epididymal obstruction, which can be avoided with early and aggressive treatment of epididymitis.

Epididymal cysts and spermatoceles are usually located at the head of the epididymis and these can be easily detected on sonography. Most epididymal cysts do not cause obstruction, however, rarely, these may compress the epididymal tubules and cause epididymal obstruction, especially if large, and produce oligo- or azoospermia, very large epididymal cysts may occasionally be difficult to differentiate from hydrocele on sonography, however, compression of epididymis and adjacent testicular margin and presence of the fluid at one end of the testis instead of surrounding the testis help to differentiate large epididymal cyst from hydrocele **(Fig. 6)**.

TRUS Evaluation of Distal Genital Ductal System

TRUS is indicated in infertile men with suspicion of obstructive pathology in distal sperm transport system. This is suggested by low-volume ejaculate with oligo- or azoospermia and palpable abnormality on digital rectal examination. The conditions that produce low-volume ejaculate with oligo- or azoospermia include agenesis of vas deferens and seminal vesicle, ejaculatory duct

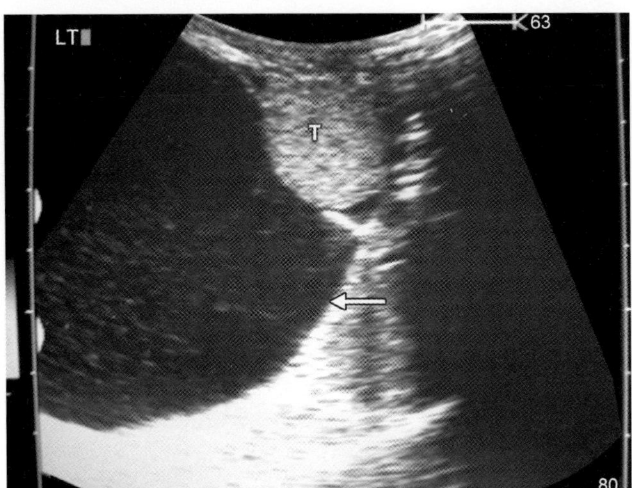

Fig. 6: Large epididymal cyst (arrow) at the upper pole of testis seen on scrotal ultrasonography pushing the testis (T) eccentrically.

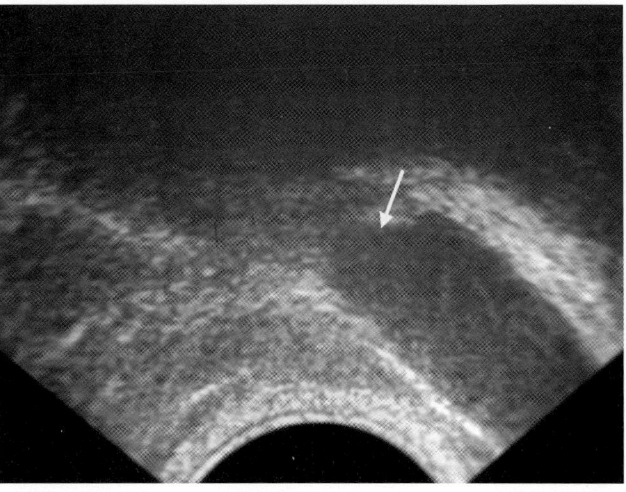

Fig. 7: Agenesis of seminal vesicle. TRUS shows absence of seminal vesicle on right side on axial scan. Normal left seminal vesicle (arrow) is seen as hypoechoic elongated structure behind the urinary bladder. (TRUS: transrectal ultrasonography).

obstruction, and urethral strictures.[1,7] Other indications of TRUS include hematospermia, painful ejaculation, severe sperm motility defects, and azoospermia in normal-volume ejaculate without testicular atrophy.[24]

On TRUS, normal prostate is a symmetric, triangular, and ellipsoid structure with homogeneous echogenicity surrounded by a thin layer of echogenic capsule. Normal seminal vesicles are paired, well-defined, saccular, elongated hypoechoic organs, situated cranial to the prostate and posterior to urinary bladder with "bow-tie" appearance on axial images. These may vary in size, shape, and degree of distention; however, usually these are symmetrical. On axial plane, ampulla of vasa deferentia are seen as round or oval tubular structures that are just cranial to prostate and medial to seminal vesicles. In sagittal plane, these can be seen behind prostate projecting medially toward seminal vesicles. Ejaculatory ducts are difficult to visualize on TRUS in normal men. These may sometimes be seen as tubular structures obliquely traversing the prostate and entering the urethra at verumontanum.[1]

Seminal Vesicles and Vas Deferens

Seminal vesicle secretions contribute about 80–90% of sperm volume. They also secrete fructose and maintain an acidic pH of semen. Congenital anomalies and obstructive lesions of seminal vesicles result in decreased semen volume, low pH, and low fructose levels.

Wolffian duct anomalies include renal agenesis, agenesis of vas deferens, agenesis or atrophy of seminal vesicles, and cysts of seminal vesicles. Seminal vesicle atrophy or agenesis may be unilateral or bilateral.[2] It occurs in all patients with agenesis of vas deferens. Bilateral absence of seminal vesicles may be seen in up to 40% of patients with low-volume azoospermia.[4] It can be diagnosed with semen analysis and clinical examination in most patients.[25] Large number of these patients also has associated renal anomalies. Another strong association is with cystic fibrosis, in which 98% of men have agenesis of seminal vesicles and vas deferens.[4] On TRUS or MRI, seminal vesicle is considered atrophic, if it measures less than 7 mm in width and dilated (as in ejaculatory duct obstruction) when it measures more than 15 mm.[2,8] Diagnosis of seminal vesicle and vas agenesis is made when these are not visualized **(Fig. 7)**.

Cysts of seminal vesicles may be congenital or acquired. Congenital cyst of seminal vesicle results from an ectopic ureter insertion into the seminal vesicle and is associated with a hypoplastic kidney on the same side. This cyst may compress ejaculatory duct and produce obstruction. Acquired cysts of seminal vesicles are secondary to infection. Chronic inflammation produces cystic dilatation with scarring and obstruction of the lumen of the seminal vesicles and causes infertility **(Fig. 8A)**. Stone formation in dilated seminal vesicles can be readily demonstrated on TRUS.[8,26] MRI also demonstrates the cystic change well due to increase in fluid content of the cyst **(Fig. 8B)**.

Ejaculatory Ducts

These are formed by confluence of seminal vesicles and terminal ampullary portion of the vas deferens and

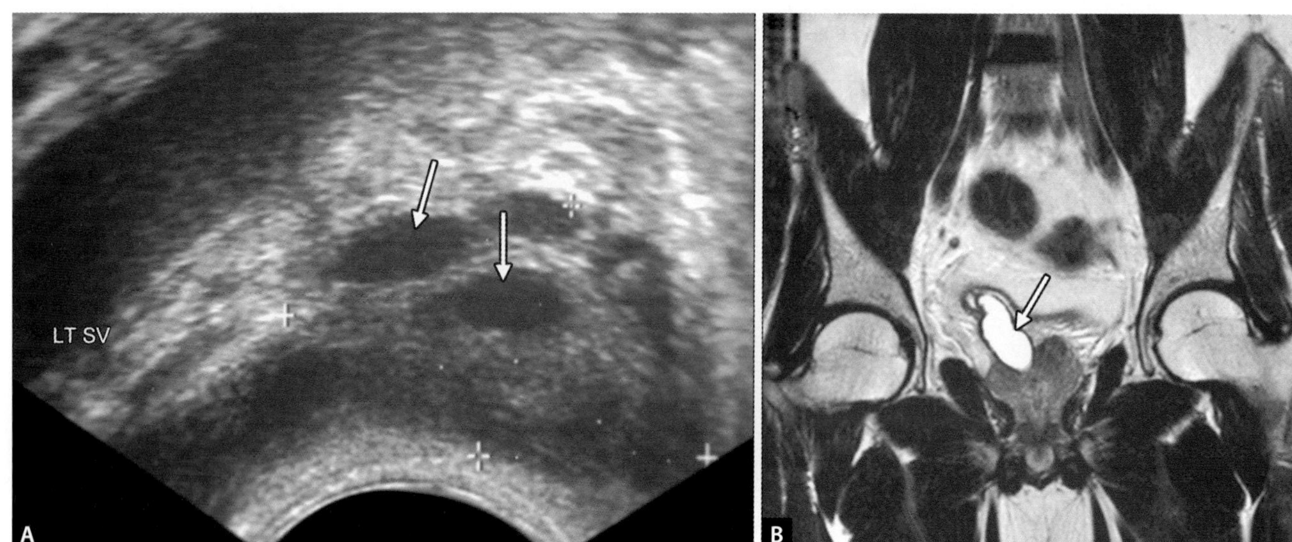

Figs. 8A and B: (A) Multiple postinflammatory seminal vesicle cysts (arrows) are seen on axial TRUS scan. (B) Coronal T2W image of a different patient showing a large hyperintense (arrow) right seminal vesicle cyst. (TRUS: transrectal ultrasonography).

hence, ejaculatory duct obstruction results in decreased semen volume with absence of seminal fructose. TRUS may demonstrate ejaculatory duct cysts, dilatation of ejaculatory ducts, or calcification in ejaculatory ducts along with dilated seminal vesicles.[4,27] Any of these findings strongly suggest ejaculatory duct obstruction. Zinner syndrome is characterized by triad of unilateral renal agenesis, ipsilateral seminal vesicle cyst, and ejaculatory duct obstruction **(Figs. 9A to D)**.

Many of these conditions can be treated with transurethral resection of the ejaculatory duct (TURED).[27] Specificity of TRUS in the diagnosis of ejaculatory duct obstruction is unsatisfactory, hence, TRUS-guided seminal vesicle aspiration followed by vesiculography is useful before TURED.[28,29] TRUS-guided seminal vesicle aspiration is performed with a 21G needle introduced transrectally. Presence of motile sperms in seminal vesicle fluid strongly suggests ejaculatory duct obstruction because sperms are not normally seen in seminal vesicles. The aspiration is followed by injection of 5–20 mL of dilute noniodinated contrast under fluoroscopic guidance and images are obtained to study the seminal vesicles and ejaculatory ducts. Pelvic and inguinal portions of vas deferens may also be visualized with this technique.[24]

Prostate

Müllerian duct cyst and utricle cyst are congenital prostatic cysts which may be indistinguishable from each other. When large, these may compress and produce ejaculatory duct obstruction.[2] On imaging, both are seen as midline cyst in prostate **(Figs. 10A to C)**. Müllerian duct cysts do not communicate with urethra and when large, may extend above the prostate. Utricle cysts communicate with urethra and do not extend above prostate. Acquired prostatic cysts like parasitic and prostatic retention cysts are usually located peripherally. These may produce obstruction to semen flow within the prostate and subsequent infertility. Chronic prostatitis may produce scarring, atrophy of seminal vesicles and strictures of ejaculatory duct, which may lead to infertility.[2] These can be identified on TRUS as disorganization of normal anatomy produced by scarring of prostatic tissue and occasional stone formation.[4]

Magnetic Resonance Imaging in Infertility

Scrotal MRI is the most important adjunct to ultrasonography in evaluation of testicular and paratesticular abnormalities. It is highly accurate in cryptorchidism, testicular tumors, trauma, and infection.

Magnetic resonance imaging is recommended for the evaluation of distal genital tract when TRUS findings are equivocal.[8,26] Various abnormalities of prostate and seminal vesicles such as cysts of seminal vesicles and ejaculatory duct, dilatation of vas deferens and seminal vesicles secondary to ejaculatory duct obstruction can be satisfactorily demonstrated. On MRI, absence or

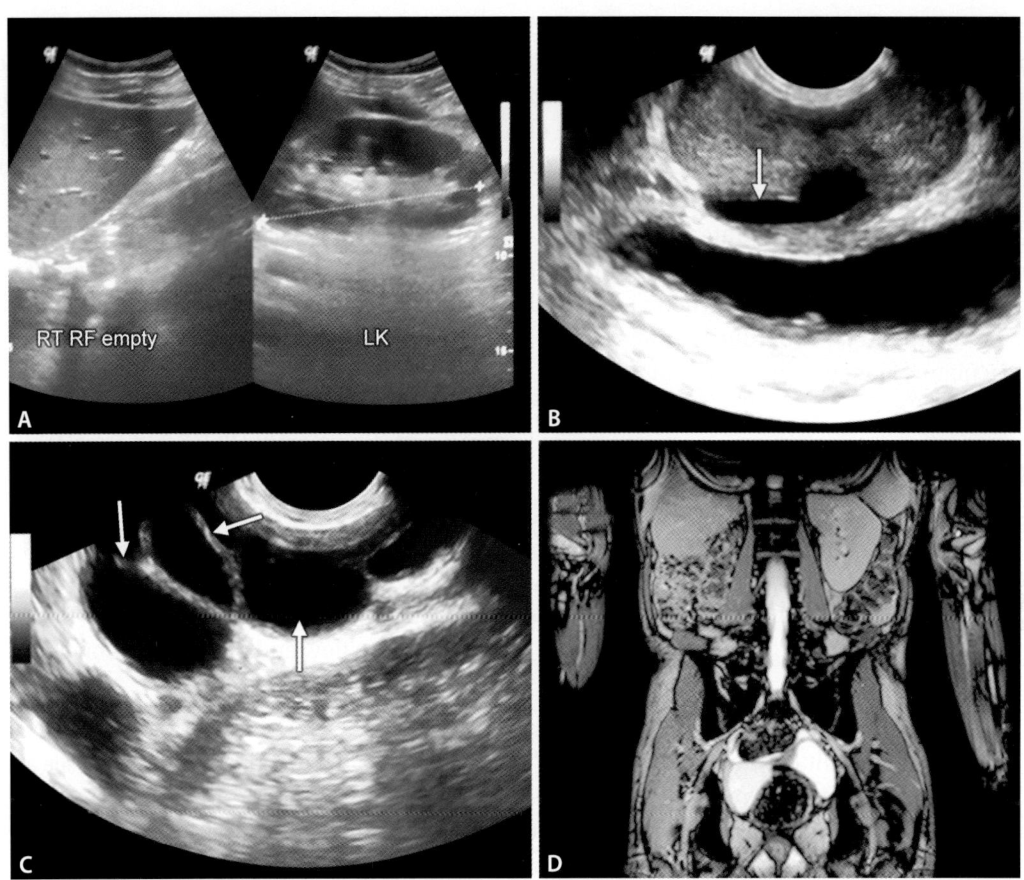

Fig. 9A to D: Zinner syndrome: (A) USG showing empty right renal fossa. (B) USG showing obstructed ejaculatory duct leading to dilatation (arrow). (C) Multiple cysts in right seminal vesicle (arrows) is also seen. (D) Coronal TRUFISP MRI image showing absent right kidney. (MRI: magnetic resonance imaging; USG: ultrasonography).

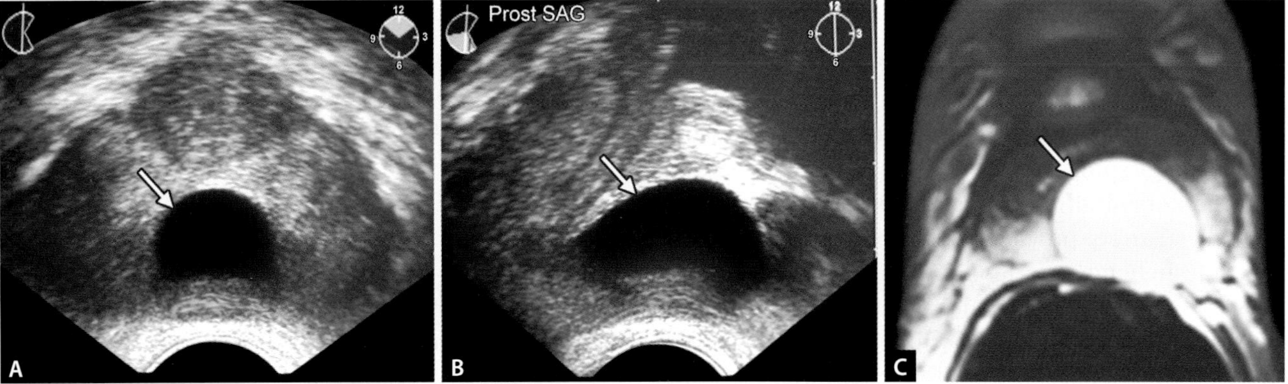

Figs. 10A to C: Prostatic cyst: (A and B) USG in axial and sagittal plane showing a cystic anechoic structure (arrow) in midline. (C) T2W axial image showing well-defined markedly hyperintense structure (arrow) in midline. (USG: ultrasonography).

atrophy of seminal vesicles with very small size and loss of normal high-signal intensity is seen in up to 40% of patients.[26] Agenesis of vas may be demonstrated. MRI is particularly advantageous in suspected case of ejaculatory duct obstruction as demonstration of normal ejaculatory ducts ruling out presence of ejaculatory duct obstruction.[30]

Imaging in Assisted Fertilization

Scrotal sonography is also useful in the work-up of assisted fertilization. Testicular volume as calculated on sonography can predict the outcome of testicular biopsies for sperm retrieval. Chances of successful sperm retrieval are significantly higher in patients with testicular volume more than 12 cc.[31] Similarly, sonography-guided testicular sperm aspiration is more accurate and it has less complications when compared with the blind aspiration, as sonography allows good visualization of testicular parenchyma, easy sampling, and avoidance of prominent vessels.[32] In patients with ejaculatory duct obstruction, sperms can also be aspirated from seminal vesicles under TRUS guidance. Intraoperative use of TRUS is helpful in identification of obstructing cyst and determining the depth of resection during transurethral resection of ejaculatory duct for the treatment of ejaculatory duct obstruction.[33]

ERECTILE DYSFUNCTION

Erectile dysfunction (ED) or impotence is defined as inability to achieve and/or maintain an erection for satisfactory sexual intercourse.[34] Its prevalence increases with age and affects up to 52% men between age group of 40–69 years.[35] ED is broadly classified into two categories: Organic and psychologic. Vasculogenic impotence is the most common cause of organic impotence and may be a marker for occult cardiovascular disease.[36] Vascular ED does not rule out the presence of contributing psychological factors, but merely means that vascular factors are predominant cause of ED. Vascular ED has two different mechanisms—obstruction in penile inflow tract, termed as arterial ED and the inability to trap the incoming blood in the cavernosa, termed as veno-occlusive ED.

Anatomy and Physiology of Penile Erection

The paired internal pudendal arteries give rise to common penile arteries which divide into four branches, one each to spongiosa, cavernosa, proximal urethra, and the dorsum of the penis (deep dorsal artery). The cavernosal artery provides blood to cavernosa through multiple helicine arteries that open directly into the cavernosal sinusoids. Venules located within the subtunical space between the periphery of erectile tissue and the tunica albugenia provide venous outflow channel from corpora cavernosa via peripheral lacunae. These vein pierce tunica albuginea and drain into cavernosal and then into deep dorsal vein.

Penile erection is a neurovascular phenomenon in which neurological stimulus via parasympathetic nerves from sacral 2, 3, and 4 leads to arterial response. It is initiated by relaxation of smooth muscles of helicine arteries leading to vasodilatation. The phase of arterial response is followed by the phase of tumescence, in which relaxation of trabecular smooth muscles and increased arterial flow lead to increase in size and length of the penis. The phase of erectile response follows when subtunical venules are compressed against tunica albuginea due to dilatation of sinusoids and increase in intracavernosal pressure. If this veno-occlusive mechanism is intact, the arterial inflow leads to increase in intracavernosal pressure to the levels of mean arterial blood pressure. Perineal muscles contractions generate further increase in pressure, which leads erectile response to rigidity.

Parameters of quality of the arterial response are peak systolic velocity (PSV) and acceleration time (AT) as measured by pharmacopenile duplex ultrasonography (PPDU) and cavernosal artery occlusion pressure as measured by cavernosometry. Parameters to assess the quality of veno-occlusive mechanism are end-diastolic velocity (EDV) and resistive index (RI) on PPDU and maintenance flow and pressure loss on cavernosometry.

Evaluation of Erectile Dysfunction

Psychological factors or systemic illnesses are responsible for erectile dysfunction in majority of patients. Careful history, clinical examination, and routine laboratory tests are extremely important for the evaluation of ED as these can identify the underlying cause in up to 80% of patients.[37] Such workup may detect reversible cause of ED or unmask the systemic illness responsible for ED. With advent of effective oral pharmacotherapy, the diagnostic approach has significantly changed over past decade. A good erectile response to these drugs excludes significant arterial or vascular disease as a cause of ED. Hence, most patients are first given a therapeutic trial and only those with failure are referred for invasive diagnostic tests like PPDU, cavernosography or angiography.[34]

Pharmacopenile Duplex Ultrasonography

Pharmacopenile duplex ultrasonography is most widely used investigation to define vascular ED and to differentiate between arterial insufficiency and defective veno-occlusive mechanism.

The different vasoactive agents used for PPDU are papaverine, and combination of papaverine, phentolamine, and prostaglandin (PG) E1 (Trimix).[3,34] Papaverine may lead to false-negative erectile response in some patients and persistent painful erection (priapism) may occur in others. PGE1 has better erection rate and less incidence of priapism.[38] Genital self-stimulation, visual erotic stimulus, or application of penoscrotal tourniquet may augment the erectile response. Gadgets like virtual glasses with facility for audiovisual erotic stimulus improve the erectile response and Doppler waveform, thereby eliminating the false-positive results of PPDU examination.[39]

Technique of PPDU: The examination must be conducted in an atmosphere of privacy. The ultrasonographic evaluation begins with scanning of flaccid penile shaft in transverse plane to measure the diameter of cavernosal artery. It ranges from 0.2 mm to 1 mm.[34] Although the arterial flow in the flaccid penis is difficult to demonstrate, Doppler flowmetry of flaccid penis has the potential to detect arteriogenic ED. PSV of less than 10 cm/s in the cavernosal artery of flaccid penis is suggestive of arteriogenic ED.[40] Later, intracavernosal injection of 60 mg of papaverine is made with 30-G needle in either of the cavernosa as cross-communications exist between both sides. Care must be taken not to inject into a vessel or urethra. The erectile response is graded visually from E0 to E5 as suggested by Broderick et al.[41] **(Box 2)**. Grade E4 and E5 are sufficient for penetration.

After evaluating the erectile response, scanning is started from the base at the penoscrotal junction to distal part, both in transverse and longitudinal planes. Dorsal scanning in sagittal plane is necessary to identify cavernosal collaterals and penile deformities such as Peyronie's disease. The postinjection diameter of both cavernosal arteries is measured. Angle-corrected flow velocities are measured as proximal as possible in cavernosal arteries. Most accurate flowmetry values are obtained at the time of peak rigidity, however, this time is highly variable. Hence, flowmetry values are normally obtained at 0, 5, 10, and 20 minutes after the injection.

Postpapaverine injection, normal spectral waveform has been described to have five phases **(Figs. 11A to D)**.[42]

Box 2: Visual grading of penile erection during PPDU.

- E0: No response
- E1: Elongation of shaft only
- E2: Moderate tumescence, no rigidity
- E3: Full tumescence, no rigidity, easily bendable
- E4: Full erection, partial rigidity
- E5: Full rigidity for at least 20 minutes

(PPDU: pharmacopenile duplex ultrasonography)

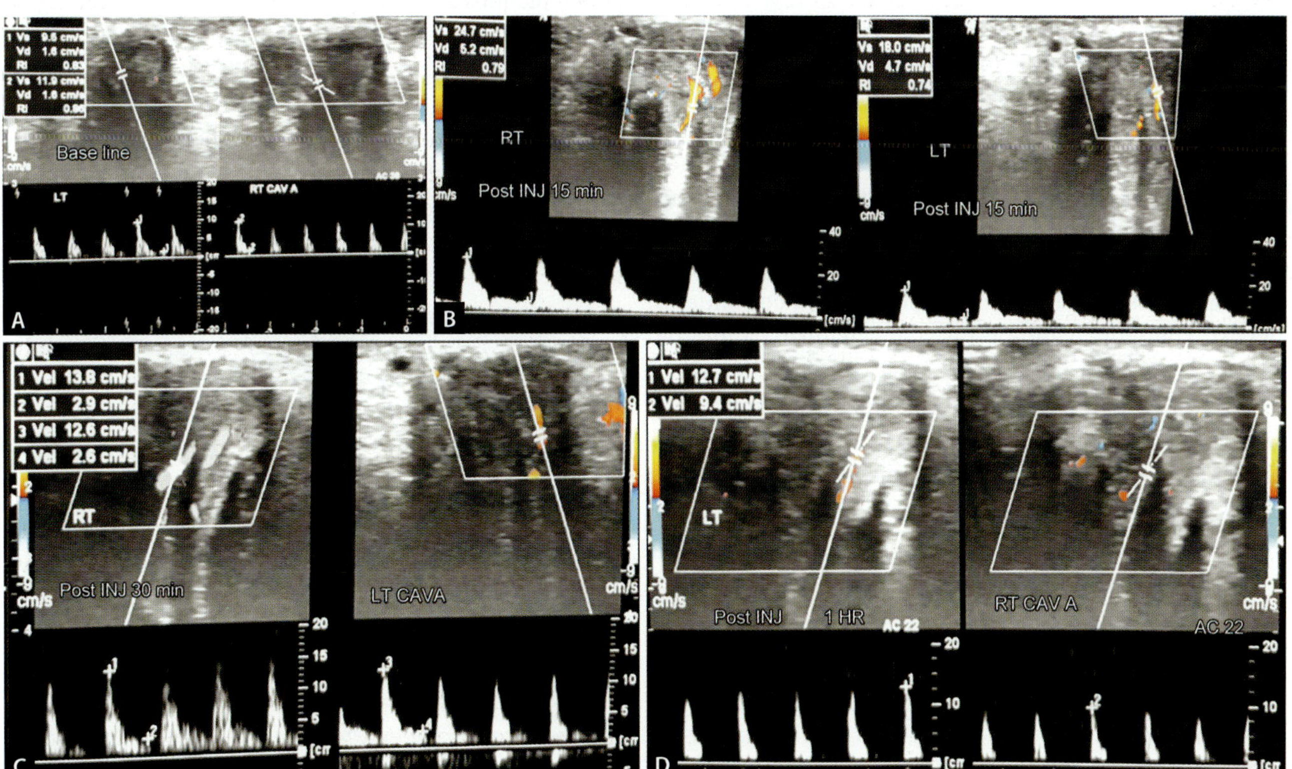

Figs. 11A to D: Normal spectral waveform progression of PPDU: (A) Baseline, (B) 15 minutes postinjection, (C) 30 minutes postinjection, (D) 1 hour postinjection. (PPDU: Pharmacopenile duplex ultrasonography).

Phase 1 is characterized by increase in both systolic and diastolic velocities. In phase 2, there is progressive decrease in EDV and appearance of a dicrotic notch. Patients with severe venous leakage do not progress beyond phase 2. In phase 3, diastolic flow approximates zero and it is reversed in phase 4. Phase 5 is characterized by eventual loss of both systolic and diastolic signals.

Various parameters studied on flowmetry are PSV, EDV, AT, and RI. Mild variations are seen in cutoff values described in different studies. PSV of more than 35 cm/s rules out arterial insufficiency and PSV of 25 cm/s is highly suggestive of the same. Lot of overlap is seen between these two values in normal and abnormal individuals.[2] Currently acceptable reference values used to interpret the examination as normal are given in **Box 3.**[34,38]

In a study of 32 men without evidence of vascular ED conducted at AIIMS, the mean PSV was 61.3 cm/s, the mean EDV was –1.2 cm (minus sign denotes flow reversal) and the mean AT was 0.06 s.[43] Mean RI was in whom diastolic flow reversal was not achieved. Another interesting observation was the linear relationship between PSV and ages of the individuals, which implies that use of single cut-off value for all ages may be debatable.

Abnormal PSV (less than 25 cm/s) and AT (more than 0.11 s) are suggestive of arterial disease. Similarly, any increase in the cavernosal artery diameter by less than 75% of the baseline diameter also indicates possibility of arterial disease. Abnormal EDV (more than 5 cm/s) and RI (<0.85) denote venous leakage. RI is considered more reliable than EDV for assessment of veno-occlusive mechanism.[43] If arterial disease is present, intracavernosal pressure remains below systemic pressure and veno-occlusion cannot occur, even if this mechanism is intact, and diastolic flow will continue to persist. Therefore, veno-occlusive mechanism cannot be assessed with EDV and RI in presence of arterial disease.

Pharmacopenile duplex ultrasonography *with oral sildenafil:* Sildenafil citrate (Viagra) has been studied as an alternative to intracavernosal injection of vasoactive drugs for PPDU, in order to make the examination noninvasive; however, the results are inconsistent.[44,45] Oral dose of 50 or 100 mg is normally used. Unlike intracavernosal agents, sildenafil alone cannot achieve erection and it must be supplemented with audiovisual sexual stimulation. Effect of sildenafil is also slow and peak erection is usually achieved between 60 minutes and 75 minutes after its oral administration. The quality of erection and the PSV achieved with sildenafil is lower than the same parameters achieved after intracavernosal injection. This may lead to false-positive PPDU results in some patients.[45] With these limitations, oral sildenafil has failed to replace intracavernosal injections of vasoactive drugs for PPDU. A recent study has suggested that best results are obtained with combination of oral sildenafil and intracavernosal injection of trimix during PPDU.[46]

Box 3: Normal reference values for PPDU.

- PSV: 25 cm/s or more
- EDV: 5 cm/s or less
- AT: 0.11 s or less
- RI: 0.85 or more

(AT: acceleration time; EDV: end-diastolic velocity; PPDU: pharmacopenile duplex ultrasonography; RI: resistive index)

Peyronie's Disease

This is a benign condition resulting from inelastic scar of tunica albuginea, which produces curvature deformities of penis and the ED. It is traumatic in origin in majority of the patients and the ED in these patients is primarily because of penile deformities, painful erection, or associated vascular disorders.[47] On sonography, the penile plaques are seen as echogenic focal thickenings of tunica, which may displace or encase dorsal vasculature. Dense plaques may contain calcifications and cause acoustic shadowing **(Fig. 12)**, however, shadowing can be seen even without evidence of calcification on plain radiographs. Most plaques are located in the middle third of the shaft of the penis.[38]

Fig. 12: Peyronie's disease: Dense echogenic plaque of tunica albuginea with distal shadowing.

Cavernosometry

Cavernosometry is a primary modality available for quantifying and mapping of veno-occlusive dysfunction. However, because of its invasive nature, it is reserved for patients with suggestion of venous leakage on PPDU if surgical repair is being considered for them. In cavernosometry, venous outflow resistance is assessed by determining the intracavernosal flow rate required to sustain an erection in a state of complete sinusoidal relaxation.

In this technique, two 19-G needles are introduced, one in each cavernosa. One needle is connected to the infusion pump and the other needle to a pressure monitor. A mixture of 30 mg of papaverine and 1 mg of phentolamine is infused. The intracavernosal pressure rises gradually and then remains steady. After this, the infusion flow rate is gradually increased to demonstrate linearly proportional increase in intracavernosal pressure. Linear relationship between cavernosal pressure and infusion rate is suggestive of a state of complete sinusoidal relaxation. If a nonlinear relationship is observed, a second dose of papaverine may be given to achieve complete sinusoidal relaxation.

Maintenance flow rate is considered as the most important parameter of cavernosometry and it involves recording of minimum flow rate, which is required to maintain intracavernous pressure at 150 mm Hg. Maintenance flow rate of more than 3 mL per minute is suggestive of venous leakage. After this, the infusion is stopped and the rate of fall of cavernosal pressure is observed for 30 seconds. The rate of fall, termed as "pressure loss," of more than 1.5 mm Hg per second is considered abnormal.[38]

Gravity cavernosometry is a simple and cost-effective modification of the above technique in which the inflow needle is connected to heparinized normal saline kept at the height of 160 cm. The infusion produces increase in cavernosal pressure, which subsequently reaches at a plateau, termed as "steady state pressure." Steady state pressure of less than 97 mm Hg is considered abnormal.[48]

Cavernosography

Patient can be taken up for cavernosography after cavernosometry in the same sitting. About 40 mL of iodinated contrast is injected in infusion line while keeping intracavernosal pressure just above mean arterial pressure. Spot films of penis and pelvis are obtained under fluoroscopic guidance in AP and both oblique projections **(Figs. 13A and B)**. Normally draining veins are not opacified. In case of venous leakage, veins are visualized draining from the veins of corpus spongiosum, the deep dorsal, cavernosal, and crural veins **(Figs. 14A and B)**. More than one site is present in most patients, with deep dorsal and cavernosal veins being the most common combination.[49]

Penile Angiography

Internal pudendal angiography is indicated in younger patients with suspected isolated arterial disease, such as post-traumatic narrowing, who may benefit from surgical repair rather than in elderly patients with diffuse atheromatous involvement. Patency of common

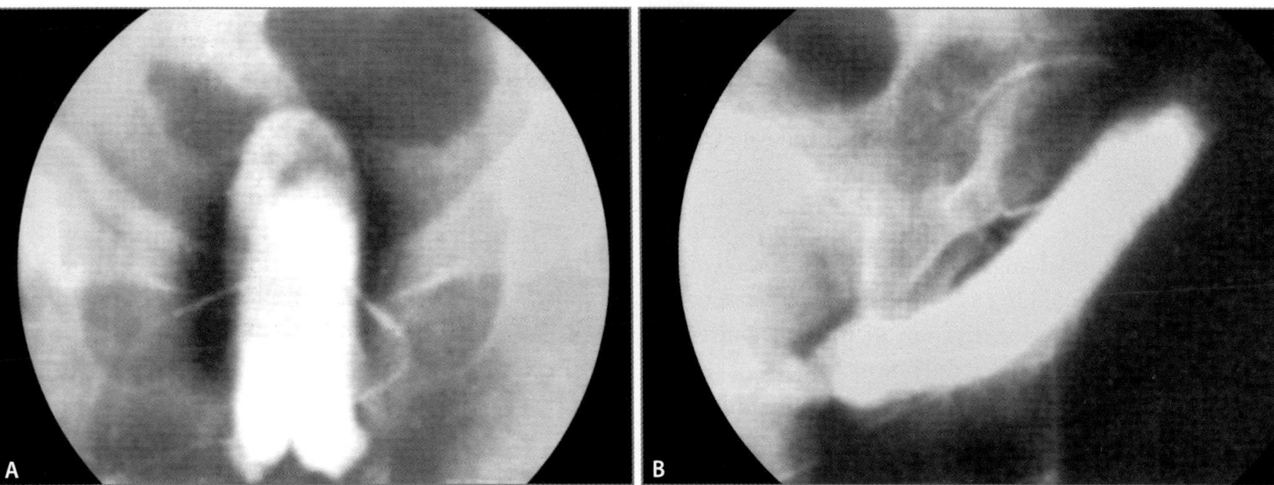

Figs. 13A and B: Normal cavernosogram: (A) AP and (B) oblique views show homogeneous opacification of bilateral cavernosa without visualization of any vein in vicinity. (AP: anteroposterior).

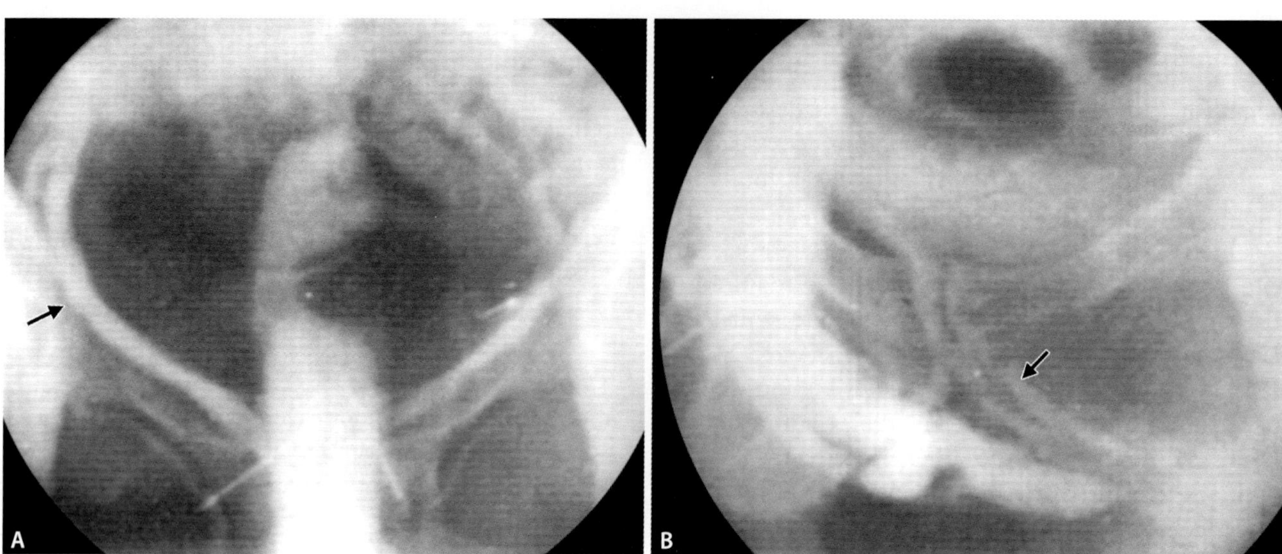

Figs. 14A and B: Cavernosogram: Veno-occlusive ED: (A) AP view shows venous leak into internal pudendal vein (arrow). (B) Oblique view (arrow) shows venous leak into deep dorsal vein in the cavernosogram of another patient. (ED: erectile dysfunction).

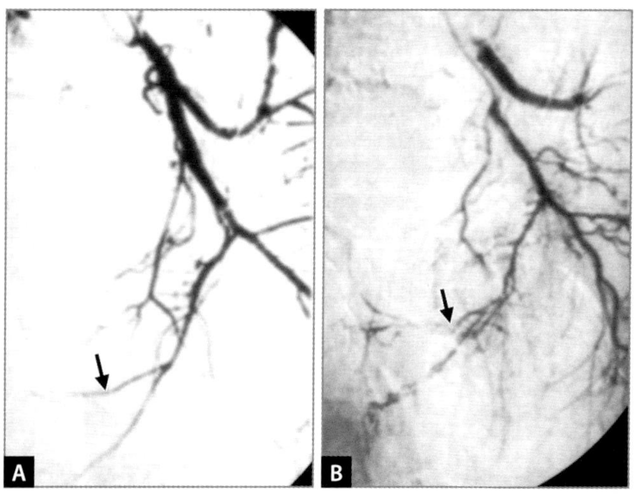

Figs. 15A and B: Internal pudendal angiogram: (A) Normal internal pudendal and common penile (arrow) arteries. (B) Internal pudendal angiogram of another patient shows post-traumatic narrowing of common penile artery (arrow) as a cause of arteriogenic ED. (ED: erectile dysfunction).

iliac, internal iliac, and internal pudendal arteries is established on initial angiographic films. Later, 60 mg of papaverine is injected in cavernosa followed by selective angiography of anterior division of internal pudendal artery. Contrast is injected at the rate of 3–4 mL per second and images are obtained in posterior oblique projection. In majority of the patients, anatomy of the penile arterial supply and the precise location of the arterial lesion is demonstrated which allows planning of appropriate surgical approach **(Figs. 15A and B)**.

Priapism

The most common complication, during the diagnostic workup and especially during PPDU and cavernosometry, is papaverine-induced prolonged and painful erection or priapism. The incidence can be as high as 11%.[34] Chances of priapism are high if PSV of more than 66 cm/s or RI of more than 1 (diastolic flow reversal) is observed.[50] It is prudent to observe the patient for at least 2 hours after the procedure. Not all priapism cases require specific treatment as penis detumescence generally occurs within few hours. In case the duration of erection exceeds 6 hours, the corpora cavernosa are drained to decrease the pressure and 10 microgram of adrenaline is injected intracavernosally to induce cavernosal smooth muscle contraction, effective venous drainage, and restriction of arterial flow. Compression bandage is also applied for few minutes. In case of recurrence of erection, the procedure is repeated.

Broadly, priapism is divided into high-flow and low-flow priapism. High-flow priapism is usually associated with trauma. The patients have painless erection and venous outflow is usually maintained. The diagnosis of high-flow priapism is usually clinical but color Doppler US may provide useful information. No cavernosal injection is required for the study.

A hypoechoic area may be seen in cavernosa on gray scale US which suggests laceration. Color Doppler study may demonstrate the cavernosal artery tear and arterial-lacunar fistula. Selective embolization of the torn artery with blood clots, coils, or polyvinyl alcohol (PVA) is the treatment of choice to treat these lesions.[51] Low-flow or ischemic priapism is seen as complication of intracavernosal injection of drugs or leukostasis in leukemic patients. The diagnosis is clinical and imaging is not required before surgical intervention. The condition is considered as an urologic emergency. US and color Doppler findings are same as that of normal rigid erection.

CONCLUSION

The diagnostic workup of male infertility should start at least 1 year after consummation of marriage and needs to be performed in a systematic and structured manner. Semen analysis should be complemented with a comprehensive medical history supplemented by imaging. Imaging has an important role in differentiating causes of obstructive azoospermia (investigation of choice is TRUS), which are potentially correctable causes of infertility from causes of nonobstructive azoospermia (investigation of choice is scrotal USG).

REFERENCES

1. Guttmacher AF. Factors affecting normal expectancy of conception. J Am Med Assoc. 1956;161:855-60.
2. World Health Organization. Towards more objectivity in diagnosis and management of male infertility. Int J Androl. 1987;(Suppl 7):1-53.
3. Colpi Ammar T, Sidhu PS, Wilkins CJ. Male infertility: the role of imaging in diagnosis and management. Br J Radiol. 2012;85(1):S59-68.
4. Cornund E, Amar E, Hamida K, et al. Ultrasound findings in male hypofertility and impotence. Eur Radiol. 2001;11:2126-36.
5. Pierik FH, Dohle GR, Muiswinkel JM, et al. Is routine scrotal ultrasonography advantageous in infertile men? J Urol. 1999; 162:1618-20.
6. Jarrow JP. Transrectal ultrasonography of infertile men. Fertil Steril. 1993;60:1035-9.
7. Raviv G, Mor Y, Levron J, et al. Role of transrectal ultrasonography in the evaluation of azoospermic men with low volume ejaculate. J Ultrasound Med. 2006;25:825-9.
8. Sihag P, Tandon A, Pal R, et al. Sonography in male infertility: a look beyond the obvious. J Ultrasound. 2018;21(3):265-76.
9. Dhabuwala CB, Parulkar BG. Doppler flow analysis and conventional ultrasonography for evaluation of the infertile male. In: Jafe R, Pierson RA, Abramowics JS (Eds). Imaging in Infertility and Reproductive Endocrinology. Philadelphia: JB Lippincot Co.; 1994. pp. 207-16.
10. Qublan HS, Al-Okoor K, Al-Ghoweri AS, et al. Sonographic spectrum of scrotal abnormalities in infertile men. J Clin Ultrasound. 2007;35:437-41.
11. Howards SS, Mittal PK, Little B, et al. Role of imaging in the evaluation of male infertility. Radiographics. 2017;37(3): 837-54.
12. Dambro TJ, Stewart RR, Carroll BA, et al. The scrotum. In: Rumack CM, Wilson SR, Charboneau JW (Eds). Diagnostic Ultrasound, 2nd edition. St Louis: Mosby; 1998. pp. 719-822.
13. Lorenc T, Krupniewski L, Palczewski P, et al. The value of ultrasonography in the diagnosis of varicocele. J Ultrason. 2016;16(67):359-70.
14. Kokacok E, Serhatlioglu S, Kiris S, et al. Colour Doppler sonographic evaluation of interrelations between diameter, reflux, and flow volume of testicular veins in varicocele. Eur J Radiol. 2003;47:251-6.
15. Chiou RK, Anderson JC, Wobig RK, et al. Color Doppler ultrasound criteria to diagnose varicoceles: correlation of a new scoring system with physical examination. Urology. 1997;50:953-6.
16. Dhamija E, Das CJ, Razik A. Intratesticular varicocele: a rare cause of male factor infertility. BMJ Case Rep. 2018;2018.
17. Dubin L, Amelar R. Varicocele size and results of varicocelectomy in selected infertile men with a varicocele. Fertil Steril. 1970;21:606-9.
18. McLure R, Kho D, Dale R, et al. Subclinical varicocele—the effectiveness of varicocelectomy. J Urol. 1991;145:786-90.
19. Gonda RL Jr, Kaw JJ, Forte KA, et al. Diagnosis of subclinical varicocele in infertility. AJR. 1987;148:71-5.
20. Gandini R, Konda D, Reale CA, et al. Male varicocele: transcatheter foam sclerotherapy with sodium tetradecyl sulfate: outcome in 244 patients. Radiology. 2008;246:612-8.
21. Halden W, White RI. Outpatient embolotherapy of varicocele. Urol Clin N Am. 1987;14:137-40.
22. Thompson ST. Prevention of male infertility: an update. Urol Clin N Am. 1994;21:365-76.
23. Simon SD, Lee RD, Mulhall PP. Should all infertile males undergo urologic evaluation before assisted reproductive technologies? Fertil Steril. 2001;75:1226-7.
24. Kim Ed, Lipshultz LI. Role of ultrasound in assessment of male infertility. J Clin Ultrasound. 1996;24:437-53.
25. Kumar R, Thulkar S, Kumar V, et al. Contributions of investigations to the diagnosis of bilateral vas aplasia. ANZ J Surg. 2005;75:807-9.
26. Kim MJ, Lee JT, Lee MS, et al. MR imaging of male infertility with an endorectal surface coil. Abdom Imaging. 1997;22: 348-53.
27. Fisch H, Lambert SM, Goluboff ET. Management of ejaculatory duct obstruction. Etiology, diagnosis and treatment. World J Urol. 2006;24:604-10.
28. Colpi GM, Negri L, Nappi RE, et al. Is transrectal ultrasonography a reliable diagnostic approach in ejaculatory duct sub obstruction? Hum Reprod. 1997;12:2186-91.
29. Purohit RS, Wu DS, Shinohara K, et al. A prospective comparison of three diagnostic methods to evaluate ejaculatory duct obstruction. J Urol. 2004;171:232-5.
30. Schnall MD, Pollack HM, Arsdalen KV, et al. The seminal tract in patients with ejaculatory dysfunction: MR imaging with an endorectal surface coil. AJR. 1992;159:337-41.
31. Toov JH, Fait G, Houser R, et al. Can Doppler ultrasonographic measurements of the testis predict spermatozoa retrieval in azoospermic patients undergoing testicular biopsy? Fertil Steril. 2001;76:1276-7.
32. Belenky A, Avrech CM, Bacher GN, et al. Ultrasound-guided testicular sperm aspiration in azoospermic patient: a new sperm retrieval method for intracytoplasmic sperm injection. J Clin Ultrasound. 2001;6:339-43.
33. Belker AM, Steinbock GS. Transrectal prostate ultrasonography as a diagnostic and therapeutic aid for ejaculatory duct obstruction. J Urol. 1990;144:356-8.

34. Mihmanli I, Kantarci F. Erectile dysfunction. Semin Ultrasound CT MRI. 2007;28:274-86.
35. Aroujo AB, Mohr BA, McKinley JB. Changes in sexual function in middle aged and older men: longitudinal data from the Massachusetts Male Aging Study. J Am Geriatr Soc. 2004;52:1502-9.
36. Montorsi F, Briganti A, Salonia A, et al. Erectile dysfunction prevalence, time of onset, and association with risk factors in 300 consecutive patients with acute chest pain, and angiographically documented coronary artery disease. Eur Urol. 2003;44:360-4.
37. Hatzichristan D, Hatzimouratidis K, Bekas M, et al. Diagnostic steps in evaluation of patients with erectile dysfunction. J Urol. 2002;168:615-20.
38. Meuleman E, Diemont WL. Investigation of erectile dysfunction. Urol Clin N Am. 1995;22:803-19.
39. Park K, Kwon DD, Oh BR, et al. Efficacy of virtual glasses in audiovisual sexual stimulation during penile colour duplex Doppler ultrasonography. Eur Urol. 2002;41:62-5.
40. Roy C, Saussine C, Tuchman C, et al. Duplex Doppler sonography of flaccid penis: potential role in the evaluation of impotence. J Clin Ultrasound. 2000;28:290-4.
41. Broderick GA, Arger P. Duplex Doppler ultrasonography: noninvasive assessment of penile anatomy and function. Semin Roentgen. 1993;28:43-56.
42. Shwartz AM, Lawe M, Berger RE, et al. Assessment of normal and abnormal erectile function: color Doppler sonography versus conventional techniques. radiology. 1991;180:105-9.
43. Bhargava R, Srivastava DN, Thulkar S, et al. Colour duplex Doppler ultrasonography evaluation of nonvasculogenic male erectile dysfunction: an Indian perspective. Australas Radiol. 2002;44:170-3.
44. Arslan D, Esen AA, Secil M. A new method for evaluation of ED: Sildenafil plus Doppler ultrasonography. J Urol. 2001;166: 181-4.
45. Copel L, Ktz R, Blacher A, et al. Clinical and duplex US assessment of effects of sildenafil on cavernosal arteries of the penis—comparison with intracavernosal injection of vasoactive agents: initial experience. Radiology. 2005;237: 986-91.
46. Park JK, Park JS, Jeon SB, et al. Why a combined intracavernosal injection with trimix and oral sildenafil is reliable therapy in ultrasonic evaluation of erectile dysfunction. BJU Int. 2008; 102:993-7.
47. Gholami SS, Lue TF. Peyronie's disease. Urol Clin N Am. 2001;28:377-90.
48. Meulman EJ, Wijkstra H, Doesbury WH, et al. Comparison of diagnostic values of pump and gravity cavernosometry in the evaluation of cavernous veno-occlusive mechanism. J Urol. 1991;146:1266-70.
49. Shabsingh R, Fishman IJ, Toombs BD, et al. Venous leaks: anatomical and physiological observations. J Urol. 1991;146:1260-4.
50. Metawea B, El-Nashar AR, Gad-Allah A, et al. Intracavernos papaverine phentolamine-induced priapism can be accurately predicted with colour Doppler ultrasonography. Urology. 2005;66:858-60.
51. Campliani S, Savoca G, Buttazi L, et al. High-flow priapism: treatment and long-term follow-up. Urology. 2002;59: 110-3.

SECTION 5

Miscellaneous

Chapter 23

Imaging of the Adrenal Gland

Devasenathipathy Kandasamy, Raju Sharma, Arun Kumar Gupta

INTRODUCTION

Thomas Addison first described a clinical entity resulting from adrenal dysfunction in 1855, but it took nearly half a century for the scientific community to accept that adrenals are essential to life. Remarkable progress has since been made in defining the structure and function of the adrenal gland. Adrenal glands are small but their common involvement in many disease processes has made cross-sectional imaging modalities essential to detect abnormal morphological and functional alterations. With the ever-increasing volume of imaging being performed, incidental adrenal nodules are detected much more than ever. Around 4% of all abdominal computed tomography (CT) scans show adrenal nodules and this number increases to 6% in autopsy studies.[1,2] The incidence also increases with age. Imaging also plays a critical role in the characterization of adrenal mass lesions. It is important to understand the normal anatomy and functional characteristics of the adrenal gland.

ANATOMY AND PHYSIOLOGY

The adrenal gland is named for its location adjacent to the kidney. It lies within perirenal fascia, embedded in perirenal fat. Each gland measures 3–5 cm in length, 2–3 cm in width, 5.0 mm in thickness and weighs around 3.5–5.0 g. Both glands differ in shape. The right adrenal is pyramidal in shape and its relations are liver laterally, upper pole of right kidney inferiorly, right crus of diaphragm posteromedially, and inferior vena cava (IVC) anteromedially. The left adrenal gland is crescent-shaped and its relations are upper pole of left kidney posterolaterally, left crus of diaphragm posteromedially, stomach in upper two-thirds anteriorly, and pancreatic body with splenic vessels in lower one-third. Each adrenal gland receives its blood supply from three arteries, namely, superior adrenal artery, a branch of inferior phrenic artery; middle adrenal artery arising from descending aorta; and inferior adrenal artery, a branch of the renal artery. There is a single adrenal vein on either side—the right adrenal vein drains into inferior vena cava and the left one into the left renal vein.

The adrenal gland is made of an outer cortex that is derived from mesoderm and an inner medulla that is derived from neural crest. The cortex forms almost 90% of the total adrenal mass; the medulla contributes only 10%. The adrenal cortex is histologically comprised of three distinct zones—zona glomerulosa, zona fasciculata, and zona reticularis from outside to inside. The adrenal cortex secretes three groups of steroid hormones. Zona glomerulosa constitutes 10–15% of the cortex and secretes mineralocorticoids; aldosterone being the most important. Zona fasciculata constitutes 80% of the cortex and secretes glucocorticoids while zona reticularis, contributing only 5–10% of cortex, secretes androgens. Zona glomerulosa is mainly involved in aldosterone biosynthesis whereas the fasciculata-reticularis zone is the site for cortisol and androgen biosynthesis.

The adrenal medulla secretes epinephrine and norepinephrine, which form an integral part of the sympathetic autonomic nervous system and play an important role in the regulation of vital functions and many metabolic processes.

IMAGING MODALITIES

A number of imaging modalities are available for evaluation of the adrenals. Before the advent of imaging modalities like ultrasound (US), CT, and magnetic resonance imaging (MRI), the radiological techniques available for evaluation of adrenals were plain radiograph of abdomen, excretory urography, invasive techniques like perirenal air insufflation, adrenal venography, and angiography. Most of these techniques have become obsolete. Angiography may be sometimes indicated to look for extra-adrenal pheochromocytoma in situations when metaiodobenzylguanidine (MIBG) scintigraphy is not available. Adrenal venous sampling may be recommended in patients with primary hyperaldosteronism, both for distinguishing unilateral from bilateral disease and for localizing unilateral tumor. According to the recommendations of the Endocrine Society, all patients with primary hyperaldosteronism of age more than 35 years should undergo preoperative adrenal venous sampling to lateralize the lesion, irrespective of the imaging findings.[3] Both the adrenal veins are sequentially catheterized and obtained samples are tested for aldosterone and cortisol levels. The right adrenal vein drains into IVC whereas the left adrenal vein drains into the left renal vein. This technique is invasive, technically difficult to perform, and needs hospitalization. Procedural complications include adrenal infarction, adrenal vein thrombosis, adrenal hemorrhage, hypotensive crises, and adrenal insufficiency.

Ultrasound is seldom used in imaging suspected adrenal pathology. CT and MRI remain the imaging modalities of choice for the evaluation of structural changes in the diseased adrenal whereas scintigraphy provides functional assessment of the gland. ^{18}F fluorodeoxyglucose positron emission tomography (^{18}F-FDG PET) has played an important role in defining physiological and pathological conditions of the adrenal glands. Integrated information obtained from anatomic and functional imaging is essential for characterization of adrenal disease.

Percutaneous biopsy of the adrenal lesion under US/CT guidance has an accuracy of 80–90%. Minor complications include abdominal pain, hematuria, or small pneumothorax. Major ones requiring treatment occur in 3–5% of the patients and include hemorrhage and pneumothorax necessitating drainage.

Ultrasound

Despite the availability of high-resolution real-time ultrasound scanners, normal adrenal gland or small adrenal lesions remain difficult to be visualized on sonography except in infants where adrenals can be well visualized on US. Therefore, ultrasonography (USG) is seldom indicated for adrenal lesion, although large adrenal mass may be detected incidentally during abdominal US examination. USG is however, useful in evaluation of suspected adrenal hemorrhage in neonates. It may also be used as a screening modality in suspected pheochromocytoma due to the easy availability. USG guidance suffices for sampling of large adrenal lesions.

Computed Tomography

Computed tomography remains the first choice of imaging modality for evaluation of the majority of adrenal diseases. The widespread availability of CT in clinical practice makes it an ideal noninvasive technique for evaluating adrenal gland morphology owing to the speed with which examination can be performed, its superior spatial resolution, and quantification of contrast washout patterns.[4,5] The introduction of multidetector-row helical CT has allowed rapid thin-slice imaging of the adrenal glands during various phases of contrast enhancement. Small adrenal lesions can be detected and accurate density measurements of lesions can be done.

The CT technique should be tailored according to the clinical indication. In general, when CT is used to study the adrenal glands, the entire abdomen through the aortic bifurcation is scanned. This is helpful for staging or for evaluating possible ectopic adrenal lesions. Oral contrast material is helpful so that unopacified loops of bowel are not confused as adrenal lesions. A nonenhanced CT examination should be done first. This may be followed by enhanced and delayed enhanced CT examination when required in a situation, where adenoma needs to be differentiated from metastasis. Currently, adrenal protocol CT is considered more accurate and is favored over MRI for the differentiation of adenoma from metastasis, unless administration of iodinated contrast is contraindicated.[6] Thin sections along with multiplanar reconstructions need to be reviewed on a workstation.

In the search for pheochromocytoma, CT should be done from lower thorax to symphysis pubis. Pericardium is a rare site but can be easily included on CT. Large sporadic pheochromocytomas are easily detected on CT. However, syndromic pheochromocytoma may be small, multiple, and extra-adrenal. In order to optimize visualization of tumors, contrast injection is necessary. It is extremely rare for the new nonionic IV contrast agents to precipitate hypertensive crisis in patients of pheochromocytoma.

The adrenal gland has a characteristic inverted Y or V shape on CT and is seen as an anteromedial ridge with two posterior limbs, the medial limb being shorter than the

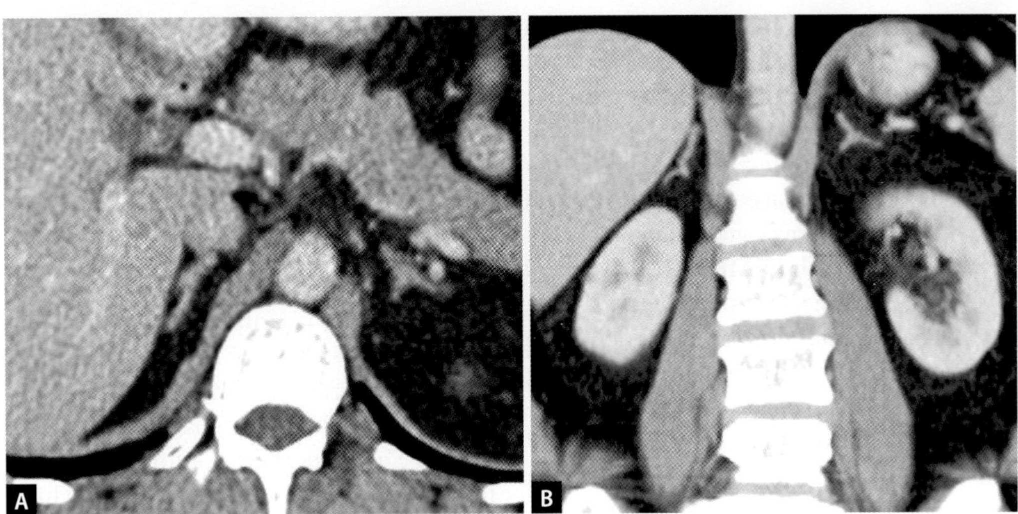

Figs. 1A and B: (A) Axial and (B) coronal CT images showing the normal adrenal glands.

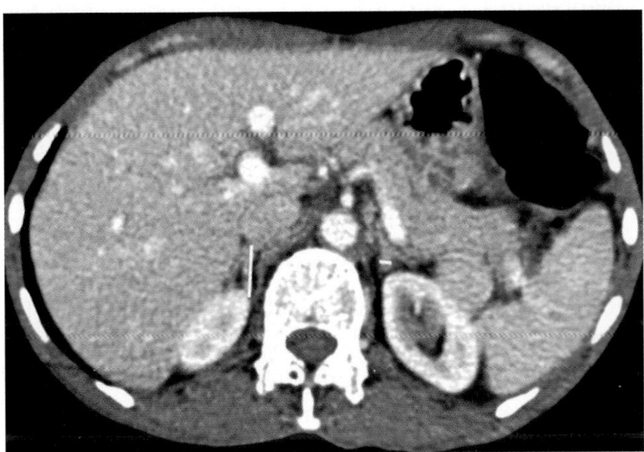

Fig. 2: Normal adrenal measurements. (1) Anteroposterior diameter and (2) limb thickness.

lateral limb. The limbs normally have a straight or concave outline **(Figs. 1A and B)**. The adrenal measurements on CT are taken as anteroposterior diameter from the tip of the anteromedial ridge to the posterior tip of the longest limb, length by calculating the number of sequential scans in which the gland is visualized **(Fig. 2)**. The criteria for enlargement of adrenal are taken as length more than 4.0 cm, anteroposterior diameter of more than 3.0 cm, and limb thickness of more than 6.0 mm or more than adjacent diaphragmatic crus. Besides these absolute measurements, any alteration in the contour, focal bulge, calcification, pattern of enhancement, CT attenuation values on nonenhanced, enhanced and delayed-enhanced techniques, and displacement of surrounding structures should be evaluated.[7]

Another advancement in the last decade is the capability of dual-energy CT (DECT) for tissue material decomposition. One of the benefits of DECT is the generation of virtual noncontrast (VNC) CT from contrast-enhanced CT (CECT) without actually acquiring the noncontrast images. In adrenal adenoma, the VNC has been found to be equally effective as true noncontrast CT (NCCT) in diagnosis.[8-10] Besides this, it can also detect the percentage of microscopic fat within the lesion to characterize them.[11,12]

Magnetic Resonance Imaging

The intention of most MRI techniques used so far has primarily been distinction of benign from malignant disease.

The most reliable in this context is the use of in-phase and out-of-phase gradient-echo (GRE) techniques (chemical shift imaging) for adenoma versus metastasis distinction. Two different echo times (TEs) (out-of-phase TE: 2.2–2.7 ms and in-phase TE: 4.2–4.5 ms) are used in each repetition time (TR) during this sequence. The shortest echo times feasible should be used to overcome the effect of T2* decay on signal. The principle behind this sequence is the ability to highlight the presence of microscopic fat, which is typically expected in adenomas. The fat and water protons are in phase at in-phase TE when the signals add up whereas at out-of-phase TE the fat and water protons are out of phase leading to cancellation of their signals. This phenomenon leads to signal drop of adenomas in out-of-phase images. It is an accurate method to diagnose adenoma, which can be helpful even when CT densitometry fails. It is because the sensitivity of MRI in detecting microscopic fat is better than CT. However, if the lipid content is very low as seen in lipopenic adenoma chemical shift imaging too will fail. CT washout technique performs better than MR chemical shift imaging in lipopenic adenomas. Another pitfall of chemical shift MRI is that it will be positive in any lesion containing microscopic fat. Metastasis from hepatocellular carcinoma and renal cell carcinoma which can have microscopic fat can show signal drop on out-of-phase imaging.[13-15] Nonetheless, both MR and CT have very high specificity (95–98%) in differentiating adenoma from metastasis.[6] The normal adrenal cortex contains abundant lipid, which however, is not enough to be demonstrated on in-phase and out-of-phase imaging.

T2-weighted images provide information on the fluid content of lesions. T2W imaging is most useful in the search for pheochromocytomas which have a high fluid content. T2W sequences also supplement benign versus malignant differentiation, although substantial overlap exists.[16] Normal adrenal gland may demonstrate corticomedullary differentiation on T2WI.

Normal adrenal glands and small adrenal masses are well demonstrated on T1-weighted fat-suppressed images **(Figs. 3A and B)**.[17] The demonstration of corticomedullary differentiation on either noncontrast T1W fat-suppressed images or immediate postgadolinium GE images is helpful in distinguishing adrenal from renal tumors.[18] The sagittal plane is more useful than coronal plane in this regard. The use of thin-section 3D-GRE sequences in one plane of acquisition allows reconstructions in other planes for defining tumor location.

Diffusion-weighted MRI provides insight into water composition and cellularity in a tumor may provide an additional tool to distinguish benign, and from malignant adrenal masses. Malignant tumors have an increased cellularity, which manifests as restricted diffusion, and a decrease in the apparent diffusion coefficient. However, even benign tumors such as adenoma and pheochromocytoma can have restricted diffusion limiting the utility of diffusion-weighted imaging (DWI) in adrenal lesion characterization.

Radionuclide Imaging

This technique is primarily used as a problem-solving modality for lesions not adequately characterized on CT and MRI. It provides functional imaging of the adrenal cortex and medulla. Radiolabeled analogs of cholesterol, e.g. 75 Se-selenomethyl-norcholesterol, NP-59 beta-iodomethyl-19-norcholesterol, can localize mass causing adrenal cortical dysfunction; the latter one is particularly useful in the workup for suspected aldosteronism. The advances in CT and MRI have largely eliminated the use of NP-59 imaging for adrenal. Iodine-131 MIBG is concentrated in sympathoadrenal tissue and is used for imaging adrenal medullary lesion, especially to evaluate for pheochromocytoma and to screen the whole body for extra-adrenal pheochromocytoma.

Positron Emission Tomography

Recently, PET has become available as a possible tool for evaluating the adrenal. ^{18}F-FDG PET imaging has been found to be a reliable noninvasive imaging technique to differentiate benign from malignant adrenal masses. It has demonstrated high sensitivity, specificity, and overall accuracy for detecting adrenal metastases in patients with malignancy. In patients with known malignancy, FDG-PET is the modality of choice to evaluate any

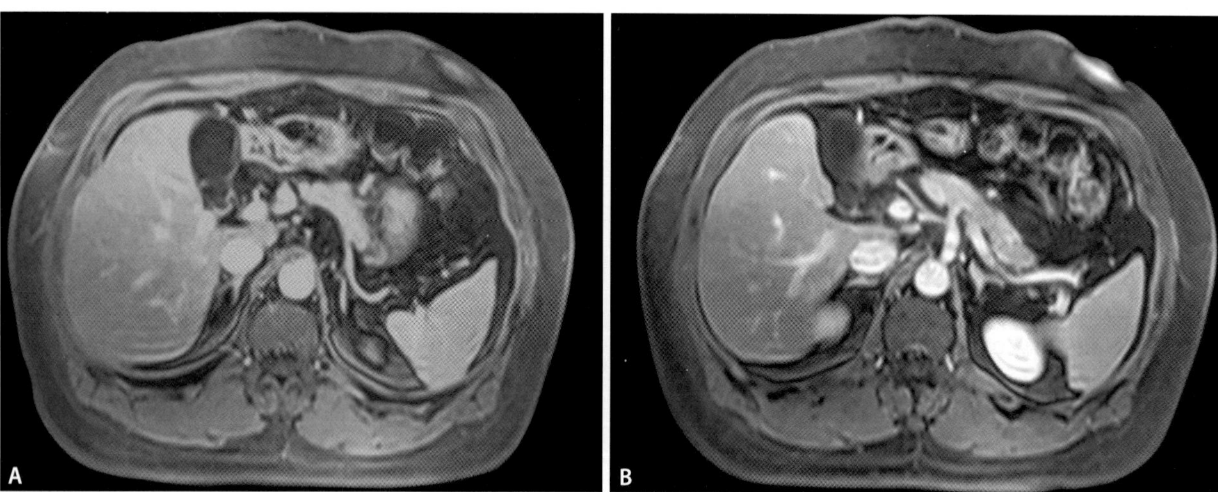

Figs. 3A and B: Gradient-echo T1W axial images showing the normal inverted "V" configuration of the adrenal gland.

adrenal lesion more than 4 cm.[19] At the same time, PET CT is not recommended in patients without a history of malignancy. The common causes of false-positive adrenal lesions on ^{18}F-FDG PET imaging are benign adenomas and pheochromocytoma.[20,21] All benign and malignant pheochromocytomas have been shown to accumulate ^{18}F-FDG, although uptake is found in a greater concentration in malignant as compared to benign pheochromocytoma.[20] The common causes of false-negative ^{18}F-FDG PET results are small-sized lesions, necrotic metastasis, and metastases from neuroendocrine tumors.[21] Small metastatic lesions can be missed because of the limited resolution of ^{18}F-FDG PET/PET-CT or the absence of sufficient tumor cells with increased glycolysis.

ADRENAL DISEASES

Diseases of the adrenal gland may manifest as a result of hormone excess or deficiency. The adrenal diseases may be considered under the following three groups.

- *Group I*: Adrenal hyperfunctional diseases
- *Group II*: Adrenal insufficiency
- *Group III*: Adrenal diseases with normal function.

Group I: Adrenal Hyperfunctional Diseases

Hyperfunctioning adrenal diseases occur either from the adrenal cortex (Cushing's syndrome, Conn's syndrome, and hyperandrogenism) or from the adrenal medulla (pheochromocytoma). The clinical features depend on the type of hormone produced and its manifestation on target organs.

Cushing's Syndrome

Cushing's syndrome is caused by adrenocorticotropic hormone (ACTH) overproduction in 75% of patients and by an excess of cortisol production from adrenal neoplasms in 25%. ACTH overproduction results from either pituitary adenoma or ectopic ACTH-producing nonendocrine tumors. Ectopic ACTH producing nonendocrine tumors include bronchial carcinoid tumor, neuroendocrine tumors of the pancreas, medullary carcinoma of thyroid, thymic carcinoid tumor, and pheochromocytoma **(Figs. 3A and B)**.

The diagnosis of Cushing's syndrome depends predominantly on the clinical features and biochemical findings. It presents an easily recognizable clinical picture of truncal obesity, moon facies, cutaneous striae, buffalo hump, hypertension, muscle weakness, fatigability, osteoporosis, profound emotional changes, and amenorrhea in women.

Appropriate workup of patients with Cushing's syndrome includes plasma cortisol and 24 hours' urine for cortisol estimation followed by dexamethasone suppression test. The abnormal test establishes the diagnosis of Cushing's syndrome. The purpose of imaging is to identify the source of excess ACTH from either a pituitary tumor or an ectopic source and to detect or exclude adrenal mass. The adrenal appearances in Cushing's syndrome depend on the etiology of the syndrome. CT is the primary modality used to evaluate adrenals in this setting. Visualization of adrenal pathology on CT is aided by the large amount of retroperitoneal fat that is usually present in these patients. MRI plays a secondary role.[22]

ACTH-dependent Cushing's syndrome: This results from a pituitary cause in 85% of patients and the rest from ectopic ACTH secretion. The adrenals show changes of hyperplasia in the form of smooth thickened limbs or multiple small nodules of varying sizes involving one or both limbs.

These changes may be seen in one or both adrenals **(Figs. 4 and 5)**. MRI signal intensity in adrenal hyperplasia closely follows that of the normal adrenal gland.

ACTH-independent Cushing's syndrome: Adrenocortical adenoma accounts for 10–20% of patients with Cushing's syndrome. It is seen as a solitary, well-defined homogeneous mass, usually around 2–3 cm in diameter **(Figs. 6A to C)**. However, when large, it shows focal areas of necrosis and hemorrhage. These adenomas are larger than those seen in Conn's syndrome and are usually lipid rich. The contralateral gland is normal but occasionally atrophic. Adrenal carcinoma accounts for 10–15% of patients with Cushing's syndrome. Also, only 10% of

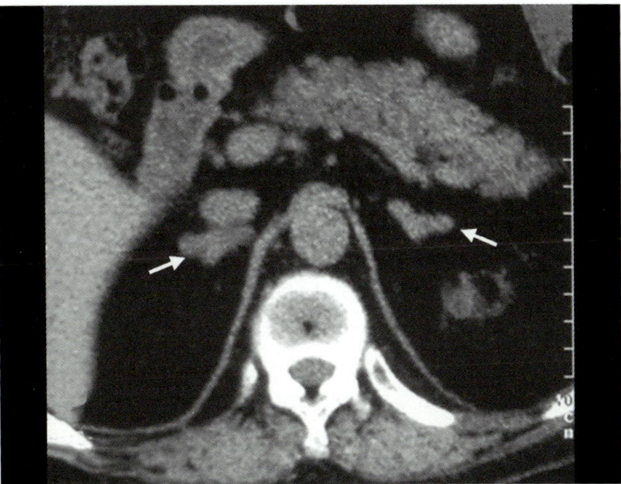

Fig. 4: Noncontrast CT of adrenal glands of a 20-year-old male patient presenting with Cushing's syndrome showing bilateral adrenal hyperplasia (arrows) with proliferation of perirenal and mesenteric fat.

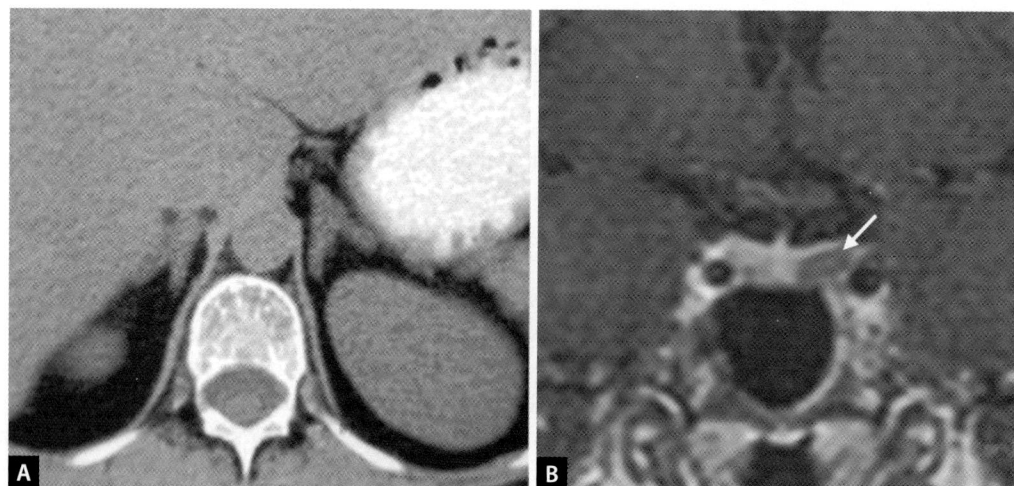

Figs. 5A and B: (A) Noncontrast CT of adrenal glands of a 32-year-old female patient presenting with Cushing's syndrome showing nodular, bilateral adrenal hyperplasia; (B) Postcontrast T1W coronal image of MRI sella of the same patient reveals a microadenoma on the left side of anterior pituitary (arrow).

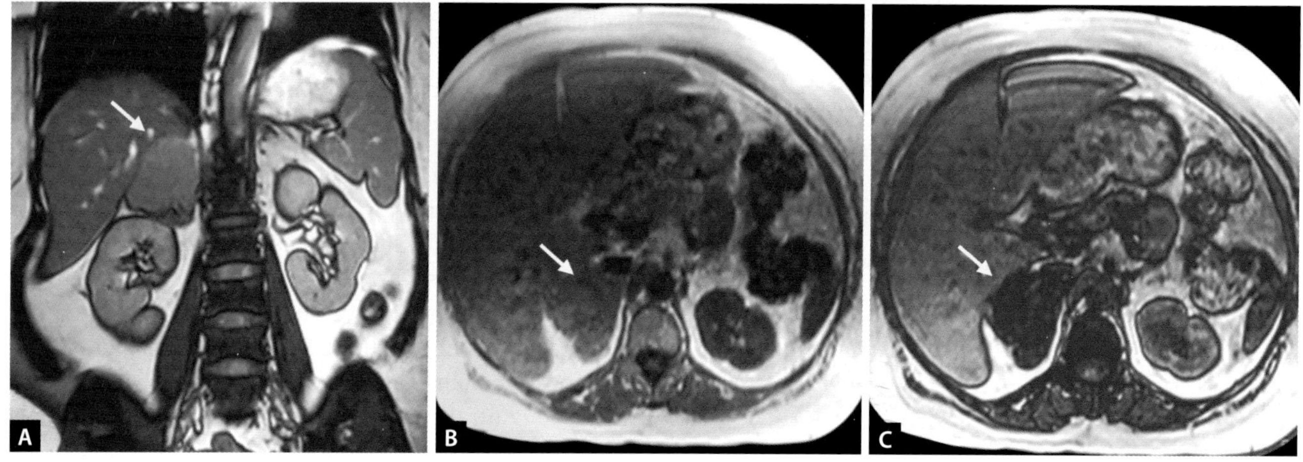

Figs. 6A to C: (A) MRI of a 44-year-old female with Cushingoid features. True-FISP coronal image shows an intermediate signal intensity mass in the right adrenal gland; T1 FLASH (B) in-phase and (C) opposed-phase images reveal significant signal drop in the opposed-phase images, suggesting adrenal adenoma.

adrenal carcinomas function to a level that results in Cushing's syndrome. It is generally seen as a large mass often more than 6.0 cm, heterogeneous with areas of necrosis and calcification, with features of local invasion, regional lymphadenopathy, and distant spread **(Figs. 7 and 8)**.

Rockall et al. while reporting findings in 37 patients with primary adrenal Cushing's syndrome found that hyperfunctioning adenomas (n = 24) and functioning carcinomas (n = 10) accounted for 92% of cases.[23]

Adenomas had a significantly smaller mean size (3.5 vs 14.5 cm) and lower mean unenhanced CT attenuation value [11 vs 28 Hounsfield unit (HU)] than did carcinomas. The presence of necrosis, hemorrhage, and calcification favored a diagnosis of carcinoma. Six of 10 carcinoma patients had metastases at presentation. Two adenomas were seen within a myelolipoma. Two adenomas were of

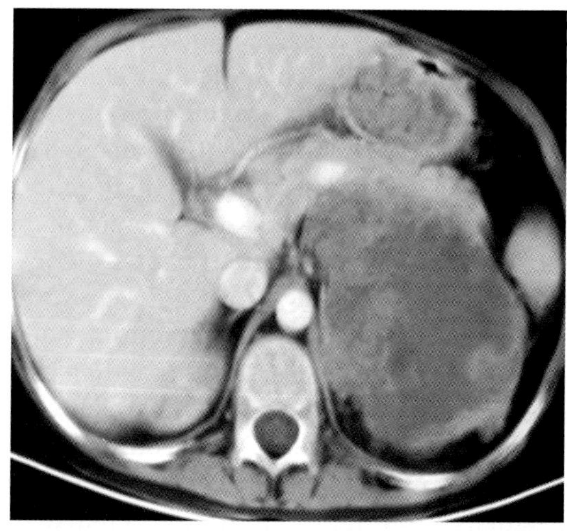

Fig. 7: Axial contrast-enhanced CT of a 12-year-old boy with Cushingoid features showing a heterogeneously enhancing mass arising from the left adrenal gland, suggesting adrenal carcinoma.

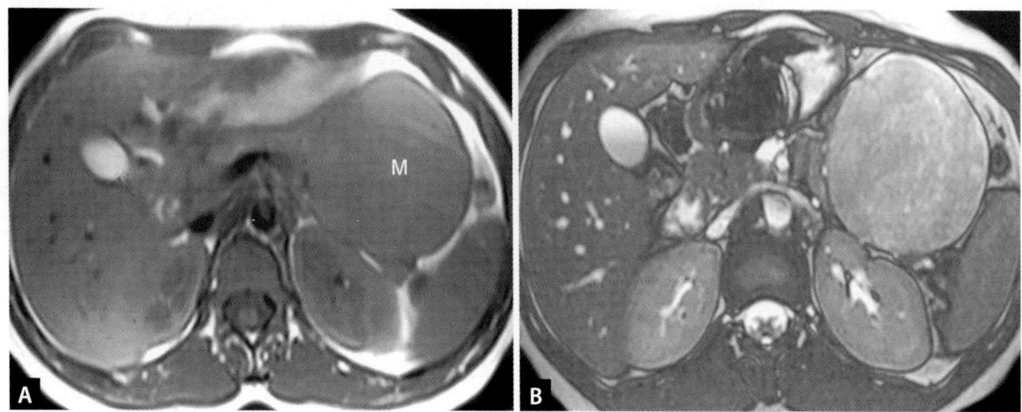

Figs. 8A and B: Axial (A) T1W and (B) T2W MR images of a 28-year-old female with clinical and biochemical features of Cushing's syndrome reveal a well-encapsulated mass (M), hypointense on T1W and heterogeneously hyperintense on T2W, arising from the left adrenal gland. On biopsy, it was a carcinoma.

uncertain malignant potential. Bilateral disease—primary pigmented nodular adrenal dysplasia (PPNAD) ($n = 2$) and ACTH-independent macronodular adrenal hyperplasia (AIMAH) ($n = 1$)—had characteristic imaging features. In PPNAD, multiple tiny (2–5 mm) nodules were visible bilaterally, with no overall glandular enlargement and normal intervening adrenal tissue. In AIMAH, both glands were grossly enlarged and contained nodules up to 3 cm in diameter.

Aldosteronism

Aldosteronism (Conn's syndrome) is associated with excess of mineralocorticoids and characterized clinically by hypertension, muscle weakness, polyuria, polydipsia, and persistent hypokalemia. It is caused by adrenal adenoma in about 80% of patients while adrenal gland hyperplasia in the rest. Adrenal carcinoma is a very rare cause of Conn's syndrome. In patients with unilateral adenoma, unilateral adrenalectomy is the treatment of choice. On the other hand, cases of bilateral adrenal gland hyperplasia are treated medically with pharmacological agents.[24] The imaging approach hence is to distinguish between these two entities. Adrenal venous sampling plays a key role in making this distinction. It is performed in all patients above 35 years to lateralize the lesion regardless of the findings on imaging.

Aldosterone-producing adenoma is small with a mean size of 1.6–1.8 cm and may have low attenuation due to high lipid content **(Fig. 9)**. A dedicated CT examination with thin sections is required for localizing the adenoma.

If CT examination is inconclusive, adrenal cortical scintigraphy with NP-59 may be done. On NP-59 scintigraphy, both adrenals are normally visualized on 5th day or later, following injection of radiopharmaceuticals. Bilateral adrenal visualization before 5th day suggests adrenal gland hyperplasia while unilateral adrenal visualization before 5th day indicates an adenoma. NP-59 scintigraphy has a long procedural time of nearly 2 weeks with an accuracy of 71% in contrast to adrenal venous sampling with an accuracy of 95–100%.

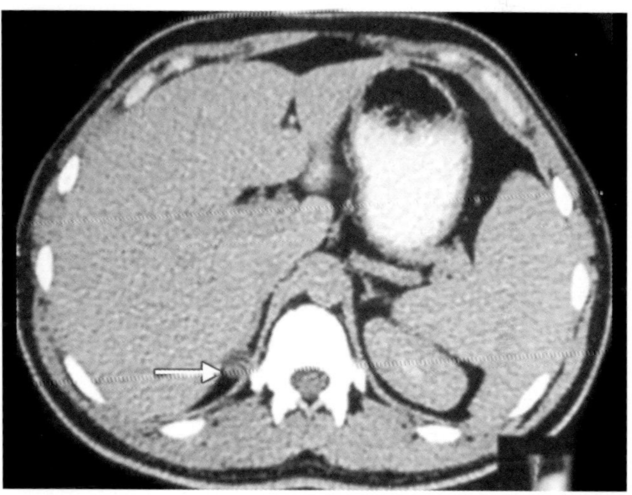

Fig. 9: Noncontrast CT of a 28-year-old male with hypertension shows a low attenuating nodule in the right adrenal (arrow) with attenuation value of 4 HU. Conn's syndrome due to adrenal adenoma.

Androgenital Syndrome

Androgenital syndrome is a consequence of excessive secretion of sex hormones. It causes virilization, feminization, or precocious puberty depending upon the age and sex of the patient. The most common form is virilization, occurring in females.

The characteristic clinical features are amenorrhea, hirsutism, clitoromegaly, and deepening of voice.

The adrenal causes of androgen excess include congenital adrenal hyperplasia (CAH) in children and virilizing tumors (adenoma or carcinoma) in adults. CAH occurs due to deficiency of enzymes involved in the synthesis of steroid hormones. Each different enzyme deficiency results in a different form of CAH. The clinical manifestations are determined by the degree of deficiency of cortisol or aldosterone and by the biological properties of the biochemical intermediates that are formed and secreted in excess.

Androgen-producing tumors are rare and include adenoma or carcinoma and occur in both males and females at a later age. In general, in adults a higher proportion of malignant tumors results in adrenogenital syndrome than benign lesions.

MRI is preferred to CT to image adrenals as well as ovaries particularly in children to detect tumors because of MRI being nonionizing. CT is, however, often the initial and only modality performed in evaluation of suspected CAH, due to the easy availability and short examination times **(Figs. 10 and 11)**.[25]

The tumors are usually more than 2.0 cm in size and show imaging characteristics described above **(Figs. 12A and B)**. Occasionally, adrenal and gonadal venous sampling may be necessary to locate the source of excessive androgens.

Pheochromocytoma

Pheochromocytomas are catecholamine-producing tumors which arise from ganglion cells anywhere in the autonomic nervous system. About 90% of pheochromocytomas originate in the adrenal medulla while 10% are extra-adrenal, the common sites being paravertebral sympathetic ganglia, organ of Zuckerkandl, urinary bladder, neck, or mediastinum. About 10% of pheochromocytomas are bilateral and 10% are malignant. About 5–10% are inherited as autosomal dominant either alone or in combination with other abnormalities such as multiple endocrine neoplasia (Type II or III), neurofibromatosis, von Hippel-Lindau's retinal, and cerebellar hemangioblastomas.

Clinical features of hypertension, paroxysmal attacks of palpitations, headache, sweating, and biochemical tests of plasma catecholamine levels and 24-hour urine vanillylmandelic acid level can provide the diagnosis. Imaging is required to locate the tumor. CT is the technique of choice to confirm adrenal mass. It is seen as soft-tissue density mass with intense contrast enhancement on CECT **(Figs. 13A to C)**. Typically on MRI, it is isointense or hypointense on T1WI and extremely hyperintense on T2WI. Although this finding is almost universally seen with pheochromocytomas, a percentage of adrenal metastases has overlapping findings.[26] In addition, a significant number of lesions may not show this typical T2 hyperintensity. Gadolinium-DTPA (diethylenetriamine penta-acetic acid) produces marked enhancement with slower washout of contrast as compared to adenoma **(Figs. 14A to D)**.

Pheochromocytomas show insignificant signal drop on out-of-phase GRE images. It may show variable necrosis but calcification in pheochromocytoma is unusual **(Figs. 15A to D)**. The initial imaging findings in benign

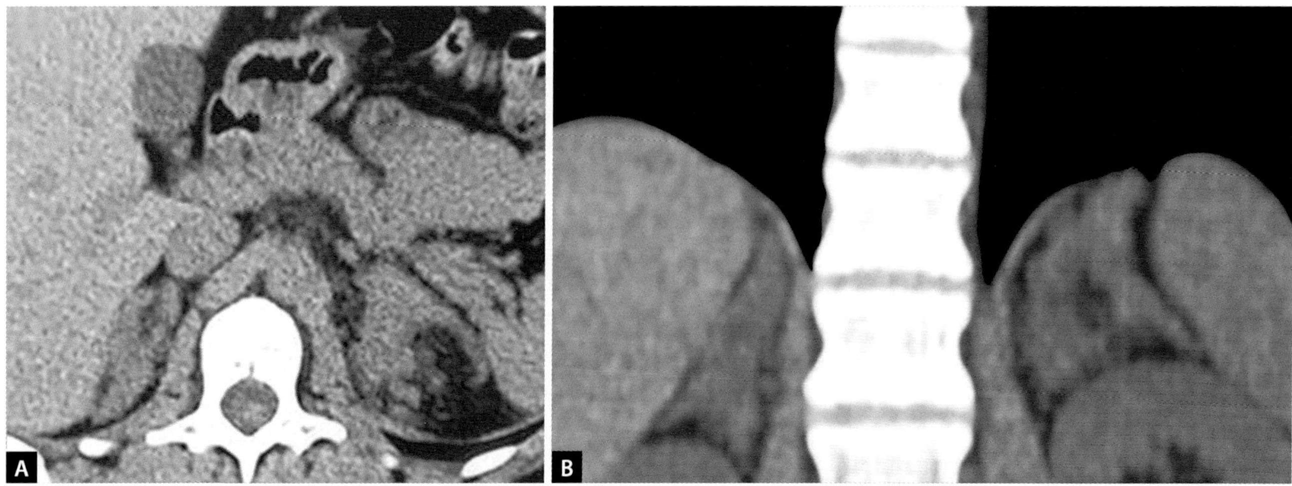

Figs. 10A and B: (A) Axial and (B) coronal noncontrast CT scans of a 13-year-old girl with features of virilization show bilateral nodular adrenal hyperplasia.

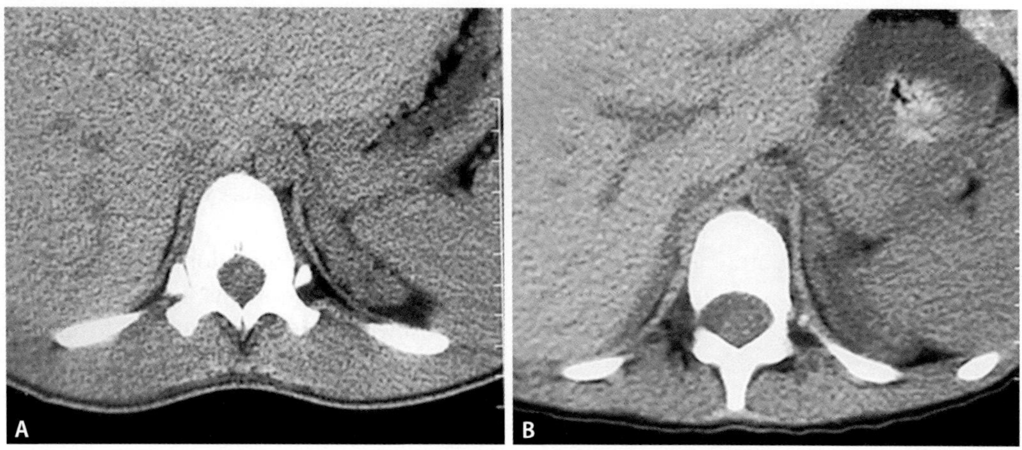

Figs. 11A and B: Axial noncontrast CT of an 11-year-old brother of the patient shown in Figure 10, presenting with precocious puberty (A), and 5-year-old sister with virilization (B) also show features of congenital adrenal hyperplasia.

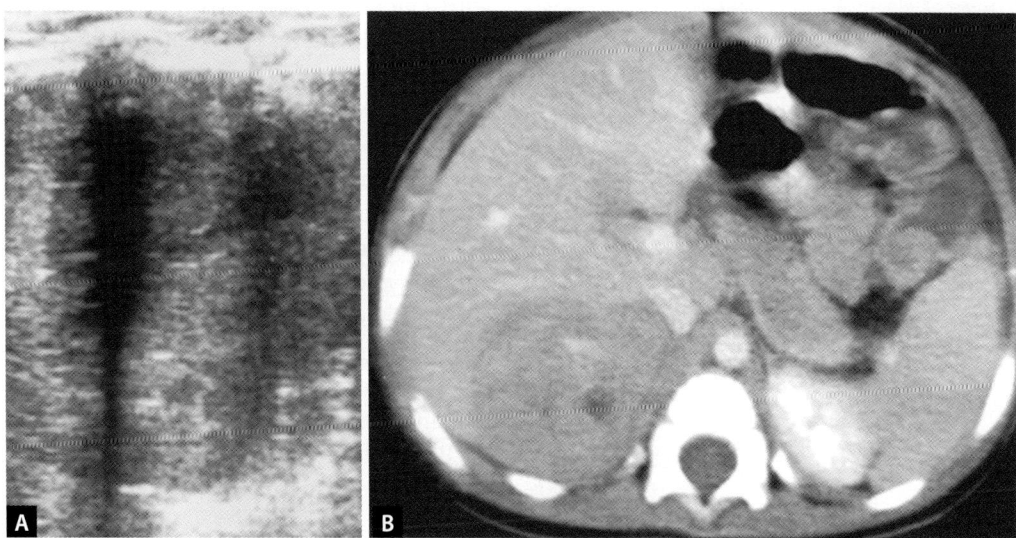

Figs. 12A and B: (A) Ultrasound and (B) axial contrast-enhanced CT of a 1.5-year-old girl child with features of virilization show a large heterogeneous mass arising from the right adrenal, suggesting a carcinoma.

and malignant pheochromocytomas are nearly identical. Only the presence of metastases can clearly define a pheochromocytoma as malignant. CT and MRI can detect adrenal pheochromocytoma equally well. However, MRI is better for detecting extra-adrenal pheochromocytoma and recurrence after surgery.

On sonography, pheochromocytoma is seen as well-defined hypoechoic mass, which may show areas of necrosis or hemorrhage. The accuracy of USG in detecting pheochromocytoma is less than CT and MRI, particularly if the tumor is small and extra-adrenal.

In patients with strongly suspected pheochromocytoma, but no adrenal mass identified on CT or MRI, MIBG scintigraphy is the technique of choice to detect ectopic location and is also indicated for metastatic or locally recurrent disease. It is seen as focal area of abnormal activity. The sensitivity of MIBG scintigraphy for detecting pheochromocytoma is 80–90% with a specificity of 90–100%, but a positive MIBG scintigraphy should always be correlated with CT or MRI.

Group II: Adrenal Insufficiency

Adrenal hypofunction refers to disorders of the adrenal cortex. It is classified as primary or secondary. The primary form is due to destruction of the adrenal cortex while the secondary form results from pituitary causes. Usually 85–90% of the adrenal cortex must be destroyed before the clinical syndrome manifests. Primary adrenal

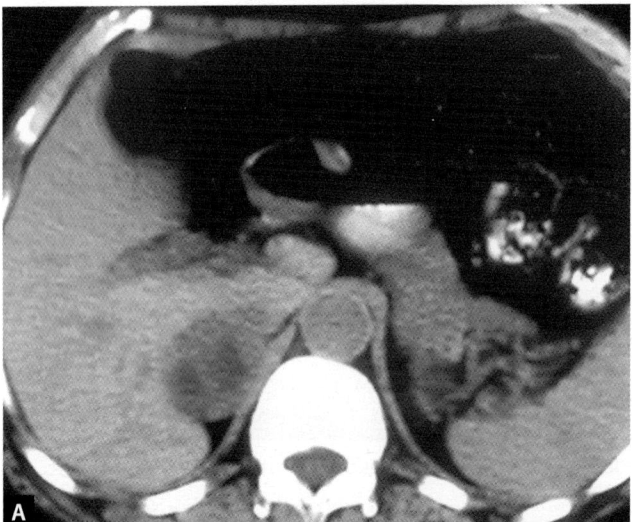

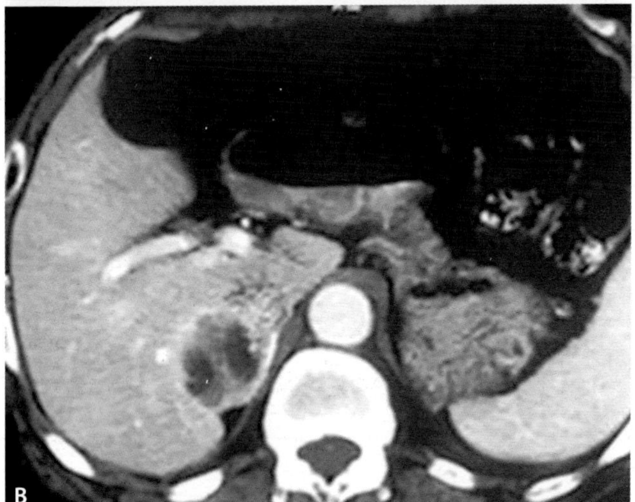

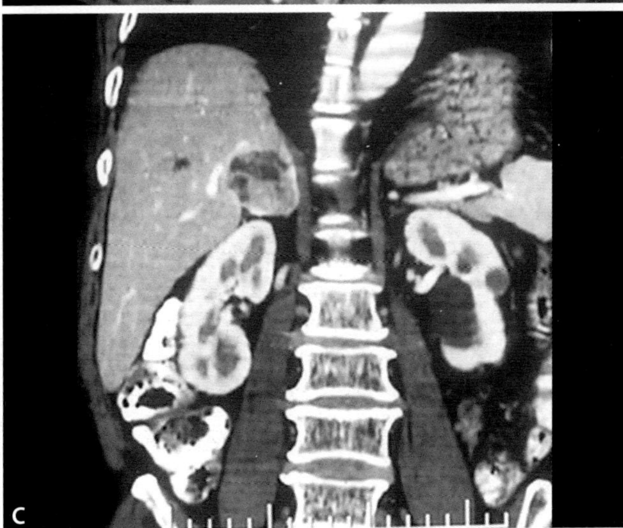

Figs. 13A to C: (A) Noncontrast CT scan of a young hypertensive male showing a mass in the right adrenal; (B) Axial and (C) coronal contrast-enhanced CT reveal intense enhancement with central areas of necrosis suggestive of pheochromocytoma.

insufficiency or Addison's disease presents with weakness, hypotension, weight loss with or without pigmentation.

The causes of Addison's disease include idiopathic atrophy, chronic granulomatous infections, e.g. tuberculosis, histoplasmosis, blastomycosis, and adrenal hemorrhage. Other causes include autoimmune diseases and drugs.

Of the chronic infections, tuberculosis accounts for more than 60% of patients in India. This is in contrast to the west where idiopathic adrenal insufficiency accounts for almost 90% of the patients. CT is an important imaging modality to define size and morphology.[27] In patients with idiopathic atrophy, the glands are often too small to be identified **(Fig. 16)**. The CT morphology in tuberculosis includes bilateral asymmetrical adrenal enlargement with or without calcification or necrosis, small gland with calcification involving one or both adrenals, or small gland with no calcification **(Figs. 17 to 19)**. There may be evidence of associated pulmonary tuberculosis. Follow-up studies in these patients on treatment have shown reduction in size of the adrenals and presence of calcification **(Figs. 17A and B)**.

In histoplasmosis, adrenals may show bilateral asymmetrical enlargement but often normal configuration and usually no calcification **(*see* Figs. 14A to D)**. Histoplasmosis in India is not as rare as reported in the Indian literature. Because of lack of awareness and investigative facilities, many of these patients are probably treated for tuberculosis.

Bilateral adrenal hemorrhage is usually associated with anticoagulant therapy or with stress caused by surgery, sepsis, or hypotension.

Less commonly, it is caused by trauma or hypoxia during delivery. CT may show asymmetrical adrenal enlargement with areas of high attenuation or blood-fluid level **(Fig. 20)**. Neonates, especially preterm infants, may also show bilateral adrenal hemorrhage **(Fig. 21)**. Follow-up studies after appropriate treatment show diminution in size and decrease in attenuation, thereby suggesting resorption **(Figs. 22A and B)**.

In the older child and adult, unilateral adrenal hemorrhage is usually caused by blunt abdominal trauma and often involves the right adrenal gland. Unilateral adrenal hemorrhage has also been recently reported in patients undergoing liver transplantation. The excision of a segment of the recipient's IVC necessitates ligation and division of the right adrenal vein. This may result in venous infarction and hemorrhage in the right adrenal gland. CT features are similar to those seen in bilateral hemorrhage.

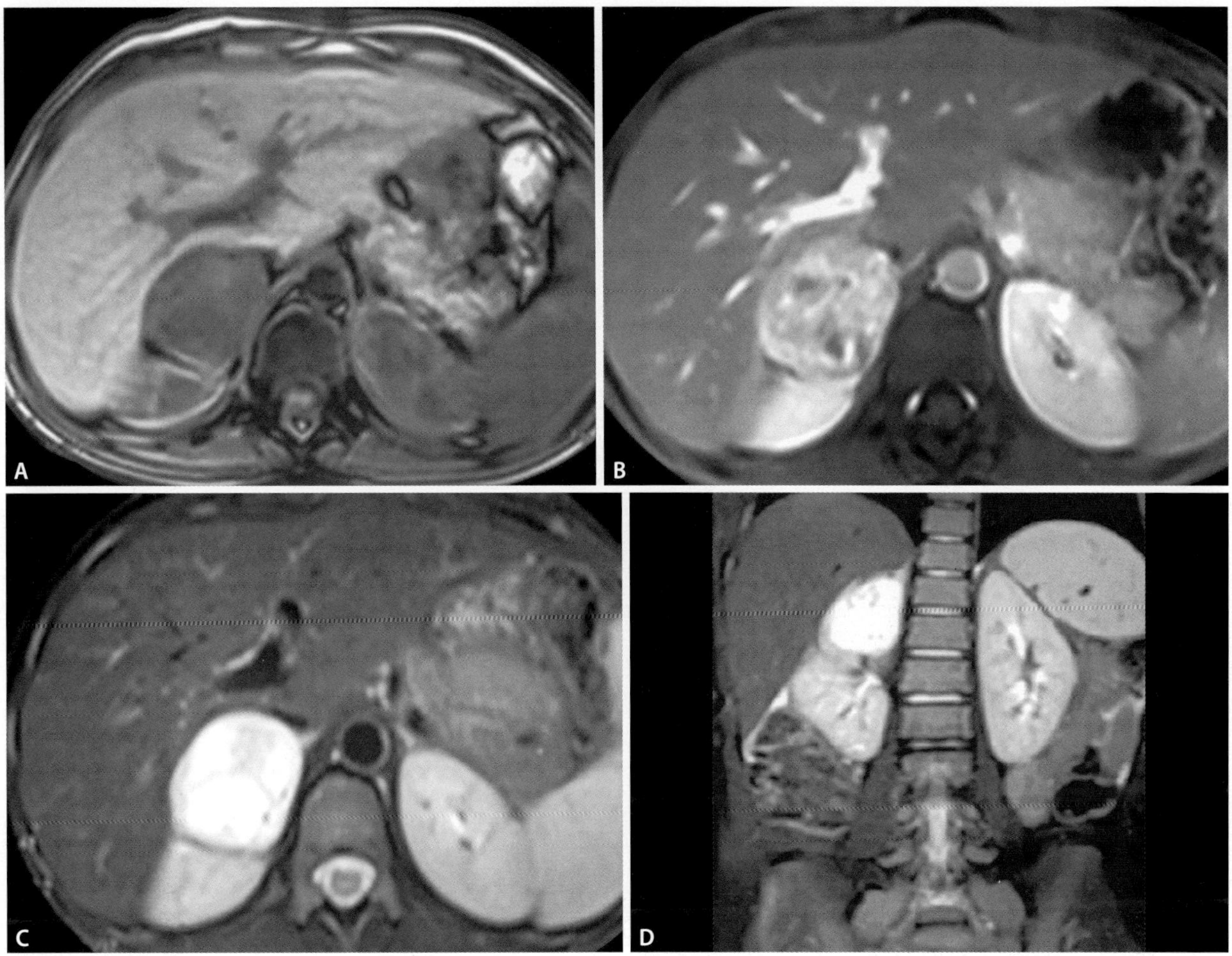

Figs. 14A to D: T1-weighted (A) pregadolinium and (B) postgadolinium axial images of a 15-year-old male with hypertension reveal an intensely enhancing right adrenal mass; T2-weighted (C) axial and (D) coronal images reveal the typical hyperintensity of a pheochromocytoma.

Group III: Adrenal Diseases with Normal Function

A number of diseases may involve the adrenals, which do not alter the adrenal function. Most of these disease entities are detected incidentally as adrenal mass or patients may present with vague abdominal pain or discomfort. These include nonfunctional adenoma or carcinoma, metastasis, lymphoma, neuroblastoma, adrenal cyst, and myelolipoma. In some of these entities, a specific diagnosis can be made from the characteristic features on CT, e.g. adrenal cyst, myelolipoma. In some, CT may show nonspecific features but correlation with clinical features may suggest the possible etiology, e.g. neuroblastoma, metastasis.

Incidentaloma

These are adrenal nodules or masses discovered during imaging done for indications other than adrenal disease **(Figs. 23 to 26)**. They are seen in 4–7% of the imaged population, and majority of them are benign in the nononcology population.[1,28] On the other hand, almost 50% of incidentally detected adrenal lesions in patients with known malignancy represent metastatic disease.[5] Characterization of such incidental masses remains an important clinical problem when a unilateral nonfunctional adrenal mass is present; the differential diagnosis rests between adenoma and carcinoma or metastasis. In a patient with known malignancy, it is very essential to differentiate such incidental adrenal mass as adenoma or metastasis because this will greatly affect the patient's management and prognosis.

Adenoma versus Metastasis

Adenomas are thought to represent non-neoplastic overgrowth of adrenocortical cells of zona fasciculata. They consist of cholesterol-laden clear cells and contribute

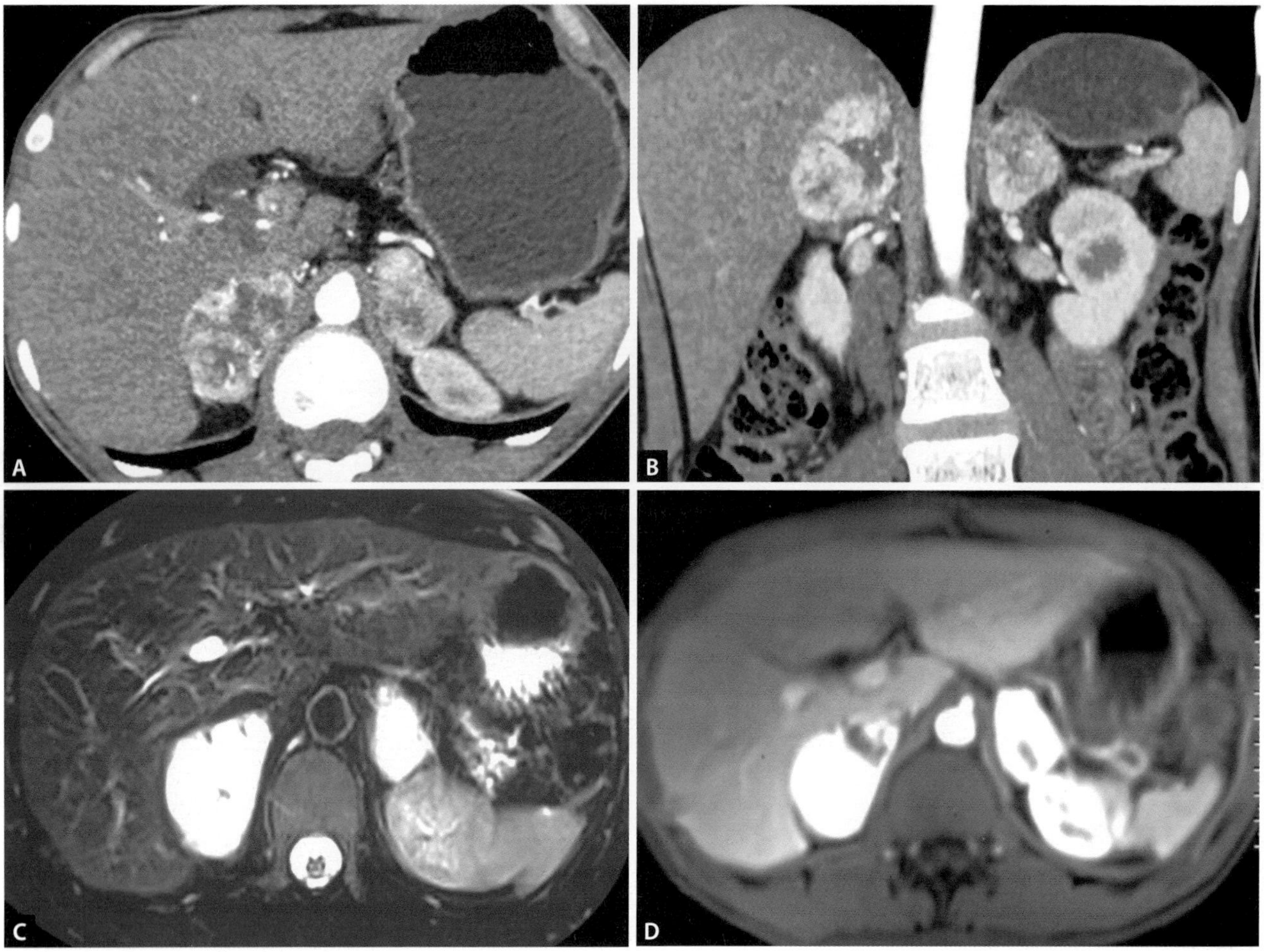

Figs. 15A to D: Bilateral pheochromocytoma. (A and B) Bilateral adrenal masses showing intense enhancement and variable necrosis on contrast-enhanced CT; (C and D) Bilateral hyperintense adrenal lesions on T2W image with intense postcontrast enhancement.

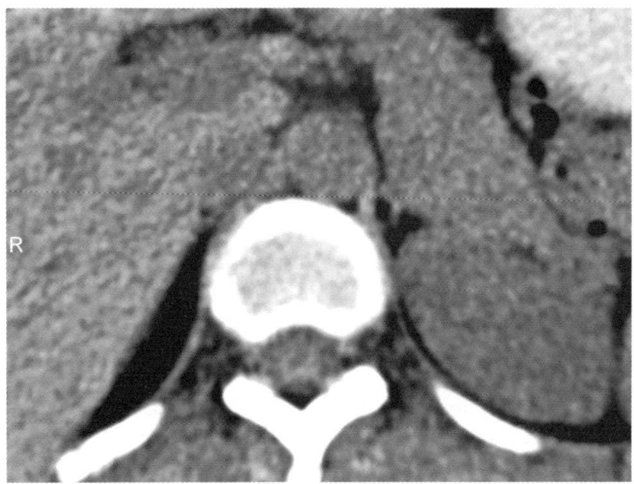

Fig. 16: Noncontrast CT scan of patient with Addison's disease showing bilateral atrophic adrenal glands.

little to steroid production. The imaging features of functional and nonfunctional adenomas on CT or MRI are similar **(Figs. 23 to 26)** except that the functional tumors are usually smaller at the time of presentation than the nonfunctional ones. They account for almost 90% of all incidentalomas.[5]

Tumors of the lung, kidney, breast, digestive tract, ovary, and melanoma are the most common primary sites to metastasize to adrenals. Metastases are well-defined with heterogeneous density and a thin, irregular enhancing rim following intravenous contrast injection, commonly unilateral and usually larger than adenoma **(Figs. 27A to D)**. On MRI, they are hypointense on T1WI and hyperintense on T2WI, relative to liver intensity.

It has been reported that 27% of patients with known malignancy have microscopic adrenal metastasis.

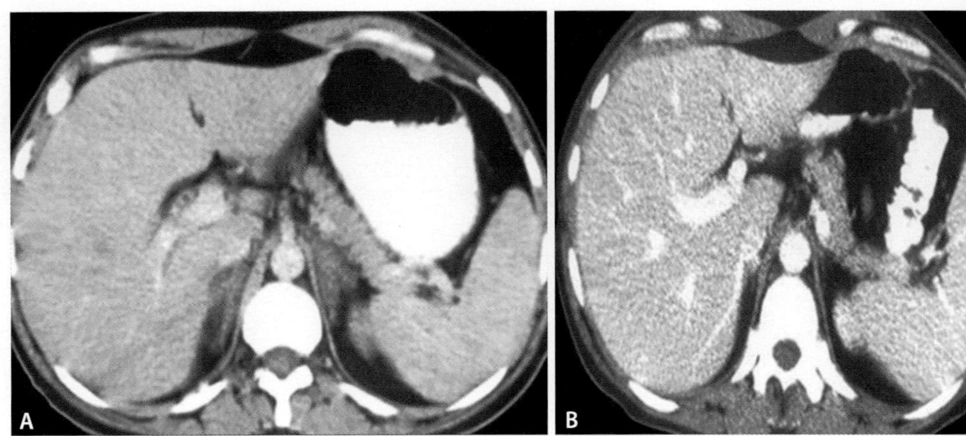

Figs. 17A and B: (A) Contrast-enhanced CT scan of a patient with fever and biochemical evidence of adrenal insufficiency shows bilateral asymmetric (left > right) enlargement of the adrenal glands. Few ill-defined focal areas are seen in the liver and spleen, also suggesting disseminated tuberculosis. Patient was put on anti-tubercular treatment; (B) Contrast-enhanced CT scan obtained 1 year later reveals small, atrophic adrenal glands.

However, the detection of an adrenal mass in a patient with known malignancy does not necessarily indicate metastatic disease and it may be a nonfunctional adenoma.

CT features of adenoma include size less than 5.0 cm and well-defined margins with smooth contour **(Figs. 23 and 24)**.

Adrenal metastasis may show large mass with heterogeneous density and irregular shape **(Figs. 27A to D)**. However, these features are not specific. It has also been reported that the size alone is a poor discriminator between benign adenoma and malignant mass.

In recent years, several studies have reported two imaging criteria based on the attenuation value and differences in the vascular enhancement pattern to differentiate benign adenoma from adrenal metastasis.[5,28]

Adenomas have abundant intracytoplasmic fat and therefore show low attenuation on NCCT **(Figs. 23A and B)**. On the other hand, metastases have little intracytoplasmic fat and thus do not show low attenuation. A large region of interest covering the adrenal mass should be used but should not include periadrenal fat for measuring the attenuation value. It has been reported that a threshold of 10 HU has 71% sensitivity and 98% specificity for characterizing adenoma versus metastasis.[29] This specificity may be increased further if other features of size, shape, and morphology are considered. Although 70% of adenomas have abundant lipid, the remaining are lipid poor and are difficult to characterize on a noncontrast scan.

If attenuation of the adrenal mass on noncontrast CT is 10 HU or less **(Figs. 9 and 23)**, the diagnosis is lipid-rich adenoma and no further evaluation is required. If attenuation is more than 10 HU, the mass is indeterminate and requires further evaluation by portal venous phase and 15-minute delayed enhanced CT scan **(Figs. 24A to C)**.[30]

Adenomas enhance rapidly with intravenous contrast media and show rapid washout. Metastasis also enhances rapidly but the washout is delayed when compared to adenoma.[26,28] It has been speculated that this difference in enhancement washout in nonadenoma is possibly due to disturbed capillary permeability, with prolonged retention of contrast in the extracellular space.

Adrenal masses with an attenuation value less than 30–40 HU on 15-minute delayed CECT are almost always adrenal adenomas.[4,31] In addition to the delayed CT attenuation itself, it is also possible to calculate the percentage washout of initial enhancement. The patient is first scanned without contrast, then again at 70 seconds, and then 15 minutes after contrast administration. Contrast washout can be quantified using relative percentage washout (RPW) and absolute percentage washout (APW) as follows:

$$\text{RPW} = 100 \times (\text{Enhanced HU} - \text{Delayed HU}) / \text{Enhanced HU}$$

$$\text{APW} = 100 \times (\text{Enhanced HU} - \text{Delayed HU}) / \text{Enhanced HU} - \text{Nonenhanced HU}$$

If the APW is greater than 60% and the RPW is greater than 40%, the lesion is labeled benign.[28,30,31] This technique has a sensitivity of 88% and a specificity of 96% for the diagnosis of adenoma.[4,28] On the other hand, metastases and adrenocortical carcinoma have relative contrast retention on delayed CECT.

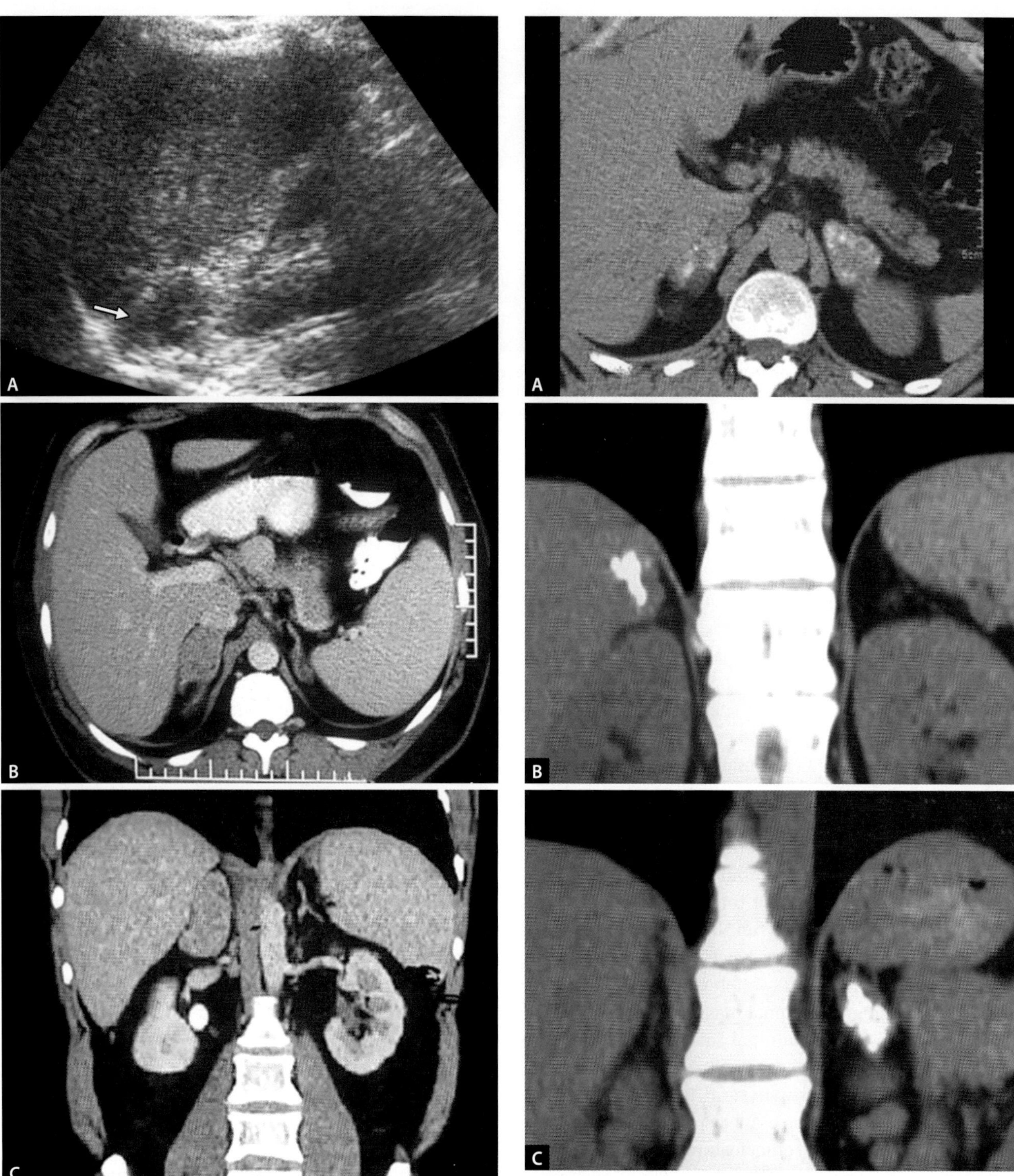

Figs. 18A to C: (A) Ultrasound, (B) axial contrast-enhanced CT, and (C) coronal multiplanar reconstruction images reveal an enlarged, heterogeneous right adrenal gland. Biopsy: Tuberculosis.

Figs. 19A to C: (A) Axial contrast-enhanced CT and (B and C) coronal multiplanar reconstructed images of two different patients with Addison's disease reveal bilateral, calcified adrenal glands, suggesting granulomatous involvement.

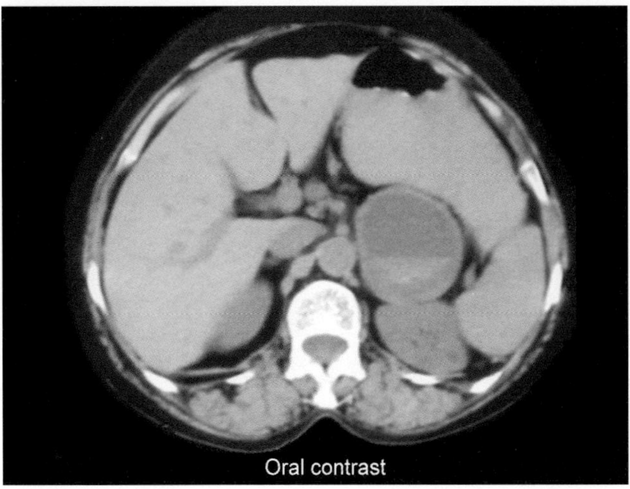

Fig. 20: Axial CT scan showing a low attenuating left adrenal mass with blood-fluid level, suggestive of adrenal hemorrhage.

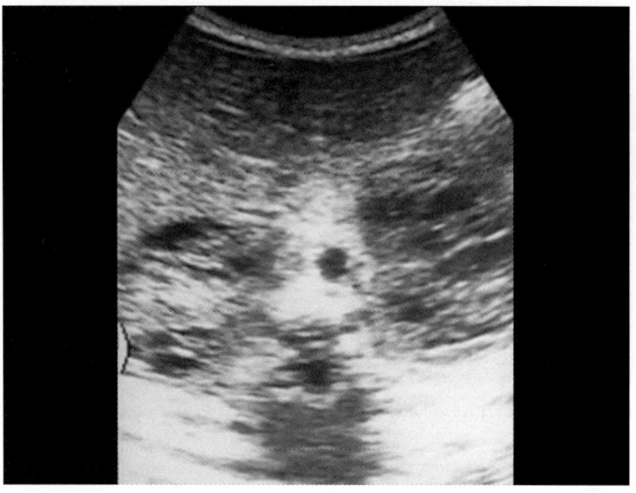

Fig. 21: Ultrasound of a preterm neonate showing bilateral enlarged adrenal glands, suggesting adrenal hemorrhage.

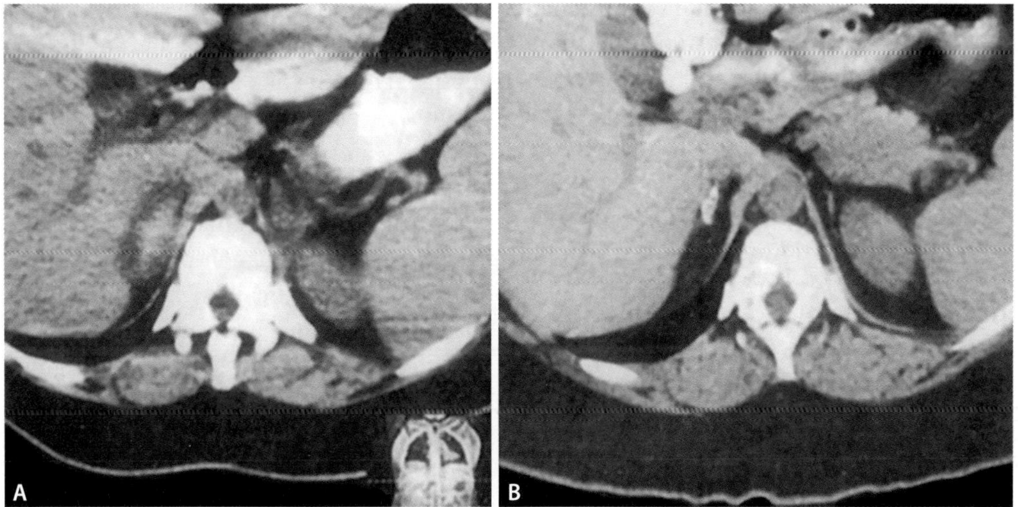

Figs. 22A and B: Adrenal hemorrhage. (A) CT scan shows asymmetrically enlarged adrenals with heterogeneous attenuation but no calcification; (B) Follow-up CT scan after 5 years shows small right adrenal with dense calcification and atrophic left adrenal.

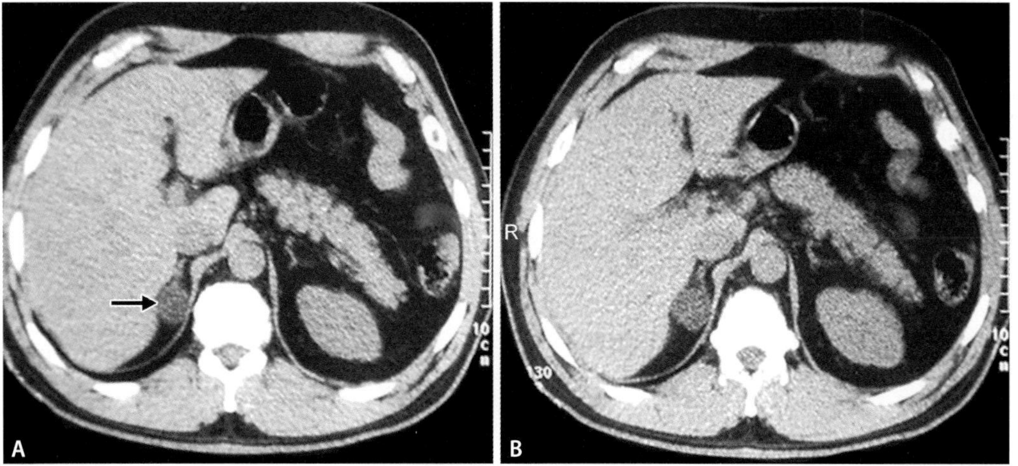

Figs. 23A and B: Adrenal adenoma. Noncontrast CT scan shows a low attenuating well-defined mass in the right adrenal (arrow). The attenuation value was 6 HU.

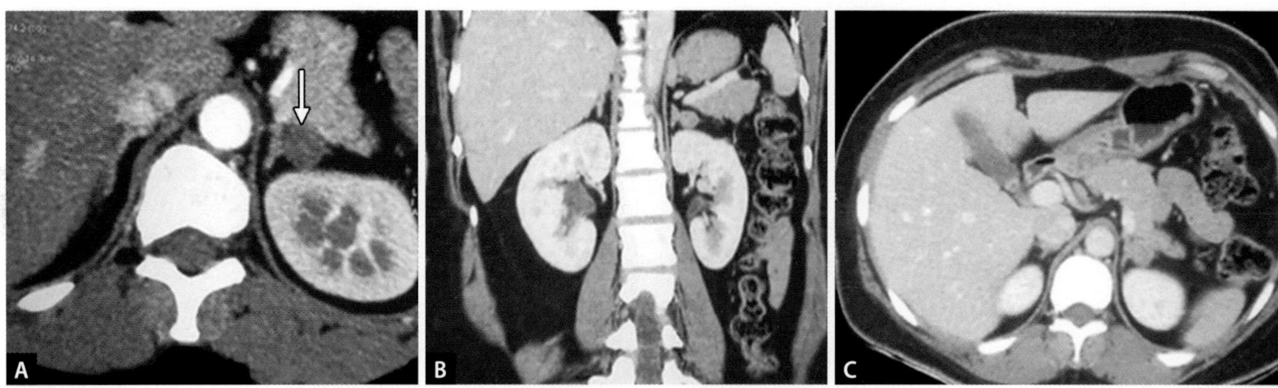

Figs. 24A to C: Adrenal adenoma. (A) Contrast-enhanced CT, (B) coronal multiplanar reconstruction, and (C) 15-minute delayed CT images show a mass in the left adrenal gland (arrow) which showed 65% washout on the delayed scan.

Dual-energy CT: The difference in CT attenuation images acquired at 140 kVp and 80 kVp is measured, and if the difference between the two kVp is more than 6 HU, it is suggestive of fat-containing lesion.[5] The cutoff values on NCCT and adrenal protocol scans are based on conventional 120 kVp scans. The values derived from VNC CT from a dual-energy scanner may not be equal to values derived from conventional scans. It has been found that the values can vary from 5 HU to 9 HU, which can be a significant confounder when the cutoff is applied.[6] However, the VNC values are usually higher than the true NCCT values which make the sensitivity lower but maintains the specificity. Hence, the traditional NCCT cutoff value of <10 HU is still valid on VNC as well irrespective of the dual-energy acquisition method (single or dual source).[8-10] It has also been found that the portal venous scan is the best phase to derive VNC for this purpose.

Magnetic resonance imaging: In recent years, MRI has become a problem-solving modality for the characterization of indeterminate adrenal masses. When results on CT examination are equivocal, MRI is the next imaging modality for characterizing the lesion. Due to increased fluid content in adrenal cancer and metastases, these appear bright on T2-weighted MRI images. However, there is significant overlap between T1W and T2W MRI images of adenoma and metastases. With the introduction of higher field strength magnets (3T), chemical shift imaging and dynamic gadolinium-enhanced MR imaging have shown promising results with adrenal gland lesions' characterization. Confident diagnosis of adenomas on MRI requires the addition of chemical shift imaging to the protocol.

Chemical shift MRI has been used to differentiate adenoma from metastasis. This technique is based on the different resonance frequency rates of protons in fat and water molecules in a magnetic field. The signal intensity (SI) on the in-phase image is derived from the signal of water plus fat protons while in the out-of-phase image; MR signal of water and lipid protons cancel each other out within a voxel. Therefore, a mass containing intracellular lipid and water will show loss of signal in the out-of-phase images when compared with the in-phase image **(Figs. 25A to C)**. Thus, adenoma appears darker on an out-of-phase image than on an in-phase image, while metastasis will show no significant signal loss on an out-of-phase image and the signal intensity remains unchanged.[16,17]

The sensitivity and specificity ranging from 81% to 100% and 94% to 100%, respectively, on chemical shift MR imaging for differentiating adenoma from metastasis have been reported.[17,28] The loss of signal can be assessed visually using spleen as the internal control **(Figs. 26A and B)**. The liver should not be used as the internal reference as it may also show signal loss on opposed-phase image when there is steatosis.

The chemical shift change can also be detected by quantitative methods. Two ratios have been defined in chemical shift imaging (CSI).

$$\text{SI index} = \frac{1 - [\text{SI(in)} - \text{SI(opp)}]}{\text{SI(in)}}\text{; and}$$

Adrenal-to-spleen ratio

$$= \frac{\text{SI adrenal (opp)}}{\text{SI spleen (opp)}} \Big/ \frac{\text{SI adrenal (in)}}{\text{SI spleen (in)}}$$

An SI index of >16.5% and an adrenal-to-spleen ratio of <0.71 are suggestive of adenoma or benign adrenal lesions. For a benign adrenal lesion characterization, the reported sensitivity and specificity using these two ratios

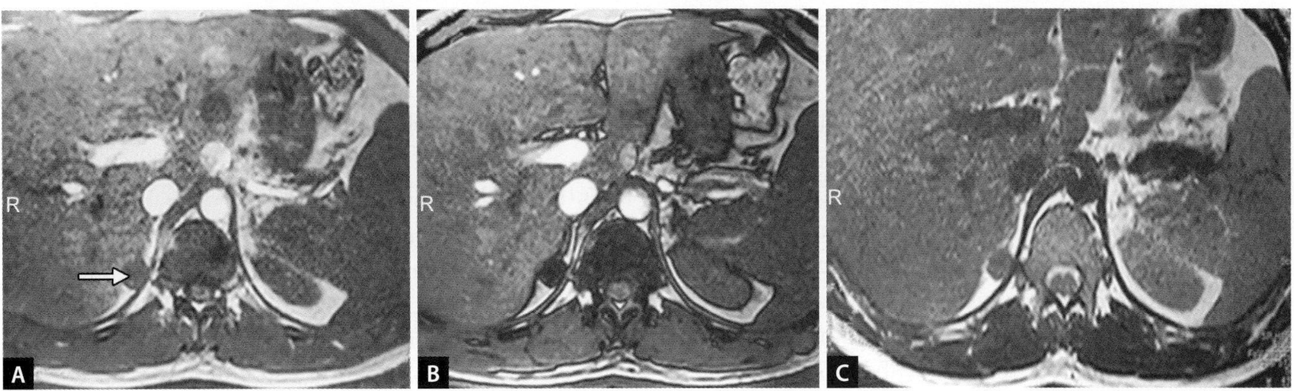

Figs. 25A to C: Incidentally detected adrenal adenoma. Gradient-echo T1W in-phase image (A) shows a hypointense nodule in right adrenal gland (arrow) which shows marked signal loss on the opposed-phase image (B). The lesion is hypointense on T2W scan (C) also.

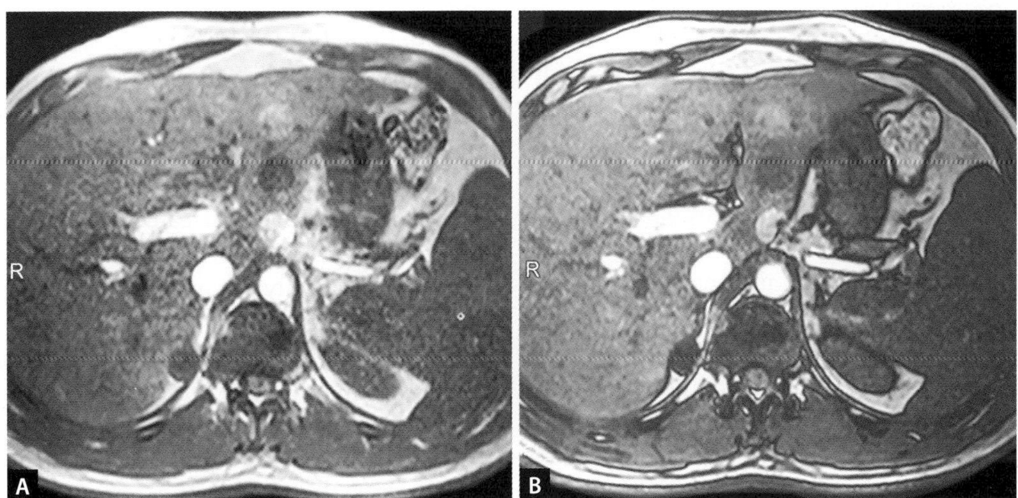

Figs. 26A and B: Adrenal adenoma. Gradient-echo T1W in-phase (A) and opposed-phase (B) images showing drop in the signal intensity of right adrenal lesion from 124 to 45 whereas spleen signal intensity changes from 83 to 80 only.

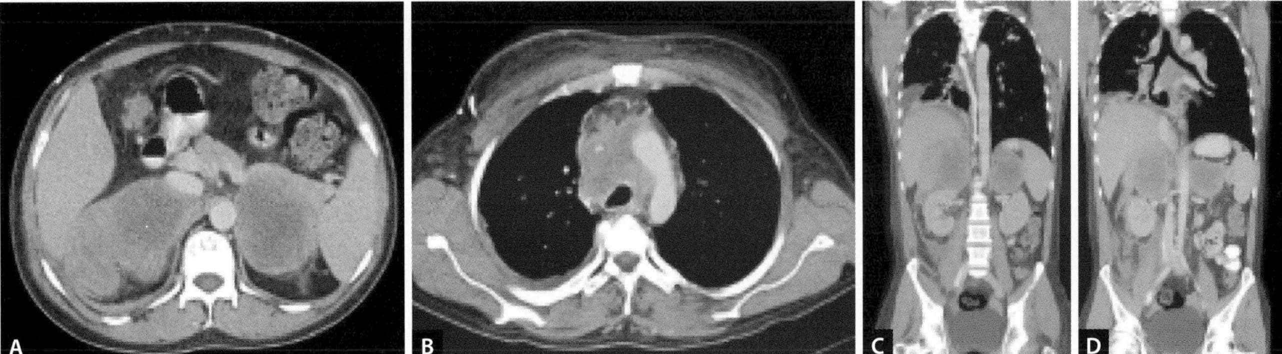

Figs. 27A to D: Adrenal metastases. (A and B) CECTs abdomen show bilateral solid adrenal masses; (C and D) CECT chest and coronal multiplanar reconstructed images show mediastinal adenopathy in a patient of bronchogenic carcinoma.

were 87–100% and 92–100%, respectively, whereas the failure rate for diagnosis of lipid-poor adenomas has been 13–17%.[28]

Positron emission tomography: Due to the limitations of CT and MR imaging, functional imaging modalities such as ^{18}F-FDG PET are now increasingly used for further characterization of an adrenal lesion. ^{18}F-FDG PET is an imaging modality that permits acquisition of functional information and when fused with CT imaging, it results in accurate localization and metabolic characterization of adrenal lesions. In PET-CT, ^{18}F is used as a glucose analog, which is taken up preferentially by malignant cells because of their increased glucose metabolism. Due to relative lack of glucose-6-phosphatase in the cancer cells as compared to cells of normal tissues, there is a focal intracellular accumulation of FDG, resulting in high tumor uptake values as compared to the background uptake values. The results of all these studies are encouraging and justify the use of PET for metastatic disease evaluation in cancer patients. Although PET results are encouraging, several inherent problems are associated with FDG-PET imaging, viz. small adrenal lesions are difficult to image owing to poor resolution, and uptake in other abdominal structures, such as renal pelvis, can obscure the adrenal gland.

^{18}F-FDG uptake is taken as abnormal when it is higher than background liver uptake.[21,32,33] If a lesion shows ^{18}F-FDG uptake less than that of the liver, or shows uptake that is significantly higher than the liver, the study can be interpreted with high confidence unless the patient has pheochromocytoma, which can be excluded by biochemical markers.[21]

In the evaluation of adrenal masses with ^{18}F-FDG PET/CT, combined information from the ^{18}F-FDG PET and unenhanced CT portions of a PET or CT study is more specific than ^{18}F-FDG PET information alone.[34] A standardized uptake value (SUV) cutoff of 3.1 has been used to differentiate malignant lesions and adenomas. PET data using a SUV cutoff of 3.1 to differentiate malignant adrenal masses from adenomas yielded a sensitivity, specificity, positive predictive value, and negative predictive value of 98.5%, 92%, 89.3%, and 98.9%, respectively.[34]

The current role of FDG PET is in the evaluation of adrenal lesions in a patient with known history of malignancy which is either enlarging or more than 4 cm in size.[6]

Adrenal Carcinoma

Adrenal carcinomas are rare neoplasms and are more common in women. They are usually larger than 10 cm at the time of presentation and are invasive. Unlike children where adrenal carcinomas are usually functional, only 10% of adult types are clinically functional which usually manifest as Cushing's syndrome or virilization in females. CT or MRI shows large solid masses with areas of degeneration and cystic changes, hemorrhage, and 33% contain calcification **(Figs. 28 and 29)**.[5,28] They tend to be locally invasive, especially into adrenal or renal veins and inferior vena cava. They are hypointense on T1-weighted and hyperintense on T2-weighted scans **(Figs. 28D to F)** and show variable enhancement. Differential diagnosis includes adenoma, metastases, lymphoma, exophytic liver tumors, or upper polar renal masses.

Adrenal Lymphoma

Primary lymphoma of the adrenal gland is unusual, but its involvement in disseminated lymphoma is common. The latter is more often seen in non-Hodgkin's lymphoma.[35] The most common presentation is diffuse bilateral enlargement of the gland, and the shape is usually maintained **(Figs. 30A to D)**. The tumor is hypovascular and shows only mild enhancement after contrast.

Adrenal Collision Tumor

This is a very rare entity characterized by the coexistence of two contiguous but histologically different tumors. Both tumors may be malignant or one may be benign and the other malignant or both may be benign. Imaging may show two distinct morphological features within the same mass. This entity should be suspected when only a focal decrease in the signal intensity of a mass is seen on opposed-phase images or a focus of bright enhancement is seen within a mass which otherwise looks like an adenoma. Such an appearance may suggest a metastatic deposit within an adrenal adenoma.[36]

Adrenal Cyst

Adrenal cysts are rare and usually seen in females. They are derived from endothelium in 45% of patients and the rest are epithelial, parasitic, or pseudocysts from prior hemorrhage. CT shows a characteristically well-defined, round, low-attenuating lesion suggesting fluid with rim enhancement **(Fig. 31A)**. Rim calcification may be noted **(Fig. 31B)**. The attenuation values may be mixed in the presence of debris or hemorrhage. On MR, adrenal cysts are hypointense on T1W and hyperintense on T2W image. The complications of adrenal cysts include hemorrhage, infection, and rupture.[28,37]

Myelolipoma

Myelolipoma is a benign tumor of the cortex, comprised of mature fat and hematopoietic elements. Patients are usually asymptomatic and the lesion is detected incidentally. It accounts for about 7–15% of all incidentalomas. The imaging appearance may vary depending on which the histological component is dominant. USG and CT features are quite characteristic and diagnostic.

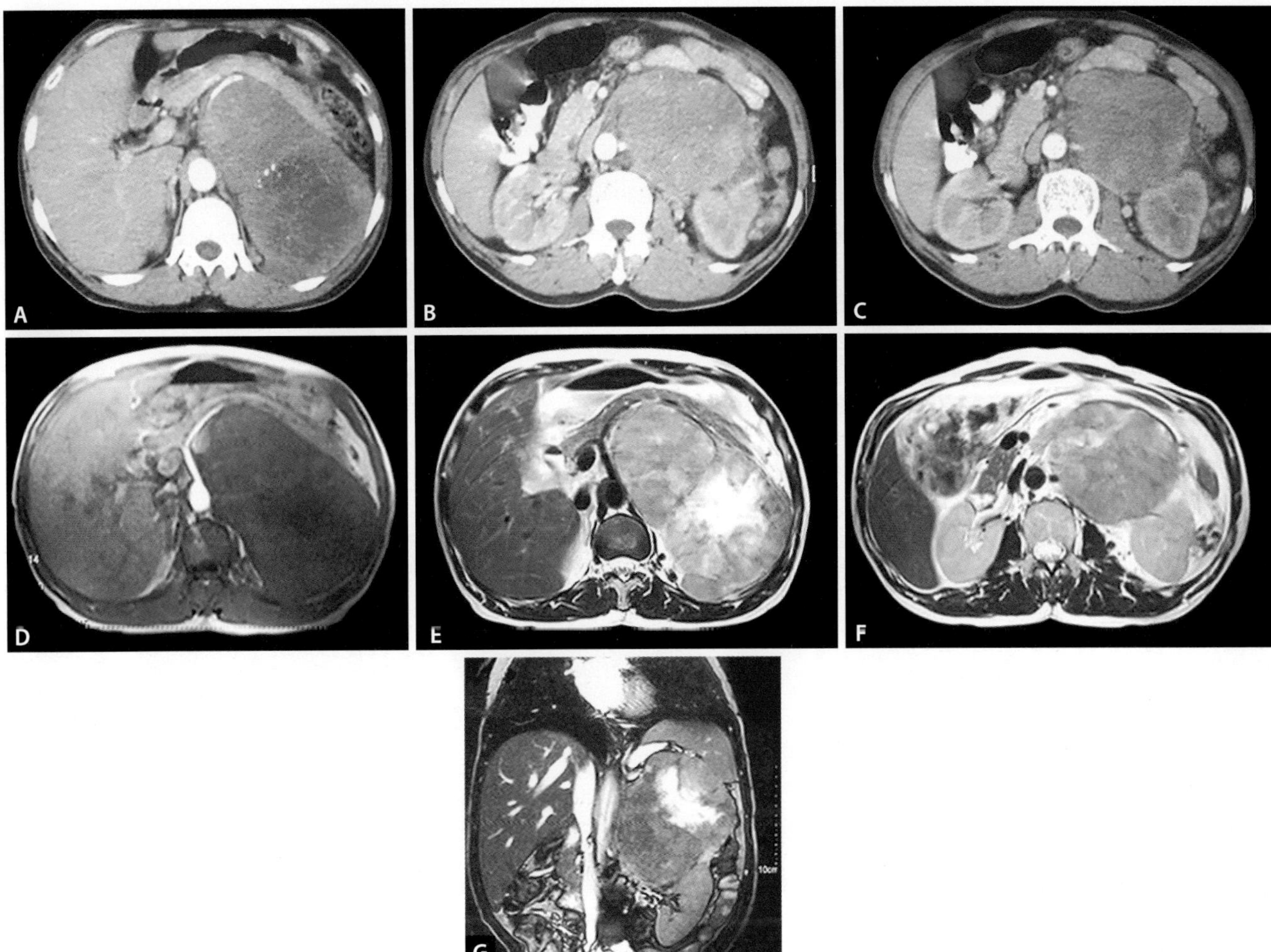

Figs. 28A to G: Adrenal carcinoma. Axial contrast-enhanced CT scans (A to C) show a large left adrenal mass with foci of calcification and areas of necrosis, encasing the left renal artery and displacing the left kidney laterally; (D) Axial T1W gradient-echo image shows a hypointense left-sided mass which is displacing the splenic artery anteriorly. The lesion is heterogeneously hyperintense on T2W scans (E and F); (G) True-FISP coronal image shows the left suprarenal mass displacing the left kidney inferolaterally.

Ultrasonography shows well-defined echogenic or heterogeneous adrenal mass, which may be associated with apparent posterior displacement of the diaphragm due to propagation speed artifact resulting from slow speed of sound through the fat. CT confirms the presence of intratumoral fat **(Figs. 32A and B)**. Punctate calcification may be seen in 20% of cases. MRI can also characterize the lesion by identification of fat which appears hyperintense on both T1W and T2W images and shows loss of signal on fat suppression techniques **(Figs. 33A to D)**. Marrow elements show low signal on T1W and moderate signal on T2W images. Differential diagnosis includes adrenal adenoma and adrenal carcinoma, and large myelolipomas may mimic retroperitoneal lipoma or liposarcoma.

Neuroblastoma

Neuroblastoma is one of the most common tumors of childhood with 80% occurring below the age of 5 years. Most neuroblastomas arise from adrenal medulla but may also arise from sympathetic chain, posterior mediastinum being the second-most common site. About 75% occur in the abdomen, and two-thirds of these are in the adrenal gland. Symptoms are related to the primary tumor and metastases, which are present in more than 50% of patients at the time of diagnosis. Children can present with a palpable mass, bone pain, and opsomyoclonus. The common sites of metastases are lymph nodes, cortical bone, marrow, skin, and liver.

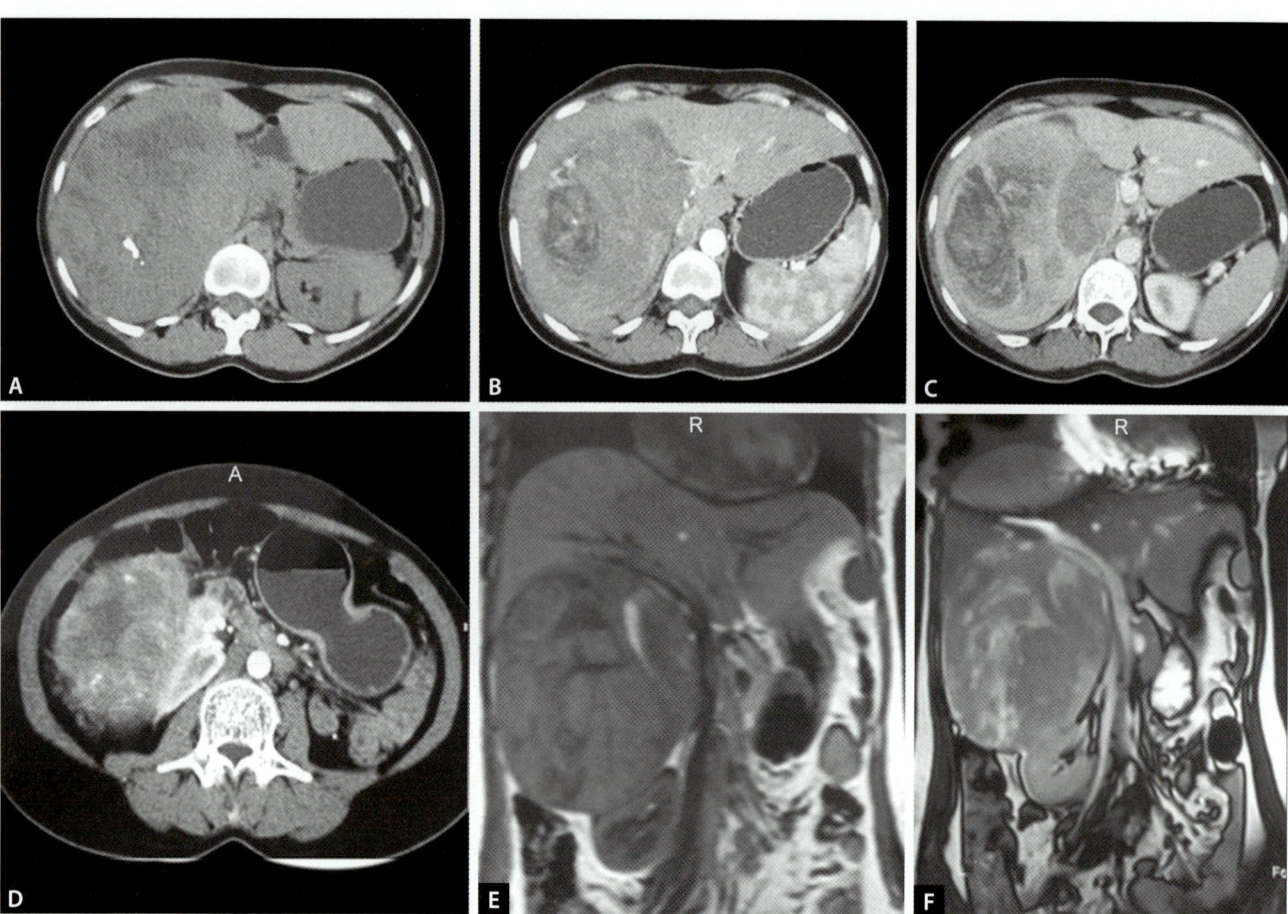

Figs. 29A to F: Adrenal carcinoma. Axial noncontrast CT scan (A) and contrast-enhanced CT scan (B to D) show a large right adrenal mass with foci of calcification. It mimics an exophytic liver mass. Gradient-echo T1W (E) and True FISP coronal (F) MR images of the same patient show the right adrenal mass displacing the kidney inferomedially.

Ultrasonography almost always shows a mass, which must be distinguished from nephroblastoma. Neuroblastoma is seen typically as large mass with heterogeneous echogenicity with scattered hyperechoic areas due to the presence of calcification. CT shows soft tissue mass with areas of low attenuation and scattered coarse or mottled calcification, seen in almost 85% of the patients. The tumor enhances with intravenous contrast. Unlike Wilm's tumor, which usually has a well-defined pseudocapsule, neuroblastoma invades adjacent structures and encases the aorta and its branches **(Fig. 34)** early in the course of the disease.

On MRI, neuroblastoma shows low signal intensity on a T1WI and increased intensity on a T2WI, relative to liver intensity. Tumor heterogeneity is seen best on T2-weighted sequence and reflects calcification and necrosis.

MRI is better than CT for defining vascular encasement, metastasis, and intraspinal extension, which occurs in 15% of patients. Therefore, MRI is the single best imaging modality for accurately staging the extent of the disease. Neuroblastoma may also take up MIBG, which may detect bony metastasis more accurately than CT or MRI. The presence of skeletal metastasis in association with an adrenal mass in a child strongly suggests the diagnosis of neuroblastoma.

CONCLUSION

With the widespread use of cross-sectional imaging techniques, detection of an adrenal mass has increased over the years. However, clinical and appropriate biochemical tests in adrenal lesions, especially for functional diseases, remain the most vital and initial mode of evaluation, followed by CT. The role of CT has continued to expand in both detection and characterization of an adrenal mass as benign or malignant. Based on size criteria and tumor morphology, it is not always possible to suggest benignity or malignancy. Follow-up studies

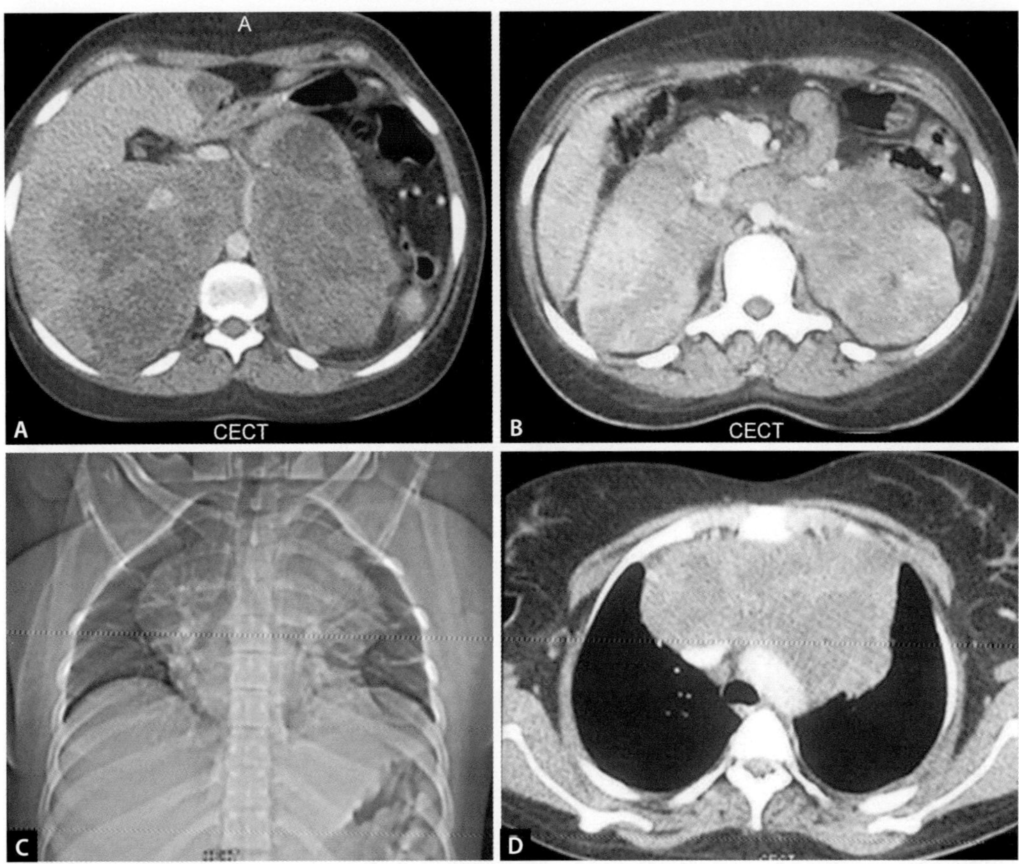

Figs. 30A to D: Adrenal involvement in non-Hodgkin's lymphoma. (A and B) Axial abdomen contrast-enhanced CT (CECT) scans show bilateral adrenal masses, retroperitoneal adenopathy, and focal renal lesions; (C) Chest radiograph and (D) CECT chest show bulky mediastinal adenopathy.

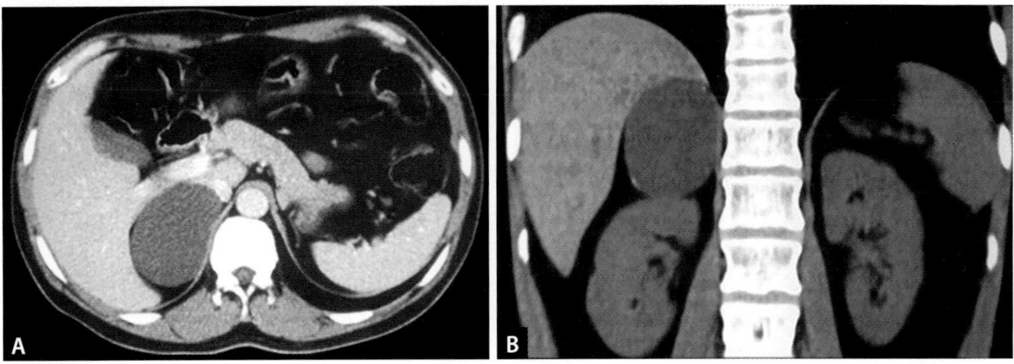

Figs. 31A and B: Adrenal cyst. (A) Axial CT and (B) coronal multiplanar reconstruction images show a fluid attenuating right adrenal mass with rim calcification.

are necessary in equivocal cases. Necrosis in the tumor is related directly to prognosis. More necrosis carries a worse prognosis. All attempts should be made to characterize an incidental adrenal mass as adenoma or metastasis in a patient with known malignancy. Lipid-rich adenoma can be characterized with attenuation value of 10 HU or less on NCCT. Lipid-poor adenoma can be differentiated from metastasis by studying the washout percentage on an adrenal protocol CT. Chemical shift MRI can be utilized as an alternative modality. If all these modalities still fail to characterize the lesion in a patient with known malignancy, having no other evidence of metastatic deposit, FDG PET or adrenal biopsy under CT guidance should be performed to establish a definitive diagnosis.

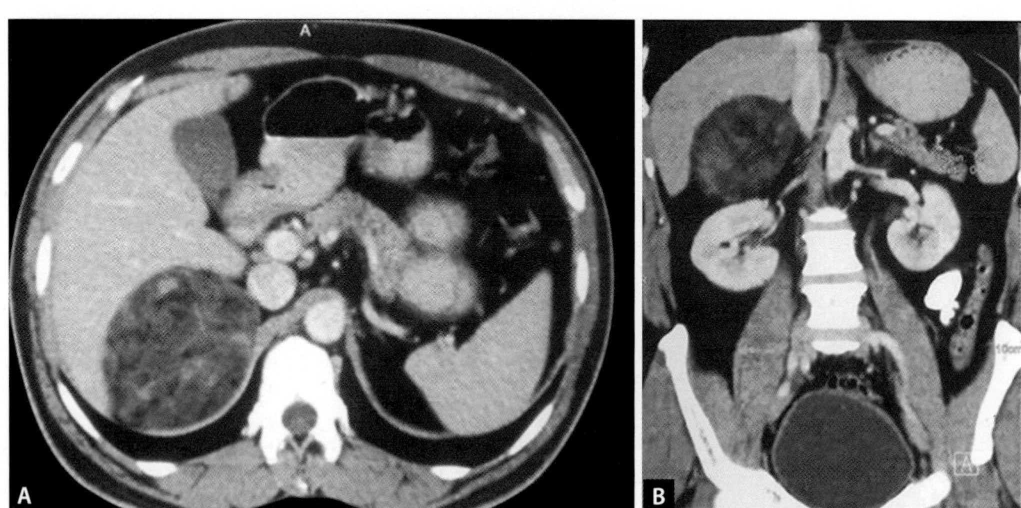

Figs. 32A and B: Adrenal myelolipoma. (A) Axial contrast-enhanced CT and (B) coronal multiplanar reconstruction images show a mixed attenuating right adrenal mass with fat and soft-tissue attenuation.

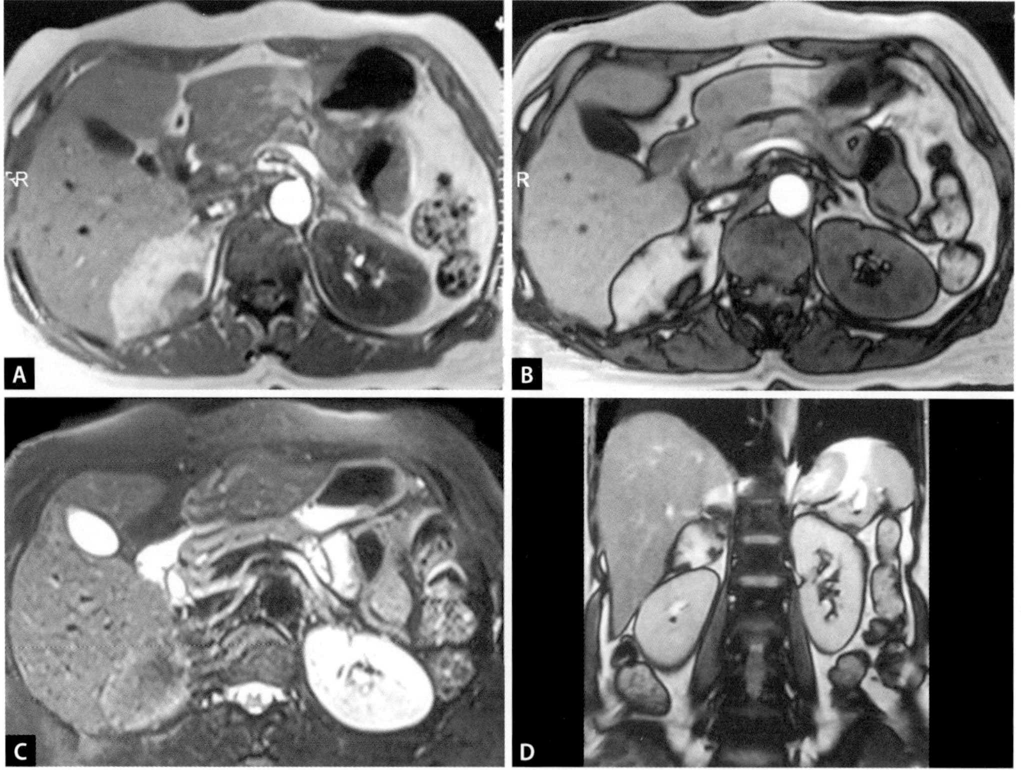

Figs. 33A to D: Adrenal myelolipoma. Gradient-echo T1W in-phase (A) and opposed-phase (B) images show a hyperintense right adrenal mass which shows no drop in signal intensity but is suppressed on T2W fat-suppressed image (C). Coronal true-FISP image (D) shows a hyperintense right adrenal mass.

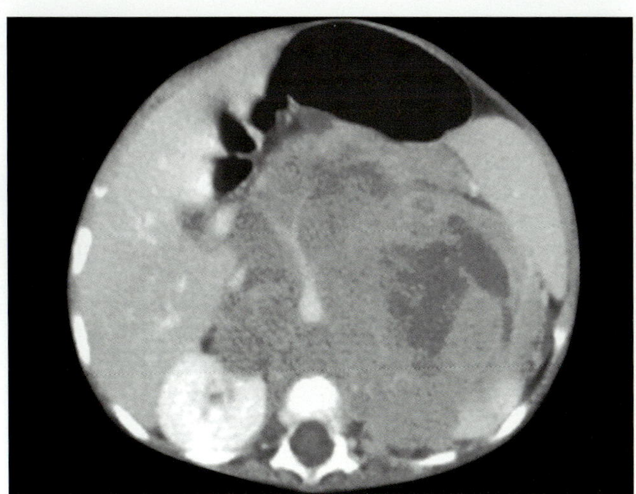

Fig. 34: Neuroblastoma. Axial contrast-enhanced CT abdomen of a 2-year-old child shows a large left adrenal mass which is extending posterior to the aorta and inferior vena cava and encasing the celiac axis.

REFERENCES

1. Young WF. The incidentally discovered adrenal mass. N Engl J Med. 2007;356(6):601-10.
2. Schieda N, Siegelman ES. Update on CT and MRI of adrenal nodules. Am J Roentgenol. 2017;208(6):1206-17.
3. Funder JW, Carey RM, Mantero F, et al. The management of primary aldosteronism: Case detection, diagnosis, and treatment: An Endocrine Society Clinical Practice Guideline. J Clin Endocrinol Metab. 2016;101(5):1889-916.
4. Korobkin M. CT characterization of adrenal masses: The time has come. Radiology. 2000;217(3):629-32.
5. Blake MA, Holalkere N-S, Boland GW. Imaging techniques for adrenal lesion characterization. Radiol Clin North Am. 2008;46(1):65-78.
6. Glazer DI, Mayo-Smith WW. Management of incidental adrenal masses: an update. Abdom Radiol (NY); 2019. https://doi.org/10.1007/s00261-019-02149-2.
7. Azoury SC, Nagarajan N, Young A, et al. Computed tomography in the management of adrenal tumors: does size still matter? J Comput Assist Tomogr. 2017;41(4):628-32.
8. Ho LM, Marin D, Neville AM, et al. Characterization of adrenal nodules with dual-energy CT: can virtual unenhanced attenuation values replace true unenhanced attenuation values? Am J Roentgenol. 2012;198(4):840-5.
9. Glazer DI, Maturen KE, Kaza RK, et al. Adrenal incidentaloma triage with single-source (fast-kilovoltage switch) dual-energy CT. Am J Roentgenol. 2014;203(2):329-35.
10. Morgan DE, Weber AC, Lockhart ME, et al. Differentiation of high lipid content from low lipid content adrenal lesions using single-source rapid kilovolt (peak)-switching dual-energy multidetector CT. J Comput Assist Tomogr. 2013;37(6):937-43.
11. Mileto A, Nelson RC, Marin D, et al. Dual-energy multidetector CT for the characterization of incidental adrenal nodules: diagnostic performance of contrast-enhanced material density analysis. Radiology. 2015;274(2):445-54.
12. Elsayes KM, Emad-Eldin S, Morani AC, et al. Practical approach to adrenal imaging. Radiol Clin North Am. 2017;55(2):279-301.
13. Sydow BD, Rosen MA, Siegelman ES. Intracellular lipid within metastatic hepatocellular carcinoma of the adrenal gland: A potential diagnostic pitfall of chemical shift imaging of the adrenal gland. Am J Roentgenol. 2006;187(5):W550-551.
14. Schieda N, Krishna S, McInnes MDF, et al. Utility of MRI to differentiate clear cell renal cell carcinoma adrenal metastases from adrenal adenomas. Am J Roentgenol. 2017;209(3):W152-9.
15. Adam SZ, Nikolaidis P, Horowitz JM, et al. Chemical shift MR imaging of the adrenal gland: principles, pitfalls, and applications. Radiogr Rev Publ Radiol Soc N Am Inc. 2016;36(2):414-32.
16. Reinig JW, Stutley JE, Leonhardt CM, et al. Differentiation of adrenal masses with MR imaging: comparison of techniques. Radiology. 1994;192(1):41-6.
17. Lee MJ, Mayo-Smith WW, Hahn PF, et al. State-of-the-art MR imaging of the adrenal gland. Radiographics. 1994;14(5):1015-29.
18. Bilbey JH, McLoughlin RF, Kurkjian PS, et al. MR imaging of adrenal masses: value of chemical-shift imaging for distinguishing adenomas from other tumors. Am J Roentgenol. 1995;164(3):637-42.
19. Mayo-Smith WW, Song JH, Boland GL, et al. Management of incidental adrenal masses: a white paper of the ACR Incidental Findings Committee. J Am Coll Radiol. 2017;14(8):1038-44.
20. Shulkin BL, Thompson NW, Shapiro B, et al. Pheochromocytomas: imaging with 2-[Fluorine-18]fluoro-2-deoxy-d-glucose PET. Radiology. 1999;212(1):35-41.
21. Yun M, Kim W, Alnafisi N, et al. 18F-FDG PET in characterizing adrenal lesions detected on CT or MRI. J Nucl Med Off Publ Soc Nucl Med. 2001;42(12):1795-9.
22. Lumachi F, Zucchetta P, Marzola MC, et al. Usefulness of CT scan, MRI and radiocholesterol scintigraphy for adrenal imaging in Cushing's syndrome. Nucl Med Commun. 2002;23(5):469-73.
23. Rockall AG, Babar SA, Sohaib SAA, et al. CT and MR imaging of the adrenal glands in ACTH-independent Cushing syndrome. Radiogr Rev Publ Radiol Soc N Am Inc. 2004;24(2):435-52.
24. Doppman JL, Gill JR, Miller DL, et al. Distinction between hyperaldosteronism due to bilateral hyperplasia and unilateral aldosteronoma: reliability of CT. Radiology. 1992;184(3):677-82.
25. Harinarayana CV, Renu G, Ammini AC, et al. Computed tomography in untreated congenital adrenal hyperplasia. Pediatr Radiol. 1991;21(2):103-5.
26. Mayo-Smith WW, Boland GW, Noto RB, et al. State-of-the-art adrenal imaging. Radiogr Rev Publ Radiol Soc N Am Inc. 2001;21(4):995-1012.
27. Ammini AC, Gupta R, Mukopadhyay C, et al. Computed tomography morphology of the adrenal glands of patients with Addison's disease. Australas Radiol. 1996;40(1):38-42.
28. Boland GWL, Blake MA, Hahn PF, et al. Incidental adrenal lesions: principles, techniques, and algorithms for imaging characterization. Radiology. 2008;249(3):756-75.

29. Boland GW, Lee MJ, Gazelle GS, et al. Characterization of adrenal masses using unenhanced CT: an analysis of the CT literature. Am J Roentgenol. 1998;171(1):201-4.
30. Caoili EM, Korobkin M, Francis IR, et al. Adrenal masses: characterization with combined unenhanced and delayed enhanced CT. Radiology. 2002;222(3):629-33.
31. Korobkin M, Brodeur FJ, Yutzy GG, et al. Differentiation of adrenal adenomas from nonadenomas using CT attenuation values. Am J Roentgenol. 1996;166(3):531-6.
32. Blake MA, Slattery JMA, Kalra MK, et al. Adrenal lesions: characterization with fused PET/CT image in patients with proved or suspected malignancy--initial experience. Radiology. 2006;238(3):970-7.
33. Shin YR, Kim KA. Imaging features of various adrenal neoplastic lesions on radiologic and nuclear medicine imaging. Am J Roentgenol. 2015;205(3):554-63.
34. Metser U, Miller E, Lerman H, et al. 18F-FDG PET/CT in the evaluation of adrenal masses. J Nucl Med Off Publ Soc Nucl Med. 2006;47(1):32-7.
35. Paling MR, Williamson BR. Adrenal involvement in non-Hodgkin lymphoma. Am J Roentgenol. 1983;141(2):303-5.
36. Schwartz LH, Macari M, Huvos AG, et al. Collision tumors of the adrenal gland: Demonstration and characterization at MR imaging. Radiology. 1996;201(3):757-60.
37. Tung GA, Pfister RC, Papanicolaou N, et al. Adrenal cysts: imaging and percutaneous aspiration. Radiology. 1989;173(1):107-10.

24

Chapter

The Retroperitoneum

Smriti Hari, Sanjay Sharma, Ekta Dhamija, Ankur Goyal

INTRODUCTION

As the name suggests, retroperitoneum (RP) is the portion of abdomen lying posterior to peritoneal cavity, located between posterior peritoneum and transversalis fascia. It extends from diaphragm superiorly to pelvis inferiorly and is divided into compartments and spaces by various fascial layers. Basic understanding of its anatomy is essential for approaching and localizing abdominal masses or collections on imaging. Computed tomography (CT) remains the workhorse of imaging of RP due to its faster acquisition and patient compliance whereas magnetic resonance imaging (MRI) serves mainly as problem solving tool. Ultrasonography (USG) on the other hand has limited role due to posterior location of the structures which get obscured by bowel gas often; however, it is the preferred modality for interventions—biopsy or fluid drainage, wherever feasible. This chapter aims to describe brief anatomy and imaging features of common retroperitoneal diseases.

ANATOMY

The RP is divided into five main compartments and three spaces by multiple fascial layers.[1,2]

- *Compartments*: There are five major compartments dividing retroperitoneal structures: (A) Lateral compartment—one on each side containing kidneys and organs; (B) Median/central or vascular compartment containing aorta, inferior vena cava (IVC), associated lymphatics, and vessels. It is located in between two perirenal spaces, anterior to the vertebra, and posterior to anterior pararenal space; and (C) Posterior compartment on both sides having psoas and iliopsoas muscles extending from T12 to lesser trochanter. It continues in pelvis bordered along transversalis fascia.
- *Spaces*: RP is divided into three spaces—the RP is divided into three spaces: An anterior pararenal space that is continuous across the midline, a perirenal space on each side, and posterior pararenal space **(Fig. 1)**.
    - The *anterior pararenal space* contains the pancreas, the second, third, and fourth segments of the duodenum, the ascending and descending colon, lymph nodes, and fat. This space is bordered anteriorly by the posterior parietal peritoneum, posteriorly by the anterior renal fascia (Gerota's fascia) and laterally by the lateroconal fascia, which is a continuation of the posterior renal fascia (Zuckerkandl fascia).[3]
    - The *perirenal space* lies between the anterior and posterior renal fascia and contains the kidney, adrenal gland, renal pelvis, proximal ureter, renal hilar vessels, lymph nodes, and fat.[4] The fascia of Gerota's blends anteriorly with the connective tissue surrounding the aorta and IVC.
    - The *posterior pararenal space* extends from the posterior renal fascia to the transversalis fascia and contains only a small amount of fat. Although it is located posterior to the kidneys, it continues anterolaterally as the properitoneal fat stripe.
- *Planes*: The renal and lateroconal fasciae are laminated, potentially expansile planes composed of apposed layers of embryonic mesentery. The *retromesenteric plane* between the leaves of the anterior pararenal fascia, the *retrorenal plane* formed by splitting

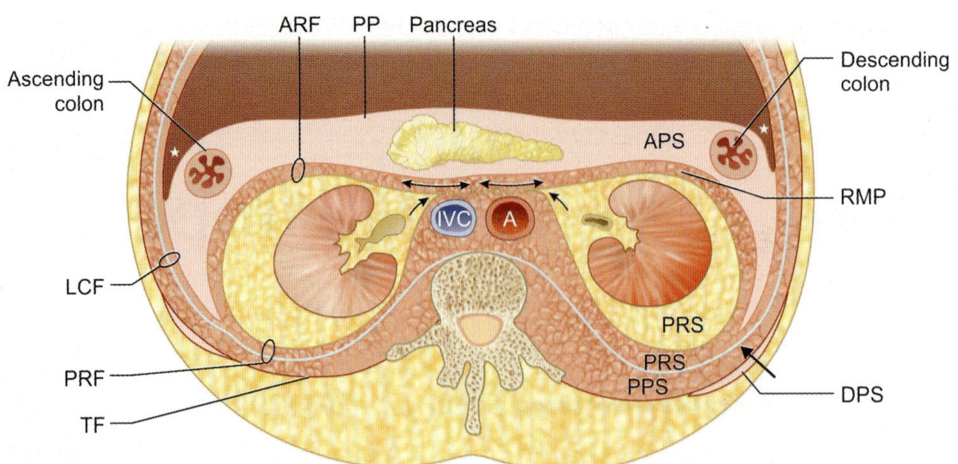

Fig. 1: Retroperitoneal and interfascial planes. Drawing at level of renal hila shows that perirenal and lateroconal fascia are laminated planes composed of apposed layers of embryonic mesentery. Note that thickness of interfascial planes is exaggerated to illustrate potentially expansile nature. Also note that perinephric spaces are closed medially (open arrows). Retromesenteric plane is continuous across midline (bidirectional arrows). Retromesenteric plane, retrorenal space, and lateroconal space communicate at fascial trifurcation (arrow). Dorsal pleural sinus may extend inferiorly to lie posterolateral to posterior pararenal space and transversalis fascia (A: aorta; APS: anterior pararenal space; ARF: anterior renal fascia; DPS: dorsal pleural sinus; IVC: inferior vena cava; LCF: lateroconal fascia; PP: parietal peritoneum; PPS: posterior pararenal space; PRF: posterior renal fascia; PRS: perinephric space; RMP: retromesenteric plane; RRS: retrorenal space; TF: transversalis fascia; *: posterior peritoneal recess).

of posterior pararenal fascia, and the *lateroconal plane* between the leaves of the lateroconal fascia.

Though most collections remain confined to the retroperitoneal compartment in which they originate; CT observations and cadaveric dissections suggest that rapidly accumulating collections can dissect and decompress through these retroperitoneal fascial planes.[5]

- *Fascia*: The anterior and posterior renal fasciae fuse inferior to the cone of renal fat, effectively sealing the caudal perinephric space, and preventing the inferior extension of perirenal fluid into the pelvis.[6] The communicating retromesenteric, retrorenal, and the lateroconal fascial planes continue downward into the true pelvis anterolateral to the psoas muscle.[7] Thus, the interfascial fluid unlike perinephric fluid can spread from the abdominal RP into the pelvis.[8] Superiorly, both layers of renal fascia blend with the diaphragmatic fascia to form the cephalic limit of the RP.

The normal anterior and posterior renal fascia measure 1–3 mm in thickness and are well-visualized on CT scan, except when abdominal fat is scanty. The posterior renal fascia is thicker and more frequently visualized than the anterior. Thickening of the retroperitoneal fascia is a sensitive but nonspecific indicator of adjacent disease, and is seen in both inflammatory **(Fig. 2)** and neoplastic disorders.

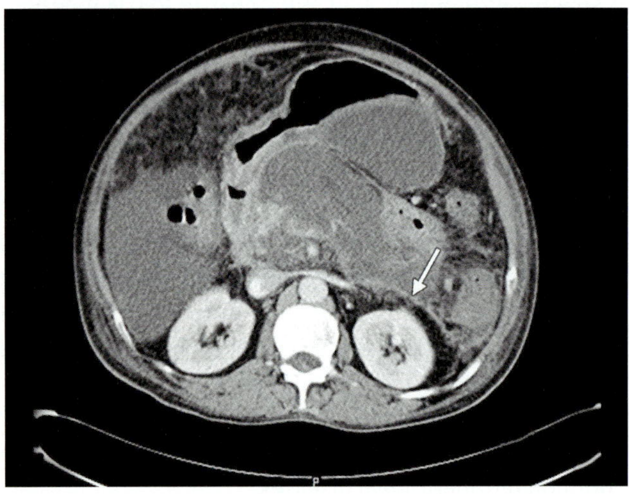

Fig. 2: Axial post contrast CT showing thickening of the left anterior renal fascia (arrow) in a patient of acute pancreatitis.

IMAGING MODALITIES

Multidetector CT is currently the preferred imaging modality for evaluating the RP. It accurately displays its anatomical limits and clearly defines individual spaces separated by various fascial layers. Isotropic multiplanar reconstructions (MPRs) of thin overlapping slices in the coronal and sagittal plane provide excellent delineation of the location and extent of retroperitoneal masses. It is a useful modality for making initial diagnosis of various pathological conditions and for follow-up. The

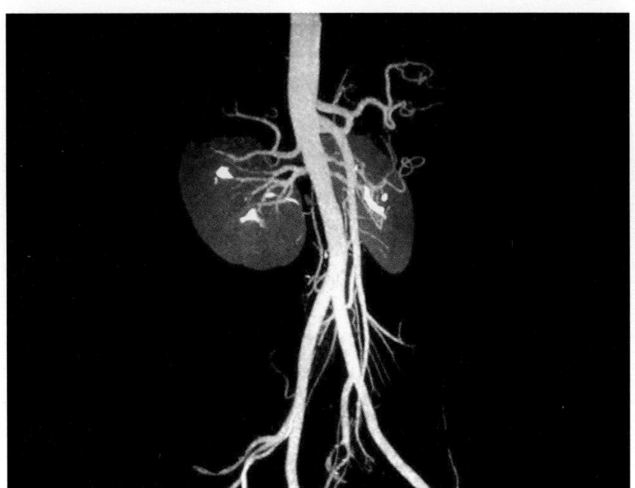

Fig. 3: Normal MDCT angiogram of the abdominal aorta. Maximum intensity projection (MIP) image shows good delineation of the entire abdominal aorta and its branches.The aorta has smooth walls and tapers gradually to the level of the aortic bifurcation.

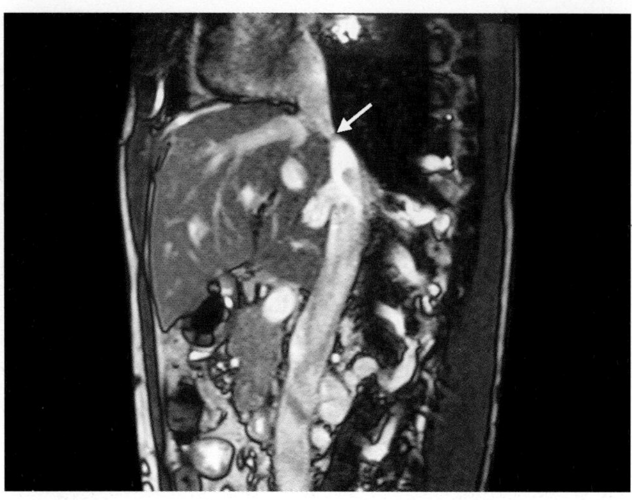

Fig. 4: Membranous obstruction of the intrahepatic IVC. Sagittal balanced steady-state (true FISP) MR image shows segmental occlusion of the IVC just below the cavoatrial junction.

introduction of multidetector technology has substantially improved the quality and ease of performing CT angiography. The simultaneous acquisition of multiple thin collimated slices in combination with enhanced gantry rotation speed offers thin slice coverage of extended volumes without any loss in spatial resolution. Multidetector computed tomography angiography (MDCTA) is increasingly being used for assessing diseases affecting the vasculature of the abdominal organs, for treatment planning, and post-therapy follow-up.[9] CT scanners with 16 or more detectors enable full abdominal coverage from the diaphragm to the groin with high spatial resolution. These scanners permit excellent evaluation of the whole arterial visceral vasculature (e.g. hepatic vessels, mesenteric vessels, and renal arteries) and the aortic-iliac axis in a single data acquisition **(Fig. 3)**.

MRI may provide additional information about retroperitoneal abnormalities because of its multiplanar capability and excellent soft tissue resolution. The MRI protocol should be devised to maximize the signal intensity differences between pathologies and the background tissues. Typical sequences used are precontrast T1-weighted spoiled gradient echo (SGE), fat-suppressed T2-weighted and postgadolinium fat-suppressed T1-weighted SGE images. In the investigation of retroperitoneal hemorrhage, precontrast fat-suppressed T1-weighted SGE sequence should be obtained because it has the greatest sensitivity for subacute hemorrhage. Both T1-weighted and T2-weighted sequences are important for delineation and characterization of retroperitoneal masses, abscesses, and fibrosis. Image acquisition in two orthogonal planes permits direct evaluation of the extent of retroperitoneal disease. Applications include evaluation of patients with suspected IVC thrombosis or Budd–Chiari syndrome **(Fig. 4)**, intravascular extension of renal, adrenal, or hepatic tumors, and evaluation of anatomic anomalies of the IVC and systemic veins.[10]

Magnetic resonance angiography (MRA) has an important role to play in the imaging of aorta and IVC. Three-dimensional (3D) gadolinium-enhanced MRA can visualize the entire aorta with a single acquisition, allowing accurate determination of the extent of aneurysm, dissection, and other abnormalities. Vascular contrast is excellent and data can be viewed in any projection, which facilitates surgical planning.[11] Typically 0.1–0.2 mmol/kg body weight of gadolinium is injected intravenously as a bolus with an automatic injector at a rate of 2–4 mL/sec, followed by 20 cc of saline to clear lines and veins. For aortic imaging, the time interval between initiating contrast injection and initiating the imaging sequence can be determined using a test bolus technique. 1–2 mL of contrast is injected as a test bolus and the aorta is scanned approximately once per second. The travel time can be directly observed and then used to calculate the correct scan delay. Alternatively, automated triggering may be employed in which the aorta is continuously scanned until the contrast material bolus is directly observed or the signal intensity reaches a specified level, at which time the 3D sequence is acquired. The dataset obtained can be postprocessed either by MPRs or by 3D maximum intensity projection (MIP) **(Fig. 5)**.

It is important to remember that arterial-phase MIP images demonstrate contrast material within the patent lumen and therefore may not accurately depict the true diameter of an aneurysm. The walls of vessels can usually be identified on source images or axial reformatted images. In addition, axial T1-weighted spoiled gradient-echo or spin-echo MR sequences following angiography are very useful in determining the diameter of the aneurysm and the extent of intra-arterial plaque or thrombus.

Likewise, it is important to scrutinize source images or thin-section reformatted images in patients who may have a dissection; an intimal flap can easily be missed if only MIP images are viewed.

Positron emission tomography (PET) scanning has shown very high sensitivity and specificity for detection of retroperitoneal diseases. PET with 2-(fluorine-18) fluoro-2-deoxy-D-glucose (FDG) allows detection of small malignant nodes not identified or not meeting size criteria for malignancy with CT **(Figs. 6A and B)** and tumor recurrences in surgical beds that are otherwise difficult to assess because of altered anatomy, surgical clip artifacts, and scar issue.[12] However, evaluation of retroperitoneal malignancies or adenopathy with FDG-PET can be complicated by urinary and colonic activity or anatomic variants. Urinary artifacts are avoided with intravenous (IV) hydration, administration of furosemide, and catheterization and retrograde filling of the bladder with saline solution. Colonic artifacts are avoided by cleansing the bowel with an iso-osmotic solution. FDG-PET is useful in assessing the RP for adenopathy in malignancies such as testicular cancer; lymphoma and rectal, ovarian or cervical cancer that spread along retroperitoneal lymphatics.

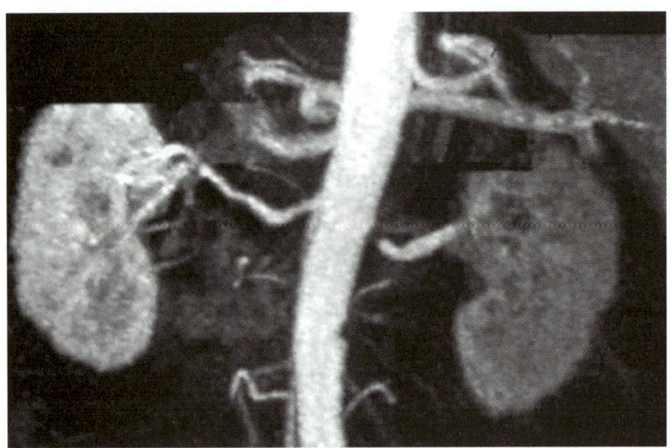

Fig. 5: Maximum intensity projection of 3D, gadolinium-enhanced MR angiogram depicting left renal artery stenosis.

Ultrasonography has role in image-guided intervention and bedside evaluation as detailed assessment of RP structures and extent of disease is limited with USG. It has advantage of portability, ease of availability, and no risk of radiation exposure.

PATHOLOGIES

Retroperitoneal pathologies may broadly be classified as neoplastic or non-neoplastic conditions. Primary retroperitoneal neoplasms are rare tumors that originate in the retroperitoneal space but outside the major organs within that compartment. These can be categorized based on their origin either from mesenchymal cells, neurogenic cells, germ cell/spermatic cord or stromal, and lymphoid

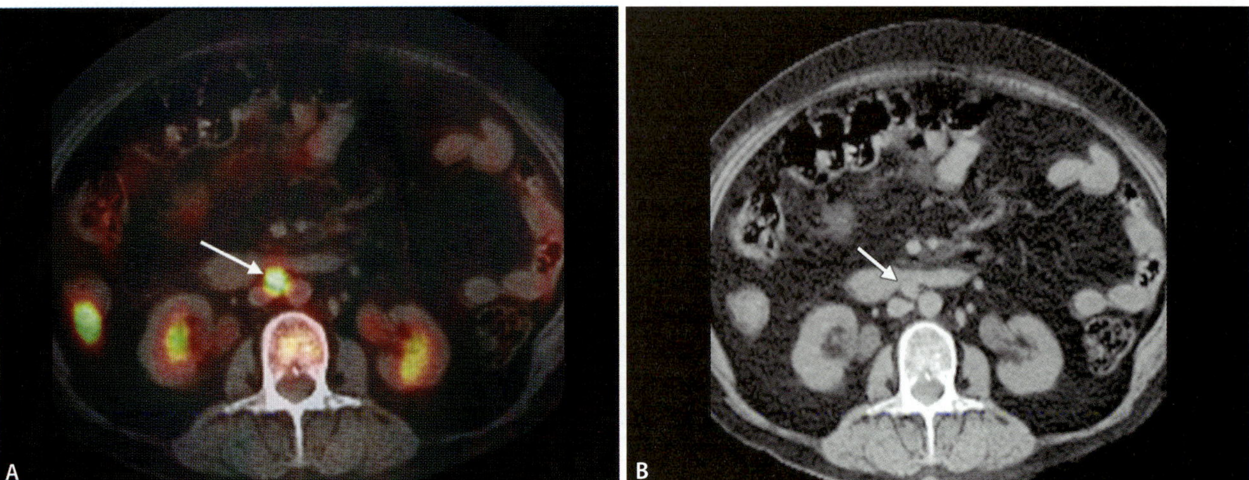

Figs. 6A and B: (A) FDG-PET image in a patient of carcinoma ovary shows increased uptake in a subcentimetric aortocaval lymph node (arrow); (B) Comparison CT image also shows the node (arrow), which was considered insignificant by the size criteria.

tissue **(Box 1)**. These can be benign or malignant. Imaging features are often overlapping and diagnosis is challenging. Imaging interpretation begins from ascertaining the location of tumor-confirming its origin from RP; followed by the organ of origin—either from a specific RP organ or primary retroperitoneal neoplasm and then recognizing specific features in terms of pattern of spread, tumor components and vascularity.[13,14]

Box 1: Common retroperitoneal pathologies.

Primary retroperitoneal neoplasms
- *Mesenchymal tumors:*
  - Liposarcoma
  - Leiomyosarcmas
  - Malignant fibrous histiocytoma
  - Desmoid
- *Neurogenic tumors:*
  - Schwannoma
  - Neurofibroma
  - Ganglioneuroma
  - Paraganglioma
  - Malignant peripheral nerve sheath tumor
- *Germ cell, sex cord or stromal tumor:*
  - Primary retroperitoneal extragonadal germ cell tumor
  - Growing teratoma syndrome
  - Primary teratoma
- *Lymphoid neoplasms:*
  - Lymphadenopathy—benign or metastatic
  - Lymphoma

Non-neoplastic conditions
- Retroperitoneal collections—infection, lymphocele, and hematoma
- Retroperitoneal fibrosis
- Erdheim-Chester disease
- Extramedullary hematopoiesis
- Lymphangioma
- Lymphangiectasis

To decide whether the tumor is located within the retroperitoneal space, it is useful to observe the displacement of normal anatomic structures. Anterior displacement of retroperitoneal organs (e.g. kidneys, adrenal glands, ureters, ascending and descending colon, pancreas, and portions of the duodenum) strongly suggests that the tumor arises in the RP **(Figs. 7A and B)**. Major vessels and some of their branches are also found in the retroperitoneal cavity, so that displacement of these vessels can be helpful as well. Before a tumor can be described as primarily retroperitoneal, the possibility that the tumor originates from a retroperitoneal organ must be excluded. Some radiologic signs that are helpful in determining tumor origin include the "beak sign", the "phantom (invisible) organ sign" and the "embedded organ sign".[15] When there is no definite sign that suggests an organ of origin, the diagnosis of primary retroperitoneal tumor becomes likely.

Beak sign—when a mass deforms the edge of an adjacent organ into a "beak" shape, it is likely that the mass arises from that organ **(Figs. 8A and B)**. On the other hand, an adjacent organ with dull edges suggests that the tumor compresses the organ but does not arise from it.

Phantom (invisible) organ sign—when a large mass arises from a small organ, the organ sometimes becomes undetectable. This is known as the phantom organ sign. However, false-positive findings do exist, as in cases of huge retroperitoneal sarcomas that involve other small organs such as the adrenal gland.

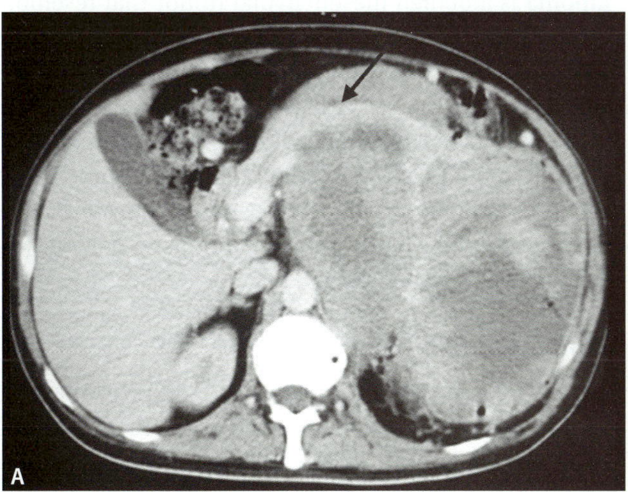

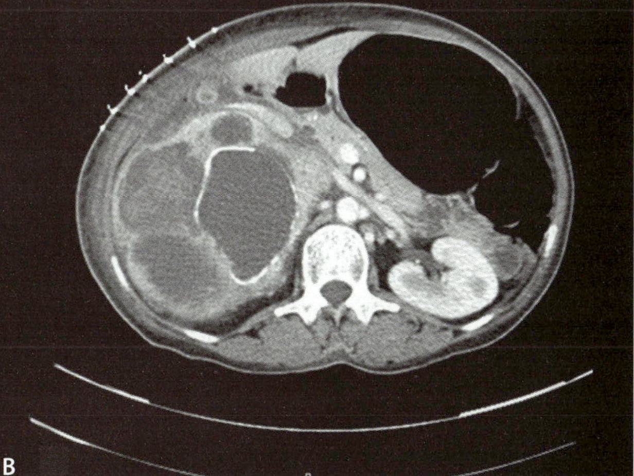

Fig. 7A and B: (A) Anterior displacement of pancreas. Axial CT image shows a large mass that is difficult to localize at first glance. However, anterior displacement of pancreas (arrow) confirms it to be in the retroperitoneal space; (B) Anterior displacement of the IVC. Axial CT image reveals a large, heterogeneous partially cystic right hypochondriac mass with septal calcification on the right. Its retroperitoneal location is suggested by the anterior displacement and stretching of the IVC (arrow). Histopathology revealed a diagnosis of paraganglioma.

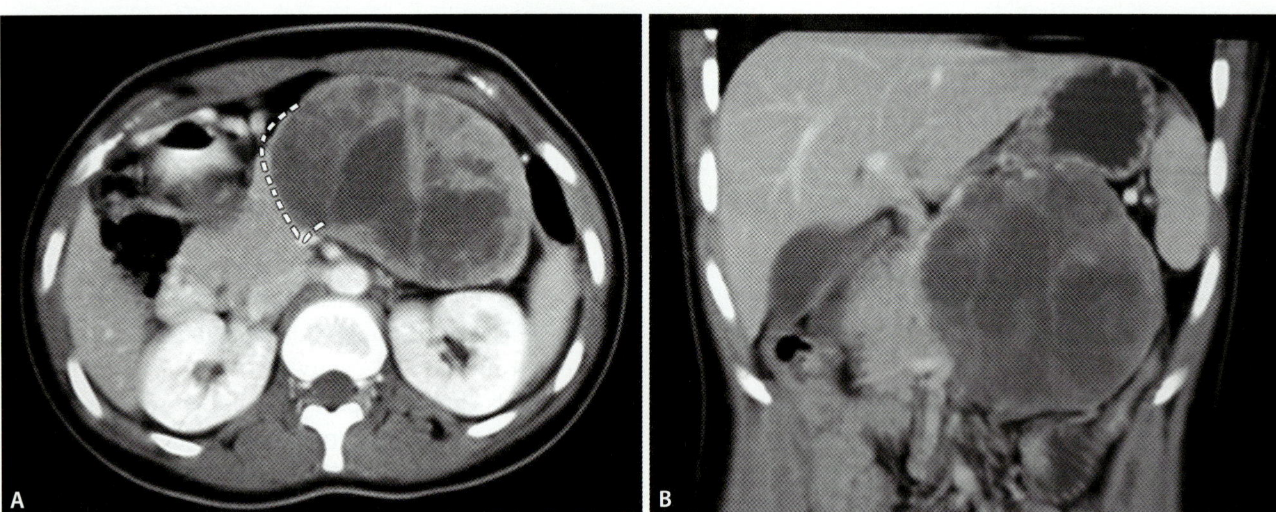

Figs. 8A and B: Beak sign. Axial CT image shows a large cystic tumor with the beak sign in its contact surface with the pancreas (dotted white line). This finding represents mucinous cystadenocarcinoma of the pancreas.

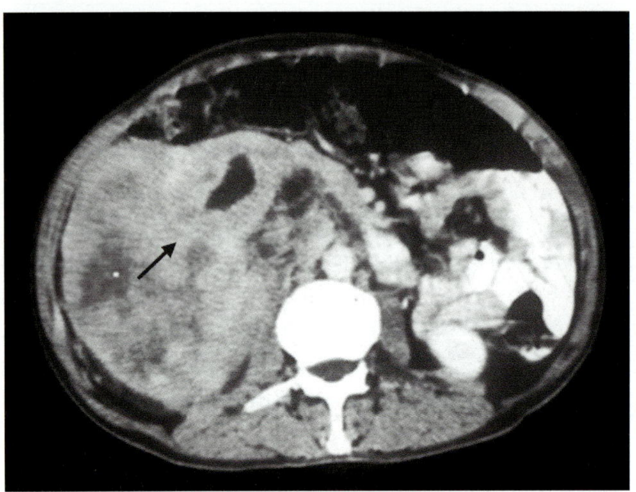

Fig. 9: Embedded organ sign. CT image shows a huge heterogeneous mass in the right side of abdomen. The lumen of the duodenum is stretched toward the mass, and the wall of the duodenum appears embedded in the mass at the contact surface (arrow). These findings represent gastrointestinal stromal tumor of the duodenum with a positive embedded organ sign.

Embedded organ sign—when a tumor compresses an adjacent plastic organ (e.g. gastrointestinal tract and IVC) that is not the organ of origin, the organ is deformed into a crescent shape. In contrast, when part of an organ appears to be embedded in the tumor (positive embedded organ sign) at the contact surface, it is likely to be the organ of origin **(Fig. 9)**.

MESODERMAL NEOPLASMS

Soft tissue sarcomas of mesenchymal origin are rare tumor accounting for less than 1%; however, around 15% occur in RP.[16] The retroperitoneal tumors often present late and with large size due to spread along the connective tissue in RP. Role of imaging is predominantly to determine the extent, spread, and resectability of the mass along with detection of lymphadenopathy and metastases. Accurate diagnosis of the tumor is not always possible; but few imaging features may assist in narrowing the differentials, e.g. presence of fat raises suspicion of liposarcoma, cystic mass may indicate lymphangioma or lymphangiectasis, spread of mass in between vessels causing displacement but not infiltration is feature of lymphoma **(Flowchart 1)**.

Lipoma

Lipoma is a benign mesenchymal tumor that resembles normal fat. Lipomas typically demonstrate homogeneous fatty (–10 to –100 HU) attenuation on CT and homogeneous signal intensity identical to that of fat on all MRI sequences. Thin (<2 mm) fibrous septa of low signal intensity on T1- and T2-weighted images may traverse the lesion. Since, lipoma is extremely rare in RP, any fat-containing lesion in this location is considered and evaluated as liposarcoma.

Liposarcomas

CT or MRI can suggest a diagnosis of liposarcoma when fat is detected within a retroperitoneal mass. The amount of fat seen in liposarcomas varies widely and depending on the histopathology and degree of fat on imaging, RP liposarcomas can be divided into—well-differentiated liposarcoma, myxoid liposarcoma, dedifferentiated, and pleomorphic liposarcomas.[16-18]

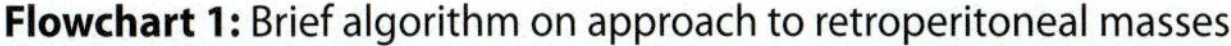

Flowchart 1: Brief algorithm on approach to retroperitoneal masses.

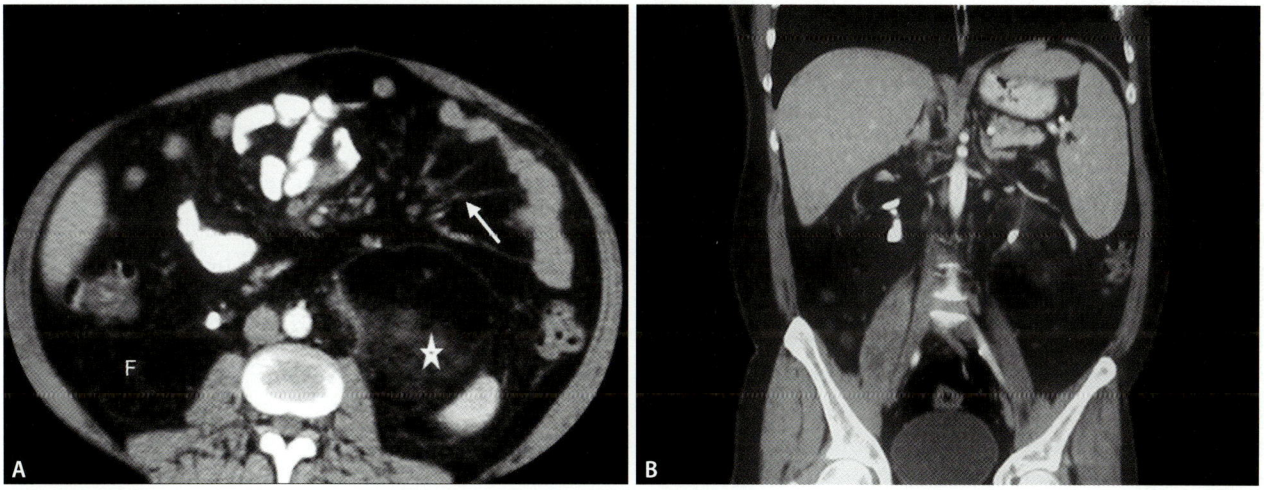

- Approach to retroperitoneal masses
  - Ascertain the location
    - Primary retroperitoneal/arising from retroperitoneal organ
      - Use beak sign, invisible organ and embedded organ sign
        - Primary retroperitoneal mass
          - *Fat present*
            - Lipoma
            - Liposarcoma
          - Fat absent
            - *Venous origin* Leiomyosarcoma
            - *Lymph nodes* Benign or metastases lymphoma
            - *Deranged serum markers* Extragonadal germ cell tumor
          - *Cystic changes*
            - Lymphangioma
            - Sometimes neurogenic and leiomyosarcoma
          - *Vascularity*
            - Paraganglioma
            - Leiomyosarcoma
          - *Pattern of spread* (In between vessels/organs)
            - Lymphoma
            - Lymphangioma

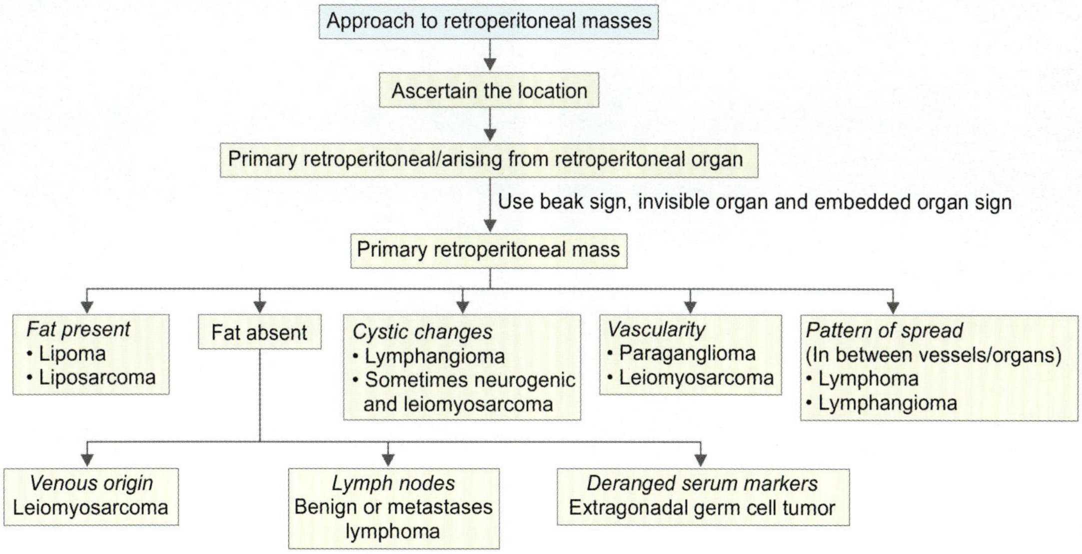

Figs. 10A and B: Retroperitoneal well-differentiated liposarcoma in a 60-year-old man with a history of increasing abdominal girth. Axial and coronal CT images show a diffusely infiltrative, retroperitoneal and abdominal mass composed of fat (F) with Hounsfield (HU) measurements of –80 to –120. There are multiple thick septa (arrow) and a posterior soft tissue component (star) with mildly higher attenuation.

The well-differentiated liposarcomas are predominantly of fat density with or without fine irregular strands of higher density **(Figs. 10A and B)**. These septations or soft tissue attenuation merge with fat component without any clear demarcation between the two components in contrast to dedifferentiated liposarcomas where soft tissue masses can be distinguishly and separately seen within the fatty tumor **(Fig. 11)**. Myxoid liposarcomas have cystic attenuation—seen as density less than muscle but greater than fat on CT. MRI will show high signal intensity within the soft tissue on T2-weighted image and heterogeneous enhancement postgadolinium administration due to presence of extracellular myxoid material within giving it a "pseudocystic" appearance. Pleomorphic liposarcoma has higher degree of anaplasia because of which it might not show minimal or no fat component on imaging and seen as heterogeneous retroperitoneal soft tissue mass.

The treatment and prognosis differ with each type of fat-containing retroperitoneal mass; hence, it is important to identify and observe internal imaging features. Few imaging findings like soft tissue septa more than 2 mm thick within a fatty retroperitoneal mass, septal irregularity or bulging, demarcated soft tissue mass within, and obvious enhancement help in approaching the RP mass appropriately.[19]

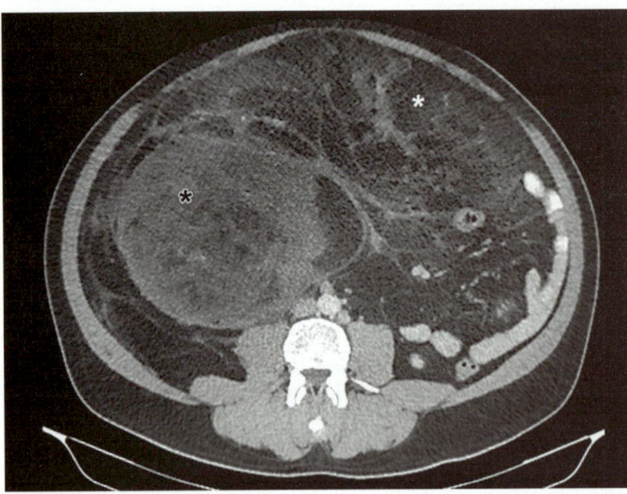

Fig. 11: Dedifferentiated liposarcoma in a 44-year-old male patient. Axial CT image shows large abdominal mass with imperceptible margins having fatty (white asterisk) as well as solid (black asterisk) component.

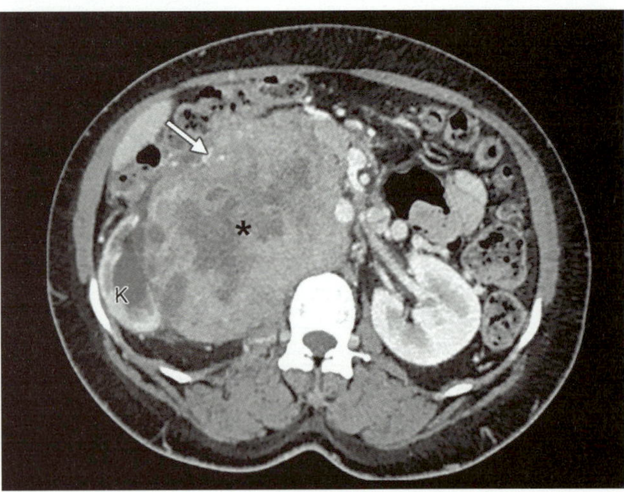

Fig. 12: Inferior vena cava (IVC) leiomyosarcoma in a 52-year-old female. Axial CT image demonstrates a large heterogeneous retroperitoneal mass (asterisk) displacing and compressing right kidney (K). The IVC is seen displaced anteriorly by the mass with luminal narrowing (arrow) indicating predominantly extraluminal component of the sarcoma.

Leiomyosarcomas

Leiomyosarcomas are the second most common retroperitoneal sarcomas with female predominance. It is the most common primary venous/IVC tumor which present as slow growing large, heterogeneous masses with foci of hemorrhage, necrosis, and cystic degeneration **(Fig. 12)**.[20] They do not contain fat or calcification. Not infrequently, retroperitoneal leiomyosarcomas extend into the adjacent veins. IVC leiomyosarcomas can have extraluminal (62%), both intraluminal as well as extraluminal (33%) and only intraluminal (5%) growth patterns from various segments of IVC.[21] Upper segment indicates extension from hepatic veins to right atrium, middle segment is from hepatic to renal veins, and lower segment involves infrarenal part of IVC.

Malignant Fibrous Histiocytomas

Malignant fibrous histiocytomas are high grade connective tissue tumors. They are multilobulated, infiltrative, unencapsulated but deceptively well-circumscribed masses. They may contain myxoid stroma, fibrous tissue, hemorrhage, and necrosis giving rise to a typical mosaic of mixed low, intermediate, and high signal intensity on T2-weighted MR images. Although both myxoid stroma and necrosis have similar T1 and T2 signal intensity, differentiation may be possible as myxoid stroma shows delayed enhancement in contrast to the nonenhancing necrotic areas. Up to 25% of malignant fibrous histiocytomas contain dystrophic calcification, a finding that is extremely uncommon in other retroperitoneal malignancies.[22]

Hemangiopericytomas

Hemangiopericytomas are highly vascular tumors thought to arise from blood vessel walls. They may demonstrate areas of intratumoral hemorrhage and multiple flow voids on MRI. Hemangiopericytomas enhance rapidly and intensely on dynamic contrast-enhanced CT or MRI.

Other Malignancies

Fibrosarcomas and neurofibrosarcomas are usually heterogeneous and thus identical in appearance to leiomyosarcomas, some liposarcomas, and malignant fibrous histiocytomas. Neuroblastomas and ganglioneuroblastomas often contain calcification. They are usually seen in children. Rhabdomyosarcomas are rare heterogeneous tumors also seen in pediatric patients.

NEUROGENIC NEOPLASMS

Neurogenic tumors may arise from paraganglionic cells (paragangliomas), ganglion cells (ganglioneuroma, ganglioneuroblastoma, and neuroblastoma), and nerve sheaths (neurofibroma and schwannoma).

Paragangliomas

Majority of paragangliomas (extra-adrenal pheochromocytoma) lie in the RP, in the immediate para-aortic region,

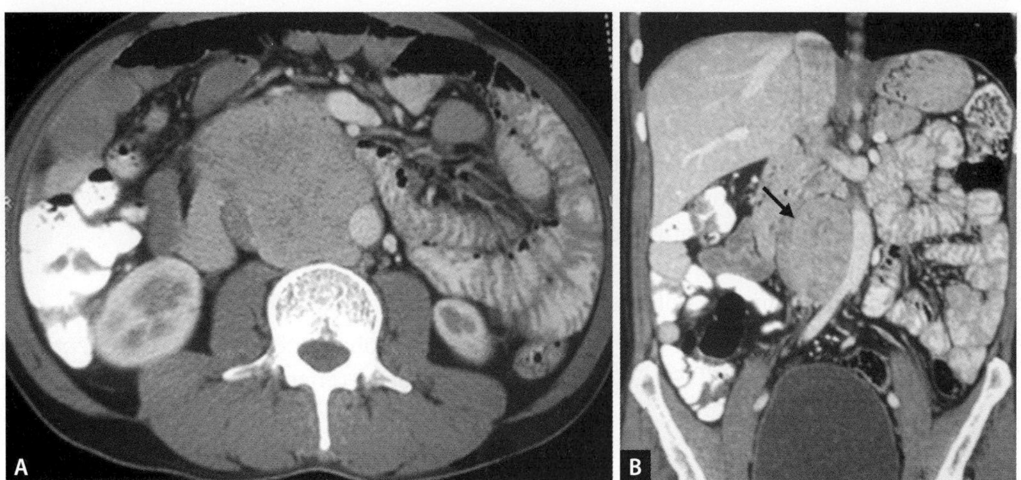

Figs. 13A and B: Retroperitoneal paraganglioma. (A) Axial CT image shows large homogeneous soft tissue density mass in the aortocaval region; (B) Coronal image shows the IVC draping around the right lateral margin of the mass (arrow).

from the level of the adrenal glands to the aortic bifurcation. Paragangliomas are well-defined soft tissue masses, usually quite large at the time of diagnosis **(Figs. 13A and B)**. Paragangliomas are homogeneous when small, but become increasingly heterogeneous as they grow due to central necrosis, hemorrhage, and even calcification.[23] On MR images, they often demonstrate extremely high signal intensity on T2-weighted images. These are generally hypervascular and most enhanced briskly after injection of IV contrast material.

Nerve Sheath Tumors

These tumors are often located adjacent to the vertebral column or deep to the psoas muscles. MRI is the imaging modality of choice for imaging of these tumors as it detects tumor extension into the neural foramina, a common feature of neurogenic tumors **(Fig. 14)**. MRI also helps in the characterization of these masses, as they tend to have high signal intensity on T2-weighted sequence due to the myxoid stroma they contain. Central low to intermediate signal intensity may be seen corresponding to fibrous tissue and is referred to as the "target sign". Sometimes, a whorled appearance consisting of linear or curvilinear structures of low signal intensity is seen on T2-weighted images. At histopathological analysis, this finding corresponds to bundles of Schwann cells and collagen fibers within the mass. Varying degrees of contrast enhancement have been reported, from slight to moderate to marked with delayed heterogeneous uptake of contrast. These enhancement features are explained by the presence of abundant myxoid material in these tumors, resulting in delayed progressive accumulation of contrast material in the extracellular space.[24]

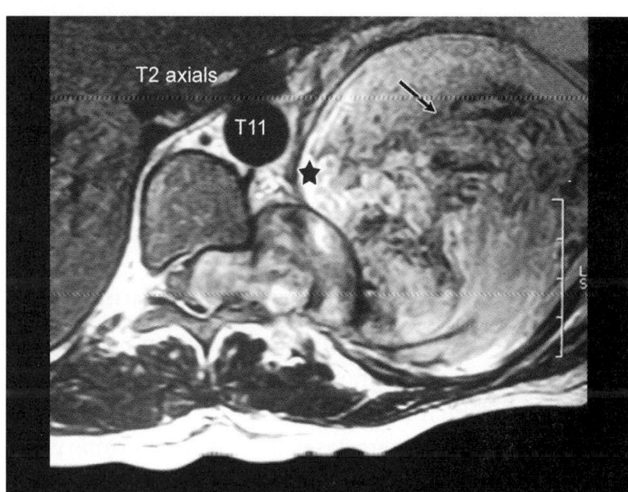

Fig. 14: Intraspinal extension of schwannoma. T2-weighted axial MR image shows a smoothly encapsulated, large heterogeneous intensity mass in the left paraspinal location. It has extended inside the extradural compartment of the spinal canal. The markedly hyperintense area (star) represents myxoid stroma. The linear, low signal intensity areas, having a somewhat whorled appearance (arrow), correspond to bundles of Schwann cells and collagen fibers within the mass.

Schwannomas usually appear as well-defined, heterogeneous soft tissue masses. Although they may contain cystic areas, they usually have large solid components. Retroperitoneal *neurofibromas* are commonly seen in patients with neurofibromatosis. On CT, neurofibromas appear as well-defined, sharply marginated, homogeneous masses that demonstrate near-water attenuation. *Ganglioneuromas* arise from sympathetic ganglia and are composed of mature Schwann cells, ganglion cells, and nerve fibers. Predominantly children and young adults (60% of cases) are affected and the prognosis is excellent, recurrence being rare after surgical resection. At CT or MRI, ganglioneuromas appear as well-circumscribed oval, crescentic, or lobulated masses. These tumors tend to partially or completely surround major blood vessels, with little or no compromise of the lumen. At unenhanced CT, the tumors appear homogeneous, with attenuation less than that of muscle. They contain calcification in about 20% of cases. The calcifications are discrete and punctate rather than amorphous and coarse as in neuroblastomas.

GERM CELL, SEX CORD OR STROMAL NEOPLASMS

Teratomas

Teratomas are congenital neoplasms containing components of all three germ layers. CT often shows calcification or even osseous elements. Fat may be seen on both CT and MRI **(Fig. 15)**. Sometimes, a dermoid plug is identifiable as a soft tissue mural nodule projecting into a cyst. The incidence of malignant degeneration is rare (<1%) and usually occurs in the dermoid plug in postmenopausal women.

Primary Extragonadal Germ Cell Tumor

Primary retroperitoneal extragonadal germ cell tumors (GCTs) arise from primordial germ cells remnants of genital ridge which fail to migrate properly. Since most of the GCTs in RP are metastases from genital primary, the patient should be evaluated for same. The retroperitoneal GCT can be seminomatous or nonseminomatous, seen as enhancing masses which are predominantly in the midline if metastasized from testicular primary neoplasm. The latter is associated with deranged serum markers and is seen as heterogeneous masses with cystic necrotic or hemorrhagic areas within. Nonseminomatous GCTs carry poor prognosis.

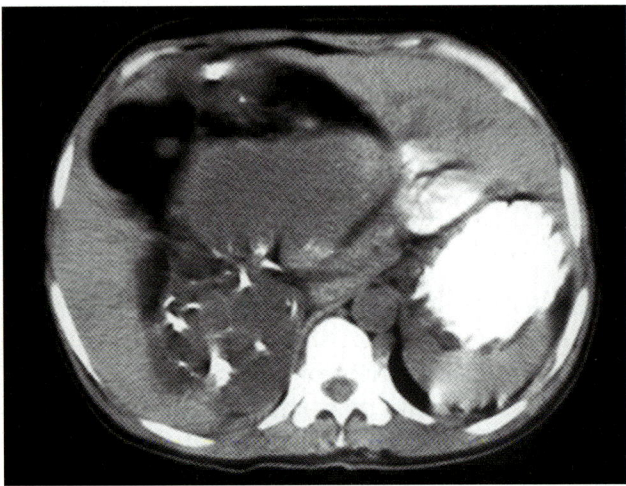

Fig. 15: Retroperitoneal teratoma. Axial CT image reveals a large heterogeneous mass containing elements that show the attenuation of fluid, fat, soft tissue and calcification.

Growing Teratoma Syndrome

It is a rare phenomenon with documentation of 1.9–7.6% rate of occurrence in literature.[16] It refers to chemorefractory retroperitoneal teratomatous mass which shows increase in size on chemotherapy despite normalization of tumor markers. Surgical resection is the treatment of choice in such patients.

LYMPHOID NEOPLASMS

Normal lymph nodes appear as small, rounded soft tissue masses adjacent to the great vessels. Retrocrural, paraceliac, gastrohepatic, para-aortic, aortocaval, periportal, peripancreatic, and external and internal iliac groups together constitute the retroperitoneal nodes. Presently, CT is the most frequently used imaging technique for evaluation of enlarged retroperitoneal nodes. The diagnosis of lymph node abnormalities on CT is based on size and image morphology. Size of a node is best determined by measuring its short-axis diameter. The retroperitoneal lymph nodes are considered abnormal if their size is more than 10 mm, except in the retrocrural space where the upper limit is 6 mm. A variety of retroperitoneal structures can be confused with enlarged lymph nodes like unopacified bowel loops, vascular collaterals, dilated lymphatics, and retroperitoneal fibrosis. Careful evaluation of serial CT images after oral and IV contrast is helpful in distinguishing between these structures.

Magnetic resonance sequences suited for detection of lymph nodes include precontrast T1-weighted spin-echo or SGE, fat-suppressed T2-weighted turbo spin-echo, and contrast-enhanced fat-suppressed sequences. The enlarged lymph nodes appear low in signal on precontrast SGE in a background of high-signal fat, and nodes are moderately high in signal on fat-suppressed T2-weighted and contrast-enhanced T1-weighted images. Fat- suppressed T2-weighted and diffusion weighted images are very sensitive for the detection of lymph nodes and perform better than CT, particularly in pediatric patients or other patients with paucity of retroperitoneal fat.

Benign Lymphadenopathy

Benign enlargement of lymph nodes may occur secondary to inflammatory or infectious disease; tuberculosis being the most common etiology in our country.[25]

The mesenteric, omental, and peripancreatic lymph nodes are most commonly involved. The nodes commonly demonstrate peripheral enhancement with central areas of low attenuation after IV contrast administration **(Fig. 16)**. Discrete homogeneous lymph nodes may also be seen in some cases. Calcification is frequently seen in tubercular lymph nodes. Enlarged lymph nodes with low density centers may also be seen in pyogenic infections, Whipple's disease, lymphomatous or metastatic nodes following radiotherapy and chemotherapy. Enlarged retroperitoneal nodes have also been observed in 30% of patients with sarcoidosis.[26] The periportal, paraceliac, and para-aortic groups are most often involved. On CT, the nodes affected by sarcoidosis generally show homogeneous soft-tissue attenuation and remain discrete. Nodal calcification is unusual in sarcoidosis.

Castleman disease is occasionally also associated with retroperitoneal lymph node enlargement. Mostly, the CT or MR appearance of these enlarged lymph nodes is not specific. However, identification of intense and uniform contrast enhancement in lymph nodes can suggest the diagnosis **(Fig. 17)**.[27]

Lymphangioleiomyomatosis is a rare cause of bulky retroperitoneal lymphadenopathy. This is a progressive disease involving the lung, lymphatic trunks, and lymph nodes, typically affecting young women of child-bearing age. Sometimes, it can primarily involve RP with or without subsequent development in the lungs.[28] The enlarged lymph nodes may show cystic, low-attenuation components on imaging.

Lymphoma

Abdominal lymph nodes are involved in 50% of the non-Hodgkin's lymphoma (NHL) patients as against 25% of those with Hodgkin's disease (HD) at presentation.[29] Mesenteric involvement is seen in more than half of the NHL patients (versus 5% of those with HD). The patterns of lymphadenopathy are also markedly different, slight enlargement of upper para-aortic nodes and contiguous spread being characteristic of HD. NHL on the other hand manifests with bulky lymph nodes in multiple locations.

The enlarged lymph nodes may appear as discrete masses or as confluent soft tissue mass obliterating the retroperitoneal fat **(Fig. 18)**. Lymphomas are "soft" tumors and frequently surround the adjacent vessels (floating aorta sign) and ureters without compressing their lumina. Lymphomas are homogeneous with minimal contrast enhancement and relatively low signal intensity at T2-weighted images representing densely packed cellular components. Nodes are rarely calcified (<1%) in untreated patients.[30]

Computed tomography is also used for follow-up of disease after treatment. Response to treatment is usually indicated by reduction in size and extent with or without appearance of dystrophic calcification within. In some patients, lymph nodes may become hypodense

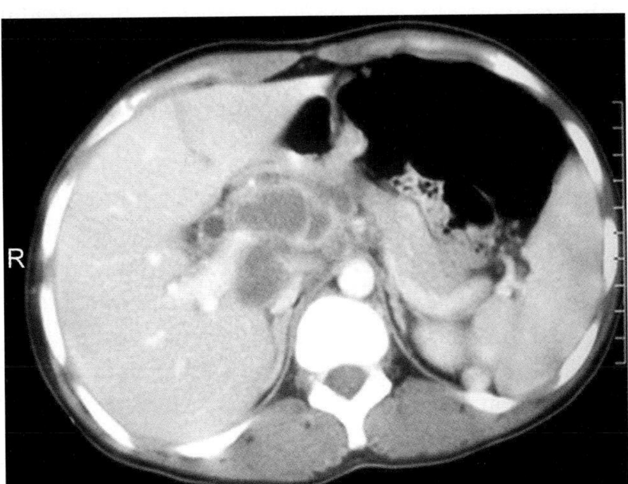

Fig. 16: Retroperitoneal tubercular lymphadenopathy. Axial CT image shows enlarged periportal and portocaval lymph nodes with characteristic central necrosis and peripheral rim enhancement.

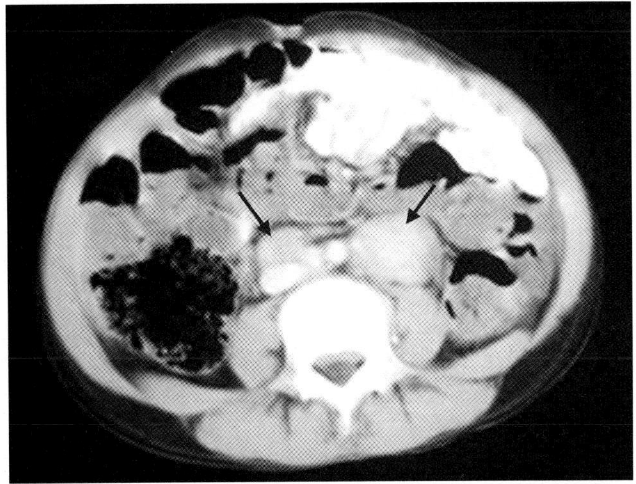

Fig. 17: Castleman disease. Contrast enhanced axial CT image shows large, well-defined, markedly enhancing para-aortic lymph nodes (arrows) compatible with the diagnosis of Castleman disease in an 8-year-old boy.

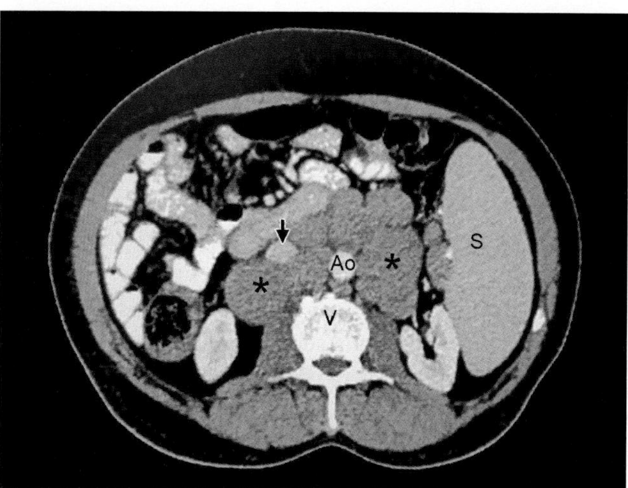

Fig. 18: Non-Hodgkin's lymphoma. Contrast-enhanced axial CT image shows large, confluent lymph nodes in pre/para-aortic, aortocaval, and retrocaval location (asterisks). Inferior vena cava (arrow) and aorta (Ao) are displaced by the mass but their patency is preserved. Note made of enlarged spleen (S) (V: vertebral body).

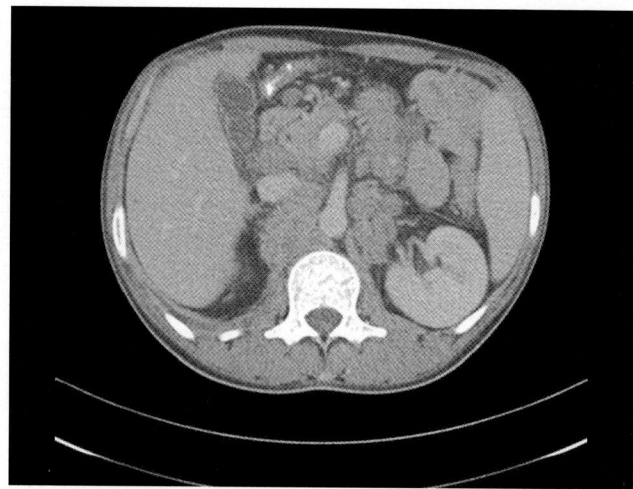

Fig. 19: *Mycobacterium tuberculosis* infection in a 35-year-old man with HIV infection. Axial CT image shows multiple, enlarged, low attenuation lymph nodes in the portocaval and paracelic regions.

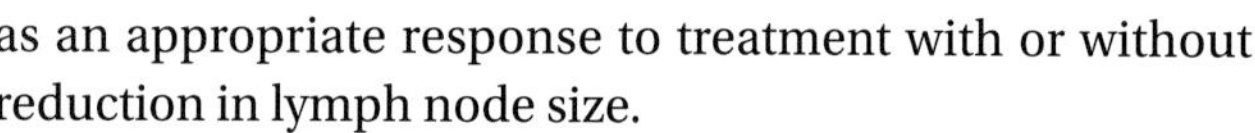

as an appropriate response to treatment with or without reduction in lymph node size.

Persistent lymph nodal masses may be seen in some patients even after treatment. These may represent residual tumor, post-treatment inflammation or fibrosis. Unfortunately, there are no reliable CT characteristics that can differentiate between malignant and benign residual masses. Several studies have suggested that MRI may be helpful in distinguishing late post-therapy fibrosis (hypointense on T2-weighted images) from viable lymph nodes (hyperintense or heterogeneous on T2-weighted images). Also, chronic fibrotic tissue shows minimal MR enhancement postcontrast while recurrence generally enhances markedly.

FDG-PET has proved to be very useful in the clinical management and follow-up of lymphomas. It is now considered the most accurate tool for the assessment of treatment response and prognosis in patients with Hodgkin's lymphoma and aggressive NHL.[31] FDG-PET can detect metabolically active disease by its increased glycolysis that is proportional to the tumor mitotic activity. It can separate high-grade from low-grade tumors and aid in prognostication. FDG-PET at the end of treatment seems to aid considerably in differentiating between residual masses with or without residual lymphoma. An early interim FDG-PET scan after 1–3 cycles of chemotherapy is a very strong predictor of outcome.[32] Like other imaging modalities, PET has its own drawbacks including inability to detect very small lesions (<5 mm) and reduced specificity due to increased uptake in metabolically active inflammatory and infective tissues.

HIV Lymphadenopathy

Enlarged lymph node are present in most (> 60%) patients with human immunodeficiency virus (HIV) infection but in more than half of these patients, the short-axis diameter of the largest node measures only 10–15 mm.[33] Although sometimes the nodal enlargement results only from reactive hyperplasia, many other diseases may be responsible. These include disseminated mycobacterial infections **(Fig. 19)**, histoplasmosis, lymphoma, and Kaposi's sarcoma. When lymph node enlargement is massive, acquired immunodeficiency syndrome (AIDS)-related lymphoma should be suspected. Intense enhancement of lymph nodes suggests a diagnosis of Kaposi's sarcoma.

Metastatic Lymphadenopathy

Metastatic lymph nodes show varied morphological patterns, but the diagnosis is usually straightforward due to the presence of a known primary. Neoplasms of the stomach, colon, pancreas, kidney, testis, ovary, uterus, bladder, and prostate may all metastasize to retroperitoneal lymph nodes. Calcification in the metastatic nodes suggests mucin producing primary from the ovary or gastrointestinal tract.

Testicular neoplasms tend to metastasize via lymphatics rather than via bloodstream. Lymphatics from the testes drain into ipsilateral lymph nodes, which follow the course of the gonadal veins. Typically, left-sided neoplasms spread to involve lymph nodes in the left renal hilum, as the left gonadal vein drains into the

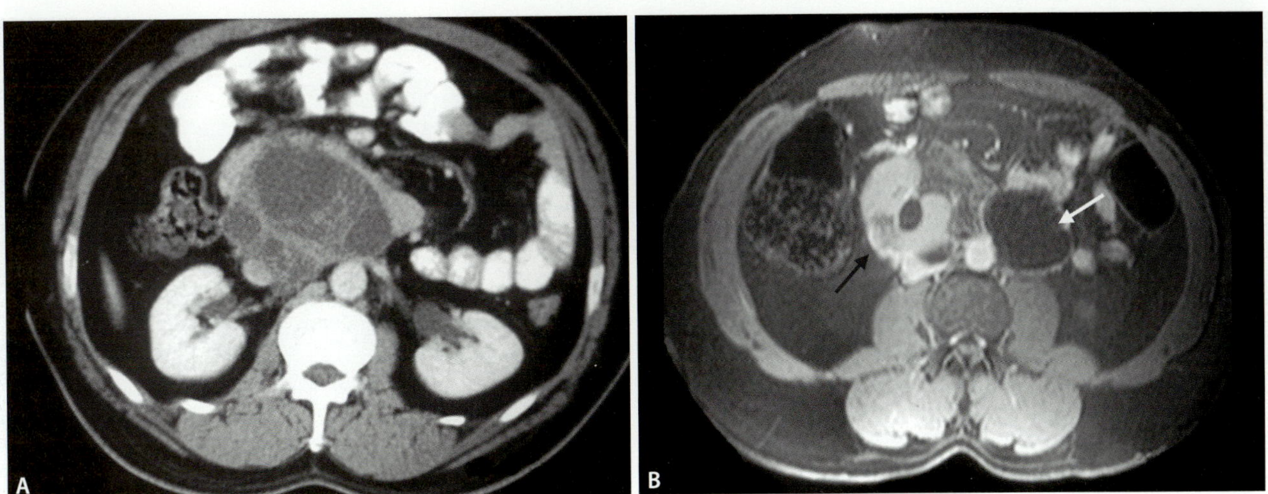

Figs. 20A and B: Metastatic testicular germ cell tumor. (A) Axial CT image shows massive, low attenuation retroperitoneal lymphadenopathy; (B) Postchemotherapy contrast-enhanced T1-weighted axial MR image in another patient shows enhancing viable tumor (black arrow) and the non-enhancing necrotic component (white arrow).

left renal vein. Right-sided neoplasms spread to paracaval lymph nodes, an area where the right gonadal vein joins the IVC. While metastatic retroperitoneal nodes from some testicular tumors appear quite homogeneous on CT, others particularly from nonseminomatous neoplasms often appear heterogeneous containing low-attenuation central areas of necrosis and rim enhancement **(Figs. 20A and B)**. Seminomas may present with bulky masses whereas nonseminomatous GCT often metastasize to normal sized nodes. On MR metastatic lymph nodes show low-intermediate signal intensity on T1-weighted images, and high signal intensity on T2-weighted images. Low signal intensity masses after treatment usually represent fibrosis.

CT and MRI use the nonspecific criterion of size and are limited in their ability to differentiate benign from malignant lymph nodes. Contrast-enhanced MR lymphography is a promising technique in differentiating benign from metastatic lymph nodes and providing information on lymph node morphology and function.

Ultrasmall super paramagnetic iron oxide (USPIO) particles with a long plasma circulation time are suitable as MR contrast agents for MR lymphography. MRI is typically performed 24–36 hours after IV infusion of USPIO particles. Normal lymph nodes decrease in signal intensity on enhanced T2-weighted and T2-weighted gradient echo images, indicating uptake of this contrast agent. Nodes infiltrated by tumor have no appreciable USPIO uptake and thus reveal no signal change on pre- and postcontrast images.[34]

FDG-PET may be more sensitive and specific than CT for certain retroperitoneal metastases depending on the primary. Nonseminomatous GCTs with well-differentiated components are not very FDG-avid.

NON-NEOPLASTIC PATHOLOGIES

Retroperitoneal Collections

Fluid collection in the RP occurs in a variety of conditions like acute pancreatitis, urinary tract disruption with urinoma formation, hematoma, and abscess. Although the clinical presentations differ, they all share a tendency to dissect within the well-defined fascial planes in the retroperitoneal space. Most of these appear on CT as water density collections and are frequently indistinguishable from one another.

Fluid collections in the anterior pararenal space often result from acute pancreatitis **(Fig. 21)**.[35] Fluid collections arise within or adjacent to the pancreas in about 40% and resolve spontaneously without leaving any clinical sequelae in over 50% of these patients. In others, the fluid collections persist, develop a fibrous capsule, and are often associated with a variety of complications including secondary infection, perforation, and erosion into the spleen, liver or vascular system. Both infected and noninfected fluid collections and pseudocysts can be treated effectively by image-guided percutaneous catheter drainage.

Abscesses, hematomas, and urinomas can all develop in the perirenal space. Perirenal hemorrhage is usually caused by blunt trauma, rupture of an aortic aneurysm, bleeding disorders, anticoagulant therapy or spontaneous bleeding within a renal tumor **(Fig. 22)**. On CT characteristically, a hyperdense, ill-defined collection

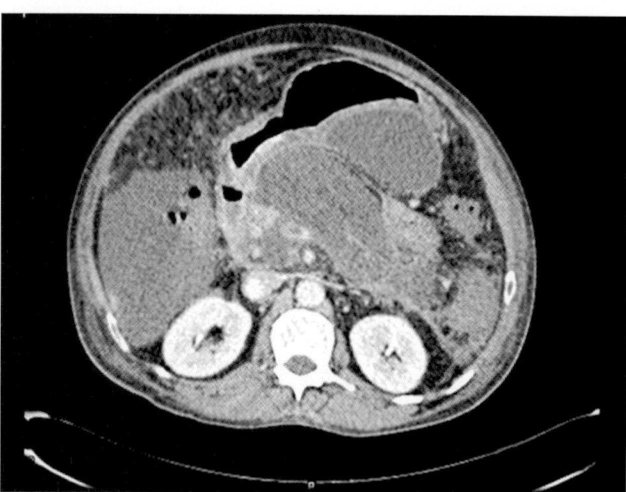

Fig. 21: Fluid collection in the anterior pararenal space. CT image in a patient with acute pancreatitis demonstrates peripancreatic fluid in the left anterior pararenal space.

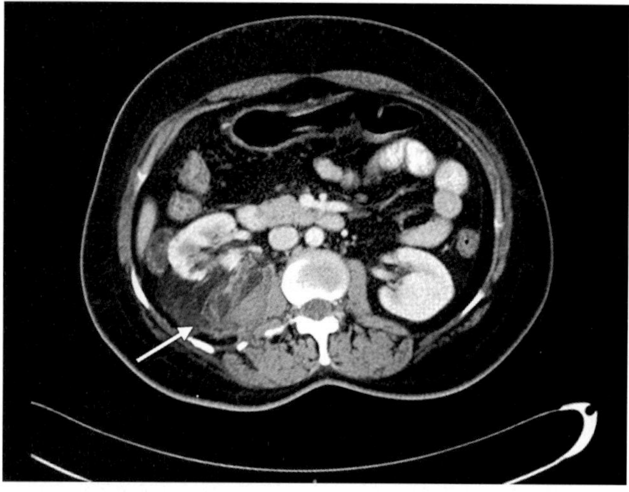

Fig. 22: Perirenal hemorrhage. Axial CT image shows right perirenal hemorrhage (arrow) that occurred spontaneously from rupture of underlying renal angiomyolipoma.

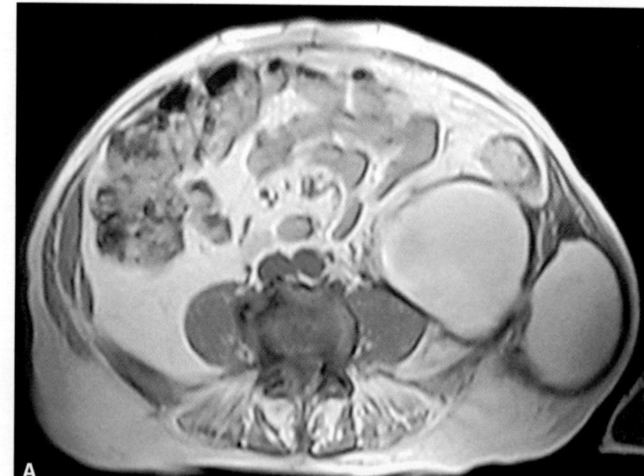

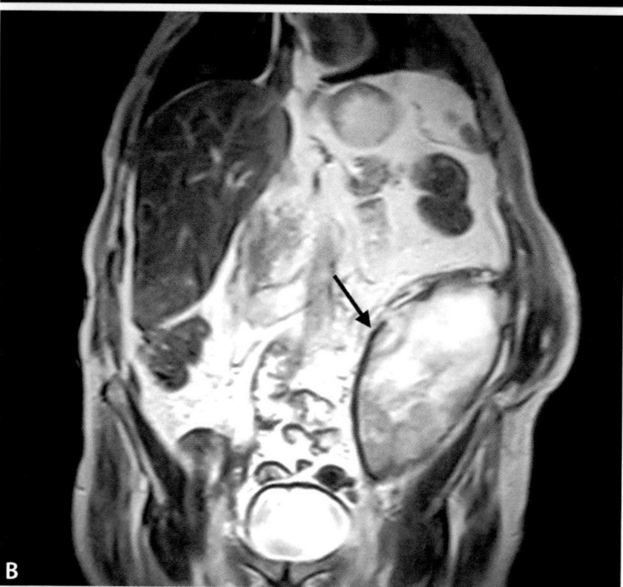

Figs. 23A and B: Spontaneous retroperitoneal hemorrhage in a patient on anticoagulant therapy. (A) Axial T1-weighted MR image shows a well-defined hyperintense lesion anterior to the left psoas. It is partially decompressing into the parietes; (B) Coronal T2-weighted image shows heterogeneous, predominantly high signal intensity within the mass. There is a markedly hypointense peripheral rim (arrow) due to hemosiderin deposition. These T1 and T2 signal intensities are diagnostic of a subacute hematoma.

originating from the disrupted vessels and extending into the interfascial planes is seen. Loculated blood can mimic a complex cyst or neoplasm. CT attenuation of hematoma varies with time, ranging from hyperdense fresh blood, typically >50 HU to near water density within several weeks. Bleeding may be intermittent resulting in a heterogeneous appearance. MRI is more useful in determining the content of retroperitoneal fluid collections as it is more sensitive and specific for detection of blood products. An acute hematoma is isointense on T1-weighted and hyperintense on T2-weighted images. Within several days, the signal gradually becomes hyperintense on T1-weighted images and a hematoma is then hyperintense on both T1- and T2-weighted images with a developing, hypointense hemosiderin rim **(Figs. 23A and B)**.

Abnormal perirenal fluid may be in either of two locations: within the renal capsule (subcapsular) or outside the capsule in the perinephric fat. Subcapsular fluid collections usually produce distortion of the renal parenchyma whereas perinephric collections do not. Urinomas result from obstructive uropathy and less frequently from abdominal trauma and surgical or diagnostic instrumentation.

Retroperitoneal abscesses are particularly difficult to diagnose, because they may not exhibit the classic clinical features, i.e. fever, chills, and an elevated white blood cell count. When an abscess is mature, its wall is thick and generally hypervascular. On contrast-enhanced CT, there is enhancement of the wall and the fluid is usually homogeneous and does not enhance. Many abscesses contain multiple septations. There may be substantial reactive inflammation in the surrounding fat.

Abnormalities in the posterior pararenal space are much less common than abnormalities in the anterior pararenal space or the perirenal space. When present, these are most commonly the result of spread of pathologic processes in the pelvis. Causes can include hematoma, infection, and neoplasm.

Aorta

The most important abdominal aortic abnormalities are aneurysm formation and aortic dissection. MDCTA and MRA have gradually replaced conventional angiography as the procedures of choice for detailed evaluation of the aorta.

Aortic Aneurysm

Most abdominal aortic aneurysms result from atherosclerosis. Other causes include trauma, infection, Takayasu's arteritis, cystic medial necrosis, and syphilis. The infrarenal aorta is the most common site of abdominal aortic aneurysms accounting for 95% of cases. If untreated, these aneurysms may enlarge and rupture with a mortality of 50–90%.[36]

The abdominal aortic aneurysm may show curvilinear calcification on plain abdominal radiography. On USG, CT, and MRI the aneurysm is identified as focal area of dilatation exceeding 3 cm in size. Spontaneous rupture is a frequent complication of aneurysms measuring 6 cm or more in diameter. Therefore, most aneurysms larger than 6 cm require surgery. Important diagnostic information needed for management includes location, diameter of aneurysm, its longitudinal length, its relationship to the renal, common iliac and femoral arteries, and assessment of the periaortic tissues for perianeurysmal fibrosis.[37] USG is a good modality for initial evaluation of aortic aneurysm. It may also be used for follow-up of patients who do not undergo surgical repair. However, CT and MRI are preferred techniques for evaluating the size, extent, and complications of aneurysms. At several centers, CT angiography has replaced conventional angiography because it is less invasive and can provide all the necessary information required for the management. Angiography frequently underestimates the dimensions of an aneurysm because it shows only the flowing blood in the lumen and does not show mural thrombus, which is detected on CT **(Fig. 24)**. Contrast-enhanced 3D gradient echo MRA demonstrates the full extent of the aneurysm and its relationship to aortic branches. Aneurysm rupture or leak is associated with a high morbidity and mortality, if not promptly treated. CT findings of ruptured abdominal aortic aneurysms are often straightforward.

Most ruptures are manifested as a retroperitoneal hematoma accompanied by an abdominal aortic aneurysm. Periaortic blood may extend into the perirenal space, the pararenal space, or both. Intraperitoneal extravasation may be an immediate or a delayed finding. Discontinuity of the aortic wall or a focal gap in otherwise continuous circumferential wall calcifications may point to the location of a rupture. There usually is a delay of several hours between the initial intramural hemorrhage and frank extravasation into the periaortic soft tissues. Contained or impending ruptures are more difficult to identify. A small amount of periaortic blood may be confused with the duodenum, perianeurysmal fibrosis or adenopathy. Imaging features suggestive of instability or impending rupture include increased aneurysm size, a low thrombus-to-lumen ratio, and hemorrhage into a mural thrombus. A peripheral crescent-shaped area of hyperattenuation within an abdominal aortic aneurysm represents an acute intramural hemorrhage and is another

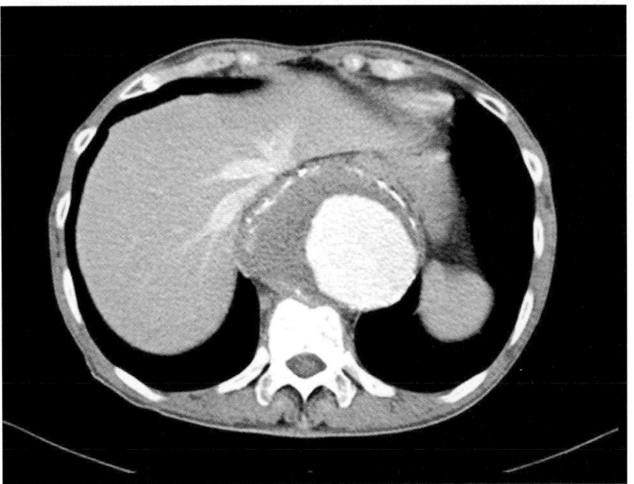

Fig. 24: Abdominal aortic aneurysm. Dynamic, contrast-enhanced axial CT image shows markedly dilated abdominal aorta with a large eccentric thrombus. A conventional angiogram on this patient would significantly underestimate the size of the aneurysm as only the patent part of the lumen containing flowing blood would be opacified.

CT sign of impending rupture. Draping of the posterior aspect of an aneurysmal aorta over the vertebrae is associated with a contained rupture.[38]

The preferred surgical treatment of abdominal aortic aneurysms is an end-to-end anastomosis with aortic graft repair. Complications of abdominal aortic surgery that can be detected on CT include graft infections, aortoenteric fistulae, anastomotic aneurysms, graft leak or rupture.

Aortic Dissection

Aortic dissection usually originates in the thorax but sometimes extends into the abdomen. Mortality rate of untreated dissection is very high approaching 25% at 1 day, 50% at 1 week, and 75% at 1 month.[39] The strategy for therapy depends on the type of dissection, the site of entry, the extent of dissection, involvement of aortic branches, patency of the false lumen, and the presence of thrombus in the false lumen.

Currently, the noninvasive modalities that are most frequently used to identify aortic dissections are USG, CT, and MRI. USG including transthoracic echocardiography and transesophageal echocardiography, is widely available and can be performed quickly and easily at the bedside. Thus, USG can be used in most patients with aortic dissections, even in relatively unstable patients. However, USG has major shortcomings, namely, a limited field of view and a diagnostic accuracy that largely depends on the investigator's experience. Furthermore, USG does not provide images that can be used to plan therapy. Multidetector CT has the advantages of shorter scanning times, wide availability, and high diagnostic accuracy and has, therefore, classically been the modality of choice for the evaluation of aortic dissection. In the past, emergency MRI evaluation of aortic dissection has been impossible owing to prolonged examination times, but the advent of 3D contrast-enhanced MRA has changed this paradigm. Contrast-enhanced MRA has largely replaced unenhanced MR angiographic techniques and has dramatically shortened the total examination time required for confident diagnosis of aortic dissections; however, it is more suitable for stable patients. In principle, contrast-enhanced MRA is similar to CT angiography. Both modalities provide excellent evaluation of aortic dissections. In patients without contraindications for either modality, at most centers, the use of each modality is based on equipment availability, the personal preference of the radiologist or referring physician, and patient acceptance. Confident diagnosis and correct classification of aortic dissection is based on the detection of an intimal flap in the aorta that separates the true and false lumina **(Fig. 25)**. Such a flap manifests as a hypointense line with a linear, arc, or "S" shape in the axial plane. The true and false lumina can be differentiated on the basis of signal intensity, morphologic features, the relationship between the lumina, and the appearance of thrombosis.

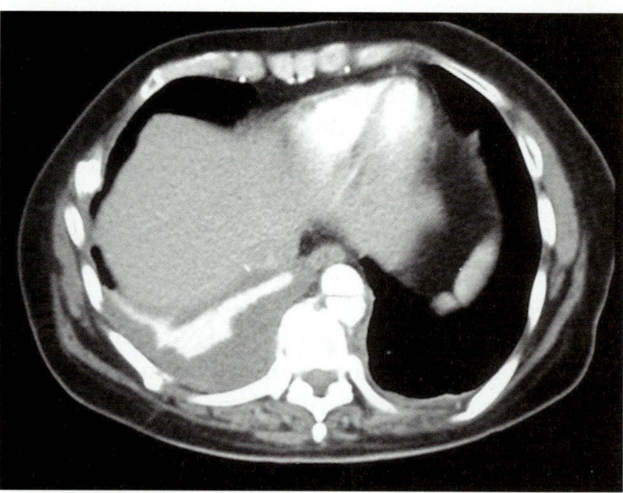

Fig. 25: Thoracoabdominal aortic dissection. Axial CT angiogram easily demonstrates the linear intimal flap between the anterior true lumen and posterior false lumen. Active extravasation into the retroperitoneum is also seen.

- *Signal intensity*: Similar to CT angiography, contrast-enhanced MRA shows the true lumen with higher signal intensity than the false lumen owing to a higher concentration of contrast material during the arterial phase.
- *Morphologic features*: The true lumen is usually smaller than the false lumen and would be thin or flat from being pressed, appearing oval in the axial plane.
- The false lumen is expanded or very large, appearing crescentic or winding around the true lumen in the axial plane.
- *Relationship between the lumina*: The lumina may be parallel to each other, the false lumen may wind around the true lumen, or the true lumen may look like a ribbon floating in the false lumen.
- *Appearance of thrombosis*: The false lumen usually contains a thrombus, especially at the retrograde end of the initial entry site, whereas the true lumen contains no thrombus in most cases.

Inferior Vena Cava

Mostly a routine CT or an MR abdominal protocol employing pre- and postcontrast SGE images provides sufficient evaluation of the IVC for patient management.

At least one MR sequence should be performed in the sagittal or coronal plane, because it permits direct visualization of the longitudinal extent of IVC. However, when detailed evaluation of retroperitoneal veins is required, it is prudent to obtain CT or MR venography.

Congenital Anomalies

Congenital abnormalities of the IVC and related veins are common. Preoperative knowledge of the presence of these anomalies is helpful, particularly in patients undergoing a portosystemic shunt procedure, aortic surgery or nephrectomy, cytoreductive surgery, and reduces the risk of major venous hemorrhage associated with these anomalies.[40]

CT and MRI are well suited to determine whether rounded or tubular retroperitoneal structures are vascular in nature. Some of the developmental anomalies of IVC are: Interruption of IVC with azygos and hemiazygos vein continuation **(Fig. 26)**, left-sided IVC, duplication of the IVC, and anomalies of the left renal vein, e.g. circumaortic or retroaortic left renal vein.[41]

Retrocaval ureter is thought to be due to persistence of right posterior cardinal vein with failure of development of the infrarenal right supracardinal vein. It occurs with a frequency of 0.2/1,000 population. In retrocaval ureter, the proximal right ureter courses medially behind the IVC, usually at L3 vertebral level and then courses anteriorly around the cava to partially encircle it. The anomaly is characterized by hydronephrosis and medial deviation (fish hook deformity) of the middle ureteral segment.

Venous Thrombosis

Inferior vena caval thrombus may result from proximal extension of thrombi from lower extremity, pelvis or renal veins. Intracaval tumor extension may occur via veins draining neoplasms such as renal cell carcinoma, hepatoma or adrenal carcinoma. CT and MRI perform well in evaluating IVC thrombosis and distinguishing tumor from bland thrombus.[42]

Tumor thrombus shows anatomic contiguity and an enhancement pattern identical to that of primary tumor **(Fig. 27)**. The bland thrombus does not enhance with contrast. Depiction of the supradiaphragmatic extent of the thrombus into the right atrium is important for surgical planning as it requires combined thoracoabdominal surgery, whereas thrombus that ends below the hepatic veins may require only an abdominal approach.[43]

In cases of chronic venous thrombosis, the affected vessel may not be identified if the thrombus is organized and contacted. In these cases careful evaluation reveals the absence of a vein in the expected location in combination with the presence of collateral vessels.

Retroperitoneal Fibrosis

Retroperitoneal fibrosis results from proliferation of fibrous tissue in the midline and para-aortic distribution. Approximately 70% cases of retroperitoneal fibrosis

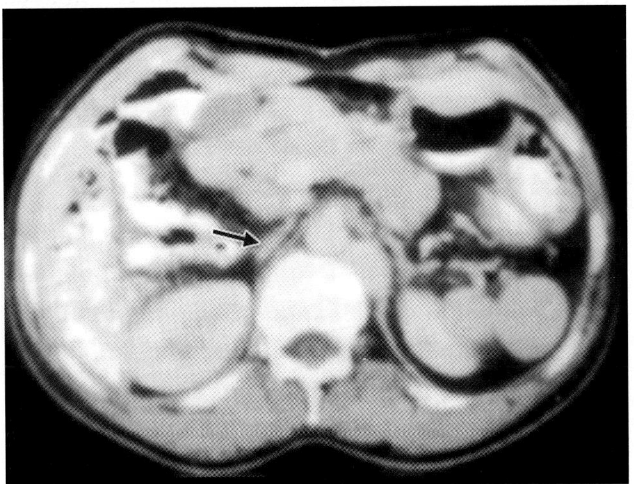

Fig. 26: Congenital polysplenia with IVC anomaly. CT scan shows multiple splenenculi and interrupted IVC with hemiazygos venous continuation. Linear density (arrow) seen lateral to the right crus is part of the right adrenal gland.

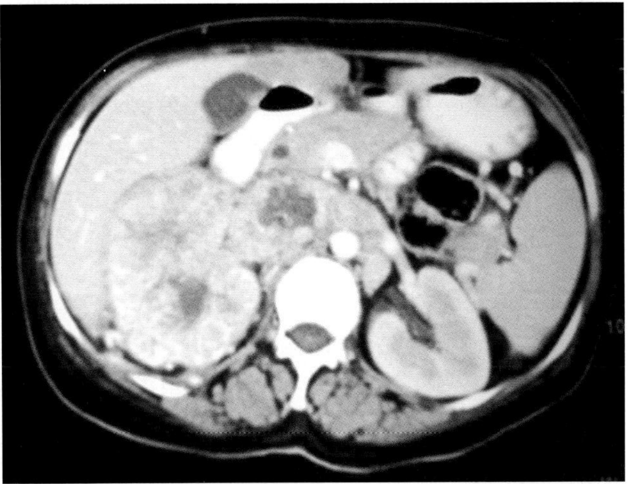

Fig. 27: IVC thrombus. Axial contrast-enhanced CT image in a 57-year-old man shows a large right renal cancer extending into the right renal vein and the IVC. The mass within the distended IVC is of the same attenuation as the primary tumor.

are idiopathic and are known as Ormond's disease. Other causes include various drugs (e.g. methysergide), previous abdominal surgery or radiation therapy, aortic hemorrhage, aortitis, aortic atherosclerosis, extravasation of urine, nonspecific gastrointestinal inflammation including appendicitis and diverticulitis, and infective pathologies including tuberculosis, histoplasmosis, syphilis, and actinomycosis. Retroperitoneal fibrosis may be a part of multifocal fibrosclerosis in which fibrous pseudotumor of the orbit, Riedel's thyroiditis, sclerosing cholangitis, and mediastinal fibrosis may also occur. Retroperitoneal malignancy especially metastases may also produce retroperitoneal fibrosis by producing a desmoplastic reaction to the tumor cells.[44]

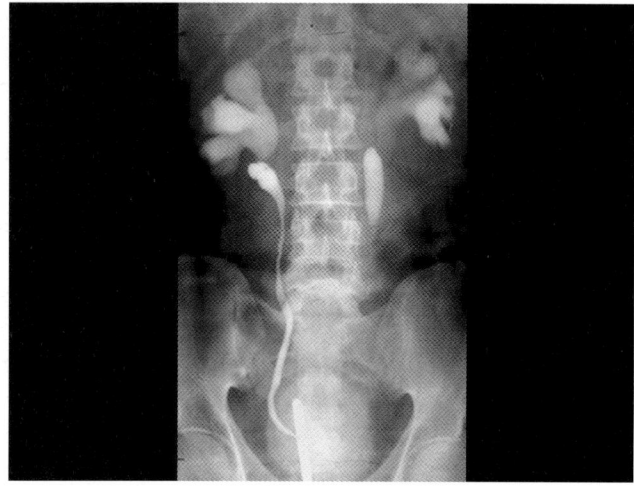

Fig. 28: Retrograde pyelography showing medial deviation of both ureters with hydroureteronephrosis in a patient with idiopathic retroperitoneal fibrosis.

Idiopathic retroperitoneal fibrosis most commonly occurs in patients between 40 years and 60 years of age. Males are affected twice as commonly as females. Fibrous plaque typically extends from below the level of the kidneys to the bifurcation of great vessels. The fibrous tissue may involve the IVC, aorta, ureters, and occasionally the iliac and renal veins in a symmetric or asymmetric distribution. Microscopically, collagen fibroblasts and inflammatory cells characterize idiopathic retroperitoneal fibrosis.

The clinical and laboratory findings of idiopathic retroperitoneal fibrosis are nonspecific and include fever, back pain, and raised erythrocyte sedimentation rate. Most patients have impaired renal functions. Excretory urography typically demonstrates bilateral hydronephrosis, which may be asymmetric and sometimes even unilateral. Retrograde studies demonstrate smooth tapering of the ureters that is most pronounced at the pelvic brim **(Fig. 28)**. The involvement may vary from focal to a long segment of ureter. Despite ureteral narrowing, there is no obstruction to retrograde passage of catheter in the ureter.

Ultrasonography demonstrates retroperitoneal fibrosis as a poorly demarcated periaortic mass that is typically echo-free or hypoechoic. Associated hydronephrosis may be seen. CT appearance of the fibrous plaque varies considerably—it can be midline or asymmetric, well circumscribed or poorly defined, localized or extensive **(Figs. 29A to C)**.

Contrast enhancement varies with the age of the process, while increased enhancement is seen in early stages due to vascularity of the immature fibrosis, chronic fibrosis does not enhance appreciably. MRI may

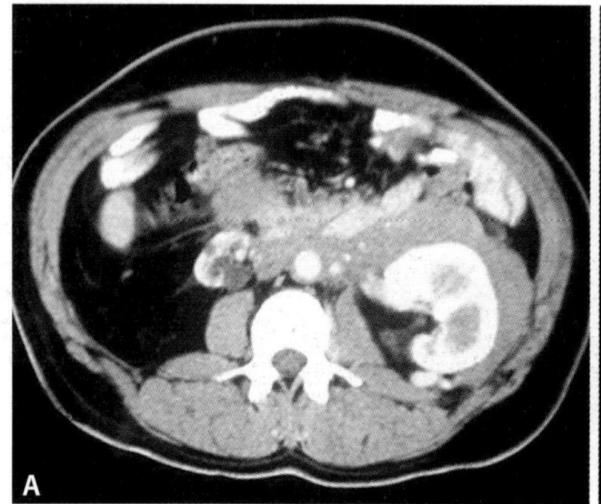

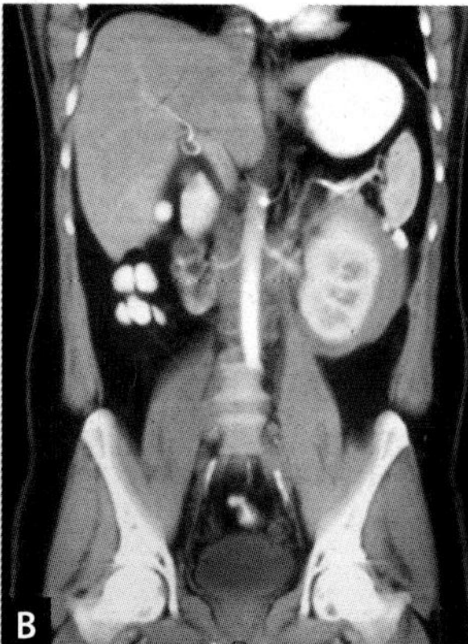

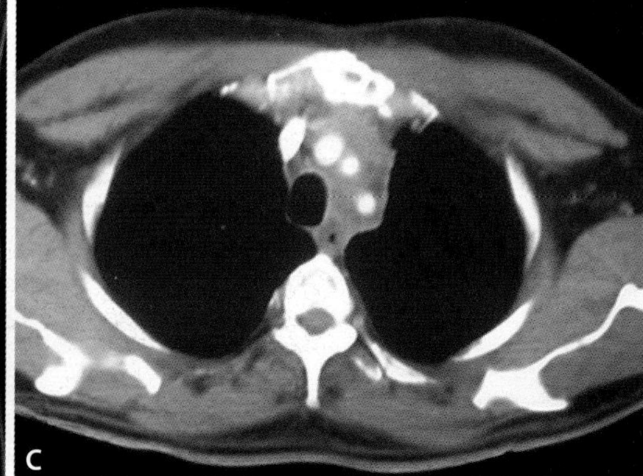

Figs. 29A to C: Retroperitoneal fibrosis. (A) Contrast-enhanced axial CT image shows hypodense, nonenhancing, infiltrating mass surrounding the aorta and IVC and extending into the left perirenal space. Right kidney is shrunken and hydronephrotic; (B) Coronal image shows the entire extent of the plaque like, perirenal soft tissue. Appearance is nonspecific, and differentials include malignancy such as lymphoma. Diagnosis was confirmed by biopsy; (C) CT scan though the chest shows evidence of mediastinal fibrosis, a frequent association of retroperitoneal fibrosis.

permit distinction between benign or non-neoplastic retroperitoneal fibrosis and malignant retroperitoneal fibrosis. In nonmalignant retroperitoneal fibrosis low or intermediate signal intensity on T1- and T2-weighted images has been reported in contrast to higher signal intensity in most malignancies on T2-weighted images **(Fig. 30)**. However, it has been recognized that benign retroperitoneal fibrosis also can have high signal intensity on T2-weighted images when it is in the active, inflammatory stage. MRI also demonstrates effect of the fibrotic mass on the aorta and IVC.

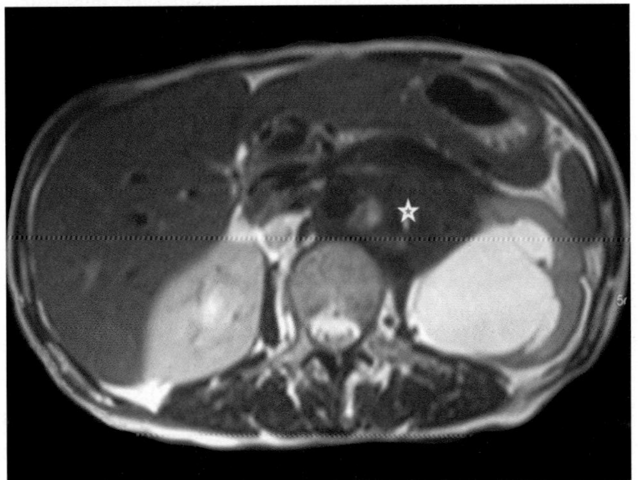

Fig. 30: Retroperitoneal fibrosis. Axial T2-weighted MR image shows a very hypointense mass (star), a finding consistent with the presence of mature fibrous tissue with little or no active inflammation.

Iliopsoas Muscle Compartment

Diseases affecting the iliopsoas muscle more commonly originate from adjacent structures and involve the muscle by direct extension. These include hemorrhage, infections, and tumors of the spine, kidneys, bowel, pancreas, and retroperitoneal lymph nodes. The iliopsoas is well evaluated by both CT and MRI. Coronal or sagittal planes provide direct evaluation of the full craniocaudal extent of the muscle.

Tuberculous spondylitis and lumbar discitis are the most common causes of an iliopsoas abscess in our country. Iliopsoas inflammatory masses display a variety of appearances, ranging from diffuse homogeneous enlargement to discrete masses containing central areas of low CT attenuation or high signal intensity on T2-weighted MR images. Postcontrast images show abscesses as expansile lesions with nonenhancing necrotic centers, intense peripheral enhancement, and enhancement of the surrounding tissues **(Figs. 31A and B)**. Calcification is detected occasionally on CT in inflammatory masses, particularly in patients with tuberculosis. MRI scores over CT in detecting intraspinal extension of the inflammatory granulation tissue and cord compression.

Neoplastic involvement of psoas muscle may occur with contiguous spread from metastatic lymph nodes from primary neoplasms (of kidney, testis, bladder, and cervix), lymphoma, renal cell carcinoma, and retroperitoneal sarcoma. Primary neoplasms of the psoas

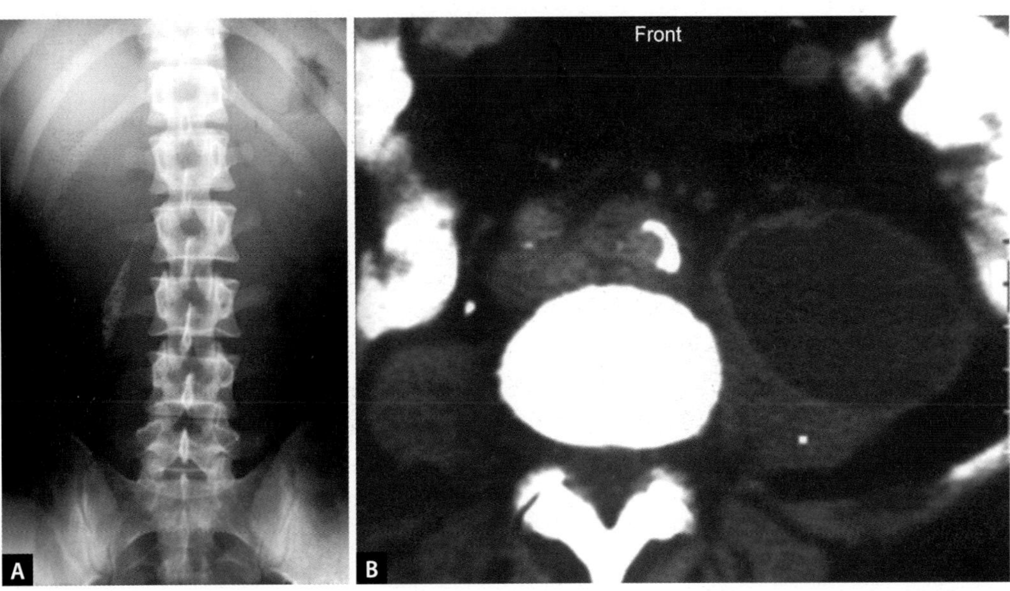

Figs. 31A and B: Psoas abscess. CT images show a well-defined, fluid density lesion in the left psoas muscle. It has a thin, peripheral enhancing rim and large necrotic center.

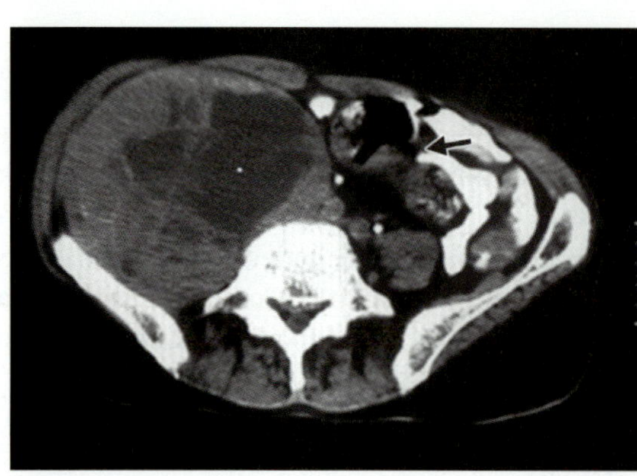

Fig. 32: Anaplastic carcinoma iliopsoas. Axial CT image shows a large heterogeneous mass involving the right iliacus muscle. The large, irregular, solid component (arrow) within the mass raises a possibility of malignancy.

muscle are rare. Iliopsoas malignancies often appear similar to other pathologies on imaging. The affected muscle is usually enlarged.

As with abscesses, iliopsoas tumor may have enhancing peripheral rims and central necrosis **(Fig. 32)**. A specific diagnosis is possible only when a large solid enhancing component is seen.

To conclude, RP is complex anatomical structure composed of multiple compartments, fascias, and planes. Better understanding of its anatomy helps in approaching retroperitoneal abnormalities and thus assist in planning further management. Sarcomas is the most common primary RP neoplasm and among non-neoplastic etiologies, inflammatory collections are the most common pathology encountered.

REFERENCES

1. Coffin A, Boulay-Coletta I, Sebbag-Sfez D, et al. Radioanatomy of the retroperitoneal space. Diagn Interv Imaging. 2015; 96(2):171-86.
2. Tirkes T, Sandrasegaran K, Patel AA, et al. Peritoneal and retroperitoneal anatomy and its relevance for cross-sectional imaging. Radiographics. 2012;32(2):437-51.
3. Korobkin M, Silverman PM, Quint LE, et al. CT of the extraperitoneal space: normal anatomy and fluid collections. Am J Roentgenol. 1992;159(5):933-42.
4. Raptopoulos V, Kleinman PK, Marks S, et al. Renal fascial pathway: posterior extension of pancreatic effusions within the anterior pararenal space. Radiology. 1986;158(2):367-74.
5. Molmenti EP, Balfe DM, Kanterman RY, et al. Anatomy of the retroperitoneum: observations of the distribution of pathologic fluid collections. Radiology. 1996;200(1):95-103.
6. Raptopoulos V, Lei QF, Touliopoulos P, et al. Why perirenal disease does not extend into the pelvis: the importance of closure of the cone of the renal fasciae. Am J Roentgenol. 1995;164(5):1179-84.
7. Aizenstein RI, Owens C, Sabnis S, et al. The perinephric space and renal fascia: review of normal anatomy, pathology, and pathways of disease spread. Crit Rev Diagn Imaging. 1997;38(4):325-67.
8. Gore RM, Balfe DM, Aizenstein RI, et al. The great escape: interfascial decompression planes of the retroperitoneum. Am J Roentgenol. 2000;175(2):363-70.
9. Kang PS, Spain JW. Multidetector CT angiography of the abdomen. Radiol Clin North Am. 2005;43(6):963-76, vii.
10. Kandpal H, Sharma R, Gamangatti S, et al. Imaging the inferior vena cava: a road less traveled. Radiogr Rev Publ Radiol Soc N Am Inc. 2008;28(3):669-89.
11. Glockner JF. Three-dimensional gadolinium-enhanced MR angiography: applications for abdominal imaging. Radiogr Rev Publ Radiol Soc N Am Inc. 2001;21(2):357-70.
12. Vesselle HJ, Miraldi FD. FDG PET of the retroperitoneum: normal anatomy, variants, pathologic conditions, and strategies to avoid diagnostic pitfalls. Radiogr Rev Publ Radiol Soc N Am Inc. 1998;18(4):805-23; discussion 823-824.
13. Messiou C, Moskovic E, Vanel D, et al. Primary retroperitoneal soft tissue sarcoma: Imaging appearances, pitfalls and diagnostic algorithm. Eur J Surg Oncol. 2017;43(7):1191-8.
14. Sanyal R, Remer EM. Radiology of the retroperitoneum: case-based review. Am J Roentgenol. 2009;192: S112-7. Available from: https://www.ajronline.org/doi/full/10.2214/AJR.07.7064. [Last accessed, October, 2019]
15. Nishino M, Hayakawa K, Minami M, et al. Primary retroperitoneal neoplasms: CT and MR imaging findings with anatomic and pathologic diagnostic clues. Radiographics. 2003;23(1):45-57.
16. Goenka AH, Shah SN, Remer EM. Imaging of the retroperitoneum. Radiol Clin North Am. 2012;50(2):333-55.
17. Craig WD, Fanburg-Smith JC, Henry LR, et al. Fat-containing lesions of the retroperitoneum: radiologic-pathologic correlation. Radiographics. 2009;29(1):261-90.
18. Kumar A, Suman SK, Kumar B, et al. Giant retroperitoneal liposarcoma: imaging and literature. Journal of Evolution of Medical and Dental Sciences. 2015;4(36):6315-22. Available from: https://www.jemds.com/latest-articles.php?at_id=7673. [Last accessed October, 2019]
19. Song T, Shen J, Liang BL, et al. Retroperitoneal liposarcoma: MR characteristics and pathological correlative analysis. Abdom Imaging. 2007;32(5):668-74.
20. Hartman DS, Hayes WS, Choyke PL, et al. From the archives of the AFIP. Leiomyosarcoma of the retroperitoneum and inferior vena cava: radiologic-pathologic correlation. Radiogr Rev Publ Radiol Soc N Am Inc. 1992;12(6):1203-20.
21. Monteagudo Cortecero J, Guirau Rubio MD, Payá Romá A. Leiomyosarcoma of the inferior vena cava: AIRP best cases in radiologic-pathologic correlation. Radiographics. 2015;35(2):616-20.
22. Cohan RH, Baker ME, Cooper C, et al. Computed tomography of primary retroperitoneal malignancies. J Comput Assist Tomogr. 1988;12(5):804-10.
23. Lee KY, Oh Y-W, Noh HJ, et al. Extraadrenal paragangliomas of the body: imaging features. Am J Roentgenol. 2006; 187(2):492-504.
24. Rha SE, Byun JY, Jung SE, et al. Neurogenic tumors in the abdomen: tumor types and imaging characteristics. Radiographics. 2003;23(1):29-43.
25. Hulnick DH, Megibow AJ, Naidich DP, et al. Abdominal tuberculosis: CT evaluation. Radiology. 1985;157(1):199-204.
26. Warshauer DM, Lee JKT. Imaging manifestations of abdominal sarcoidosis. Am J Roentgenol. 2004;182(1):15-28.

27. Gossios K, Nikolaides C, Bai M, et al. Widespread Castleman disease: CT findings. Eur Radiol. 1996;6(1):95-8.
28. Kehagias D, Pafiti A, Vaos N, et al. Retroperitoneal lymphangioleiomyomatosis: CT appearance. Eur Radiol. 1998;8(3):471-3.
29. Sheth S, Fishman EK. Non-Hodgkin lymphoma: pattern of disease at spiral CT. Crit Rev Diagn Imaging. 2001;42(6):307-56.
30. Apter S, Avigdor A, Gayer G, et al. Calcification in lymphoma occurring before therapy: CT features and clinical correlation. Am J Roentgenol. 2002;178(4):935-8.
31. Schöder H, Moskowitz C. PET imaging for response assessment in lymphoma: potential and limitations. Radiol Clin North Am. 2008;46(2):225-41, viii.
32. Specht L. 2-[18F]fluoro-2-deoxyglucose positron-emission tomography in staging, response evaluation, and treatment planning of lymphomas. Semin Radiat Oncol. 2007;17(3):190-7.
33. Radin R. HIV infection: analysis in 259 consecutive patients with abnormal abdominal CT findings. Radiology. 1995;197(3):712-22.
34. Bellin MF, Lebleu L, Meric JB. Evaluation of retroperitoneal and pelvic lymph node metastases with MRI and MR lymphangiography. Abdom Imaging. 2003;28(2):155-63.
35. Ishikawa K, Idoguchi K, Tanaka H, et al. Classification of acute pancreatitis based on retroperitoneal extension: application of the concept of interfascial planes. Eur J Radiol. 2006;60(3):445-52.
36. Missiroli C, Singh AK. Nontraumatic emergencies of abdominal aorta. Semin Ultrasound CT MR. 2008;29(5):369-77.
37. Taneja K, Sharma S, Das B, et al. Aortic aneurysm and dissection: Imaging with computerised axial tomography. Indian J Thorac Cardiovasc Surg. 1994;10(1):52-6.
38. Rakita D, Newatia A, Hines JJ, et al. Spectrum of CT findings in rupture and impending rupture of abdominal aortic aneurysms. Radiogr Rev Publ Radiol Soc N Am Inc. 2007;27(2):497-507.
39. Anagnostopoulos CE, Prabhakar MJ, Kittle CF. Aortic dissections and dissecting aneurysms. Am J Cardiol. 1972;30(3):263-73.
40. Aljabri B, MacDonald PS, Satin R, et al. Incidence of major venous and renal anomalies relevant to aortoiliac surgery as demonstrated by computed tomography. Ann Vasc Surg. 2001;15(6):615-8.
41. Onbaş O, Kantarci M, Koplay M, et al. Congenital anomalies of the aorta and vena cava: 16-detector-row CT imaging findings. Diagn Interv Radiol Ank Turk. 2008;14(3):163-71.
42. Cuevas C, Raske M, Bush WH, et al. Imaging primary and secondary tumor thrombus of the inferior vena cava: multidetector computed tomography and magnetic resonance imaging. Curr Probl Diagn Radiol. 2006;35(3):90-101.
43. Lawrentschuk N, Gani J, Riordan R, et al. Multidetector computed tomography vs magnetic resonance imaging for defining the upper limit of tumour thrombus in renal cell carcinoma: a study and review. BJU Int. 2005;96(3):291-5.
44. Cronin CG, Lohan DG, Blake MA, et al. Retroperitoneal Fibrosis: A Review of Clinical Features and Imaging Findings. Am J Roentgenol. 2008;191(2):423-31.

Chapter 25

Urinary Tract Trauma

Atin Kumar, Shivanand Gamanagatti

INTRODUCTION

Approximately 10% of all traumatic injuries involve the urinary tract, most often the kidney.[1] Although trauma to the urinary tract is seldom the cause of death, serious morbidity can result, if such injuries are missed. An accurate radiographic and imaging evaluation is important to determine the presence and extent of injury for the proper management of the patients. Evaluation of the urinary tract trauma should be integrated into the overall management of the trauma patient.

Blunt trauma accounts for 80–90% of all renal injuries.[1] These are primarily due to deceleration injuries in motor vehicle accidents, falls, or assault. In approximately 10–20% of the patients, penetrating injuries result due to gunshot or knife wounds. The penetrating injuries are much more likely to result in high-grade renal injuries compared with blunt trauma. Pre-existing kidney lesions, e.g. renal tumors, hydronephrosis, polycystic kidney disease, and horseshoe kidneys, make the kidney more susceptible to the injury. In 80% of the patients with penetrating trauma and 75% of blunt trauma patients, associated injuries, e.g. splenic rupture, liver laceration, and injuries to the small and large bowel, are seen.[2] In about 50% of these patients, bone fractures are present. Iatrogenic causes such as surgery, interventional procedures, and biopsies are also associated with trauma to the urinary tract.

RENAL TRAUMA

Since the late 1980s, the prevailing techniques of imaging and clinical management of renal trauma have changed dramatically. Consensus has been building toward a conservative approach and successful clinical management must be based on an accurate assessment of the extent of injury.

Imaging Work-up in a Patient with Suspected Renal Trauma

Trauma to the kidney may be suspected to be minor or significant on the basis of clinical picture, nature, and site of injury. An unstable patient may undergo no imaging work-up, if an immediate surgery is indicated on clinical grounds. In a clinically stable patient with abdominal trauma and with suspected abdominal organ injury and/or hypotension, kidneys are imaged as part of a standard abdomen and pelvic computed tomography (CT). The current globally accepted indications specifically for radiological evaluation of urinary tract in trauma patients are as follows:[2–6]

- Macroscopic hematuria (visible to human eye)
- Microscopic hematuria (>5 RBC/high power field) with hypotension (systolic BP < 90 mm Hg at any time during evaluation) or other significant abdominal injuries which necessitate imaging
- Injuries associated with renal injury such as direct contusion or hematoma of flank soft tissues, fractures of lumbar spine, lower rib, and transverse process
- Penetrating trauma with any degree of hematuria in stable patients.

Earlier, children with any degree of hematuria were also an indication for radiological evaluation, but recently there has been a trend to have an approach similar to an adult patient. Renal imaging is not required in a patient with minor trauma having microhematuria without shock.

An approach to a patient having significant trauma can be outlined as shown in **Flowchart 1**.

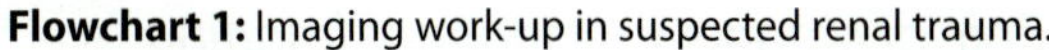

Flowchart 1: Imaging work-up in suspected renal trauma.

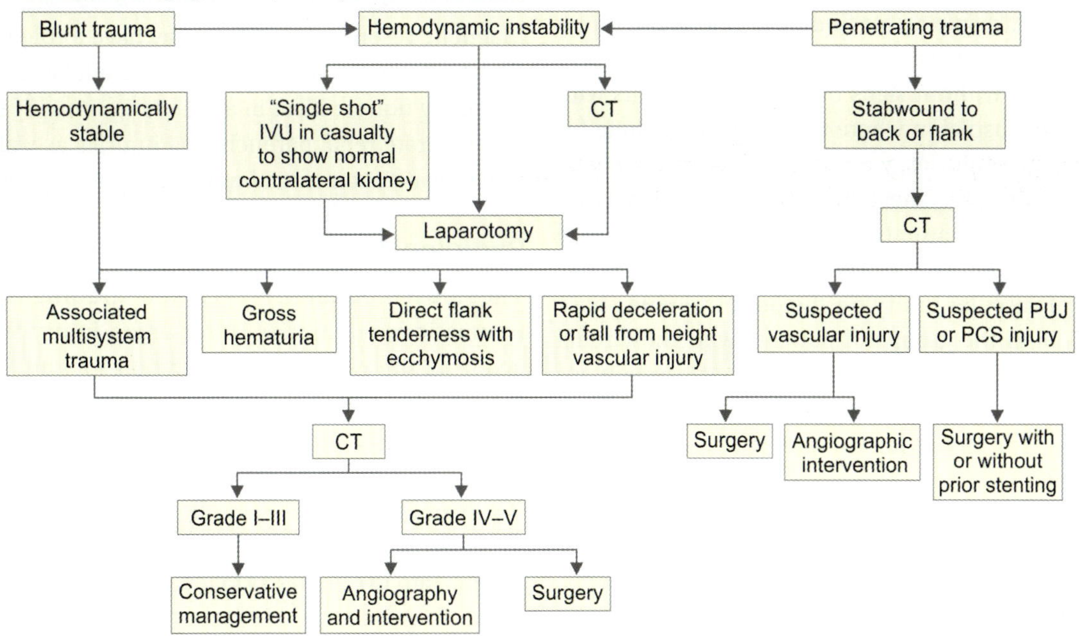

(PUJ: pelviureteric junction; PCS: postconcussion syndrome)

Role of Radiography (Plain Radiographs)

Widespread availability and use of CT and ultrasound have replaced abdominal radiography for evaluation of renal trauma. However, radiographs have a role in the setting of penetrating abdominal trauma.

Role of Ultrasound

Specific visceral injuries are poorly assessed on ultrasonography. The value of sonography lies primarily in the rapid establishment of the presence of hemoperitoneum in an unstable patient.

In the setting of abdominal trauma, it is usually done with Focused Assessment with Sonography in Trauma (FAST) protocol. It is insensitive to detect retroperitoneal blood and renal parenchymal injuries.

Role of Intravenous Urography

The role of intravenous urogram (IVU) in suspected renal trauma is limited. It has been replaced by CT which is now easily available and is more sensitive than IVU for parenchymal injuries, urinary contrast extravasation, and other abdominal injuries. However, IVU still has a role, depending on the preference of the surgeon, to establish gross function and evaluation of the uninjured contralateral kidney in hemodynamically unstable patients going for surgery and for urological evaluation of patients who are already in the operating room.[2,3] The technique followed is usually a tailored "single-shot" study with a radiograph obtained 10 minutes after administration of intravenous contrast. However, if time and condition of the patient permit, a precontrast plain radiograph, and delayed radiographs may be taken for assessment of urinary contrast extravasation and for delayed function.

Role of Computed Tomography

The contrast-enhanced CT (CECT) scan is currently the investigation of choice for radiological evaluation of patients with blunt abdominal trauma.[4,5] It has replaced IVU for evaluation of renal trauma. The current trend of conservative management of blunt renal trauma has further enhanced the role of CT because 80% of renal injuries seen on CT are self-limiting.

Computed tomography accurately assesses all the criteria essential for the management of renal trauma, viz. extent of damaged nonviable tissue, amount of perirenal hemorrhage, extravasation of urine, and evidence of renal pedicle or vascular injury.

The CT of abdomen and pelvis (along with chest) is usually done in a hemodynamically stable patient who is being evaluated for any suspected abdominal injury. Many institutions routinely do a dual-phase CECT with arterial and portal venous phase. However, some other institutions follow the practice of doing a standard portal venous phase after contrast administration with another delayed phase, if indicated, based on the findings on this phase for suspected vascular injury. At our institution which is a grade 1 trauma center, we routinely do a dual

(arterial and venous) phase CT in all patients in whom the index of clinical suspicion for finding a solid organ injury is high. Essentially, these patients are those who are FAST positive with or without signs of shock. In patients with a low index of suspicion where the CT is being done for ruling out organ injuries, we routinely perform a single portal venous phase. These are most commonly FAST negative. In these patients, we acquire an immediate delayed phase after the portal venous phase if we find any suspicion of vascular injury on the portal venous phase images. In both the groups of patients who show renal lacerations extending up to the pelvicalyceal system, we acquire a 3–5 min delayed limited acquisition through the kidneys for detection of pelvicalyceal contrast extravasation.

Multiplanar reformatted images and three-dimensional images including CT urographic images can significantly aid in the evaluation.

Role of Angiography

Catheter angiography is not indicated as a diagnostic test in patients with renal trauma. However, in the last two decades, there is an increasing role of therapeutic angiographic interventions as a nonsurgical therapy in the form of transcatheter embolization of ongoing hemorrhage in renal trauma in hemodynamically stable patients. Angioembolization is indicated for vascular complications of injury including post-traumatic pseudoaneurysms and arteriovenous fistulas. In certain situations of acute traumatic main renal artery thrombosis, thrombolysis of renal artery thrombus with vascular stent placement can be done provided the time to injury is very short (less than 2 hours) or there is a solitary functioning kidney.

Role of Retrograde Pyelography

Retrograde pyelography has a role in the specific setting of suspected renal pelvic, ureteropelvic junction (UPJ), or ureteral injury, which has not been adequately excluded on CT. However, it is often not practically possible in an emergent situation and also does not characterize renal injuries.

Role of Radionuclide Renal Scintigraphy

With widespread availability of CT, radionuclide scintigraphy is rarely used in an acute trauma setting. It may have a role in demonstrating the function of an injured kidney in patients allergic to iodinated contrast and in follow-up of repair of renovascular trauma.

Role of Magnetic Resonance Imaging

Magnetic resonance imaging may have a role in patients where CT is contraindicated or not available. However, it is usually not practical in an acute trauma setting. It can demonstrate renal parenchymal injuries as well as renal function after contrast administration.

Radiological Findings

The most commonly accepted grading system of traumatic renal injuries is the Organ Injury Scale (OIS) given by the American Association for the Surgery of Trauma (AAST). The original grading scale for renal injuries was given in 1989 and has been revised in 2018.[7,8] The grading is based on the depth of injury and involvement of vessels or the collecting system.[7] The AAST 2018 OIS for renal injuries[8] classifies the renal trauma into five grades as follows.

Grade 1

Grade 1 renal injuries account for approximately 75–80% of all renal injuries. They include the following:

- *Contusion:* Focal ill-defined area of hypodensity, which shows decreased enhancement as compared to adjacent normal renal parenchyma **(Figs. 1A and B)**. These are better appreciated on the portal venous phase which corresponds to the parenchymal phase for the kidneys. On the arterial phase images (which correspond to the corticomedullary phase for the kidneys), the detection of contusion may be limited as there is suboptimal enhancement of renal pyramids. They need to be differentiated from segmental infarcts which constitute grade 4 renal injury. Contusions generally are rounded in shape with ill-defined margins and show some contrast enhancement, especially on the delayed phase. In contrast, segmental infarcts are wedge shaped with well-defined margins and do not show any contrast enhancement even on the delayed phase. A global contusion may show a striated nephrogram or spidery collecting system (due to parenchymal edema).[9,10]
- *Subcapsular hematoma:* A hyperattenuating [40–60 Hounsfield unit (HU)] fluid collection lying between the renal parenchyma and the renal capsule. It leads to mass effect over the underlying renal parenchyma resulting in flattening of its contour **(Figs. 2A and B)**. It does not enhance on contrast administration.

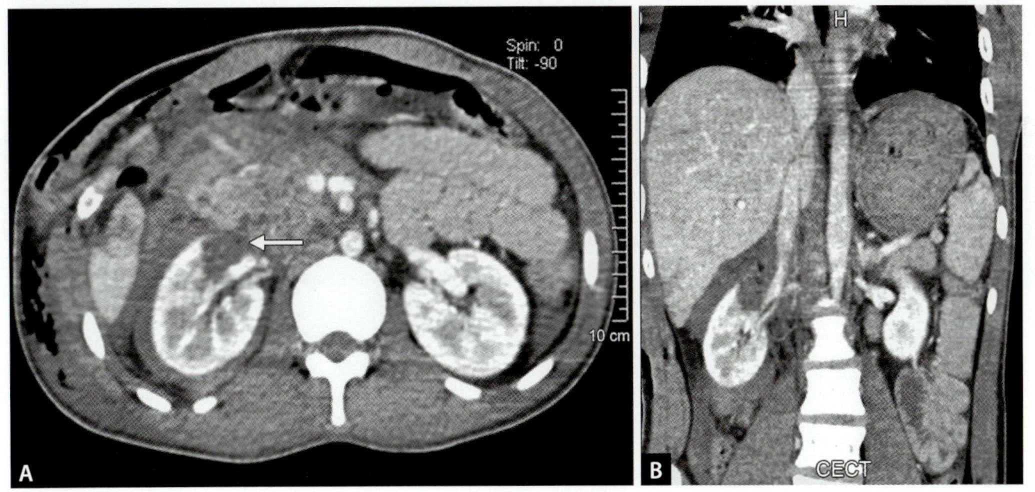

Figs. 1A and B: Axial (A) and multiformatted coronal (B) CECT shows a focal hypodense area (arrow) in anterior part of right kidney suggestive of contusion.

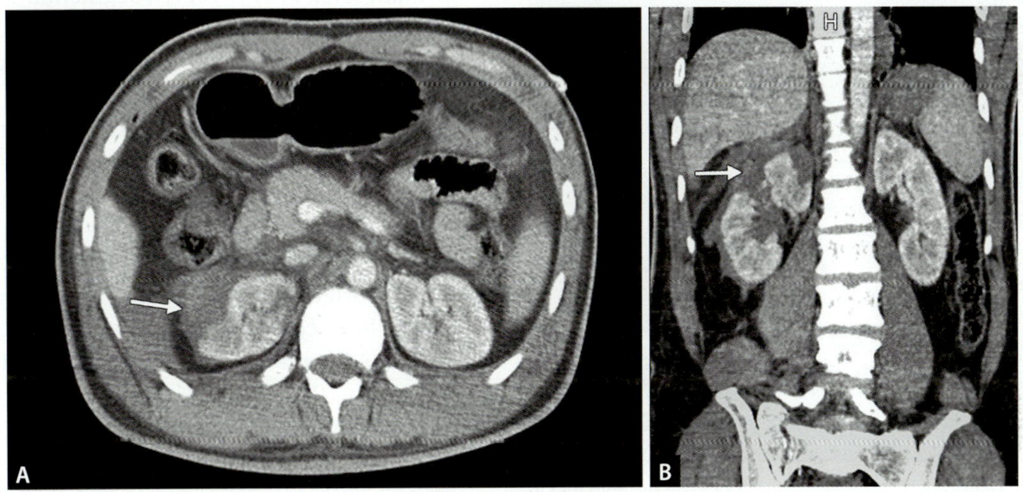

Figs. 2A and B: Axial (A) and multiformatted coronal (B) CECT shows a hyperdense nonenhancing subcapsular hematoma (arrows).

Grade 2

Grade 2 renal injuries include the following:

- *Perirenal hematoma:* An ill-defined hyperattenuating fluid collection in perinephric space between the renal parenchyma and Gerota's fascia **(Figs. 3A and B)**. It occurs after laceration of the renal capsule.
- *Laceration:* A superficial (<1 cm deep), irregular or linear, low-attenuation area within the renal parenchyma which may contain blood or clot. It does not enhance after contrast administration. The laceration does not extend to the collecting system.

Grade 3

Grade 3 renal injuries include the following:

- *Lacerations:* >1 cm in depth but do not involve the collecting system **(Fig. 4)**. The lacerations may be reaching very close to the collecting system. The integrity of the collecting system can be ascertained by evaluating the excretory phase images which do not show extravasation of urinary contrast.
- *Vascular injury:* A contained vascular injury (pseudoaneurysm or arteriovenous fistula) or active bleeding limited within Gerota's fascia. The vascular injury is classified under grade 3, if there are no other associated features to upgrade the renal injury. These injuries are included new in the revised 2018 version and were not present in an earlier version of the OIS scale.

Grade 4

Grade 4 renal injuries include the following:

- *Lacerations:* Deep lacerations extending through the kidney parenchyma into the collecting system.

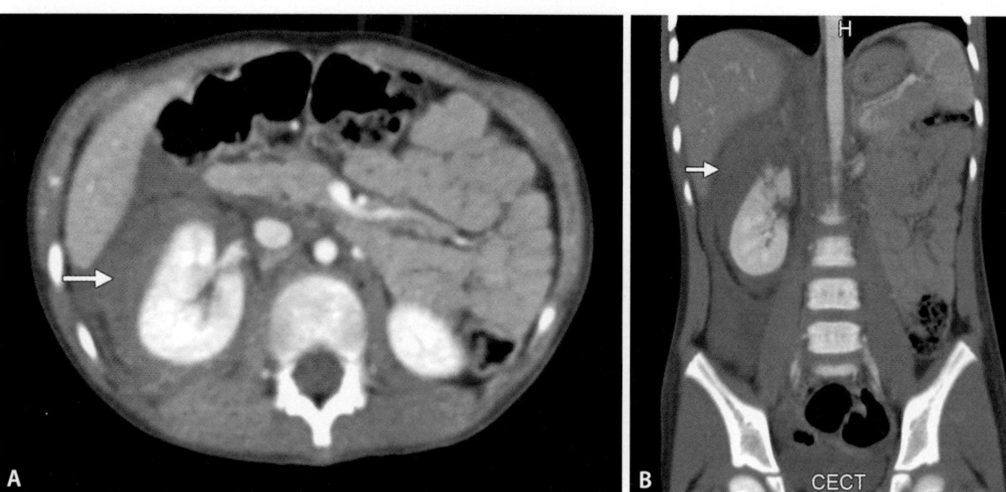

Figs. 3A and B: Axial (A) and multiformatted coronal (B) CECT shows perinephric hematoma (arrows) around right kidney.

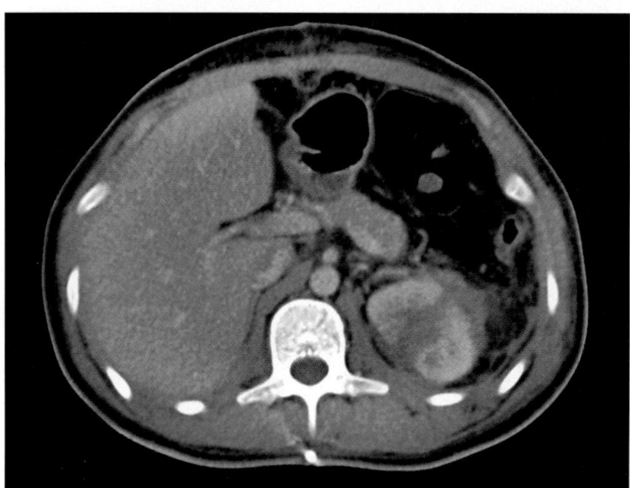

Fig. 4: Axial CECT abdomen shows a linear hypodense nonenhancing laceration involving upper pole of left kidney.

It leads to extravasation of urine and urinary contrast. Delayed phase CT in the excretory phase is important to demonstrate urinary contrast extravasation **(Figs. 5A to D)**. The lacerations may also involve the renal pelvis or the UPJ. If there is complete ureteropelvic avulsion, then urinary contrast extravasation is seen medial to the kidney without opacification of the ureter **(Figs. 6A and B)**. Opacification of the ureter in this setting would indicate a partial disruption of the pelviureteric junction (PUJ). Retrograde pyelography may be required for definitive diagnosis to demonstrate the distal ureter if CT or IVU fail to demonstrate distal ureteric filling.

- *Vascular injury:* Segmental renal artery or vein intimal injury/thrombus
- *Infarction:* Segmental or complete. It occurs due to dissection, thrombosis, or laceration of the segmental or main renal artery. On CT, segmental infarct is seen as a peripheral-based, well-circumscribed, wedge-shaped focal nonenhancing area through the renal parenchyma in a radial or segmental orientation **(Figs. 7A and B)**. The main renal artery thrombosis occurs due to stretching of the renal artery between the artery origin anchored to aorta and mobile kidney. This leads to an intimal tear with subsequent thrombosis. CT reveals abrupt termination of the renal artery after its origin with nonenhancing renal parenchyma except for a cortical rim sign, which usually appears few days later, and retrograde opacification of renal vein from IVC **(Figs. 8A and B)**. Devascularization without active bleeding adjacent to the kidney should be classified as grade 4. The role of renal angiography with thrombolysis is not well established. It may be done in selected cases, ideally within a couple of hours after trauma.[9] The time window can be extended till 12–24 hours in a patient with only one kidney or bilateral renal artery thrombosis.
- *Active bleeding:* Uncontained hemorrhage secondary to injury of segmental or main renal vessels extending outside the confines of Gerota's fascia into the retroperitoneum or peritoneum.

Grade 5

Grade 5 renal injuries include the following:

- *Shattered kidney:* It refers to gross renal parenchymal disruption secondary to multiple renal lacerations associated with devitalized areas due to renal infarction **(Figs. 9A and B)**. There is often loss of identifiable renal parenchymal anatomy.
- Main renal artery or vein laceration or avulsion injuries at hilum.

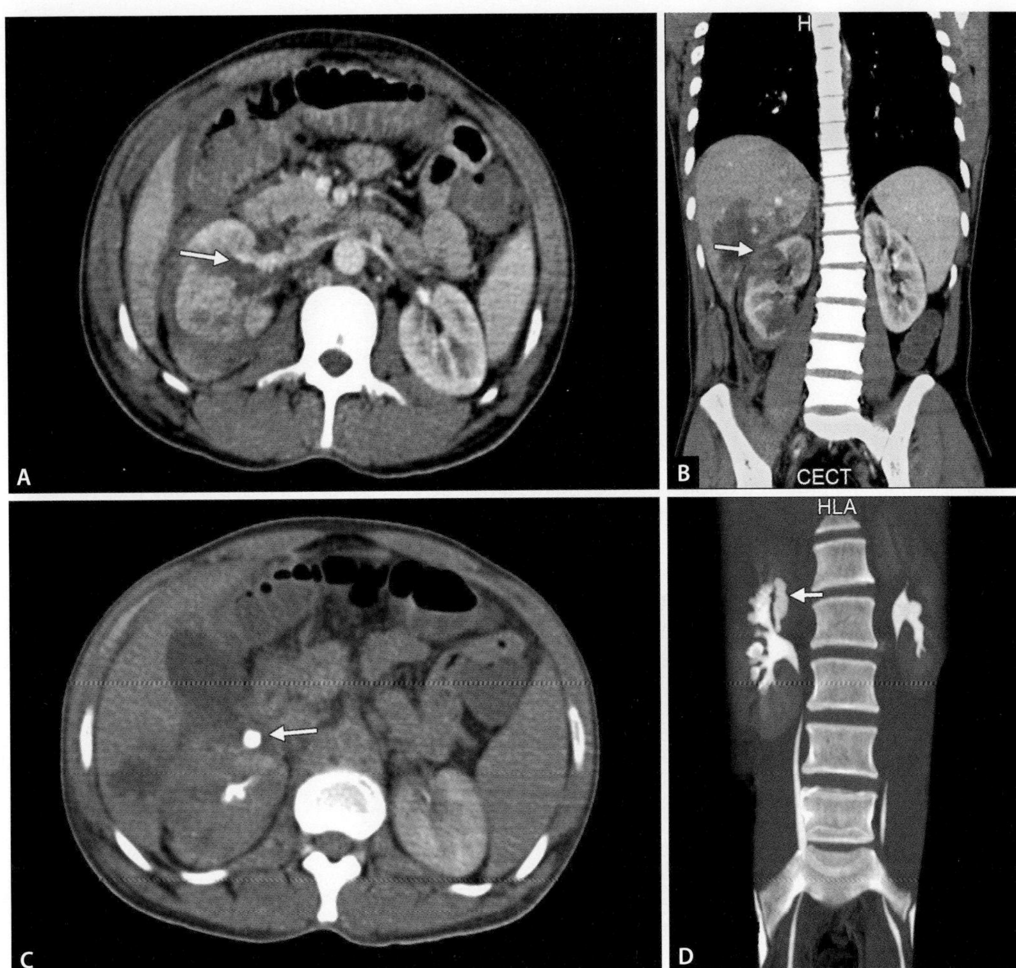

Figs. 5A to D: Axial (A) and multiformatted coronal (B) CECT shows a deep laceration (arrows) in upper pole of right kidney extending into pelvicalyceal system with perinephric hematoma. Delayed phase axial CT (C) shows contrast lying outside the kidney on its anterior aspect signifying urinary contrast extravasation. Reformatted coronal MIP image (D) clearly shows the extravasated contrast from upper calyceal injury.

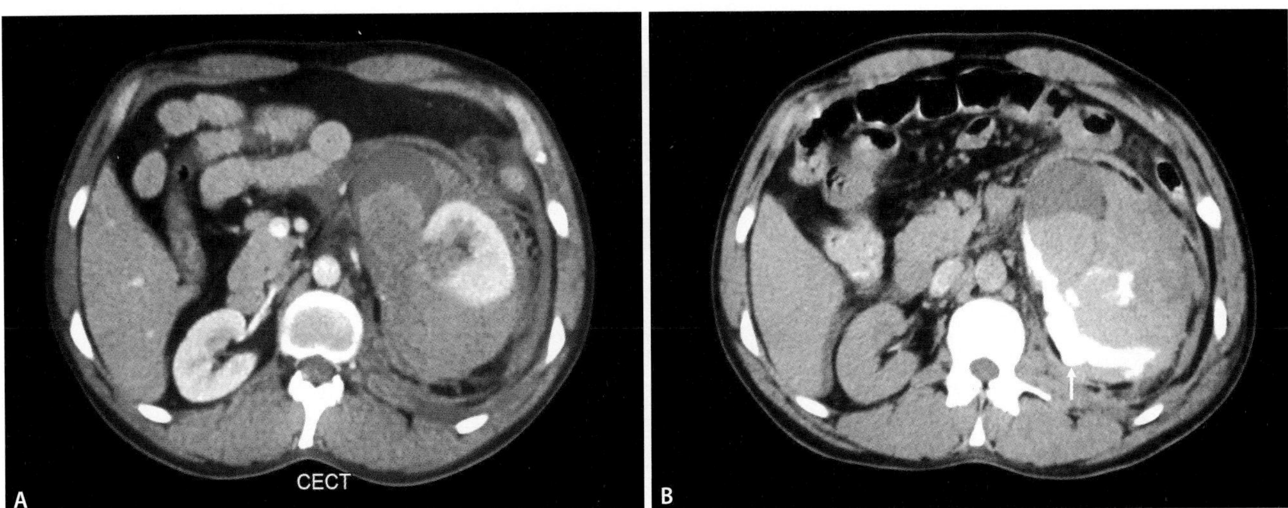

Figs. 6A and B: Axial CECT abdomen (A) shows extensive left perirenal hematoma/fluid collection. Delayed phase axial image (B) shows urinary contrast extravasation in medial perinephric space (arrow) signifying renal pelvic avulsion.

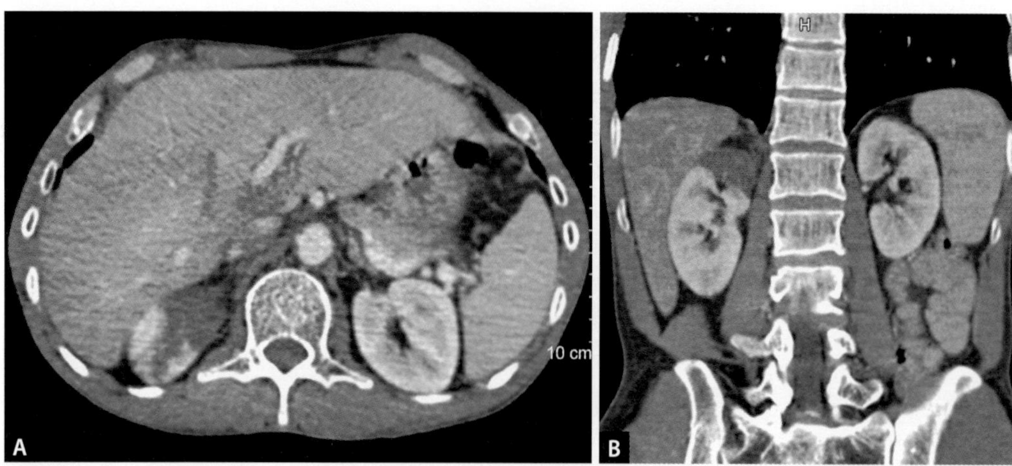

Figs. 7A and B: Axial (A) and multiformatted coronal (B) CECT shows a well-defined peripheral based wedge-shaped nonenhancing area in upper pole of right kidney suggestive of a segmental infarct.

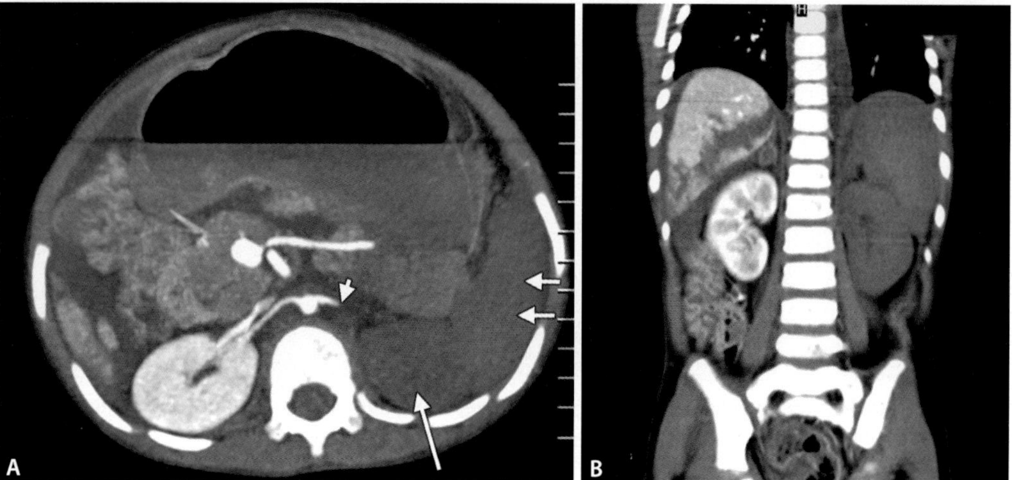

Figs. 8A and B: Axial MIP (A) and multiformatted coronal (B) CECT shows nonenhancing left kidney (long arrow) with abrupt termination of left renal artery (short arrow). Also note devascularized spleen [medium arrows in (A) and large liver laceration (B)].

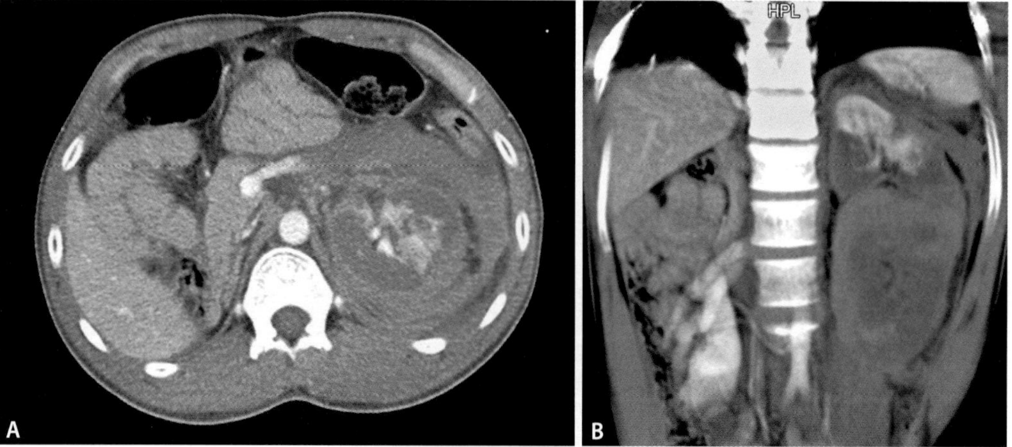

Figs. 9A and B: Axial (A) and multiformatted coronal (B) CECT shows completely shattered left kidney with large devitalized (nonenhancing) areas.

- *Devascularized kidney with active bleeding:* It occurs secondary to the main renal arterial laceration or avulsion. This is seen on imaging as extravasation of vascular contrast into the perirenal region with a large hematoma in the medial compartment close to the hilum **(Figs. 10A to C)**. It is important to differentiate it from the main renal artery thrombosis without laceration or avulsion which also leads to devascularized kidney and is classified under grade 4 injury. Presence of active bleed/hematoma adjacent to the main renal artery signifies avulsion making it grade 5 injury. Renal vein injury is seen on CT as intraluminal thrombus with features of renal vein occlusion including increased size of kidney, diminished or delayed enhancement and delayed excretion **(Figs. 11A and B)**.

For bilateral injuries, one grade has to be advanced up to grade 3.

Renal Trauma with Pre-existing Abnormality

A kidney harboring a preexisting abnormality is at more risk for injury in blunt abdominal trauma, especially in children.[11] Hydronephrosis or extrarenal pelvis is at more risk of rupture. Cysts and tumors can also frequently hemorrhage after trauma.

An ectopic or horseshoe kidney is also more prone to trauma because it is less protected **(Figs. 12A and B)**.

Management

The classification of renal trauma into grades correlates with the need for surgery. In general, the trend is toward

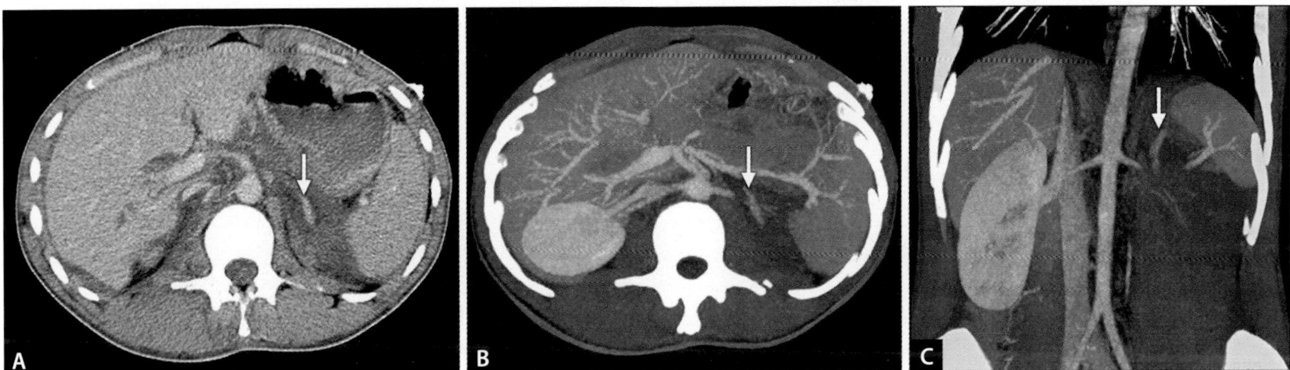

Figs. 10A to C: Axial CECT abdomen (A) shows a focal hyperattenuating area (arrow) in left suprarenal location within a hypodense hematoma. Axial (B) and reformatted coronal (C) MIP images clearly shows the arterial contrast extravasation (arrows) within the left perinephric hematoma. Note the abrupt termination of transected left renal artery and nonenhancing left kidney.

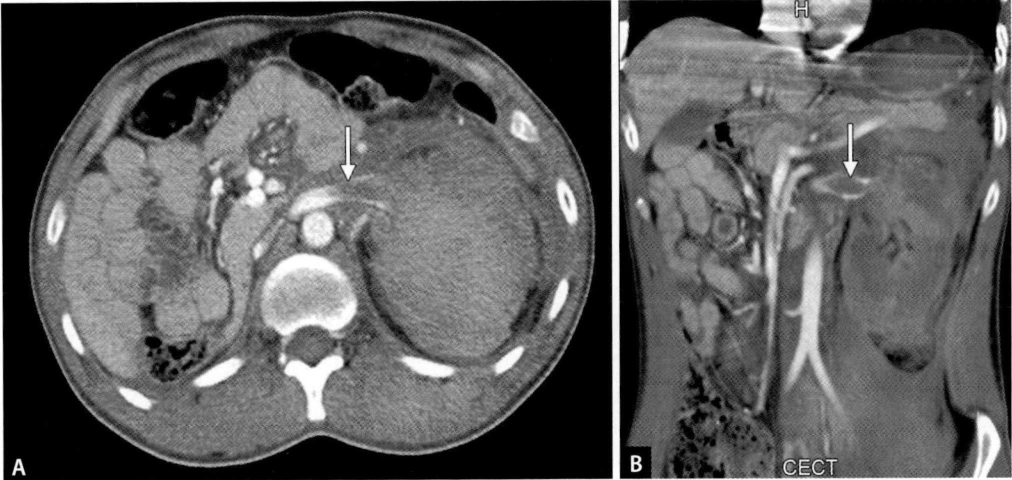

Figs. 11A and B: Axial (A) and multiformatted coronal (B) CECT shows an enlarged nonenhancing left kidney with large perinephric hematoma with a hypodense thrombus in the left main renal vein (arrows).

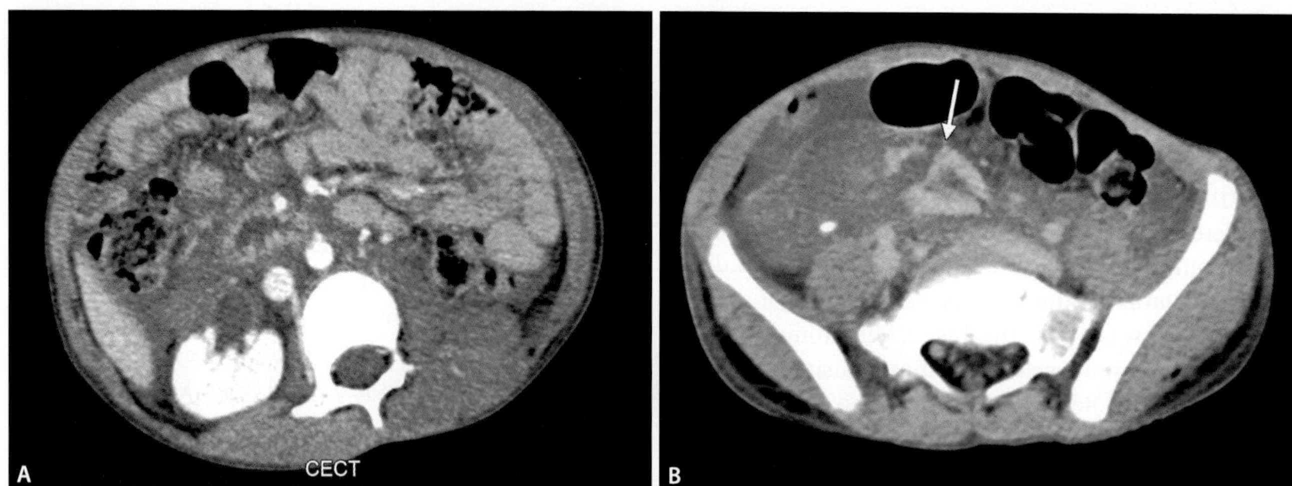

Figs. 12A and B: Axial CECT (A) at the level of kidneys shows left kidney is not present in left renal fossa. Axial image through the pelvis (B) shows extensive lacerations of ectopic left kidney (arrow).

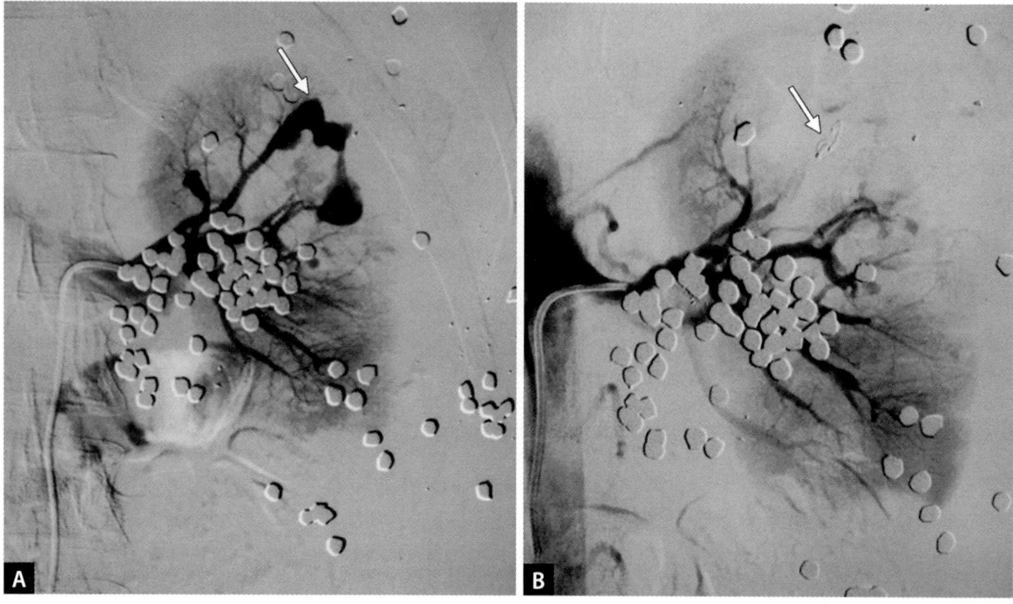

Figs. 13A and B: DSA image (A) of selective left renal artery injection in a patient injured with multiple pellets shows pseudoaneurysm formation with active bleed (arrow) in upper pole of left kidney. The involved upper polar segmental branch was selectively embolized with coil (arrow in B) resulting in thrombosis of pseudoaneurysm.

nonoperative management for all but most severe injuries.[12] Grade 1–3 injuries are classified as low-grade injuries. These constitute >90% of all renal injuries and are almost always managed conservatively. The only absolute indication for active intervention in these grade patients is presence of life-threatening active hemorrhage which may be dealt with angiographic embolization **(Figs. 13A and B)** or surgical exploration.[4]

Most of grade 4 injuries can also be managed conservatively. Even large urinary extravasations resolve spontaneously on conservative management. Drainage is required in cases of increasing symptoms of pain, fever, or ileus. It is also indicated if the urinary collections are increasing in size or get infected. Ureteric stent placement is the preferred method for drainage and can be supplemented, if required, by percutaneous drainage of these collections with or without percutaneous nephrostomy.[3,13] If they fail to resolve, surgical repair may be warranted. Grade 4 injuries with significant devitalized tissue (>50%), especially with concomitant injuries or urine leak, usually require surgical debridement or repair to prevent the later development of urinoma, abscess, or infection which may warrant nephrectomy.

Active contrast extravasation limited to Gerota's fascia would often heal spontaneously due to tamponade effect. However, if there is a breach in Gerota's fascia with bleed extending beyond its confines, then angiographic embolization is often required, especially if the size of the hematoma is increasing.[6,9]

With aggressive monitoring and increasing use of angiographic embolization and percutaneous drainage, overall <10% of grade 4 injuries require surgical intervention.[13] Grade 5 injuries with complete avulsion of the ureteropelvic junction require surgical repair whereas partial tears may resolve on conservative management or stenting and proximal drainage.[2,3] Devascularization of the kidney may be managed conservatively in a stable patient but requires nephrectomy in case of active bleed or major parenchymal disruption. Surgical repair or angiographic thrombolysis of acute renal artery thrombosis can be done to try to preserve the renal function but is shown to have best results, usually within few hours of injury.[14] Renal hypertension developing weeks to months after renal trauma is a frequent finding which usually can be managed medically but may occasionally require nephrectomy.

To summarize, the only absolute indication for surgical exploration (or angiographic embolization) is life-threatening active hemorrhage.[4] Relative indications for operative management include the presence of (1) >50% of renal parenchyma devitalization, (2) arterial thrombosis, and (3) urinary extravasation which is not controlled by conservative management including proximal drainage and stenting.

Follow-up Imaging

Low-grade renal injuries do not require follow-up imaging unless there is a clinical worsening. High-grade renal injuries should be followed up with repeat imaging including the excretory phase after 48–72 hours. This has been shown to detect many urinary leaks or vascular injury, which were not detected earlier.[6]

Penetrating injuries have a lower threshold for repeat imaging and also for surgical repair.[6]

URETERAL TRAUMA

Iatrogenic surgical trauma accounts for 95% of all ureteral injuries and usually occurs in association with gynecological procedures.[15] In gynecological surgery, majority of ureteral injuries are discovered postoperatively (84%) with an average delay of 65 days after the procedure. The patients present with flank pain, fever, hematuria, and occasionally anuria. The emergence of endoscopic and laparoscopic surgery and endourological diagnostic and therapeutic interventions in the last two decades has further contributed to the increased incidence of iatrogenic ureteral trauma.[16] Iatrogenic ureteral injuries occur in 21% of patients undergoing open urological surgery and in 79% of patients undergoing endoscopic urological procedures. Recognition of the injury during surgery or the endoscopic procedure leads to immediate repair or placement of double J-stent for conservative management.

Gunshot wound, stabbing, and blunt trauma account for the remaining 5% of the ureteral injuries. Penetrating trauma to ureter is frequently associated with injuries to other organs.[17] Hematuria is usually present but may be absent. Blunt trauma in children with deceleration injury may occasionally lead to ureteral avulsion.

Imaging Work-up

Role of Intravenous Urogram

Traditionally, IVU has been used as a follow-up study to identify ureteric injury following trauma. However, with widespread availability of CT, its role has become limited. IVU still has a role in the form of one-shot study in unstable patients who require emergency surgery.[18] IVU demonstrates extravasation at the site of injury or obstruction proximal to the site of injury **(Fig. 14)**. Patients in whom ureteral injury is missed, urinary extravasation, hydronephrosis, and abscess formation can

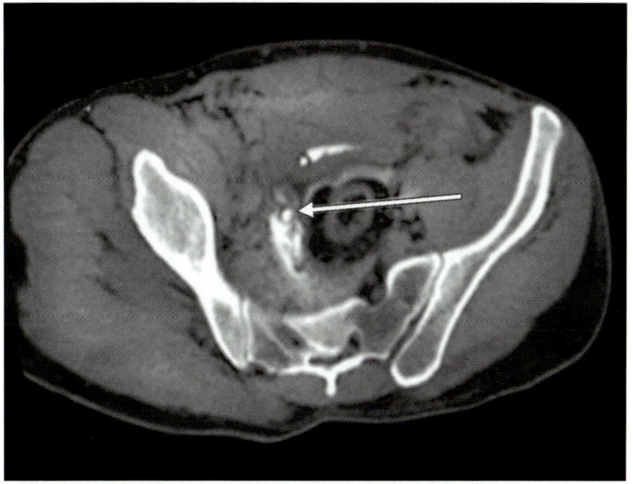

Fig. 14: Postcontrast delayed axial CT scan image at the level of pelvis shows extravasated urinary contrast material adjacent to the right ureter (arrow) suggesting ureteric injury.

result. Demonstration of a mature fistulous tract or a large urinoma at a later stage is much more likely (90–100%). Hydronephrosis is seen at a later stage in 90% patients after ureteral injury. Ureteral avulsion may be diagnosed by contrast extravasation medial to the kidney.

Role of CT

Delayed phase CT has an important role in detection of ureter avulsion at UPJ in acute blunt trauma.[19] The diagnosis depends on the demonstration of contrast extravasation medial to the kidney and lack of distal ureter opacification. CT is also useful in accurate assessment of the size of the associated perirenal hematoma which helps the surgeon in deciding on the need for surgery.

Role of Antegrade and Retrograde Ureterograms

Ureterograms obtained *via* the antegrade or retrograde route are considered the gold standard for confirming the presence of ureteral injury. The ureterogram clearly defines the type and location of the injury as also its magnitude. Any associated fistulae and communicating urinomas are also delineated.

Classification

Ureteral injuries have been classified into the following AAST grades:[20]

- *Grade 1*: Hematoma or contusion without devascularization.
- *Grade 2:* Laceration or transection involving <50% of circumference.
- *Grade 3:* Laceration or transection involving >50% of circumference.
- *Grade 4:* Complete tear or transection with <2 cm of devascularization.
- *Grade 5:* Avulsion with >2 cm of devascularization.

Management

Injuries detected during surgery are treated immediately by either surgical repair or endourologic interventions.[20,21] Injuries recognized later are treated by percutaneous nephrostomy for urinary diversion and antegrade or retrograde stent placement. Stenting may be preceded by balloon dilatation or endoureterectomy for strictures. In ureteral avulsion, stenting is coupled with drainage of urinoma which prevents fibrosis and facilitates passage of guidewire antegradely across the dehiscence. Fistulae are also managed with nephrostomy and stenting. Disruption of the pelvic ureter can be managed by antegrade uretero-neocystostomy and stenting for 1–3 months for which a curved transjugular intrahepatic portosystemic shunt needle sheath can be used.

URINARY BLADDER TRAUMA

Urinary bladder injury is relatively rare and constitutes only 2% of all abdominal injuries that require surgical repair. It may be due to blunt, penetrating, or iatrogenic trauma. Majority of the patients of bladder trauma have associated fracture of pelvis most commonly of the anterior pubic arch.[22] A distended bladder is more prone to injury.

The patient presents with suprapubic pain or tenderness and/or hematuria. In such cases, the recommendation is to first exclude urethral injury by a retrograde urethrography (RGU) followed by insertion of Foley's catheter. If a urethral injury is found, a suprapubic cystostomy is usually done. This is followed by cystography which may be conventional technique or CT cystography. However, with increasing use of CT scan, CT cystography has become the investigation of choice which can be done at the same sitting if the patient is undergoing CT scan for abdominal injuries.[23] Delayed scanning of the bladder after intravenous contrast administration so as to allow the contrast excreted by kidneys to opacify the bladder is not a substitute for CT cystography as it has been shown to miss a significant number of bladder ruptures.[23,24] Conventional cystography may be done, if CT is not available.

Cystography

Conventional Cystography

Technique:

- 300–400 mL of dilute contrast is instilled into the bladder *via* the urethral (if urethral injury excluded) or the suprapubic route. The ideal way is by a gravity-dip infusion and not injection. It allows adequate contrast to be instilled without chances of forceful worsening of the bladder injury.
- The initial film is taken after 100 mL contrast is instilled to check gross extravasation.
- Films are then taken after the entire contrast is instilled.
- A postdrainage film excludes extravasation hidden by a distended bladder.

CT Cystography

The technique recommended is retrograde filling of the bladder with contrast (same as with conventional cystography) by gravity-dip infusion followed by a computed tomogram of the pelvis. With this technique, the diagnostic accuracy is comparable to that of conventional cystography. The CT cystography is best done as a separate phase immediately after acquisition of images of abdomen and pelvis after intravenous contrast administration. If done simultaneously with the routine phases, there may be a diagnostic pitfall in the interpretation of extravasated contrast material in the abdomen. It may be from intraperitoneal urinary bladder rupture or extravasation from vessels. Postdrainage scans are not required. According to the current recommendations, CT cystography is indicated in the following situations:

- Unexplained pelvic-free fluid with or without pelvic fractures.
- Gross or significant microscopic hematuria with nonacetabular pelvic fractures.

Classification

Blunt Trauma

The AAST classification for urinary bladder (UB) injury has five injury grades. However, it involves measuring the size of lacerations which is a potential pitfall on imaging as the size of defect varies with the distension of the bladder. Hence, the AAST classification for UB is not much used radiologically.[25] The classification based on imaging which is most widely followed was described by Sandler et al.[22]

- *Type 1:* Bladder contusion
- *Type 2:* Intraperitoneal bladder rupture
- *Type 3:* Interstitial bladder injury
- *Type 4: Extraperitoneal injury*:
  - Simple
  - Complex
- *Type 5:* Combined UB injury.

Bladder contusion (Type 1): This consists of a self-limiting, incomplete mural tear with localized ecchymosis. CT cystography is normal, showing a well-distended uniformly hyperattenuating thin-walled bladder with no contrast leakage. No specific therapy is required. A perivesical hematoma may be associated with major pelvic fractures even when no evidence of actual bladder tear is seen on cystography. Accumulated blood compresses upon the extraperitoneal part of the bladder narrowing it at the base. An "inverted tear drop" or "inverted pear sign" may be seen on cystogram.

Intraperitoneal injury (Type 2): Intraperitoneal rupture usually occurs after a blow to the lower abdomen in the presence of distended bladder. Rupture occurs at the dome due to increased intravesical pressure. This is the weakest point of the bladder and also the peritonealized portion of the bladder wall. Urine will thus enter the peritoneal cavity. On cystography, contrast material may be seen outlining the abdominal viscera, loops of bowel, mesenteric folds, paracolic gutters, or pouch of Douglas **(Figs. 15A and B)**. The contrast material may track to upper abdomen also. The locations of free intraperitoneal contrast are predictable with well-defined boundaries as compared to extraperitoneal rupture.

Interstitial injury (Type 3): This represents a dissecting rupture of the bladder wall without frank perforation. On CT cystography, a mural hematoma/defect may be seen. Occasionally, intramural contrast may be seen. However, there is no contrast extravasation outside the bladder. Such defects may involve both extraperitoneal and intraperitoneal portions of the bladder wall. Hence,

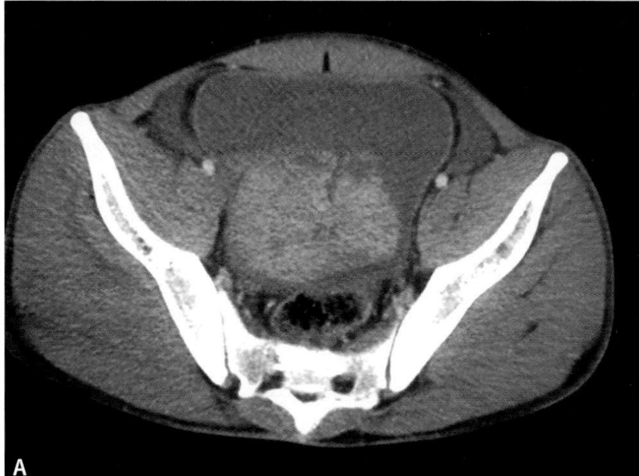

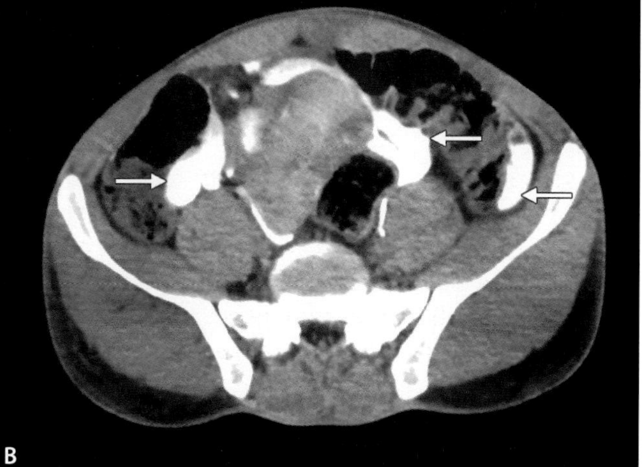

Figs. 15A and B: Axial CECT image (A) through urinary bladder shows a hyperdense clot within the bladder. Axial CT cystography image (B) shows extravasation of contrast outside the bladder in the peritoneal cavity outlining the bowel loops (arrows).

interstitial rupture was designated as a separate category in this classification.

Extraperitoneal injury (Type 4): This is the most common injury to the bladder (80–90% of cases) and usually occurs in association with a fractured pelvis or in penetrating trauma. Earlier, it was thought that the tear was caused by direct penetration of the bladder by bone fragments. However, now it is postulated that this type of injury may be either a type of bursting or shearing injury resulting from the force of pelvic ring disruption.

In simple (Type 4A), extraperitoneal rupture extravasation is confined to the perivesical space.

On CT cystography, flame-shaped areas of extravasation are noted in the perivesical spaces and in the prevesical space (space of Retzius) where it can track cranially up to umbilicus. The ill-defined contrast in the prevesical space is said to have a "molar tooth" appearance.

A complex (Type 4B) extraperitoneal rupture is diagnosed when contrast extravasation extends beyond the perivesical space into the scrotum, thigh, perineum, hip joint, and anterior abdominal wall **(Fig. 16)**. It occurs secondary to rupture of urogenital diaphragm. Contrast may also track upward into the paranephric spaces.

It is important to differentiate intraperitoneal rupture from extraperitoneal rupture of bladder because the former requires surgical repair where the latter is usually managed conservatively with Foley's catheter placement.

Combined extra- and intraperitoneal bladder injury (Type 5): An injury may result in rupture of both intraperitoneal and extraperitoneal portions of the bladder wall. On CT cystography, both patterns of contrast extravasation may be seen.

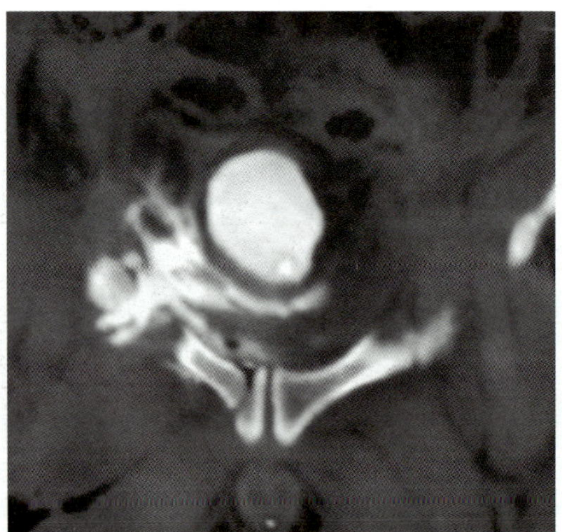

Fig. 16: Reformatted coronal MIP CT cystography image shows complex extraperitoneal rupture of urinary bladder with contrast lying in extraperitoneal spaces in perineum extending into right hip joint.

Penetrating Bladder Trauma

Injury may result from gunshot or knife wounds and may result in extraperitoneal, intraperitoneal, or combined bladder injury. There is a high incidence of associated bowel or other visceral injury, and exploratory surgery is required in virtually every patient.

Iatrogenic Bladder Trauma

Bladder injuries may be due to urologic, gynecologic, or obstetric procedures. Bladder perforations or vesicovaginal and vesicouterine fistulae may form. Cystography and hysterosalpingography help in the diagnosis. Migration of surgical devices such as drains, catheters, contraceptives, or orthopedic prostheses can sometimes perforate the bladder.

Management

Types 1, 3, and 4 injuries are managed conservatively with placement of Foley's catheter. However, intraperitoneal rupture of bladder requires surgical repair. Hence, Types 2 and 5 injuries are managed surgically.

URETHRAL TRAUMA

Posterior urethral injuries result from pelvic fractures and gunshot wounds. Injury associated with pelvic fracture mostly involves the urethra near the urogenital diaphragm. Anterior urethral injuries are much less common and are more commonly due to iatrogenic cause, straddle injury, or gunshot wound. The lifelong consequences in males include incontinence, strictures, and impotence. Female urethra injury is rare.

The clinical signs suggestive of urethral injury in a male patient with pelvic trauma include gross hematuria, blood at urethral meatus, inability to void, swelling or hematoma of the perineum or penis, and a high-riding prostate on per rectal examination associated with pelvic fracture.[26] The clinical signs in a female patient include difficulty in micturition, blood at meatus, hematuria, labial edema, vaginal bleeding, or urine leak per rectum. If the above signs are present in a patient with pelvic trauma, urethrography should be done for evaluation of urethra before insertion of Foley's catheter.

Radiology

The urethra is best evaluated with RGU or voiding cystourethrography.

Technique of Urethrography

- Dynamic RGU, ideally under fluoroscopy, is used for the evaluation of urethral injury.
- Steep oblique films are obtained, at the end of injection of 25–30 mL of 50% contrast.
- If the urethra appears intact, a catheter is passed into the bladder for cystography and a voiding urethrogram is obtained.

Blunt Urethral Trauma

Urethral injuries are classified anatomically as anterior or posterior urethral injuries. Posterior urethral injury occurs in 4–14% of patients with pelvic fracture and up to 20% of these have associated bladder laceration.[27] Anterior urethral injury commonly results from straddle pelvic injury secondary to the patient falling astride a blunt object or direct blow to the perineum. However, more commonly, anterior urethral injuries may be iatrogenic due to instrumentation.

Posterior Urethral Injuries Associated with Pelvic Fracture

- Commonly, prostatomembranous urethral injury above the urogenital diaphragm results.
- A high riding urinary bladder is seen on excretory urography. This is due to disruption of puboprostatic ligaments and hematoma in retropubic and perivesical spaces.
- Contrast extravasation will be seen adjacent to the posterior urethra and sometimes into the pelvic extraperitoneal space.

Anterior Urethral Injury

Straddle injuries resulting from the patient falling astride a blunt object or direct blow to the perineum may lead to anterior, mostly bulbous, urethral injuries. More commonly, anterior urethral injuries may be iatrogenic due to instrumentation. In partial rupture, extravasation of contrast occurs on urethrogram but continuity of the urethra is preserved. In complete rupture, no contrast is seen in the proximal urethra. Venous intravasation is seen commonly. Treatment is by suprapubic urinary diversion and delayed surgery.

Classification

Based on findings of urethrography, the following types of urethral injuries have been described by Goldman, et al.[28] who have modified the initial classification given by Colapinto and McCallum.[29]

- *Type I:*
  - Stretched, but intact posterior urethra is seen **(Fig. 17)**.
  - In this type of injury, the prostate is detached from the urogenital diaphragm with an elevated bladder seen on cystography due to retropubic hematoma and rupture of puboprostatic ligaments.
  - No extravasation is seen on the urethrogram.
- *Type II:*
  - Seen in around 15% of cases.
  - Urethra is ruptured at the membranoprostatic junction above the urogenital diaphragm which is intact **(Fig. 18)**.

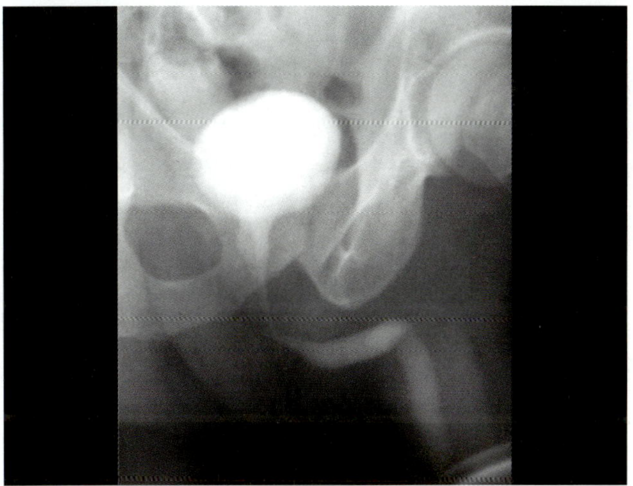

Fig. 17: MCU shows a stretched posterior urethra in a patient with multiple pelvic fractures.

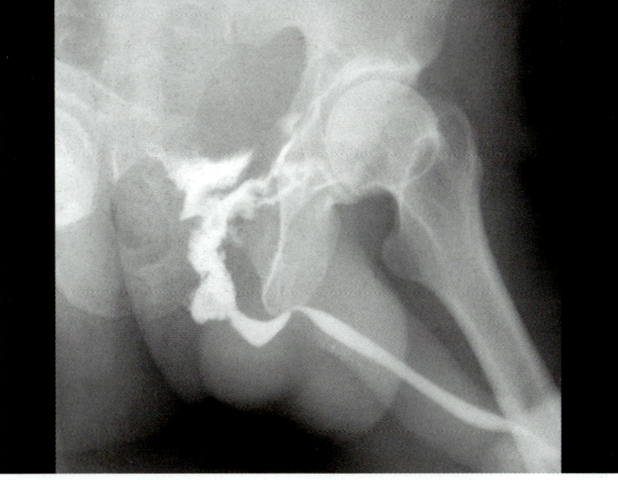

Fig. 18: RGU shows a type II urethral injury with contrast extravasation from posterior urethra above the urogenital diaphragm.

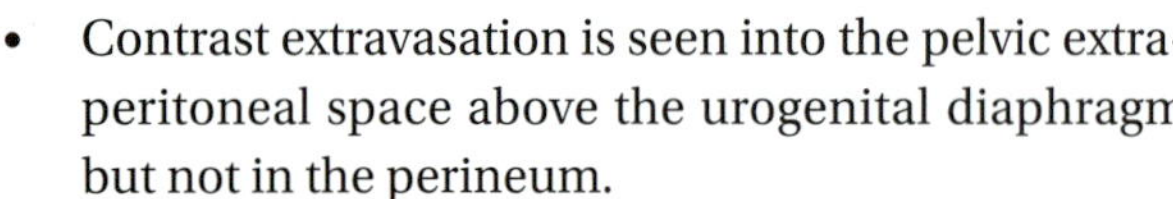

- Contrast extravasation is seen into the pelvic extraperitoneal space above the urogenital diaphragm but not in the perineum.

- *Type III:*
  - Most common type.
  - Membranobulbous urethral rupture is seen with disruption of urogenital diaphragm.
  - Contrast extravasation both above and below urogenital diaphragm, i.e. into pelvis and the perineum **(Fig. 19)**.

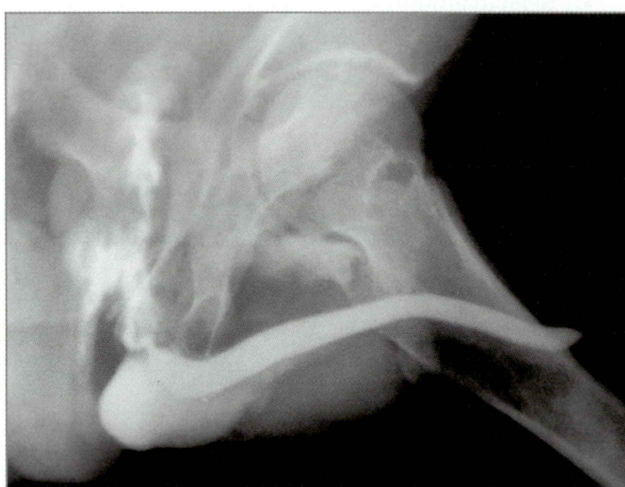

Fig. 19: RGU shows a type III urethral injury with contrast extravasation from posterior urethra both above and below the urogenital diaphragm.

- *Type IV:*
  - There is bladder neck injury with extension into the posterior urethra.
  - Contrast extravasation is seen in the pelvic extraperitoneal space with disruption of bladder neck **(Fig. 20)**.
- *Type IVa:*
  - Extraperitoneal bladder base injury simulating a bladder neck injury.
  - Radiologically indistinguishable from type IV injury
- *Type V:*
  - Caused by straddle injury.
  - Anterior urethra, most commonly bulbous urethra, injury is seen which may be partial or complete.
  - Contrast extravasation is seen into the penile soft tissues **(Fig. 21)**.

Management

Type I injuries are managed conservatively with placement of a urethral or suprapubic catheter. In general, partial disruptions are also managed conservatively with suprapubic or urethral catheterization whereas complete disruptions of the urethra are managed either by endoscopic realignment or by delayed urethroplasty.

Bladder neck injuries involve internal sphincter and hence are treated surgically to prevent development of incontinence. However, Type IVa injury may be treated conservatively since it does not involve the bladder neck.

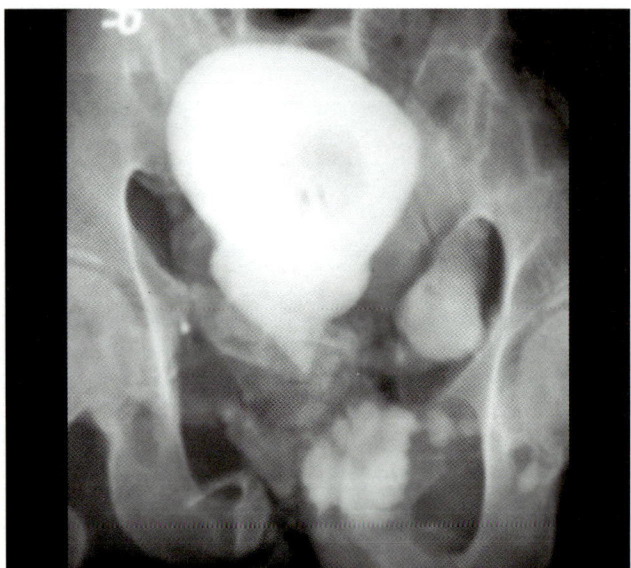

Fig. 20: MCU showing elongated injured bladder neck with contrast extravasation around the prostatic urethra.

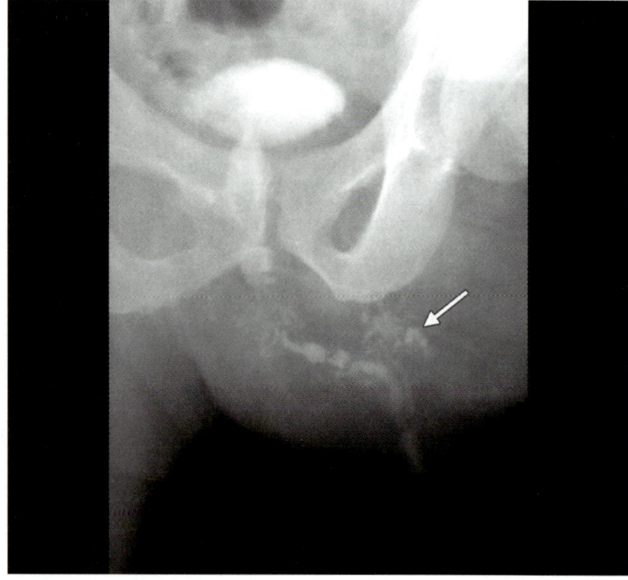

Fig. 21: RGU showing contrast extravasation in penile tissues from anterior urethral injury (arrow).

Evaluation before Delayed Urethroplasty

- A combined voiding cystourethrogram and a retrograde urethrogram are obtained.
- The bladder is filled with 30% dilute contrast through the suprapubic cystostomy.
- The patient is then asked to void.
- A simultaneous retrograde urethrogram is performed.
- This technique demonstrates the proximal and distal extent of the stricture. This enables the surgeon to decide between a transperineal and a transpubic approach for urethroplasty.
- Recently, reports have shown the potential of MRI to demonstrate the length of the urethral injury along with the amount of displacement of the prostatic apex. This information is helpful in preoperative planning of the surgical approach.

Penetrating Injury

Penetrating trauma to the urethra may be secondary to knife or gunshot wounds. The diagnosis is established by RGU. Early surgery is the treatment of choice.

Iatrogenic Injury

Iatrogenic urethral injury may result from pelvic surgery, urethral instrumentation, or indwelling catheters.

Female Urethra

Injury to the female urethra is rare because of its mobility. Excretory urography or cystourethrography may show extravasation of contrast at the site of rupture.

REFERENCES

1. McAninch JW. Renal injuries. In: Gillenwater JY, Grayhack JT, Howards SS, et al. (Eds). Adult and Pediatric Urology, 3rd edition. St. Louis, MO: Mosby; 1996. pp. 539-53.
2. Kawashima A, Sandler CM, Corl FM, et al. Imaging of renal trauma: a comprehensive review. Radiographics. 2001;21(3): 557-74.
3. Smith JK, Kenny PJ. Imaging of renal trauma. Radiol Clin N Am. 2003;41(5):1019-35.
4. Harris AC, Zwirewich CV, Lyburn ID, et al. CT findings in blunt renal trauma. Radiographics. 2001;21:S201-14.
5. Park SJ, Kim JK, Kim KW, et al. MDCT findings of renal trauma. Am J Roentgenol. 2006;187(2):541-7.
6. Baghdanian AH, Baghdanian AA, Armetta A, et al. Utility of MDCT findings in predicting patient management outcomes in renal trauma. Emerg Radiol. 2017;24(3):263-72.
7. Moore EE, Shackford SR, Patcher HL, et al. Organ injury scaling: spleen, liver and kidney. J Trauma. 2001;50:195-200.
8. Kozar RA, Crandall M, Shanmuganathan K, et al. Organ injury scaling 2018 update: spleen, liver, and kidney. J Trauma Acute Care Surg. 2018;85(6):1119-22.
9. Chien LC, Vakil M, Nguyen J, et al. The American Association for the Surgery of Trauma Organ Injury Scale 2018 update for computed tomography-based grading of renal trauma: a primer for the emergency radiologist. Emerg Radiol. 2019 doi: 10.1007/s10140-019-01721-z. [Epub ahead of print].
10. Dayal M, Gamanagatti S, Kumar A. Imaging in renal trauma. World J Radiol. 2013;5(8):275-84.
11. Pollack HM, Wein AJ. Imaging of renal trauma. Radiology. 1989;172:297-308.
12. Knudson MM, Maull KI. Nonoperative management of solid organ injuries: past, present and future. Surg Clin N Am. 1999;79(6):1357-71.
13. Brandes SB, McAninch JW. Reconstructive surgery for trauma of the upper urinary tract. Urol Clin N Am. 1999;26(1): 183-99.
14. Peterson NE. Genitourinary trauma. In: Feliciano DV, Moore EE, Mattox KL (Eds). Trauma, 3rd edition. Stamford, CT: Appleton & Lange; 1996. pp. 661-94.
15. Assimos DG, Patterson LC, Taylor CL. Changing incidence and etiology of iatrogenic ureteral injuries. J Urol. 1994; 152(6 Pt 2):2240-6.
16. Campbell EW, Jr, Filderman S, Jacobs SC. Ureteral injury due to blunt and penetrating trauma. Urology. 1992;40(3): 216-20.
17. Pitts JC, Peterson NE. Penetrating injuries of the ureter. J Trauma. 1981;21:978-82.
18. Lynch TH, Matnz-NL, Las, et al. European Association of urology: guidelines on urological trauma. Eur Urol. 2005;47: 1-15.
19. Kenney PJ, Panicek DM, Witanowski LS. Computed tomography of ureteral disruption. J Comput Assit Tomogr. 1987;11(3):480-4.
20. Bent C, Iyngkaran T, Power N, et al. Urological injuries following trauma. Clin Radiol. 2008; 63(12):1361-71.
21. Lask D, Abarbanel J, Luttwak Z, et al. Changing trends in the management of iatrogenic ureteral injuries. J Urol. 1995; 154(5):1693-5.
22. Sandler CM, Hall JT, Rodriguez MB, et al. Bladder injury in blunt pelvic trauma. Radiology. 1986;158:633-8.
23. Vaccaro JP, Brody JM. CT cystography in the evaluation of major bladder trauma. Radiographics. 2000;20(5):1373-81.
24. Power N, Ryan S, Hamilton P. Computed tomographic cystography in bladder trauma: pictorial essay. Can Assoc Radiol J. 2004;55(5):304-8.
25. Joshi G, Kim EY, Hanna TN, et al. CT cystography for suspicion of traumatic urinary bladder injury: indications, technique, findings, and pitfalls in diagnosis: Radiographics Fundamentals|Online Presentation. Radiographics. 2018; 38(1):92-3.
26. Patel U. Lower urinary tract trauma. In: Patel U, Rickards D (Eds). Imaging and Urodynamics of the Lower Urinary Tract. London, Taylor & Francis; 2005. pp. 115-21.
27. Kawashima A, Sandler CM, Wasserman NF, et al. Imaging of urethral disease: a pictorial review. Radiographics. 2004;24(Suppl 1):S195-216.
28. Goldman SM, Sandler CM, Corriere JN, Jr, et al. Blunt urethral trauma: a unified anatomical mechanical classification. J Urol. 1997;157(1):85-9.
29. Colapinto V, McCallum RW. Injury to the male posterior urethra in fractured pelvis: a new classification. J Urol. 1977;118(4):575-80.

SECTION 6

Interventions

Chapter 26

Nonvascular Interventions in the Urinary Tract

Mandeep Kang, Naveen Kalra, Ujjwal Gorsi, Sreedhara BC

INTRODUCTION

The past few decades have witnessed a revolution in the development of minimally invasive procedures, with interventional radiology being in the forefront of these advances. The development of percutaneous procedures under image guidance was based on the knowledge that a fine, thin needle of 21–22 gauge (G) can be safely and accurately positioned within the human body in most organ parts. Nonvascular interventions in the urinary tract are well-established procedures with the first description of a percutaneous nephrostomy (PCN) being published in literature more than 70 years ago.[1] Propelled by technological advances, minimally invasive uroradiological interventional therapies have completely changed the present day practice of urology.

PERCUTANEOUS NEPHROSTOMY

Percutaneous nephrostomy is the first step in image-guided urointerventional procedures, which secures an access into the urinary tract.[2] It involves image-guided placement of a catheter into the pelvicalyceal system.[3] Besides urinary diversion in an obstructed system, the access can be used to create large-bore tracks through which various endourological procedures can be safely performed with fewer complications than open surgical procedures.[4]

Indications

- *Supravesical urinary tract obstruction:* Obstruction of the upper urinary tract can be due to extrinsic or intrinsic causes and is the most common indication for PCN (85–90% of cases).

  Benign causes of obstruction include:
  - Calculous disease (most common)
  - Ureteral/anastomotic stricture
  - Blood clots
  - Sequestered papillae
  - Fungal balls
  - Retroperitoneal fibrosis.

  Malignant causes of obstruction include neoplasms of the urinary bladder, cervix, and prostate. Percutaneous nephrostomy (PCN) should be offered to patients with tumors, which are potentially responsive to therapy or have stable disease and to improve the overall quality of life.
- Providing an alternative pathway for drainage as part of the management of urinary leaks or fistulas.
- *Access for subsequent interventions:*
  - Antegrade ureteric stenting
  - Nephrolithotomy/lithotripsy
  - Stone dissolution
  - Ureteral occlusion for treating an urinary fistula
  - Urothelial lesion: Tissue diagnosis/treatment by fulguration
  - Removal of a foreign body such as fungal ball
  - Whitaker test
  - Upper urinary tract instillation (medications or cooling pyeloperfusion for ablative procedures).

There is no absolute contraindication for PCN with the only relative contraindication being coagulopathy, which should be corrected prior to the procedure.

Anatomy for Percutaneous Renal Entry

Knowledge of anatomy of the kidneys is basic to understanding how to safely gain access to the collecting system for performing a PCN under image guidance. The main renal artery usually bifurcates into anterior and posterior divisions with further segmental branches. The anterior division supplies the anterior two-thirds of the renal parenchyma while the posterior division supplies the posterior third. A zone of relative avascularity, known as Brödel's line or zone of bloodless incision exists between these two vascular territories, which runs just posterior to the lateral convex border of the kidney **(Fig. 1)**. The best route to access the collecting system lies through this relatively avascular plane.[4] Because the kidneys are normally rotated about their horizontal axis with the pelvis facing anteromedially, the posterior calyces are directed posterolaterally with their long axis aligned with this avascular zone; these calyces should ideally be targeted at PCN. In the renal hilum, the renal artery is the most anterior structure followed by the renal vein with the renal pelvis being the most posterior structure. Placement of the puncture needle centrally for accessing the collecting system should not be done, only the calyces (which anatomically are completely surrounded by renal parenchyma) should be punctured.

Central puncture can lead to two problems. First, a hilar vessel can be injured leading to severe bleeding; second, there may be urinary leakage from the catheter tract due to absence of renal tissue around the renal pelvis leading to inadequate sealing of the track.[5]

The site of access to the pelvicalyceal system depends upon the indication for nephrostomy. A lower pole

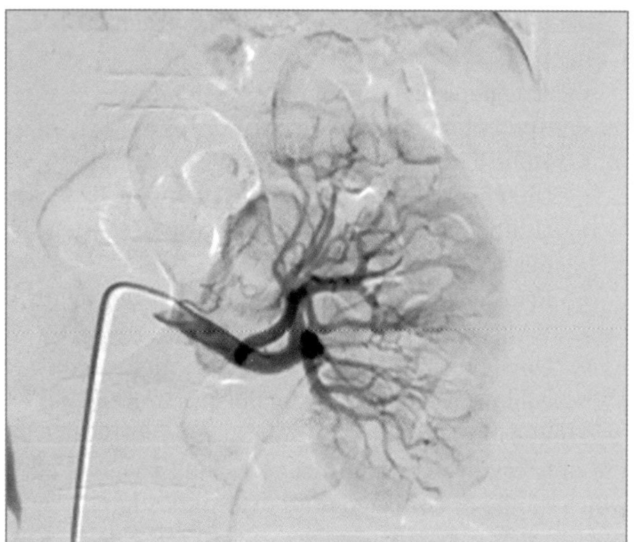

Fig. 1: Vascular anatomy of the kidney. Selective left renal arteriogram 25° left posterior oblique view shows bifurcation of the main renal artery into dorsal and ventral branches. The avascular plane of Brödel lies along the plane of division of these vascular territories.

posterior calyx can be safely accessed using a subcostal approach to avoid transgression of the pleura.[5] However, puncturing a posterior calyx in the upper pole or interpolar region provides the easiest access to the pelviureteric junction for subsequent ureteral interventions. In cases of complex stone disease, entry through the upper polar posterior calyx allows visualization of most parts of the collecting system.[4]

Technique

A detailed evaluation of the patient must be performed including the clinical history, laboratory parameters, and relevant radiology. The patient should also be evaluated on ultrasound (US) or fluoroscopy as body habitus can change your choice of image guidance. Coagulation parameters [prothrombin time index (PTI) > 75%, international normalized ratio (INR) < 1.5] and the hemogram (Hb >7 g/dL, platelet count > 75,000) should be checked and abnormalities, if any, must be corrected prior to the procedure. Patients with azotemia may have profound metabolic disturbances. Any metabolic acidosis or hyperkalemia should be corrected prior to performing the intervention as these imbalances can cause systemic complications such as cardiac arrhythmias or even cardioplegia.[3] Urine analysis to screen for possible urinary infection should also be performed. Prophylactic broad-spectrum antibiotics should be started prior to the procedure in patients with known or potentially infected system (urinary conduit diversions, obstruction with or without fever, and urinary leaks). An informed consent must be obtained from the patient after explaining in detail the need for the procedure, the procedure itself, and the potential complications, which can occur.

Percutaneous nephrostomy is usually performed under fluoroscopic or US guidance. In certain cases, CT guidance may be used, for example, in emphysematous pyelonephritis when air in the collecting system obscures visualization on US. In addition, in patients with different body habitus such as kyphoscoliosis or morbid obesity, CT may be the only modality, which can provide adequate image guidance.[6] The use of MR guidance has also been described.[7]

The patient is placed prone on the fluoroscopy table with a bolster under the abdomen to fix the kidneys against the posterior abdominal wall and prevent their anterior displacement during the procedure. If the patient is unable to lie in prone position, a prone-oblique position can be used with the side to be punctured in the dependent position.

The back and flanks are cleansed and draped. The calyx to be punctured is chosen depending upon the indication. The chosen site of puncture is infiltrated with local anesthetic not only into the skin and subcutaneous tissues, but also deeper through the perirenal fat up till the renal capsule, therefore a long 9–10 cm needle maybe required.[5] This is generally adequate for pain relief during the procedure; however, conscious sedation may be required in apprehensive or noncooperative patients. Infants and young children will require general anesthesia.

The chosen calyx can be punctured with an 18-G needle under US guidance in a dilated system **(Figs. 2A and B)**. After removing the stylet, a urine sample should be aspirated for culture. A small volume of iodinated contrast is then injected to opacity the collecting system. A 0.035" stiff guidewire is then passed through the needle and negotiated into the pelvis. After a stab incision along the needle, the cannula is removed and the tract dilated using fascial dilators. For drainage of noninfected urine, catheters of 8–10 F size are usually sufficient. The catheter is placed over the guidewire and coiled in the pelvis **(Figs. 3A to D)**. A check injection of contrast should be done to confirm position of all side holes of the catheter within the collecting system.

Pigtail catheters with or without locking devices may be used. The catheter is fixed to the skin using sutures or other retention devices, connected to a urine collection bag and allowed to drain under gravity.

A variety of techniques may be used for the initial puncture. Some workers inject intravenous iodinated contrast to opacify the collecting system followed by direct puncture of the pelvis under fluoroscopic guidance with a 22-G needle. Iodinated contrast (with or without room air or carbon dioxide) is then injected under fluoroscopic control to better opacify the collecting system and find a suitable calyx. The selected calyx can then be punctured from the posterolateral aspect with an 18-G needle, with the subsequent steps being the same as described before. Another variation of this "two-stick" technique, particularly when the collecting system is only mildly dilated, is to use a 22-G needle for the second puncture as well, through which a 0.014" hydrophilic guidewire can be passed, over which a 5-F percutaneous access set is placed and the guidewire exchanged for a 0.035" stiff or super-stiff Amplatz guidewire.[5,7-9] Regardless of the technique used, care has to be taken not to overdistend the collecting system so as to avoid pyelovenous reflux, particularly in infected systems.

Occasionally, external urinary diversion is necessary in nondilated collecting systems (e.g. in urinary leak or fistulas). These kidneys can be punctured using the double-stick technique with initial opacification of the collecting system with intravenous injection of iodinated contrast.[10] Alternatively, these kidneys can be accessed using sonographic guidance after intravenous injection of frusemide. Even if the calyces do not dilate adequately to be visualized on US, the renal pelvis can be seen and punctured with a skinny needle, iodinated contrast, or saline injected to distend the calyces so that a definitive calyceal puncture can be made with fluoroscopic or US guidance.[11]

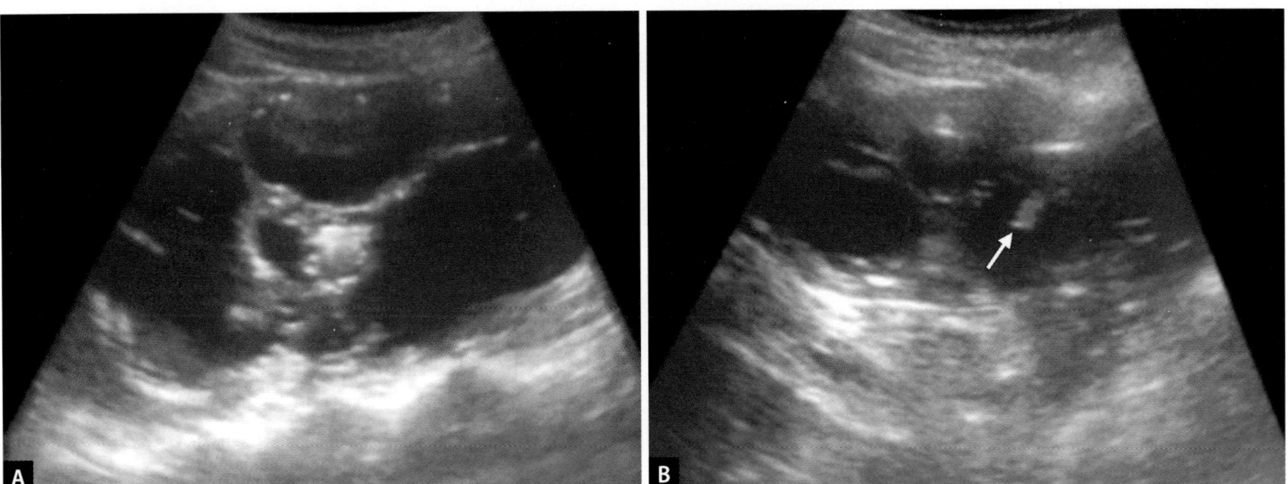

Figs. 2A and B: Percutaneous nephrostomy. (A) Longitudinal sonogram shows gross hydronephrosis with internal echoes suggestive of pyonephrosis. (B) The lower pole calyx has been punctured using an 18-gauge needle. Needle tip is seen *in situ* (arrow).

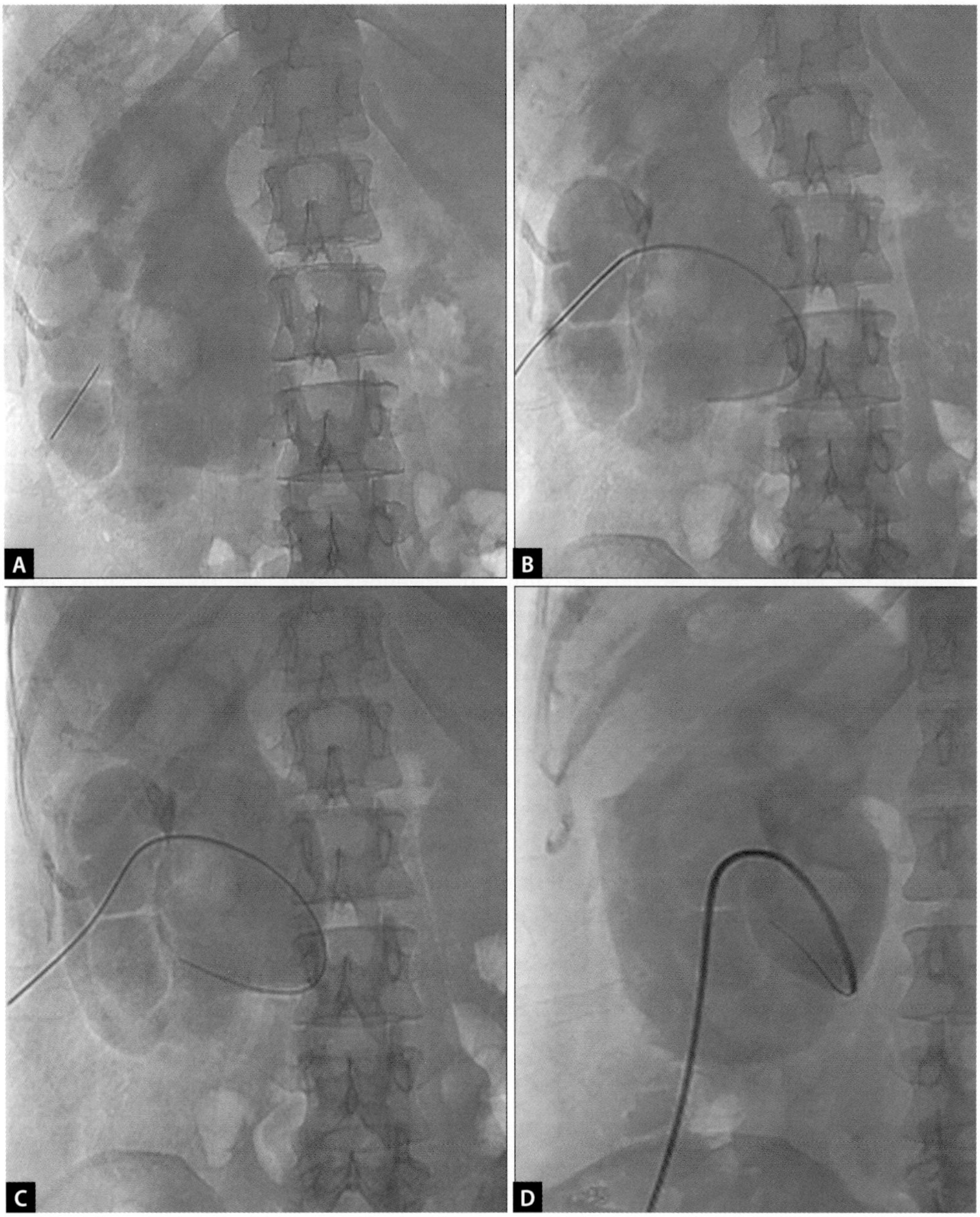

Figs. 3A to D: Percutaneous nephrostomy. (A) The grossly dilated calyces are opacified due to a CECT abdomen done the previous day. These have been directly punctured by an 18-gauge needle under fluoroscopic guidance. (B) A stiff guidewire has been negotiated into the pelvis. (C) The puncture needle has been withdrawn and the track is being dilated using fascial dilators. (D) An 8-F catheter is being threaded over the guidewire to coil in the pelvis. (CECT: contrast-enhanced computed tomography).

Postprocedure Care

Vital signs need to be carefully monitored in the immediate postprocedure period as there is a potential for ongoing blood loss or the development of septicemic shock (due to pyelovenous reflux and bacteremia) in patients at risk. Ideally, the patient should be admitted overnight for observation after the procedure, during which time the tube should be gently flushed with saline every 4 hours. Hematuria is initially present after PCN in virtually all patients, this usually gradually settles within 24–48 hours. The PCN tube output should be recorded to assess for adequacy of drainage. Appropriate analgesics, including narcotics, if required (particularly for patients with intercostal entry), should be provided. The patients should be instructed regarding tube care, especially if long-term drainage is anticipated. The dressing around the catheter should be changed daily. The catheters need to be changed every 8–10 weeks, if long-term drainage is required.[12]

Results

Placement of a nephrostomy tube is technically successful in 84–99% of cases in dilated systems. The success rate will be lower in patients with nondilated systems, complex stone disease such as staghorn calculi, anatomical variants, and renal cysts.[3,5] Use of CT guidance may improve the technical success in patients with anatomical variants or renal cysts.[6,13]

Complications

These may be divided into systemic and local complications.

Systemic Complications

The most common systemic complication that can at times be fatal is sepsis. Every obstructed system should be considered as potentially infected. Manipulation of guidewires, catheter, and injection of contrast all lead to an increase in the pressure in the collecting system, which can lead to pyelovenous reflux. The incidence of septic complications is reported between 1% and 2.5%.[13,14] The incidence rises to 7–9% in the setting of pyonephrosis.[3] One should avoid overdistention of the system by limiting the amount of contrast injected and also keeping manipulation to a minimum in the initial procedure. Complicated or prolonged procedures should be avoided in an infected system; further manipulation should be undertaken only 48–72 hours after the initial procedure when the system is adequately decompressed.[4,5,15]

Prone positioning of the patient during the PCN procedure can lead to respiratory insufficiency, especially in infants or young children under sedation. Close patient monitoring is therefore of utmost importance.[5]

Local Complications

The most common procedure site complication is bleeding, which may occur from the renal parenchymal vessels or the intercostal vessels. Transient hematuria is observed in almost every patient. Severe bleeding that requires transfusion or further intervention is seen in 1–3% of patients.[3] Bleeding noticed at the time of PCN can often be controlled by placement of a larger-bore nephrostomy catheter to tamponade the track.[16] If bleeding persists for 2–3 days, a nephrostogram should be obtained to check for the position of the catheter. If the tip of the catheter is abutting the calyceal or pelvic wall or all the side holes are not lying within the PCN, repositioning can be done. Severe bleeding developing after catheter insertion requires further evaluation.

A track fistulogram can be obtained by exchanging the nephrostomy catheter with an introducer sheath over a stiff guidewire. The sheath is then gradually withdrawn while injecting contrast. At times, the venous or arterial source of bleed may fill with contrast. Angiographic evaluation for identification of any complication such as formation of a renal arteriovenous fistula, pseudoaneurysm, or vessel laceration should be scheduled without delay in patients with persistent or severe bleeding. Most of these vascular injuries can be managed by the endovascular route; surgical intervention is rarely necessary.[16,17] Bleeding can lead to a perinephric hematoma, which can cause a page kidney with subsequent deterioration in renal function. This should be drained percutaneously.

Adjacent organs may be inadvertently punctured. A retrorenal colon, an uncommon anatomic variant (more common on the right side), may be transgressed (0.2–0.5%) leading to a nephrocolic fistula. Treatment is conservative and consists of ensuring adequate urinary drainage by placement of an antegrade or retrograde ureteric stent, and withdrawing the nephrostomy catheter into the colon to allow the nephrocolic track to heal.[10] Pleural complications in the form of pneumothorax, pleural effusion, emphysema, or hemothorax may occur in 0.1–0.6% of cases. The incidence rises with intercostal entry or complex endourologic procedures.[5] If pleural transgression has occurred, the PCN catheter should be left in place to allow a mature track to form. The catheter can then be removed and a new access obtained into the kidney if required.[16]

Catheter blocks or dislodgements are technical complications, which may occur. The blocked catheter should be cleaned with a guidewire and changed. Replacement of a dislodged catheter is usually possible through the previous tract. Many times the whole tract can be opacified by injecting a small amount of dilute contrast via a sheath placed at the site of urine leak on the skin. A hydrophilic guidewire is then used to probe the tract which usually finds its way into the collecting system.[5,16]

Overall, considering both major and minor complications, the complication rate is around 10%. The mortality rate for PCN varies from 0.046% to 0.3%.[3-5]

Extended Applications of Percutaneous Nephrostomy

Antegrade Ureteric Stenting

The most common extended application of PCN is placement of a ureteric stent for urinary obstruction or fistula. It is often much easier to negotiate areas of narrowing, fistulae, or discontinuity in the ureter in an antegrade rather than a retrograde manner. The stenting is usually performed under local anesthesia and conscious sedation. After the initial PCN, a safety guidewire is placed through an access sheath to avoid losing renal access during the subsequent manipulation of the working guidewire. The obstructed segment is negotiated using different types of angiographic catheters and hydrophilic guidewires. Once the stricture has been negotiated, the guidewire–catheter combination can be advanced into the urinary bladder and coiled within its lumen. The hydrophilic guidewire is then exchanged for a super-stiff Amplatz wire **(Figs. 4A to D)**. Determination of the correct length of the ureteric stent required can be done by using the bent guidewire technique. Balloon dilatation of strictures, placement of ureteric stents, postprocedure drainage of the upper urinary tract, and subsequent nephrostograms can all be performed via the initial PCN tract. The percutaneous external urinary

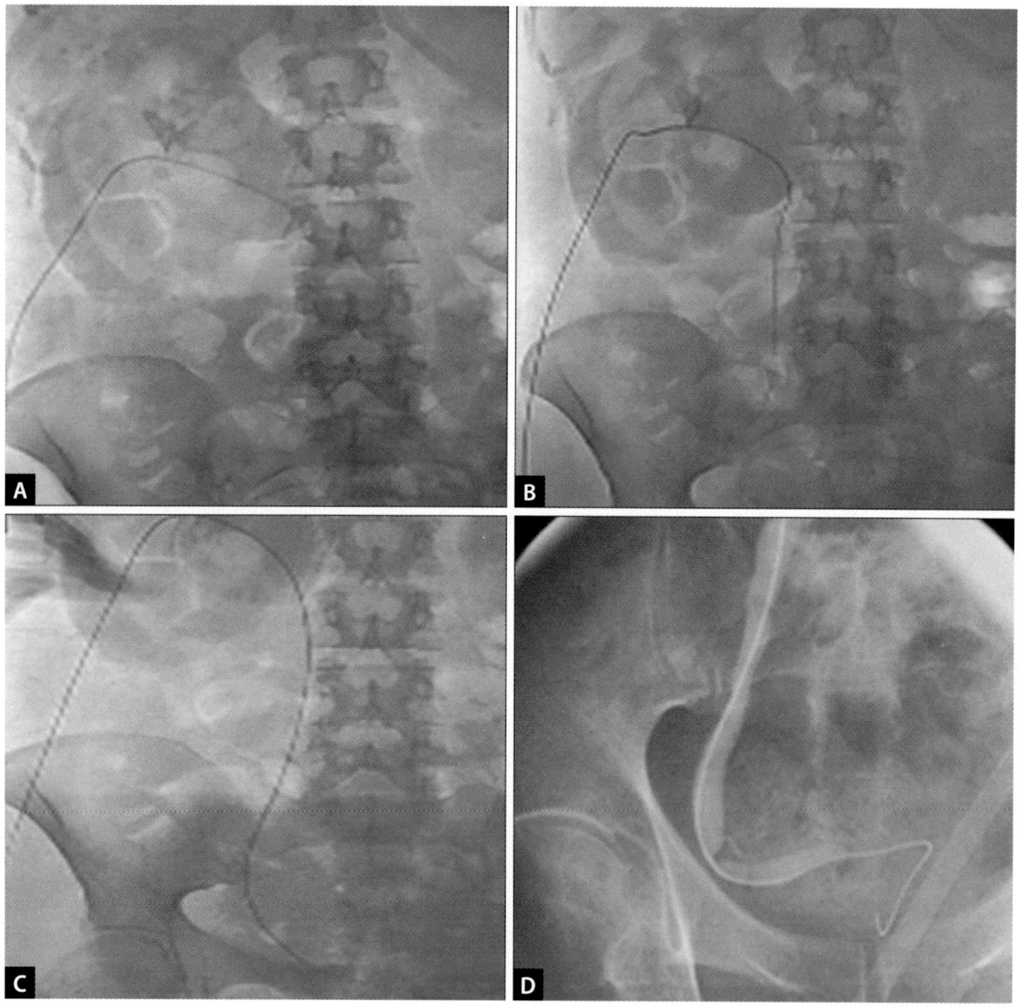

Figs. 4A to D: Antegrade stenting in a patient with carcinoma of the urinary bladder. (A) The PCN catheter has been exchanged for a curved angiographic catheter over a stiff guidewire. (B) A hydrophilic guidewire has been introduced through the catheter and is being negotiated down the ureter. (C) The catheter guidewire combination has been advanced into the urinary bladder. (D) The hydrophilic guidewire has been exchanged for a super-stiff Amplatz guidewire after negotiating a tight stricture at the ureterovesical junction. The ureteric stent is then placed over the stiff guidewire. (PCN: percutaneous nephrostomy).

catheter is left in place for 24 hours after the procedure, after which it is capped to check for free flow of urine into the bladder. Thereafter, if there is no hydronephrosis on sonography and contrast injection shows free flow down the double J stent, the external catheter is removed under fluoroscopic control to ensure that there is no inadvertent pulling back of the proximal loop of the stent.[5,19]

Balloon dilatation of benign ureteric strictures may provide durable relief in up to 50% of cases. Following the dilatation, the ureter is buttressed with a stent. In cases where repeated entry into the ureter may be required, a percutaneous nephroureteral catheter (internal-external stent) can be placed for providing mechanical support as well as preserving percutaneous access.[12] Anastomotic strictures after cystectomy and ureteric diversion to an ileal conduit can also be managed through an antegrade percutaneous approach.[20]

Internal-external stents are also placed in cases of ureteric leaks or fistulas because of the anticipated need for multiple percutaneous ureteral interventions and prolonged urinary drainage to allow healing. One should ensure that a solid portion of the tube traverses the site of leak with side holes above and below.

In patients with fistulas of the ureters or lower urinary tract associated with advanced inoperable pelvic malignancies, external drainage with a PCN catheter and a drainage catheter placed in the associated urinoma can at times, not provide adequate urinary diversion. In such cases, ureteral occlusion can be done using stainless steel or platinum coils deployed in the ureter proximal to the leak along with a PCN to provide relief from the distressing symptoms.[21] Other materials that can be used for ureteral occlusion include gelatin sponge, *n*-butyl cyanoacrylate, detachable balloons, or radiofrequency (RF) electrocautery.[22] The major drawback is the need for a life-long nephrostomy catheter due to the permanent occlusion.

Large-bore Track Creation

Percutaneous nephrostomy forms the first step for creation of a large-diameter track, which may be indicated for performing percutaneous stone therapy, nephroscopy, or antegrade ureteroscopy.[23] Tracks up to the size of 30F or larger can be created by using a combination of balloon dilatation systems and coaxial dilators.

SCLEROTHERAPY FOR RENAL CYSTS

Benign renal cysts (cortical or parapelvic) are found in approximately 50% of males above the age of 50 years. Renal cysts can vary greatly in size and are frequently multiple. They are usually silent, but large, infected, or hemorrhagic cysts can cause symptoms. Large cysts can also cause obstruction of the pelvicalyceal system with formation of calculi, and pressure atrophy of the adjacent renal parenchyma.[8,24]

A renal cyst that is symptomatic requires treatment. They can be managed percutaneously with a combination of sclerotherapy and drainage. Various agents can be used to induce sclerosis of the epithelial lining of the cyst. These include hypertonic dextrose or water-soluble contrast, iophandylate, absolute alcohol, tetracycline, and sodium tetradecyl sulfate. The procedure consists of puncture of the cyst under sonographic guidance and aspiration of the cyst contents. Contrast is then injected to demonstrate the internal appearance of the cyst and to rule out any communication of the cyst with the collecting system. If no communication is demonstrated and the cyst is small, sclerosant can be injected amounting to about one-third of the aspirated contents of the cyst. The sclerosant is left in place for 15–20 minutes with frequent postural changes of the patient to ensure contact with all the walls of the cyst and then reaspirated. If the cyst is larger, a 5F percutaneous drainage catheter can be placed in the cyst and left to drain for 24–48 hours before sclerotherapy. Larger cysts may require multiple sessions of sclerotherapy.

If a cyst is communicating with the renal collecting system, injection of sclerosant is not advisable as it can cause strictures in the pelvicalyceal system. An infected cyst is managed like an abscess with percutaneous catheter drainage. Good outcomes of sclerotherapy in renal cysts have been reported in literature with success rates varying between 75% and 100%.[8,24]

PERCUTANEOUS CATHETER DRAINAGE

Percutaneous catheter drainage can be done to drain renal or perirenal abscesses, collections, lymphoceles, or urinomas. The basic technique is similar to PCN consisting of needle puncture under imaging guidance, insertion and dilatation of the track followed by catheter placement **(Figs. 5A to C)**. The caliber and type of drainage catheter needs to be tailored according to the nature of fluid to be drained.

BIOPSIES

Core biopsy using automated guns is more common than fine-needle aspiration (FNA) in the genitourinary tract. Renal biopsy with a 16–18-G gun is used for identifying the cause of renal parenchymal disease. Biopsy or FNA can be performed for genitourinary tumors. Transrectal

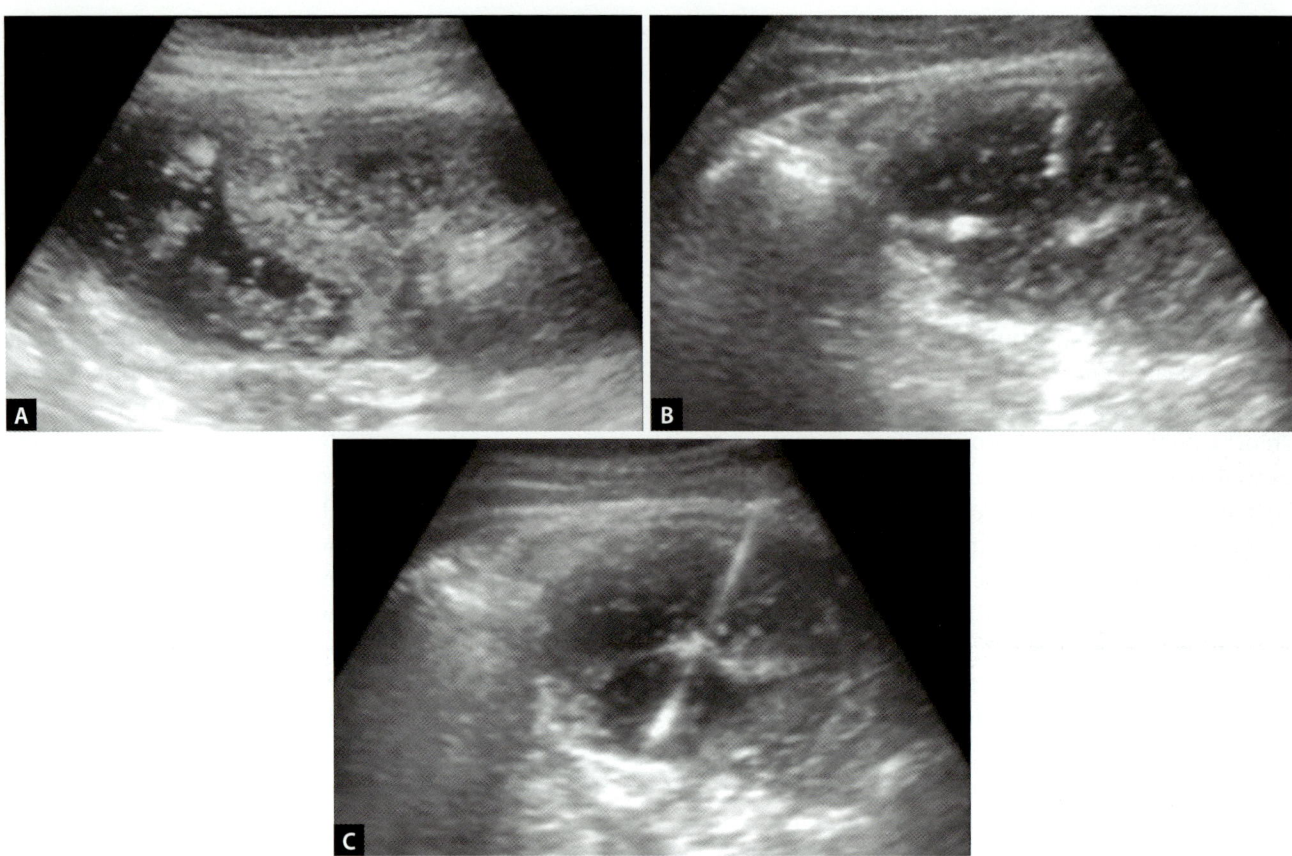

Figs. 5A to C: (A) An irregular collection with debris and internal echoes is seen in the upper pole of the kidney, suggestive of renal abscess. (B) The abscess has been punctured with an 18-gauge needle. (C) Guidewire is seen coiled in the abscess.

US-guided biopsy of the prostate is useful in suspected cases of prostatic carcinoma.

THE COMPLICATED RENAL TRANSPLANT

Common complications in renal transplant recipients include graft rejection, perigraft, or pelvic fluid collections (urinomas, lymphoceles, etc.), ureterovesical anastomotic strictures and focal parenchymal lesions. The percutaneous procedures required in this group of patients are similar to those required in native kidneys. The transplant kidney is approached from the lateral aspect with the patient supine **(Figs. 6A to D)**. These patients are usually very sick and immunocompromised; therefore, meticulous attention should be paid to asepsis.

ABLATION OF RENAL TUMORS

The incidence of renal cell carcinoma (RCC) has been seen to rise over recent years. This is probably due to the increased abdominal imaging and improvements in CT and MR technology resulting in the incidental detection of small, asymptomatic renal tumors in patients undergoing imaging for other indications. Recent studies have indicated that RCC may be incidentally detected during cross-sectional imaging in up to 60% of patients.[25,26] Patients with RCC limited to renal parenchyma have an excellent prognosis for cure, if the RCC can be resected. In the past, radical nephrectomy had been the conventional treatment for RCC. However, over last three decades, nephron-sparing surgery has become a viable alternative to radical nephrectomy and shown to be equally effective curative surgery for patients with a small (<5 cm), single, and well-defined RCC with a contralateral normal kidney.[25] However, nephron-sparing surgery requires more technical skills than radical nephrectomy with higher intraoperative blood loss. Many patients may be poor surgical candidates due to presence of significant comorbidities and advanced age. In addition, some patients may have multiple, bilateral tumors or poor renal function. In these patients, minimally invasive nephron-sparing surgical techniques have been applied including laparoscopic partial nephrectomy and percutaneous ablative techniques. Percutaneous ablative techniques for the treatment of RCC include thermal ablative techniques such as radiofrequency ablation (RFA), microwave ablation (MWA), and high-intensity

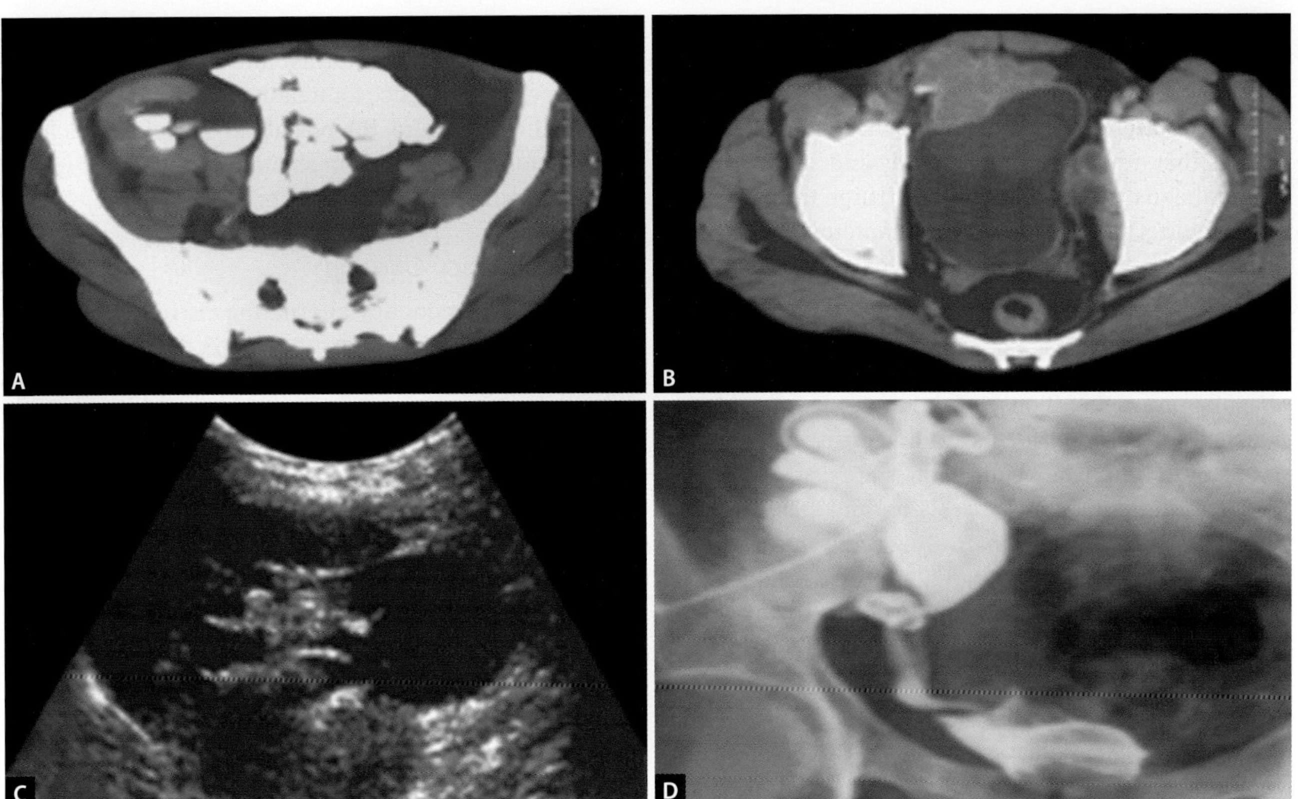

Figs. 6A to D: Anastomotic stricture in a transplant kidney. (A) CECT abdomen axial image showing hydroureteronephrosis in the transplant kidney. (B) There is a large, lobulated mass involving the ureterovesical anastomotic site engulfing the ureter. (C) Ultrasound image showing dilatation of the pelvis with minimal dilatation of the calyces. (D) Nephrostogram obtained after percutaneous nephrostomy demonstrates the stricture at the anastomotic site. This was successfully stented later.

focused US, which are based on heating the tissue, cryoablation (based on the freezing the tissue), and non thermal ablative technique irreversible electroporation (IRE). The first reports on the use of RFA in the treatment of renal tumors appeared in 1997 and it is widely used as an effective curative treatment option today.[27]

Indications

The American Urological Association guidelines support use of thermal ablative techniques in the treatment of T1a disease (<4 cm).[28] Indications for thermal ablation according to European Association of Urology guidelines include small renal masses in elderly comorbid patients unfit for surgery, increased risk of multiple tumors due to genetic predisposition (e.g. Von Hippel–Lindau syndrome), and in patients with tumors in both kidneys or with a single kidney and increased risk of complete loss of renal function following surgery (partial nephrectomy).[29,30]

The advantages of ablative therapies over surgery include decreased morbidity, better renal parenchymal volume preservation,[31] faster recovery, shorter hospital admission, and probably being the only treatment option for patients with comorbidities, unfit for surgery.[32] Meta-analysis of surgical (open or laparoscopic) and percutaneous ablative techniques reveal a lesser major complication rate for percutaneous ablative techniques.[33] The major disadvantage of ablative therapies over partial nephrectomy is higher local recurrence rate.[28] This difference may be overstatement due to a lack of significant data on long-term disease-free survival following percutaneous ablation of small RCCs. Short- and medium-term published study results[34-37] indicate that proper patient selection can yield good outcome comparable to that of partial nephrectomy, with added benefit of improved renal function preservation. The advantages and risks of each technique should be compared and contrasted with patient, and decision to ablate over surgery requires careful consideration.

Patient Selection and Preprocedure Evaluation

Large tumor size, tumors located near the hilum (renal sinus fat) or ureter were earlier not considered for ablative therapies due to the risk of complications and higher recurrence rate. However, with improved ablation devices, technical skills, and displacement of vital structures from the tumor, there has been significant increase in renal masses that are treated successfully and safely through percutaneous ablative techniques. Large tumors (up to 5 cm), central tumors, tumors in the anteromedial kidney, adjacent to bowel loops, and ureter have all been treated percutaneously, with cryoablation in particular.

Laboratory investigations to be performed prior to the procedure include serum creatinine, platelet count, and coagulation profile. Biopsy of the tumor before ablation is usually performed for tissue diagnosis, or just prior to ablation. Prophylactic antibiotics are usually administered. Contraindications are relative and include uncorrected coagulopathy and an ongoing acute illness.

All patients must undergo a contrast-enhanced CT or magnetic resonance imaging (MRI) of the abdomen before the procedure. The tumor should still be Robson's stage I or II to achieve curative results. Spread of the tumor beyond the renal fascia, into renal vein, or lymph nodes or distant metastases are contraindications for ablation. There is no absolute size criterion; however, the likelihood of complete ablation increases in smaller tumors. Tumors larger than 7 cm are unlikely to be successfully ablated and should only be considered for cytoreduction. ABLATE, a practical planning algorithm for percutaneous renal tumor ablation has been proposed, which takes into account: A—axial diameter of the tumor, B—proximity to bowel loops, L—location of the tumor within the kidney, A—adjacency or proximity to the ureter, T—touching the collecting system/renal sinus fat, and E—exophytic or endophytic location of the tumor.[38] Another commonly used algorithm is the RENAL nephrometry score (R—radius, E—endophytic or exophytic location of tumor, N—nearness to the renal sinus or collecting system, A—anterior or posterior location of the tumor, and L—location of the tumor in relation to polar line), a standardized classification system for quantifying the anatomic characteristics of renal masses. Higher score correlates with higher tumor grade, pathological stage, and increased risk of complications.[39,40]

Technical Considerations: Different Ablation Devices

Radiofrequency ablation, cryoablation, and MWA are the most commonly used thermal ablative devices for percutaneous ablation of renal tumors, and each has its own merits and demerits, which requires careful consideration. Irreversible electroporation (IRE) and high-intensity focused ultrasound are less commonly used in clinical practice for treating renal tumors. Regardless of the procedure, the postablative goal is to achieve a predictable and complete ablation of the tumor with at least 5–10 mm tumor-free margin.[41]

Radiofrequency Ablation

In RFA, high-frequency alternating current with wavelength ranging from 350 to 500 kHz is passed through a RF electrode placed in the target tumor. Grounding pads placed around the patient's thigh complete the electrical circuit. RF energy results in the heating of cells near the RF electrode/site of energy deposition. When human tissue is heated beyond 49°C, cell death occurs within minutes due to loss of enzymatic function, destruction of cell membranes, and cytoplasm. Temperatures more than 60°C cause immediate cell death. When the temperature exceeds 100°C, the cells boil releasing gas vapors, which cause tissue charring. These in turn inhibit the dispersion of RF energy decreasing the effectiveness of the procedure. Hence, ideal RFA devices should produce prolonged heating of the target tissue between 50°C and 100°C.[27] Various modifications developed toward this purpose include: (1) Pulsed energy deployment; (2) expansion of electrode surface; (3) intraparenchymal injection of iron compounds or saline before and during RF application; and (4) internal cooling of the needle electrode with saline.

Microwave Ablation

In microwave ablation (MWA), oscillating microwave electromagnetic field causes agitation of water molecules, which increases kinetic energy and, in turn increase in temperature inducing cell death via coagulation necrosis. Unlike RFA, microwaves transmit through all types of tissues and nonmetallic materials including water vapor, dehydrated, desiccated, and charred tissues created during the ablation. Hence, microwave produces larger zone of ablation, faster ablation with relatively less heat sink effect. Microwave systems have evolved significantly over the years through generator power optimization and optimization of cooling capabilities of antenna. Performance of each MWA differs as a function of power and time, as supported by the particular system. This affects size and shape of ablation zone created by different devices, hence requires careful attention by the interventional radiologists during device and patient selection.

Cryoablation

Cryoablation relies on rapid cooling of the tissue to induce cell death. Argon gas is used to rapidly freeze cryoprobe to achieve temperature up to –140°C, with critical temperature for cell death being between –20°C and –40°C. It is followed by passive thawing and second session of freeze for over 6–10 minutes depending on the size of the lesion. Rapid cooling leads to formation of ice crystals both intra- and extracellularly, leading to cell dehydration and rupture. Thawing of this frozen tissue leads to microvascular thrombosis and occlusion, and cell hypoxia, causing indirect ischemic injury.[42]

In contrast to RFA and MWA, cryoablation allows direct visualization of the ice ball and ablation zone approximately. The shape and size of the ice ball, there by ablative area can be manipulated by using multiple cryoprobes. During real-time assessment of ablation zone, the true ablation zone of irreversible cell death is approximately 5–10 mm deep to visualized ice ball edge, with temperature at the edge of the ice ball being 0°C approximately, which is a nonlethal temperature.[43] The ice ball must extend at least 5 mm beyond the margin of tumor to avoid residual lesion. In contrast to other thermal ablative therapies, cryoablation induces the maximum postablative immunomodulatory effect by releasing pro-inflammatory cytokines and dendritic cells (antigen-presenting cells) activation subsequently.[44]

Choice of Ablative Therapy: Clinical Consideration

Radiofrequency ablation, MWA, and cryoablation are established thermal ablative techniques for renal tumor ablation, and success of the procedure is a function of patient selection and method used for ablation, rather than ablation technology.[45] While the merits and drawbacks within a particular patient context are considered for choice of ablative therapy, one must also consider whether cooling or heating is the most appropriate mechanism to induce cell death. Ablation with heating mechanism has lower risk of hemorrhage compared to cryoablation. Between RFA and MWA, RFA is sensitive to heat sink effect with longer ablation duration compared to MWA. Hence, MWA may be a good choice for larger tumors and exophytic tumors as fewer applicators are required for complete ablation **(Figs. 7A to D)**.[46]

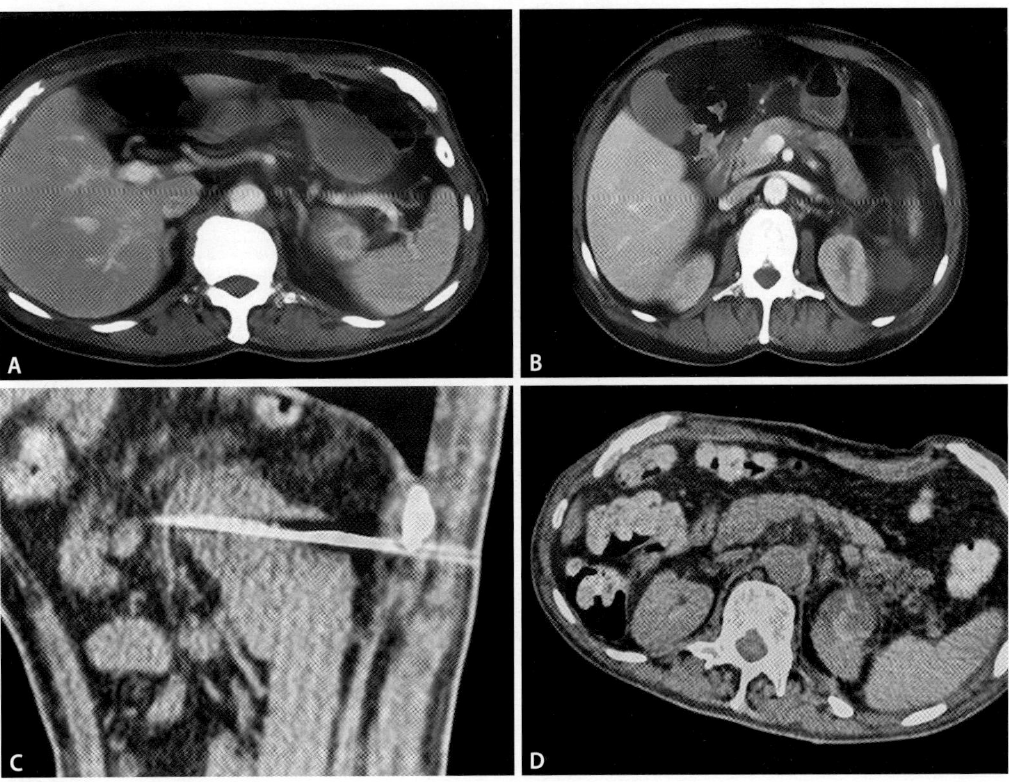

Figs. 7A to D: Microwave ablation (MWA) of a renal cell carcinoma. (A and B) Preprocedure axial CT image shows heterogeneously enhancing mass in upper pole of left kidney. (C) Intraprocedural CT sagittal reformatted image shows MWA probe *in situ* (D) Post-MWA ablation NCCT image shows ablated area with hemorrhage. (NCCT: noncontrast computed tomography).

Relative to the RFA and MWA, cryoablation is less painful to the patient and allows real-time visualization of the ablation zone **(Figs. 8A to D)**. Cryoablation is ideal for centrally placed tumors, as it is not associated with increased risk of bleeding from hilar vessels compared to MWA and RFA. In addition, ablation margin visualization in real time decreases the risk of ureteral damage.

All these procedures can be performed on an outpatient basis, and usually under local anesthesia with conscious sedation. General anesthesia may be required in certain cases such as deep seated, difficult to access lesions where precise respiratory control is required and large lesions where multiple probes need to be placed. The technique of placing cryoprobe or an electrode is similar to that of performing an imaging-guided biopsy of a focal lesion. The goal is to ablate the target tumor tissue as well as a 0.5–1 cm circumferential rim of adjacent normal parenchyma; therefore, an appropriate electrode size should be selected. The electrode is advanced till the deepest margin of the tumor as the ablation beyond the electrode tip is less.

Postprocedure and Follow-up

All patients should be kept under observation for 4–6 hours after the procedure. Antibiotics should be continued for at least 5 days postprocedure. Appropriate analgesics should be prescribed for ensuring adequate analgesia. Few complications have been reported after percutaneous ablation in renal lesions. Hematuria occurs rarely, is usually self-limited and commonly resolves

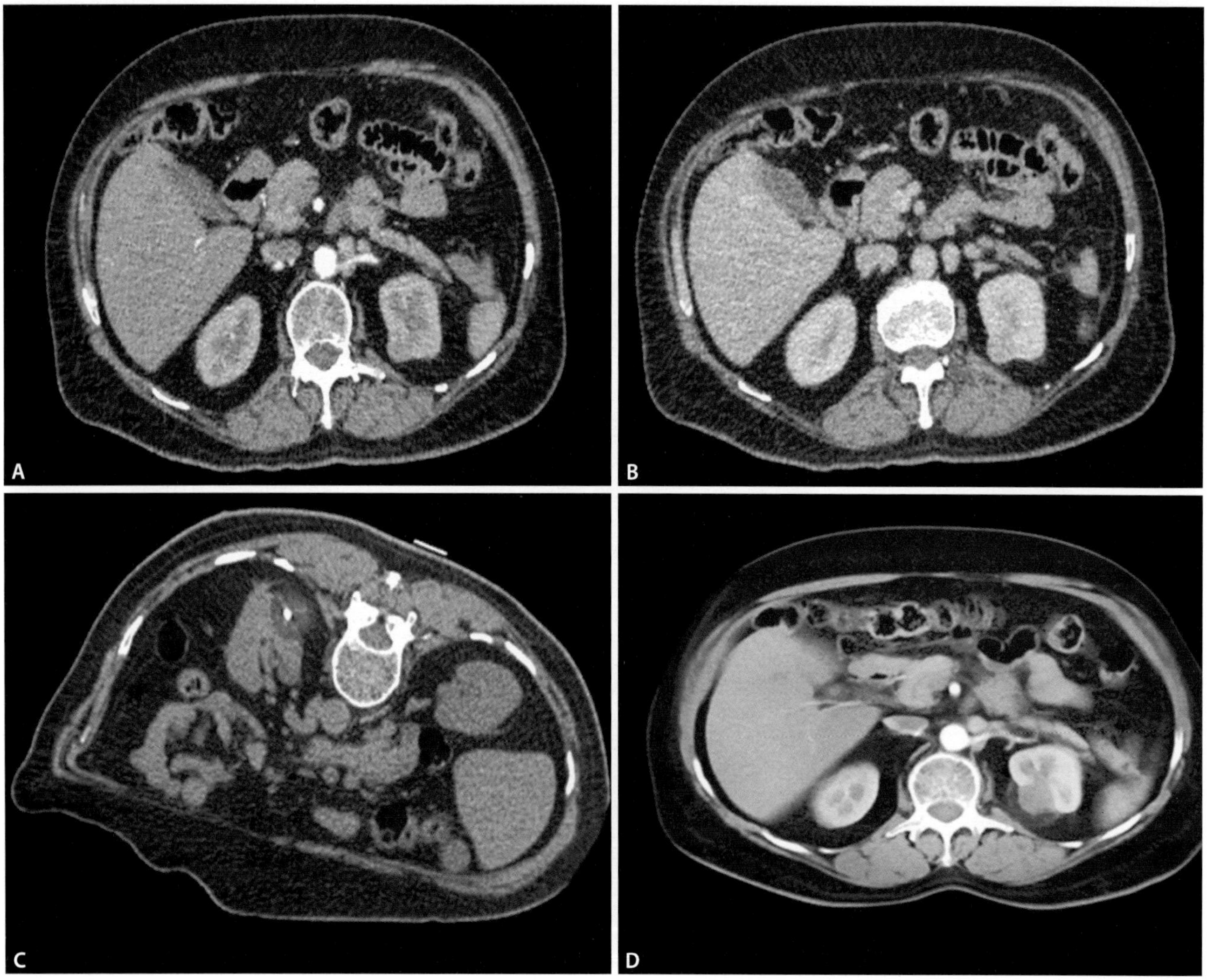

Figs. 8A to D: Cryoablation of a renal cell carcinoma. (A and B) Preprocedure axial CT images in arterial and venous phases show heterogeneously enhancing mass in upper pole of left kidney. (C) Intraprocedural CT image show cryoprobe *in situ* with formation of ice ball. (D) Post-cryoablation arterial phase CT image shows nonenhancing ablated area.

within 1–2 days. Thermal necrosis of adjacent bowel has been reported. There should be at least 5 mm of intervening gap or fat between the target tumor and bowel to avoid injury. If bowel abuts the target, sterile water/dextrose or air can be injected for bowel loops displacement and ensure safe ablation of the tumor (hydrodissection). RFA of lesions adjacent to the adrenal gland can cause release of vasoactive catecholamines, which requires administration of alpha-blockers. Perirenal hemorrhage is common but is rarely clinically significant. Needle-track seeding and development of ureteric strictures are other rare complications.

A contrast-enhanced biphasic CT should be obtained immediately after the procedure to determine adequacy of ablation. Thereafter a contrast-enhanced CT or MRI should be obtained at 1-, 3-, 6-, and 12-month intervals to look for residual or recurrent tumor. Imaging after the first year can be done at 6–9-month intervals. CT is more often used for postablation follow-up because of its wider availability and lower cost; however, MRI may be used in patients with renal insufficiency **(Figs. 9A to C)**.

Immediately after ablation, the tumor usually appears larger because of ablation of 0.5–1 cm of adjacent normal tissue. On follow-up imaging, ablated tumors appear as focal, nonenhancing masses, which show decrease in size with time. Soft tissue stranding may be seen in the perinephric fat. At times, a curvilinear, hyperattenuating area or halo is seen surrounding the ablated lesion.[24]

Nodular enhancement in the ablated tumor or an increase in the size of lesion represent residual or recurrent tumor. On MR, the area of necrosis appears hypointense on T2-weighted images. On T1-weighted images, it usually appears hyperintense compared to the renal cortex, and occasionally it may appear iso- to hypointense. Peripheral smooth enhancement of the rim may be seen early after ablation but this gradually resolves

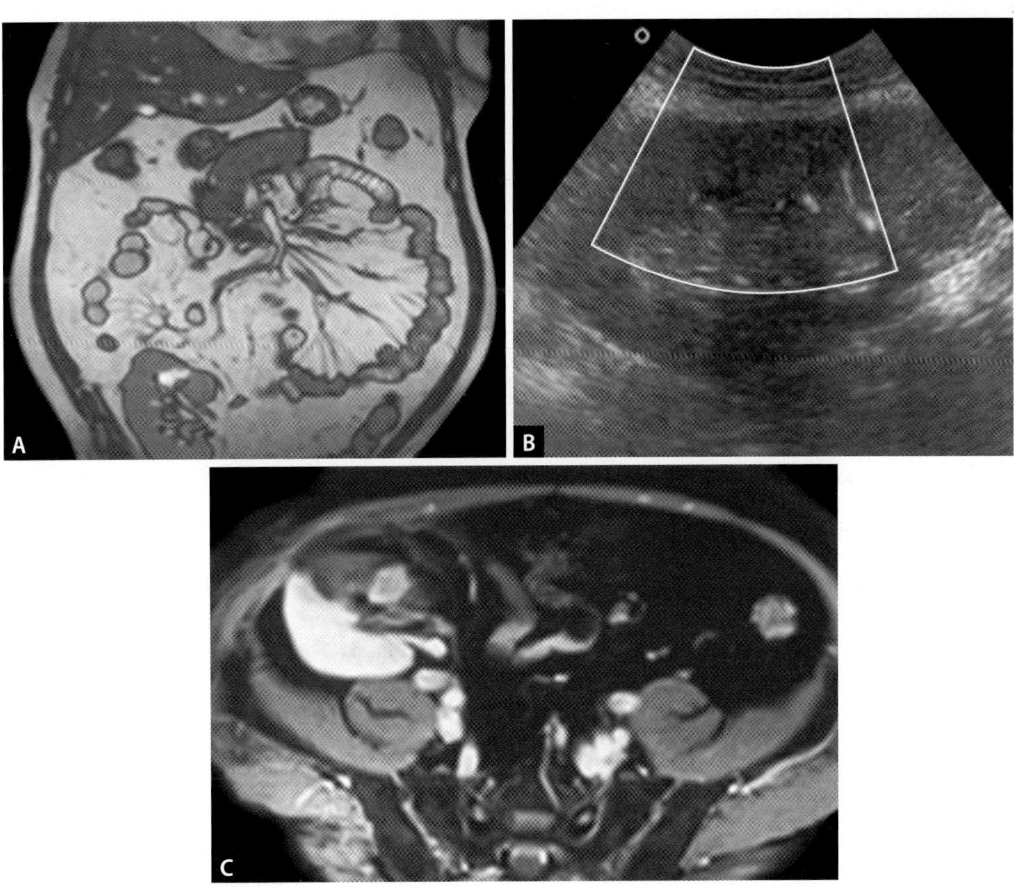

Figs. 9A to C: Radiofrequency ablation of a renal cell carcinoma in a transplant kidney. (A) Preprocedure MR coronal T2-weighted image shows a focal area of hyperintensity in the upper pole of the transplant kidney. (B) Follow-up Doppler image after 6 weeks shows absence of flow to the region of the ablated tumor. (C) MR axial postgadolinium T1 image 1 month after radiofrequency ablation shows absence of enhancement of the renal parenchyma in the region of ablation. Note the defect is larger than the original tumor size due to ablation of a rim of normal parenchyma around the tumor. (RFA: radiofrequency ablation).

over 3 months. Residual viable tumor tissue appears hyperintense on T2-weighted images and shows nodular enhancement postgadolinium on T1 images.[26]

To summarize, percutaneous ablative therapies are an effective treatment option in patients with early-stage renal cell carcinoma (RCC) who are poor surgical candidates, patients with increased risk of multiple tumors due to genetic predisposition, and in patients with bilateral tumors or with a solitary kidney. The choice of ablative technique is governed by preprocedural assessment and operative experience.

REFERENCES

1. Goodwin WE, Casey WL, Woolf W. Percutaneous trocar (needle) nephrostomy in hydronephrosis. J Am Med Asso. 1955;157(11):891-4.
2. Banner MP, Ramchandani P, Pollack HM. Interventional procedures in the upper urinary tract. Cardiovascular Intervent Radiol. 1991;14(5):267-84.
3. Pabon-Ramos WM, Dariushnia SR, Walker TG, et al. Quality improvement guidelines for percutaneous nephrostomy. J Vasc Interv Radiol. 2016;27(3):410-4.
4. Dyer RB, Regan JD, Kavanagh PV, et al. Percutaneous nephrostomy with extensions of the technique: step by step. Radiographics. 2002;22(3):503-25.
5. Hausegger KA, Portugaller HR. Percutaneous nephrostomy and antegrade ureteral stenting: technique–indications–complications. Eur Radiol. 2006;16(9):2016-30.
6. Meira MS, Barbosa PNVP, Bitencourt V, et al. Retrospective analysis of computed tomography guided percutaneous nephrostomies in cancer patients. Radiol Bras. 2019;52(3): 148-54.
7. Kariniemi J, Sequeiros RB, Ojala R, et al. MRI guided percutaneous nephrostomy: a feasibility study. Eur Radiol. 2009;19(5):1296-301.
8. Park BK, Kim SH, Moon MH. Nonvascular interventions of the urinary tract. J Korean Med Sci. 2002;17(6):727-36.
9. Funaki B, Vatakencherry G. Comparison of single-stick and double-stick techniques for percutaneous nephrostomy. Cardiovasc Intervent Radiol. 2004;27(1):35-7.
10. Ray CR, Brown AC, Smith MT, et al. Percutaneous access of nondilated renal collecting systems. Semin Intervent Radiol. 2014;31(1):98-100.
11. Gupta S, Gulati M, Suri S. Ultrasound guided percutaneous nephrostomy in nondilated pelvicalyceal system. J Clin Ultrasound. 1998;26(3):177-9.
12. Adamo R, Saad WEA, Brown DB. Management of nephrostomy drains and ureteral stents. Tech Vasc Interv Radiol. 2009: 12(3):193-204.
13. Farrell TA, Hicks ME. A review of radiologically guided percutaneous nephrostomies in 303 patients. J Vasc Intervent Radiol. 1997;8(5):769-74.
14. Wah TM, Weston MJ, Irving HC. Percutaneous nephrostomy insertion: outcome data from a prospective multi-operator study at a UK training centre. Clin Radiol. 2004;59(3):255-61.
15. Zagoria RJ, Dyer RB. Do's and don'ts of percutaneous nephrostomy. Acad Radiol. 1999;6(6):370-77.
16. Krohmer SJ, Pillai AK, Guevara CJ, et al. Image-guided nephrostomy interventions: How to recognize, avoid, or get out. Tech Vasc Intervent Radiol. 2018;21(4):261-6.
17. Vignali C, Lonzi S, Bargellini I, et al. Vascular injuries after percutaneous renal procedures: treatment by transcatheter embolization. Eur Radiol. 2004;14(4):723-9.
18. Gerspach JM, Bellman GC, Stoller ML, et al. Conservative management of colon injury following percutaneous renal surgery. Urology. 1997;49(6):831-6.
19. Kahriman G, Ozcan N, Dogan A, et al. Percutaneous antegrade ureteral stent placement: single centre experience. Diagn Interv Radiol. 2019;25(2):127-33.
20. Tal R, Bachar GN, Baniel J, et al. External Internal nephro-ureteral-ileal stents in patients with an ileal conduit: long-term results. Urology. 2004;63(3):438-41.
21. Titton RL, Gervais DA, Hahn PF, et al. Urine leaks and urinomas: diagnosis and imaging-guided intervention. Radiographics 2003;23(5):1133-47.
22. Avritscher R, Madoff DC, Ramirez PT, et al. Fistulas of the lower urinary tract: Percutaneous approaches for the management of a difficult clinical entity. Radiographics. 2004;24(Suppl 1): S217-36.
23. Bhattacharya T, Kumaradevan J, Watkinson AF. Percutaneous nephrolithotomy: state of the art. Semin Intervent Radiol. 2000;17(4):341-9.
24. Hanna RM, Dahniya MH. Aspiration and sclerotherapy of symptomatic simple renal cysts: value of two injections of a sclerosing agent. Am J Roentgenol. 1996;167(3):781-3.
25. Kawamoto S, Permpongkosol S, Bluemke DA, et al. Sequential changes after radiofrequency ablation and cryoablation of renal neoplasms: role of CT and MR imaging. Radiographics. 2007;27(2):343-55.
26. Farrell MA, Charboneau WJ, DiMarco DS, et al. Imaging-guided radiofrequency ablation of solid renal tumours. Am J Roentgenol. 2003;180(6):1509-13.
27. Zagoria RJ. Imaging-guided radiofrequency ablation of renal masses. Radiographics. 2004;24(Suppl 1):S59-71.
28. Campbell SC, Novick AC, Belldegrun A, et al. Guideline for management of the clinical T1 renal mass. J Urol. 2009;182(4): 1271-9.
29. Ljungberg B, Bensalah K, Canfield S, et al. EAU guidelines on renal cell carcinoma: 2014 update. Eur Urol. 2015;67(5): 913-24.
30. Van Poppel H, Becker F, Cadeddu JA, et al. Treatment of localised renal cell carcinoma. Eur Urol. 2011;60(4): 662-72.
31. Woldu SL, Thoreson GR, Okhunov Z, et al. Comparison of renal parenchymal volume preservation between partial nephrectomy, cryoablation, and radiofrequency ablation. J Endourol. 2015;29(8):948-55.
32. Higgins LJ, Hong K. Renal ablation techniques: state of the art. Am J Roentgenol. 2015;205(4):735-41.
33. Hui GC, Tuncali K, Tatli S, et al. Comparison of percutaneous and surgical approaches to renal tumor ablation: metaanalysis of effectiveness and complication rates. J Vasc Interv Radiol 2008;19(9):1311-20.
34. Katsanos K, Mailli L, Krokidis M, et al. Systematic review and meta-analysis of thermal ablation versus surgical nephrectomy for small renal tumours. Cardiovasc Intervent Radiol. 2014;37(2):427-37.

35. Chang X, Liu T, Zhang F, et al. Radiofrequency ablation versus partial nephrectomy for clinical T1a renal cell carcinoma: long-term clinical and oncologic outcomes based on a propensity score analysis. J Endourol. 2015;29(5):518-25.
36. Thompson RH, Atwell T, Schmit G, et al. Comparison of partial nephrectomy and percutaneous ablation for cT1 renal masses. Eur Urol. 2015;67(2):252-9.
37. Yu J, Liang P, Yu X, et al. US-guided percutaneous microwave ablation versus open radical nephrectomy for small renal cell carcinoma: intermediate-term results. Radiology. 2014; 270(3):880-7.
38. Schmit GD, Kurup AN, Weisbrod AJ, et al. ABLATE: a renal ablation planning algorithm. Am J Roentgenol. 2014;202(4): 894-903.
39. Kutikov A, Uzzo RG. The RENAL nephrometry score: a comprehensive standardized system for quantitating renal tumor size, location and depth. J Urol. 2009;182(2):844-53.
40. Parsons RB, Canter D, Kutikov A, et al. Renal nephrometry scoring system: the radiologist's perspective. Am J Roentgenol. 2012;199(3):W355-9.
41. Clark TWI, Millward SF, Gervais DA, et al. Reporting standards for percutaneous thermal ablation of renal cell carcinoma. J Vasc Interv Radiol. 2009;20(7 Suppl):S409-16.
42. Brian CA, Erick MR. Percutaneous cryoablation of renal tumors: patient selection, technique, and postprocedural imaging. Radiographics. 2010;30(4):887-902.
43. Georgiades C, Rodriguez R, Azene E, et al. Determination of the nonlethal margin inside the visible "ice-ball" during percutaneous cryoablation of renal tissue. Cardiovasc Intervent Radiol. 2013;36(3):783-90.
44. Jansen MC, van Hillegersberg R, Schoots IG, et al. Cryoablation induces greater inflammatory and coagulative responses than radiofrequency ablation or laser induced thermotherapy in a rat liver model. Surgery. 2010;147(5):686-95.
45. Cadeddu JA, Raman JD. Renal tumor ablation is a function of patient selection and technique—not the ablation technology. Cancer. 2008;113:2623-26.
46. Lubner MG, Brace CL, Hinshaw JL, et al. Microwave tumor ablation: mechanism of action, clinical results, and devices. J Vasc Interv Radiol. 2010;21(8 Suppl):S192-203.

27

Chapter

Vascular Interventions in the Genitourinary Tract

Shivanand Gamanagatti, Ankur Goyal, Deep Narayan Srivastava

INTRODUCTION

Interventional vascular radiology has grown over the past two to three decades and the radiologist has an important role to play in patient's management. With the current advances in technology allowing more accurate and controlled deployment of embolic agents, embolotherapy has now become the procedure of choice for the management of visceral and solid organ aneurysms and also percutaneous renal revascularization has become an accepted procedure of choice for renal artery stenosis (RAS).

Various vascular interventional procedures in genitourinary practice are directed toward vascular dilatation or vascular embolization. The commonly performed procedures include:

- Renal artery angioplasty
- Renal artery stenting
- Renal artery embolization
- Uterine artery embolization (UAE)
- Vaginal arteriovenous malformation (AVM) embolization
- Varicocele embolization
- Scrotal AVM embolization
- Prostatic artery embolization (PAE)
- Transjugular renal biopsy (TJRB)
- Prophylactic balloon placement in adherent placenta.

RENAL ARTERY ANGIOPLASTY

Renal artery stenosis is the most common cause of secondary hypertension, seen with a 14% prevalence among patients with chronic renal failure. Among the various causes of RAS, atherosclerosis is the most common etiology, others being fibromuscular dysplasia, Takayasu's arteritis, neurofibromatosis, etc. Medical therapy and surgical treatment including renal vascularization and nephrectomy are traditional methods of treatment for renovascular hypertension. These methods, however, have several disadvantages. The lowering of blood pressure by medical therapy further reduces renal blood flow and further deterioration of renal function even in controlled blood pressure. The surgical revascularization methods are considerably beneficial to most patients but considering the associated morbidity and operative mortality rate of 8%, surgery should be done only on carefully selected patients. Presently, percutaneous transluminal renal angioplasty (PTRA) is the first line of treatment for RAS due to its relatively lower morbidity and mortality compared to surgical methods. The Society of Cardiovascular and Interventional Radiology (SCVIR) has laid down guidelines for the renal artery angioplasty. Various pathological lesions are shown in **Table 1**.

Table 1: Various pathological lesions.

Cause	*Affected segment*	*Incidence (%)*
Atherosclerosis	Ostium and proximal 1/3	90
Fibromuscular dysplasia	Mid and distal 1/3	10
Takayasu's arteritis	Ostium and proximal part	<1
NF-1	All	<1
Radiation	All	<1
Trauma	All	<1

According to the SCVIR guidelines, the above lesions can be divided into four categories as follows:[1]

- *Category I: Lesions* are those for which balloon angioplasty alone is the procedure of choice. It includes fibromuscular dysplasia of the renal artery and unilateral short (<3 cm) and nonostial atherosclerosis **(Figs. 1 and 2)**.
- *Category II: Lesions* are well suited for angioplasty and are atherosclerotic bilateral nonostial stenosis, postoperative anastomotic stenosis, and stenoses associated with worsening renal function **(Fig. 3)**.
- *Category III: Lesions* have a moderate chance of technical success or long-term benefits compared to bypass surgery and are atherosclerotic renal ostial stenosis, nonatheromatous lesions involving the proximal renal arteries.
- *Category IV: Lesions* have a low technical success rate. This includes renal artery stenoses in vessels that arise from an aneurysmal or severely diseased aortic segment or stenoses associated with renal artery aneurysm.

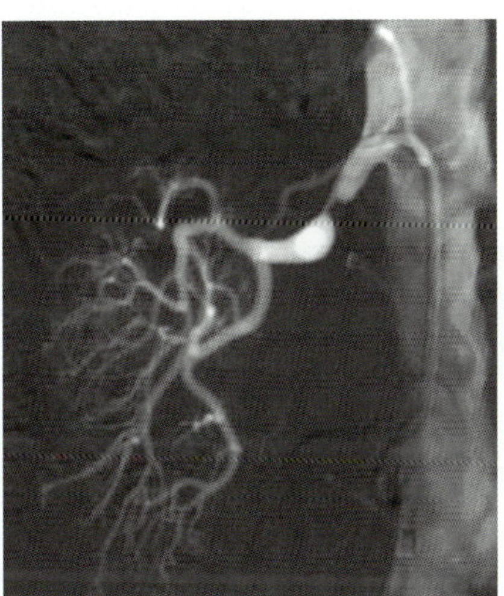

Fig. 1: Selective renal angiogram showing nonostial short segment narrowing with post-stenotic dilation of right renal artery (category I lesions).

Imaging the Renal Arteries

Conventional angiography has been conventionally considered the best anatomic study for evaluating patients with RAS. Duplex ultrasonography can be very helpful and should be the first imaging study in patients suspected of having RAS. The quality of renal ultrasonography depends on the operator and on other variables such as body habitus, but even so, the sensitivity of duplex scanning has been reported to be 98%, with 98% specificity and high positive and negative predictive values.[2]

Computed tomography angiography (CTA) has now replaced conventional angiography for evaluating renal arteries. The images are comparable to those of conventional angiography, vessels can be evaluated in three dimensions, and CTA offers options for clarifying anatomy which may be better than with conventional angiography. Exposure of the patient to radiation from renal CTA is comparable to that of catheter angiography.[2]

Magnetic resonance angiography (MRA) is also used to evaluate the anatomy of the renal arteries. It has lower resolution than CTA or conventional angiography but is excellent for patients with impaired renal function, especially with the availability of noncontrast angiography sequences.[2,3]

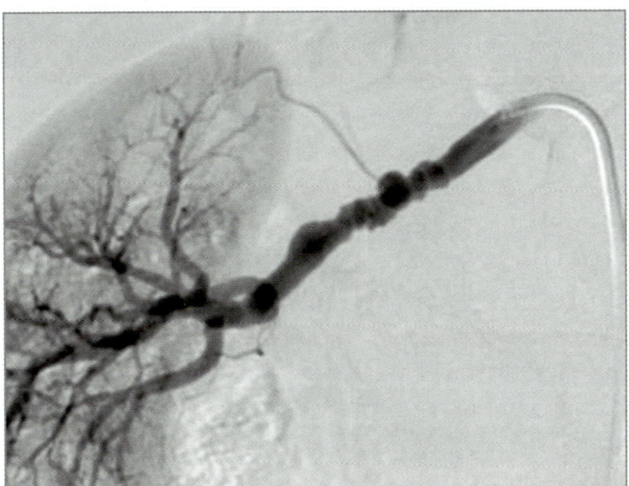

Fig. 2: Selective renal angiogram showing classic string of pearls appearance of right renal artery suggestive of fibromuscular dysplasia (category I lesions).

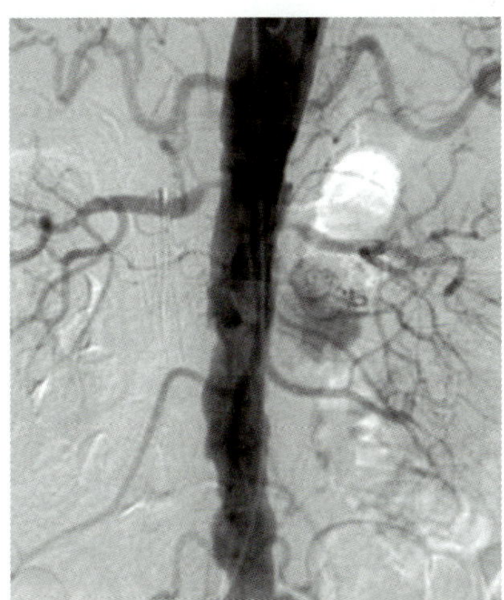

Fig. 3: Flush aortogram showing diffuse atherosclerotic abdominal aorta and ostial narrowing of bilateral renal arteries (category II lesions).

Technique[4-6]

Endovascular treatment of RAS involves either percutaneous transluminal angioplasty or a combination of angioplasty and stent placement.

Renal Artery Angioplasty

The procedure is most commonly performed through a femoral artery approach. However, if indicated by the patient's anatomy (e.g. presence of iliac artery occlusions or a very steeply angled renal artery), the brachial approach can be used. A 6-F sheath is inserted into the femoral artery. It will be very helpful if a long (typically 35 cm) sheath is used as a guiding catheter. A preshaped catheter is then used to access the renal artery. The catheter is used in combination with a guidewire to cross the lesion. A hydrophilic guidewire such as a Terumo can be very helpful, especially in lesions that are difficult to cross, though many would also use the soft-tipped Bentson guidewire. Having crossed the lesion, heparin and an antispasmodic drug are administered. The author uses 3000 units of heparin and 300 mg of isosorbide dinitrate.

With the catheter across the stenosis, the guidewire is changed to a specialist guidewire such as the roadrunner. The guidewire itself is very stiff, providing good support for the angioplasty balloon. The atraumatic nature of the tip is very important, as it can be placed in a cortical branch without a significant danger of causing spasm. An angioplasty balloon is then introduced over the guidewire and angioplasty is performed **(Figs. 4A to E)**. After confirming the proper position of balloon, it is inflated and left for 30 seconds.

Balloons are not oversized but should instead be of the same diameter as the artery distal to the stenosis. Typical balloon diameters will vary between 5 mm and 7 mm. Loin pain with balloon inflation is common but should not be severe. In the event of the latter, vessel rupture may occur,

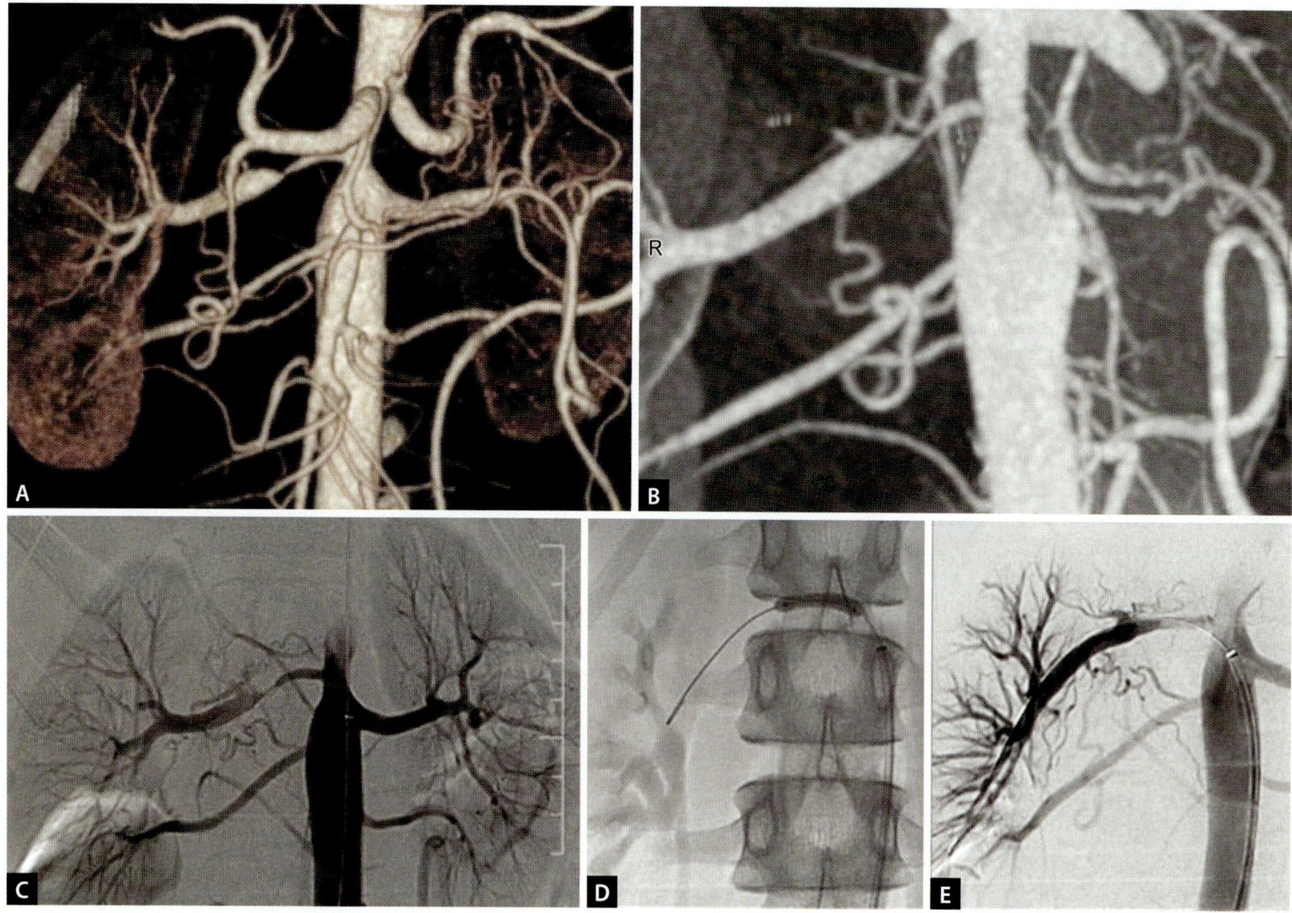

Figs. 4A and E: A case of renal artery stenosis treated by angioplasty: (A and B) CT images showing narrowing of juxtarenal part of abdominal aorta and right main renal artery with post-stenotic dilatation; (C) Flush aortogram confirming the CT findings of narrowing of juxtarenal part of abdominal aorta and right main renal artery; (D) Angioplasty spot image showing dilatation of narrowed segment of main renal artery using 6 mm balloon catheter; (E) Post-angioplasty angiogram showing <10% percent residual narrowing of angioplasty segment.

and dilation should be stopped and a smaller balloon should be used. After dilation, the balloon is removed, the guidewire is left in place, and a check angiogram is performed through the long sheath or guiding catheter. If there has been a complication or further dilation is required, access has thus been maintained to allow additional intervention. The angioplasty is considered technically successful if after the angioplasty, the arterial lumen had less than 30% residual stenosis and the pressure gradient is less than 10 mm Hg. The clinical results can be assessed by the effect on blood pressure control and improvement of renal function.

RENAL ARTERY STENTING

The renal artery stent placement is now an established method of adjunctive treatment to renal angioplasty. Several problems related to renal angioplasty, such as flow-compromising dissection, residual stenosis greater than 30% with a trans-stenotic pressure gradient greater than 20 mm Hg or restenosis, can be successfully treated with stenting. The renal artery stenting has shown better technical results, long-term patency, and a lower rate of restenosis than that of PTRA. Stents are almost exclusively placed in the renal arteries by using an angioplasty balloon (balloon-expandable rather than self-expanding stents). In many respects, insertion of renal artery stents is performed in a similar way to renal angioplasty. However, stents are normally inserted at the ostium of the renal artery because they are used for the treatment of atheromatous disease. It is therefore essential to have a clear idea of the exact location of the ostium to facilitate accurate stent placement. Prior to stent insertion, it is of value to predilate the stenosis with a 4-mm balloon to ease the passage of the stent across the stenosis. Although many recommend the use of a guiding catheter, modern long sheaths also perform very well. Use of either allows angiograms to be performed while finally positioning the stent prior to deployment. There are no reported adverse consequences associated with leaving the stent projecting 2 mm or so into the aorta.

Positioning the stent in this manner ensures that the entire lesion is stented. Sometimes it may be necessary to perform renal arterial intervention from a brachial approach, for example, when femoral access is not possible or if the renal arteries are sharply angulated inferiorly **(Figs. 5A and B)**.

Outcome

Compared with the relatively good outcomes after angioplasty for fibromuscular dysplasia, balloon angioplasty alone has not been as successful in treating atherosclerotic RAS. This is most likely because of the high degree of elastic recoil in atherosclerotic arteries compared with that encountered in fibromuscular webs.

The restenosis rate after angioplasty alone varies widely but has been reported to be from 10% to 46%.[5] Angioplasty (without stent placement) has a higher technical success rate when applied to atherosclerotic lesions in the midportion of the main renal artery (72–82%) than in ostial lesions (success rate ≈ 60%).

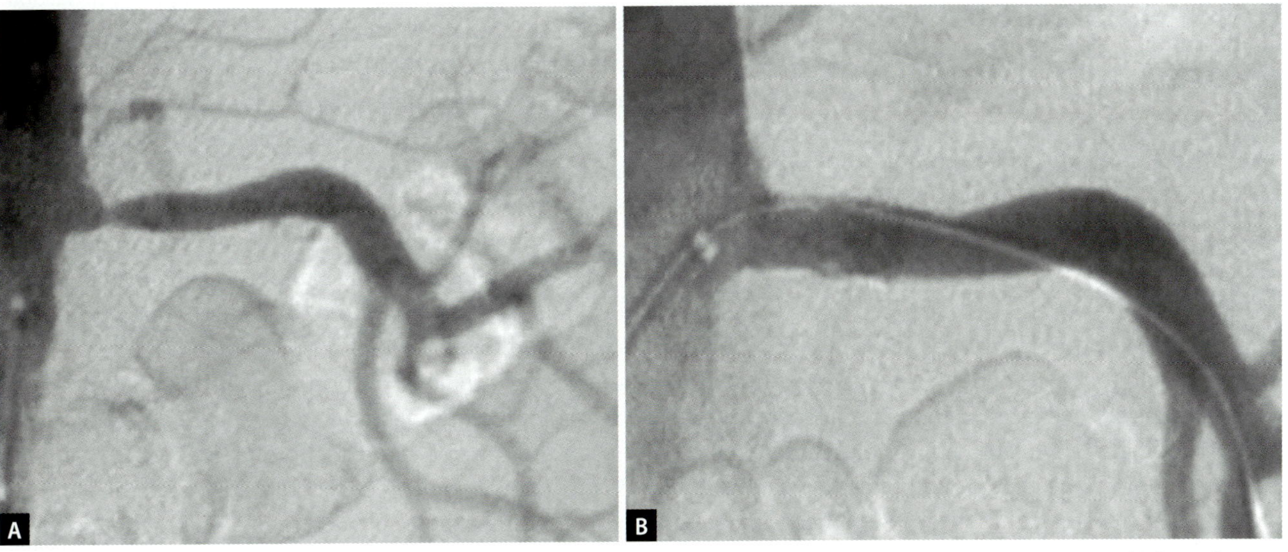

Figs. 5A and B: A case of renal artery ostial narrowing treated by stenting: (A) Renal angiogram showing ostial narrowing of left renal artery. (B) Post-stenting angiogram showing 0% residual stenosis.

Stents are now almost uniformly used for all ostial lesions and almost all atherosclerotic RAS. One current report quotes a technical success rate for stents of 94–100% and a restenosis rate of 11–23%, with an improvement in blood pressure control in 50–80% and stabilization of renal function in 60–70%.[5,6]

Renal function at the time of stent placement strongly predicts patency and expected survival after intervention. In patients with normal renal function, 3-year survival is 94%, 74% if serum creatinine is between 1.5 mg/dL and 2.0 mg/dL, and 52% if serum creatinine is > 2.0 mg/dL.[6] It is important to understand that though renal artery revascularization in atherosclerosis seldom cures the disease, it brings down the blood pressure and/or the requirement of antihypertensive medication modestly.

Renal Artery Intervention in Renal Transplants

Although technically angioplasty and stenting are similar in many ways to procedures in native kidneys, the management of transplant RAS involves some important differences. Cadaveric transplants are generally anastomosed to the recipient external iliac artery, because it is possible to obtain the full length of renal artery and renal vein stump. These procedures are separately described in the chapter on Imaging of Renal Transplant.

Complications

The complications can be divided into major (renal insufficiency, renal artery occlusion, renal artery damage including rupture, etc.) and minor (temporary renal insufficiency, retroperitoneal hematoma, femoral artery complications, etc).

RENAL ARTERIAL EMBOLIZATION

The various indications are embolization of renal neoplasms, renal pseudoaneurysms (secondary to either traumatic or iatrogenic injury), end-stage kidney, etc.

Technique

There are three different types of renal embolization: (1) proximal (occlusion of main or segmental renal artery), (2) distal (occlusion of lobular or arcuate arteries), and (3) capillary (occlusion of arterioles and glomeruli). Depending upon the type of embolization, the catheter is advanced into the renal artery branches. The superselective embolization with a coaxial catheter can save part of renal parenchyma. The selection of embolizing material also depends upon the purpose of occlusion (temporary or permanent). The various materials used for embolization are particles (gelfoam, polyvinyl alcohol), liquid agents (alcohol, sclerosants), coils, and detachable balloons.

Transcatheter Embolization of Renal Neoplasms

The current role of renal embolization in carcinoma of the kidney is uncertain.

The most important aim of preoperative embolization of the renal artery is to prevent migration of tumor cells from being flooded out.

The various indications are:

- To relieve symptoms such as pain, hematuria, polycythemia, congestive heart failure
- To facilitate surgical resection by preoperative embolization to reduce the tumor vascularity
- To inhibit tumor growth and to reduce tumor mass
- To stimulate an immune response by decreasing the tumor load
- Prophylactic embolotherapy in angiomyolipomas to avoid risk of hemorrhage.

The impact of renal embolization as the palliative method of treatment on the survival time is difficult to estimate, but improvement in local symptoms such as hematuria and pain is evident.

Varieties of embolizing agents have been used such as gelatin sponge, stainless steel coil, *n*-butyl cyanoacrylate, absolute alcohol, and autologus blood clot. But the embolization material of choice is ethanol. Ethanol is widely used for permanent embolization. The optimal dose is 0.5 mL/kg of body weight with an upper limit of 1 mL/kg and at the rate of 2 mL/sec. The advantages of alcohol over other permanent embolizing material are complete tissue necroses with permanent arterial occlusion, milder postinfarction syndrome, less chances of infection, and simple to use.

The technique for delivery of absolute alcohol to renal artery includes the balloon occlusion technique and superselective technique.[7,8] The balloon occlusion technique serves several purposes like it prevents reflux of alcohol into aorta and prolongs the contact period of alcohol with endothelium.

In the superselective technique, an endhole catheter is advanced superselectively into lobar braches and the alcohol is injected to prevent reflux. This is then followed by large vessel embolization with coils. The mechanism of action of alcohol is proposed to be a combination of perivascular necrosis, sludging of erythrocytes in small arteries, and glomeruli and endothelial damage.

The rate of injection has serious impact over the success of embolization. An injection rate of 1–5 mL/sec leads to perivascular necrosis, sludging of erythrocytes in small arteries, and glomeruli indicating direct tissue toxicity. A slow rate of injection of 0.1 mL/sec causes endothelial damage and less tissue toxicity. Hence, a slow rate of injection is desirable in benign conditions such as AVM and angiomyolipomas, where permanent arterial occlusion with minimal tissue damage is desirable.[7]

All arteries smaller than major segmental arteries must be occluded. Angiographic findings of successful embolization include stagnation of flow and extravasation of contrast material into adjacent renal parenchyma **(Figs. 6A to F)**.

Care must be taken when embolizing with absolute ethanol as it causes vigorous thrombosis due to denaturing proteins. Ethanol can cause seizures and intoxication if it reaches the systemic circulation. It can also permeate the tissues and cause injury to adjacent structures such as bowel and nerves.

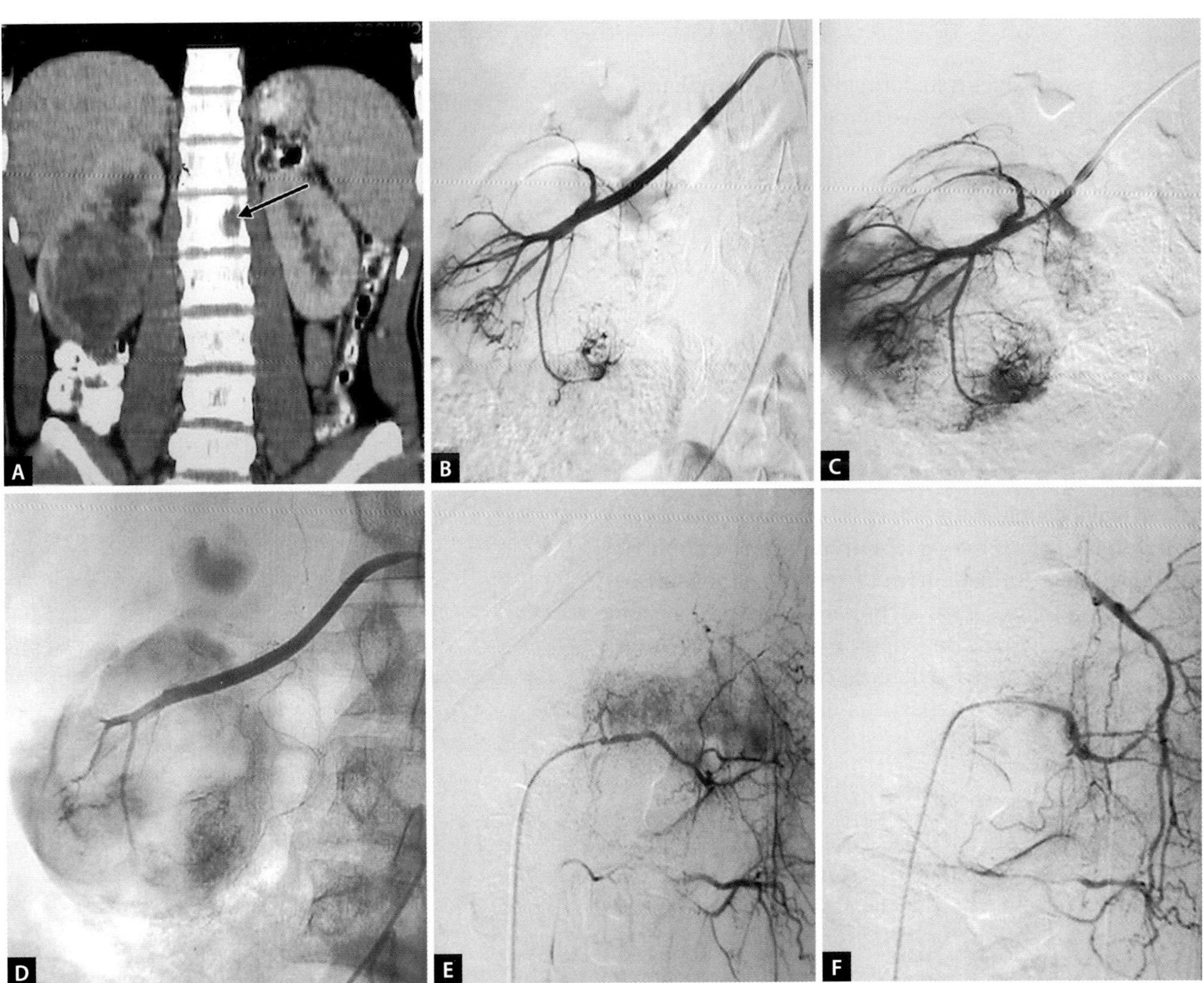

Figs. 6A to F: A case of renal cell carcinoma with vertebral metastasis treated by absolute alcohol. (A) Coronal MPR image showing large mass lesion in lower pole of right kidney. Note: destructive lytic lesion in L1 vertebra (arrow); (B) Selective angiogram showing tumor neovascularity in lower polar region; (C) Delayed angiogram showing tumor blush and no arteriovenous shunting; (D) Postembolization angiogram showing stasis of contrast, persistent tumor staining and obliteration of tumor vascularity; (E) Selective angiogram of paraspinal artery showing tumor blush supplying the L1 vertebral lesion; (F) Following embolization with polyvinyl alcohol (PVA) particles (500–700 μ) showing obliteration of tumor vascularity.

Transcatheter Embolization of Renal Pseudoaneurysms

Incidence

Incidence of aneurysm formation differs for the various etiologies of renal artery aneurysms. However, literature suggests that incidence ranges between 0.015% and 9.7%.[9] Poutasse have classified renal artery aneurysms into saccular, fusiform, dissecting and pseudoaneurysms.[10] The natural history of these aneurysms is not well-defined in the literature. However, the incidence of rupture rate ranges from 0% to 14%.[10] Renal artery aneurysms that are treated surgically are approached by nephrectomy, ex vivo repair and reimplantation.[9-11]

Causes

Typically, pseudoaneurysm formation in the renal artery distribution is either iatrogenic or traumatic. Other causes of aneurysm formation include fibromuscular dysplasia, polyarteritis nodosa, amphetamine abuse, angiomyolipoma (either with or without associated tuberous sclerosis) and neurofibromatosis.

Risks Posed by the Aneurysm

Rupture is a rare risk of these aneurysms. However, pregnant women are more prone to rupture which is similar to splenic artery aneurysms rupture.

Anatomic/Physiologic Considerations

The vascular supply to the kidney is considered endorgan, and hence infarction is common after embolization. Therefore, in patients with renal insufficiency or underlying diseases such as tuberous sclerosis or von Recklinghausen's disease, nephron-sparing procedures are vital. Superselective embolization is advisable in all cases of renal artery embolization unless partial or total nephrectomy is planned.

Technique

The renal arteries arise at the L2 level from the abdominal aorta. A left anterior oblique view during a flush injection of the aorta will often provide the best view of the origins. Careful examination for accessory renal arteries is necessary.

A renal double curve or Cobra catheter will easily engage the main renal ostium. A Rosen wire is an atraumatic guidewire that allows for secure exchange or upsizing to a guiding catheter or Balkin sheath. Selective injection should be performed to identify the feeding vessel or vessels. This can be done through the sheath. Many embolization techniques can be used in this setting depending on the type, number and location of the aneurysms. Commonly pseudoaneurysms are embolized superselectively by using coils **(Figs. 7A to D)**. Sometimes, aneurysms of the main renal artery maybe amenable to stent graft placement, thus allowing distal perfusion to be maintained. Alternative management options include surgical repair by resection, aneurysmorraphy and autotransplantation.

More peripherally located aneurysms can be selectively coil embolized using microcatheter technique **(Figs. 8A to F)**. Both distal and proximal control is not always possible and may not be necessary due to the vascular anatomy.

In the presence of multiple aneurysms from a lesion such as an angiomyolipoma, a combination of particle and coil embolization can be performed. If actively bleeding, the aneurysms are coiled first, followed by occlusion of the feeding vessels to the tumor with polyvinyl alcohol (PVA) or embospheres. Gelfoam can be sandwiched between coil nests to assist thrombosis.[12-15]

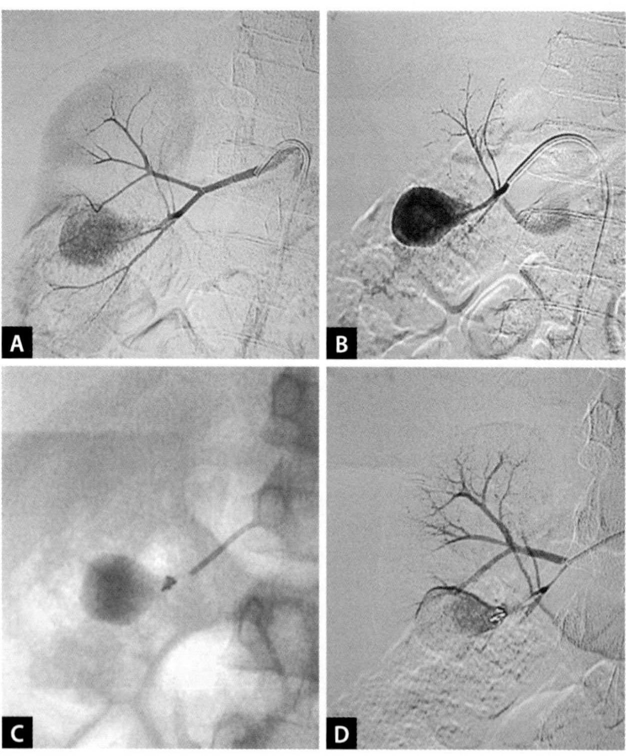

Figs. 7A to D: Post-percutaneous nephrolithotomy (PCNL) renal artery pseudoaneurysm treated by coil embolization. (A and B) Selective renal angiogram showing large pseudoaneurysm arising from lower polar artery; (C) Spot image showing coil at the neck of pseudoaneurysm; (D) Post-embolization angiogram showing nonfilling of pseudoaneurysm.

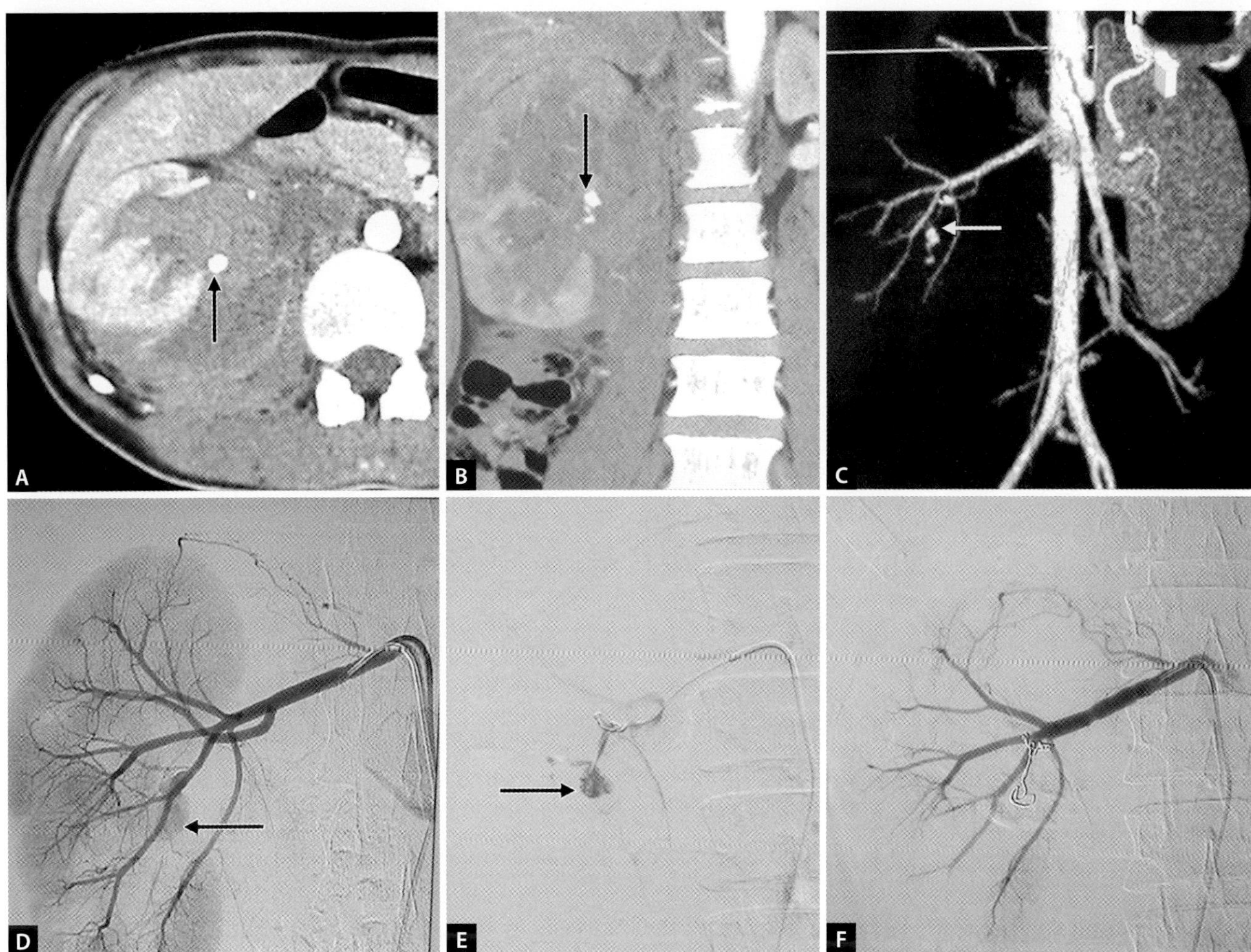

Figs. 8A to F: Post-PCNL renal artery pseudoaneurysm treated by microcoils using microcatheter coaxial technique. (A to C) Contrast-enhanced CT images showing small extrarenal pseudoaneurysm with surrounding large hematoma formation; (D) Selective renal angiogram showing filling of pseudoaneurysm supplied by lower polar branch of right renal artery; (E) Superselectively getting access into the branch supplying pseudoaneurysm using microcatheter; (F) Post-embolization angiogram showing nonfilling of pseudoaneurysm.

Results of Embolization

The technical success is quite high once the renal artery is securely accessed. If super- selective techniques are used, very little ischemia results and there is very little chance of inducing renal failure.

Complications

Although rare, dissection or perforation of the renal arteries and their branches can occur. Rupture may lead to rapid development of retroperitoneal hemorrhage. Both dissection flaps and rupture can be immediately controlled with balloon tamponade. Although dissection flaps can often be tacked down, rupture typically requires emergent surgery. Even perforation of smaller branch vessels can occur if a guidewire is passed too far into the periphery.

Embolization of End-stage Kidney

The nonfunctional kidney may manifest with pain, hypertension, albuminuria and other symptoms. In such cases embolization procedure can replace surgical nephrectomy **(Figs. 9A to D)**.

Technique

Absolute alcohol is a very effective "permanent" agent for occluding capillaries. The embolization material is injected cautiously through an endhole catheter under fluoroscopic control to avoid reflux into the aorta. The embolization is considered complete when there is stasis of contrast medium in the major renal arteries without any flow of contrast material into the distal branches. There is therefore residual opacification of the parenchyma of the embolized kidney. During the embolization,

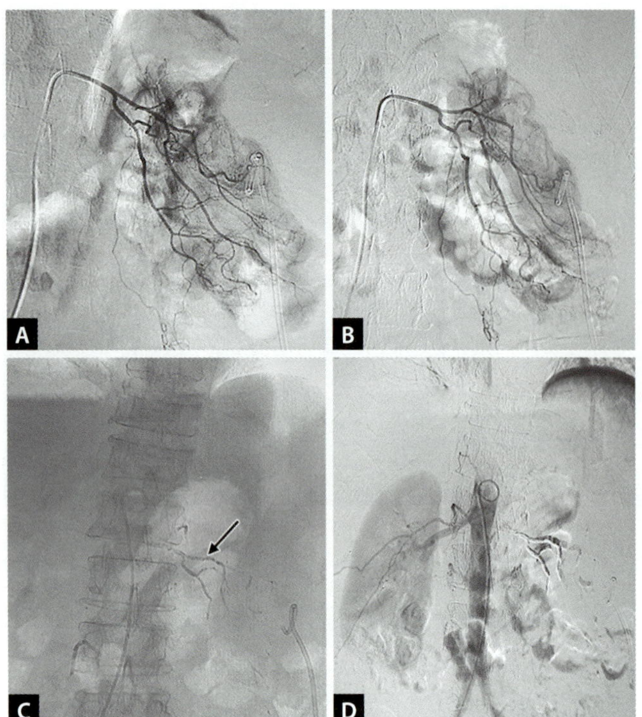

Figs. 9A to D: Glue embolization of nonfunctioning kidney. (A and B) Selective renal angiogram showing tortuous intrarenal branches; (C) Spot image showing glue cast in the intrarenal branches; (D) Post-embolization flush aortogram showing complete obliteration of left renal artery and no parenchymal blush seen.

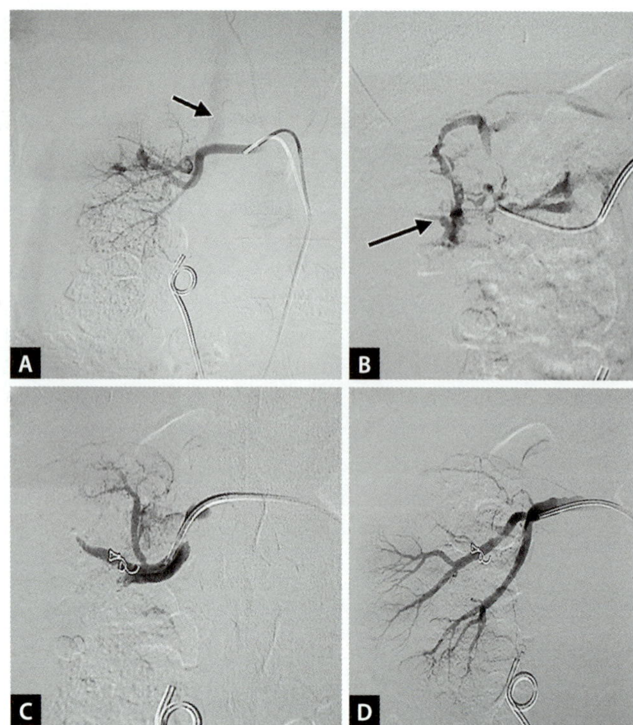

Figs. 10A to D: Post-PCNL arteriovenous (AV) fistula treated by coil embolization. (A) Selective right renal angiogram showing small contrast-filled structure supplied by upper polar artery with early draining vein; (B) Superselective angiogram showing getting close to the site of AV fistula (arrow); (C) Coil embolization of the AV fistula site; (D) Post-embolization angiogram showing obliteration of the AV fistula.

patients commonly experience severe flank pain on the side of the kidney being infarcted and intravenous opiate analgesia is required for pain control. This limits the procedure to embolization of a single kidney at any one sitting. Patients must be then carefully monitored for 24 hours and kept in the hospital until their pain and any associated pyrexia has settled.[7,8]

The complications are mainly postembolization syndrome in the form of flank pain for few days, fever, nausea, vomiting, etc. There may be hypertension in the first few hours. Majority of these symptoms are self-limited and are resolve without any specific treatment. Rarely there may be major complications like renal failure, renal abscess and testicular infarction. The results of embolization are quite encouraging in most of the clinical situations.

Arteriovenous fistulas and malformations: Acquired arteriovenous fistulas in the kidney are usually the result of trauma, especially percutaneous biopsy. Massive renal arteriovenous (AV) fistulas can cause high-output heart failure. Congenital AVMs of the kidney are exceedingly rare. These lesions consist of numerous dilated, tortuous vessels within the subepithelium of the collecting system. When symptomatic, they usually present with gross hematuria and less commonly are associated with hypertension or an abdominal bruit. Color Doppler sonography, CT and MRI are useful in detecting some of these lesions.

At angiography, an AV fistula produces dilatation of the feeding branch and early filling of the draining vein. Numerous segmental or interlobar arteries feed the renal AVM, which is composed of dilated, tortuous channels with rapid shunting into renal vein and inferior vena cava.

Transcatheter embolization is the first-line of treatment for most of these lesions. Coils are effective for treatment of fistulas **(Figs. 10A to D)**. In AVMs, the nidus should be obliterated using a liquid agent such as cyanoacrylate (glue).[16-19]

UTERINE ARTERY EMBOLIZATION

Indications

Uterine artery embolization has become an extremely valuable therapy for patients with gynecological and obstetric diseases.

The various indications where it can be used are uterine leiomyoma, uterine AVMs, and postpartum and postoperative hemorrhage (PPH). UAE can also control bleeding following radiotherapy treatment in cases of carcinoma cervix.

Uterine Leiomyoma

Uterine artery embolization is the minimally invasive therapy in the management of uterine fibroids. The common indications for treatment are menorrhagia leading to anemia, abdominal pain, uterine enlargement with mass effect, infertility and late miscarriages. The advantages of UAE compared to operative therapies are that the patient retains the uterus, all the myomas are treated together in the same sitting and therapy is less invasive **(Figs. 11 and 12)**.

The disadvantages are vaginal expulsion of necrotic fibroid if the fibroid is submucosal, postembolization syndrome and a procedure which is not a fully curative treatment since the mean reduction of fibroid is about 40% or so.

Uterine Arteriovenous Malformations

The AVMs may either be congenital due to faulty development of arteries, veins, capillaries or are acquired as a result of intervillous space enlargement at the site of myometrial scar. The predisposing factors for acquired AVMs are previous uterine surgery, dilatation and curettage, intrauterine contraceptive devices, previous pregnancy, genital tuberculosis and trophoblastic disease.

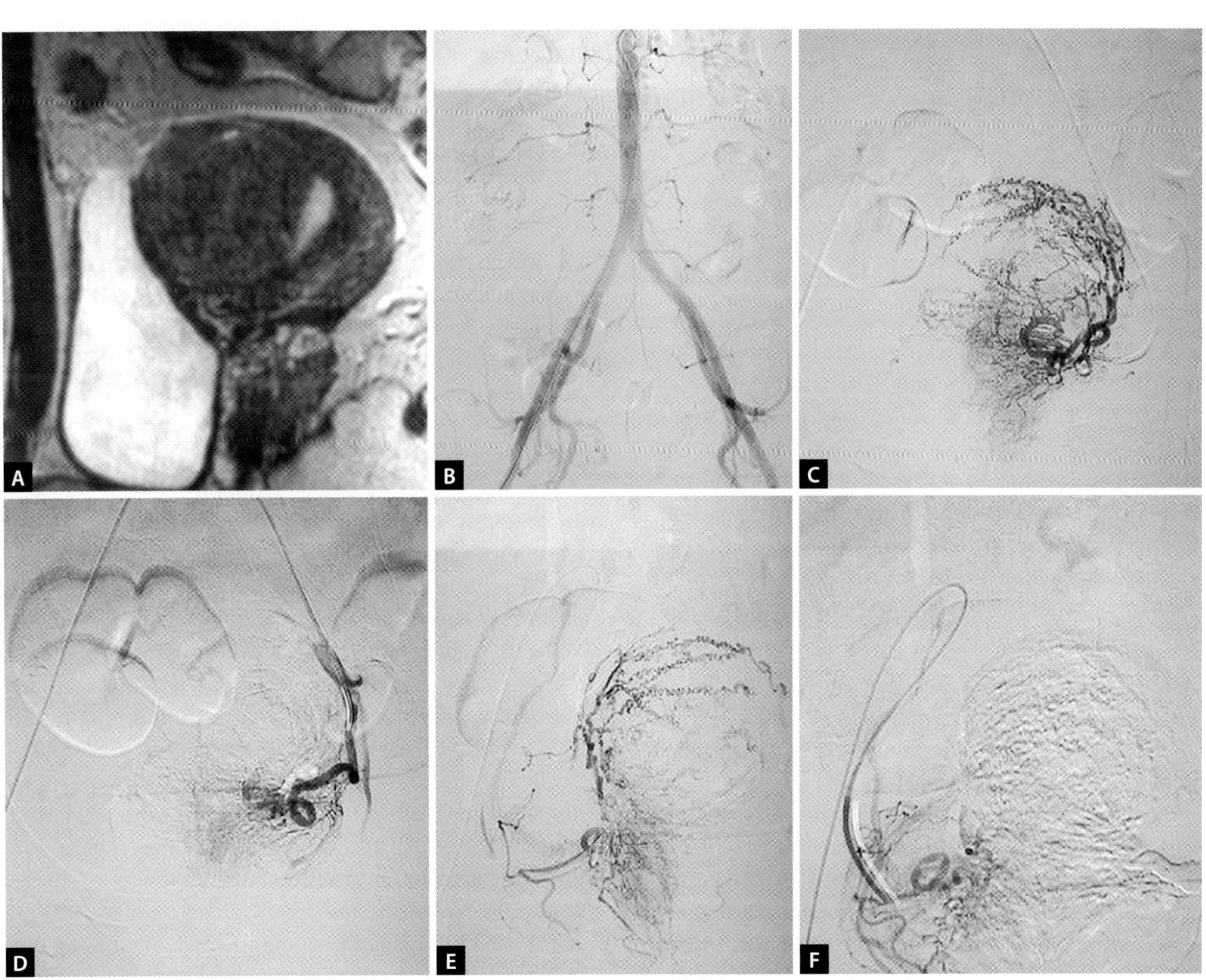

Figs. 11A to F: Uterine artery embolization of uterine fibroid. (A) Sagittal T2W MR image showing fibroid in fundal region; (B) Flush aortogram to look for any ovarian artery supply; (C) Selective left uterine artery angiogram showing increased vascularity supplying the fibroid; (D) Post-embolization angiogram showing reduction in vascularity following embolization with PVA particles (500–700 μ); (E and F) Right uterine angiogram followed by embolization using PVA particles and Robert's uterine catheter.

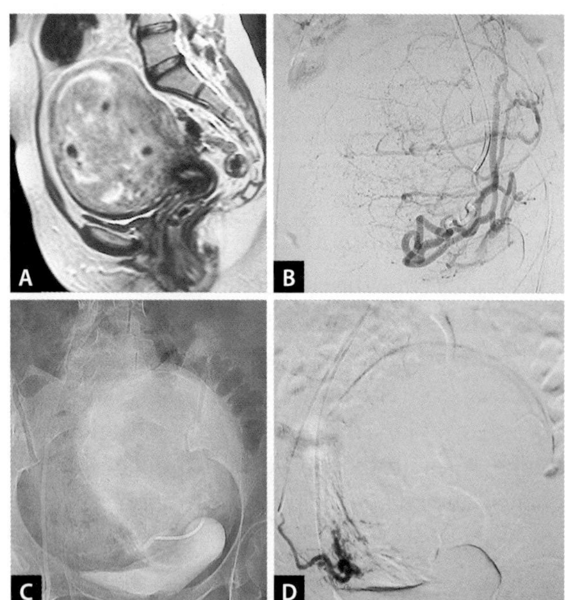

Figs. 12A to D: Uterine artery embolization of large uterine fibroid. (A) Sagittal T2W MR image showing large fibroid in fundal region; (B) Selective left uterine artery angiogram showing increased vascularity supplying the fibroid and splaying of branches by the large fibroid; (C) Post-embolization angiogram showing reduction in vascularity and stasis following embolization with PVA particles (500–700 µ); (D) Right uterine angiogram after the embolization showing reduction in vascularity.

AVMs are usually seen in women of child-bearing age with congenital ones presenting with spontaneous abortion because of bleeding. The clinical presentation in acquired AVMs is profuse, intermittent repetitive bleeding.

UAE has shown good results in the treatment of these lesions with the added advantage that patient also maintains fertility **(Figs. 13A to F)**.

Postsurgical and Postpartum Hemorrhage (Figs. 14A to D)

Role of interventional radiology in the management of PPH has gained wide acceptance in the obstetric-gynecologic community as an alternative to uterine artery ligation or hemostatic hysterectomy.

The postsurgical hemorrhage due to vascular leak can be treated with gelfoam embolization of uterine or anterior division of internal iliac artery (IIA). The various causes of postpartum hemorrhage are abnormal placentation, retained products of conception, birth canal laceration, uterine atony or rupture of uterus. All such catastrophic bleeding conditions can be treated by angiographic embolization of uterine artery by using various embolizing materials.

Patient selection: The choice between endovascular and operative treatment should be made jointly by the patient, gynecologist and intervention radiologist after the current status of all available treatment modalities has been considered and presented in a forthright fashion. Only symptomatic patients in whom other causes for disease have been excluded (including a recent Papanicolaou test) should undergo this treatment. The intervention radiologist is obligated to become the primary physician caring for the patient in preprocedure consultation, hospital recovery and all outpatient management. Adenomyosis also may respond to UAE.[20,21]

Absolute or relative contraindications include pregnancy, active or chronic pelvic infection, gynecologic malignancy (unless palliative or as an adjunct to operation), uncorrectable coagulopathy, severe contrast allergy, and prior pelvic surgery or radiation therapy. The effect of UAE on fertility has not been established, although pregnancy can occur after the procedure. Pedunculated fibroids with relatively narrow stalks are prone to detachment after UAE and may require operative removal.

Technique

Uterine artery embolization for fibroids was first reported by Ravina and coworkers.[22] A pelvic arteriogram with the catheter positioned in the infrarenal abdominal aorta is obtained as a road map, especially to identify any ovarian artery supply. Selective catheterization of the anterior divisions of the IIAs is performed with a cobra or ultralong reverse-curve (e.g. Roberts) catheter.

Once the uterine artery is identified and selected, angiography shows the markedly dilated spiral arteries feeding the uterus. Tumor hypervascularity and vessel displacement is seen. In some cases, the descending portion of the uterine artery can be engaged with the 5-French diagnostic catheter. However, vasospasm may be a problem, so that coaxial placement of a microcatheter directed well into the uterine artery often is required. The preferred agents for embolization are small—caliber particulate matter, including PVA particles (500–700 µm), tris-acryl gelatin microspheres (Embospheres, 700–900 µm) and gelfoam pieces. There does not appear to be any significant difference in clinical efficacy between the two agents. Particle size <500 µm is not used because of the potential risk of crossing over to ovaries through utero-ovarian anastomoses. Proximal embolization (e.g. with coils) is inadvisable, because collateral vessels are very likely to develop and which will continue to feed the tumor. Embolization with particulate

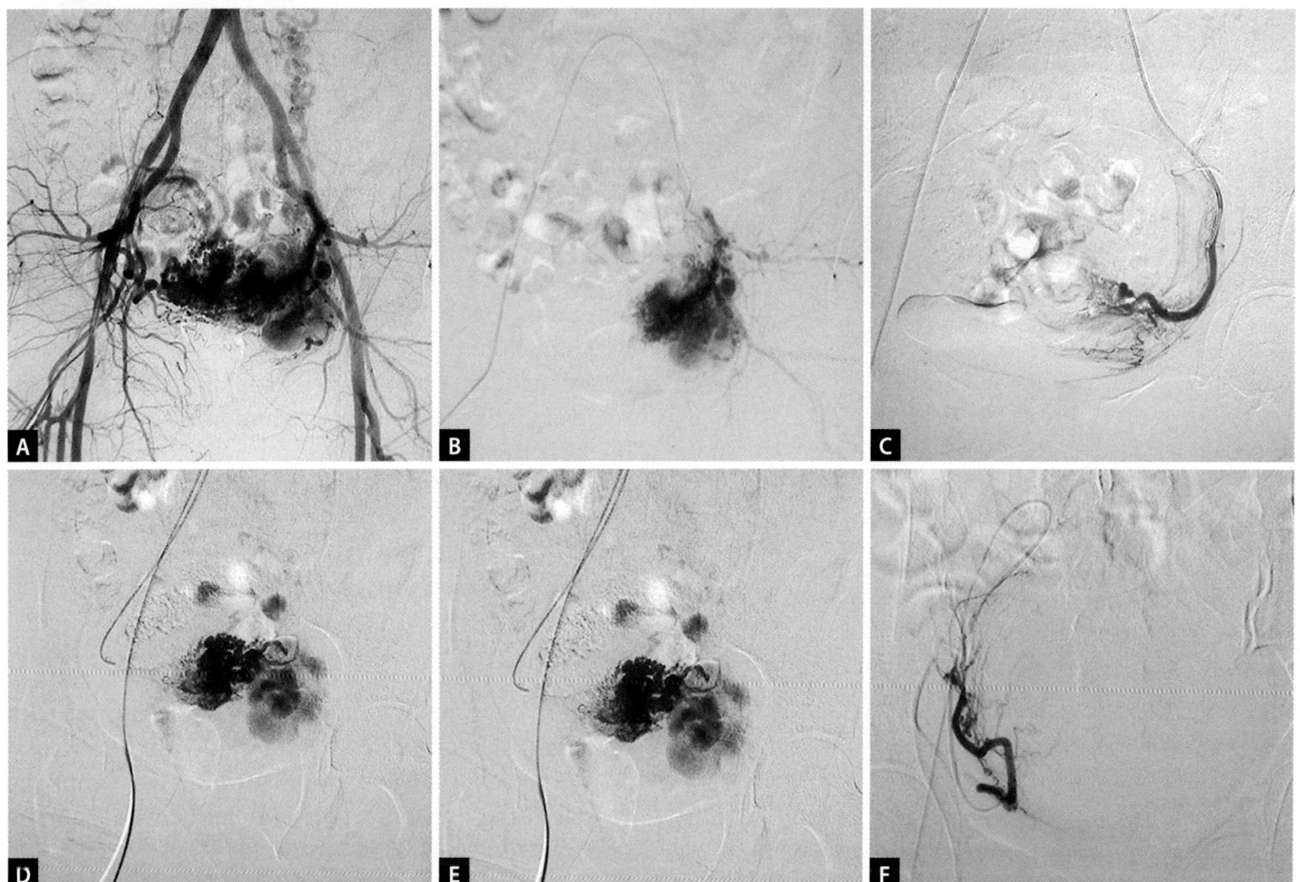

Figs. 13A to F: Uterine arteriovenous malformation treated by angioembolization. (A) Flush aortogram showing large vascular blush in the pelvis; (B) Selective angiogram of left uterine artery showing large vascular blush with nidus; (C) Post-embolization angiogram following embolization with PVA particles 700–1000 μ showing complete obliteration of the vascular blush on left side; (D and E) Selective angiogram of right uterine artery showing residual vascular blush with nidus which was obliterated with PVA particle embolization (F).

slurry (made with diluted contrast material) is continued until there is no flow in uterine artery branches ("pruned-tree" appearance). Regardless of the location of fibroids, bilateral embolization is necessary to prevent development of collateral vessels.[23-26]

Bilateral completion internal iliac arteriograms are obtained to identify any additional vessels feeding the tumors. The interventionalist should be observant of variant arterial anatomy and important collateral vessels. In most cases, the ovarian arteries contribute to fibroids through anastomoses with the main uterine artery. In about 10% of patients, the uterine artery is the major blood supply to the ovary, or the ovarian artery has significant direct communication with the fibroid. Embolization of these vessels theoretically increases the risk of ovarian infarction and infertility. Any other collateral vessels that feed the tumor must also be occluded. This is particularly true in women who have undergone prior pelvic surgery, had other tubal pathology or have fundal fibroids. Postprocedure care should be directed by the interventionalist who performed the UAE. A postembolization syndrome consisting of pain, nausea and vomiting, and low-grade fever is to be expected. Most patients require overnight hospitalization. Pain must be aggressively managed with IV, and later with oral narcotic. Antiemetics are given prophylactically or as needed. Discharge medications include anti-inflammatory drugs (e.g. ketorolac) and potent oral narcotics. Follow-up is done by the interventionalist, including routine clinic evaluation at 1–3 weeks after the procedure.[27]

Results

Bilateral UAE is successful in about 95% of cases. Incomplete infarction of fibroids may be associated with the potential for continued growth. Clinical success with substantial improvement in symptoms is seen in about

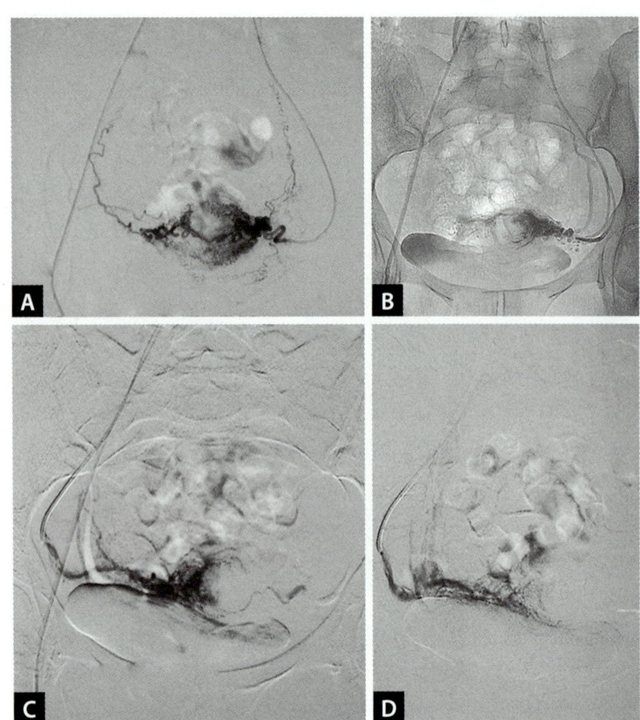

Figs. 14A to D: Post MTP continuous uterine bleeding treated by angioembolization. (A) Selective angiogram of left uterine artery showing vascular blush; (B) Post-embolization angiogram following embolization with PVA particles 700–1000 μ showing complete obliteration of the vascular blush and stasis of contrast; (C) Selective angiogram of right uterine artery showing vascular blush which was obliterated with PVA particle embolization (D).

80–90% of women. Submucosal lesions and small lesions seem to respond better than other tumors. Failure or recurrence is noted in about 6% of cases. If symptoms continue and leiomyomas persist or enlarge on imaging studies, repeat UAE (with aggressive search for collateral vessels including the ovarian arteries) is often warranted.

Complications

Intra- and postprocedure pain is a common problem after UAE. Important complications after UAE are intrauterine infection, uterine ischemia and necrosis, pulmonary embolism, and expulsion of pedunculated submucosal lesions. The overall complication rate is about 5% while major complications occur in about 1%. Most patients do not have a significant change in follicle-stimulating hormone level after the procedure though this is more likely to occur in women older than 45 years of age. Amenorrhea (which is often transient) occurs in less than 10% of cases, but it is much more likely in patients older than 45–50 years of age. Serious infections as complications are observed in 1% of treated women. Less than 2% require subsequent hysterectomy for any complications of UAE.[28-30]

The reasons for UAE failure are incomplete embolization, presence of important collaterals (e.g. ovarian arteries), large fibroids and recanalization of embolized arteries.

VAGINAL ARTERIOVENOUS MALFORMATION EMBOLIZATION

Vaginal AVMs are rare entities, and their most common presentation is vaginal hemorrhage and rarely dyspareunia. These lesions can be successfully treated by angioembolization of the supplying vessels using glue depending upon the angiographic flow dynamics. Angioembolization being safe and effective should be the first treatment of choice for symptomatic vaginal vascular malformation **(Figs. 15A to F)**.

SCROTAL ARTERIOVENOUS MALFORMATION AND TESTICULAR TUMOR EMBOLIZATION

Scrotal AVMs are rare entity. The scrotal AVMs and the paratesticular masses may occasionally present with uncontrollable bleeding. These lesions can be successfully treated by angioembolization of the supplying vessels using either Glue or PVA particles depending upon the situations **(Figs. 16 and 17)**. Angioembolization being safe and effective should be considered as choice of treatment for the treatment of symptomatic scrotal vascular malformation.

VARICOCELE EMBOLIZATION (FIGS. 18A TO C)

Varicocele is an important cause of male infertility. Varicocele embolization is indicated in an individual who have been infertile for at least 2 years and having oligoasthenospermia without an apparent cause of infertility. The embolization is done after placing catheter deep into the internal spermatic vein. Various embolizing materials like steel coils, PVA particles, gelfoam are used.[31-33]

PROSTATIC ARTERY EMBOLIZATION

Prostatic artery embolization is a new minimally invasive treatment modality for benign prostatic hyperplasia. Transurethral resection of prostate or surgical enucleation is associated with risk of urinary incontinence and increased risk of erectile dysfunction. The thin prostatic arteries branch from anterior division of IIAs and require expertise to selectively catheterize because of small caliber, arteriosclerosis and variations in anatomy.[34] A CT angiography or 3D rotational angiogram are often done

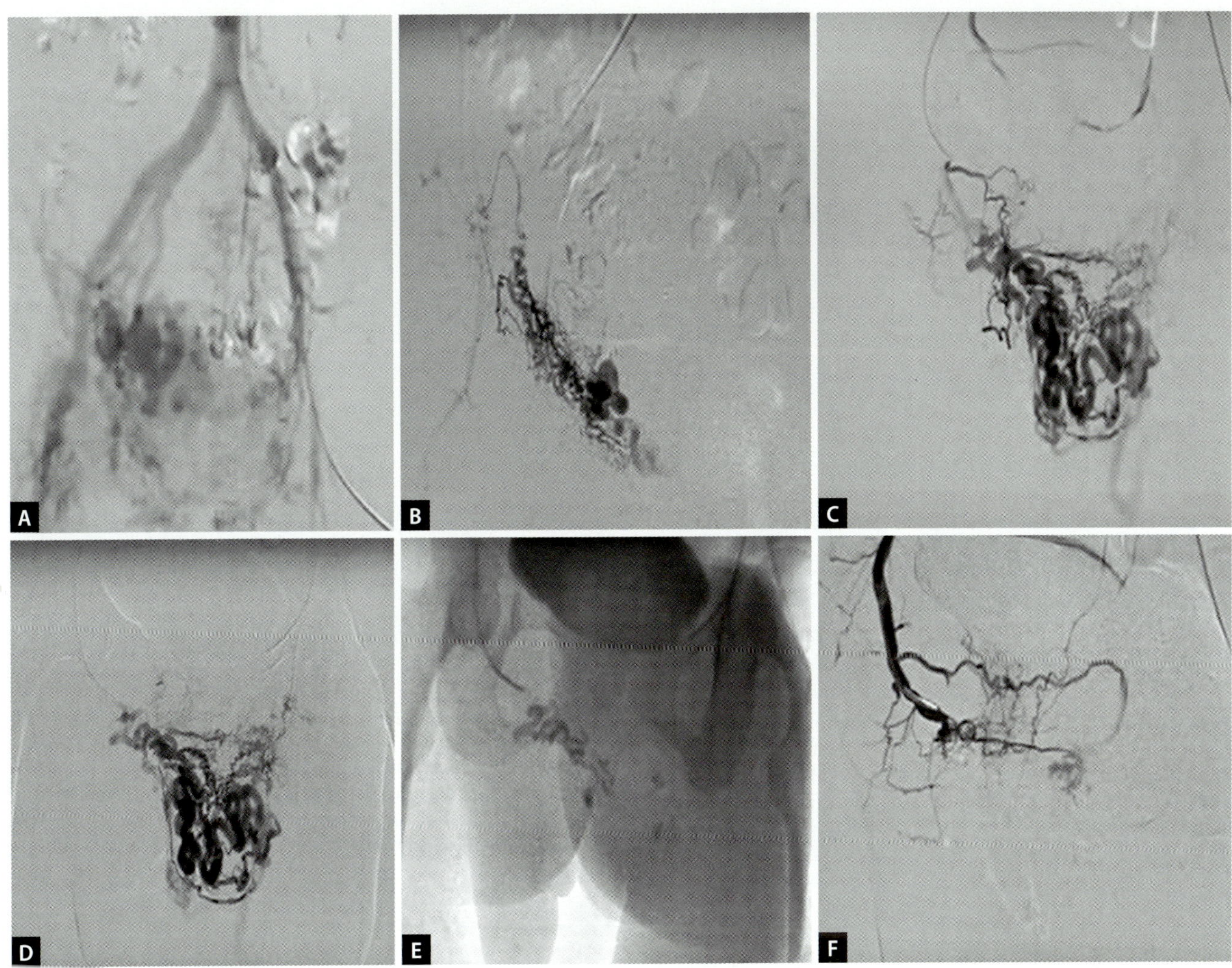

Figs. 15A to F: Vaginal arteriovenous malformation (AVM) treated by angioembolization. Selective angiogram of right internal pudendal artery showing multiple feeders supplying the nidus of AVM (A to D), which was obliterated using glue (E and F).

to delineate the anatomy and oblique projections are helpful in digital subtraction angiography to identify the prostatic arteries. PVA particles of size <300 μ or gelatin microspheres are commonly used for embolization. Shrinkage of the prostate volume starts about 1 month after the embolization.

TRANSJUGULAR RENAL BIOPSY (FIGS. 19A TO C)

Transjugular renal biopsy is indicated in the presence of coagulopathy, patient unable to lie prone or small kidneys.[35] During this procedure, renal vein is accessed via transjugular route and then needle is directed into a lower pole renal vein branch, away from larger vessels into the parenchyma so that bleeding, if any, would be into the vein itself. This procedure has not got much acceptance because of technically demanding nature and high incidence of complications like arterial puncture and capsular perforation.[36]

PROPHYLACTIC BALLOON PLACEMENT IN ADHERENT PLACENTA (FIGS. 20A TO D)

Placenta accreta spectrum (PAS) is a term used to describe placenta accreta, increta and percreta. It results due to placental implantation at an area of abnormal decidualization.

Spectrum of adherent placenta:

- *Accreta vera:* Placental villi attach to myometrium
- *Increta:* Villi penetrate into the myometrium
- *Percreta:* Villi penetrate through the placental villi through the myometrium to the uterine serosa or adjacent organs.

Incidence of these entities are 79%, 14% and 7%, respectively, for accreta , increta and percreta.[6] The most

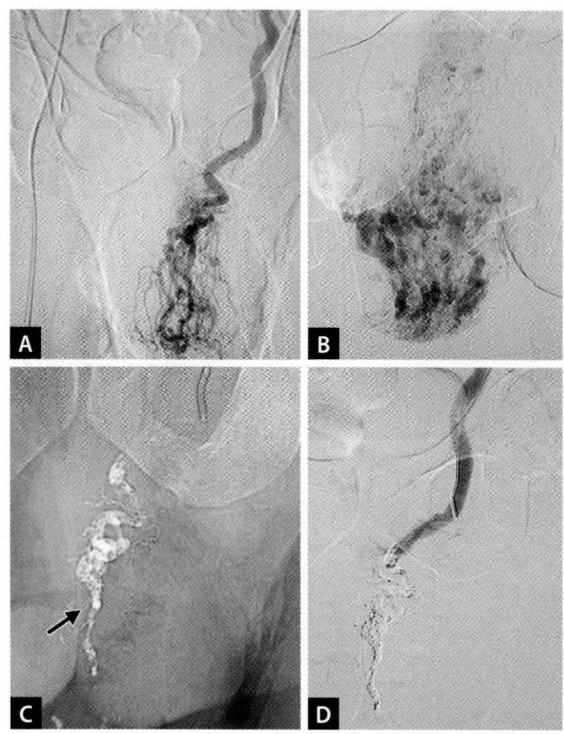

Figs. 16A to D: Scrotal arteriovenous malformation treated by glue embolization. (A and B) Selective left internal pudendal artery angiogram showing hypertrophied artery and large nidus; (C) Spot image showing glue cast obliterating the nidus; (D) Post-embolization angiogram showing complete obliteration of the vascular nidus.

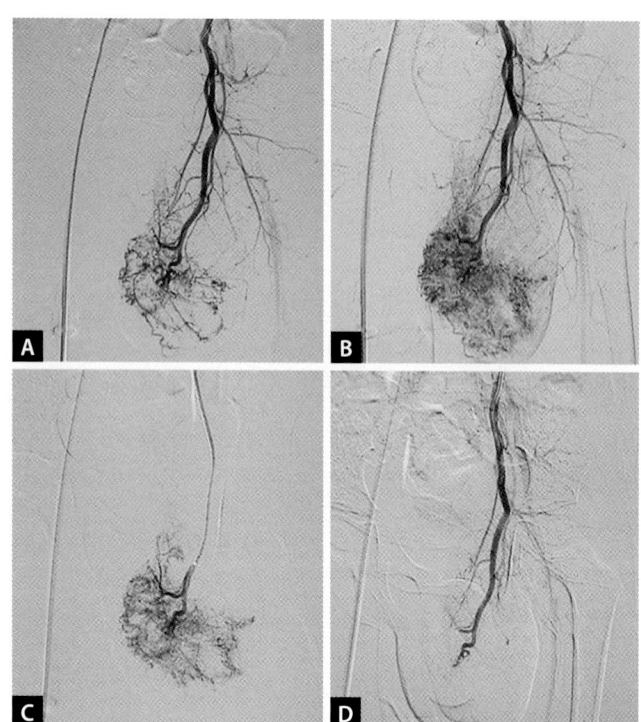

Figs. 17A to D: Left paratesticular mass in 5-year-old child with scrotal bleeding treated by angioembolization. (A and B) Selective left internal pudendal artery angiogram showing hypertrophied artery and large tumor blush; (C) Catheter brought close to the tumor blush; (D) Post-embolization angiogram following embolization using PVA particles 300–500 μ, showing complete obliteration of tumor blush.

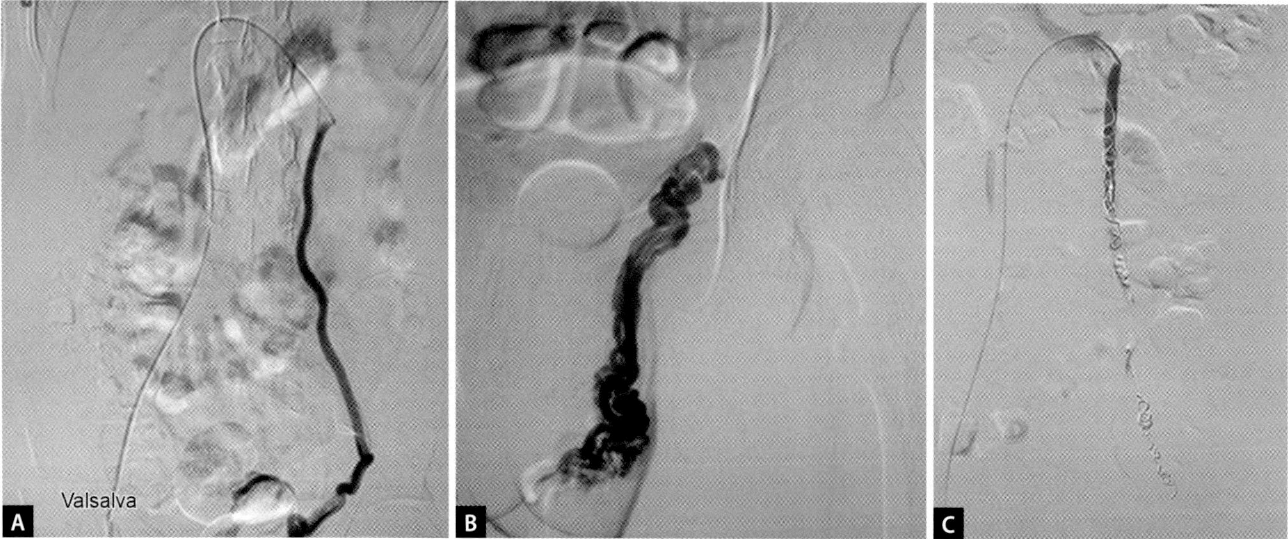

Figs. 18A to C: Technique of varicocele embolization: (A) Left gonadal vein was accessed through transfemoral venous route; (B) Catheter was advanced as distally as possible to the point of formation of gonadal vein from pampiniform plexus; (C) Entire left gonadal vein was embolized using combination of coils and glue till the point just proximal to draining into left renal vein.

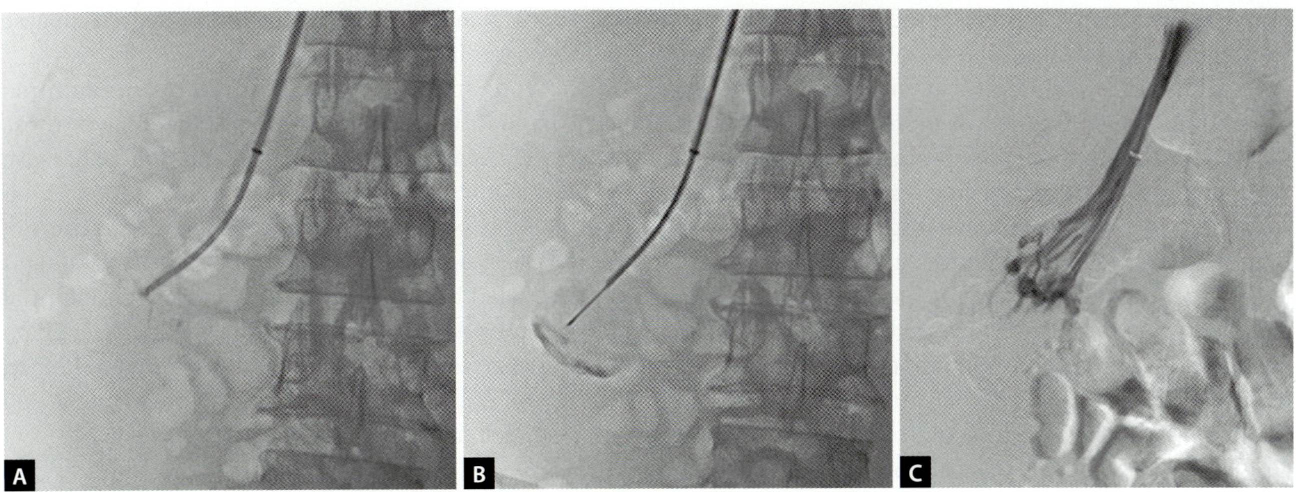

Figs. 19A to C: Spot images showing technique of transjugular renal biopsy (TJRB): TJLB needle placed inside lower polar branch of renal vein (A) through right transjugular route and biopsy is being taken from posterolateral cortex (B) followed by postbiopsy venogram showing free flow of contrast without any leak (C). (TJLB: transjugular liver biopsy).

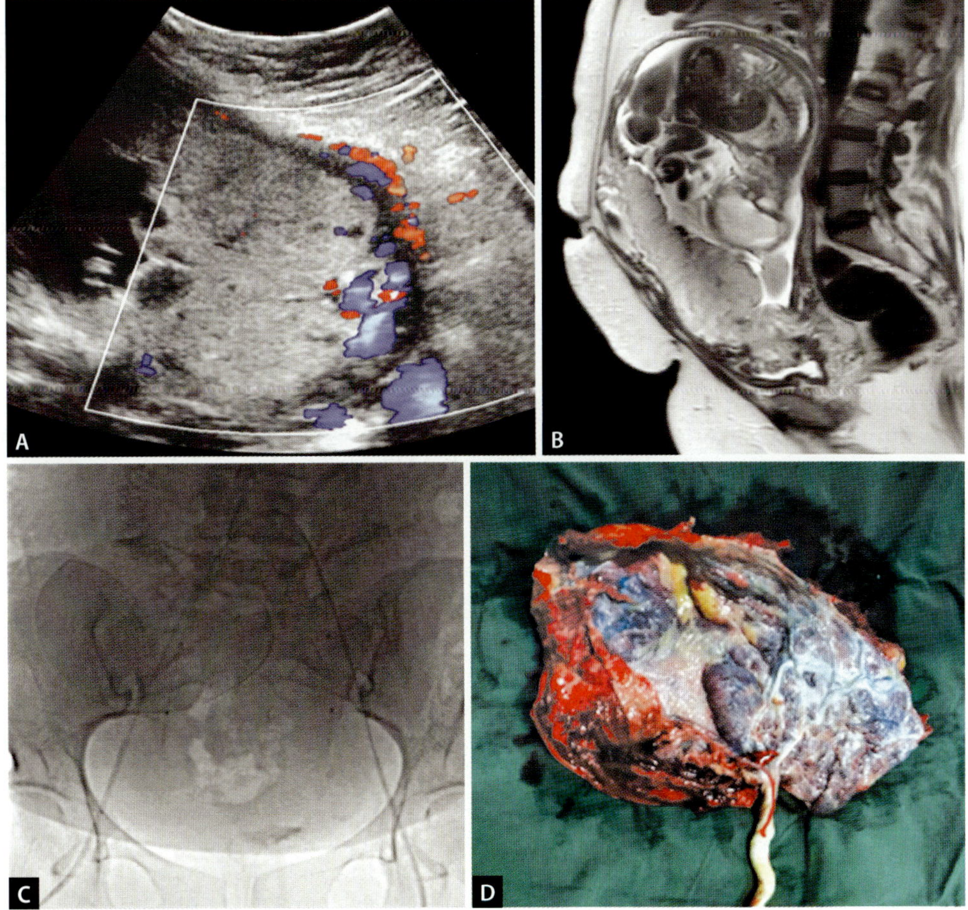

Figs. 20A to D: Technique of preoperative balloon placement in adherent placenta: (A) Ultrasonographic image showing low-lying heteroehoic placenta with thick interplacental bands and loss of retroplacental clear space. The planes with urinary bladder are ill defined with highly increased vascularity at bladder placenta interface; (B) T2-weighted sagittal image of same patient showing grossly heterointense placenta which is seen invading into bladder as well as scar site; (C) Patient was taken up for prophylactic balloon placement in bilateral internal iliac arteries before taking up for C-section. After delivery of baby, balloons were inflated and hysterectomy was done; (D) Image shows hysterectomy specimen showing adherent placenta attached to it. Intraoperative blood loss was 6.8 L.

important risk factor for development of PAS is placenta previa after a previous cesarean delivery.[37] It is usually asymptomatic and detected at the time of placental separation. The consequences of this is that at the time of placental separation, lack of normal cleavage plane between the uterus and placenta results in major hemorrhage and is a very common indication of peripartum hysterectomy.[38,39] After diagnosis, it is very important to develop a preoperative plan for the patient with a high likelihood of PAS. It should have a multidisciplinary team on board. The common treatment is usually cesarean hysterectomy with placenta left undisturbed *in situ* at 34–35 weeks. There are two possible management options. One is either to go for total abdominal hysterectomy with placenta *in situ*. In the other case scenario, uterus is preserved with placenta left *in situ*. Interventional radiology has an important role in both the clinical scenarios. In the first scenario of hysterectomy, balloon is placed in both IIAs and embolization is performed postcesarean delivery. As a result, there is a bloodless surgical field for hysterectomy, and it also reduces the blood loss during surgery. In the second scenario of uterine preservation, balloons are inflated in both IIA after delivery and embolization of both arteries is done immediately or the balloons can be deflated. If there is no bleeding, balloons can be removed.

Procedure (Figs. 20A to D)

On the day of delivery of patient with placenta accreta (by cesarean section), patient is first taken to interventional lab. Bilateral common femoral arteries are accessed with a 7F arterial sheath. Using minimum radiation and contrast, balloon catheters (10 mm × 4 cm) are placed in anterior divisions of bilateral IIAs (preoperative balloon placement). Patient is then shifted to maternity operation theater with sheaths and balloon catheters secured to skin by sutures. Baby is delivered by fundal incision and decision of hysterectomy is taken intraoperatively according to blood loss. Bilateral balloons are inflated after the delivery of the baby to occlude the anterior divisions of the IIAs. Hysterectomy is done with inflated balloons *in situ*. Keeping the balloons inflated, additional embolization can be done with gelfoam or coils, if the bleeding persists. Balloons are deflated after completion of hysterectomy, and the patient is shifted to the recovery room. Vascular sheaths are removed in the recovery room, if there is no persistent bleeding after a few hours. In the scenario of uterine preservation, balloons are inflated in both IIA after delivery and embolization of both arteries is done immediately or the balloons can be deflated in case there is no significant bleeding.

Many people have used infrarenal abdominal aortic balloon inflation for control of bleeding in these patients.[40,41] Apart from these, balloon placement has also been done in common iliac and uterine arteries. Other than balloon placement, postdelivery embolization of uterine arteries and IIAs can be done in case bleeding is not controlled during surgery. The primary endpoint of the procedure is estimated blood loss volume. Secondary endpoints are total number of units of packed red blood cells (PRBCs) transfused, number of patients transfused and hysterectomy rate.

CONCLUSION

In conclusion, renal artery aneurysms can be life-threatening if hemorrhage occurs. Following aneurysm rupture, surgical morbidity and mortality are fairly high. Aggressive management by the interventional radiologist, therefore is paramount since these patients are in any case too sick for major revascularization procedures, making endovascular techniques a more desirable approach. Embolization of dysfunctioning kidneys using various embolization techniques and regimens in the management of hypertension or protein wasting in end-stage renal disease has replaced surgical nephrectomy. The evolution of uterine fibroid embolization has established the role of embolotherapy as a viable alternative to hysterectomy, and undoubtedly revolutionized the management of postpartum bleeding. A variety of methods for embolization are described in the literature. The type of treatment should be tailored to each individual case as the anatomy and flow dynamics will typically dictate the therapy best suited.

REFERENCES

1. Cicuto KP, McLean GK, Oleaga JA, et al. Renal artery stenosis: Anatomical classification for percutaneous transluminal angioplasty. Am J Roentgenol. 1981;137:599-601.
2. Rountas C, Vlychou M, Vassiou K, et al. Imaging modalities for renal artery stenosis in suspected renovascular hypertension: Prospective intraindividual comparison of color Doppler US, CT angiography, GD-enhanced MR angiography, and digital substraction angiography. Ren Fail. 2007;29(3):295-302.
3. Tan KT, van Beek EJ, Brown PW, et al. Magnetic resonance angiography for the diagnosis of renal artery stenosis. A metaanalysis. Clin Radiol. 2002;57:617-24.
4. Hoffman O, Carreres T, Sapoval MR, et al. Ostial renal artery stenosis angioplasty. Immediate and mid-term angiographic and clinical results. J Vasc Interv Radiol. 1998;9:65-73.
5. Matsumoto AH, Tegtmeyer CJ, Fitzgerald EK, et al. Percutaneous transluminal angioplasty of visceral arterial

stenoses: results and long-term clinical follow-up. J Vasc Interv Radiol. 1995;6:165-74.
6. Moss JG, Hamilton G. Renal and visceral artery intervention. In: Dyet JF, Nicholson AA, Ettles DF, Wilson SE (Eds), Textbook of Endovascular Procedures. Philadelphia: Churchill Livingston; 2000. pp. 151-73.
7. Park JH, Kim WS, Han MC, et al. Renal arterial embolization with absolute ethanol. J Korean Med Sci. 1987;2(1):13-8.
8. Park JH, Kim SH, Han JK, et al. Transcatheter arterial embolization of unresectable renal cell carcinoma with a mixture of ethanol and iodized oil. Cardiovasc Intervent Radiol. 1994 ;17(6):323-7.
9. Martin RS 3rd, Meacham PW, Ditesheim JA, et al. Renal artery aneurysm: selective treatment for hypertension and prevention of rupture. J Vasc Surg. 1989;9:26-34.
10. Poutasse EF. Renal artery aneurysms. Their natural history and surgery. J Urol. 1966;95:297- 306.
11. Poutasse EF. Renal artery aneurysms. J Urol. 1975;113:443-49.
12. Liguori G, Trombetta C, Bucci S, et al. Percutaneous management of renal artery aneurysm with a stent-graft. J Urol. 2002; 167:2518-19.
13. Pershad A, Heuser R. Renal artery aneurysm: successful exclusion with a stent graft. Catheter Cardiovasc Interv. 2004;61:314-16.
14. Rundback JH, Rizvi A, Rozenblit GN, et al. Percutaneous stent-graft management of renal artery aneurysms. J Vasc Interv Radiol. 2000;11:1189-93.
15. Schneidereit NP, Lee S, Morris DC, et al. Endovascular repair of a ruptured renal artery aneurysm. J Endovasc Ther. 2003;10:71-4.
16. Crotty KL, Orihuela E, Warren MM. Recent advances in the diagnosis and treatment of renal arteriovenous malformations and fistulas. J Urol. 1993;150:1355-9.
17. Takebayashi S, Aida N, Matsui K. Arteriovenous malformations of the kidneys: Diagnosis and follow-up with color Doppler sonography in six patients. Am J Roentgenol. 1991;157:991-5.
18. Allione A, Pomero F, Valpreda S, et al. Worsening of hypertension in a pregnant women with renal arteriovenous malformation: a successful superselective embolization after delivery. Clin Nephrol. 2003;60:211-3.
19. Takebayashi S, Hosaka M, Ishizuka E, et al. Arteriovenous malformations of the kidneys: Ablation with alcohol. Am J Roentgenol. 1988;150:587-90.
20. Andrews RT, Spies JB, Sacks D, et al. Patient care and uterine artery embolization for leiomyomata. J Vasc Interv Radiol. 2004;15:115-20.
21. Siskin GP, Tublin ME, Stainken BF, et al. Uterine artery embolization for the treatment of adenomyosis: clinical response and evaluation with MR imaging. Am J Roentgenol. 2001;177:297-302.
22. Ravina JH, Herbreteau D, Ciraru-Vigneron N, et al. Arterial embolisation to treat uterine myomata. Lancet. 1995;346:671-2.
23. Worthington-Kirsch RL, Andrews RT, et al. Uterine fibroid embolization: technical aspects. Tech Vasc Intent Radiol. 2002;5:17-34.
24. Banovac F, Ascher SM, Jones DA, et al. Magnetic resonance imaging outcome after uterine artery embolization for leiomyomata with use of tris-acryl gelatin microspheres. J Vasc Interv Radiol. 2002;13:681-8.
25. Pelage JP, Le Dref O, Beregi JP, et al. Limited uterine artery embolization with tris-acryl gelatin microspheres for uterine fibroids. J Vasc Interv Radiol. 2003;14:15-20.
26. Pelage JP, Le Dref O, Soyer P, et al. Arterial anatomy of the female genital tract: Variations and relevance to transcatheter embolization of the uterus. Am J Roentgenol. 1999;172:989-94.
27. Siskin GP, Bonn J, Worthington-Kirsch RL, et al. Uterine fibroid embolization: pain management. Tech Vasc Interv Radiol. 2002;5:35-43.
28. Pelage JP, Walker WJ, Dref OL. Uterine necrosis after uterine artery embolization for leiomyoma. Obstet Gynecol. 2002;99:676-7.
29. Spies JB, Spector A, Roth AR, et al. Complications after uterine artery embolization for leiomyomas. Obstet Gynecol. 2002;100:873-80.
30. Spies JB, Roth AR, Gonsalves SM, et al. Ovarian function after uterine artery embolization for leiomyomata: assessment with use of serum follicle stimulating hormone assay. J Vasc Interv Radiol. 2001;12:437-42.
31. Lima SS, Castro MP, Costa OF. A new method for the treatment of varicocele. Andrologia. 1978;10:103-06.
32. Trombetta C, Salisci E, Deriu M, et al. Echo-flowmetric control 6 years after percutaneous treatment of varicocele. Arch Ital Urol Androl. 1993;65:363-67.
33. Usuki N, Nakamura K, Takashima S, et al. Embolization of varicocele with ethanol. Nippon Igaku Hoshasen Gakkai Zasshi 1994;54:870-5 (Japanese).
34. Teichgräber U, Aschenbach R, Diamantis I, et al. Prostate artery embolization: indication, technique and clinical results. Rofo. 2018;190(9):847-55.
35. Rathod KR, Popat BA, Pandey A, et al. Safety and effectiveness of transjugular renal biopsy: a single center study. Indian J Nephrol. 2017;27(2):118-123.
36. Thompson BC, Kingdon E, Johnston M, et al. Transjugular kidney biopsy. Am J Kidney Dis. 2004;43(4):651-62.
37. Silver RM, Landon MB, Rouse DJ, et al. Maternal morbidity associated with multiple repeat cesarean deliveries. Obstet Gynecol. 2006;107(6):1226-32.
38. Mehrabadi A, Hutcheon JA, Liu S, et al. Contribution of placenta accreta to the incidence of postpartum hemorrhage and severe postpartum hemorrhage. Obstet Gynecol. 2015;125(4):814-21.
39. Zelop CM, Harlow BL, Frigoletto FD, et al. Emergency peripartum hysterectomy. Am J Obstet Gynecol. 1993;168(5):1443-8.
40. Zeng C, Yang M, Ding Y, et al. Preoperative infrarenal abdominal aorta balloon catheter occlusion combined with Bakri tamponade reduced maternal morbidity of placenta increta/percreta. Medicine (Baltimore). 2017;96(38):e8114.
41. Luo F, Xie L, Xie P, et al. Intraoperative aortic balloon occlusion in patients with placenta previa and/or placenta accreta: a retrospective study. Taiwan J Obstet Gynecol. 2017;56(2):147-52.

Index

Page numbers followed by *b* refer to box, *f* refer to figure, *fc* refer to flowchart, and *t* refer to table.

A

D

E

F

M

N

O

P

S

U

V

W

X

Y

Z